Diagnostic Pulmonary Pathology

LUNG BIOLOGY IN HEALTH AND DISEASE

Executive Editor

Claude Lenfant

Former Director, National Heart, Lung, and Blood Institute
National Institutes of Health
Bethesda, Maryland

1. Immunologic and Infectious Reactions in the Lung, *edited by C. H. Kirkpatrick and H. Y. Reynolds*
2. The Biochemical Basis of Pulmonary Function, *edited by R. G. Crystal*
3. Bioengineering Aspects of the Lung, *edited by J. B. West*
4. Metabolic Functions of the Lung, *edited by Y. S. Bakhle and J. R. Vane*
5. Respiratory Defense Mechanisms (in two parts), *edited by J. D. Brain, D. F. Proctor, and L. M. Reid*
6. Development of the Lung, *edited by W. A. Hodson*
7. Lung Water and Solute Exchange, *edited by N. C. Staub*
8. Extrapulmonary Manifestations of Respiratory Disease, *edited by E. D. Robin*
9. Chronic Obstructive Pulmonary Disease, *edited by T. L. Petty*
10. Pathogenesis and Therapy of Lung Cancer, *edited by C. C. Harris*
11. Genetic Determinants of Pulmonary Disease, *edited by S. D. Litwin*
12. The Lung in the Transition Between Health and Disease, *edited by P. T. Macklem and S. Permutt*
13. Evolution of Respiratory Processes: A Comparative Approach, *edited by S. C. Wood and C. Lenfant*
14. Pulmonary Vascular Diseases, *edited by K. M. Moser*
15. Physiology and Pharmacology of the Airways, *edited by J. A. Nadel*
16. Diagnostic Techniques in Pulmonary Disease (in two parts), *edited by M. A. Sackner*
17. Regulation of Breathing (in two parts), *edited by T. F. Hornbein*
18. Occupational Lung Diseases: Research Approaches and Methods, *edited by H. Weill and M. Turner-Warwick*
19. Immunopharmacology of the Lung, *edited by H. H. Newball*
20. Sarcoidosis and Other Granulomatous Diseases of the Lung, *edited by B. L. Fanburg*
21. Sleep and Breathing, *edited by N. A. Saunders and C. E. Sullivan*
22. *Pneumocystis carinii* Pneumonia: Pathogenesis, Diagnosis, and Treatment, *edited by L. S. Young*

23. Pulmonary Nuclear Medicine: Techniques in Diagnosis of Lung Disease, *edited by H. L. Atkins*
24. Acute Respiratory Failure, *edited by W. M. Zapol and K. J. Falke*
25. Gas Mixing and Distribution in the Lung, *edited by L. A. Engel and M. Paiva*
26. High-Frequency Ventilation in Intensive Care and During Surgery, *edited by G. Carlon and W. S. Howland*
27. Pulmonary Development: Transition from Intrauterine to Extrauterine Life, *edited by G. H. Nelson*
28. Chronic Obstructive Pulmonary Disease: Second Edition, *edited by T. L. Petty*
29. The Thorax (in two parts), *edited by C. Roussos and P. T. Macklem*
30. The Pleura in Health and Disease, *edited by J. Chrétien, J. Bignon, and A. Hirsch*
31. Drug Therapy for Asthma: Research and Clinical Practice, *edited by J. W. Jenne and S. Murphy*
32. Pulmonary Endothelium in Health and Disease, *edited by U. S. Ryan*
33. The Airways: Neural Control in Health and Disease, *edited by M. A. Kaliner and P. J. Barnes*
34. Pathophysiology and Treatment of Inhalation Injuries, *edited by J. Loke*
35. Respiratory Function of the Upper Airway, *edited by O. P. Mathew and G. Sant'Ambrogio*
36. Chronic Obstructive Pulmonary Disease: A Behavioral Perspective, *edited by A. J. McSweeny and I. Grant*
37. Biology of Lung Cancer: Diagnosis and Treatment, *edited by S. T. Rosen, J. L. Mulshine, F. Cuttitta, and P. G. Abrams*
38. Pulmonary Vascular Physiology and Pathophysiology, *edited by E. K. Weir and J. T. Reeves*
39. Comparative Pulmonary Physiology: Current Concepts, *edited by S. C. Wood*
40. Respiratory Physiology: An Analytical Approach, *edited by H. K. Chang and M. Paiva*
41. Lung Cell Biology, *edited by D. Massaro*
42. Heart–Lung Interactions in Health and Disease, *edited by S. M. Scharf and S. S. Cassidy*
43. Clinical Epidemiology of Chronic Obstructive Pulmonary Disease, *edited by M. J. Hensley and N. A. Saunders*
44. Surgical Pathology of Lung Neoplasms, *edited by A. M. Marchevsky*
45. The Lung in Rheumatic Diseases, *edited by G. W. Cannon and G. A. Zimmerman*
46. Diagnostic Imaging of the Lung, *edited by C. E. Putman*
47. Models of Lung Disease: Microscopy and Structural Methods, *edited by J. Gil*
48. Electron Microscopy of the Lung, *edited by D. E. Schraufnagel*
49. Asthma: Its Pathology and Treatment, *edited by M. A. Kaliner, P. J. Barnes, and C. G. A. Persson*
50. Acute Respiratory Failure: Second Edition, *edited by W. M. Zapol and F. Lemaire*

51. Lung Disease in the Tropics, *edited by O. P. Sharma*
52. Exercise: Pulmonary Physiology and Pathophysiology, *edited by B. J. Whipp and K. Wasserman*
53. Developmental Neurobiology of Breathing, *edited by G. G. Haddad and J. P. Farber*
54. Mediators of Pulmonary Inflammation, *edited by M. A. Bray and W. H. Anderson*
55. The Airway Epithelium, *edited by S. G. Farmer and D. Hay*
56. Physiological Adaptations in Vertebrates: Respiration, Circulation, and Metabolism, *edited by S. C. Wood, R. E. Weber, A. R. Hargens, and R. W. Millard*
57. The Bronchial Circulation, *edited by J. Butler*
58. Lung Cancer Differentiation: Implications for Diagnosis and Treatment, *edited by S. D. Bernal and P. J. Hesketh*
59. Pulmonary Complications of Systemic Disease, *edited by J. F. Murray*
60. Lung Vascular Injury: Molecular and Cellular Response, *edited by A. Johnson and T. J. Ferro*
61. Cytokines of the Lung, *edited by J. Kelley*
62. The Mast Cell in Health and Disease, *edited by M. A. Kaliner and D. D. Metcalfe*
63. Pulmonary Disease in the Elderly Patient, *edited by D. A. Mahler*
64. Cystic Fibrosis, *edited by P. B. Davis*
65. Signal Transduction in Lung Cells, *edited by J. S. Brody, D. M. Center, and V. A. Tkachuk*
66. Tuberculosis: A Comprehensive International Approach, *edited by L. B. Reichman and E. S. Hershfield*
67. Pharmacology of the Respiratory Tract: Experimental and Clinical Research, *edited by K. F. Chung and P. J. Barnes*
68. Prevention of Respiratory Diseases, *edited by A. Hirsch, M. Goldberg, J.-P. Martin, and R. Masse*
69. *Pneumocystis carinii* Pneumonia: Second Edition, *edited by P. D. Walzer*
70. Fluid and Solute Transport in the Airspaces of the Lungs, *edited by R. M. Effros and H. K. Chang*
71. Sleep and Breathing: Second Edition, *edited by N. A. Saunders and C. E. Sullivan*
72. Airway Secretion: Physiological Bases for the Control of Mucous Hypersecretion, *edited by T. Takishima and S. Shimura*
73. Sarcoidosis and Other Granulomatous Disorders, *edited by D. G. James*
74. Epidemiology of Lung Cancer, *edited by J. M. Samet*
75. Pulmonary Embolism, *edited by M. Morpurgo*
76. Sports and Exercise Medicine, *edited by S. C. Wood and R. C. Roach*
77. Endotoxin and the Lungs, *edited by K. L. Brigham*
78. The Mesothelial Cell and Mesothelioma, *edited by M.-C. Jaurand and J. Bignon*
79. Regulation of Breathing: Second Edition, *edited by J. A. Dempsey and A. I. Pack*
80. Pulmonary Fibrosis, *edited by S. Hin. Phan and R. S. Thrall*
81. Long-Term Oxygen Therapy: Scientific Basis and Clinical Application, *edited by W. J. O'Donohue, Jr.*

82. Ventral Brainstem Mechanisms and Control of Respiration and Blood Pressure, *edited by C. O. Trouth, R. M. Millis, H. F. Kiwull-Schöne, and M. E. Schläfke*
83. A History of Breathing Physiology, *edited by D. F. Proctor*
84. Surfactant Therapy for Lung Disease, *edited by B. Robertson and H. W. Taeusch*
85. The Thorax: Second Edition, Revised and Expanded (in three parts), *edited by C. Roussos*
86. Severe Asthma: Pathogenesis and Clinical Management, *edited by S. J. Szefler and D. Y. M. Leung*
87. *Mycobacterium avium*–Complex Infection: Progress in Research and Treatment, *edited by J. A. Korvick and C. A. Benson*
88. Alpha 1–Antitrypsin Deficiency: Biology • Pathogenesis • Clinical Manifestations • Therapy, *edited by R. G. Crystal*
89. Adhesion Molecules and the Lung, *edited by P. A. Ward and J. C. Fantone*
90. Respiratory Sensation, *edited by L. Adams and A. Guz*
91. Pulmonary Rehabilitation, *edited by A. P. Fishman*
92. Acute Respiratory Failure in Chronic Obstructive Pulmonary Disease, *edited by J.-P. Derenne, W. A. Whitelaw, and T. Similowski*
93. Environmental Impact on the Airways: From Injury to Repair, *edited by J. Chrétien and D. Dusser*
94. Inhalation Aerosols: Physical and Biological Basis for Therapy, *edited by A. J. Hickey*
95. Tissue Oxygen Deprivation: From Molecular to Integrated Function, *edited by G. G. Haddad and G. Lister*
96. The Genetics of Asthma, *edited by S. B. Liggett and D. A. Meyers*
97. Inhaled Glucocorticoids in Asthma: Mechanisms and Clinical Actions, *edited by R. P. Schleimer, W. W. Busse, and P. M. O'Byrne*
98. Nitric Oxide and the Lung, *edited by W. M. Zapol and K. D. Bloch*
99. Primary Pulmonary Hypertension, *edited by L. J. Rubin and S. Rich*
100. Lung Growth and Development, *edited by J. A. McDonald*
101. Parasitic Lung Diseases, *edited by A. A. F. Mahmoud*
102. Lung Macrophages and Dendritic Cells in Health and Disease, *edited by M. F. Lipscomb and S. W. Russell*
103. Pulmonary and Cardiac Imaging, *edited by C. Chiles and C. E. Putman*
104. Gene Therapy for Diseases of the Lung, *edited by K. L. Brigham*
105. Oxygen, Gene Expression, and Cellular Function, *edited by L. Biadasz Clerch and D. J. Massaro*
106. $Beta_2$-Agonists in Asthma Treatment, *edited by R. Pauwels and P. M. O'Byrne*
107. Inhalation Delivery of Therapeutic Peptides and Proteins, *edited by A. L. Adjei and P. K. Gupta*
108. Asthma in the Elderly, *edited by R. A. Barbee and J. W. Bloom*
109. Treatment of the Hospitalized Cystic Fibrosis Patient, *edited by D. M. Orenstein and R. C. Stern*
110. Asthma and Immunological Diseases in Pregnancy and Early Infancy, *edited by M. Schatz, R. S. Zeiger, and H. N. Claman*
111. Dyspnea, *edited by D. A. Mahler*

112. Proinflammatory and Antiinflammatory Peptides, *edited by S. I. Said*
113. Self-Management of Asthma, *edited by H. Kotses and A. Harver*
114. Eicosanoids, Aspirin, and Asthma, *edited by A. Szczeklik, R. J. Gryglewski, and J. R. Vane*
115. Fatal Asthma, *edited by A. L. Sheffer*
116. Pulmonary Edema, *edited by M. A. Matthay and D. H. Ingbar*
117. Inflammatory Mechanisms in Asthma, *edited by S. T. Holgate and W. W. Busse*
118. Physiological Basis of Ventilatory Support, *edited by J. J. Marini and A. S. Slutsky*
119. Human Immunodeficiency Virus and the Lung, *edited by M. J. Rosen and J. M. Beck*
120. Five-Lipoxygenase Products in Asthma, *edited by J. M. Drazen, S.-E. Dahlén, and T. H. Lee*
121. Complexity in Structure and Function of the Lung, *edited by M. P. Hlastala and H. T. Robertson*
122. Biology of Lung Cancer, *edited by M. A. Kane and P. A. Bunn, Jr.*
123. Rhinitis: Mechanisms and Management, *edited by R. M. Naclerio, S. R. Durham, and N. Mygind*
124. Lung Tumors: Fundamental Biology and Clinical Management, *edited by C. Brambilla and E. Brambilla*
125. Interleukin-5: From Molecule to Drug Target for Asthma, *edited by C. J. Sanderson*
126. Pediatric Asthma, *edited by S. Murphy and H. W. Kelly*
127. Viral Infections of the Respiratory Tract, *edited by R. Dolin and P. F. Wright*
128. Air Pollutants and the Respiratory Tract, *edited by D. L. Swift and W. M. Foster*
129. Gastroesophageal Reflux Disease and Airway Disease, *edited by M. R. Stein*
130. Exercise-Induced Asthma, *edited by E. R. McFadden, Jr.*
131. LAM and Other Diseases Characterized by Smooth Muscle Proliferation, *edited by J. Moss*
132. The Lung at Depth, *edited by C. E. G. Lundgren and J. N. Miller*
133. Regulation of Sleep and Circadian Rhythms, *edited by F. W. Turek and P. C. Zee*
134. Anticholinergic Agents in the Upper and Lower Airways, *edited by S. L. Spector*
135. Control of Breathing in Health and Disease, *edited by M. D. Altose and Y. Kawakami*
136. Immunotherapy in Asthma, *edited by J. Bousquet and H. Yssel*
137. Chronic Lung Disease in Early Infancy, *edited by R. D. Bland and J. J. Coalson*
138. Asthma's Impact on Society: The Social and Economic Burden, *edited by K. B. Weiss, A. S. Buist, and S. D. Sullivan*
139. New and Exploratory Therapeutic Agents for Asthma, *edited by M. Yeadon and Z. Diamant*
140. Multimodality Treatment of Lung Cancer, *edited by A. T. Skarin*
141. Cytokines in Pulmonary Disease: Infection and Inflammation, *edited by S. Nelson and T. R. Martin*
142. Diagnostic Pulmonary Pathology, *edited by P. T. Cagle*

143. Particle–Lung Interactions, *edited by P. Gehr and J. Heyder*
144. Tuberculosis: A Comprehensive International Approach, Second Edition, Revised and Expanded, *edited by L. B. Reichman and E. S. Hershfield*
145. Combination Therapy for Asthma and Chronic Obstructive Pulmonary Disease, *edited by R. J. Martin and M. Kraft*
146. Sleep Apnea: Implications in Cardiovascular and Cerebrovascular Disease, *edited by T. D. Bradley and J. S. Floras*
147. Sleep and Breathing in Children: A Developmental Approach, *edited by G. M. Loughlin, J. L. Carroll, and C. L. Marcus*
148. Pulmonary and Peripheral Gas Exchange in Health and Disease, *edited by J. Roca, R. Rodriguez-Roisin, and P. D. Wagner*
149. Lung Surfactants: Basic Science and Clinical Applications, *R. H. Notter*
150. Nosocomial Pneumonia, *edited by W. R. Jarvis*
151. Fetal Origins of Cardiovascular and Lung Disease, *edited by David J. P. Barker*
152. Long-Term Mechanical Ventilation, *edited by N. S. Hill*
153. Environmental Asthma, *edited by R. K. Bush*
154. Asthma and Respiratory Infections, *edited by D. P. Skoner*
155. Airway Remodeling, *edited by P. H. Howarth, J. W. Wilson, J. Bousquet, S. Rak, and R. A. Pauwels*
156. Genetic Models in Cardiorespiratory Biology, *edited by G. G. Haddad and T. Xu*
157. Respiratory-Circulatory Interactions in Health and Disease, *edited by S. M. Scharf, M. R. Pinsky, and S. Magder*
158. Ventilator Management Strategies for Critical Care, *edited by N. S. Hill and M. M. Levy*
159. Severe Asthma: Pathogenesis and Clinical Management, Second Edition, Revised and Expanded, *edited by S. J. Szefler and D. Y. M. Leung*
160. Gravity and the Lung: Lessons from Microgravity, *edited by G. K. Prisk, M. Paiva, and J. B. West*
161. High Altitude: An Exploration of Human Adaptation, *edited by T. F. Hornbein and R. B. Schoene*
162. Drug Delivery to the Lung, *edited by H. Bisgaard, C. O'Callaghan, and G. C. Smaldone*
163. Inhaled Steroids in Asthma: Optimizing Effects in the Airways, *edited by R. P. Schleimer, P. M. O'Byrne, S. J. Szefler, and R. Brattsand*
164. IgE and Anti-IgE Therapy in Asthma and Allergic Disease, *edited by R. B. Fick, Jr., and P. M. Jardieu*
165. Clinical Management of Chronic Obstructive Pulmonary Disease, *edited by T. Similowski, W. A. Whitelaw, and J.-P. Derenne*
166. Sleep Apnea: Pathogenesis, Diagnosis, and Treatment, *edited by A. I. Pack*
167. Biotherapeutic Approaches to Asthma, *edited by J. Agosti and A. L. Sheffer*
168. Proteoglycans in Lung Disease, *edited by H. G. Garg, P. J. Roughley, and C. A. Hales*
169. Gene Therapy in Lung Disease, *edited by S. M. Albelda*
170. Disease Markers in Exhaled Breath, *edited by N. Marczin, S. A. Kharitonov, M. H. Yacoub, and P. J. Barnes*
171. Sleep-Related Breathing Disorders: Experimental Models and Therapeutic Potential, *edited by D. W. Carley and M. Radulovacki*

172. Chemokines in the Lung, *edited by R. M. Strieter, S. L. Kunkel, and T. J. Standiford*
173. Respiratory Control and Disorders in the Newborn, *edited by O. P. Mathew*
174. The Immunological Basis of Asthma, *edited by B. N. Lambrecht, H. C. Hoogsteden, and Z. Diamant*
175. Oxygen Sensing: Responses and Adaptation to Hypoxia, *edited by S. Lahiri, G. L. Semenza, and N. R. Prabhakar*
176. Non-Neoplastic Advanced Lung Disease, *edited by J. R. Maurer*
177. Therapeutic Targets in Airway Inflammation, *edited by N. T. Eissa and D. P. Huston*
178. Respiratory Infections in Allergy and Asthma, *edited by S. L. Johnston and N. G. Papadopoulos*
179. Acute Respiratory Distress Syndrome, *edited by M. A. Matthay*
180. Venous Thromboembolism, *edited by J. E. Dalen*
181. Upper and Lower Respiratory Disease, *edited by J. Corren, A. Togias, and J. Bousquet*
182. Pharmacotherapy in Chronic Obstructive Pulmonary Disease, *edited by B. R. Celli*
183. Acute Exacerbations of Chronic Obstructive Pulmonary Disease, *edited by N. M. Siafakas, N. R. Anthonisen, and D. Georgopoulos*
184. Lung Volume Reduction Surgery for Emphysema, *edited by H. E. Fessler, J. J. Reilly, Jr., and D. J. Sugarbaker*
185. Idiopathic Pulmonary Fibrosis, *edited by J. P. Lynch III*
186. Pleural Disease, *edited by D. Bouros*
187. Oxygen/Nitrogen Radicals: Lung Injury and Disease, *edited by V. Vallyathan, V. Castranova, and X. Shi*
188. Therapy for Mucus-Clearance Disorders, *edited by B. K. Rubin and C. P. van der Schans*
189. Interventional Pulmonary Medicine, *edited by J. F. Beamis, Jr., P. N. Mathur, and A. C. Mehta*
190. Lung Development and Regeneration, *edited by D. J. Massaro, G. Massaro, and P. Chambon*
191. Long-Term Intervention in Chronic Obstructive Pulmonary Disease, *edited by R. Pauwels, D. S. Postma, and S. T. Weiss*
192. Sleep Deprivation: Basic Science, Physiology, and Behavior, *edited by Clete A. Kushida*
193. Sleep Deprivation: Clinical Issues, Pharmacology, and Sleep Loss Effects, *edited by Clete A. Kushida*
194. Pneumocystis Pneumonia: Third Edition, Revised and Expanded, *edited by P. D. Walzer and M. Cushion*
195. Asthma Prevention, *edited by William W. Busse and Robert F. Lemanske, Jr.*
196. Lung Injury: Mechanisms, Pathophysiology, and Therapy, *edited by Robert H. Notter, Jacob Finkelstein, and Bruce Holm*
197. Ion Channels in the Pulmonary Vasculature, *edited by Jason X.-J. Yuan*
198. Chronic Obstructive Pulmonary Disease: Cellular and Molecular Mechanisms, *edited by Peter J. Barnes*

199. Pediatric Nasal and Sinus Disorders, *edited by Tania Sih and Peter A. R. Clement*
200. Functional Lung Imaging, *edited by David Lipson and Edwin van Beek*
201. Lung Surfactant Function and Disorder, *edited by Kaushik Nag*
202. Pharmacology and Pathophysiology of the Control of Breathing, *edited by Denham S. Ward, Albert Dahan and Luc J. Teppema*
203. Molecular Imaging of the Lungs, *edited by Daniel Schuster and Timothy Blackwell*
204. Air Pollutants and the Respiratory Tract: Second Edition, *edited by W. Michael Foster and Daniel L. Costa*
205. Acute and Chronic Cough, *edited by Anthony E. Redington and Alyn H. Morice*
206. Severe Pneumonia, *edited by Michael S. Niederman*
207. Monitoring Asthma, *edited by Peter G. Gibson*
208. Dyspnea: Mechanisms, Measurement, and Management, Second Edition, *edited by Donald A. Mahler and Denis E. O'Donnell*
209. Childhood Asthma, *edited by Stanley J. Szefler and Søren Pedersen*
210. Sarcoidosis, *edited by Robert Baughman*
211. Tropical Lung Disease, Second Edition, *edited by Om Sharma*
212. Pharmacotherapy of Asthma, *edited by James T. Li*
213. Practical Pulmonary and Critical Care Medicine: Respiratory Failure, *edited by Zab Mosenifar and Guy W. Soo Hoo*
214. Practical Pulmonary and Critical Care Medicine: Disease Management, *edited by Zab Mosenifar and Guy W. Soo Hoo*
215. Ventilator-Induced Lung Injury, *edited by Didier Dreyfuss, Georges Saumon, and Rolf D. Hubmayr*
216. Bronchial Vascular Remodeling In Asthma and COPD, *edited by Aili Lazaar*
217. Lung and Heart–Lung Transplantation, *edited by Joseph P. Lynch III and David J. Ross*
218. Genetics of Asthma and Chronic Obstructive Pulmonary Disease, *edited by Dirkje S. Postma and Scott T. Weiss*
219. *Reichman and Hershfield's* Tuberculosis: A Comprehensive, International Approach, Third Edition (in two parts), *edited by Mario C. Raviglione*
220. Narcolepsy and Hypersomnia, *edited by Claudio Bassetti, Michel Billiard, and Emmanuel Mignot*
221. Inhalation Aerosols: Physical and Biological Basis for Therapy, Second Edition, *edited by Anthony J. Hickey*
222. Clinical Management of Chronic Obstructive Pulmonary Disease, Second Edition, *edited by Stephen I. Rennard, Roberto Rodriguez-Roisin, Gérard Huchon, and Nicolas Roche*
223. Sleep in Children, Second Edition: Developmental Changes in Sleep Patterns, *edited by Carole L. Marcus, John L. Carroll, David F. Donnelly, and Gerald M. Loughlin*
224. Sleep and Breathing in Children, Second Edition: Developmental Changes in Breathing During Sleep, *edited by Carole L. Marcus, John L. Carroll, David F. Donnelly, and Gerald M. Loughlin*

225. Ventilatory Support for Chronic Respiratory Failure, *edited by Nicolino Ambrosino and Roger S. Goldstein*
226. Diagnostic Pulmonary Pathology, Second Edition, *edited by Philip T. Cagle, Timothy C. Allen, and Mary Beth Beasley*

The opinions expressed in these volumes do not necessarily represent the views of the National Institutes of Health.

Diagnostic Pulmonary Pathology

Second Edition

Edited by
Philip T. Cagle
Weill Medical College of Cornell University
New York, New York, USA
The Methodist Hospital
Houston, Texas, USA
Timothy C. Allen
The University of Texas Health Science Center at Tyler
Tyler, Texas, USA
Mary Beth Beasley
Mount Sinai Medical Center
New York, New York, USA

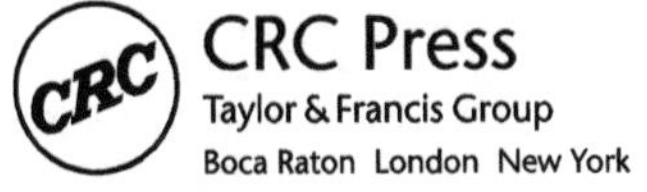

CRC Press is an imprint of the
Taylor & Francis Group, an **informa** business

First published 2008 by Informa Healthcare, Inc.

Published 2019 by CRC Press
Taylor & Francis Group
6000 Broken Sound Parkway NW, Suite 300
Boca Raton, FL 33487-2742

First issued in paperback 2019

ISBN 13: 978-0-367-45263-6 (pbk)
ISBN 13: 978-1-4200-6595-4 (hbk)

Visit the Taylor & Francis Web site at
http://www.taylorandfrancis.com

and the CRC Press Web site at
http://www.crcpress.com

Library of Congress Cataloging-in-Publication Data

Diagnostic pulmonary pathology / edited by Philip T. Cagle, Timothy C. Allen, Mary Beth Beasley.—2nd ed.
p. ; cm.—(Lung biology in health and disease ; 226)
Includes bibliographical references and index.
ISBN-13: 978-1-4200-6595-4 (hardcover : alk. paper)
ISBN-10: 1-4200-6595-5 (hardcover : alk. paper) 1. Lungs—Histopathology.
2. Lungs—Diseases—Diagnosis.
I. Cagle, Philip T. II. Allen, Timothy C.
III. Beasley, Mary Beth. IV. Series: Lung biology in health and disease ; v. 226.
[DNLM: 1. Lung Diseases—diagnosis. 2. Biopsy—methods.
3. Lung Diseases—pathology. 4. Lung Neoplasms—diagnosis.
5. Lung Neoplasms—pathology. W1 LU62 v.226 2008 / WF 600 D5355 2008]

RC711.D53 2008
616.2′4—dc22

2008000761

Introduction

The history of medicine tells us that postmortem dissection of human tissues was practiced by the Arabians as early as the 11th century. Muslim physicians, in particular, have been noted for their pioneering work. However, the main focus of this work was mostly to learn about anatomy. The 19th century brought a new page in the history of pathology. Indeed, work of Carl Rokitansky (1804–1878), Rudolf Virchow (1821–1902), and Julius Cohnheim (1839–1884) among others introduced pathology as we know it today—to correlate symptoms and clinical manifestations with tissue alterations. Virchow took this a step further by adapting the microscope to uncover tissue alterations at the cellular level. This really opened the door to modern pathology and to a medical discipline that gives the clinicians ultimate direction for diagnosis and therapeutic approaches.

Since World War II, pulmonary medicine has emerged as a strong and foremost specialty, which from its very beginning recognized the importance of anatomical and clinical pathology. These two medical specialties, pulmonary medicine and pathology, have worked in an effective synergistic manner at both the fundamental and clinical investigative levels and at the level of clinical medicine as well. In the 1950s, the study of disease was greatly enhanced by the use of electron microscopy.

In the later years of the 1990s, the series of monographs Lung Biology in Health and Disease recognized that the synergistic relationship of pulmonary medicine and pathology should be demonstrated to medical students, fellows, practicing pulmonologists, and pathologists. This led to the production and publication of *Diagnostic Pulmonary Pathology* in 2000 by Dr. Philip Cagle and outstanding experts in one, or even both, of the disciplines of pulmonary medicine and pathology. The idea behind the book was that if the practice of the physicians would be enhanced by this monograph, then their patients would benefit even more.

As Dr. Cagle points out in the preface of this new edition "many advances have taken place in pulmonary pathology, radiology, and pulmonary medicine" since the development and publication of the first edition of *Diagnostic Pulmonary Pathology*. Not least was the publication of the Human Genome in 2001; as we see almost every day, we move closer to major advances in pulmonary medicine and pathology from this new science. Thus, it should be no surprise that a new edition should be developed. While many of the chapters have the same title, all have new contents and, in some cases, new authors. In addition, six new chapters are included: three of them provide the readers a practical view of molecular diagnoses of some conditions and others present new opportunities to further refine the diagnosis of some diseases by radiology.

As the editor of this series of monographs, it is my privilege to thank Drs. Cagle, Allen, Beasley, and all the contributors for allowing us to present this volume to our readership with the confidence that ultimately patients will benefit.

Claude Lenfant, MD
Vancouver, Washington, U.S.A.

Preface

The first edition of *Diagnostic Pulmonary Pathology* provided a practical, user-friendly approach to the diagnosis of both neoplastic and non-neoplastic lung diseases that differed from most traditional textbooks. The theme was one of problem solving and the organization paralleled the actual strategy used by pathologists and pulmonologists in arriving at a patient's diagnosis in daily clinical practice. As is the first edition, the new edition will be valuable to residents in pathology and internal medicine, fellows specializing in pulmonology and pulmonary pathology, academic physicians with an interest in lung and pleural disease, and private practice pulmonologists and pathologists with active pulmonary practices. As with the first edition, the new edition's organization will lend itself to use for board study, both for pathologists in training and for pulmonologists in training.

Since the first edition of *Diagnostic Pulmonary Pathology* was published in 2000, many advances have taken place in pulmonary pathology, radiology, and pulmonary medicine. There has been considerable progress in classification of pulmonary disease since 2000: including the new 2004 World Health Organization classification of lung tumors, new classification schemes for interstitial lung diseases in both adult and pediatric patients and for pulmonary hypertension and evolution of our understanding of pre-neoplastic lesions. New understanding about chronic hypersensitivity pneumonitis, asthma, air pollution, transplant-related pathology, and tobacco-related lung diseases has emerged in recent years. There have been advances in technology in histopathology, diagnostic molecular pathology, and diagnostic thoracic radiology, including the widespread use of PET scans, in the past few years. These rapid advancements give reason and scope to a new edition of *Diagnostic Pulmonary Pathology*. Since 2000, important new pulmonary infectious agents, such as severe acute respiratory syndrome (SARS), have been recognized and some familiar ones have had a resurgence, including Pulmonary Tuberculosis, with its worldwide implications. Information regarding agents of chemical and biological warfare that affect the lungs, such as sarin gas, small pox, and anthrax, has become increasingly important. The clinical course, radiological features, and pathological findings of these infections and weaponized chemical and biological agents will be widely discussed in the second edition.

The new edition will maintain the format of the first edition: beginning with histopathological or clinical findings as they actually occur in daily practice, then providing the differential diagnosis of these findings and the process for eliminating possibilities from the differential diagnosis to arrive at the final diagnosis, etiology, and appropriate treatment. This unique approach differs from traditional pulmonary disease textbooks, most of which provide encyclopedic knowledge on different diseases but require that the pathologist or clinician already know what the diagnosis is likely to be. Instead, *Diagnostic Pulmonary Pathology* starts with the patient's clinical, radiologic, and biopsy findings and directs the pathologist or clinician to the proper diagnosis. The new edition will incorporate new classifications and new diagnostic techniques that have become available in the past six years.

The new edition retains the streamlined accessibility to information and enhancement of communication between medical specialties that characterized in the previous edition. Traditional textbooks on pulmonary pathology and pulmonary medicine categorize diseases according to etiology or mechanism, an approach that is the opposite of daily medical practice. In daily medical practice, patients present with a histopathological or clinical finding and the pathologist and pulmonologist must rule out possibilities from the differential diagnosis to determine the etiology and treatment. Rather than ask the reader to hunt through multiple chapters to identify the possible diagnoses that might fit a particular histopathological or clinical finding, *Diagnostic Pulmonary Pathology* provides information in the same manner that patients present in daily medical practice.

The audience for the second edition of *Diagnostic Pulmonary Pathology* is the same as for the first edition: pulmonary pathologists, pulmonologists, thoracic surgeons in both private and academic practices as well as fellows training in pulmonary pathology and pulmonary medicine. Due to its unique organization, the second edition will retain its value to those with less specific background in lung diseases but who must diagnose them nevertheless, including general pathologists, general medicine practitioners, general pathology residents, and general medicine residents.

Philip T. Cagle
Timothy C. Allen
Mary Beth Beasley

Contributors

Timothy C. Allen The University of Texas Health Science Center at Tyler, Tyler, Texas, U.S.A.

Rose C. Anton Weill Medical College of Cornell University, New York, New York, and The Methodist Hospital, Houston, Texas, U.S.A.

Mary Beth Beasley Mount Sinai Medical Center, New York, New York, U.S.A.

Shanda Blackmon The Methodist Hospital, Houston, Texas, U.S.A.

Alain C. Borczuk Columbia University Medical Center, New York, New York, U.S.A.

Elisabeth Brambilla Centre Hospitalier Universitaire de Grenoble, INSERM U823, University UJF, Grenoble, France

Brett Burbridge Oregon Health and Science University, Portland, Oregon, U.S.A.

Philip T. Cagle Weill Medical College of Cornell University, New York, New York, and The Methodist Hospital, Houston, Texas, U.S.A.

Joe M. Chan Oregon Health and Science University, Portland, Oregon, U.S.A.

Andrew Churg University of British Columbia, Vancouver, British Columbia, Canada

Thomas V. Colby Mayo Clinic Arizona, Scottsdale, Arizona, U.S.A.

Sanja Dacic University of Pittsburgh, Pittsburgh, Pennsylvania, U.S.A.

Megan K. Dishop Baylor College of Medicine, Texas Children's Hospital, Houston, Texas, U.S.A.

John C. English Vancouver General Hospital and The University of British Columbia, Vancouver, British Columbia, Canada

Michael C. Fishbein David Geffen School of Medicine, University of California, Los Angeles, California, U.S.A.

Armando E. Fraire Department of Pathology, University of Massachusetts Medical School, Worcester, Massachusetts, U.S.A.

Adaani E. Frost Baylor College of Medicine, Houston, Texas, U.S.A.

Françoise Galateau-Sallé *MESONAT Registry/ERI 3 INSERM CHU* Caen University of Medicine, Caen, France

Marc V. Gosselin Oregon Health and Science University, Portland, Oregon, U.S.A.

Donald G. Guinee, Jr. Virginia Mason Medical Center, Seattle, Washington, U.S.A.

Ruta Gupta Cedars Sinai Medical Center, Los Angeles, California, U.S.A.

Abida K. Haque Weill College of Cornell University, New York, New York; The Methodist Hospital, Houston; and San Jacinto Methodist Hospital, Baytown, Texas, U.S.A.

Philip S. Hasleton Clinical Sciences Block, Manchester Royal Infirmary, Manchester, U.K.

John G. Hay New York University School of Medicine, New York, New York, U.S.A.

Kirk D. Jones Department of Anatomic Pathology, University of California San Francisco, San Francisco, California, U.S.A.

Keith M. Kerr Department of Pathology, Aberdeen University Medical School and Aberdeen Royal Infirmary, Aberdeen, U.K.

Andras Khoor Mayo Clinic, Jacksonville, Florida, U.S.A.

Talmadge E. King, Jr. Department of Medicine, University of California San Francisco, San Francisco, California, U.S.A.

Steven H. Kirtland Virginia Mason Medical Center, Seattle, Washington, U.S.A.

Lisa Kopas Baylor College of Medicine, Houston, Texas, U.S.A.

Chi K. Lai David Geffen School of Medicine, University of California, Los Angeles, California, U.S.A.

Faqian Li David Geffen School of Medicine, University of California, Los Angeles, California, U.S.A.

Kevin O. Leslie Mayo Clinic Arizona, Scottsdale, Arizona, U.S.A.

Richard W. Light Vanderbilt University Medical Center, Nashville, Tennessee, U.S.A.

Alberto M. Marchevsky Cedars Sinai Medical Center, Los Angeles, California, U.S.A.

John R. Muhm Mayo Clinic Arizona, Scottsdale, Arizona, U.S.A.

N. Paul Ohori UPMC-Presbyterian, Pittsburgh, Pennsylvania, U.S.A.

Soumya Parimi Virginia Mason Medical Center, Seattle, Washington, U.S.A.

Helmut H. Popper Institute of Pathology, Medical University of Graz, Graz, Austria

Gary W. Procop Cleveland Clinic Foundation and the Cleveland Clinic Lerner College of Medicine, Cleveland, Ohio, U.S.A.

Kirtee Raparia The Methodist Hospital, Houston, Texas, U.S.A.

Victor L. Roggli Department of Pathology, Duke University Medical Center, Durham, North Carolina, U.S.A.

David J. Ross David Geffen School of Medicine, Ronald Reagan UCLA Medical Center, University of California, Los Angeles, California, U.S.A.

Lewis J. Rubin University of California, San Diego School of Medicine, La Jolla, California, U.S.A.

Zeenat Safdar Baylor College of Medicine, Houston, Texas, U.S.A.

Rajeev Saggar David Geffen School of Medicine, Ronald Reagan UCLA Medical Center, University of California, Los Angeles, California, U.S.A.

Harald Sauthoff New York University School of Medicine, New York, New York, U.S.A.

Anu Sharma Department of Cytopathology, Pittsburgh VA Medical Center and Department of Pathology, University of Pittsburgh, Pittsburgh, Pennsylvania, U.S.A.

Om P. Sharma Keck School of Medicine, Los Angeles, California, U.S.A.

Anna E. Sienko The Methodist Hospital, Houston, Texas, U.S.A.

Thomas Sporn Department of Pathology, Duke University Medical Center, Durham, North Carolina, U.S.A.

Henry D. Tazelaar Mayo Clinic, Scottsdale, Arizona, U.S.A.

Jeffrey Truell David Geffen School of Medicine, University of California, Los Angeles, California, U.S.A.

W. Dean Wallace Cedars-Sinai Medical Center, Los Angeles, California, U.S.A.

Chih-Wei Wang Chang Gung Memorial Hospital, Taoyuan, Taiwan

Eunhee S. Yi Mayo Clinic, Rochester, Minnesota, U.S.A.

Leslie H. Zimmerman Veterans Administration Medical Center, San Francisco, California, U.S.A.

Contents

1
Transbronchial Biopsies: Clinical Perspective

ADAANI E. FROST
Baylor College of Medicine, Houston, Texas, U.S.A.

I. Introduction

A transbronchial biopsy (TBBx) of the lung provides a limited amount of tissue from a limited sampling area but with reduced morbidity and mortality as compared with surgical biopsy. Its clinical utility, therefore, is determined by the following:

1. The likelihood of successfully sampling the area of interest
2. The likelihood, in a given disease state, of being able to make a positive pathological diagnosis
3. The likelihood that an appropriate diagnosis will have a significant impact on treatment or outcome
4. The likelihood of morbidity or mortality with the procedure—a determination based on the nature of the underlying disease process and patient-specific risks

Successful sampling as well as morbidity and mortality are to a certain extent affected by operator skill, the assessment of which, except in very broad terms, is beyond the scope of this handbook.

Pulmonary disease processes can be broadly categorized into those that are focal versus diffuse and those affecting immunocompetent versus immunosuppressed patients. In the following pages, an attempt to assess the clinical utility of TBBx in various disease processes is undertaken.

A. Procedural Risks: Morbidity and Mortality

The procedural risks of TBBx are well established for the procedure in general and for certain high-risk groups specifically. In stable immunocompetent outpatients (1) and in the general patient population, bronchoscopy with TBBx has been reported as a relatively benign procedure (2). A retrospective review in 1983 of 40,000 bronchoscopies with transbronchial biopsies performed in the United Kingdom revealed a mortality of 0.12% and a major complication rate of 2.7% (3). These major complications included bleeding and pneumothorax requiring intervention. The use of fluoroscopy in decreasing the likelihood of complications is controversial, though it does increase diagnostic yield in focal disease (4), and some data suggest that while it does not alter the frequency of pneumothorax, it may decrease the likelihood of pneumothorax requiring drainage. Patients on mechanical ventilation (5) as well as those with bullous emphysema, thrombocytopenia (6), coagulation disorders, and possibly acquired immunodeficiency syndrome (AIDS) (7) are at significantly increased risk for complications. While pulmonary hypertension (PH) is theoretically a risk factor, it is unclear that it has any impact on the risks of bleeding with TBBx. One small study of risks and benefits of biopsy in cardiac transplant recipients suggested that a mean pulmonary artery pressure greater than 16 mmHg was associated with a higher incidence of bleeding; this was however not statistically significant (8). A recent survey of patterns of practice conducted at the American College of Chest Physicians suggested that factors generally considered risks for transbronchial lung biopsy included thrombocytopenia, uremia, hypoxemia, and PH. Mean pulmonary artery pressures greater than 30 were considered to be unsafe for TBBx by 96% of respondents (9). Guidelines published by the British Thoracic Society state that "some patients are known to be at increased risk of bleeding, including those who have uraemia, immunosuppression, PH, liver disease, coagulation disorders, or thrombocytopenia (10)." No reliable data is offered in support for increased risk of bleeding conferred by PH; however, the frequency of substantial bronchial collateral hypertrophy provides physiological rationale for such a risk.

B. Novel Techniques Increasing Bronchoscopic Yield

Several novel techniques to increase diagnostic yield with TBBx have been developed. A brief review of the literature on these techniques is included here as these techniques are not widely available, and are very operator/facility dependent and require extensive training.

Endobronchial Ultrasound

Endobronchial ultrasound (EBUS) is a diagnostic technique permitting visualization of the tracheobronchial wall and the immediately adjacent structures. The ERS/ATS consensus statement on interventional pulmonology recommends that this technique should be reserved for experienced bronchoscopists who have participated in approximately 40 supervised procedures and undertake 25 procedures per year. Currently, EBUS-assisted transbronchial lung biopsy has been used to evaluate peripheral or fluoroscopically occult pulmonary nodules. The procedure involves advancing a thin ultrasound probe through a working channel of the bronchoscope (using anatomical cues based on prior CT estimation of site of lesion). An EBUS picture consistent with a proximate lesion identifies the sampling site. The prior addition of a guide sheath surrounding the probe permits control of the site (for bleeding) and repeat sampling of the site to increase yield. Diagnostic yield for otherwise bronchoscopically occult lesions has been reported to be as high as 84% when an EBUS image is acquired (11). Lesions smaller than 2 cm continue to have a relatively low diagnostic yield (29%) (12).

CT Guidance and Ultrathin Bronchoscopic Biopsy

Ultrathin bronchoscopes aided by CT-guided navigation have been utilized to improve yield in the evaluation of the small (<2 cm) peripheral pulmonary nodule (13). Diagnostic sensitivity as high as 65% has been reported (14) using this technique. Lesions in the left superior segment of the lower lobe have been found to be less amenable to this diagnostic approach even in expert centers. The presence of a pulmonary artery and/or a bronchus leading to the lesion increases the likelihood of diagnosis using this very specialized and center-specific technique (15).

Electromagnetic Navigation Diagnostic Bronchoscopy

Electromagnetic navigation diagnostic bronchoscopy (ENB) is designed to guide bronchoscopic biopsy using a sensor probe that picks up the electromagnetic field generated by a localization system, a processor, an amplifier, and a location board. The position of the sensor can be identified, and its position and orientation displayed on a monitor and superimposed on previously acquired CT images. This image-guided localization device guides TBBx of predetermined targets in the bronchial tree. Because of the size of the bronchoscope needed for the working channel, this technique has so far required general anesthesia. This methodology has resulted in overall diagnostic yields in these hard-to-reach lesions of 62.5% (16). Combinations of ENB with EBUS have yielded higher diagnostic yield than either methodology alone (17).

For the general pulmonologist, however, these diagnostic methods are not routinely available. In high-risk patients where diagnosis is potentially critical for survival and comorbidities (as discussed below) impart unacceptable risk to surgical biopsy, consideration of referral to centers expert in these novel techniques should be considered.

II. The Immunocompetent Patient

A. Focal Radiological Abnormalities

This category includes progressive or persistent infiltrates (localized to one area of the lung), nodules, and masses.

Likelihood of Successful Sampling and Positive Diagnosis

The likelihood of successful sampling and diagnosis depends on the size and position of the lesion. When an endobronchial lesion is seen, the diagnostic yield is high (90–100%) (18–21), with little additional diagnostic benefit from brushing or bronchoalveolar lavage (BAL).

Bronchoscopy is useful in the diagnosis of peripheral lung lesions. Transbronchial biopsies assisted by biplane fluoroscopy and additional cytological sampling by BAL, and cytological brushing can yield a diagnosis in between 40% and 80% of lung cancers (22–25). Benign lesions are diagnosed with greater difficulty, since this is in part a diagnosis of exclusion (26). Diagnostic yield in peripheral lesions is predicated largely on the size of the lesion; lesions less than 2 cm in diameter have only a 15% to 35% diagnostic yield with routine bronchoscopy and biopsy unaided by specialized techniques discussed earlier. Other factors have been implicated in lower yields, although none have been substantiated (e.g., distance from the hilum, cell type).

Likelihood That TBBx Diagnosis Will Have a Significant Impact on Treatment or Outcome

The physician has an obligation to the patient to perform the least invasive procedure to achieve the desired outcome (in this case, a diagnosis that will facilitate treatment). However, in the presence of a nodule or mass, if malignancy is highly suspected and if the patient is an acceptable surgical candidate (no evidence of metastatic disease or an extrapulmonary primary, acceptable pulmonary function tests (PFTs), and a surgically approachable lesion), an excisional open lung biopsy with intraoperative frozen section using a minithoracotomy or thoracoscopic approach is preferred to a bronchoscopic biopsy. The rationale for this is that an established diagnosis of malignancy (including a localized small cell tumor) would require surgical excision. Similarly, failure to make a diagnosis or making a diagnosis not compatible with the clinical appearance would result in the patient proceeding to surgical biopsy. Since virtually all roads lead to surgery, there is little clinical value in attempting to make a less invasive diagnosis.

In a patient with medical risk factors for surgery (e.g., severe pulmonary disease, cardiac disease, etc.), the risks of any procedure should be tempered by a rational approach to treating the underlying lesion. Since the only primary pulmonary malignancy amenable to nonsurgical treatment is small cell carcinoma, consideration of *no* diagnostic intervention in this high-risk population or a diagnostic intervention limited to BAL (to rule out a treatable benign lesion) should be entertained. Again referral to centers with expertise in the EBUS, or ENB guidance should be considered.

B. Diffuse Radiological Abnormalities

This category includes heterogeneous and homogeneous infiltrates.

Likelihood of Successful Sampling and Positive Diagnosis

The overall diagnostic yield for diffuse lung disease with TBBx in the immunocompetent patient is approximately 37% (27). Diseases that are peribronchial in their distribution (sarcoid, lymphangitic carcinoma) and those with specific definable histology (alveolar proteinosis, malignancy, eosinophilic granuloma) are particularly amenable to diagnosis by TBBx. Mucosal and parenchymal biopsy will provide a definite diagnosis in 85% to 97% of patients with sarcoid (28). Langerhans' histiocytosis can be diagnosed by routine histology as well as the finding of the characteristic X bodies on electron microscopy (EM) (these may also be detected in BAL sampling; and by S100 stains identifying Langerhans cells). Similarly, TBBx has a high diagnostic yield in lymphangitic carcinoma, pulmonary alveolar proteinosis, and Goodpasture's disease. The diagnosis of Wegener's has been made by TBBx, but the size of the lesions and the limitation of sampling usually require a larger piece of tissue that can be afforded by TBBx; even in the presence of an open lung biopsy, sampling may have an effect on successful diagnosis (29).

Likelihood That a TBBx Diagnosis Will Have a Significant Effect on Treatment or Outcome

Interstitial lung diseases within certain broad categories in the immunocompetent host can have vastly different potential treatments. Sarcoidosis responds well to steroids, as do some forms of pulmonary fibrosis. Goodpasture's disease and Wegener's granulomatosis require careful scrutiny of kidney function, high-dose and prolonged pulse cyclophosphamide therapy and/or oral mycophenolate mofetil maintenance and occasionally plasmapheresis. Lymphangitic carcinoma carries a dismal prognosis, with therapy and potential response to therapy largely dependent on the underlying malignancy. Infectious etiologies such as tuberculosis and histoplasmosis clearly require organism-specific therapy. Alveolar proteinosis is both a biopsy and lavage diagnosis. Langerhans histiocytosis has no known treatment, although its diagnosis would initiate family screening, registry or study enrollment, and smoking cessation. Lymphangioleiomyomatosis has many other associated features and variable responses to limited therapeutic options (leuprolide, progesterone) that differ radically from the characteristics of previously mentioned diagnoses. Occupational/environmental lung diseases usually require a combination of histology, lavage, and history to make the diagnosis, and therapy may involve removing the patient from his or her domestic or occupational environment.

Therefore, in a well individual with a diffuse interstitial infiltrates, bronchoscopy and TBBx are well tolerated and may provide a clear-cut histological diagnosis (76%) (4) that may direct therapy. In a patient compromised by severe lung disease or other complicating diseases, a less invasive diagnosis by exclusion using BAL alone may be a wiser choice. BAL is as useful as biopsy for most infectious etiologies. The X bodies of Langerhans histiocytosis have been found in BAL samples. Alveolar proteinosis has a characteristic, cloudy BAL with the consistency of cream soup. Wegener's and Goodpasture's and the other alveolar hemorrhage syndromes have pathognomonic serological markers and other systemic findings. Alveolar hemorrhage can be differentiated from other "alveolar filling" disorders based on the characteristics of the BAL; the immediate therapy is similar once infection has been ruled out. In the critically ill patient and in the presence of diffuse alveolar hemorrhage with a normal pulmonary capillary wedge pressure and no evidence of infection, one article recommends that therapy (steroids) should be initiated even while diagnostic evaluations are being undertaken (30). Therefore, TBBx provides a definitive diagnosis with reliability in diffuse interstitial lung disease. However, in severely ill individuals where the main differential includes an infectious process versus an idiopathic or autoimmune disease (where steroids may be the only viable intervention), this differential can be achieved with BAL alone without the added risks of TBBx.

Patients with acute respiratory distress syndrome (ARDS) on the ventilator are a critically ill group of patients in whom bronchoscopy with BAL has proven useful in diagnosis and treatment. A review (31) of the role of transbronchial lung biopsy in these patients suggests that earlier in the disease in patients who are immunocompetent, TBBx with fluoroscopic control is a useful adjunct and permitted specific diagnosis with good pathological correlation with open lung biopsy. A combined procedure (that is BAL and TBBx) was helpful in obtaining a specific diagnosis in up to 74% of patients resulting in significant modification of therapy in 63% of patients. Only one side should be biopsied (due to the risk of bilateral pneumothoraces), multiple samples need to be obtained, and the biopsies have to be of adequate size. TBBx in conjunction with BAL was contraindicated in the ARDS patients with bleeding diathesis, hemodynamic instability, oxygen saturation less than 90% on high FiO_2, and clinical evidence of severe PH.

III. The Immunocompromised Patient

This category comprises an increasingly broad group of patients including those immunosuppressed by the nature of their disease or its treatment (e.g., diabetes, autoimmune disease), transplant patients (solid organ, bone marrow, hematopoietic stem cell), those with profound but intermittent immunosuppression for treatment of hematological and other malignancies, and patients with AIDS. Broad diagnostic possibilities in the immunocompromised patient include infections (usual or opportunistic), manifestations of the primary disease process (recurrence of a primary malignancy, autoimmune pneumonitis), adverse consequences of therapy [radiation pneumonitis, drug toxicity, lung transplant rejection, bronchiolitis obliterans with organizing pneumonia (BOOP) after bone marrow transplant], ARDS, or new malignancy [Kaposi's sarcoma in AIDS, second tumors, posttransplant lymphoproliferative disease (PTLD), and immunosuppression induced tumors].

A. Focal Radiological Abnormalities

The differentiation of focal versus diffuse infiltrates in this patient population is becoming less critical with modern methods of serological and noninvasive surveillance/sampling and with routine prophylaxis of immunosuppressed patients for commonly recognized pathogens [*Nocardia*, *Pneumocystis carinii* (PCP), cytomegalovirus (CMV)].

Likelihood of Successful Sampling and Positive Diagnosis

The likelihood of successful sampling in this group is equivalent to that in immunocompetent patients.

Likelihood That a TBBx Diagnosis Will Have a Significant Effect on Treatment or Outcome

Focal radiological abnormalities can occur as a consequence of malignancy or infection in this patient population. PTLD occurs in recipients of solid organ transplants as both focal nodules (single or multiple) or as an infiltrate (focal or diffuse). Recurrent or immunosuppression precipitated malignancies can present as solitary or multiple nodules. Infections in this patient population not infrequently present as nodular lesions. A bronchoscopy and a biopsy in a patient posttransplant or with AIDS might obviate the need for a surgical lung biopsy—the approach of choice in the immunocompetent patient with a solitary nodule or mass.

The finding of elevated polymerase chain reaction (PCR) for Epstein-Barr virus (EBV) (the virus responsible for PTLD) while suggestive of the disease is not diagnostic. Many infectious entities (notably *Nocardia*, *Cryptococcus*, and *Aspergillus*) can present as nodules. Though the yield is poor if the lesions are smaller and peripheral, if the patient is otherwise stable the possibility of finding a diagnosis that would spare the patient a surgical lung biopsy makes TBBx coupled with BAL a useful endeavour. No diagnosis or one not consistent with the clinical picture should precipitate surgical lung biopsy.

B. Diffuse Radiological Abnormalities

The approach to diffuse radiological abnormalities in the immunosuppressed patient population has changed with the routine use of both prophylaxis regimens (for CMV and *Pneumocystis*), and serological screening tools (CMV antigenemia, CMV-PCR, Human Herpes Virus (HHV) screening on nasal swabs, influenza antigen on nasal swabs; EBV-PCR, *Aspergillus* galactomannan) and significantly altered the diagnostic utility of BAL and TBBx.

Likelihood of Successful Sampling and Positive Diagnosis

A retrospective review of 169 bronchoscopies in over 1100 hematopoietic stem cell transplant recipients (HSCT's) was undertaken in the context of current standards of prophylaxis and serologic monitoring. This review concluded that diagnostic bronchoscopy is useful for determining the etiology of pulmonary infiltrates in 50% of adult allogenic and 34% of autologous HSCT recipients; this information *often* influences therapy (in allo-HCST 50% of the time and in 36% of auto-HCST recipients). However, BAL alone provided most diagnoses whereas TBBx provided additional specific information in less than 10% of cases. Complications occurred in 9% of all HSCT patients and were associated with a significantly higher in-hospital mortality rate (38% mortality for allo-HSCT vs. 27% for auto-HSCT recipients). Importantly a specific diagnosis by bronchoscopy was not associated with an improved in-hospital mortality in either group (32). The surprising lack of benefit of bronchoscopy may reflect variable timing of the procedure, delay in bronchoscopy relative to onset of symptoms, or the limited sensitivity of diagnostic bronchoscopy. It would certainly support a role for isolated BAL without the additional risk of TBBx in this patient population. Similar conclusions were reported in a review of 101 bronchoscopies performed in 1651 HSCT recipients. This review called into question the utility of bronchoscopy at all in this patient population where diagnostic yield was only 50%, where additional therapy was administered in only 20%, and where there was no detectable survival benefit (33). Given these dismal results, pending a large multicenter study, it should be recognized that the onset of pulmonary complications in the HSCT population is associated with inordinately high mortality and that bronchoscopy may confer only limited benefit on diagnosis or therapy. When these patients proceed to either autopsy or surgical lung biopsy rarely is a treatable/reversible condition identified. The rarely reported (four) cases of pulmonary alveolar proteinosis in recipients of bone marrow (34) and stem cell transplantation (35) make it hard to justify TBBx in this patient population particularly as its outcome is either relatively benign (resolution with reconstitution of marrow associated with use of GCSF) or catastrophic when associated with multisystem organ failure.

Newly recognized and increasingly important pathogens such as HHV6 viruses, and metapneumovirus, can be identified on BAL (culture or PCR) and do not require the additional risk of a TBBx.

Likelihood That a TBBx Diagnosis Will Have a Significant Effect on Treatment or Outcome

The impact of diagnosis on treatment and outcome is dependent on the cause of the immuno-incompetence. This recent data suggests that transbronchial lung biopsy for diffuse pulmonary infiltrates in the HSCT patient population is likely to yield little and confer a substantial risk.

In contrast, this data review does not reflect the tremendous utility of transbronchial lung biopsy in lung transplant recipients where it is used to monitor transplant rejection, response to therapy, and onset of unexpected pathology (primary disease recurrence, viral or bacterial pathogens, malignancy). The latter are a unique patient population but one where newer methods of monitoring for adequate immunosuppression may ultimately discriminate between acute cellular rejection and some of these other entities.

Though the poor diagnostic yield of BAL in, for example, leukemic infiltrates is quoted as a rationale for proceeding to TBBx early in the diagnosis and evaluation period, there is conflicting data on its practical utility. In one review (36), in no cases of leukemic infiltrate was the pulmonary lesion the only evidence of active leukemia with blast crisis. Therefore, the only really important diagnostic decision prior to embarking on chemotherapy for these patients is to ascertain that infection is not partly responsible for the diffuse pulmonary infiltrates—a decision that can be arrived at with BAL alone. A retrospective review of 107 fiberoptic bronchoscopies with and without transbronchial lung biopsy in 98 consecutive patients with hematological malignancies and pulmonary infiltrates demonstrated that the combination of BAL and TBBx was superior to BAL alone in the diagnosis of neoplastic infiltrates—however no comment was made about other manifestations of malignancy—but most importantly it was useful for discriminating toxic pneumonitis (37). The utility of TBBx in making a diagnosis of toxic pneumonitis in patients treated for malignancy is therefore potentially important therapeutically and in discriminating this entity from malignancy. Again operator judgment and clinical scenario need to be considered in the decision to biopsy the nontransplant patient treated for malignancy with pulmonary infiltrates.

In HIV/AIDS in the presence of diffuse pulmonary infiltrates, a multilobar BAL will make a reliable diagnosis of PCP; however, TBBx improves the sensitivity for diagnoses of tuberculosis and fungal pneumonias and is necessary to confirm invasive aspergillosis. Tissue confirmation with TBBx is necessary for noninfectious disorders such as non-Hodgkin's lymphoma, lymphocytic and nonspecific pneumonitis. Visualization of endobronchial Kaposi's is usually sufficient for the diagnosis of that entity though diagnostic yield is enhanced by the detection of HHV8 in BAL samples (38).

References

1. Hernandez Blasco L, Sanchez Hernandez IM, Villen Garrido V, et al. Safety of the transbronchial biopsy in outpatients. Chest 1991; 99:562–565.
2. Shure D. Bronchoscopy: transbronchial biopsy and needle aspiration. Chest 1989; 95: 1130–1138.
3. Simpson FG, Arnold AG, Purvis A, et al. Postal survey of bronchoscopic practice by physicians in the United Kingdom. Thorax 1986; 41:311–317.
4. Anders GT, Johnson JE, Bush BA, et al. Transbronchial biopsy without fluoroscopy: a seven-year perspective. Chest 1988; 94:557–560.
5. Papin TA, Gram CM, Weg JC. Transbronchial biopsy during mechanical ventilation. Chest 1986; 89:168–170.
6. Papin TA, Lynch JP III, Weg JG. Transbronchial biopsy in the thrombocytopenic patient. Chest 1985; 88:549–552.
7. Milligan SA, Luce JM, Golden U, et al. Transbronchial biopsy without fluoroscopy in patients with diffuse roentgenographic infiltrates and the acquired immunodeficiency syndrome. Am Rev Respir Dis 1988; 137:486–488.
8. Schulman LL, Smith CR, Drusin R, et al. Utility of airway endoscopy in the diagnosis of respiratory complications of cardiac transplantation. Chest 1988; 93:960–967.
9. Wahidi M, Rocha A, Hollingsworth J, et al. Contraindications and safety of transbronchial lung biopsy via flexible bronchoscopy. Respiration 2005; 72:285–295.
10. British Thoracic Society Bronchoscopy Guidelines Committee. British Thoracic Society guidelines on diagnostic flexible bronchoscopy, Thorax 2001; 56(suppl 1):i1–i21.
11. Dooms CA, Verbeken E, Becker H, et al. Endobronchial ultrasonography in bronchoscopically occult pulmonary lesions. J Thorac Oncol 2007; 2:121–124.

12. Yoshikawa M, Sukoh N, Yamazaki K, et al. Diagnostic value of endobronchial ultrasonography with a guide sheath for peripheral pulmonary lesions without X-ray fluoroscopy. Chest 2007; 131:1788–1793.
13. Asano F, Matsuno Y, Matsushita T, et al. Transbronchial diagnosis of a pulmonary peripheral small lesion using an ultrathin bronchoscope with virtual bronchoscopic navigation. J Bronchol 2002; 9:108–111.
14. Shinagawa N, Yamazaki K, Onodera Y, et al. CT-guided transbronchial biopsy using an ultrathin bronchoscope with virtual bronchoscopic navigation. Chest 2004; 125: 1138–1143.
15. Shinagawa N, Yamazaki K, Onodera Y, et al. Factors related to diagnostic sensitivity using an ultrathin bronchoscope under CT guidance. Chest 2007; 131:549–553.
16. Makris D, Scherpereel A, Leroy S, et al. Electromagnetic navigation diagnostic bronchoscopy for small peripheral lung lesions. Eur Respir J 2007; 29:1187–1192.
17. Eberhardt R, Anantham D, Ernst A, et al. Multimodality bronchoscopic diagnosis of peripheral lung lesions. A randomized controlled trial. Am J Respire Crit Care Med 2007; 176:36–41.
18. Shure D, Astarita RW. Bronchogenic carcinoma presenting as an endobronchial mass. Chest 1983; 6:865–867.
19. Popovich J, Kvale PA, Eichenhorn MS, et al. Diagnostic accuracy of multiple biopsies from flexible fiberoptic bronchoscopy. Am Rev Respir Dis 1982; 125:521–523.
20. Martini N, Mccormich PM. Assessment of endoscopically visible bronchial carcinomas. Chest 1978; 73:718–720.
21. Zaval DC. Diagnostic fiberoptic bronchoscopy: techniques and results of biopsy in 600 patients. Chest 1975; 68:12–19.
22. Cortese DA, McDougall JC. Biopsy and brushing of peripheral lung cancer with fluoroscopic guidance. Chest 1979; 75:141–145.
23. Kvale PA, Bode FR, Kini S. Diagnostic accuracy in lung cancer: comparison of techniques used in association with flexible fiberoptic bronchoscopy. Chest 1976; 69:752–757.
24. Radke JR, Conway WA, Eyler WR, et al. Diagnostic accuracy in peripheral lung lesions: factors predicting success with flexible fiberoptic bronchoscopy. Chest 1979; 76:176–179.
25. Arroliga AC, Matthay RA. The role of bronchoscopy in lung cancer. Clin Chest Med 1993; 14:87–98.
26. Wallace JM, Deutsch AL. Flexible fiberoptic bronchoscopy and percutaneous needle lung aspiration for evaluating the solitary pulmonary nodule. Chest 1982; 81:665–671.
27. Wall CP, Gaensler EA, Carrington CB, et al. Comparison of transbronchial and open biopsies in chronic infiltrative lung diseases. Am Rev Respir Dis 1981; 123:280–285.
28. Armstrong JR, Radke JR, Kvale PA, et al. Endoscopic findings in sarcoidosis: characteristics and correlations with radiographic staging and bronchial mucosal biopsy yield. Ann Otol Rhinol Laryngol 1981; 90:339–343.
29. Myers JL, Katzenstein AA. Wegener's granulomatosis presenting with massive pulmonary hemorrhage and capillaritis. Am J Surg Pathol 1987; 11:895–898.
30. Green RJ, Ruoss SJ, Kraft SA, et al. Pulmonary capillaritis and alveolar hemorrhage: update on diagnosis and management. Chest 1996; 110:1305–1316.
31. Terminella L, Sharma G. Diagnostic studies in patient with acute respiratory distress syndrome. Semin Thorac Cardiovasc Surg 2006; 18:2–7.
32. Patel NR, Lee P-S, Kim JH, et al. The influence of diagnostic bronchoscopy on clnical outcomes comparing adult autologous and allogeneic bone marrow transplant patients. Chest 2005; 127:1388–1396.
33. Hofmeister CC, Czerlanis C, Forsythe S, et al. Retrospective utility of bronchoscopy after hematopoietic stem cell transplant. Bone Marrow Transplant 2006; 38:693–698.
34. Cordonnier C, Fleury-Feith J, Escudier E, et al. Secondary alveolar proteinosis is a reversible cause of respiratory failure in leukemia patients. Am J Respir Crit Care Med 1994; 149:788–794.

35. Tomonari A, Shirafuji J, Iseki T, et al. Acquired pulmonary alveolar proteinosis after umbilical cord blood transplantation for acute myeloid leukemia. Am J Hematol 2002; 70:154–157.
36. Kovalski R, Hansen-Flaschen J, Lodata RF, et al. Localized leukemic pulmonary infiltrates: diagnosis by bronchoscopy and resolution with therapy. Chest 1990; 97:674–678.
37. Mulabecirovic A, Gaulhofer P, Auner HW, et al. Pulmonary infiltrates in patients with hematologic malignancies: transbronchial lung biopsy increases the diagnostic yield with respect to neoplastic infiltrates and toxic pneumonitis. Ann Hematol 2004; 83:420–422.
38. Narayanswami G, Salzman SH. Bronchoscopy in the human immunodeficiency virus-infected patient. Semin Respir Infect 2003; 18(2):80–86.

2
Endobronchial and Transbronchial Biopsies

KIRTEE RAPARIA
The Methodist Hospital, Houston, Texas, U.S.A.

PHILIP T. CAGLE
Weill Medical College of Cornell University, New York, New York,
and The Methodist Hospital, Houston, Texas, U.S.A.

I. Introduction

Endobronchial and transbronchial biopsies are useful in diagnosing neoplasms, infections, and certain interstitial lung diseases (Table 1). The diagnostic yield is often increased when the biopsy information is combined with simultaneously obtained cytological examination and microbiological cultures (1–4). Knowledge of the clinical context, radiological distribution of abnormalities, and histopathological patterns is essential for appropriate diagnosis, especially in the setting of diffuse or multifocal lung disease (5). Advances in diagnostic imaging such as high-resolution CT scans have made the transbronchial biopsy part of a new collaborative multidisciplinary process in diagnosing lung diseases.

There is a wide disparity in the diagnostic yield—ranging from 36% to 90%—reported in the literature for endobronchial and transbronchial biopsies (1–4). Multiple factors that are beyond the control of the pathologist affect the diagnostic yield of endobronchial and transbronchial biopsies, particularly sampling errors and the amenability of the pathological process to diagnosis by these procedures (Table 2). The diagnostic yield is also affected by the use of fluoroscopy, the type of forceps, the skill and experience of the bronchoscopist, and the number of samples obtained. Complications such as bleeding may confound even the best bronchoscopists.

The pathologist should not attach a specific diagnosis to artifacts, nonspecific or normal changes, or inadequate samples (5) despite the desire to "give a diagnosis" from self-expectations or pressure from the clinician. Therefore, the pathologist should be familiar with these artifacts and nonspecific or normal changes (Table 3).

II. Procedural Artifacts

Altered histological appearance could be caused by events during or immediately after the bronchoscopic procedure, initial fixation, or subsequent processing. Use of the biopsy forceps not uncommonly results in so-called crush artifact—compression of the tissue, especially the parenchyma. The compression of alveolar septa may give a false impression of interstitial fibrosis or increased interstitial cellularity, which may be confused with an interstitial pneumonia. The compression may also create rounded spaces, so-called bubble artifact,

Table 1 Diseases Diagnosable by Endobronchial/Transbronchial Biopsies

Neoplasms
Primary pulmonary carcinoma (including carcinoid tumors and rare types of carcinomas)
Metastases including lymphangiitic spread
Lymphoma/lymphoproliferative disorders
Infections
Virus
Mycoplasma
Bacteria
Mycobacteria
Fungus
Pneumocystis jiroveci
Other (parasites, etc.)
Inflammatory/interstitial diseases
Sarcoidosis
Diffuse alveolar damage/acute interstitial pneumonia
Constrictive bronchiolitis obliterans
Organizing pneumonia (bronchiolitis obliterans organizing pneumonia)
Hypersensitivity pneumonitis (extrinsic allergic alveolitis)
Eosinophilic pneumonia
Diffuse alveolar hemorrhage syndromes (Wegener's granulomatosis, Churg-Strauss syndrome, etc.)
Acute rejection (in lung transplants)
Collagen-vascular disease
Intravenous drug abuse microangiopathy
Alveolar proteinosis
Pulmonary langerhans cell histiocytosis
Lymphangioleiomyomatosis

Table 2 Reasons for Failure to Diagnose by Bronchoscopic Biopsy

Nature and location of the disease process
Skill and experience of the bronchoscopist
Type of forceps
Use of fluoroscopy
Number and size of samples
Procedural complications
Overinterpretation of procedural artifacts, normal or nonspecific findings

which may be confused with lipid vacuoles or fungal organisms (5,11) (Fig. 1). In addition to compression by the forceps, peribronchial anchoring fibers and limited sample size may contribute to the false impression of interstitial fibrosis on transbronchial biopsy. With a few specific exceptions, diffuse, mature interstitial fibrosis, like that seen in usual interstitial pneumonia or asbestosis, cannot be diagnosed on transbronchial biopsy and requires larger samples of lung tissue (at least a wedge biopsy) to determine its extent and distribution.

Compression of large bronchial vessels or other components of the bronchial wall may be misinterpreted as scarring. Crush artifact of lymphocytes or other cells may lead to

Table 3 Artifacts, Nonspecific Changes, and Normal Variants in Bronchoscopic Biopsies

Procedural artifacts
Crush artifact
Parenchyma
Lymphocytes
Bronchial structures
Atelactasis
Bubble artifact/ Rounded intraparenchymal spaces
Intra-alveolar hemorrhage
Glove starch, cotton fibers, sponge artifact, etc.
Normal variations
Peribronchial anchoring fibers
Bronchial-associated lymphoid tissue
Submucosal fat
Calcification and ossification of bronchial cartilage
Oncocytic change of mucosal gland epithelium
Endogenous structures
Anthracotic pigment
Nonspecific findings
Peribronchial fibrosis
Focal scars
Intraalveolar macrophages
Reactive changes of mucosal gland epithelium
Endogenous structures

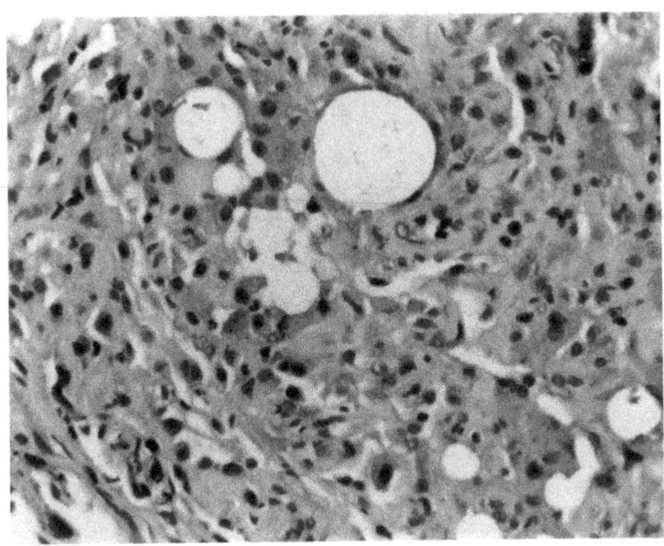

Figure 1 Rounded holes created by forceps compression artifact in parenchyma of transbronchial biopsy.

a false impression of small cell carcinoma; for this reason, diagnoses of malignancy should be made only on intact cells. Intra-alveolar hemorrhage often results from the biopsy procedure and should not be overinterpreted as a pathological process.

The sponge artifact consists of triangular-shaped spaces in the lung parenchyma without granulomas or polarizable foreign material. This results from rigid spikes of synthetic material in the foam biopsy sponges that pierce into soft, unfixed tissues (11).

III. Normal Structures and Normal Variations

Normal structures and normal variations of structures may sometimes be misleading. Bundles of smooth muscle, nerves, and nerve ganglia in the bronchial wall should not be confused with discrete pathological structures like granulomas. Submucosal fat may be present in the bronchial wall. With advancing age, bronchial walls may show calcification or ossification (with or without bone marrow) of their cartilage (6) and oncocytic change of the bronchial mucous glands (Fig. 2). Reactive changes in the mucous gland epithelium may result in cytological atypia and even mitoses that suggest cancer.

The anthracotic pigment in bronchial lymph nodes may occasionally give the gross impression of a pigmented lesion, like melanoma, to the bronchoscopist (Fig. 3). Pleura with reactive mesothelial cell proliferation may sometimes be obtained on transbronchial biopsy. The various endogenous and exogenous structures discussed in chapter 24 may appear in transbronchial biopsies. Occasionally, blue bodies (7) or corpora amylacea (8)

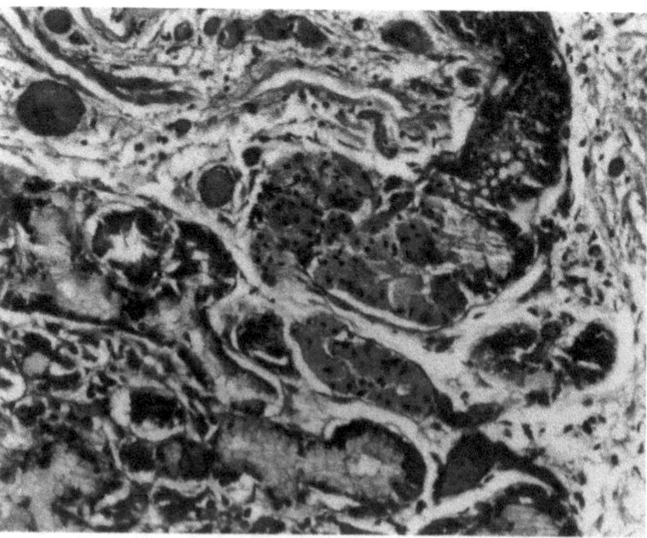

Figure 2 Oncocytic change in the epithelium of bronchial mucous glands.

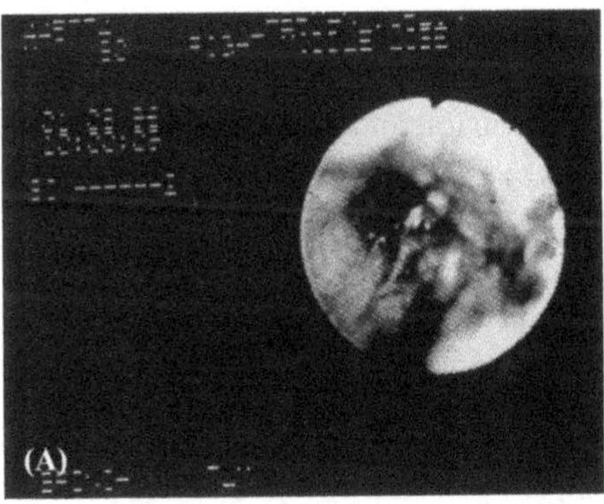

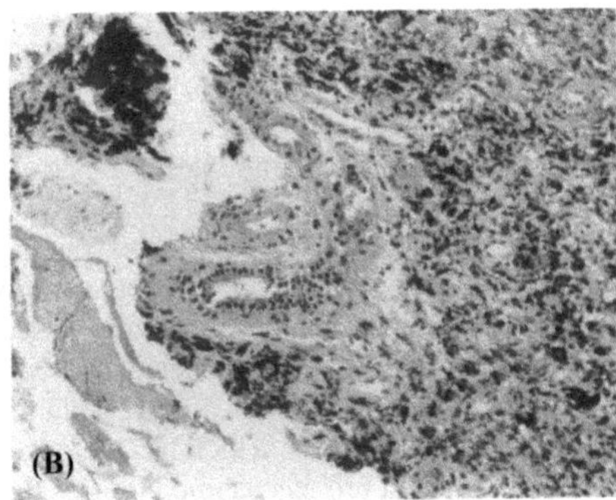

Figure 3 (**A**) Pigmented lesion of bronchial mucosa suggestive of metastatic melanoma on bronchoscopy. (**B**) Submucosal lymph node with leakage of anthracotic pigment into the submucosa accounts for the appearance seen at bronchoscopy.

may be numerous on transbronchial biopsy, so that exposure to inorganic dusts is erroneously suspected.

IV. Special Stains

Transbronchial biopsies may sometimes sample membranous bronchioles. When these are obscured by crush artifact, trichrome stains may provide recognition of these airways by highlighting the bundles of smooth muscle (9). Intra-alveolar foamy macrophages may be found in small airways obstruction, offering indirect evidence of bronchiolitis even when no bronchioles are sampled.

Iron stains may be helpful in identifying hemosiderin from previous hemorrhage. Deposits of hemosiderin may be round and/or in clusters, suggesting specific structures like asbestos bodies or other ferruginous bodies on iron stains. Close examination of the iron-stained material and comparison with the hematoxylin and eosin stains typically resolves this issue. Smoker's pigment, found in macrophages, also stains with iron stain, but the stain is fairly light compared with hemosiderin.

Special stains may be helpful in diagnosing specific diseases, particularly infections. It should be noted that acid-fast and methenamine silver stains are negative for organisms in about half of the mycobacterial and fungal infections demonstrated by cultures; therefore, such infections should not be ruled out when the stains are negative. Many rounded to elongated structures will appear black with silver stains, including mucin, hemosiderin, elastic fibers, and cotton fibers, which should not be mistaken for fungal organisms. Likewise, anthracotic pigment should not be mistaken for yeast on silver stains.

Immunohistochemistry may assist in diagnosing certain infections (e.g., cytomegalovirus, Epstein-Barr virus) and malignancies (e.g., cytokeratin to identify small blue cells as small cell carcinoma, B- and T-cell markers for lymphoma). DNA may also be extracted from biopsies for amplification by polymerase chain reaction.

V. Specific Diagnoses

In general, correlation of the biopsy results with the clinical information will help to avoid overinterpretation of sampling errors, artifacts, and nonspecific findings. As already noted, making the diagnoses listed in Table 1 is dependent on the sampling by the bronchoscopist and the confidence with which the findings on the small bronchoscopic sample may be applied to the entire lungs. Whereas peribronchial mature fibrosis cannot be assumed to be a specific finding, active granulation tissue in the alveolar spaces with incorporation into the interstitium can be expected to represent a pathological process, like organizing pneumonia or organizing diffuse alveolar damage. On the other hand, we have seen failure to diagnose sarcoidosis, which has the potential to be diagnosed by bronchoscopic biopsies, despite repeated bronchoscopic biopsies over a period of time because of fortuitous failure to sample the granulomas. Katzenstein and Askin emphasized the nonspecificity of many histological patterns, including interstitial fibrosis, diffuse alveolar damage, and alveolar hemorrhage (12). The specifics for diagnosing various diseases can be found in the respective chapters of this book. Generally, bronchoscopic biopsies permit diagnosis of diseases with unique, specific findings provided that there is sampling of those findings. As previously noted, processes that require evaluation of the extent and distribution of mature fibrosis—such as usual interstitial pneumonia, asbestosis, etc.—require larger samples of tissue than can be provided by bronchoscopic biopsies for a histopathological diagnosis. Idiopathic interstitial pneumonias are low-power architectural diagnoses, and that low-power architecture cannot, by definition, be achieved with transbronchial biopsy (13). Increasingly, however, transbronchial biopsies are used in conjunction with current sophisticated imaging techniques to rule out other interstitial lung diseases in specific clinical settings, for example in the diagnosis of idiopathic interstitial pneumonias.

Bronchioloalveolar carcinoma is currently defined as carcinoma in situ growing in a lepidic pattern on the alveolar septa without invasion of underlying lung parenchyma or other tissues. Therefore, a diagnosis of bronchioloalveolar carcinoma requires that the entire tumor be sampled, and a diagnosis of bronchioloalveolar carcinoma cannot be made on a transbronchial biopsy (14).

In addition to its traditional diagnostic roles, currently the transbronchial biopsy is often used in combination with diagnostic imaging for the evaluation of diffuse lung diseases. The transbronchial biopsy is a powerful tool for diagnosis; however, close interaction between pulmonologist, radiologist, and pathologist enhances the utility of transbronchial biopsy and improves the quality of patient care.

References

1. Smith CS, Murray GF, Wilcox BR, et al. The role of transbronchial lung biopsy in diffuse pulmonary disease. Ann Thorac Surg 1977; 24(1):54–58.
2. Jenkins R, Myerowitz RL, Kavic T, et al. Diagnostic yield of transbronchoscopic biopsies. Am J Clin Pathol 1979; 72:926–930.
3. Gilman MJ, Wang KP. Transbronchial, lung biopsy in sarcoidosis: an approach to determine the optimal number of biopsies. Am Rev Respir Dis 1980; 122:721–724.
4. Wall CP, Gaensler EA, Carrington CB, et al. Comparison of transbronchial and open biopsies in chronic infiltrative lung diseases. Am Rev Respir Dis 1981; 123:280–285.

5. Leslie KO, Gruden JF, Parish JM, et al. Transbronchial biopsy interpretation in the patient with diffuse parenchymal lung disease. Arch Pathol Lab Med 2007; 131:407–423.
6. Colby TV, Yousem SA. Pulmonary histology for the surgical pathologist. Am J Surg Pathol 1988; 12:223–239.
7. Ashley DJ. Bony metaplasia in trachea and bronchi. J Pathol 1970; 102(3):186–188.
8. Koss MN, Johnson FB, Hochholzer L. Pulmonary blue bodies. Hum Pathol 1981; 12:258–266.
9. Michaels L, Levene C. Pulmonary corpora amylacea. J Pathol Bacteriol 1957; 74:49–56.
10. Cagle PT, Brown RW, Frost A, et al. Diagnosis of chronic lung transplant rejection by transbronchial biopsy. Mod Pathol 1995; 8:137–142.
11. Kendall DM, Gal AA. Interpretation of tissue artifacts in transbronchial lung biopsy specimens. Ann Diagn Pathol 2003; 7:20–24.
12. Katzenstein AL, Askin FB. Interpretation and significance of pathologic findings in transbronchial lung biopsy. Am J Surg Pathol 1980; 4:223–234.
13. Churg A. Transbronchial biopsy: nothing to fear. Am J Surg Pathol 2001; 25:820–822.
14. Travis WD, Brambilla E, Müller-Hermelink HK, et al. Pathology and Genetics: Tumours of the Lung, Pleura, Thymus and Heart. Lyon: IARC; 2004.

3
Pediatric Lung Disease

MEGAN K. DISHOP
Baylor College of Medicine, Texas Children's Hospital, Houston, Texas, U.S.A.

I. Role of Diagnostic Lung Biopsy

A. Overview

Open lung biopsy was initially developed for adults in the late 1940s and was not applied for children until the mid-1950s. In the period through the mid 1960s, lung biopsy in children was still largely an ancillary procedure done at the time of surgery for a variety of cardiac malformations to evaluate the pulmonary vasculature. Only very few children, mostly older children, underwent lung biopsy for diagnosis of primary lung disease (1). By the 1970s and 1980s, with improved treatment modalities for childhood cancer, the advent of organ transplantation, a better understanding of the congenital primary immunodeficiency syndromes, and the increasing pediatric AIDS population, lung biopsy was increasingly applied for diagnosis of acute and rapidly progressive pulmonary disease in immunocompromised pediatric patients. Although not without controversy, diagnostic lung biopsy became an increasingly accepted procedure in this population, due in part to the use of trimethoprim/sulfamethoxazole as an effective agent for *Pneumocystis* treatment and the advent of effective antiviral and antifungal agents (2–5). Since then, lung biopsy has also been increasingly applied to young infants as a consequence of improved modalities for respiratory support and more successful therapeutic measures in this population (6). Diagnostic lung biopsy is now frequently employed also to characterize chronic respiratory disease in both infants and children, to determine prognosis and guide further choices in therapy, including consideration of lung transplantation.

B. Biopsy Procedures

Video-assisted thoracoscopic lung biopsy and open lung biopsy through a limited thoracotomy are the most widely accepted procedures for diagnostic lung biopsy in children. Lung biopsy may also be performed at the time of cardiovascular surgery for assessment of pulmonary vascular disease, although this is not as routinely employed as in the past. Alternative modalities, including transbronchial biopsy and percutaneous needle aspiration/biopsy, have had their advocates but have not been widely accepted for pediatric patients (7–9). Transbronchial biopsy is currently used most commonly in pediatric lung transplant recipients for the assessment of rejection and infection and can be used even in infants with more recent availability of smaller instruments (10). Transbronchial biopsy has a limited role, however, in the diagnosis of diffuse developmental or interstitial lung disease in

Table 1 Pediatric Wedge Lung Biopsy: Guidelines for Tissue Handling

Culture	Microbiology cultures (bacterial, fungal, acid-fast) and viral culture (~1/3 biopsy)
Rapid diagnosis/special stains	Imprint preparations (3 air dried, 3 alcohol fixed)
Electron microscopy	Glutaraldehyde (small portion)
Molecular study	Freeze and hold (small portion)
Immunofluorescence	Inflate with 1:1 mixture of 50% sucrose and cryomatrix. Freeze and hold (one section)
Histology	Remove staple line, inflate with formalin, fix 20 min, section perpendicular to margin (at least 1/2 biopsy)

children, as this biopsy method precludes evaluation of both alveolar architecture and vascular disease. Video-assisted thoracoscopic biopsy is now a widely available surgical technique and has largely replaced open thoracoscopic biopsy for children in our center. The diagnostic yield and safety of thoracoscopic biopsy in children appears to be similar to open lung biopsy in experienced hands and is superior to transbronchial or percutaneous biopsy in most diagnostic settings (11–15).

C. Biopsy Handling

Open and video-assisted thoracoscopic biopsies yield a wedge of peripheral lung tissue, which should be handled in a standard fashion to gain the maximum benefit (Table 1) (16). Ideally, the lung biopsy should be a wedge of tissue at least 1.5-cm deep and approximately 2 to 3 cm in length. The size should provide sufficient lung tissue for both histologic sampling and special studies, and the depth of the biopsy is important to allow examination of the terminal bronchioles and accompanying muscular pulmonary arteries. While these special studies may not be utilized for diagnosis in every case, it is not always possible to identify in advance which studies will be most helpful, and as a result, we find it prudent to follow a standard protocol in all cases and retain tissue for special studies, if later indicated.

The lung should be received fresh from the operating room in a sterile container and is initially handled with sterile instruments to allow collection of bacterial, mycobacterial, and fungal cultures, as well as a sample for viral culture. The surgical staples are removed and the stapled margin may be submitted for culture in addition to a lateral section of tissue. Certainly, a focal lesion such as a granuloma should be sampled directly. In the setting of an immunosuppressed child with acute respiratory failure, preparation of touch imprint slides allows special stains for infectious organisms to be performed on the same day of biopsy and may expedite diagnosis and therapy for these patients. In all cases, a small portion of lung tissue (1- to 2-mm pieces) is placed in glutaraldehyde fixative for possible electron microscopy (EM). Although this tissue is processed only to resin blocks in the majority of cases, complete ultrastructural examination has proven most useful in evaluating the genetic disorders of surfactant metabolism, pulmonary interstitial glycogenosis (PIG), storage disorders, and viral infection. The small amount of tissue required, low cost of initial fixation and processing, and the inherent difficulty in predicting which patients will benefit from this study are all factors which support routine collection of tissue for EM. One section perpendicular to the surgical margin is frozen in cryomatrix and may be used for immunofluorescence study in immune-mediated processes or frozen section for lipid staining (17). A sucrose-cryomatrix mixture (1:1 mixture of 50% sucrose and cryomatrix) allows inflation of the lung tissue with a tuberculin syringe and acts to support the alveolar walls during sectioning. The sucrose-cryomatrix mixture can be held indefinitely under refrigeration but should be warmed to room temperature to decrease the viscosity prior to use. A small portion of lung tissue may be frozen also without cryomatrix for molecular study or other tissue assay.

The remaining portion of the biopsy (approximately half) should be inflated with formalin by transpleural injection using a tuberculin syringe, repositioning the needle as necessary to produce complete expansion (18). The inflated lung should then be immersed in formalin for at least 20 minutes prior to sectioning. The tissue should be sectioned perpendicular to the surgical margin so that both central tissue and peripheral pleural angle are represented in each plane of section submitted for microscopic study. Although transbronchial biopsies can be successfully processed the same day if necessary, the amount of lung tissue in a typical wedge biopsy precludes rapid processing.

D. Patient Characteristics and Indications for Lung Biopsy in Children

Age at biopsy ranges from a few days to late adolescence (Table 2, Figure 1). There has been an increase in the proportion of infants and young children who come to diagnostic lung biopsy, with almost half of biopsies from children younger than five years, and nearly one-fourth from those younger than two years. Approximately one-third of pediatric lung biopsies are from immunosuppressed or immunocompromised children, and another one-third are for diagnosis of nodules in children with newly diagnosed or recurrent malignancy (Table 3). Other underlying diseases leading to lung biopsy may include cardiac disease, chromosomal disorders, collagen vascular disease, neuromuscular disease, and metabolic disease. A significant proportion of children who undergo diagnostic lung biopsy (15–20%) have no other known extrapulmonary disease.

As pediatric lung biopsy has become increasingly available as a diagnostic tool, the indications for such biopsies have evolved rapidly over time. Current indications include the diagnosis of infection in the immunocompromised host with acute respiratory deterioration, evaluation of focal lesions in patients with malignancy, diagnosis of acute respiratory

Table 2 Pediatric Lung Biopsy: Age at Biopsy

Age	Number	Percentage
Age 0 to 4 yr	106	40%
Less than 12 mo	37	14%
12 to 23 mo	20	7.5%
2 to 4 yr	49	18.5%
Age 5 to 9 yr	49	18.5%
Age 10 to 14 yr	61	23%
Age 15 to 18 yr	49	18.5%

265 wedge lung biopsies (age 0–18 years), 10-year period (1997–2007).
Source: Texas Children's Hospital, Houston, Texas, U.S.A.

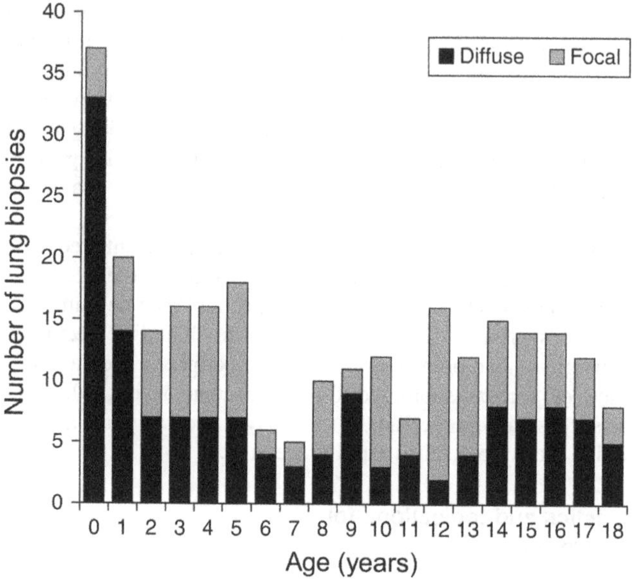

Figure 1 Pediatric lung biopsy: Age distribution by indication for diffuse vs. focal lung disease.

disease in other children, and diagnosis of chronic progressive lung disease. Children with chronic lung disease typically present with nonspecific signs and symptoms, such as tachypnea, respiratory distress, and oxygen desaturation, as well as diffuse nonspecific radiologic abnormalities. Although now a less common indication, lung biopsies are still occasionally performed for evaluation of the pulmonary vasculature in patients with underlying cardiovascular disease, typically during palliative or corrective surgery. A few other specific indications for lung biopsy in infancy are addressed below.

Approximately half of pediatric lung biopsies are performed for evaluation of diffuse lung disease, including patients with and without immunocompromise, presenting with either acute or chronic respiratory symptoms (Table 4). A significant proportion are done in immunocompromised children with acute decompensation and suspected opportunistic infection, accounting for approximately three-quarters of biopsies for diffuse lung disease in this population. The range of pathogens and reaction patterns are similar to adults, and impaired host response and/or partial treatment may produce atypical histologic patterns. While many of the chronic lung diseases seen in adults may also affect infants and children, they occur with a very different frequency (19–27). Infants and children are more likely than adults to have pulmonary disease related to developmental abnormalities, poor lung growth, and genetic disease. Interstitial lung disease is uncommon in children. While nonspecific interstitial pneumonia (NSIP) and lymphoid interstitial pneumonia (LIP) are not uncommon patterns in children, usual interstitial pneumonia (UIP) is exceedingly rare, if it occurs at all (28). Desquamative interstitial pneumonia (DIP) has been described in

Table 3 Pediatric Lung Biopsy: Patient Characteristics

Clinical characteristics	Number		Percentage
Immunocompromised	**84**		**31.7%**
Malignancy, with chemotherapy (no BMT)	27		10.2%
BMT	21		7.9%
Solid organ transplant	12		4.5%
Lung transplant		9	
Other (renal, liver)		3	
Congenital immunodeficiency	16		6.0%
Chronic granulomatous disease		9	
Severe combined immunodeficiency		3	
Common variable immunodeficiency		2	
Other		2	
HIV infection	1		0.4%
Collagen vascular disease	1		0.4%
Other	6		2.3%
Normal host (Immunocompetent)	**181**		**68.3%**
Malignancy (off chemotherapy, no BMT)	82		30.9%
Leukemia/lymphoma/histocytosis		14	
Solid tumor		68	
Cardiac abnormality	10		3.8%
Congenital heart disease		9	
Cardiomyopathy		1	
Chronic neonatal lung disease	11		4.2%
Prematurity and its complications		8	
Pulmonary hypoplasia, other		3	
Chronic airway disease	13		4.9%
Cystic fibrosis		3	
Bronchiectasis or suspected BOS		7	
Suspected NEHI		3	
Chromosomal disorders	6		2.3%
Down syndrome		4	
Other		2	
Collagen vascular disease/IBD, chronic	12		4.5%
Pulmonary hemorrhage syndrome/hemosiderosis	13		4.9%
Other	5		1.9%
Neuromuscular disorders		2	
Metabolic disease		1	
Marfan syndrome		1	
Pulmonary hypertension, NOS		1	
No known underlying disorder	41		15.5%
Pneumonia, suspected bacterial/viral infection		13	
Nodular disease, suspected granulomatous infection		7	
Pneumonia, suspected aspiration syndrome		6	
Suspected genetic disorder of surfactant metabolism		1	
Suspected hypersensitivity drug reaction		1	
Other		13	

265 wedge lung biopsies (age 0–18 years), 10-year period (1997–2007).

Abbreviations: BMT, bone marrow transplant; HIV, human immunodeficiency virus; BOS, bronchiolitis obliterans syndrome; NEHI, neuroendocrine cell hyperplasia of infancy; IBD, inflammatory bowel disease; NOS, not otherwise specified.

Source: Texas Children's Hospital, Houston, Texas, U.S.A.

Table 4 Pediatric Lung Biopsy: Indications for Wedge Lung Biopsy

Clinical indication	Biopsies ($n = 265$)		Percent of total	
Diffuse lung disease	**143**		**54%**	
Acute respiratory failure	74		27.9%	
Immunocompromised		40		15.1%
Normal host		34		12.8%
Chronic lung disease	69		26%	
Immunocompromised		14		5.3%
Normal host		55		20.8%
Focal lesions	**122**		**46%**	
Systemic disease	110		41.5%	
Malignancy (solid tumor)		69		26.0%
Leukemia/lymphoma		20		7.5%
Bone marrow transplant		7		2.6%
Chronic granulomatous disease		8		3.0%
Other systemic disease				
Autoimmune disease, CVID, SCID, CF		6		2.3%
No underlying disease	12		4.5%	
Diagnoses: granulomas, abscess, infarction, calcification				

265 wedge lung biopsies (age 0–18 years), 10-year period (1997–2007).
Abbreviations: CVID, common variable immunodeficiency; SCID, severe combined immunodeficiency; CF, cystic fibrosis.
Source: Texas Children's Hospital, Houston, Texas, U.S.A.

children, but is a different disease than adults, as it appears to be unrelated to smoking exposure and is more often a manifestation of the genetic disorders of surfactant metabolism.

E. Special Indications for Lung Biopsy in Infants

The interpretation of lung biopsies from neonates and infants is currently the greatest challenge in the histopathologic diagnosis of pediatric lung disease. The number of infant lung biopsies has increased in recent years and they present special problems in assessment. While the biopsies may be done for any of the general indications discussed above, they are usually done for one of a very limited number of indications specific to infancy (Table 5). Histologic assessment of infant lung biopsies should include a similar approach as in other settings, but must also include assessment for intrinsic developmental abnormalities and evaluation of the adequacy of alveolar growth. The widespread use of extracorporeal membrane oxygenation (ECMO) and nitric oxide as supplements to conventional ventilatory therapy for neonatal respiratory failure has resulted in biopsies to assess the lungs of infants who either do not respond to or cannot be weaned from such therapies. Conditions to consider in these infants include genetic disorders of surfactant metabolism, alveolar capillary dysplasia with misalignment of pulmonary veins (ACD/MPV), and other abnormalities affecting lung growth.

Table 5 Infant Lung Biopsy: Special Indications

1.	Failure to respond or failure to wean term or near-term infant from ventilatory support/ECMO/ nitric oxide
2.	Late-onset tachypnea or respiratory failure in a term or near-term infant, with or without underlying disease
3.	Recurrence of respiratory symptoms in former preterm infant
4.	Evaluation of the pulmonary vasculature in the setting of congenital heart disease, usually at the time of surgical repair

Abbreviation: ECMO, extracorporeal membrane oxygenation.

II. Diffuse Lung Disease

A. Alveolar Capillary Dysplasia with Misalignment of Pulmonary Veins

ACD/MPV is a rare developmental lung abnormality resulting in severe pulmonary hypertension of the newborn (29). These infants usually present early in the first days of life, and most die before one month of age, although there are also reports of later onset and longer survival. Many infants with ACD/MPV have congenital abnormalities in other organs, particularly the heart and gastrointestinal tract, but no consistent pattern of association has been identified. Although ACD/MPV may be familial, the genetic basis remains unknown (30,31).

ACD/MPV was initially diagnosed only at autopsy, but is now being sought by lung biopsy in neonates and young infants with persistent pulmonary hypertension who do not have a sustained response to ventilatory support, ECMO, and/or nitric oxide therapy (30,32). Lung biopsy is used in this setting to determine etiology of pulmonary hypertension and to prognosticate regarding the utility or futility of continued medical management. As there is no other effective therapy for ACD/MPV, lung transplantation remains the only potential therapeutic option for survival and would require early diagnosis and referral.

Lung biopsies in ACD/MPV show striking abnormalities of both the pulmonary vasculature and the lobular architecture. The small pulmonary artery branches show extreme medial hypertrophy, with prominent muscularization of the tiny intralobular arterioles also. The veins and venules, both in the bronchovascular region and in the lobular parenchyma, are dilated and may be a clue to diagnosis at low power (Fig. 2). Although the largest pulmonary veins are normally located in the interlobular septa, the smaller dilated veins and venules are abnormally positioned, accompanying the artery branches (Fig. 3). There is also a striking reduction in the capillary bed (ACD), with most capillaries in the center of the widened alveolar walls and lacking the usual juxtaposition with the alveolar epithelium. A number of cases also show prominence of the pulmonary lymphatics, either as a generalized or as a patchy process (29,33). In addition to this constellation of vascular abnormalities, the lobules are abnormally developed having a somewhat simplified appearance and decreased radial alveolar count. Despite the histologic evidence of lobular hypoplasia, the lungs are not typically small, and indeed their weights are often increased.

As more experience is gained with ACD/MPV, it is becoming clear that there is variable severity, particularly of the capillary deficiency component, which may account for the delayed onset and prolonged survival of some infants. Although the combination of

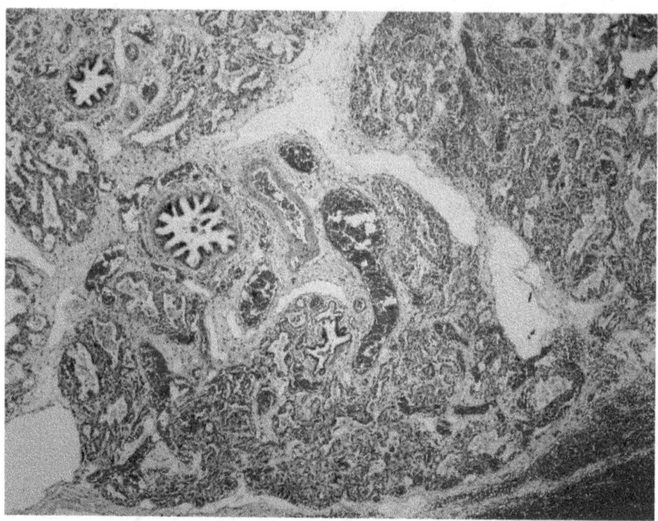

Figure 2 Alveolar capillary dysplasia with misalignment of pulmonary veins. Four-week-old term infant with respiratory distress, cyanosis, and severe persistent pulmonary hypertension, unresponsive to conventional therapies. Lung biopsy shows abnormal architecture with small lobules and markedly distended veins and intralobular venules. Hematoxylin and eosin stain, 2 ×.

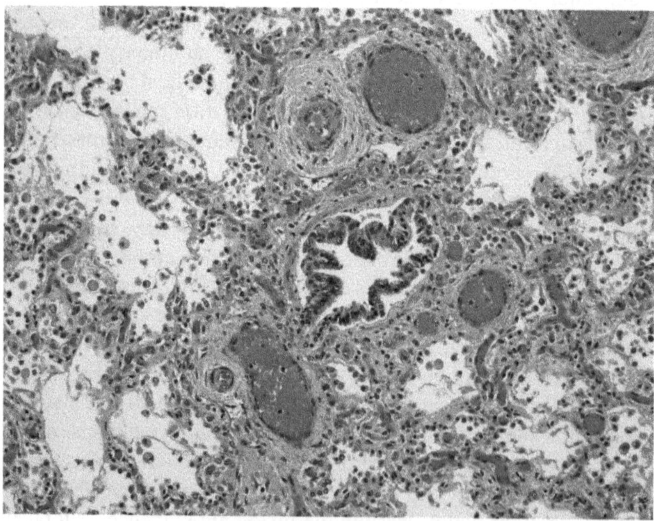

Figure 3 Alveolar capillary dysplasia with misalignment of pulmonary veins. Thick-walled pulmonary arteries are accompanied by malpositioned dilated and congested veins in the bronchovascular bundles. The airspace walls also contain thick-walled small arteries, dilated congested veins, and relatively few capillaries. Hematoxylin and eosin stain, 10 ×.

changes is quite distinctive when specifically sought, the diagnosis can be elusive initially, particularly in the uninflated lung and when only the arteriopathy is recognized. For example, ACD/MPV has been misinterpreted as pulmonary arterial smooth muscle hyperplasia only, with the lobular changes thought to be acquired injury from therapeutic measures, and with the abnormally positioned veins being misinterpreted as dilated arteries or blood-filled lymphatics.

B. Genetic Disorders of Surfactant Metabolism

The surfactant dysfunction disorders are a group of lung diseases occurring predominantly in infants and children that are caused by mutations in three proteins affecting surfactant metabolism: surfactant protein B (SP-B) (*SFTPB* gene on chromosome 2p12-p11.2), surfactant protein C (SP-C) (*SFTPC* gene on chromosome 8p21), and the ATP-binding cassette subfamily A member 3 protein (*ABCA3* gene on chromosome 16p13.3) (34–36). Mutations in *SFTPB* and *ABCA3* genes have an autosomal recessive pattern of inheritance, while *SFTPC* mutations are autosomal dominant, in some cases manifesting as chronic lung disease in successive generations (37–39). It should be noted that a subset of cases with typical histologic features of the genetic surfactant disorders have no mutations detected in these three genes, suggesting the presence of other currently unknown causative genes.

The histologic manifestations of the surfactant disorders appear to vary depending on the severity and age at biopsy. In infancy, a number of overlapping histologic patterns have been described, including pulmonary alveolar proteinosis (PAP), chronic pneumonitis of infancy (CPI), and DIP. SP-B deficiency typically results in a variant PAP pattern with granular eosinophilic proteinaceous alveolar material, prominent uniform alveolar epithelial hyperplasia, and relatively little evidence of lobular remodeling with only mild to moderate widening of alveolar walls (Fig. 4) (40–43). Inflammation is generally inconspicuous, and the vasculature appears normal. The alveolar proteinosis material is highlighted by periodic acid–Schiff (PAS) stain, which may be helpful in distinguishing it from edema or hyaline membranes. SP-B deficiency is typically fatal in the neonatal period or early infancy, but early diagnosis allows evaluation for lung transplantation.

In contrast to the PAP pattern of SP-B deficiency, lung biopsies from infants with SP-C deficiency typically show a pattern of CPI, characterized by less conspicuous proteinosis material and more prominent cholesterol clefts and lobular remodeling (Fig. 5) (44,45). While significant fibrosis is not a manifestation in infancy, lobular remodeling is reflected by irregular enlargement of airspaces, diffuse interstitial widening, and prominent interstitial extension of airway smooth muscle. These patients tend to be biopsied later than infants with SP-B deficiency and generally have a much wider range of age at presentation and diagnosis. *SFTPC* mutations have been recognized in some families as a cause of chronic interstitial pneumonia and pulmonary fibrosis in adults (46,47).

Despite its relatively recent description in 2004 as a cause of fatal lung disease in infants, mutations in the *ABCA3* gene now account for the greatest proportion of infants and children with abnormalities of surfactant metabolism (48). Like SP-C deficiency, *ABCA3* mutations have been recognized also as a cause of chronic interstitial lung disease in older children, adolescents, and young adults (49). ABCA3 deficiency often results in a variant PAP pattern in infancy, which is similar histologically to SP-B deficiency (Fig. 6). Other described patterns include DIP in some infants and NSIP pattern in older infants and

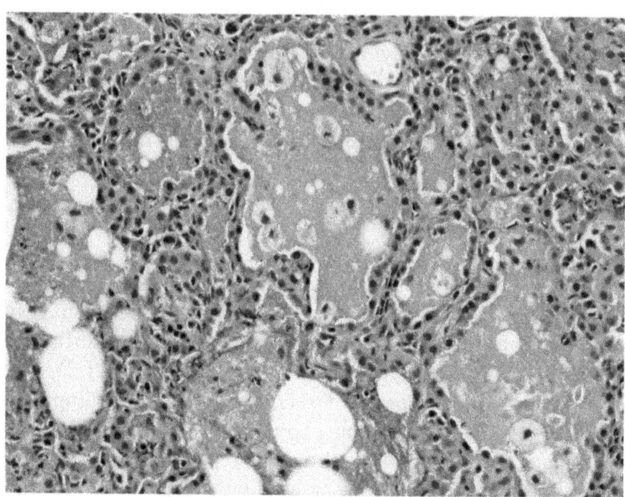

Figure 4 Genetic disorders of surfactant metabolism. Pulmonary alveolar proteinosis, SP-B mutations. Three-month-old term infant girl with tachypnea, oxygen requirement, and bilateral diffuse lung disease, later diagnosed with SP-B gene mutations. Lung biopsy shows homogenous proteinosis material filling the airspaces, associated with increased foamy macrophages, mild interstitial widening, and diffuse alveolar epithelial hyperplasia. Hematoxylin and eosin stain, 20 ×. *Abbreviation*: SP-B, surfactant protein B.

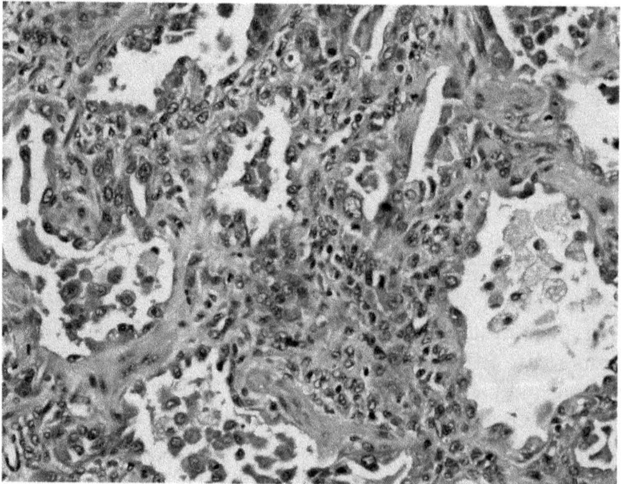

Figure 5 Genetic disorders of surfactant metabolism. Chronic pneumonitis of infancy, SP-C mutation. Three-month-old infant boy with hypoxia and tachypnea since birth, later found to have a mutation in the surfactant protein C gene. Lung biopsy shows a pattern of "chronic pneumonitis of infancy," characterized by extensive lobular remodeling with interstitial widening, interstitial extension of airway smooth muscle, variable interstitial chronic inflammation, diffuse alveolar epithelial hyperplasia, and increased foamy alveolar macrophages. Cholesterol clefts and focal granular and globular alveolar proteinosis material (not shown) are also typical features. Hematoxylin and eosin stain, 20 ×. *Abbreviation*: SP-C, surfactant protein C.

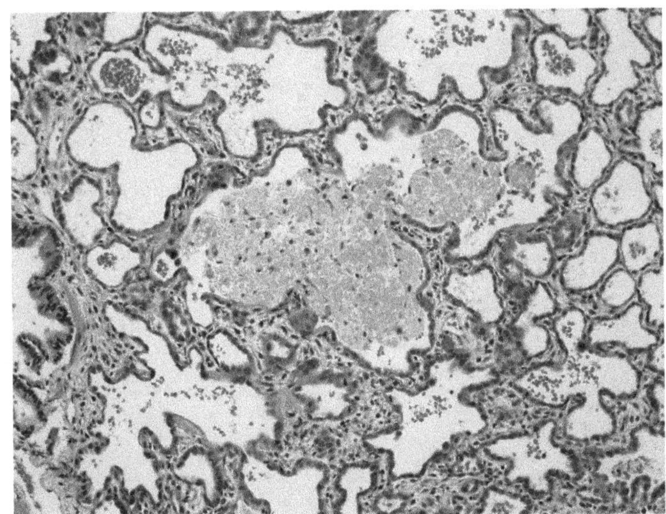

Figure 6 Genetic disorders of surfactant metabolism. Pulmonary alveolar proteinosis, *ABCA3* mutations. Six-day-old term neonate with respiratory failure, persistent pulmonary hypertension of the newborn, and diffuse granular disease on chest X ray resembling hyaline membrane disease, later diagnosed with mutations in both alleles of the *ABCA3* gene. Lung biopsy shows early lobular remodeling with aggregates of amorphous and coarse granular alveolar proteinosis material, admixed with foamy macrophages and cellular debris. Diffuse alveolar epithelial hyperplasia and interstitial widening are also prominent. Hematoxylin and eosin stain, 10 ×.

children. As with SP-C deficiency, cholesterol clefts (endogenous lipoid pneumonia pattern) may be a conspicuous feature, particularly in older patients (Fig. 7).

Although definitive diagnosis relies on mutation testing, EM is an important adjunct to diagnosis in suspected cases and may even suggest the affected gene. Ultrastructural examination may allow identification of lamellar body abnormalities described in either *SFTPB* or *ABCA3* mutations, although "normal" lamellar bodies do not exclude the presence of an underlying genetic defect. Typically, SP-B deficiency results in deficient mature lamellar bodies and increased multivesicular bodies and multilamellated structures (50). *ABCA3* mutations are associated with distinctive round electron-dense bodies within structures resembling small abortive and condensed lamellar bodies (Figs. 8 and 9) (51–53). Absence of lamellar bodies has also been described with *ABCA3* mutations. No consistent abnormalities of lamellar bodies have been associated with SP-C deficiency.

Prognosis of the surfactant dysfunction disorders varies to some degree with the gene affected and age at presentation. SP-B and ABCA3 deficiency appear to have the earliest and most severe presentation, although prolonged survival is possible in both SP-C and ABCA3 deficiency. There is currently no effective therapy for this group of disorders, and patients are managed supportively and with lung transplantation. Administration of surfactant in the neonatal period does not typically result in clinical improvement.

C. Pulmonary Alveolar Proteinosis

The differential diagnosis of genetic disorders of surfactant metabolism includes the form of PAP similar to that seen in adults. This "acquired" pattern is characterized by patchy or

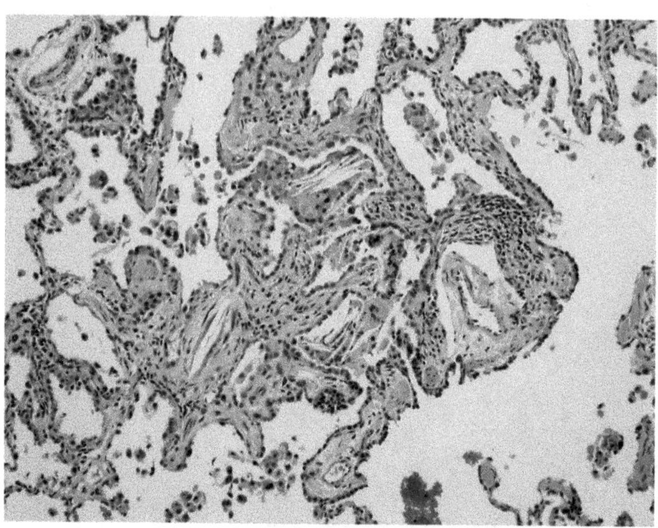

Figure 7 Genetic disorders of surfactant metabolism. Nonspecific interstitial pneumonia and endogenous lipoid pneumonia pattern in older children, *ABCA3* mutations. Nine-year-old boy with chronic lung disease. Lung biopsy shows patchy mild interstitial lymphocyte infiltrates associated with areas of mild fibrosis and collections of cholesterol clefts surrounded by increased alveolar macrophages (cholesterol granulomas). Rare globules of proteinosis material were also noted (not shown). Relative to infants, older children and adolescents with genetic abnormalities of surfactant metabolism (SP-C or *ABCA3* mutations) typically have less prominent reactive features and less conspicuous proteinosis material on lung biopsy. Hematoxylin and eosin stain, 10 ×.

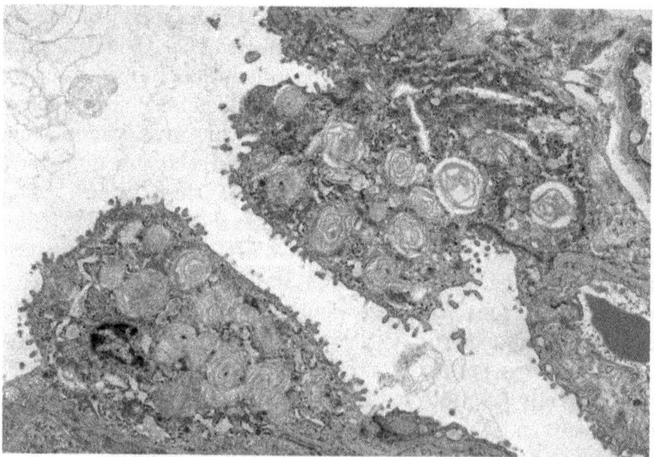

Figure 8 Normal lamellar body ultrastructure. Electron microscopy of two-month-old infant. Type II alveolar epithelial cells show adequate number, size, and ultrastructure of lamellar bodies. Original magnification, 4000 ×.

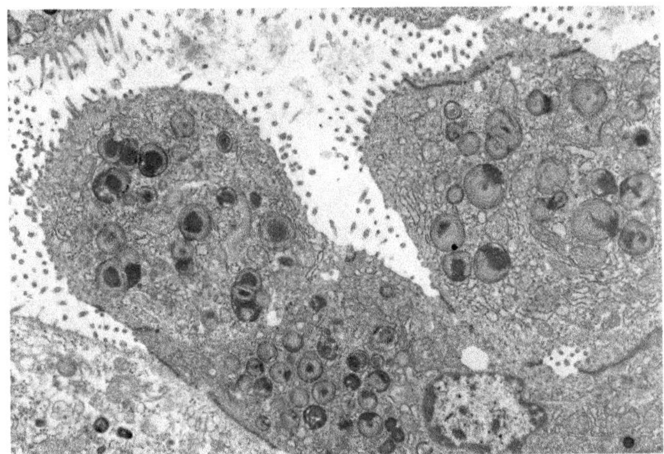

Figure 9 Genetic disorders of surfactant metabolism. Electron microscopy, *ABCA3* mutations. Two-month-old infant with respiratory failure. The type II alveolar epithelial cells show characteristic dense bodies associated with *ABCA3* mutations. Many lamellar bodies are small and contain large central and eccentric round electron dense bodies. Original magnification, 4000 ×.

diffuse alveolar infiltrates of smooth or finely granular eosinophilic proteinosis material admixed with occasional cholesterol clefts (Fig. 10). The prominent alveolar epithelial hyperplasia and lobular remodeling associated with the genetic disorders of surfactant metabolism are typically absent. This form of PAP occurs both spontaneously and in the setting of infection and is typically associated with an underlying systemic disease or alteration of the immune system, for example, patients undergoing chemotherapy, bone marrow transplant recipients, children with rheumatologic disorders, or patients who are immunosuppressed due to steroids. The accumulation of intra-alveolar proteinosis material is likely related to macrophage dysfunction and poor degradation and recycling of surfactant. As in adults, PAP in otherwise healthy children may be associated with serum antibodies to granulocyte macrophage colony-stimulating factor (GM-CSF). The differential diagnosis includes *Pneumocystis jiroveci* infection in immunocompromised patients, as well as the genetic disorders of surfactant metabolism, particularly in neonates and young infants.

D. Alveolar Growth Abnormalities

Alveolar growth abnormalities encompass a broad spectrum of pediatric lung disease characterized by insufficient alveolar growth and/or development, reflected histologically by variable airspace enlargement and simplification due to deficient alveolar septation. When mild, these features are often subtle and easily overlooked, particularly in unexpanded lung biopsies (Figs. 11 and 12). When severe, the airspace enlargement is more obvious, manifesting as cystic change, which is often accentuated in the subpleural regions

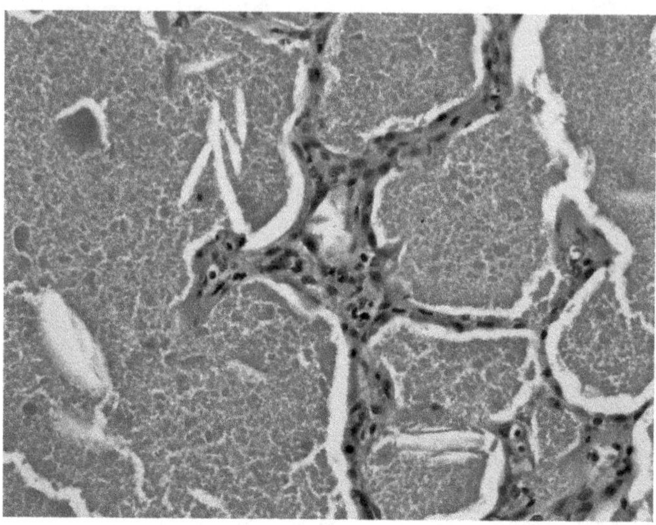

Figure 10 Pulmonary alveolar proteinosis, acquired pattern. Alveolar proteinosis may occur occasionally in children due to antibodies to GM-CSF and in immunosuppressed patients, which is thought to result from macrophage dysfunction. In contrast to the genetic disorders of surfactant protein metabolism, this form of alveolar proteinosis produces areas of smooth and granular proteinosis material, uniformly distending airspaces admixed with rare cholesterol clefts. Similar to the pattern of pulmonary alveolar proteinosis seen in adults, alveolar epithelial hyperplasia and chronic lobular remodeling are typically absent. Hematoxylin and eosin stain, 20 ×. *Abbreviation*: GM-CSF, granulocyte macrophage colony-stimulating factor.

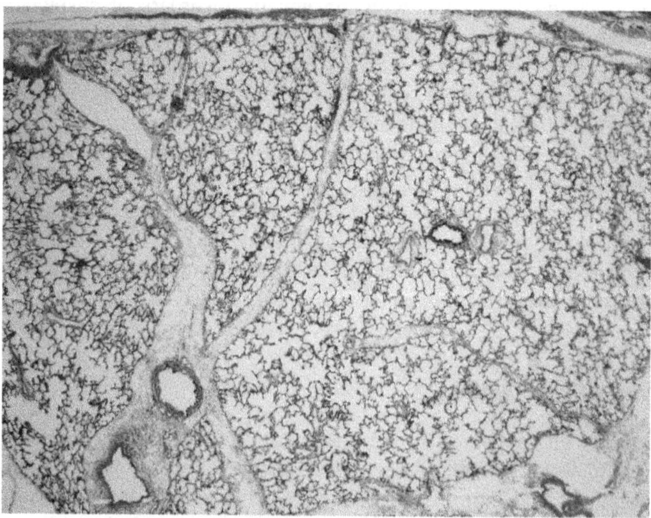

Figure 11 Normal alveolar architecture in five-month-old term infant. The alveoli are uniform in size, thin walled, and show appropriate delicate septations. Hematoxylin and eosin stain, 2 ×.

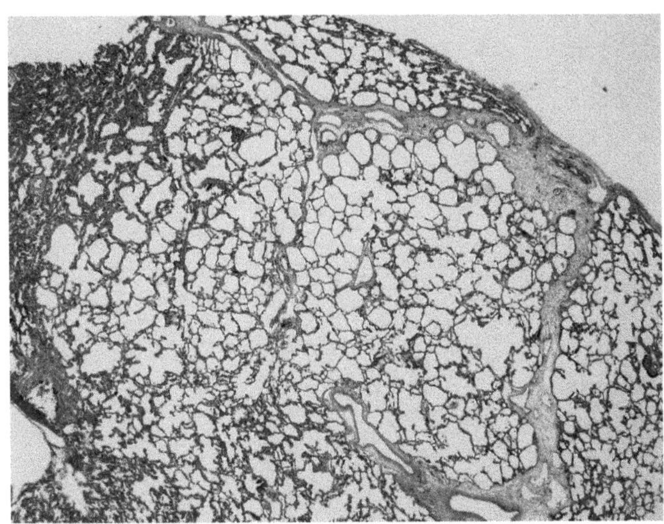

Figure 12 Alveolar growth abnormality, chronic neonatal lung disease. Three-month-old former premature infant, delivered at 30 weeks' gestation, with chronic neonatal lung disease. In contrast to the normal infant lung (see Fig. 11, same magnification), the airspaces are larger, irregular in size and shape, and simplified, showing rounded contours and deficient septation. Hematoxylin and eosin stain, 2 ×.

(Fig. 13). Most commonly, alveolar enlargement and simplification reflects the effects of insufficient prenatal development (pulmonary hypoplasia) or the effects of prematurity and associated hyaline membrane disease (chronic neonatal lung disease/bronchopulmonary dysplasia). Hypoplastic lungs may show continued development postnatally; however, this phase of lung growth is often incomplete, resulting in persistent deficiency of alveoli (54). The airspace remodeling and interstitial fibroplasia that occurs during repair from hyaline membrane disease may result in similar alveolar deficiency. While the degree of lung development differs initially between a term infant with pulmonary hypoplasia and a preterm infant with neonatal respiratory distress syndrome, their postnatal course is often similar clinically, requiring aggressive ventilatory support and oxygen therapy, and it is not surprising then that the histopathologic manifestations are indistinguishable on biopsy once there has been progression to chronic lung disease.

Other factors that contribute to poor alveolarization may include underlying congenital heart disease, chromosomal disorders, and/or superimposed respiratory illness in the first months of life during the period of most rapid postnatal alveolarization. For example, children with Down syndrome, with or without associated congenital heart disease, typically have an underlying structural abnormality of lung growth, which consists of airspace enlargement and widened alveolar ducts, classically manifesting as a subpleural zone of small cysts (Fig. 14). While history of prematurity and risk factors leading to pulmonary hypoplasia are usually easily elicited by clinical history, the group of alveolar growth abnormalities because of postnatal growth failure is more difficult to correlate clinically. These infants often have history of only mild respiratory insufficiency at birth and the

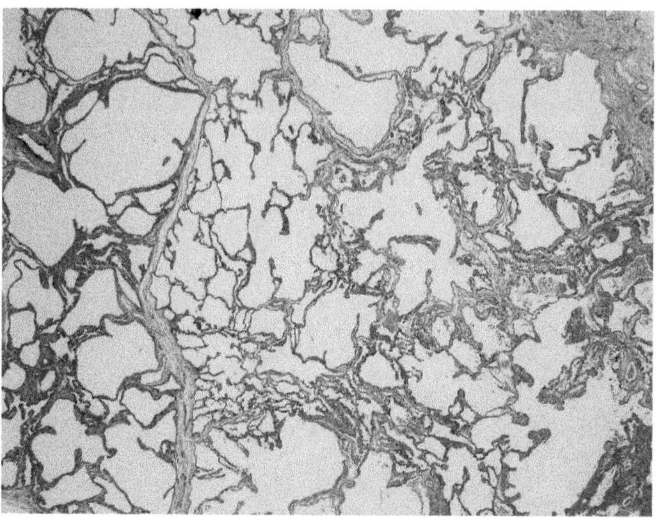

Figure 13 Alveolar growth abnormality, chronic neonatal lung disease. Nine-month-old former premature infant, delivered at 27 weeks' gestational age, with severe bronchopulmonary dysplasia. In contrast to the normal infant (see Fig. 11, same magnification), the airspaces are markedly distorted and enlarged with highly variable size and shape and many large round poorly septated airspaces. Some alveoli are distended, while others are collapsed, and there is also patchy interstitial widening by fibrosis. Hematoxylin and eosin stain, 2 ×.

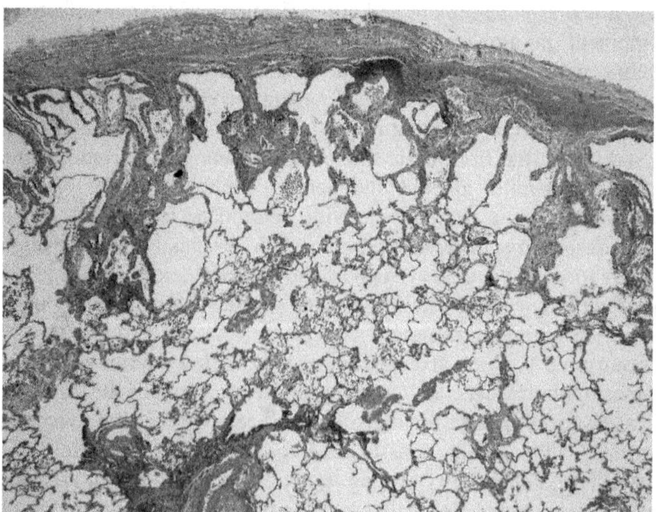

Figure 14 Alveolar growth abnormality, Down syndrome. Five-year-old term infant with trisomy 21, atrioventricular septal defect repaired at 7 months of age, failure to thrive, and gastroesophageal reflux. Poor alveolarization and distended alveolar ducts are typical in these children and often result in subpleural cystic airspace enlargement, also recognizable on chest CT imaging. Hematoxylin and eosin stain, 4 ×.

resultant histologic features also tend to be mild. Complete expansion of the lung biopsies is critical in accurately assessing overall alveolar architecture and irregular elastin deposition in such cases (55).

It should be noted that lungs with incomplete alveolar growth and development may also have superimposed airway injury and muscularization and are susceptible to the compounded effects of air trapping and hyperinflation (56). Although air trapping certainly causes alveolar enlargement, appropriate alveolar septation and accompanying alveolar duct distention helps to distinguish this as an isolated process from the round, simplified, poorly septated airspaces in the alveolar growth abnormalities. In practice, the morphologic distinction between hyperinflation and mild alveolar growth abnormalities can be difficult and may in fact reflect concurrent features of both processes.

Regardless of etiology, alveolar growth abnormalities are often accompanied by some degree of secondary pulmonary arterial changes due to the increased vascular resistance resulting from the deficient capillary bed. As expected, the pulmonary arterial changes are most severe in cases with severe airspace enlargement and may also be modified by overcirculation or chronic congestive changes in the setting of congenital heart disease.

E. Pulmonary Interstitial Glycogenosis (Infantile Cellular Interstitial Pneumonia)

First reported in 2002, PIG has also been described as infantile cellular interstitial pneumonia (ICIP), cellular interstitial pneumonitis of infancy, and histiocytoid interstitial pneumonitis (57–60). It is a poorly understood entity of the infant lung characterized by increased interstitial cellularity and expansion of alveolar septa by a proliferation of structural cells (Fig. 15). These cells have bland uniform ovoid nuclei with pale chromatin and are highlighted only by vimentin. The interstitial cellularity may be misinterpreted as histiocyte infiltrates or other inflammatory processes, such as NSIP pattern, but are negative for lymphoid and histiocyte markers by immunohistochemistry. The initial description as "glycogenosis" reflects the presence of glycogen in the cytoplasm of these cells, a feature that can be demonstrated by PAS stain or EM, if necessary. There is typically minimal, if any, alveolar epithelial hyperplasia, no alveolar exudate, and no interstitial fibrosis.

This phenomenon is vastly underrecognized and underreported in the medical literature. PIG is commonly a feature of biopsies for diffuse lung disease in infants younger than six months of age, and is not present beyond one year of age. Although it has been described as an isolated abnormality, PIG is seen most often as a background change in association with other well-recognized conditions, such as the alveolar growth abnormalities, pulmonary arteriopathy, and in the compressed lung adjacent to congenital lung malformations. While PIG may be diffuse, many cases show only a patchy distribution, perhaps leading to underrecognition of this process.

Clinically, infants with isolated PIG are reported to have been well for days to weeks and then present with tachypnea, hazy lung fields on chest X ray, and mild desaturation. PIG may also explain clinical exacerbation of known chronic neonatal lung disease or severity of clinical symptoms, which is disproportionate to that expected for gestational age, presumably due to the widened alveolar walls and impaired oxygen diffusion. These infants usually improve with time, and the prognosis is generally good, although largely dependent on the severity and/or reversibility of any associated lung disease. The

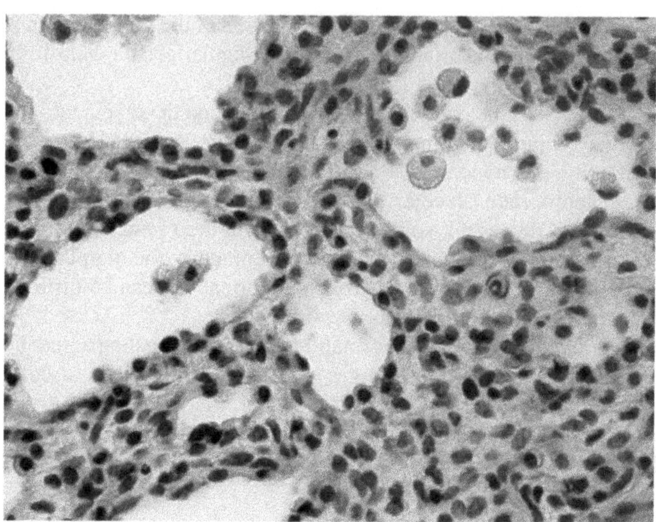

Figure 15 Pulmonary interstitial glycogenosis (infantile cellular interstitial pneumonia). Four-week-old former premature infant delivered at 27 weeks' gestation with chronic neonatal lung disease. Pulmonary interstitial glycogenosis is a pattern of interstitial widening and cellularity in infant lungs characterized by increased interstitial glycogen-rich mesenchymal cells. It is thought to be a reactive phenomenon unique to the infant lung and is often associated with abnormalities of alveolar growth. Hematoxylin and eosin stain, 40 ×.

pathogenesis remains unclear, although it likely represents a secondary reactive proliferation of cells in the rapidly growing and remodeling infant lung as a response to a variety of lung insults. PIG may be considered a unique reaction pattern of the infant lung and probably does not reflect a specific etiologic agent or genetic disorder.

F. Neuroendocrine Cell Hyperplasia of Infancy

Neuroendocrine cell hyperplasia of infancy (NEHI) is an entity described in 2005 as a pathologic correlate to the clinical syndrome of persistent tachypnea of infancy (61,62). These patients typically have nonspecific signs and symptoms of interstitial lung disease (tachpnea, hypoxia, retractions), without cough, wheeze, or response to bronchodilators. Chest X ray shows hyperexpansion and interstitial prominence, and chest computed tomography (CT) typically demonstrates minor peribronchial thickening and patchy ground-glass opacities, most prominently in the central regions of the right middle lobe and lingula (Fig. 16) (62,63). Lung biopsy in these patients is surprisingly "normal" by hematoxylin and eosin (H&E) stain, with only minimal, if any, airway changes (Fig. 17). Nonspecific airway abnormalities may include a mild increase in airway-associated lymphoid tissue, mild reactive epithelial hyperplasia, mildly increased airway smooth muscle, and increased numbers of clear cells in the bronchioles. Increased free alveolar macrophages have also been noted. Diagnosis is confirmed by using immunohistochemistry

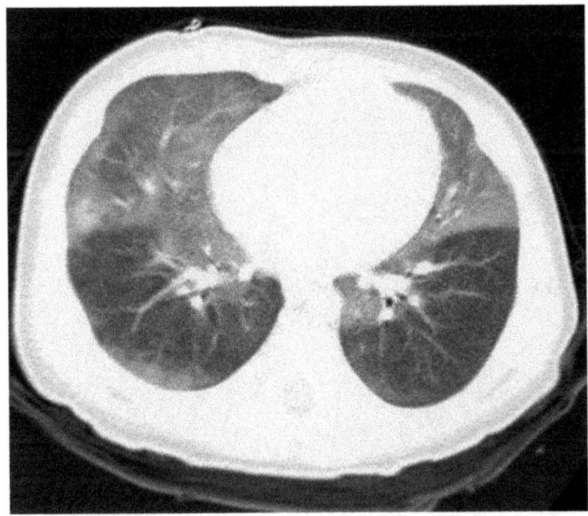

Figure 16 Neuroendocrine cell hyperplasia of infancy. Chest CT. Five-month-old boy with tachypnea and persistent oxygen requirement. Chest CT imaging demonstrates typical regions of perihilar ground-glass opacity, most accentuated in the right middle lobe and lingula.

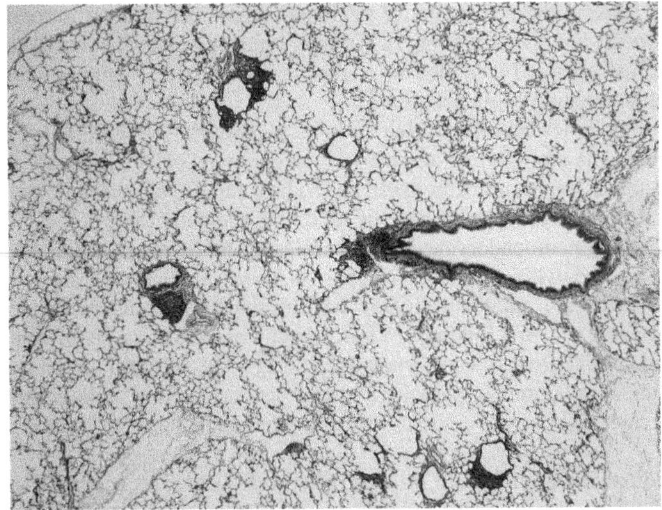

Figure 17 Neuroendocrine cell hyperplasia of infancy. Nine-month-old term infant with chronic tachypnea and failure to thrive. Lung biopsy shows appropriate alveolar architecture and near-normal bronchioles, with only a minimal increase in airway-associated lymphoid tissue. Hematoxylin and eosin stain, 2 ×.

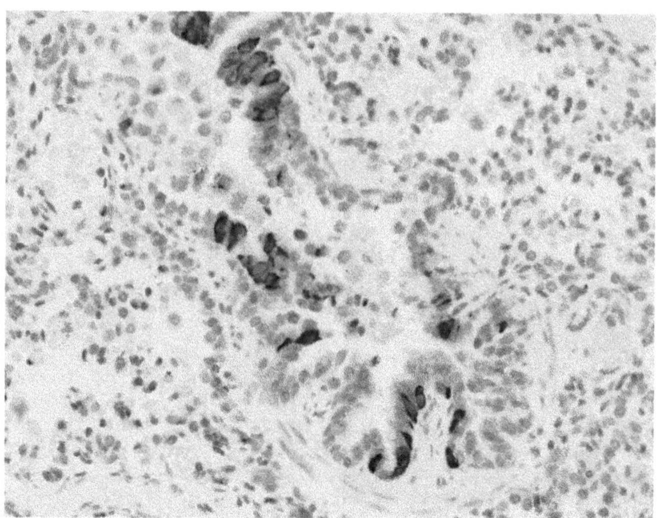

Figure 18 Neuroendocrine cell hyperplasia of infancy. Bombesin immunohistochemistry highlights increased numbers of neuroendocrine cells in this bronchiole, including groups of cells as well as scattered individual cells. Bombesin, 40 ×.

for neuroendocrine cells, with both an increase in the percentage of airways with neuroendocrine cells and an increase in the percentage of neuroendocrine cells relative to total airway epithelial cells in individual airways (Fig. 18). While a number of antibodies have been applied for immunohistochemistry, bombesin is the one most widely studied and provides the basis for standardization of diagnosis.

Diagnostic criteria include (*i*) neuroendocrine cells in at least 75% of total airway profiles, (*ii*) neuroendocrine cells representing at least 10% of epithelial cells in individual airway profiles, (*iii*) large and/or numerous neuroepithelial bodies, and (*iv*) absence of other significant airway or interstitial disease. The absence of superimposed pathologic processes is an important criterion, since neuroendocrine cell hyperplasia per se is not a specific finding and has been associated with a number of lung disorders, including bronchopulmonary dysplasia, cystic fibrosis, pulmonary hypoplasia, mechanical ventilation, acute lung injury, and smoke exposure (64–67). Findings of lymphocytic bronchiolitis, significant airway fibrosis, or other interstitial process would exclude the diagnosis. It is also important to note that NEHI is a clinical-radiographic-pathologic diagnosis, and definitive diagnosis should be made only in the appropriate clinical setting and with supportive imaging characteristics.

Similar to chronic idiopathic bronchitis of infancy (68) and follicular bronchitis (69), NEHI is on the mild end of the spectrum of diffuse lung disease in infancy, with slow symptomatic improvement over time and no associated risk of respiratory failure or mortality. While NEHI patients typically come to medical attention in infancy, symptoms may persist in toddlers and older children.

The pathogenesis of this disorder is poorly understood, and it is not clear whether NEHI represents an intrinsic abnormality of airway development influenced by genetic factors, or whether it is secondarily induced by preceding pulmonary injury, environmental influences, or chronic hypoxia. Sibling pairs with NEHI might suggest a genetic component, although common environmental influences are also possible. The role of preceding viral illness and high altitude environment in some patients remains unknown.

G. Congenital Heart Disease

Abnormalities of the pulmonary vasculature in patients with congenital heart disease reflect the altered hemodynamics produced by the abnormal flow through the heart and lungs (70,71). While some generalizations about pulmonary vascular disease can be made according to the type of cardiac malformation, the morphology of the pulmonary vasculature in any individual patient is subject to a number of concurrent variables affecting hemodynamics over time, including the size of shunt lesions or valvular lesions, complexity of multiple malformations, chronicity, and presence and timing of cardiac surgery for both palliation and definitive repair. Recurrence of a given hemodynamic abnormality may also occur after repair, as in the setting of recurrent pulmonary vein stenosis or poor valve function. Furthermore, it is recognized that the degree of histologic abnormality of the pulmonary arterial circulation generally correlates poorly with clinical findings and physiologic measures of pulmonary arterial hypertension. Specifically, mild medial hypertrophy of the pulmonary arteries is often associated with normal mean pulmonary artery pressures (70). The pulmonary vascular alterations may also be modified or exacerbated by the presence of other associated lung disease, such as bronchopulmonary dysplasia, pulmonary hypoplasia, structural lung abnormalities associated with Down syndrome, or ACD/MPV. With those caveats in mind, the vasculopathies associated with congenital heart disease can be divided into two basic types: (*i*) pulmonary arteriopathy due to overcirculation, and (*ii*) chronic congestive vasculopathy due to impaired pulmonary venous outflow.

First, pulmonary arteriopathy due to overcirculation is associated with cardiac lesions resulting in left to right shunting, increased volume and pressure of blood flow delivered to the lungs, and a progressive increase in pulmonary vascular resistance if unrepaired. Examples include atrial septal defect, ventricular septal defect, atrioventricular septal defect (atrioventricular canal), large patent ductus arteriosus, and D-transposition of the great arteries with ventricular septal defect (70,71). Over time, the pulmonary arteries show medial hypertrophy, intimal proliferation, and concentric intimal fibroplasia, as well as extension of arterial smooth muscle into the normally nonmuscularized intra-acinar arterioles (Figs. 19 and 20). A reduction in the number of small peripheral arteries has also been reported in the setting of severe medial hypertrophy and pulmonary arterial hypertension (70). By the Heath-Edwards classification, severe grades of pulmonary arteriopathy are associated with necrotizing arteritis, plexogenic arterial lesions, and dilatation lesions.

Second, chronic congestive vasculopathy is a histologic pattern associated with cardiovascular lesions resulting in increased pulmonary venous pressures (venous hypertension). Examples include pulmonary vein stenosis, total anomalous pulmonary venous return, and left-sided valvular obstruction (mitral valve stenosis and/or aortic valve stenosis). The constellation of findings in the lung include venous thickening and dilation, lymphatic dilation and muscularization, capillary congestion, alveolar hemorrhage, increased hemosiderin-laden macrophages, and secondary pulmonary arteriopathy, primarily with medial hypertrophy (Fig. 21). Because pulmonary overcirculation may result in similar arterial changes as well as chronic microhemorrhages and focal hemosiderin, the

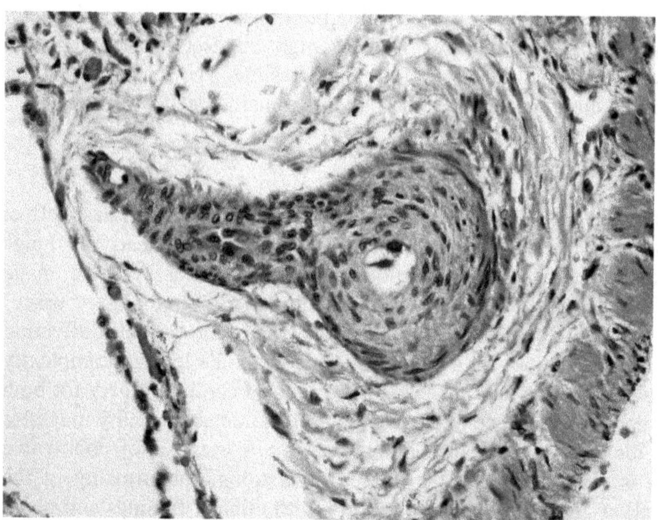

Figure 19 Congenital heart disease. Pulmonary arteriopathy due to overcirculation. Increased blood volumes are delivered to the lungs in patients with left-to-right shunt lesions, such as a large atrial septal defect, ventricular septal defect, atrioventricular canal, or patent ductus arteriosus. The associated progressive arteriopathy is characterized by medial hypertrophy with variable cellular and concentric intimal fibrosis, as in this patient with Down syndrome and complete atrioventricular canal. Hematoxylin and eosin stain, 20 ×.

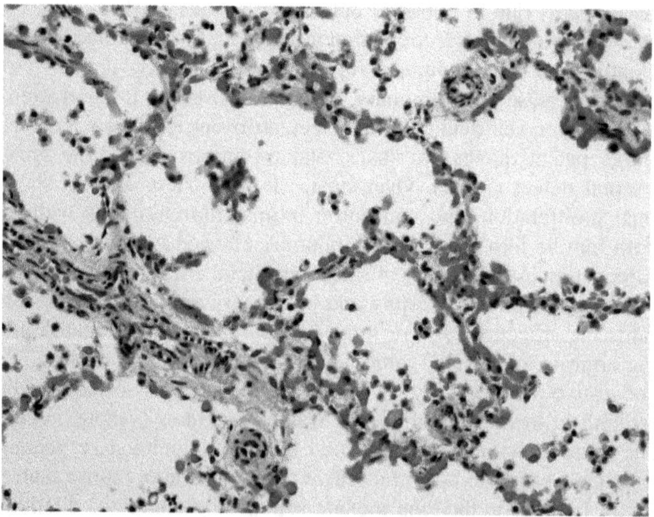

Figure 20 Congenital heart disease. Pulmonary arteriopathy due to overcirculation. The small intra-acinar arterioles are normally thin walled, but may become thickened and muscularized in the setting of chronic pulmonary overcirculation and reflect the increased pulmonary vascular resistance in these patients. Hematoxylin and eosin stain, 20 ×.

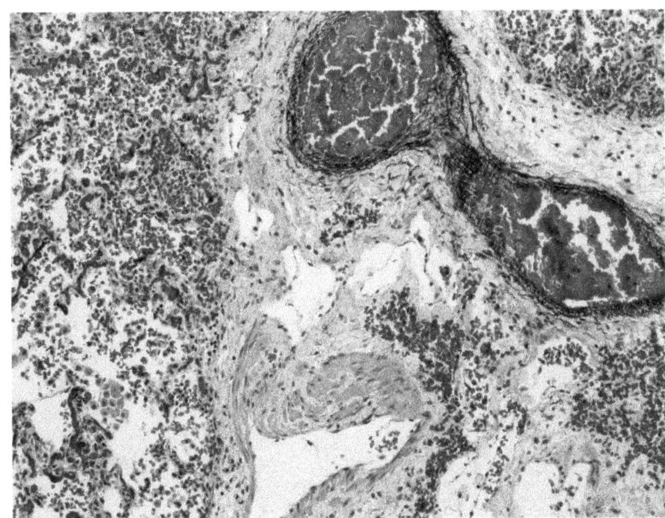

Figure 21 Congenital heart disease. Chronic congestive vasculopathy. Four-month-old girl with total anomalous pulmonary venous return and recurrent severe pulmonary vein obstruction after surgical repair. The vein (*upper right*) is thickened ("arterialized") and the adjacent lymphatics (*lower central*) are dilated with muscularization of their walls. The alveolar parenchyma is congested with extensive alveolar hemorrhage. An associated pulmonary arteriopathy and numerous hemosiderin-laden macrophages (not shown) are also typical features of chronic congestive vasculopathy. Hematoxylin and eosin stain, 10 ×.

chronic venous thickening and lymphatic muscularization are critical clues to diagnosis of chronic congestive vasculopathy. Pulmonary vein stenosis may not be easily detected by echocardiogram, and histologic features on lung biopsy, which suggest chronic venous hypertension, should prompt further clinical investigation by cardiac catheterization to exclude pulmonary vein abnormalities as a cause of pulmonary hypertension.

H. Respiratory Viral Infection

Respiratory viruses are a common cause of both acute illness and chronic lung disease in children (72,73). Although they cause only a minority of pneumonias in adults, viruses are the most common etiology of lower respiratory infection in children, including up to 90% of pneumonias in infants. Of these, the most common viral pathogens are respiratory syncytial virus (RSV), parainfluenza virus (PIV), metapneumovirus, influenza, adenovirus, and measles (particularly in developing countries). Lung biopsy is rarely performed in previously healthy children for diagnosis of viral infection because of the widespread availability of rapid diagnostic tests for RSV and influenza, and the typically mild and self-limited nature of symptoms. However, in immunocompromised patients, such as those with a history of bone marrow transplantation, chemotherapy, or solid organ transplantation, viral infection may result in acute respiratory failure and overwhelming infection. Lung

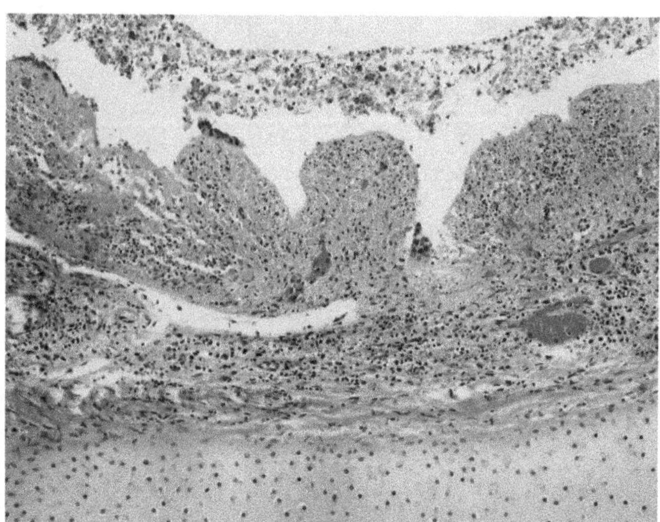

Figure 22 Infectious disease. Necrotizing bronchitis, influenza virus. An 18-month-old boy with a 5-day history of upper respiratory symptoms, diagnosed with influenza A virus infection complicated by bacterial sepsis. At autopsy, the lungs showed extensive tracheal and bronchial mucosal necrosis, as well as lymphocytic bronchiolitis and patchy diffuse alveolar damage. Hematoxylin and eosin stain, 10 ×.

biopsy may be performed in such cases to confirm diagnosis and evaluate other etiologies, such as *P. jiroveci* or other fungal disease.

Histologic features of viral respiratory tract infection typically include lymphocytic bronchitis and bronchiolitis, with or without mucosal necrosis, intraluminal mucus and debris, and interstitial lymphocyte infiltrates (pneumonitis). Extensive necrosis of airway mucosa is common in influenza and adenovirus infections (Fig. 22), and severe infections may also result in diffuse alveolar damage. Airway mucosal hyperplasia and squamous metaplasia may be prominent features. Epstein-Barr virus infection typically results in lymphocytic bronchiolitis with large lymphoid follicles containing secondary germinal centers (follicular bronchiolitis) (Fig. 23). A pattern of giant cell pneumonia reflects the viral cytopathic effect caused by RSV, parainfluenza, or measles virus. It should be noted that the multinucleate epithelial giant cells associated with these viruses may be particularly florid in immunocompromised patients. Other cytopathic changes associated with specific viruses include "smudged" or "ground-glass" nuclei in adenovirus infection, small globular eosinophilic cytoplasmic inclusions in RSV infection, Cowdry A and Cowdry B inclusions in herpesvirus infection, and large nuclear inclusions and small granular cytoplasmic inclusions in cytomegalovirus infection (Fig. 24). Herpes simplex virus and varicella-zoster virus pneumonia typically cause a miliary pattern of zonal parenchymal necrosis, surrounded by degenerating cells showing multinucleation and viral cytopathic effect. Immunohistochemistry and molecular methods are useful adjuncts for diagnosis of viral agents from tissue. Long-term sequelae of viral infection in both healthy and immunocompromised patients may include chronic cough and obliterative bronchiolitis [clinically,

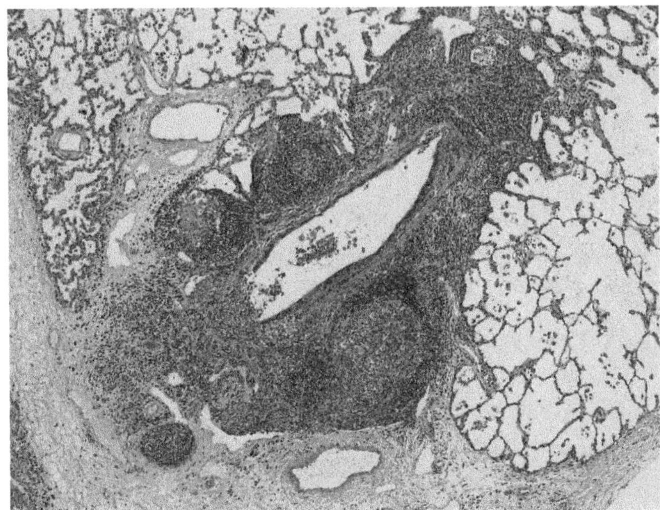

Figure 23 Infectious disease. Follicular bronchiolitis, EBV infection. Peribronchiolar lymphocyte infiltrates with large reactive germinal centers characterize EBV infection in this 20-month-old previously healthy boy. Hematoxylin and eosin stain, 4 ×. *Abbreviation*: EBV, Epstein-Barr virus.

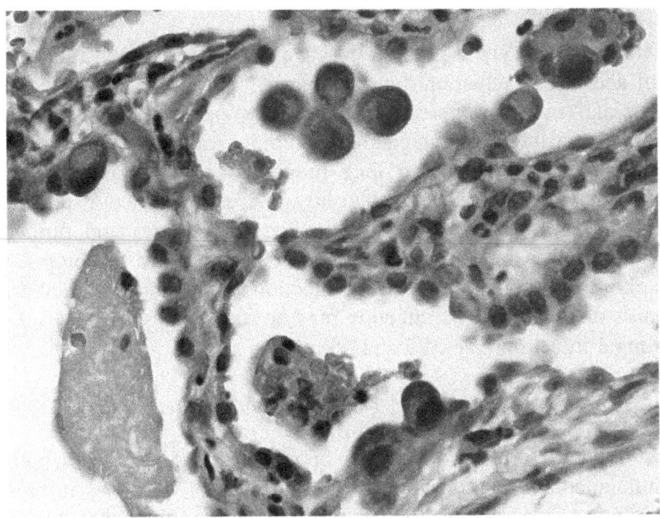

Figure 24 Infectious disease. Cytomegalovirus pneumonitis. Four-month-old infant with vertically acquired human immunodeficiency virus infection and acute respiratory distress due to *Pneumocystis* and cytomegalovirus pneumonia. Several alveolar epithelial cells and alveolar macrophages show characteristic viral cytopathic effect of cytomegalovirus, including cell enlargement, large nuclear inclusions, and small granular cytoplasmic inclusions. Hematoxylin and eosin stain, 40 ×.

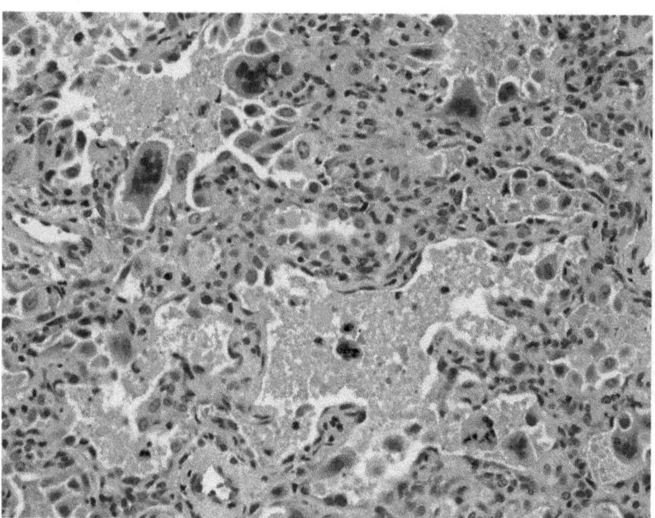

Figure 25 Infectious disease. Respiratory syncytial virus and *Pneumocystis jiroveci* pneumonia. Six-month-old infant presenting with rotavirus diarrhea and respiratory insufficiency, newly diagnosed with severe combined immunodeficiency. Lung biopsy shows florid syncytial giant cells with small globular cytoplasmic inclusions, typical of respiratory syncytial virus infection in the immunocompromised patient. Frothy proteinaceous alveolar exudate also led to diagnosis of *Pneumocystis* pneumonia. Hematoxylin and eosin stain, 20 ×.

bronchiolitis obliterans syndrome (BOS)], a process which evolves most often after the severe mucosal necrosis of adenovirus infection, for example.

Immunocompromised and immunosuppressed patients are susceptible to a wide spectrum of lower respiratory tract infections, including bacterial, viral, fungal, and parasitic etiologies, and these patients may undergo lung biopsy for evaluation of acute respiratory failure or nodular disease. If bronchoalveolar lavage does not reveal a specific infectious etiology, lung biopsy allows direct tissue sampling for cultures and further morphologic evaluation of fungal and viral infection. It should be emphasized that biopsies from these patients may harbor more than one concurrent infectious agent, and in particular, cytomegalovirus pneumonitis or *Pneumocystis* infection may be superimposed on a background of other viral or fungal infection (Figs. 25 and 26).

I. Granulomatous Disease

Diagnostic lung biopsy is often performed for nodular or multinodular disease in both immunocompetent and immunocompromised children. The differential diagnosis in previously healthy children include primarily infectious disease, including granulomas due to tuberculosis (Fig. 27), atypical mycobacteria, fungal, or yeast organisms (e.g., histoplasmosis, blastomycosis, or coccidiomycosis). Other noninfectious causes of granulomas in the pediatric population include sarcoidosis, Wegener's granulomatosis, and, rarely, foreign body granulomas due to intravenous drug injection. *Pneumocystis* infection is increasingly recognized as a cause of granulomatous pneumonitis in immunosuppressed

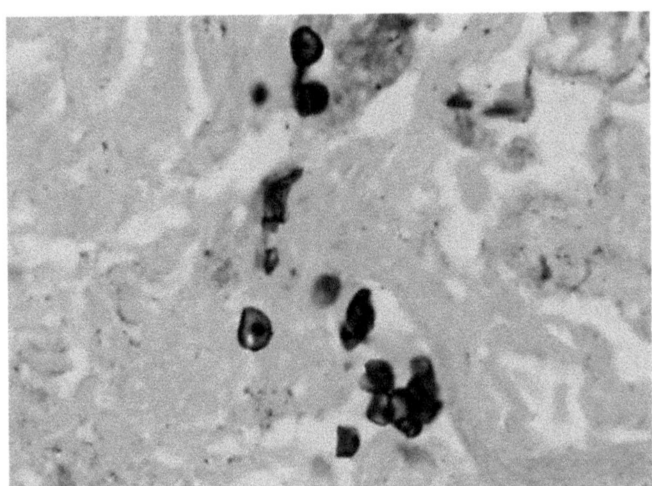

Figure 26 Infectious disease. *Pneumocystis jiroveci* pneumonia. Silver stain on the same lung biopsy highlights clusters of *Pneumocystis* organisms within the alveolar spaces. Methenamine silver nitrate stain, 40 ×.

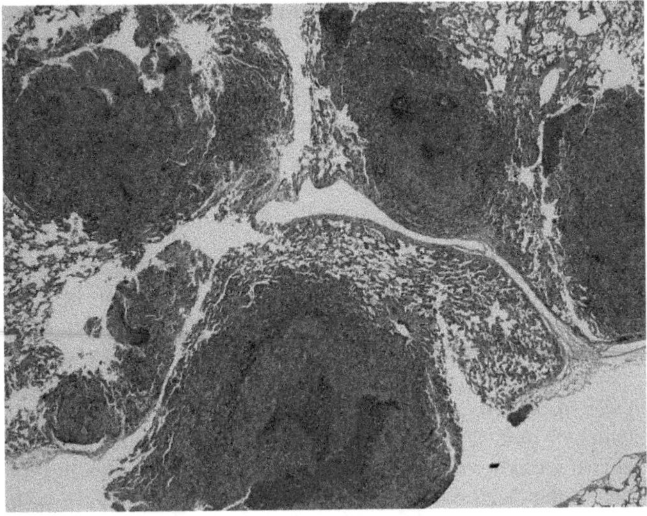

Figure 27 Infectious disease. Granulomatous pneumonitis. Four-week-old girl diagnosed with neonatal tuberculosis. Lung biopsy showed a miliary pattern of multiple scattered necrotizing granulomas. Frequent acid-fast bacilli were seen on special stains. Hematoxylin and eosin stain, 2 ×.

patients. Patients with chronic granulomatous disease often have recurrent pulmonary infections, which may manifest as nodular zones of typically necrotizing granulomatous inflammation (Fig. 28). Special stains should be performed to exclude fungal and acid-fast organisms, including mycobacteria and *Nocardia*. The primary differential diagnosis for

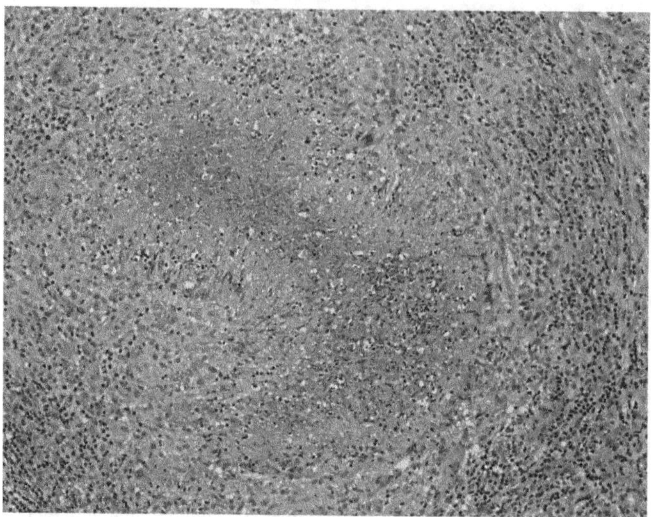

Figure 28 Infectious disease. Chronic granulomatous disease. A 15-year-old boy with chronic granulomatous disease and recurrent pulmonary infections, including *Aspergillus* species. Lung biopsy shows necrotizing granulomatous inflammation with rare acid-fast bacilli identified on special stains. Hematoxylin and eosin stain, 10 ×.

nodular disease in immunosuppressed or immunocompromised patients is angioinvasive fungal infection, such as *Aspergillus* species, resulting in spherical zones of parenchymal hemorrhage and necrosis.

J. Aspiration Injury

The diagnosis of aspiration injury in children is a problematic area, as there is currently no conclusive clinical test and only very few specific histologic clues to the diagnosis. Most investigations of aspiration injury include a bronchoalveolar lavage for lipid-laden macrophages. It is important to remember that while the absence of lipid-laden macrophages or their rare presence militates against the diagnosis of aspiration, their presence, even in large numbers, is not diagnostic or specific for aspiration. Lipid-laden macrophages may be found in any active inflammatory disease with cell breakdown (for example, resolving bacterial pneumonia), in patients receiving intravenous lipid preparations, fat embolization related to bone fracture, and a number of other processes. Various indices have been developed in an attempt to improve the diagnostic utility of the lavage findings; however, none of these is completely reliable (74). The import of lipid-laden macrophages must be considered in the clinical setting.

On biopsy, aspiration syndromes may show one or a mixture of several histopathologic features. Airway-associated lymphoid hyperplasia or follicular bronchiolitis is frequently present in aspiration, but may be found in other settings as well. Additional features of aspiration may include focal organizing pneumonia, lipoid pneumonia (cholesterol clefts and increased foamy macrophages) (Fig. 29), and granulomas containing identifiable foreign debris or hyalinized material. Certainly, absence of these findings does not exclude the

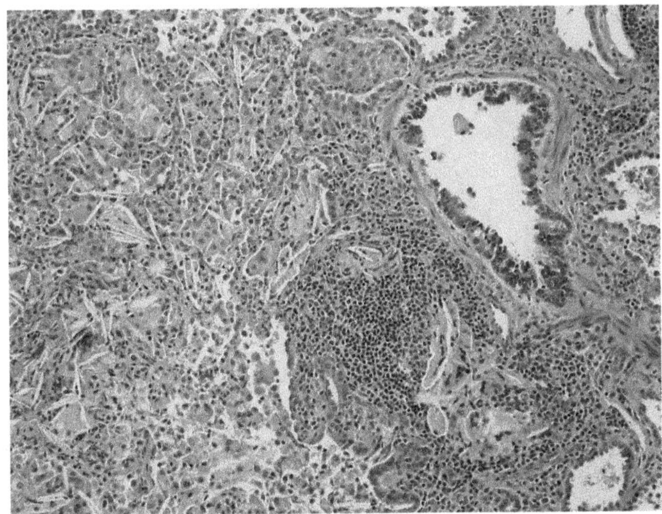

Figure 29 Aspiration injury. Cholesterol granulomas. Two-year-old girl with bronchopulmonary dysplasia and history of gastroesophageal reflux with recurrent aspiration episodes. Lung biopsy shows increased periairway alveolar macrophages and cholesterol clefts. Mildly increased airway-associated lymphoid tissue is also a common but nonspecific finding. Hematoxylin and eosin stain, 10×.

diagnosis, and correlation with clinical findings is important in each case. Another distinctive histologic pattern of aspiration is exogenous lipoid pneumonia, classically due to aspiration of mineral oil. In addition to foamy and vacuolated alveolar macrophages, there are vacuoles in the interstitium and interlobular septa of the lung (Fig. 30).

K. Obliterative Bronchiolitis

Obliterative (or constrictive) bronchiolitis is the pathologic process underlying BOS, a constellation of clinical and diagnostic imaging findings including an obstructive pattern on pulmonary function tests and evidence of mosaic perfusion and air trapping on expiratory chest CT. The differential diagnosis of BOS in children includes prior viral infection, especially adenovirus, chronic aspiration injury, Stevens-Johnson syndrome, chronic airway rejection in lung transplant recipients, chronic graft-versus-host disease in bone marrow transplant recipients, and occasionally asthma and cystic fibrosis. Histologically, obliterative bronchiolitis is characterized by varying degrees of airway fibrosis, ranging from mild subepithelial fibrosis with luminal constriction to complete fibrosis with obliteration of the airway lumen (Fig. 31). Inflammation may be present if there is ongoing injury, but is typically absent in end-stage disease and in cases resulting from remote episodes of airway injury. Connective tissue stains, such as trichrome stain, elastic stain, and Movat pentachrome stain, or immunohistochemistry for smooth muscle actin, may be helpful in discriminating the subtle residual components of the airway wall after fibrous obliteration (Fig. 32). "Unpaired" pulmonary artery branches may suggest bronchiolar obliteration on routine H&E stained sections. Other histologic findings, which suggest airway obstruction and/or chronic

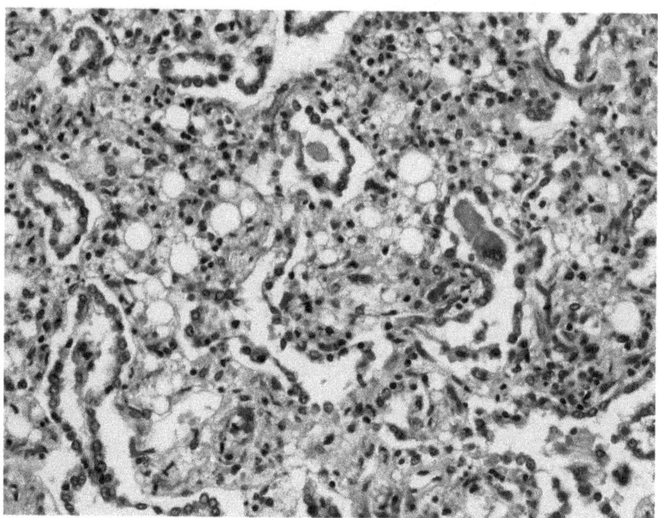

Figure 30 Aspiration injury. Exogenous lipoid pneumonia. Four-year-old former premature boy with mental retardation and cerebral palsy. Aspiration events resulted in a pattern of interstitial widening and large interstitial vacuoles (exogenous lipoid pneumonia). Reactive alveolar epithelial hyperplasia is also prominent in this example. Hematoxylin and eosin stain, 20 ×.

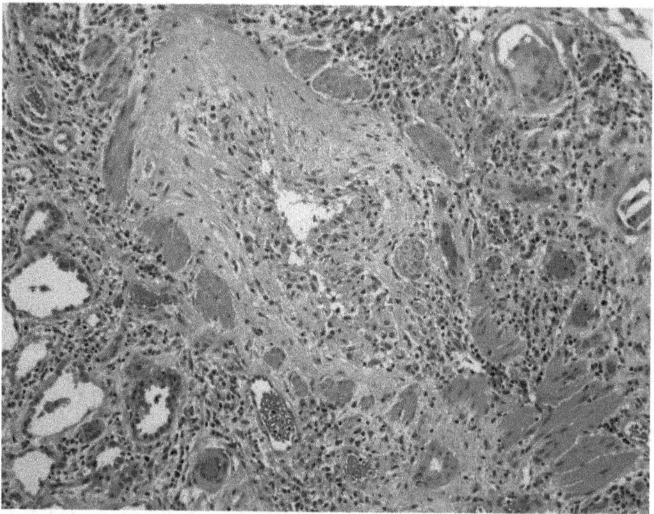

Figure 31 Obliterative bronchiolitis. Postviral injury. Four-year-old lung transplant recipient with history of adenovirus bronchiolitis and pneumonia, resulting in bronchiolitis obliterans syndrome two years after transplant. This bronchiole shows near-complete luminal obliteration by fibroconnective tissue. Hematoxylin and eosin stain, 10 ×.

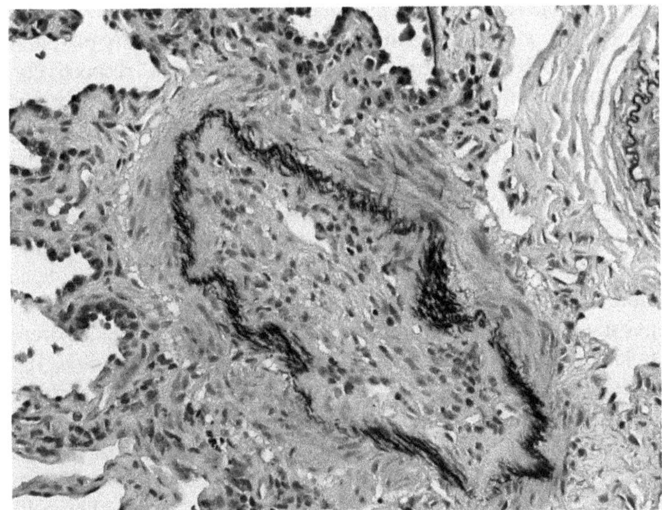

Figure 32 Obliterative bronchiolitis. Postaspiration injury. Five-year-old girl with mental retardation, cerebral palsy, and chronic recurrent aspiration. Connective tissue stains are helpful in highlighting obliterated airways, as in this example in which a thick layer of elastin separates the outer smooth muscle wall from the inner fibrotic airway lumen. Movat pentachrome stain, 20 ×.

airway injury, include mucus stasis within bronchiolar lumens and adjacent airspaces, distention of airspaces and alveolar ducts, increased periairway foamy macrophages and cholesterol clefts, and interstitial extension of airway smooth muscle. Sampling error may be a problem because of the variable degree of fibrosis in individual airways. Because histologic diagnosis depends on evaluation of terminal and respiratory bronchioles, wedge biopsies should be at least 1.5-cm deep to maximize the diagnostic yield. Shallow biopsies of the peripheral alveoli and alveolar ducts are inadequate for evaluation of obliterative bronchiolitis. Recognizing the variable distribution of airway involvement, any evidence of remote airway fibrosis helps to support the diagnosis of BOS in the proper clinical setting, even in the absence of complete airway obliteration histologically.

L. Hemorrhage Syndromes

Diffuse alveolar hemorrhage syndromes typically present with anemia, pulmonary infiltrates, and hemosiderin-laden macrophages on bronchoalveolar lavage cytology. Pulmonary hemorrhage episodes may lead to lung biopsy to assist in determining etiology and guiding further management. Classification of hemorrhage syndromes is divided broadly into disorders with capillaritis, hemorrhage secondary to cardiovascular disease, and other causes (75). Hemorrhage related to capillaritis may be seen in an idiopathic form and also secondary to a wide variety of systemic autoimmune processes, including Wegener's granulomatosis, microscopic polyangiitis, systemic lupus erythematosus, Goodpasture's syndrome (antiglomerular basement membrane disease), antiphospholipid antibody syndrome, Henoch-Schonlein purpura, IgA nephropathy, polyarteritis nodosa, and Behcet syndrome (76). Capillaritis may also be drug induced or associated with cryoglobulinemia.

In Wegener's granulomatosis and microscopic polyangiitis, the pulmonary microvascular injury is mediated by antineutrophil cytoplasmic antibodies (ANCA), specifically c-ANCA (antiproteinase 3 antibody) and p-ANCA (antimyeloperoxidase antibody), respectively. Cardiovascular causes of pulmonary hemorrhage include pulmonary hypertension, chronic heart failure, left-sided obstructive lesions such as mitral stenosis or pulmonary vein stenosis, pulmonary veno-occlusive disease, arteriovenous malformation, and vascular thrombosis with pulmonary infarction. Noncardiovascular disorders associated with pulmonary hemorrhage include bone marrow transplantation, immunodeficiency, coagulation disorders, and when there is no known etiology clinically or on biopsy, idiopathic pulmonary hemosiderosis.

If the etiology of pulmonary hemorrhage is not clear from clinical history or serologic studies, further diagnostic evaluation may require a wedge biopsy of lung parenchyma, as bronchoalveolar lavage and transbronchial biopsy are insufficient to allow full characterization of the vasculature. In addition to nonspecific features of hemorrhage (extravasated red blood cells, hemosiderin-laden macrophages, mineralization of elastic fibers, focal organizing pneumonia), the biopsy should be assessed for indicators of specific etiology, including capillaritis, pulmonary arteriopathy, and chronic congestive vasculopathy. Even in wedge biopsies, pulmonary capillaritis may be a relatively subtle diagnosis, which is easily missed if not carefully sought. The diagnosis of capillaritis rests on identification of increased neutrophils in the interstitium of alveolar walls, often associated with patchy foci of alveolar fibrin, alveolar neutrophils (acute alveolitis), and/or necrosis of alveolar walls (Fig. 33). While occasional neutrophils are seen normally circulating in capillaries, linear infiltrates or aggregates of neutrophils within alveolar walls should suggest the diagnosis. Increased number and size of lymphoid aggregates in many cases

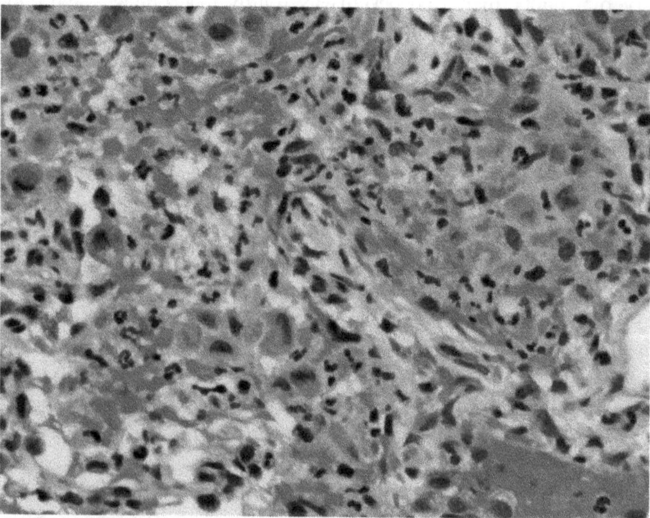

Figure 33 Hemorrhage syndromes. Capillaritis. Four-year-old girl with isolated pulmonary hemorrhage. Pulmonary capillaritis is indicated by neutrophil infiltrates within the interstitium, extending into the adjacent alveolar spaces (alveolitis), admixed with hemorrhage and intra-alveolar fibrin. Hematoxylin and eosin stain, 20 ×.

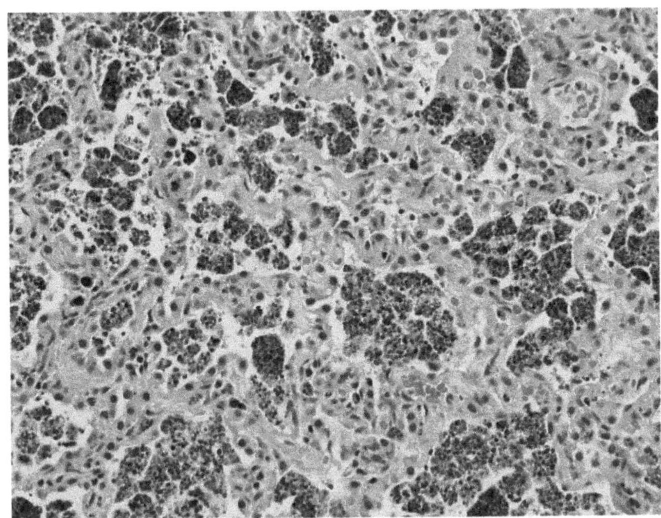

Figure 34 Hemorrhage syndromes. Idiopathic pulmonary hemosiderosis. Six-year-old boy with recurrent pulmonary hemorrhage, initially presenting with anemia and bilateral pulmonary infiltrates. Rheumatology evaluation and serologic studies were negative. Lung biopsy shows abundant hemosiderin-laden macrophages without evidence of inflammation or associated vasculopathy. Hematoxylin and eosin stain, 10 ×.

reflects immunologic activation and is a helpful diagnostic clue that prompts search for other diagnostic features of capillaritis. Immunofluorescence study of lung tissue may aid in identifying immunoglobulin or complement deposits, but this study is often negative in spite of morphologic evidence of capillaritis, perhaps because of transient immune deposits. Similarly, ANCA serologic titers are helpful diagnostically when elevated, but normal titers would not exclude the diagnosis of capillaritis. Indeed, ANCA titers may fluctuate and do not always correspond directly to disease activity. It should also be noted that steroid therapy prior to lung biopsy may modify the degree of inflammation in capillaritis, and definitive diagnosis may be more difficult in such cases.

After excluding pulmonary capillaritis, histologic features related to congenital heart disease should be sought, including the pulmonary arteriopathy resulting from pulmonary overcirculation and the vasculopathy resulting from chronic congestion (see sect. II.G). Idiopathic pulmonary hemosiderosis is a clinical diagnosis of exclusion, but histologically correlates with increased hemosiderin-laden macrophages, without other evidence of inflammation or chronic vascular disease (Fig. 34).

III. Nodules, Cysts, and Lung Tumors in Children

A. Nodules and Evaluation for Metastatic Tumor

Biopsy of focal lesions is a less common procedure in children than in adults. In children, the most common impetus for the biopsy of a focal lesion is the assessment and treatment of metastatic disease in patients with known malignancy. The most common metastatic lesions excised in the pediatric population are Wilms tumor and osteosarcoma, although a wide variety of solid tumors and hematopoietic neoplasms may produce focal nodules in the lung. Such lesions do not ordinarily present a diagnostic problem; however, in a significant proportion of cases, the lung biopsy shows another focal process rather than metastasis. Studies have shown that at least 10% and up to 30% of lesions detected by screening CT do not show tumor on biopsy (77). A wide variety of both infectious and noninfectious focal lesions may be identified, including granulomatous lesions due to mycobacteria and fungi and nongranulomatous lesions including pleural-based lymph nodes and small scars. Such scars may result from obliteration of tumor after therapy or resolved infarction related to embolization from central lines or other venous access.

B. Cysts and Developmental Lesions

Most cystic masses of the lung in infants and children represent developmental lesions. The differential diagnosis of pediatric lung cysts includes bronchogenic cyst, bronchial atresia (BA), intralobar sequestration (ILS), extralobar sequestration (ELS), congenital pulmonary airway malformation (CPAM) (previously called congenital cystic adenomatoid malformation, CCAM), as well as cystic pleuropulmonary blastoma (PPB) (see sect. III.C) and various acquired cystic lesions (persistent pulmonary interstitial emphysema, pneumatocele) (Table 6). Congenital lobar overinflation shows clinical and diagnostic imaging overlap with BA also and may have a somewhat cystic appearance. The most common developmental cystic lesions have been reviewed elsewhere and diagnostic features are discussed briefly below (78).

Bronchogenic Cyst

Bronchogenic cysts are unilocular cystic lesions typically filled with mucus or fluid material and lined by ciliated respiratory epithelium. Smooth muscle and occasional cartilage plates are typically present in the wall, replicating normal bronchial architecture (Fig. 35). While these cysts are most often outside of the lung parenchyma and positioned adjacent to the tracheobronchial tree, intrapulmonary examples may also occur.

Bronchial Atresia, Intralobar Sequestration, and Extralobar Sequestration

BA is a congenital lesion, which may be lobar, segmental, or subsegmental. It may be isolated or associated with systemic arterial connection (ILS). Isolated segmental BA most

Table 6 Pediatric Cystic Lung Lesions: Differential Diagnosis

Developmental	Neoplastic	Acquired
Bronchogenic cyst	Pleuropulmonary blastoma	Persistent PIE
Bronchial atresia	cystic (type I)	Pneumatocele
Intralobar sequestration	solid and cystic (type II)	Abscess/necrotizing pneumonia
Extralobar sequestration		
CPAM, large cyst type		
Congenital lobar overinflation		
Lymphatic cyst/malformation		

Abbreviations: CPAM, congenital pulmonary airway malformation; PIE, pulmonary interstitial emphysema.

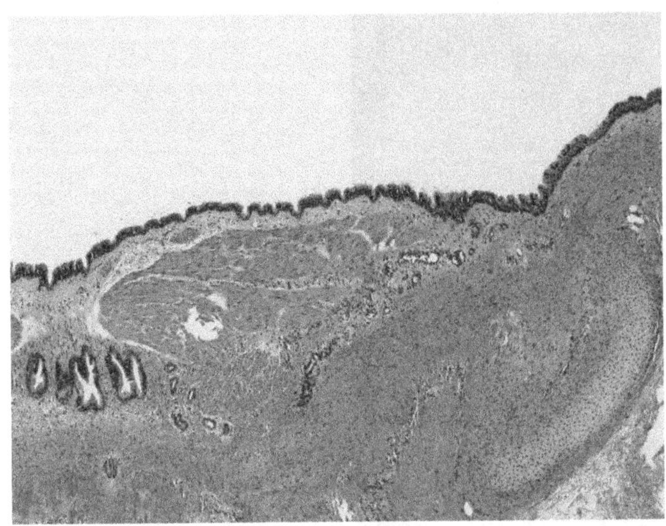

Figure 35 Developmental lesions. Bronchogenic cyst. Six-month-old girl with left mediastinal cyst. This bronchogenic cyst replicates normal airway structure, including a ciliated respiratory epithelial lining, a few submucosal glands, a smooth muscle wall, and a cartilage plate (*lower right*). Hematoxylin and eosin stain, 2 ×.

often results in a central mucocele at the site of the atretic bronchus, distal mucus stasis, and parenchymal maldevelopment in the distribution of the affected bronchus (Fig. 36). This pattern of distal microcystic maldevelopment is composed of increased density and complexity of bronchiolar structures and distension and/or elongation of surrounding alveolar spaces. Histologically identical to Stocker type II CPAM, this pattern of parenchymal maldevelopment implies pathogenesis from intrauterine bronchial obstruction, and has been described in BA, ILS, ELS, and rarely, in congenital lobar overinflation (79). In some cases, the parenchymal maldevelopment is relatively mild, corresponding to alveolar distension and elongation, with less conspicuous abnormality of the bronchiolar profiles (Fig. 37). While many BAs are now detected by prenatal ultrasound, some present in older children as incidental findings on imaging or with symptoms referable to infection or extrinsic compression of unaffected airways.

Extralobar and intralobar pulmonary sequestrations both refer to lung malformations in which the parenchyma is "sequestered," or isolated, from the remaining lung by virtue of the lack of bronchial connection and lack of normal pulmonary arterial connection. ELSs are typically pyramidal structures detached from the remaining lung and invested completely in pleura, often seen at the base of the left thoracic cavity, and in some cases identified incidentally at the time of diaphragmatic hernia repair. Grossly, there is a vascular pole at the hilum including systemic arterial supply, usually from the thoracic or abdominal aorta, but no patent bronchus (Fig. 38). Microscopic features are typically similar to the pattern described as Stocker type II CPAM (Fig. 39). As mentioned above, ILS is equivalent to a combination of BA and aberrant systemic arterial supply. In contrast to ELS, ILS is confined within a lobe, sharing the same pleural investment as the adjacent unaffected lung. A large elastic artery

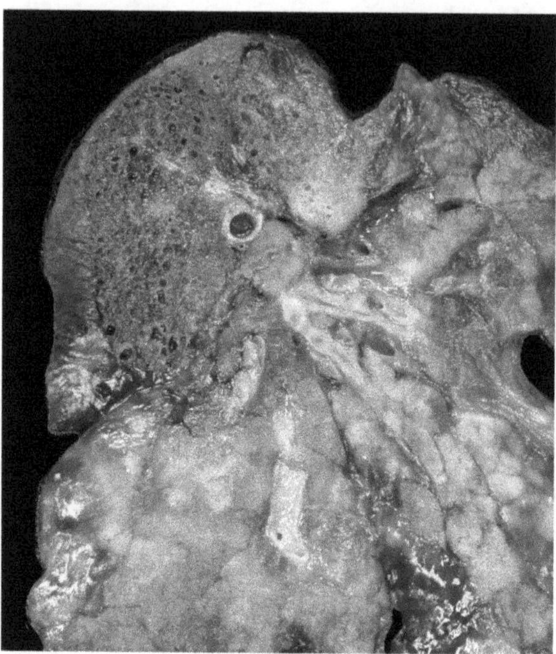

Figure 36 Developmental lesions. Bronchial atresia. Six-month-old girl with a fetal lung mass identified at four months' gestation. Postnatally, there was hyperaeration of the left upper lobe with mediastinal shift and multiple small cystic spaces (up to 5-mm diameter) on imaging. The lung parenchyma in the left upper lobe is maldeveloped with a segmental microcystic pattern. A central dilated bronchus containing mucus reflects bronchial obstruction due to atresia.

typically enters the pleura away from the hilum, often at the medial basal angle of a lower lobe (Fig. 40). ILS shares a similar pattern of parenchymal development as in BA and ELS. Unbalanced hemodynamics within an ILS may result in vascular shunting and alveolar hemorrhage in some cases (Fig. 41). Like BA, ILSs may come to attention because of recurrent infection, as bacteria may gain access to the sequestered parenchyma via the pores of Kohn between alveolar spaces. While ELSs are certainly malformations, the origin of ILSs is more controversial. The lesions detected in infants and young children are likely congenital malformations, and occasional association with other malformations supports this assertion. ILS in adults has been theorized to represent an acquired lesion resulting from airway obliteration and ingrowth of collateral arterial supply, although late presentation of an occult congenital malformation is also possible.

Congenital Lobar Overinflation

Congenital lobar overinflation (also called congenital or infantile lobar emphysema) refers to marked enlargement of a lobe, typically an upper lobe, which is most often detected postnatally with respiratory distress or unilateral hyperinflation and mediastinal shift on chest X ray in the first month of life. The underlying pathogenesis is typically partial airway

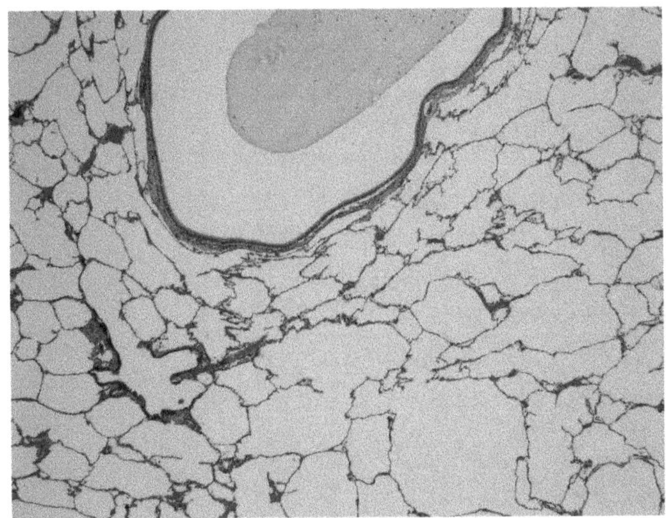

Figure 37 Developmental lesions. Bronchial atresia, postobstructive pattern. A 13-year-old boy with wheezing and dyspnea on exertion, found to have left upper lobe "emphysema" and a mass corresponding to a mucocele in the suprahilar region on chest CT imaging. Examination of the left upper lobe after lobectomy confirmed the presence of segmental bronchial atresia. Microscopically, the parenchyma shows a mucus-filled ectatic bronchiole surrounded by distended, elongated, and poorly septated airspaces. Hematoxylin and eosin stain, 4 ×.

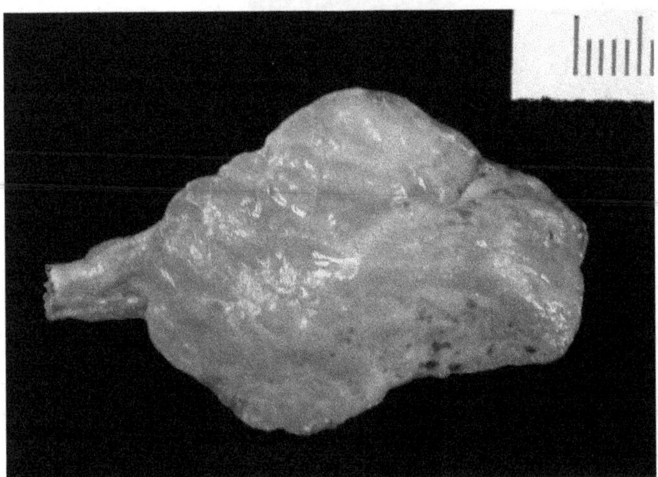

Figure 38 Developmental lesions. Extralobar sequestration. Seven-year-old boy with a small incidental lung lesion identified during lobectomy for segmental bronchial atresia. Similar small extralobar sequestrations are more commonly identified incidentally in infants during repair of congenital diaphragmatic hernia.

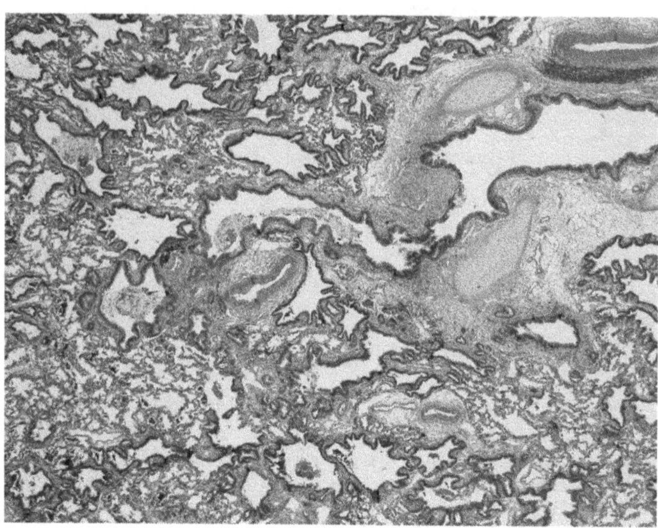

Figure 39 Developmental lesions. Extralobar sequestration. Microscopically, extralobar sequestration shows microcystic change of the parenchyma with increased numbers of branching, complex bronchiolar profiles containing a small amount of mucus and surrounded by incompletely developed airspaces, a histologic constellation indicating bronchial obstruction during intrauterine development. Hematoxylin and eosin stain, 4 ×.

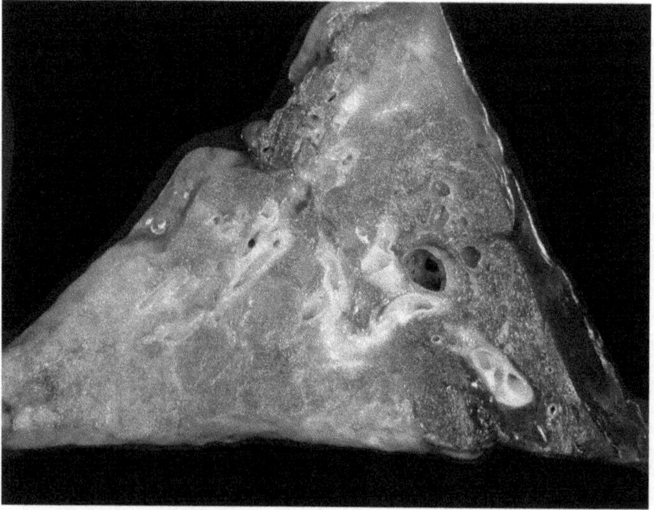

Figure 40 Developmental lesions. Intralobar sequestration. Seven-month-old girl with a right lower lobe mass. Systemic arterial supply from the thoracic aorta is indicated by a large elastic artery entering the lung at the basal angle and dilated arterial profiles extending through the surrounding congested and microcystic parenchyma of the posterior basal segment of the lung.

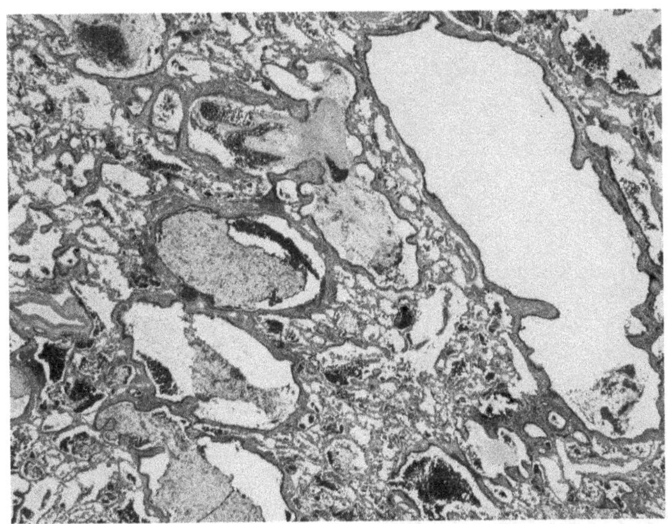

Figure 41 Developmental lesions. Intralobar sequestration. A 14-month-old term infant with VACTERL association, tracheoesophageal fistula, congenital heart disease, and a cystic lung lesion of the left lower lobe. A large systemic artery supplied the lobe from the infradiaphragmatic aorta. Dilated branching bronchiolar profiles contain mucus and are surrounded by poorly developed airspaces, indicating a component of bronchial obstruction due to atresia. The patchy areas of hemorrhage within airspaces also reflect the abnormal high-pressure flow to this segment of the intralobar sequestration. Hematoxylin and eosin stain, 4 ×.

obstruction due to bronchomalacia, in which the deficiency in cartilage causes collapse during expiration and progressive distal air trapping, or bronchial stenosis, as by an anatomic variation such as "kinking," web formation, or extrinsic compression. Grossly, the lobe is markedly enlarged, pale, and spongy, but typically without gross cyst formation (Fig. 42). Microscopically, the alveoli appear well developed with delicate walls and normal septation, but marked overdistension. In contrast to BA and ILS, the proportion of bronchioles relative to surrounding alveoli is appropriate. Only rare cases arising in utero show a component of microcystic maldevelopment histologically similar to that seen in BA. Such cases support the theory of microcystic change occurring as a manifestation of "bronchial obstruction sequence," whether due to bronchial stenosis or BA.

CPAM, Large Cyst Type

The large cyst type of CPAM is of uncertain pathogenesis and is distinguished from the small cyst type more commonly associated with bronchial obstruction. This cystic lesion is composed of a large cyst with multiple septations or a coarsely trabeculated wall, defined as greater than 2 cm in greatest dimension, but typically measuring several centimeters in diameter (Fig. 43). Histologically, the cystic spaces are lined by respiratory type epithelium and, despite gross circumscription, these lesions show interdigitation of the cyst wall with surrounding airspaces (Fig. 44). Small foci of mucigenic epithelium, resembling gastric

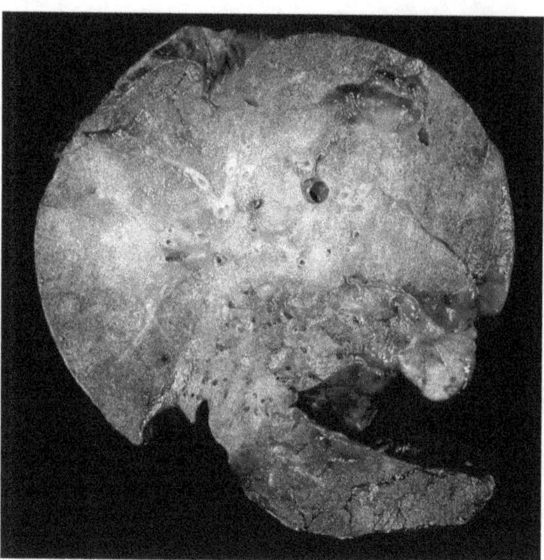

Figure 42 Developmental lesions. Congenital lobar overinflation. Six-week-old term infant girl with history of respiratory distress and marked hyperinflation of the left lung with mediastinal shift. The left upper lobe shows a large region of pale, markedly overinflated spongy parenchyma, sparing the lingula.

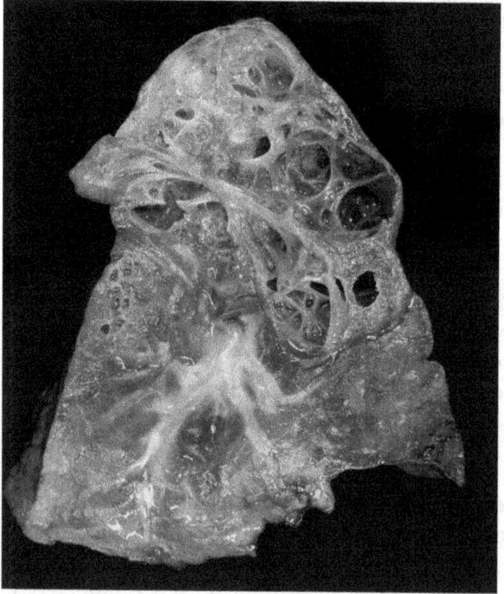

Figure 43 Developmental lesions. Congenital pulmonary airway malformation, large cyst type. Eight-week-old term infant girl with a large cystic lung lesion detected prenatally at 28 weeks' gestation. The lesion is composed of large complex cystic spaces with thick trabeculations.

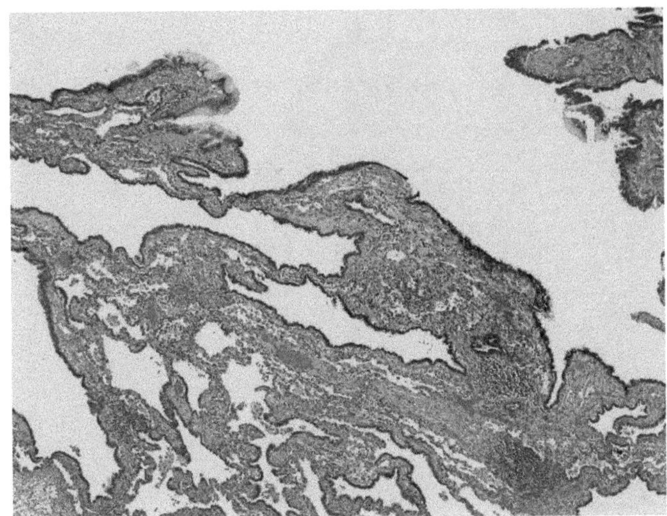

Figure 44 Developmental lesions. Congenital pulmonary airway malformation, large cyst type. Four-month-old girl with a large cystic lesion of the right middle lobe. Microscopically, this congenital pulmonary airway malformation shows a cyst wall lined by respiratory-type epithelium and showing interdigitation with the surrounding lung parenchyma. Mucigenic epithelium resembling gastric foveolar epithelium (*upper left*) is a characteristic, but inconstant, finding in this lesion. Hematoxylin and eosin stain, 4 ×.

foveolar epithelium, are distinctive for this lesion, but this finding is not present in all cases. The mucigenic epithelium is thought to be the precursor for rare reports of bronchioloalveolar carcinoma arising from preexisting cysts in older children and adults.

C. Primary Lung Tumors

Primary benign and malignant lung tumors are rare in childhood, and most neoplasms involving the lung are metastatic (80,81). Nevertheless, the possibility of a primary pulmonary neoplasm should not be dismissed in the evaluation of an isolated lung mass in a child. Inflammatory myofibroblastic tumor is one of the most common benign pulmonary tumors occurring in childhood and may be endobronchial or intraparenchymal (Fig. 45). Other benign tumors of the pediatric tracheobronchial tree and lung include squamous papillomas related to human papillomavirus infection, infantile hemangioma, chondroma or hamartoma, congenital peribronchial myofibroblastic tumor, and leiomyoma.

Carcinoid tumor is the most common malignant endobronchial tumor in children (Fig. 46), with a differential diagnosis also including mucoepidermoid carcinoma and other tumors arising from the bronchial submucosal glands. Primary sarcomas involving the lung include synovial sarcoma, bronchopulmonary fibrosarcoma, and leiomyosarcoma. Ewing's sarcoma most commonly involves the lung by direct extension from the thoracic wall. Special considerations for lung masses in the immunocompromised population include the Epstein-Barr virus–associated neoplasms: posttransplant lymphoproliferative disorders and smooth muscle tumors.

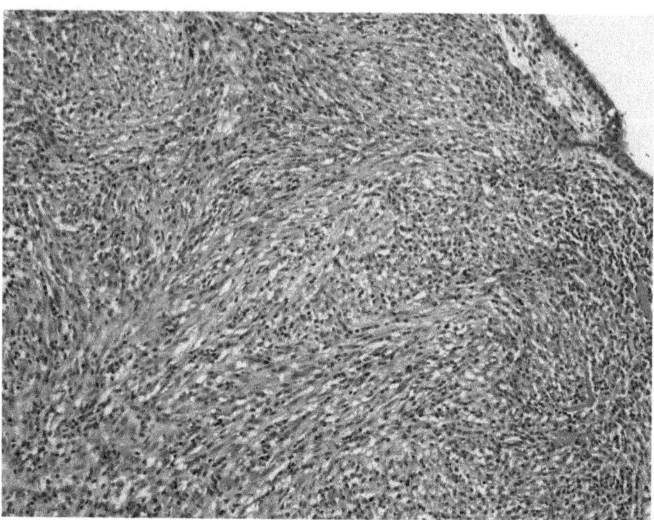

Figure 45 Lung neoplasms. Inflammatory myofibroblastic tumor. Four-year-old otherwise healthy boy with an obstructive right upper lobe bronchus mass. The submucosal proliferation of spindled cells shows haphazard fascicular arrangement with increased infiltrating lymphocytes, with morphology typical of inflammatory myofibroblastic tumor. Hematoxylin and eosin stain, 10 ×.

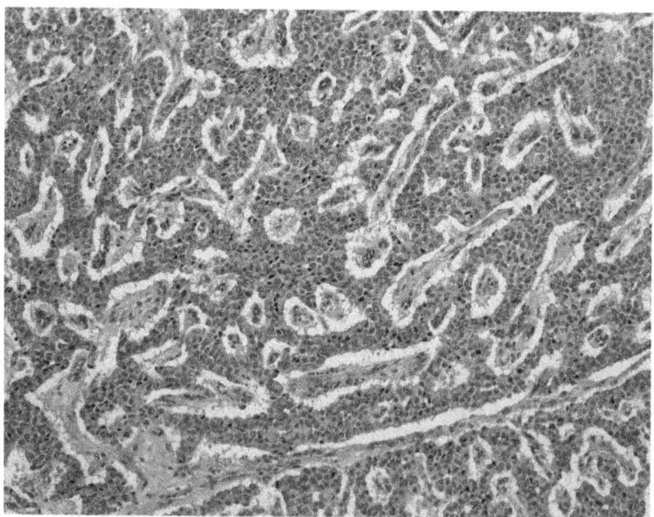

Figure 46 Lung neoplasms. Carcinoid tumor. A 11-year-old boy with hemoptysis and an obstructive mass of the right mainstem bronchus. The microscopic features are typical of a carcinoid tumor, including anastomosing cords of cells with uniform round nuclei and stippled chromatin, as well as a highly vascular supporting stroma. Hematoxylin and eosin stain, 10 ×.

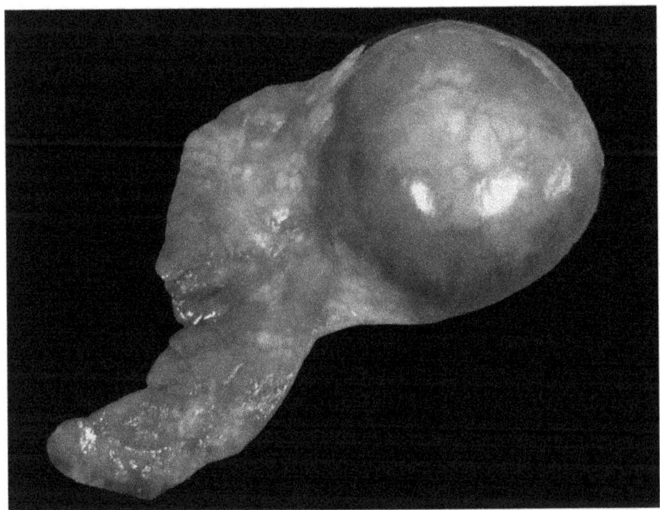

Figure 47 Lung neoplasms. Pleuropulmonary blastoma, cystic type. Four-month-old term infant boy with a 5.2-cm cystic mass of the left upper lobe and a presumptive diagnosis of congenital pulmonary airway malformation. Cut section showed a purely cystic lesion with thick and thin septae and microscopic features of pleuropulmonary blastoma. A second small 5-mm cyst was identified in the right lower lobe and showed similar histologic features.

PPB is the most common primary malignancy of the lung parenchyma in children. It is a relatively recently recognized embryonal malignancy with a spectrum of gross and microscopic morphology, from low-grade cystic lesions to high-grade overtly malignant solid forms (82). PPB is classified by gross features as type I (cystic), type II (solid and cystic), and type III (solid). It should be emphasized that PPB is distinct from pulmonary blastoma (PB), a tumor more common in adults that has malignant epithelial and stromal components. Although there may be entrapped alveolar and respiratory epithelial elements in PPB, the malignant component is exclusively a primitive stromal cell type. The purely cystic type I lesions are intraparenchymal lesions covered by pleura, but may protrude from the pleural surface (Fig. 47), leading in some cases to simple amputation of a small pedicle and risk of incomplete resection and recurrence as a higher grade lesion. Type I cystic PPB is typically indistinguishable grossly from the large cyst type of CPAM and is a diagnosis which may be subtle microscopically. Cystic PPB is composed of multiple thick and thin septa lined predominantly by flat to cuboidal alveolar-type epithelium, similar to that described in type IV (peripheral-type) CPAM (Fig. 48). The key to recognition of cystic PPB is the identification of immature-appearing undifferentiated spindled mesenchyme in the septa, a feature that may require careful search and additional sectioning in the proper setting. These foci of undifferentiated mesenchyme often form a highly vascular "cambium" layer beneath the alveolar epithelium (Fig. 49). Other mesenchymal elements, most frequently immature cartilage (Fig. 50) or plump and eosinophilic rhabdomyoblasts, may also be present. The PPBs with solid components (type II and type III) contain sheets of malignant mesenchymal cells (Fig. 51), some of which may display ultrastructural and

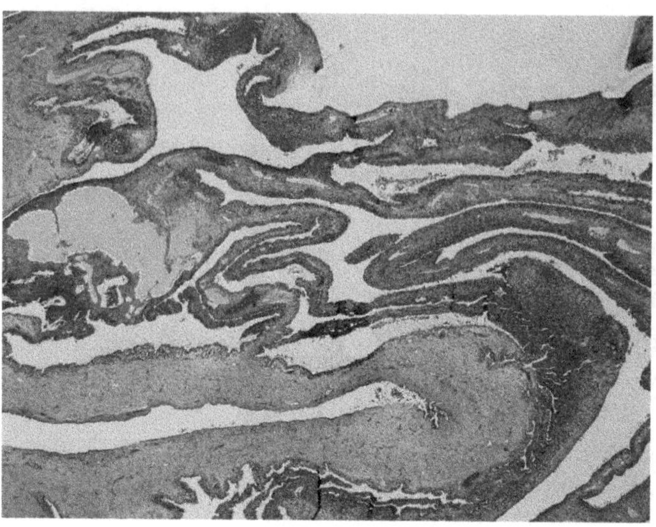

Figure 48 Lung neoplasms. Pleuropulmonary blastoma, cystic type. One-and-a-half-month-old infant with acute respiratory distress due to left tension pneumothorax. A left upper lobe multicystic lesion was resected, showing complex variably thickened and cellular septa. Hematoxylin and eosin stain, 2 ×.

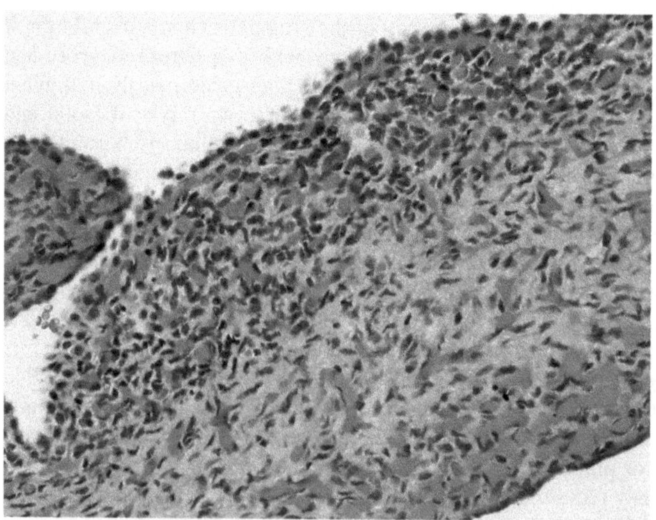

Figure 49 Lung neoplasms. Pleuropulmonary blastoma, cystic type. The regions of primitive round and spindled cells are often highly vascular and form a cambium-like layer under the alveolar epithelium. Hematoxylin and eosin stain, 20 ×.

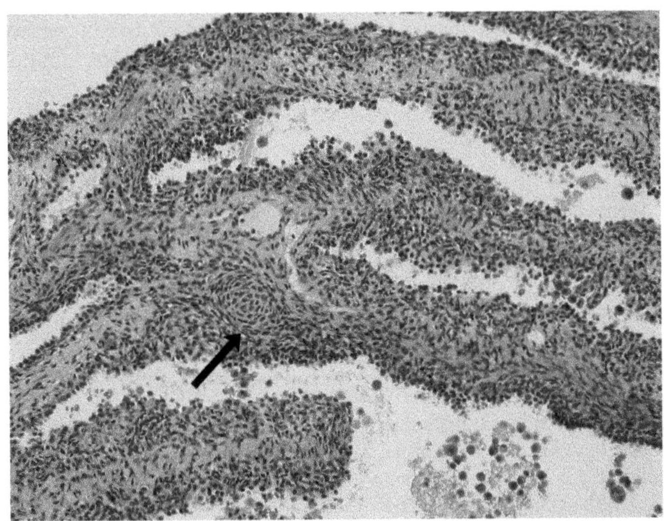

Figure 50 Lung neoplasms. Pleuropulmonary blastoma, cystic type. The septa are lined by alveolar type cuboidal epithelium and are expanded by hyperchromatic primitive cells as well as occasional small immature islands of cartilage (*arrow*). Hematoxylin and eosin stain, 4 ×.

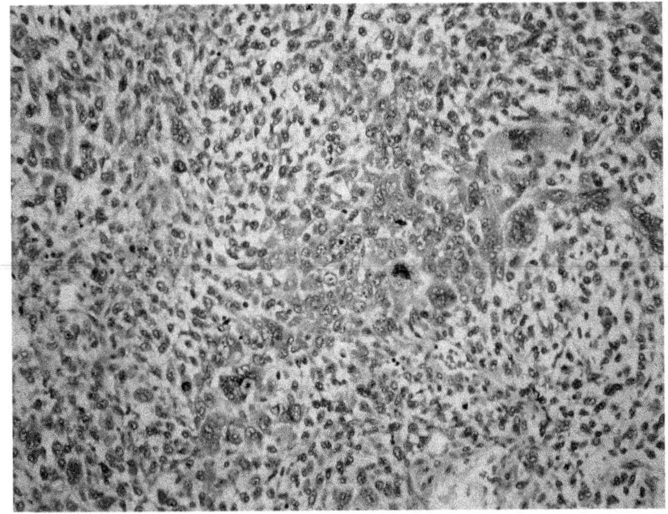

Figure 51 Lung neoplasms. Pleuropulmonary blastoma, solid type. Four-year-old with recurrence of a right upper lobe pleuropulmonary blastoma two years after initial resection. This high-grade solid lesion shows sheets of primitive spindled cells with focal areas showing eosinophilic cytoplasm similar to rhabdomyoblast differentiation, as well as severe cytologic atypia and prominent mitoses. Hematoxylin and eosin stain, 10 ×.

immunohistochemical markers of rhabdomyosarcoma. A diagnosis of PPB has important implications for other family members as well as for the affected child, as there is a familial association with other embryonal tumors and with cystic renal lesions (83).

References

1. Weng TR, Levison H, Wentworth P, et al. Open lung biopsy in children. Am Rev Respir Dis 1968; 97:673–684.
2. Prober CG, Whyte H, Smith CR. Open lung biopsy in immunocompromised children with pulmonary infiltrates. Am J Dis Child 1984; 138:60–63.
3. Doolin EJ, Luck SR, Sherman JO, et al. Emergency lung biopsy: friend or foe of the immunosuppressed child? J Pediatr Surg 1986; 21:485–487.
4. Foglia RP, Shilyansky J, Konkalsrud EW. Emergency lung biopsy in immunocompromised pediatric patients. Ann Surg 1989; 210:90–92.
5. Joshi VV, Oleske JM, Minnefor AB, et al. Pathologic pulmonary findings in children with the acquired immunodeficiency syndrome: a study of ten cases. Hum Pathol 1985; 16:241–246.
6. Bond SJ, Lee DJ, Stewart DL, et al. Open lung biopsy in pediatric patients on extracorporeal membrane oxygenation. J Pediatr Surg 1996; 31:1376–1378.
7. Muntz HR, Wallace M, Lusk RP. Pediatric transbronchial lung biopsy. Ann Otol Rhinol Laryngol 1992; 101:135–137.
8. Smyth RL, Carty H, Thomas H, et al. Diagnosis of interstitial lung disease by a percutaneous lung biopsy sample. Arch Dis Child 1994; 10:143–144.
9. Spencer DA, Alton HM, Raafat F, et al. Combined percutaneous lung biopsy and high-resolution computed tomography in the diagnosis and management of lung disease in children. Pediatr Pulmonol 1996; 22:111–116.
10. Mullins D, Livne M, Mallory GB, et al. A new technique for transbronchial biopsy in infants and small children. Pediatr Pulmonol 1995; 20:253–257.
11. Rothenberg SS, Wagner JS, Chang JHT, et al. The safety and efficacy of thoracoscopic lung biopsy for diagnosis and treatment in infants and children. J Pediatr Surg 1996; 31:100–104.
12. Fan LL, Kozinetz CA, Wojtczak HA, et al. Diagnostic value of transbronchial, thoracoscopic, and open lung biopsy in immunocompetent children with chronic interstitial lung disease. J Pediatr 1997; 131:565–569.
13. Fan LL, Kozinetz CA, Deterding RR, et al. Evaluation of a diagnostic approach to pediatric interstitial lung disease. Pediatrics 1998; 101(1):82–85.
14. Bush A. Diagnosis of interstitial lung disease. Pediatr Pulmonol 1996; 22:81–82.
15. Flake AW. Is a CT guided needle better than a knife? Pediatr Pulmonol 1996; 22:83–84.
16. Langston C, Patterson K, Dishop MK, et al. A protocol for the handling of tissue obtained by operative lung biopsy: recommendations of the chILD pathology co-operative group. Pediatr Dev Pathol 2006; 9:173–180.
17. Gianoulis M, Chan N, Wright JL. Inflation of lung biopsies for frozen section. Mod Pathol 1988; 1:357–358.
18. Churg A. An inflation procedure for open lung biopsies. Am J Surg Pathol 1988; 7:69–71.
19. Howenstine MS, Eigen H. Current concepts on interstitial lung disease in children. Curr Opin Pediatr 1999; 11(3):200–204.
20. Clement A, Henrion-Caude A, Fauroux B. The pathogenesis of interstitial lung diseases in children. Paediatr Respir Rev 2004; 5:94–97.
21. Hilman BC, Amaro-Galvez R. Diagnosis of interstitial lung disease in children. Paediatr Respir Rev 2004; 5:101–107.
22. Fan LL, Mullen AL, Brugman SM, et al. Clinical spectrum of chronic interstitial lung disease in children. J Pediatr 1992; 121:867–872.

23. Langston C, Fan LL. The spectrum of interstitial lung disease in childhood. Pediatr Pulmonol 2001; S23:70–71.
24. Fan LL, Deterding RR, Langston C. Pediatric interstitial lung disease revisited. Pediatr Pulmonol 2004; 38:369–378.
25. Clement A, ERS Task Force. Task force on chronic interstitial lung disease in immunocompetent children. Eur Respir J 2004; 24:686–697.
26. Langston C, Fan LL. Diffuse interstitial lung disease in infants. Pediatr Pulmonol 2001; S23:74–76.
27. Deutsch GH, Young LR, Deterding RR, et al. Diffuse lung disease in young children: application of a novel classification scheme. Am J Respir Crit Care Med 2007; 176(11):1120–1128.
28. Fan LL, Langston C. Chronic interstitial lung disease in children. Pediatr Pulmonol 1993; 16:184–196.
29. Wagenvoort CA. Misalignment of lung vessels: a syndrome causing persistent neonatal pulmonary hypertension. Hum Pathol 1986; 17:727–730.
30. Boggs S, Harris MC, Hoffman DJ, et al. Misalignment of pulmonary veins with alveolar capillary dysplasia: variable phenotypic expression and the presumptive pre-mortem diagnosis in an affected sibling. J Pediatr 1994; 124:125–128.
31. Simonton S, Chrenka B. Familial persistent pulmonary hypertension in two siblings with phocomelia and alveolar capillary dysplasia (ACD): a new syndrome? Mod Pathol 1993; 6:9P (abstr).
32. Sirkin W, O'Hare BP, Cox PN, et al. Alveolar capillary dysplasia: lung biopsy diagnosis, nitric oxide responsiveness, and bronchial generation count. Pediatr Pathol Lab Med 1997; 17:125–132.
33. Langston C. Misalignment of pulmonary veins and alveolar capillary dysplasia. Pediatr Pathol 1991; 11:163–170.
34. Tredano M, de Blic J, Griese M, et al. Clinical, biological, and genetic heterogeneity of the inborn errors of pulmonary surfactant metabolism. Clin Chem Lab Med 2001; 39(2):90–108.
35. Cole FS, Hamvas A, Nogee LM. Genetic disorders of neonatal respiratory function. Pediatr Res 2001; 50(2):157–162.
36. Whitsett JA, Wert SE, Xu Y. Genetic disorders of surfactant homeostasis. Biol Neonate 2005; 87:283–287.
37. Nogee LM, Dunbar AE, Wert SE, et al. A mutation in surfactant protein C gene associated with familial interstitial lung disease. N Engl J Med 2001; 344(8):573–579.
38. Amin RS, Wert SE, Baughman RP, et al. Surfactant protein deficiency in familial interstitial lung disease. J Pediatr 2001; 139:85–92.
39. Tredano M, Griese M, Brasch F, et al. Mutation in SFTPC in infantile pulmonary alveolar proteinosis with or without fibrosing lung disease. Am J Med Genet A 2004; 126(1):18–26.
40. Nogee LM, de Mello DE, Dehner LP, et al. Brief report: deficiency of pulmonary surfactant protein B in congenital alveolar proteinosis. N Engl J Med 1993; 328:406–410.
41. deMello DE, Nogee LM, Heyman S, et al. Molecular and phenotypic variability in the congenital alveolar proteinosis syndrome associated with inherited surfactant protein B deficiency. J Pediatr 1994; 124:43–50.
42. deMello DE, Lin Z. Pulmonary alveolar proteinosis: a review. Pediatr Pathol Mol Med 2001; 20:413–432.
43. Trapnell BC, Whitsett JA, Nakata K. Mechanisms of disease: pulmonary alveolar proteinosis. N Engl J Med 2003; 349(26):2527–2539.
44. Katzenstein AA, Gordon LP, Oliphant M, et al. Chronic pneumonitis of infancy. A unique form of interstitial lung disease occurring in early childhood. Am J Surg Pathol 1995; 19(4):439–447.
45. Cameron HS, Somaschini M, Carrera P, et al. A common mutation in the surfactant protein C gene associated with lung disease. J Pediatr 2005; 146:370–375.
46. Chibbar R, Shih F, Baga M, et al. Nonspecific interstitial pneumonia and usual interstitial pneumonia with mutation in surfactant protein C in familial pulmonary fibrosis. Mod Pathol 2004; 17:973–980.

47. Lawson WE, Grant SW, Ambrosini V, et al. Genetic mutations in surfactant protein C are a rare cause of sporadic cases of IPF. Thorax 2004; 59:977–980.
48. Shulenin S, Nogee LM, Annilo T, et al. ABCA3 gene mutations in newborns with fatal surfactant deficiency. N Engl J Med 2004; 350(13):1296–1303.
49. Bullard JE, Wert SE, Whitsett JA, et al. ABCA3 mutations associated with pediatric interstitial lung disease. Am J Respir Crit Care Med 2005; 172:1026–1031.
50. deMello DE, Heyman S, Phelps DS, et al. Ultrastructure of lung in surfactant protein B deficiency. Am J Respir Cell Mol Biol 1994; 11:230–239.
51. Tryka AF, Wert SE, Mazursky JE, et al. Absence of lamellar bodies with accumulation of dense bodies characterizes a novel form of congenital surfactant defect. Pediatr Dev Pathol 2000; 3:335–345.
52. Cutz E, Wert SE, Nogee LM, et al. Deficiency of lamellar bodies in alveolar type II cells associated with fatal respiratory disease in a full-term infant. Am J Respir Crit Care Med 2000; 161:608–614.
53. Edwards V, Cutz E, Viero S, et al. Ultrastructure of lamellar bodies in congenital surfactant deficiency. Ultrastruct Pathol 2005; 29:503–509.
54. Thurlbeck W, Kida K, Langston C, et al. Postnatal lung growth after a repair of diaphragmatic hernia. Thorax 1979; 34:338–343.
55. Margraf LR, Tomashefski JF, Bruce MC, et al. Morphometric assessment of the lung in bronchopulmonary dysplasia. Am Rev Respir Dis 1991; 143:391–400.
56. Hislop AA, Haworth SG. Airway size and structure in the normal fetal and infant lung and the effect of premature delivery and artificial ventilation. Am Rev Respir Dis 1989; 140:1717–1726.
57. Canakis AM, Cutz E, Manson D, et al. Pulmonary interstitial glycogenosis: a new variant of neonatal interstitial lung disease. Am J Respir Crit Care Med 2002; 165:1557–1565.
58. Schroeder SA, Shannon DC, Mark EJ. Cellular interstitial pneumonitis in infants. A clinicopathologic study. Chest 1992; 101:1065–1069.
59. Smets K, Dhaene K, Schelstraete P, et al. Neonatal pulmonary interstitial glycogen accumulation disorder. Eur J Pediatr 2004; 163:408–409.
60. Onland W, Molenaar JJ, Leguit RJ, et al. Pulmonary interstitial glycogenosis in identical twins. Pediatr Pulmonol 2005; 40:362–366.
61. Deterding RR, Fan LL, Morton R, et al. Persistent tachypnea of infancy (PTI)—a new entity. Pediatr Pulmonol 2001; S23:72–73.
62. Deterding RR, Pye C, Fan LL, et al. Persistent tachypnea of infancy is associated with neuroendocrine cell hyperplasia. Pediatr Pulmonol 2005; 40:157–165.
63. Brody AS, Crotty EJ. Neuroendocrine cell hyperplasia of infancy (NEHI). Pediatr Radiol 2006; 36(12):1328.
64. Johnson DE, Anderson WR, Burke BA. Pulmonary neuroendocrine cells in pediatric lung disease: alterations in airway structure in infants with bronchopulmonary dysplasia. Anat Rec 1993; 236:115–119, 172–173.
65. Johnson D, Wobken J, Landrum B. Changes in bombesin, calcitonin and serotonin immunoreactive pulmonary neuroendocrine cells in cystic fibrosis and after prolonged mechanical ventilation. Am Rev Respir Dis 1988; 137:123–131.
66. Asabe K, Tsuji K, Handa N, et al. Immunohistochemical distribution of bombesin-positive pulmonary neuroendocrine cells in a congenital diaphragmatic hernia. Surg Today 1999; 29:407–412.
67. Johnson DE, Georgieff MK. Pulmonary neuroendocrine cells. Their secretory products and their potential roles in health and chronic lung disease in infancy. Am Rev Respir Dis 1989; 140:1807–1812.
68. Hull J, Chow CW, Robertson CF. Chronic idiopathic bronchiolitis of infancy. Arch Dis Child 1997; 77:512–515.

69. Kinane BT, Mansell AL, Zwerdling RG, et al. Follicular bronchitis in the pediatric population. Chest 1993; 104:1183–1186.
70. Rabinovitch M, Haworth SG, Castaneda AR, et al. Lung biopsy in congenital heart disease: a morphometric approach to pulmonary vascular disease. Circulation 1978; 58:1107–1122.
71. Haworth SG. Pulmonary vascular disease in different types of congenital heart disease: implications for interpretation of lung biopsy findings in early childhood. Br Heart J 1984; 52:557–571.
72. Zuppan CW, Robinson CC, Langston C. Viral pneumonia in infants and children. In: Askin FB, Langston C, Rosenber HS, et al., eds. Pulmonary Disease. Perspectives in Pediatric Pathology. Vol 18. Basel, Switzerland: Karger, 1995:111–153.
73. Hammond S, Chenever E, Durbin JE. Respiratory virus infectio in infants and children. Pediatr Dev Pathol 2007; 10:172–180.
74. Langston C, Pappin A. Lipid-laden alveolar macrophages as an indicator of aspiration pneumonia (letter). Arch Pathol Lab Med 1996; 120:326–327.
75. Susarla SC, Fan LL. Diffuse alveolar hemorrhage syndromes in children. Curr Opin Pediatr 2007; 19:314–320.
76. Fullmer J, Langston C, Dishop MK, et al. Pulmonary capillaritis in children: a review of eight cases with comparison to other alveolar hemorrhage syndromes. J Pediatr 2005; 146:376–381.
77. Robertson PL, Boldt DW, DeCampo JF. Paediatric pulmonary nodules: a comparison of computed tomography, thoracotomy findings and histology. Clin Radiol 1988; 39:607–610.
78. Langston C. New concepts in the pathology of congenital lung malformations. Semin Pediatr Surg 2003; 12:17–37.
79. Riedlinger WF, Vargas SO, Jennings RW, et al. Bronchial atresia is common to extralobar sequestration, intralobar sequestration, congenital cystic adenomatoid malformation, and lobar emphysema. Pediatr Dev Pathol 2006; 9:361–373.
80. Cohen MC, Kaschula RO. Primary pulmonary tumors in childhood: a review of 31 years' experience and the literature. Pediatr Pulmonol 1992; 14:222–232.
81. Hartman GE, Schochat SJ. Primary pulmonary neoplasms of childhood: a review. Ann Thorac Surg 1983; 36:108–119.
82. Dehner LP, Watterson J, Priest J. Pleuropulmonary blastoma: a unique intrathoracic pulmonary neoplasm of childhood. Perspect Pediatr Pathol 1995; 18:214–226.
83. Priest JR, Watterson J, Strong L, et al. Pleuropulmonary blastoma: a marker for familial disease. J Pediatr 1996; 128:220–224.

4
Interstitial Lymphocytic Infiltrates

ANU SHARMA
Department of Cytopathology, Pittsburgh VA Medical Center and Department of Pathology, University of Pittsburgh, Pittsburgh, Pennsylvania, U.S.A.

I. Introduction

Interstitial lymphocytic infiltrates probably represent the commonest manifestation of subacute and chronic lung injury. The following content highlights the diverse disease entities presenting with this histopathological manifestation.

II. Background

A. Normal Lymphoid Tissue in the Lung: Bronchus-Associated Lymphoid Tissue

Organized aggregates of lymphoid cells are normally associated with the walls of the terminal airways. These are quite prominent in children and rather sparse in an otherwise healthy adult, presenting only as focal submucosal aggregates. The bronchus-associated lymphoid tissue (BALT) represents a reactive process illustrated by these lymphoid aggregates secondary to infections and other pathological states.

B. Histological Patterns of Pulmonary Lymphoid Infiltrates

The pattern of lymphoid infiltration in the lung can provide clues to the diagnosis and underlying disease association.

Nodular, Solitary/Multifocal: These are 1- to 2-mm-diameter nodules present in a peribronchiolar location, usually benign, representing follicular hyperplasia/follicular bronchitis/bronchiolitis, and are commonly associated with chronic infections including HIV, postobstructive changes, rheumatoid arthritis, and systemic lupus erythematosus (SLE).

Solitary: Solitary nodules comprising of lymphoid cells in lung, 2 to 5 cm in size, can be seen in infections, inflammatory pseudotumors/plasma cell granulomas, rarely in nodular lymphoid hyperplasia (previously “pseudolymphoma”) or atypical presentation of a collagen vascular disease or a drug reaction. Lymphomas and posttransplantation lymphoproliferative processes typically present as solitary or multiple large nodules.

Interstitial: Lymphocytic interstitial pneumonia (LIP) represents a primary lymphoproliferative lesion of the lung with this distinct presentation. Diffuse interstitial lymphoid infiltrates are also seen as part of interstitial lung diseases like hypersensitivity pneumonitis (HP) and nonspecific interstitial pneumonia (NSIP). Certain infections, in particular *Pneumocystis carinii*, illustrate this pattern. Other less common causes include drug reaction and rarely viral illnesses.

Combined: This represents a combination of nodular and interstitial pattern, commonly encountered in mucosa-associated lymphoid tissue (MALT) lymphomas, diffuse lymphoid hyperplasia (DLH), drugs, infections, and certain autoimmune disease such as rheumatoid arthritis and SLE.

On the basis of these patterns, various disease entities associated with interstitial lymphoid infiltrates can now be considered. An exhaustive list is tabulated below.

I. Interstitial lymphoid infiltrates as part of primary pulmonary lymphoproliferative disorders
   A. Benign lymphoproliferative disorders
      Follicular bronchiolitis
      Nodular lymphoid hyperplasia (pseudolymphoma)
      LIP
   B. Malignant lymphoproliferative disorders
      Extranodal marginal zone B-cell lymphomas (MALT lymphoma)
      Intermediate/high-grade non-Hodgkin's lymphomas
      Lymphomatoid granulomatosis/angioinvasive lymphomas
      Posttransplantation lymphoproliferative disorder

II. Interstitial lymphoid infiltrate as a secondary presentation or as a component of specific disease entities
   A. Infections
      P. carinii
      Viral
      Mycoplasma
   B. Chronic interstitial lung diseases
      Hypersensitivity pneumonitis
      Nonspecific interstitial pneumonitis
      Collagen vascular diseases with secondary pulmonary involvement
         Rheumatoid arthritis
         Systemic lupus erythematosus
         Sjögren's disease
         Polymyositis
   C. Drug toxicity
   D. Graft-versus-host disease (GVHD)

III. Interstitial Lymphoid Infiltrates as Part of Primary Pulmonary Lymphoproliferative Disorders

A. Benign Lymphoproliferative Disorders

These represent a spectrum of inflammatory lesions ranging from hyperplasia of the pulmonary lymphoid tissue (BALT) to a diffuse expansion of the interstitium (1). The following three distinct entities are described in this category.

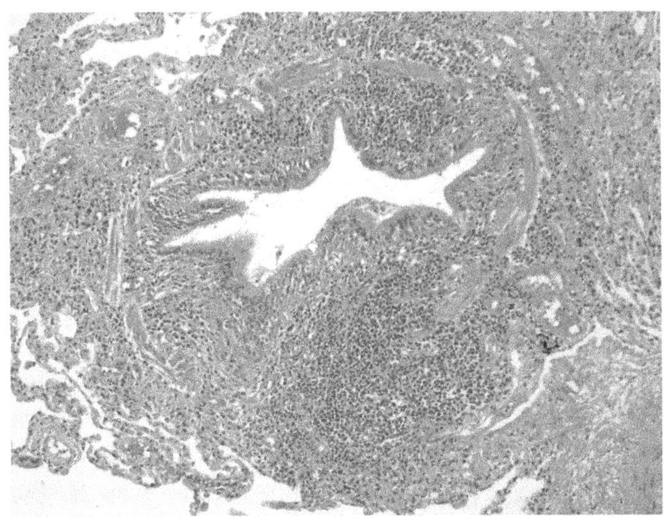

Figure 1 Follicular bronchiolitis in a patient with rheumatoid arthritis.

Follicular Bronchiolitis

Follicular bronchitis/bronchiolitis consists of nodular proliferation of polyclonal lymphoid cells in a peribronchial/bronchiolar location organized as lymphoid follicles with reactive germinal centers adjacent to large airways. It occurs in both pediatric and adult population. It is highly associated with underlying immunodeficiency in children, either acquired (AIDS) or familial like congenital immune deficiency disorders. In adults, barring chronic infectious states associated with bronchiectasis, it represents (*i*) a manifestation of collagen vascular diseases like rheumatoid arthritis (Fig. 1) or (*ii*) a poorly defined hypersensitivity reaction. Microscopically, a biopsy specimen shows aggregates of lymphoid cells 1 to 2 mm in size, with an occasional germinal center formation, located adjacent to pulmonary airways. The infiltrate may spill over into the surrounding interstitium, but the predominant component is airway centered. Immunohistochemically, these lymphoid aggregates/follicles comprise of polyclonal B cells, bcl-2-positive germinal centers. A rim of $CD3^+$ mature T cells is evident at the periphery (2–4).

Nodular Lymphoid Hyperplasia

Nodular lymphoid hyperplasia (NLH), previously called pseudolymphoma, has a relatively benign clinical course and is seen more commonly in adults. This is a rare condition, often discovered incidentally on radiological studies. Earlier studies have loosely incorporated this lesion under "inflammatory pseudotumors." Histologically, the lesion illustrates a lymphoid aggregate, usually subpleural in location, obliterating the underlying pulmonary parenchyma (Fig. 2). Pleural invasion is distinctly absent. The lesion is made up of lymphoid follicles with prominent germinal centers, predominantly comprising of B cells. The lymphocytes are predominantly small, rarely with accompanying admixture of eosinophils

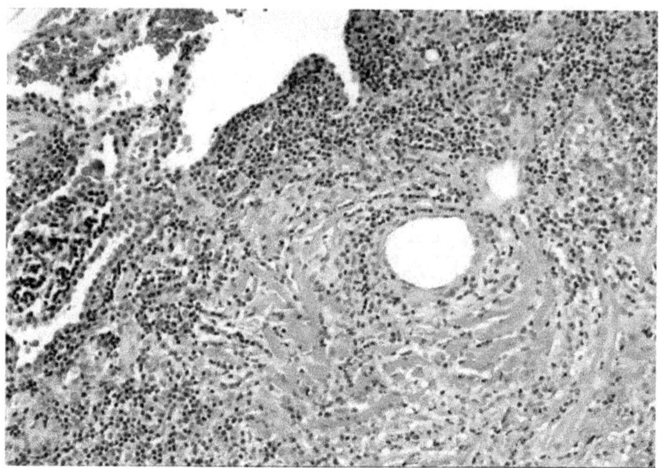

Figure 2 Nodular lymphoid hyperplasia (pseudolymphoma).

and histiocytes. Reactive T cells and polytypic plasma cells are frequently encountered within the interfollicular regions. A dense sclerosis sometimes dominates these interfollicular areas (5).

The diseases associated with NLH are Sjögren's disease and SLE, although the majority of the cases show no evidence of an underlying pathology.

Lymphocytic Interstitial Pneumonia

LIP presents as a diffuse infiltration of the pulmonary interstitium by mature small lymphocytes, plasma cells that expand the interstitium with focal peribronchial/bronchiolar distribution (Fig. 3). Scattered multinucleated giant cells and ill-defined granulomas are also seen. The lymphoid population shows an admixture of B cells with variable numbers of polytypic plasma cells. The T cells could either be CD4 or CD8 type depending on the underlying condition clinically presenting as LIP.

Although LIP may represent the histological manifestation in varying infections or drug-related pulmonary disorders, this diagnosis is particularly significant in two distinct patient populations: (*i*) pediatric and (*ii*) patients with acquired (HIV-associated) or congenital immunodeficiency. In the HIV population, LIP afflicts both pediatric and adult subjects, although prevalence is much higher in children. Chest radiography shows bilateral miliary to fine nodular interstitial infiltrates. Upon exclusion, underlying infectious etiology, particularly *P. carinii* and *Mycobacterium tuberculosis*, which may present quite similarly, a diagnosis of LIP can be made (6).

In the non-AIDS pediatric population, LIP is associated with familial immunodeficiency, i.e., congenital immune deficiency syndrome (7). In immunocompetent adults, underlying autoimmune disorders particularly Sjögren's syndrome, Hashimoto's thyroiditis, myasthenia gravis, primary biliary cirrhosis, chronic active hepatitis, and amyloidosis are implicated.

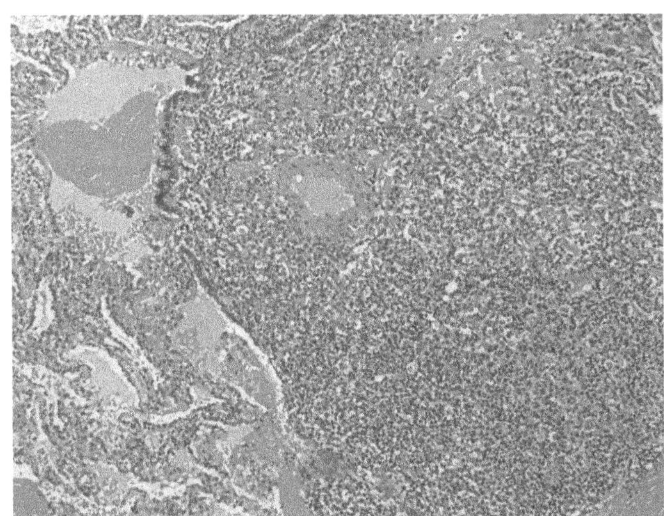

Figure 3 Lymphocytic interstitial pneumonia in a patient infected with HIV.

Laboratory analysis in patients with LIP reveals dysproteinemia in more than 80% of the cases either as hypergammaglobulinemia (usually immunoglobulin M) or, rarely, as hypogammaglobulinemia (in 10% cases) (8). In the HIV population, a persisting circulating CD8 lymphocytosis is evident. It is hypothesized that Epstein-Barr virus (EBV) is related to the pathogenesis of non-AIDS related LIP. EBV genome has been found in the lungs of patients with LIP, suggesting that EBV may be the antigen that promotes the proliferation of B cells within the interstitium. However, the author believes that LIP is a morphological expression of a variety of different disease processes, given the diversity of the involved cell populations, variable clinical course of this disease, and its association with a wide variety of systemic disorders (9,10).

B. Malignant Lymphoproliferative Disorders

Primary pulmonary lymphomas are relatively rare extranodal forms of lymphoid neoplasia. They arise from the BALT and are morphologically similar to MALT lymphomas arising in stomach, small and large intestines, and salivary glands. They are best considered originating from a single putative progenitor B cell (the centrocyte-like cell) of BALT origin.

Microscopically, a diagnosis of lymphoma is entertained on the basis of the following:

1. Architectural patterns (low power)
    a. Lymphangitic distribution along the pulmonary lymphatic channels: peribronchiolar, subpleural, and interstitial
    b. Angiodestructive lesion with or without necrosis
    c. Consolidative mass

2. Microscopic features (intermediate and high power)
   a. Polymorphous cellular lymphoid infiltrate with large atypical cells
   b. Presence of "lymphoepithelial" lesions
   c. Presence of vasculitis or angioinvasion

Since there are many nonneoplastic mimics of malignant lymphomas in the lung, pertinent clinical history especially prior history of pneumonia, allergies, collagen vascular disease and any drug use should be actively sought. Laboratory workup can also be of great assistance in this regard. Analysis for viral serologies and HIV status is quite pertinent. Assays for rheumatoid factor, antineutrophil cytoplasmic antibody, and antinuclear antibody further assist in a diagnostic determination.

MALT Lymphomas

MALT lymphomas present as solitary or multiple mass lesions with a distinctive extension along the lymphatic channels (lymphangitic tracking). There is obliteration of underlying pulmonary parenchymal architecture with frequent invasion into the pleura or bronchial cartilage. Sometimes, a LIP-like diffuse interstitial pattern is also identified. The predominant cell population in this group of lymphomas is the monocytoid B cell with admixed plasmacytoid cells, small lymphocytes, and immunoblasts. Unlike reactive lymphoid conditions, plasma cells in lymphomas typically show "Dutcher bodies." Invasion of the bronchial epithelium ("lymphoepithelial lesions") is frequently identified, as is "angiitis." Both of these findings are nonspecific and can be seen in other lymphoproliferative disorders. Germinal centers are infrequently seen in these lymphomas, and rare ill-defined granulomas and areas of organizing pneumonia are also identified (Fig. 4).

Evidence of monoclonality assists in making a diagnosis of lymphoma. These low-grade lymphomas illustrate the phenotype of marginal zone lymphocytes expressing B-cell markers (CD20, CD79a, and PAX-5) with a kappa (κ) or lambda (λ) light chain restriction

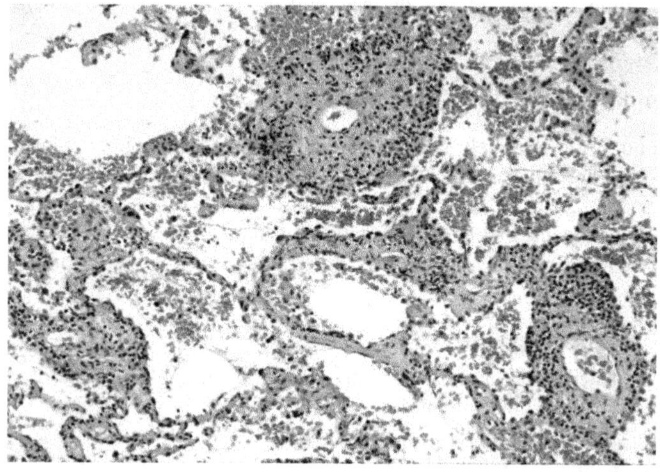

Figure 4 MALT lymphoma (4×). *Abbreviation*: MALT, mucosa-associated lymphoid tissue.

in case of a prominent plasmacytic component. Surface markers like CD5, CD10, bcl-1, and bcl-2 are prominently absent. These lymphomas may express CD21 and CD35. Molecular analysis may show clonal immunoglobulin gene rearrangement. Other pertinent molecular alterations associated with MALT lymphomas include trisomy 18 and trisomy 3. About half the cases will have a t(14:18) (API2/MALT1).

Clinically, patients with low-grade lymphomas of the lung have a mean age of presentation in the sixth decade. Common associations include HIV, EBV-related viral etiology, and Sjögren's disease (11). A small percentage of cases transform into more aggressive lymphomas, representing a poorer prognosis.

Intermediate/High-Grade Non-Hodgkin's Lymphomas

These may be either B-cell or T-cell type. They are relatively infrequent and have a five-year survival of about 50%. Most of the B-cell lymphomas arise from a preexisting low-grade lymphoma. These lesions are distinctively more aggressive, with large atypical cells, vasculitis, and areas of necrosis. An angiocentric distribution is classically seen in lymphomas with a T-cell phenotype.

Lymphomatoid Granulomatosis

Lymphomatoid granulomatosis (LYG) was first described by Liebow (8) as an angiocentric/angiodestructive lymphoreticular proliferation, with a characteristic triad of histological findings: granulomatosis/necrosis, secondary to angiitis, with infiltration of lymphocytes with the walls of small- and medium-sized vessels and an associated polytypic lymphoid infiltrate comprising of abundant small T lymphocytes and a smaller population of atypical lymphocytes with a B-cell immunophenotype (Fig. 5). LYG is now recognized as an EBV-related B-cell lymphoproliferative disorder with abundant associated T cells. As reported by Guinee et al., the small population of CD20-positive B cells illustrated EBV genome and

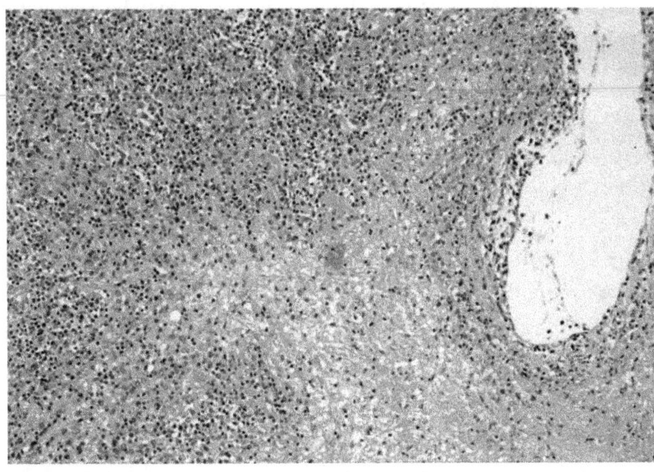

Figure 5 Lymphomatoid granulomatosis.

was associated with clonal gene rearrangement of the immunoglobulin heavy chain (12,13). Immunohistochemical studies reveal the dominant population of cells to be T-cell type expressing CD3. A smaller percentage of cells carry a B-cell phenotype (CD20-positive), as described above. Identification of EBV within the atypical B cells by in situ hybridization studies or immunohistochemistry is further helpful in diagnosis.

The differential diagnosis of LYG would include infections, HP, sarcoidosis, and drug reactions, particularly methotrexate.

Key points that assist in this differential are as follows:

1. LYG presents as an angiodestructive lymphoid infiltrate, typically with a lymphangitic distribution. (Vascular infiltration without destruction of vessel walls may be seen in reactive conditions).
2. It can present as a consolidated mass with prominent necrosis.
3. It consists of dominant T-cell infiltrate with clusters of large atypical B cells.
4. It shows absence of necrotizing granulomatous reaction.

IV. Interstitial Lymphoid Infiltrates as a Secondary Presentation or as a Component of Specific Clinical Entities

A. Infections

P. carinii

P. carinii is a commonly encountered infection in immunocompromised states, in particular HIV and posttransplant population. Since these patient subgroups show a higher association with primary pulmonary lymphoproliferative disorders such as LIP, DLH, and posttransplant lymphoproliferative disorders, this distinction is of high clinical significance. *P. carinii* infection presents as patchy interstitial lymphoplasmacytic infiltrate with associated alveolar frothy exudate (Fig. 6A). Areas of organizing pneumonias may be seen with scattered nonnecrotizing granulomas (14). Confirmatory methenamine silver stain highlights the characteristic cysts (Fig. 6B).

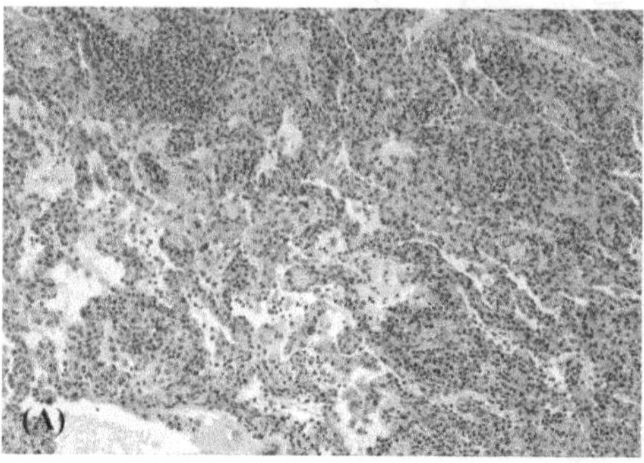

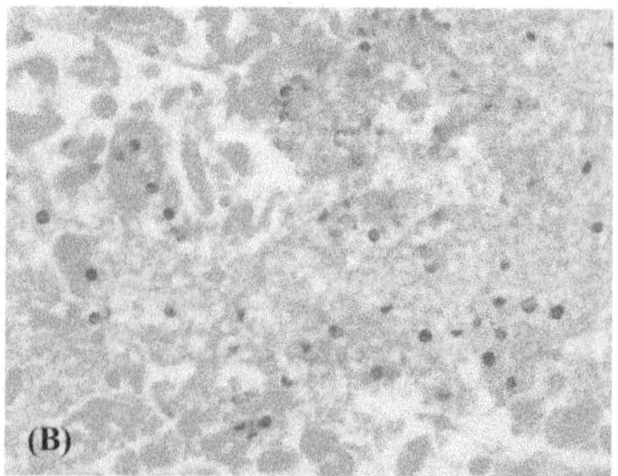

Figure 6 (**A**) Interstitial lymphoid infiltrates secondary to *P carinii* infection (4×). (**B**) Gomori's methenamine silver stain highlighting the *P. carinii* cysts within the frothy alveolar exudate.

Key features assisting in differentiating *P. carinii* infection from LIP are as follows

1. Lack of lymphangitic pattern of distribution of the lymphoid infiltrate
2. Absence of destruction of underlying pulmonary architecture
3. Failure of the interstitial infiltrate to expand the interstitium
4. Presence of characteristic intra-alveolar frothy exudate

Viral

Viral infections in the adult population can be seen in immunocompetent or immunosuppressed patients. The conditions commonly associated are AIDS, corticosteroid therapy, and immunosuppressive therapy in posttransplant patients, and less frequently in diabetes mellitus. The following viral infections commonly present with prominent lymphoid interstitial infiltrates.

Cytomegalovirus

Most common clinical presentation of cytomegalovirus (CMV) pneumonitis is a diffuse interstitial lymphocytic infiltrate and associated variable numbers of cells with the characteristic CMV inclusions (Fig. 7A). The infected cells have a characteristic peribronchiolar distribution (Fig. 7B). In cases of high clinical suspicion, immunohistochemical staining for CMV antigen highlights the infected cells. This is particularly helpful in cases where the inclusions are rather smudged due to pretreatment with ganciclovir. However, isolated cells with immunoreactivity could represent an incidental finding and may not be clinically relevant.

Adenovirus

Adenovirus infection mainly occurs in children, presenting as necrotizing bronchitis or bronchopneumonia. Classically, the bronchial and alveolar lining cells show a large eosinophilic to amphophilic inclusion occupying the entire cell in some cases. These cells are termed "smudge cells." A clear halo may surround these inclusions in some cases, closely simulating a CMV inclusion. Diffuse alveolar damage, bronchiectasis, or a bronchiolitis obliterans organizing pneumonia (BOOP)-like pattern may also occur.

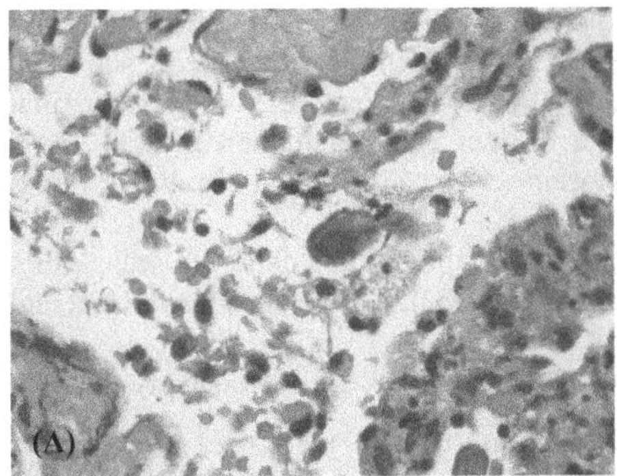

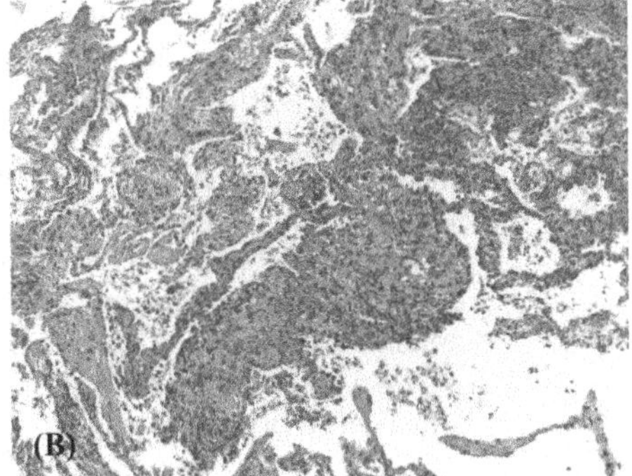

Figure 7 (**A**) Characteristic "CMV inclusion". (**B**) Cytomegalovirus (CMV) pneumonitis.

Influenza/Parainfluenza

Cellular interstitial lymphoid infiltrates are the most common finding in mild cases of influenza/parainfluenza infection. Associated diffuse alveolar damage and organizing pneumonia is seen. Rarely, giant cells may be seen. The fulminant form of this disease presents with necrotizing bronchitis and bronchiolitis with prominent hemorrhage and hyaline membranes.

Mycoplasma pneumoniae

Typically biopsied in immunocompromised patients, mycoplasma pneumonia presents as acute and chronic lymphocytic infiltrate accentuated around the bronchioles with associated plasma cells in the bronchiolar walls. The diagnosis is confirmed by serological studies.

B. Chronic Interstitial Lung Diseases

The disease entities in this category that pose a diagnostic challenge in the evaluation of lymphocytic interstitial infiltrates are

1. hypersensitivity pneumonitis,
2. NSIP, and
3. autoimmune diseases with pulmonary manifestations.

Hypersensitivity Pneumonitis

HP, also called extrinsic allergic alveolitis, is classically described as a type III/IV immune-mediated reaction to inhaled antigens in the environment (e.g., fungal/molds, bacterial, animal protein). Presentation may be *acute,* following exposure to massive amounts of antigen, or *chronic* (or *subacute*), resulting from a prolonged low-level exposure. The former is a self-limiting disease; therefore, the cases are rarely biopsied. Chronic exposure results in the classical presentation of HP, in some cases leading to irreversible lung injury. There are three major histological components of this disease, present in varying degrees in different cases (Fig. 8).

1. *Interstitial inflammation*: The inflammatory infiltrate is predominantly lymphoplasmacytic, with a conspicuous absence of eosinophils and neutrophils. These lymphocytes show an increase in suppressor T cells with an inversion of CD4/8 ratio (up to >2.0). The bronchoalveolar lavage fluid in these patients shows an increase in plasma cells and mast cells. On a microscopic section, the interstitial inflammation appears patchy, with a distinct centrilobular predilection. It is classically described as "bronchiolocentric" in distribution, as it surrounds smaller airways preferentially.
2. *Granuloma formation*: Granulomas, with or without giant cells, are seen within the alveolar walls or clustered around the bronchioles. They are nonconfluent and nonnecrotizing.
3. *BOOP*: Airspace granulation tissue with bronchiolitis is frequently seen in hypersensitivity pneumonia.

Although the differential diagnosis of HP includes sarcoidosis, nonspecific interstitial pneumonitis, and in more advanced cases usual interstitial pneumonias, in the context of lymphocytic interstitial infiltrates, a differentiation from LIP would be critical.

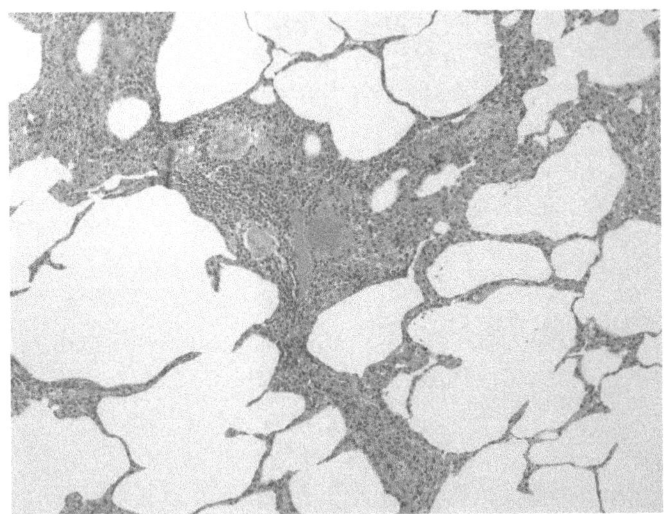

Figure 8 Interstitial infiltrates in hypersensitivity pneumonitis.

Key points to consider are as follows:

- LIP lacks the bronchiolocentric distribution of the lymphoid infiltrate typical for HP.
- HP lacks the diffuse interstitial expansion by the mononuclear infiltrate as seen in LIP.

Nonspecific Interstitial Pneumonia

NSIP is a chronic idiopathic interstitial pneumonia that may occur in cellular, fibrotic, or mixed pattern. In cellular pattern NSIP, lymphoplasmacytic infiltrates expand alveolar septa forming a "linear" pattern with preserved, recognizable lung architecture (Fig. 9). Alveolar pneumocyte hyperplasia may occur. The severity of the infiltrate is variable, and lymphoid nodules may occur. The infiltrate may be patchy, with intervening normal lung present. The differential diagnosis of cellular pattern NSIP includes HP. Cellular pattern NSIP may be accentuated around bronchioles; however, NSIP lacks the poorly formed granulomas characteristic of HP. Other differential diagnoses of cellular pattern NSIP include collagen vascular diseases and drug reactions. Cellular pattern NSIP may also be found in patients with acute respiratory distress syndrome, probably as a pattern of resolving diffuse alveolar damage. Differentiating cellular pattern NSIP from LIP may prove to be quite challenging in some cases. This is particularly true in the case of HIV-infected patients, who may present with LIP, NSIP, or lymphocytic infiltrates secondary to drugs and opportunistic infections (15).

Autoimmune Diseases

Autoimmune diseases with pulmonary manifestations commonly illustrate a cellular NSIP–like pattern with associated follicular bronchiolitis. The following diseases are most commonly considered in this differential.

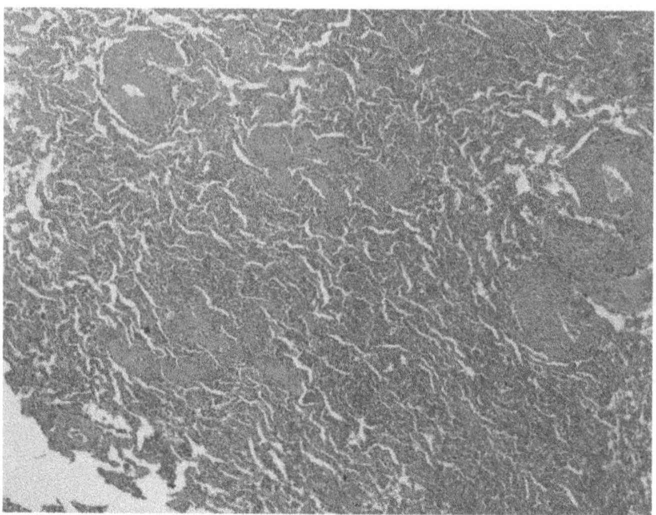

Figure 9 Nonspecific interstitial pneumonia, cellular type, with prominent interstitial inflammation.

Rheumatoid Arthritis

Rheumatoid arthritis in lung illustrates varying histomorphology. It can present as an interstitial pneumonitis with a distinct NSIP pattern. The inflammatory infiltrate is predominantly lymphocytic with a significant plasma cell population. Follicular bronchitis and bronchiolitis is commonly observed.

Systemic Lupus Erythematosus

Lupus pneumonitis also illustrates chronic interstitial inflammation with a cellular NSIP pattern. Association with follicular bronchiolitis is observed commonly.

Sjögren's Syndrome

Systemic manifestations of Sjögren's syndrome are commonly encountered in the lung. The findings in the lung closely correlate with those in salivary glands—namely, atrophy of the mucous glands in the tracheobronchial tree as well as a lymphocytic infiltration of the interstitium. Sjögren's syndrome is also associated with numerous primary lymphoproliferative disorders of the lung like LIP (Fig. 10), follicular bronchitis, as well as primary pulmonary lymphomas (16,17). These are sometimes associated with EBV infection (11). Additionally, NSIP is the most common form of interstitial lung disease seen in these patients.

Polymyositis/Dermatomyositis

These usually present as interstitial lymphoid infiltrates and fibrosis. Other changes may include diffuse alveolar damage (DAD), BOOP, pulmonary hemorrhage, and rarely usual interstitial pneumonias. Some cases with pulmonary hypertension have also been reported.

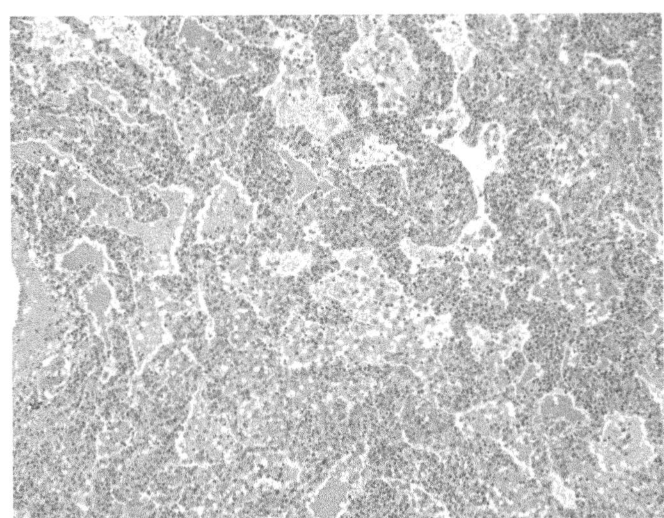

Figure 10 LIP-like presentation in Sjögren's syndrome. *Abbreviation*: LIP, lymphocytic interstitial pneumonia.

C. Drug Toxicity

Numerous drugs have been known to cause pulmonary toxicity. However, before a drug can be implicated, it is important to exclude all other possible causes that could cause pulmonary manifestations in the patient. Upon such exclusion, further support for this underlying etiology is rendered if drug discontinuation causes abatement in pulmonary symptoms and a recurrence upon rechallenge.

The histological findings for most pulmonary drug toxicities are somewhat nonspecific. In the context of this chapter, historically, the following drugs have been associated with lymphocytic/chronic interstitial infiltrates: amiodarone, BCNU, busulfan, carboplatin, chlorambucil, cocaine, cyclophosphamide, fluoxetin, gold, melphalan, nitrofurantoin, phenytoin, pindolol, procarbazine, quinidine, sulfasalazine, tocainide, tryptophan, methylphenidates, and amphetamines. Of particular note is the pulmonary toxicity secondary to methotrexate (18), which presents with a component of lymphocytic interstitial infiltrates in about 71% of the biopsied patient. Azathioprine-induced interstitial pneumonia (19) has been reported in patients under treatment for ulcerative colitis. Interstitial lymphoid infiltrates have also been reported in a series of patients with rheumatoid arthritis secondary to etanercept therapy (20). A hypersensitivity-like reaction has been reported in cases treated with Sirolimus (21) and Lanalidomide (22).

In this context, it is important to note that the underlying conditions being treated, i.e., ulcerative colitis, rheumatoid arthritis, myelodysplastic syndrome, and immunosuppressive therapy secondary to transplantation, each in their own way can also be associated with lymphocytic interstitial infiltrates. Differentiating the underlying etiology for the interstitial lung infiltrate would require strict criteria for diagnosis of drug reactions as previously illustrated.

D. As a Manifestation of Acute Graft-Versus-Host Disease in the Lung

Pulmonary GVHD typically presents with a BOOP-like pattern or in more chronic cases as bronchiectasis. Rarely may it illustrate lymphocytic bronchitis with patchy interstitial lymphocytic infiltrate and a characteristic perivascular accentuation. In these cases, exclusion of underlying infectious etiologies would be critical (23).

References

1. Nicholson AG, Wotherspoon AC, Diss TC, et al. Reactive pulmonary lymphoid disorders. Histopathology 1995; 26(5):405–412.
2. Joshi VV, Gagnon GA, Chadwick EG, et al. The spectrum of mucosa-associated lymphoid tissue lesions in pediatric patients infected with HIV: a clinicopathologic study of six cases. Am J Clin Pathol 1997; 107(5):592–600.
3. Koss MN. Pulmonary lymphoid disorders. Semin Diagn Pathol 1995; 12(2):158–171.
4. Yousem SA, Colby TV, Carrington CB. Follicular bronchitis/bronchiolitis. Hum Pathol 1985; 16(7): 700–706.
5. Abbondanzo SL, Rush W, Bijwaard KE, et al. Nodular lymphoid hyperplasia of the lung: a clinicopathologic study of 14 cases. Am J Surg Pathol 2000; 24(4):587–597.
6. Marcy TW, Reynolds HY. Pulmonary consequences of congenital and acquired primary immunodeficiency states. Clin Chest Med 1989; 10(4):503–519.
7. Popa V. Lymphocytic interstitial pneumonia of common variable immunodeficiency. Ann Allergy 1988; 60(3):203–206.
8. Liebow AA, Carrington CB. Diffuse pulmonary lymphoreticular infiltrations associated with dysproteinemia. Med Clin North Am 1973; 57(3):809–843.
9. Swigris JJ, Berry GJ, Raffin TA, et al., Lymphoid interstitial pneumonia: a narrative review. Chest 2002; 122(6):2150–2164.
10. Koss MN, Hochholzer L, Langloss JM, et al. Lymphoid interstitial pneumonia: clinicopathological and immunopathological findings in 18 cases. Pathology 1987; 19(2):178–185.
11. Yum HK, Kim ES, Ok KS, et al. Lymphocytic interstitial pneumonitis associated with Epstein-Barr virus in systemic lupus erythematosus and Sjogren's syndrome. Complete remission with corticosteriod and cyclophosphamide. Korean J Intern Med 2002; 17(3):198–203.
12. Guinee D Jr., Jaffe E, Kingma D, et al. Pulmonary lymphomatoid granulomatosis. Evidence for a proliferation of Epstein-Barr virus infected B-lymphocytes with a prominent T-cell component and vasculitis. Am J Surg Pathol 1994; 18(8):753–764.
13. Medeiros LJ, Jaffe ES, Chen YY, et al. Localization of Epstein-Barr viral genomes in angiocentric immunoproliferative lesions. Am J Surg Pathol 1992; 16(5):439–447.
14. Ognibene FP, Masur H, Rogers P, et al. Nonspecific interstitial pneumonitis without evidence of Pneumocystis carinii in asymptomatic patients infected with human immunodeficiency virus (HIV). Ann Intern Med 1988; 109(11):874–879.
15. Travis WD, Fox CH, Devaney KO, et al. Lymphoid pneumonitis in 50 adult patients infected with the human immunodeficiency virus: lymphocytic interstitial pneumonitis versus nonspecific interstitial pneumonitis. Hum Pathol 1992; 23(5):529–541.
16. Quismorio FP Jr. Pulmonary involvement in primary Sjogren's syndrome. Curr Opin Pulm Med 1996; 2(5):424–428.
17. Parambil JG, Myers JL, Lindell RM, et al. Interstitial lung disease in primary Sjogren syndrome. Chest 2006; 130(5):1489–1495.
18. Imokawa S, Colby TV, Leslie KO, et al. Methotrexate pneumonitis: review of the literature and histopathological findings in nine patients. Eur Respir J 2000; 15(2):373–381.

19. Nagy F, Molnar T, Makula E, et al. A case of interstitial pneumonitis in a patient with ulcerative colitis treated with azathioprine. World J Gastroenterol 2007; 13(2):316–319.
20. Yousem SA, Dacic S. Pulmonary lymphohistiocytic reactions temporally related to etanercept therapy. Mod Pathol 2005; 18(5):651–655.
21. McWilliams TJ, Levvey BJ, Russell PA, et al. Interstitial pneumonitis associated with sirolimus: a dilemma for lung transplantation. J Heart Lung Transplant 2003; 22(2):210–213.
22. Thornburg A, Abonour R, Smith P, et al. Hypersensitivity pneumonitis-like syndrome associated with the use of lenalidomide. Chest 2007; 131(5):1572–1574.
23. Workman DL, Clancy J Jr. Interstitial pneumonitis and lymphocytic bronchiolitis/bronchitis as a direct result of acute lethal graft-versus-host disease duplicate the histopathology of lung allograft rejection. Transplantation 1994; 58(2):207–213.

5
Predominantly Mature Interstitial Fibrosis

THOMAS SPORN and VICTOR L. ROGGLI
Department of Pathology, Duke University Medical Center, Durham, North Carolina, U.S.A.

I. Introduction

Mature fibrosis, defined as heavily cross-linked collagen fibers appearing as fibrillar, eosinophilic material on conventionally stained sections, results from numerous forms of parenchymal injury to the lungs. This pattern is frequently encountered in biopsy specimens, and its recognition generates a long list of differential diagnostic possibilities. Fortunately, recognition of the histologic pattern of fibrosis can be of considerable aid in narrowing the differential diagnosis. Fibrosis may be predominantly nodular or predominantly linear and reticular, distributed predominantly within peripheral or basilar locations, within the upper lung zones, or distributed focally or more randomly within the lungs. The relationship between these patterns of mature fibrosis and the most common associated pathologic entities is summarized in Figure 1. The salient microscopic features permitting the distinction of these entities are the subject of this chapter. As a rule, the approach to this type of lung biopsy generally obliges careful correlation with the clinical issues germane to the case to reach the correct diagnosis. Of particular importance is the radiographic appearance, as chest X rays or computed tomography of the thorax may be the only source of information regarding some of the patterns of disease illustrated in Figure 1.

The identification of fibrosis in biopsy specimens may be considerably hindered by poor expansion of the alveoli as an artifact of processing in the surgical pathology laboratory. Airless and collapsed lung parenchyma that is otherwise normal may be misinterpreted as showing mature fibrosis. Accordingly, the interpretation of patterns of fibrosis within the lungs is best facilitated by proper inflation and fixation of the specimen. Although these procedures are most readily accomplished on whole lung or lobectomy specimens, techniques for inflation fixation of open or thoracoscopic lung biopsy specimens have been described and are recommended by the authors (1). Examination of sections using Masson's trichrome stain may be useful in problematic cases. Transbronchial lung biopsies generally provide insufficient information to permit a secure diagnosis in cases typified by the pattern of mature fibrosis in the lung (2). Generous sampling by means of surgical lung biopsy is generally preferred and is often a requisite for an accurate diagnosis.

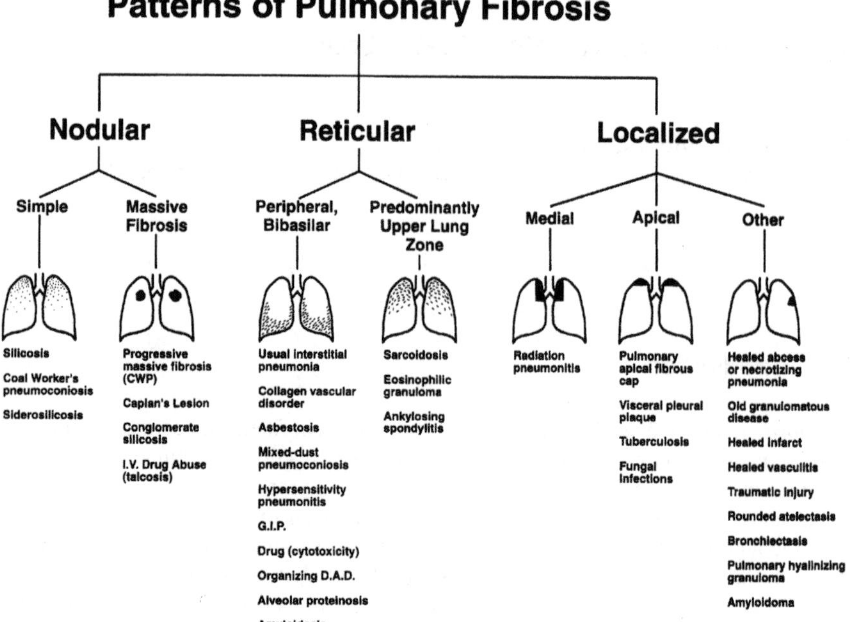

Figure 1 Diagram illustrating the various patterns of pulmonary fibrosis. These patterns can be of great assistance in making the correct diagnosis. See text for details.

II. Mature Fibrosis, Predominantly Reticular Pattern

This pattern represents the most common and difficult diagnostic problem regarding mature pulmonary fibrosis encountered by the surgical pathologist. It is useful to divide this pattern into disorders manifested by predominantly peripheral and basilar patterns of fibrosis and those with predominantly upper lung zone distribution. The former is more common and offers the broadest range of differential diagnostic possibilities. The following section addresses the histopathologic points of distinction among the diagnostic entities comprising this category.

A. Mature Fibrosis, Predominantly Reticular, with Peripheral and Bibasilar Distribution

The major entities in this category and their distinguishing characteristics are listed in Table 1. The single most common entity in this group is usual interstitial pneumonia (UIP, idiopathic pulmonary fibrosis), a progressive fibrotic disease of unknown etiology. The histologic features of this disorder are characterized by geographic and temporal heterogeneity, incorporating predominantly mature fibrosis, immature fibrosis with conspicuous fibroblast foci, and areas of much spared lung tissue containing normal or near normal alveolar architecture. Variable numbers of chronic inflammatory cells are observed within

Table 1 Differential Diagnosis of Reticular, Predominantly Peripheral and Bibasilar, Mature Pulmonary Fibrosis

Disease	Comments
Usual interstitial pneumonia	Spatially and temporally variable, with areas of mature fibrosis, foci of immature fibrosis, and areas of near normal lung. Honeycomb changes frequent.
Nonspecific interstitial pneumonia	Spatially and temporally uniform, typically collagenization and loose fibroblastic tissue without linear fibroblast arrays (fibroblast foci). Honeycomb changes infrequent.
Collagen vascular disorders	Rheumatoid arthritis, polymyositis/dermatomyositis, scleroderma, systemic lupus erythematosus, some cases of Sjogren's syndrome. Histologically indistinguishable from UIP.
Asbestosis	Same as UIP except that asbestos bodies are present in histologic sections. Parietal pleural plaques often present.
Mixed-dust pneumoconiosis	Same as UIP with additional finding of dust deposits and numerous birefringent particulates by polarizing microscopy.
Hypersensitivity pneumonitis	Chronic nonspecific interstitial pneumonia pattern in late phase, variable lymphocytic interstitial infiltrate, may find interstitial giant cells and small granulomas.
Drug cytotoxicity	Chronic nonspecific interstitial pneumonia pattern, may find marked alveolar type II cell hyperplasia with atypical type II pneumocytes.
Giant cell interstitial pneumonia	Diffuse fibrosis, abundant epithelial proliferation, numerous intra-alveolar macrophages, numerous giant cells lining alveoli or free within alveolar spaces.
Organizing diffuse alveolar damage	Alveolar duct-centered fibrosis pattern. Marked type II cell hyperplasia, hyaline membrane remnants. May progress to honeycombing.
Alveolar proteinosis	End-stage fibrosis with focal residual intra-alveolar deposits of granular proteinaceous PAS-positive eosinophilic material.
Amyloidosis	Smudgy or waxy eosinophilic deposits involving alveolar septa and vascular walls. Congo red positive. Frequent concomitant cardiac amyloidosis.

Abbreviations: UIP, usual interstitial pneumonia; PAS, periodic acid–Schiff.

the interstitium, and hyperplastic type II pneumocytes line the fibrotic alveolar septa. Honeycomb changes, characterized by cystic spaces with fibrotic walls lined by a metaplastic and generally cuboidal epithelium with mucostasis and inflammatory debris, are frequently observed. Variable numbers of macrophages are present within the alveolar spaces (3).

Nonspecific interstitial pneumonia (NSIP) is another form of chronic interstitial pneumonia that may be idiopathic or arise in the setting of underlying systemic inflammatory disorders. NSIP is characterized by the cellular and fibrosing variants. The latter features scant chronic inflammation and a diffuse pattern of interstitial fibrosis that lacks the typical variegation, conspicuous fibroblast foci, and honeycombing that typifies UIP. The fibrosis in NSIP is generally loosely fibroblastic or collagenized without distortion of the native lung architecture. The fibrosing variant of NSIP may be misdiagnosed as UIP, particularly on small biopsies. The distinction is important, as NSIP has a generally more favorable prognosis and response to therapy than UIP (4–6).

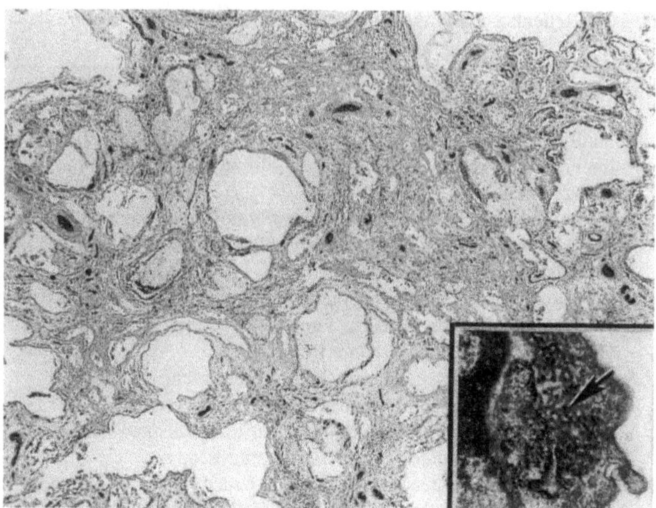

Figure 2 Diffuse pulmonary fibrosis with honeycomb changes in a patient with dermatomyositis. H&E stain, ×25. Inset: Tubuloreticular inclusions (*arrowhead*) in the cytoplasm of pulmonary endothelial cell in a patient with scleroderma.

A variety of connective tissue disorders, typically rheumatoid arthritis, scleroderma, polymyositis/dermatomyositis, systemic lupus erythematosus, and Sjogren's syndrome, may be complicated by the development of diffuse and severe pulmonary fibrosis (7). The pattern of pulmonary fibrosis in these disorders may be histologically indistinguishable from that of UIP or the fibrosing variant of NSIP, although Sjogren's syndrome is most often associated with a pattern that closely resembles lymphocytic interstitial pneumonia. The diagnosis of rheumatoid interstitial lung disease is only possible in the clinical setting of a patient with the histologic features of UIP and clinical or laboratory evidence of rheumatoid arthritis. In this regard, it is of interest that some patients with UIP have an elevated serum fluorescent antinuclear antibody level and arthropathy, but no other manifestations of a systemic inflammatory disorder. Although the patterns of pulmonary fibrosis within these disorders may be histologically indistinguishable, patients with rheumatoid lung are more likely to have pleural fibrosis than patients with UIP. Rheumatoid nodules, though rare in patients with interstitial fibrosis, may also aid in the distinction when present. Finally, some studies have indicated that tubuloreticular inclusions are often observed by electron microscopy in endothelial cells and even epithelial cells in lung biopsies from patients with collagen vascular disorders (Fig. 2), whereas they are rarely, if ever, observed in patients with UIP unassociated with these disorders (8).

The distinction between UIP and certain pneumoconioses may be problematic in some cases. The histologic appearance of late-stage asbestosis may resemble UIP histologically, except for the requisite finding of asbestos bodies in histologic sections (Fig. 3). Fibroblast foci are also typically far less conspicuous in asbestosis than in UIP. The question frequently arises as to how many asbestos bodies are necessary to make the diagnosis of asbestosis in a patient with pulmonary fibrosis. In most cases of asbestosis,

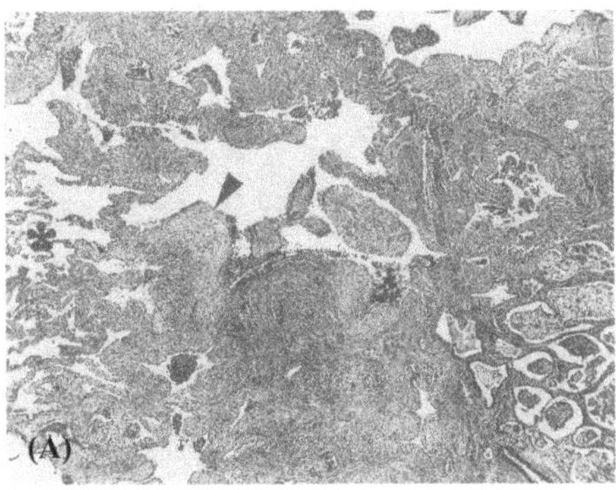

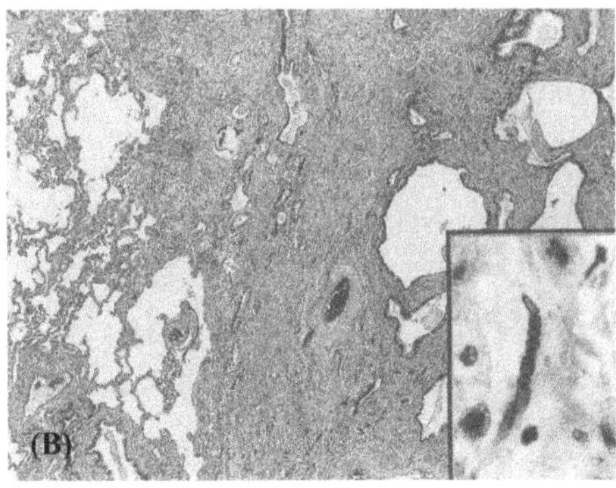

Figure 3 (**A**) Usual interstitial pneumonia with areas of old fibrosis, new fibrosis (*arrowhead*), and nearly normal lung parenchyma (*asterisk*). Honeycomb changes are apparent at lower right. H&E stain, ×32. (**B**) Diffuse pulmonary fibrosis with honeycomb changes (right half of field) in a patient with asbestosis. Inset: Asbestos bodies associated with pulmonary fibrosis. H&E stain, ×32; Inset ×680.

asbestos bodies are readily identified on hematoxylin and eosin (H&E)-stained sections. Occasionally, iron stains are necessary to facilitate their identification. In the vast majority of cases, several asbestos bodies should be observed on most 2 × 2 cm histologic sections stained for iron and examined systematically (9). A few cases of "occult" asbestosis have been described in which asbestos bodies were not seen in histologic sections. However, in a series of 24 cases of diffuse interstitial fibrosis lacking asbestos bodies on H&E-stained sections, we were unable to identify by electron microscopy a lung fiber burden within the range observed in bona fide cases of asbestosis, even when there was a history of exposure (10). Accordingly, analytic studies using tissue digestion techniques and electron microscopy are not necessary in cases where asbestos bodies are not identified histologically. The presence of parietal pleural plaques, identified pathologically in 83% of our cases of asbestosis, may point to asbestosis, but are not diagnostic of this entity per se. Moreover, plaques may occur with much lower levels of asbestos exposure than are required to induce asbestosis and were, in fact, observed in 3 of the 24 UIP cases noted above in asbestos-exposed individuals (10).

Difficulty may also arise in trying to distinguish UIP from mixed dust pneumoconiosis (MDP). The latter occurs in some individuals with inhalational exposure to an admixture of high levels of silicate minerals with lower concentrations of crystalline silica (11,12). A linear or reticular pattern of fibrosis may predominate in MDP with potential for confusion with UIP, especially on smaller biopsy specimens. If scattered silicotic nodules are present in the biopsy specimen, which may not always be seen in cases of MDP, this may alert the pathologist to the possibility of pneumoconiosis. Dust deposits, predominantly in a perivascular and peribronchiolar distribution, are also more prominent in MDP, and the presence of dust macules should alert the pathologist to this possibility. Fibroblastic foci are uncommon in MDP. Polarizing microscopy is particularly useful in making this distinction, as numerous birefringent particles within the interstitium are typically seen in MDP (Fig. 4). There is potential for overinterpretation of material identified on polarizing microscopy, as a few scattered birefringent particles are observed even in normal lungs, and

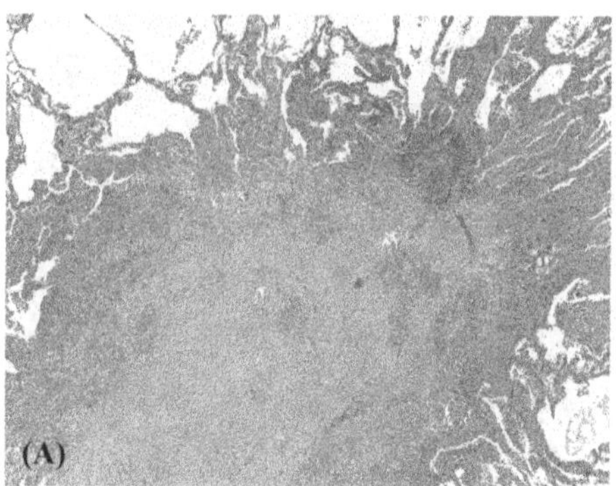

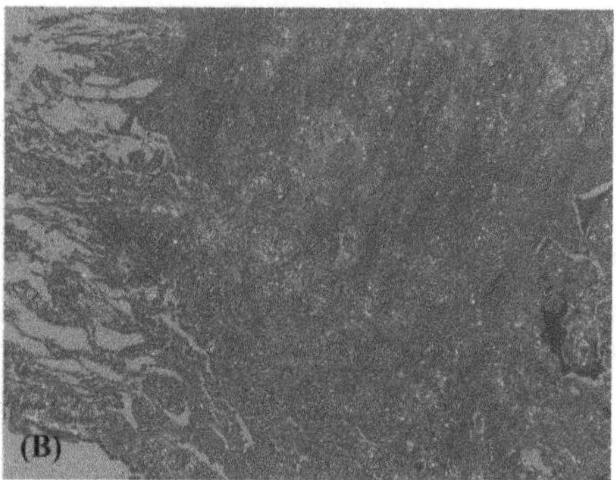

Figure 4 Mixed dust pneumoconiosis examined by (**A**) light and (**B**) polarizing microscopy. Peribronchiolar fibrotic lesion shows peripheral accumulation of dust and numerous birefringent particulates with optical characteristics typical of silicates. H&E stain, ×100.

patients with UIP have impaired clearance of their particulate burden. Such particles may not be foreign and are typically calcified organic material derived from endogenous cellular metabolism.

The histologic features of hypersensitivity pneumonitis (HP, extrinsic allergic alveolitis) are those of a bronchocentric lymphoid interstitial infiltrate, minute and usually poorly formed interstitial granulomas, organizing pneumonia, and giant cells. In comparison with the idiopathic fibrosing interstitial pneumonitides, HP is accompanied by a rapid onset of clinical symptoms (see also chap. 3). However, in the advanced stages, HP may show primarily a linear or reticular pattern of interstitial fibrosis and hence the potential for confusion with UIP. In this circumstance, HP generally shows a pattern of chronic NSIP and lacks the spatial and temporal heterogeneity typical for UIP (13). The history of exposure to inhaled organic antigens can assist in making the distinction as can residual areas of intense lymphocytic interstitial infiltrates associated with multinucleate giant cells or minute and incomplete granulomas.

Giant cell interstitial pneumonia (GIP), also known as hard metal lung disease, must also be distinguished from UIP. This disorder, caused by inhalation of hard metal dusts containing tungsten carbide and cobalt in the occupational setting of manufacture or use of industrial cutting tools and drilling equipment, is characterized histologically by interstitial fibrosis with marked epithelial hyperplasia and numerous alveolar macrophages. The most characteristic finding is numerous multinucleate giant cells, both free within the alveoli and lining the alveolar spaces (Fig. 5A). Occasional cases may be histologically indistinguishable from UIP, NSIP, or desquamative interstitial pneumonia (DIP), and the correct diagnosis in that circumstance depends on proper occupational history and analysis of lung samples for hard metal dust particles (tungsten, tantalum, vanadium) (11). While it is cobalt that is actually believed to be the principal etiologic agent in such cases, the element's water solubility may preclude its detection in pathologic specimens. A similar pattern of fibrosing interstitial pneumonia with giant cells has been described as a complication of chronic nitrofurantoin therapy (14).

Diffuse lung injury from cytotoxic drug therapy may be reflected in a variety of histologic patterns, including cellular interstitial fibrosis with marked alveolar type II cell

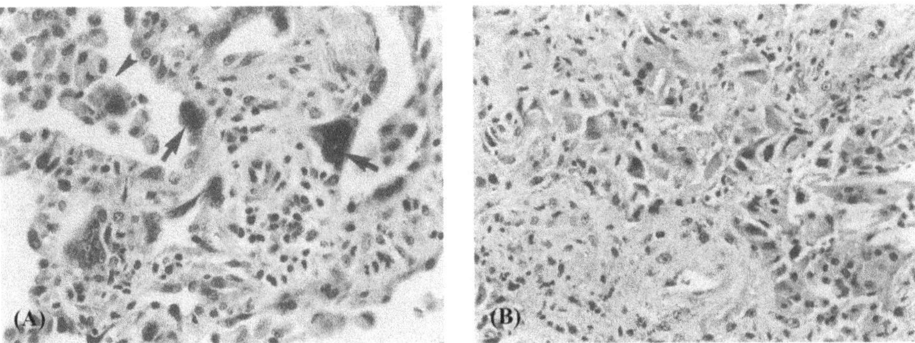

Figure 5 (**A**) Giant cell interstitial pneumonia associated with exposure to hard metal dust. Multinucleate giant cells are observed both within the alveolar spaces (*arrowhead*) as well as lining alveolar septa (*arrows*). H&E stain, ×400. (**B**) Drug induced pulmonary cytotoxicity associated with high-dose chemotherapy in a breast cancer patient who subsequently underwent bone marrow transplantation. There is marked interstitial fibrosis, alveolar collapse, and marked alveolar type II cell proliferation, many of which are atypical. H&E stain, ×170.

hyperplasia. A wide variety of agents have been implicated in causing this reaction within the lungs. Antineoplastic agents, typically busulfan and bleomycin have been the most thoroughly studied of these drugs (Table 2) (15–17). The finding of markedly atypical alveolar type II cells, sometimes with nucleoli so prominent as to suggest viral inclusions, should prompt the pathologist to inquire into the patient's history of drug treatment (Fig. 5B).

Organizing phase diffuse alveolar damage (DAD), the histologic correlate to late progressive adult respiratory distress syndrome (ARDS), may also be confused with UIP. The early stages of diffuse alveolar organization are followed by predominantly immature fibrosis (chap. 7) that in some instances of long-term patient survival may become more mature and even resemble the end stages of honeycomb change (18). One other factor that may be useful in the distinction is the predominance of fibrosis centered on alveolar ducts in DAD (19). In these cases, the distinction from UIP may be quite difficult and requires

Table 2 Pharmacologic Agents Associated with Mature Pulmonary Fibrosis

Cytotoxic drugs	Noncytotoxic drugs
Antibiotics (e.g., bleomycin)	Antibacterial agents (e.g., nitrofurantoin)
Alkylating agents (e.g., busulfan)	Analgesics
Nitrosoureas	Opiates
Antimetabolites	Sedatives
Miscellaneous	Anticonvulsants
	Diuretics
	Major tranquilizers
	Antiarrhythmics
	Miscellaneous

Source: From Ref. 12.

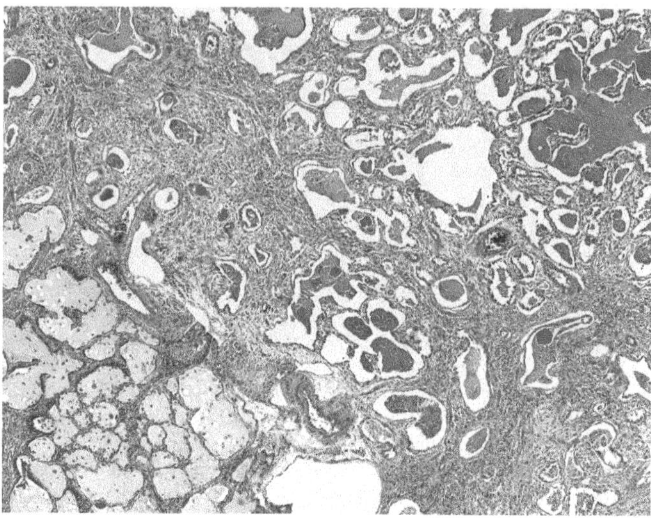

Figure 6 End-stage pulmonary fibrosis in a patient with alveolar proteinosis undergoing lung transplantation having developed disease refractory to whole lung lavage therapy. Residual eosinophilic proteinaceous material is focally present within alveolar spaces adjacent to confluent areas of fibrosis. H&E stain, ×200.

careful correlation with the clinical history. Such clinical distinction is usually apparent; UIP has an insidiously progressive course, whereas ARDS has a precipitous onset, frequently arising in the setting of critical illness, systemic inflammation, or trauma. Cases of accelerated UIP have superimposed features of DAD (20).

Pulmonary alveolar proteinosis (PAP) is an alveolar filling process in which eosinophilic, granular, and periodic acid–Schiff (PAS)-positive proteinaceous material accumulates within the alveolar spaces. This disorder has both primary and secondary forms and may follow infection and immunosuppression, and is discussed further in chapter 8. Treatment is with whole lung lavage that may be curative. Some patients, however, become refractory to lavage treatments and develop a more reticular fibrotic pattern on chest X ray in contrast to the predominantly airspace pattern early in the disease. The later stages are predominated by mature fibrosis and the histologic findings may be difficult to distinguish from UIP or fibrotic NSIP. Careful examination will usually disclose residual areas of alveolar filling by the characteristic PAS-positive material (Fig. 6), indicating the true underlying disease process resulting in late-stage fibrosis.

Amyloidosis is not strictly a mature fibrotic process, as the interstitium of the lungs is expanded by the deposition of fibrillar amyloid rather than collagen. This disorder may sufficiently resemble pulmonary interstitial fibrosis clinically and pathologically so as to be confused with the true fibrosing disorders, therefore it is discussed in this section. Systemic amyloidosis may result in the deposition of amyloid within alveolar septal walls as well as the walls of small pulmonary vessels (Fig. 7A), giving a reticular pattern on chest X ray. Histologically, these deposits have a homogeneous, waxy appearance that differs from the fibrillar nature of collagen. Collagen is weakly birefringent on H&E-stained sections when viewed with polarizing microscopy and not congophilic, whereas amyloid shows positive

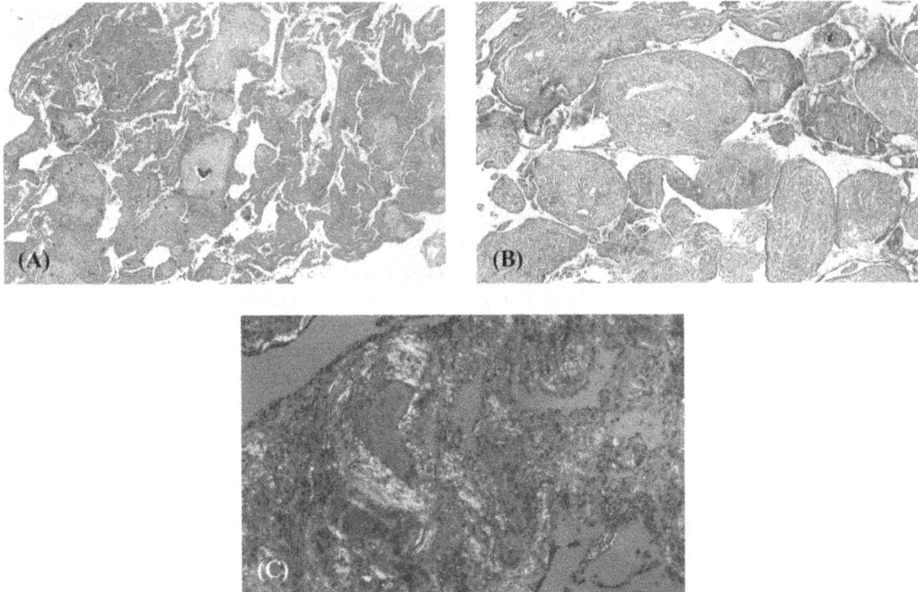

Figure 7 (**A**) Alveolar septal amyloidosis. There is thickening of alveolar septa and vasculature with amorphous eosinophilic material that may be mistaken for collagen deposition. (**B**) Positive Congo red staining and (**C**) apple green birefringence under polarized light confirms this is amyloid protein deposition.

staining with Congo red (Fig. 7B) and characteristic apple green birefringence with polarizing microscopy (Fig. 7C), or staining with thioflavin T, which secures the diagnosis. In problematic cases, electron microscopy may be useful to identify the characteristic deposits of randomly oriented amyloid fibrils. Pulmonary interstitial amyloidosis is typically associated with cardiac amyloidosis pathologically.

B. Mature Fibrosis, Predominantly Reticular, with Upper Lung Zone Distribution

The major entities in this category and their distinguishing characteristics are listed in Table 3. Sarcoidosis is the most common entity in this group, a systemic and idiopathic granulomatous disease with characteristic involvement of the lungs and bilateral hilar and mediastinal lymph nodes. The early stages of this disease are characterized by non-necrotizing granulomatous inflammation with primary distribution along the lymphovasculature (chap. 15). Progression to diffuse interstitial fibrosis with honeycomb change characterizes late-stage disease. Unlike the fine reticular pattern of fibrosis in UIP that imparts a micronodular pattern resembling cirrhotic liver, the pattern of fibrosis in advanced sarcoidosis is more coarse and coalescent, resulting in traction bronchiectasis and paracicatricial emphysema as well as large cystic spaces within the lungs, often in the upper lung zones (Fig. 8A). These contrast with the more basilar, smaller, and more uniform cystic structures of honeycomb changes characteristic of UIP, and may be colonized with

Table 3 Differential Diagnosis of Reticular, Predominantly Upper Lung Mature Pulmonary Fibrosis

Disease	Comments
Sarcoidosis	Coarse pattern of fibrosis distorting secondary lobular structure. Cystic spaces common. Residual giant cells, Schauman bodies, or scattered granulomas often present. Hilar lymph nodes contain conglomerate fibrotic nodules, often with scattered giant cells and/or granulomas.
Eosinophilic granuloma (histiocytosis X)	Markedly distorted parenchyma with bronchiectasis and paracicatricial emphysema. Residual active lesions with Langerhans histiocytes and eosinophils may be present and are the key to the correct diagnosis.
Ankylosing spondylitis	Interstitial fibrosis with chronic inflammation, mucous retention, and bronchiectasis. History of axial skeletal arthritis. Strong linkage with HLA-B27 haplotype.

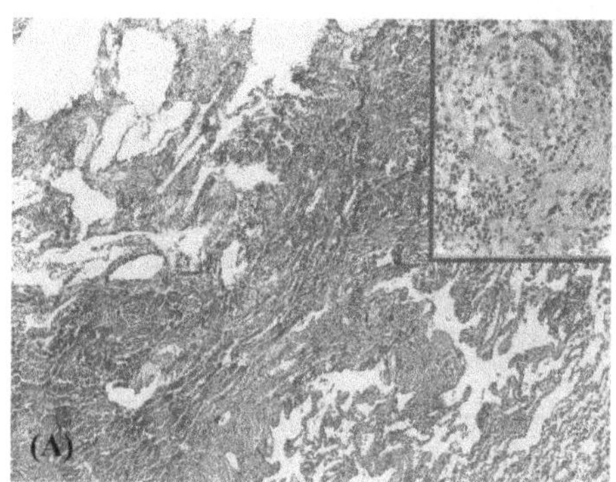

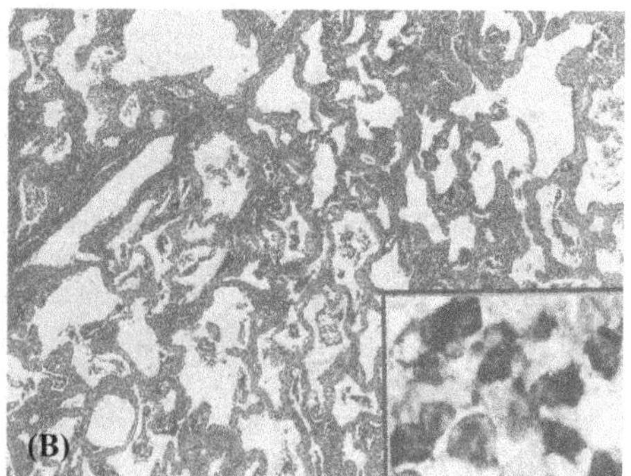

Figure 8 (**A**) End-stage sarcoidosis with broad zone of fibrous tissue distorting the lung parenchyma. There are adjacent areas of near normal lung. Inset: Careful search in such cases may sometimes disclose scattered nonnecrotizing granulomas and/or giant cells. H&E stain, ×25, Inset ×125. (**B**) End-stage pulmonary fibrosis in a patient with eosinophilic granuloma shows thickened and fibrotic alveolar septa with architectural distortion. Inset: Careful search of S-100-stained sections in such cases may disclose residual clusters of positive-staining Langerhans histiocytes. H&E stain, ×25; Inset: immunoperoxidase stain, ×680.

fungi such as *Aspergillus*, leading to mycetoma formation or chronic necrotizing aspergillosis.

Histologically, advanced sarcoidosis shows broad bands of hyalinized collagen, often distorting the secondary lobular architecture of the lung. Residual granulomatous inflammation may be difficult to find, but scattered giant cells or Schaumann bodies are often identified (Fig. 8A). Conglomerate fibrotic nodules and giant cells with or without residual granulomas are virtually always present in the hilar nodes. Birefringent particles may be seen in association with giant cells. These represent endogenous calcium carbonate or calcium oxalate crystals, and should not be confused with exogenous particulates indicative of pneumoconiosis (Fig. 9).

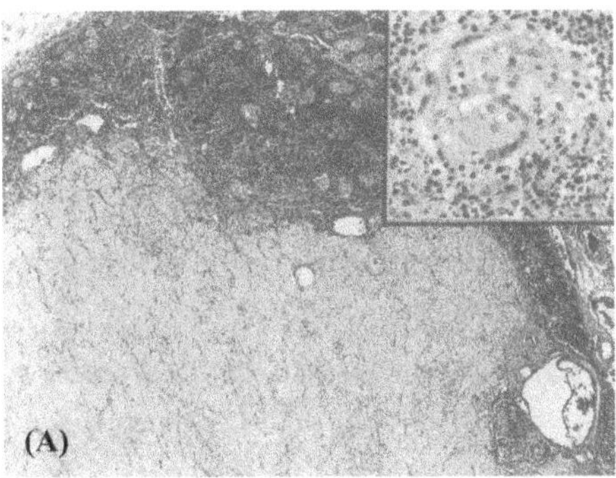

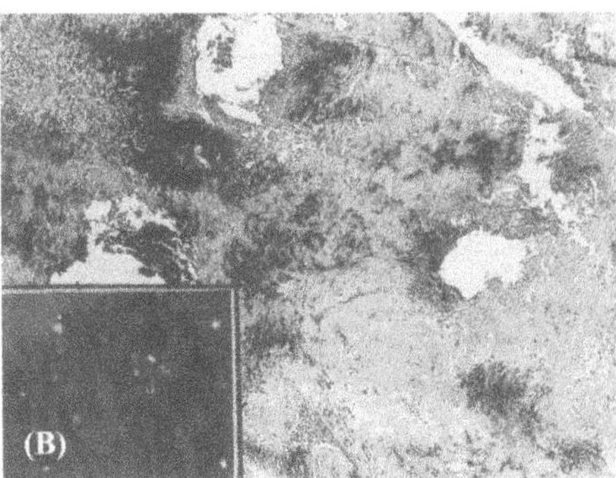

Figure 9 (**A**) Hilar lymph node in a patient with end-stage sarcoidosis. Much of the node is replaced by sheets of fibrous tissue derived from coalescent nonnecrotizing granulomas. Note the relative absence of pigment. Inset: Careful search in such cases may disclose residual nonnecrotizing granulomas. H&E stain, ×25; Inset: ×250. (**B**) Lymph node from a patient with silicosis, showing replacement by much of the node by fibrous tissue. Note the abundance of pigment within the node. Inset: Examination with polarizing microscopy demonstrates numerous birefringent particulates. H&E stain, ×25; Inset: × 400.

Eosinophilic granuloma of the lung, also termed pulmonary Langerhans cell histiocytosis, is a form of lung disease highly associated with cigarette smoking that also tends to involve predominantly the upper lung zones. In its early stages, this disorder presents with stellate interstitial accumulations of Langerhans histiocytes associated with variable numbers of eosinophils (21). These lesions are often associated with bronchioles, imparting a cavitary appearance. In the adult, treatment is based on smoking cessation and corticosteroids, but some of these patients either present with or progress to advanced fibrosis, which must then be distinguished from the other disorders discussed in this chapter. The lung parenchyma may be markedly distorted with areas of paracicatricial emphysema and traction bronchiectasis. The diagnosis may be made on careful searching for residual active lesions containing Langerhans histiocytes and eosinophils (Fig. 8B). CD1A and S-100 label the Langerhans histiocytes, but not alveolar macrophages, and are thus useful diagnostic immunostains.

Pulmonary interstitial fibrosis associated with ankylosing spondylitis may also feature predominantly upper lung zone involvement, but is found in only about 1% of patients with the disease (22). The histologic appearance includes interstitial fibrosis with epithelial metaplasia, chronic inflammatory infiltrates, and bronchiectasis with mucostasis. The typical history of arthritis involving the axial skeleton clinches the diagnosis. There is also a strong association between the HLA B27 haplotype and this disorder.

III. Mature Fibrosis, Predominantly Nodular Pattern

This pattern is strongly associated with mineral dust pneumoconioses, especially following exposure to dusts containing silica and silicates. The major entities in this category and their distinguishing characteristics are listed in Table 4. It is useful to divide this category into

Table 4 Differential Diagnosis of Nodular Mature Fibrosis

Disease	Comments
Simple nodular fibrosis	
Silicosis	Silicotic nodules in lung and in multiple lymph nodes bilaterally show dense, concentric, acellular, whorled collagen. Dust deposits primarily at periphery of nodule, and fine birefringent particles seen throughout nodule. No giant cells or necrosis.
Coal worker's	Same as silicosis, but with greater amounts of black pneumoconiosis pigment often forming collarettes around nodules resembling "Medusa heads."
Siderosilicosis	Same as silicosis plus perivascular and peribronchiolar deposits of iron oxides (particles with dark brown to black centers and golden brown rim or halo).
Massive nodular fibrosis	
Progressive massive fibrosis	Dense bundles of haphazardly arranged hyalinized collagen of coal worker's fibers separated by large amounts of black pigment. Central pneumoconiosis necrosis secondary to ischemia or mycobacterial superinfection is common. Birefringent particulates abundant.
Caplan's syndrome (Rheumatoid pneumoconiosis)	Large smooth-bordered fibrotic lesions with necrobiotic rheumatoid nodules, palisading fibroblasts, and laminated dust deposits. Collar of lymphocytes, plasma cells, and histiocytes at periphery.
Conglomerate silicosis	Similar to progressive massive fibrosis with less pigment deposition. Fused whorled silicotic nodules frequently visible within lesions.
IV drug abuse talcosis	Fibrotic areas contain foreign body giant cells and numerous brightly birefringent needle-like particulates. Foreign body granulomas with similar particulates within alveolar septa of adjacent nonfibrotic lung.

disorders characterized by bilateral small nodules (simple nodular fibrosis pattern) and disorders characterized by irregular masses of fibrosis, usually bilaterally distributed (massive fibrosis pattern). The differential diagnostic features of these disorders are addressed in the following sections.

A. Mature Fibrosis, Simple Nodular Pattern

The prototypic disease in this group is silicosis, a pneumoconiosis caused by the inhalation of crystalline silica. Typical occupations associated with exposure to excessive amounts of crystalline silica include sandblasting, quarry work, stone masonry, pottery and ceramic manufacture, boiler scaling, firebrick manufacture, abrasive powder manufacture, foundry work, and mining (11). The hallmark of such exposure is the silicotic nodule, which consists of concentric, whorled bundles of densely hyalinized and acellular collagen. Dust deposits may be seen at the periphery of the nodule, depending on the precise composition of the dust inhaled. Fine birefringent particles are observed within the nodules when viewed with polarized light (23). In simple silicosis, the lung parenchyma between nodules is normal or near normal. Giant cells are seldom seen in association with silicotic nodules.

Silicotic nodules are frequently observed in hilar lymph nodes in patients exposed occupationally to crystalline silica. These nodules may be confused with fibrosis of healed granulomas in advanced or quiescent sarcoidosis or with ancient fibrocalcific granulomas secondary to tuberculosis or fungal infections. Further confusion may occur due to the presence of birefringent calcium carbonate or oxalate particles in association with the granulomas of sarcoidosis. Distinguishing features include the frequent presence of giant cells in association with fibrotic nodules of sarcoidosis and the scant number of birefringent particles in the fibrotic nodules. In contrast, silicosis typically lacks giant cells, is associated with more dust deposits in the node, and contains numerous tiny birefringent particles within the fibrotic nodules (Fig. 9B). Healed infectious granulomas usually involve only one or at most a few lymph nodes, whereas silicotic nodules involve multiple lymph nodes bilaterally. The presence of necrosis strongly favors infectious granulomas. Yeast forms are frequently seen in necrotic areas of old histoplasma granulomas, but acid-fast bacilli are seldom seen in ancient granulomas due to tuberculosis.

Coal miners are often exposed to silica from the rock around the coal seam. Therefore, silicotic nodules may be observed in the lungs of individuals with coal worker's pneumoconiosis (CWP). These nodules are classified as either micronodules or macronodules, depending on whether they are more or less than 7 mm in maximum dimension (24). The silicotic nodules in CWP are similar to those in silicosis, except that greater amounts of black pigment are typically seen in the former, often forming collarettes around the silicotic nodules resembling "Medusa heads."

Hematite miners and welders may be exposed to excessive amounts of crystalline silica in their work and thus may have silicotic nodules within their lungs. The iron oxides from welding fumes and from hematite have a characteristic appearance and are usually distributed in a perivascular and peribronchiolar pattern. The particles have dark brown to black centers and are often surrounded by a golden brown rim or halo. The combination of silicotic nodules and iron deposits within the lungs is sometimes referred to as siderosilicosis.

B. Mature Fibrosis, Massive Forms

Massive fibrosis is defined by the irregular deposition of collagen measuring at least 2 cm in one or more dimensions, usually involving the upper lung zones. These fibrotic deposits are often bilateral and asymmetrical. The prototypic lesion is progressive massive fibrosis (PMF) of CWP, an uncommon but devastating complication of this disease. The collagen bundles in PMF are characteristically arranged in a haphazard fashion and separated by large amounts of coal dust. Central necrosis is common, usually caused by local ischemia or concomitant infection with *Mycobacterium tuberculosis*. Examination with polarizing microscopy shows numerous birefringent particulates of varying size and magnitude of brightness, the typical optical features of silicates.

Caplan's syndrome (rheumatoid pneumoconiosis) is characterized by massively fibrotic lesions in the lungs of coalminers with rheumatoid arthritis. These lesions have smooth borders and measure up to 5 cm or more in maximum dimension. Microscopically, they show a combination of necrobiotic rheumatoid nodules in association with laminated deposits of dust, palisading of fibroblasts at the periphery of necrotic areas, and a peripheral collar of lymphocytes, plasma cells, and histiocytes. Giant cells may be observed. Vasculitis in the form of endarteritis obliterans is common (25).

Massive fibrosis may also result from coalescence of silicotic nodules to form conglomerate silicosis. The appearance is similar to that of PMF in CWP, although the pigmentation is typically less in conglomerate silicosis. Massive fibrosis may be seen in other pneumoconioses as well, including kaolin worker's pneumoconiosis, hematite miner's pneumoconiosis, and dental technician's pneumoconiosis (11). Important factors in the progression to massive fibrosis include the silica content of the inhaled dust and the presence of superimposed tuberculosis. The correct diagnosis depends on obtaining an accurate occupational history, the characteristics of the dust by light microscopy, or in some cases, analysis of the inorganic particulate content of the tissue by electron microscopic techniques (11).

Long-term follow-up studies of intravenous drug abusers with intravascular pulmonary talcosis have shown that some of these patients progress to develop massive fibrosis (26). Paracicatricial emphysema in the vicinity of the fibrotic lesions can be extensive, and spontaneous pneumothorax is a clinical problem. The characteristic features of this disease are foreign body granulomas within the alveolar septa containing large numbers of needle-like brightly birefringent particulates, typical of talc. Talc is actually a platiform silicate structure that has a needle-like appearance when viewed on edge. The identity of the particulates can be confirmed by analytic electron microscopy. Embolization of talc particles, crospovidone, and microcrystalline cellulose derived from parenteral injection of crushed pills or tablets is also a well-recognized cause of severe pulmonary hypertension and interstitial scarring among such users.

IV. Mature Fibrosis, Localized Patterns

Disorders associated with localized patterns of mature fibrosis and their distinguishing characteristics are summarized in Table 5. In some of these disorders, such as radiation pneumonitis and pulmonary apical fibrous caps, the distribution within the lungs is a major factor in the correct diagnosis. The remaining entities in this category may have a more random distribution within the lungs, and the correct diagnosis depends on histologic features and correlation with the clinical history. If no factor or factors initiating lung injury are discovered, then a diagnosis of pulmonary scar of unspecified nature is appropriate.

A. Mature Fibrosis, Medial Distribution

The pattern of fibrosis in radiation pneumonitis depends on the ports used to deliver radiation to the thorax. Quite often the radiation is delivered to the mediastinal lymph nodes, and the medial aspects of one or both lungs are included incidentally in the fields. A clue to the diagnosis in such cases is that the pattern of fibrosis does not follow anatomic boundaries but is rather confined to the radiation zone. Microscopically, there is obliteration of the alveolar architecture by mature fibrosis that often has a faintly basophilic, fibrillar nature to it. Vascular changes with intimal fibrosis and luminal narrowing are characteristic features that support the diagnosis. A history of radiation at least six months prior to obtaining the tissue samples clinches the diagnosis (Fig. 10A).

Table 5 Differential Diagnosis of Localized Mature Pulmonary Fibrosis

Disease	Comments
Radiation pneumonitis	Does not follow anatomic boundaries, but rather fits the distribution of radiation ports. Alveolar architecture obliterated by mature, slightly basophilic fibrillar fibrosis. Arterial intimal fibrosis and luminal narrowing.
Apical fibrous cap	Fibrosis involving one or both apices and extending into lung parenchyma. Histologically similar to radiation pneumonitis, with obliteration of alveolar architecture and entrapment of bronchioles. Vascular changes less prominent.
Visceral pleural plaque	Thickened pleura, consisting of layers of acellular hyalinized collagen arranged in a "basket-weave" pattern.
Tuberculosis	Fibrosis with cavitation, caseous necrosis, and granulomatous inflammation. Calcification and ossification common.
Fungal infections	Similar to tuberculosis. Fungal organisms often detectable with silver stains.
Mycetomas	Apical fibrosis and cavity with intracavitary mass of fungal hyphae. Adjacent pleural fibrosis common.
Healed abscess or necrotizing pneumonia	Mature fibrosis with no distinguishing features.
Healed infarct	Pleural-based wedge-shaped fibrosis, often with obliterated vessel at apex of scar. Most common location is posterior basal segment of right lower lobe.
Healed vasculitis	Similar to healed infarct, but may have multiple irregular areas of localized fibrosis.
Traumatic injury	Mature fibrosis with no distinguishing features. May find foreign body on gross or microscopic examination.
Rounded atelectasis	Atelectasis adjacent to area of pleural thickening with infolding of fibrotic pleura. Usually located in lower lobe, may be bilateral.
Bronchiectasis	Fibrosis and honeycomb changes distal to ectatic bronchi, may be confused with UIP (see Table 1). Small airways disease changes with mucous plugging and foamy macrophages in alveoli.
Pulmonary hyalinizing granuloma	Dense lamellar collagen in irregular parallel or serpentine arrangement with concentric pattern around granuloma large vessels. Chronic inflammatory cells surround periphery of sharply circumscribed nodule.
Amyloidoma	Waxy, homogeneous eosinophilic appearance, Congo red positive, apple green birefringence. Foreign body giant cells and ossification are common.
Neoplasms	Neoplastic cells between, or in vicinity of, collagen bundles.

Abbreviation: UIP, usual interstitial pneumonia.

B. Mature Fibrosis, Apical Distribution

Pulmonary apical fibrous caps consist of mature fibrosis extending irregularly into the lung, occur primarily in smokers, and are associated rather inexplicably with chronic bronchitis (27). They may be either unilateral or bilateral and occur at the apex of the upper lobe or,

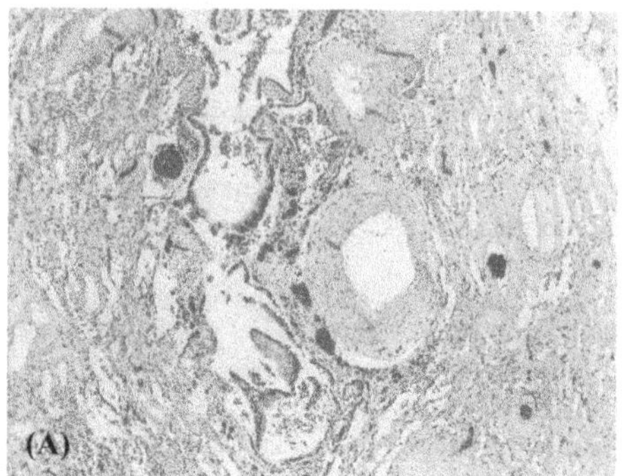

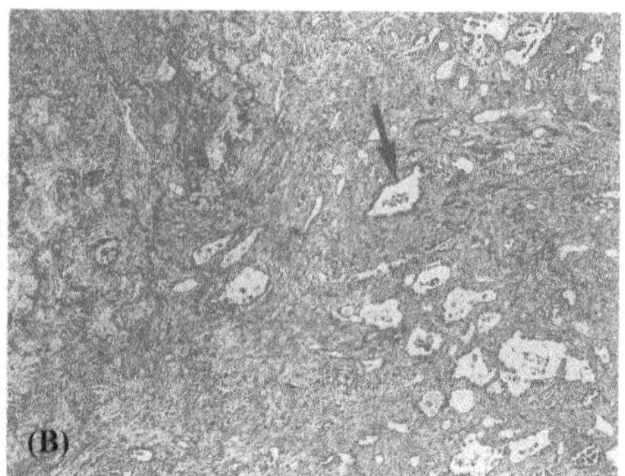

Figure 10 (**A**) Chronic radiation pneumonitis showing interstitial fibrosis and alveolar septal collapse. Notice the prominent thick-walled pulmonary arteries. H&E stain, ×52. (**B**) Pulmonary apical fibrous cap showing obliteration of alveolar spaces by bundles of wavy fibrillar collagen. At higher magnification, these are seen to be interspersed with numerous wavy basophilic elastic fibers. Residual entrapped bronchioles (*arrow*) are also present. H&E stain, ×52.

less commonly, in the apical portion of the superior segment of the lower lobe. The fibrosis often has a slightly basophilic, fibrillar appearance. On close inspection, elastic fibers are easily observed in most cases. Alveolar architecture is obliterated, although scattered entrapped bronchioles are present. The histologic similarity to radiation pneumonitis is rather striking (Fig. 10B), except that vascular changes are less prominent in the apical caps. The relatively poor perfusion of apical lung and the histologic similarities to radiation pneumonitis raises the possibility that these lesions are somehow related to local tissue ischemia.

Visceral pleural plaques can sometimes involve the apices and must be distinguished from apical fibrous caps. The former is associated with fibrosis in the visceral pleural, whereas the latter is in the lung parenchyma, with little if any pleural thickening. In addition, pleural plaques histologically consist of layers of acellular hyalinized collagen arranged in a "basket-weave" pattern, whereas the fibrosis in apical caps is less compact and less organized. Pleural plaques are frequently associated with prior history of asbestos exposure, especially when they are bilateral. They more often involve the parietal pleura (28).

Reactivation tuberculosis usually involves the pulmonary apices, and therefore must be distinguished from apical fibrous caps. Cavitation, caseous necrosis, and granulomatous inflammation are frequently associated with reactivation tuberculosis, whereas these features are not observed in the apical fibrous cap. Focal calcification and even ossification may be seen in either healed apical tuberculosis or in apical fibrous caps.

In addition to tuberculosis, fungal infections can also produce apical fibrosis that may be unilateral or bilateral. Histoplasmosis, blastomycosis, and coccidioidomycosis must be considered in the differential diagnosis of such lesions. The histologic features are similar to those of tuberculosis, except that fungal organisms can frequently be identified in silver stains. Mycetomas most commonly contain *Aspergillus* species and may also be associated with extensive apical fibrosis and pleural thickening. The diagnosis depends on the finding of a cavity and an intracavitary mass of fungal mycelia.

C. Mature Fibrosis, Localized Forms

A variety of conditions can be associated with localized areas of fibrosis within the lungs. The most frequent causes of these lesions are healed infections. Old healed tuberculosis, fungal infections, and necrotizing pneumonias or abscesses can result in scar formation, the extent of which is dependent on the degree of destruction of lung architecture during the original infectious process. The appearance of the scars is generally nonspecific, although those related to healed tuberculosis or fungal infections may show residual necrosis or granuloma formation. Calcification and even ossification are common in these healed foci of necrotizing granulomatous inflammation. Organisms may still be identified in such lesions due to fungi, but histologic identification of acid-fast bacilli in these areas is not common.

Vascular diseases may also result in localized scars, mostly resultant from infarcts secondary to thromboemboli. These occur subpleurally and are wedge shaped, with the most common location being the posterior basal segment of the right lower lobe. The histologic findings are nonspecific, although an obliterated medium-sized pulmonary artery at the apex of the scar may serve as a clue to the diagnosis. A similar pattern may be seen in cases of healed vasculitis involving the lung. Patients who have recovered from treatment of Wegener's granulomatosis, for example, may show multiple areas of irregular, localized fibrosis throughout the lungs (Fig. 11).

Traumatic injuries such as gunshot wounds, shrapnel, or fractured ribs may also result in localized scars within the lung. The findings are nonspecific unless a foreign body

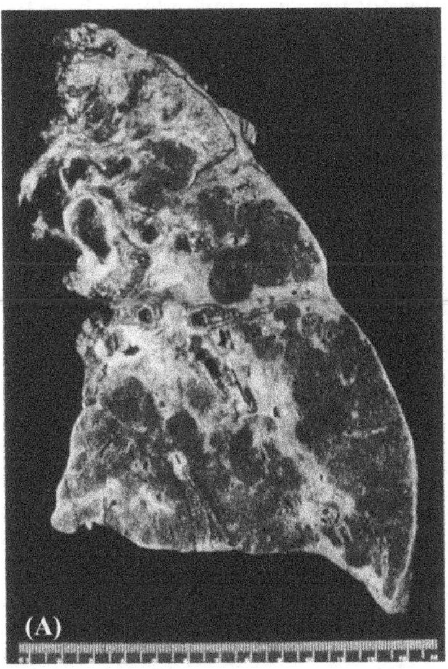

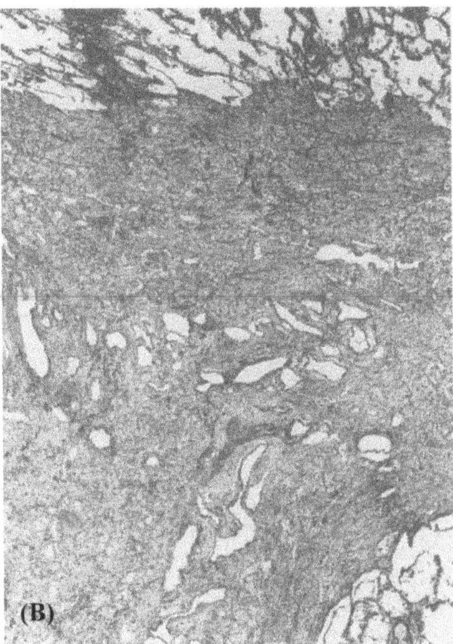

Figure 11 (**A**) Coronal section of autopsy lung in a patient with treated Wegener's granulomatosis. Numerous pale, irregular scars are present in the lung parenchyma. (**B**) Histologic section shows broad, nonspecific scars, with no evidence of active inflammation or vasculitis. H&E stain, ×25.

can be identified on gross or microscopic examination. An overlying fractured rib on radiologic examination may provide a clue to the diagnosis.

Rounded atelectasis is an area of atelectatic lung subjacent to an area of localized pleural thickening, often with invagination or buckling of the fibrotic pleura (28). The process appears as a subpleural mass lesion on chest X-ray, and may uncommonly be resected, mistaken for a neoplasm clinically and radiographically. Rounded atelectasis is strongly associated with a history of prior exposure to asbestos. It has a characteristic appearance on computed tomography of the thorax, including a pleural-based mass lesion, usually in the lower lung zones and posteriorly, with adjacent pleural thickening and a "comet tail" pointed toward the hilar region. Rounded atelectasis may be unilateral or bilateral (28).

Bronchiectasis may be associated with considerable fibrosis in the lungs, especially distal to the areas of bronchial ectasia. Such areas when sampled by the surgeon can look strikingly similar to the honeycomb changes and fibrotic lung of UIP. Thus a diagnosis of UIP should only be made with some knowledge of the patient's clinical and radiographic findings.

Pulmonary hyalinizing granuloma is an unusual lesion producing localized fibrosis within the lung. Most patients have multiple, bilateral lesions (29). This disorder has a characteristic histologic appearance featuring dense lamellar collagen strands in an irregular parallel arrangement, concentrically around larger vessels, and in a serpentine pattern (Fig. 12). The periphery of the nodules is surrounded by more intense chronic inflammation with lymphocytes, sometimes accompanied by lymphoid follicles, plasma cells, and occasional eosinophils. Localized nodular masses of amyloid (amyloidoma) may occur in the lung, and these must be distinguished from true areas of fibrosis. Amyloidomas have the

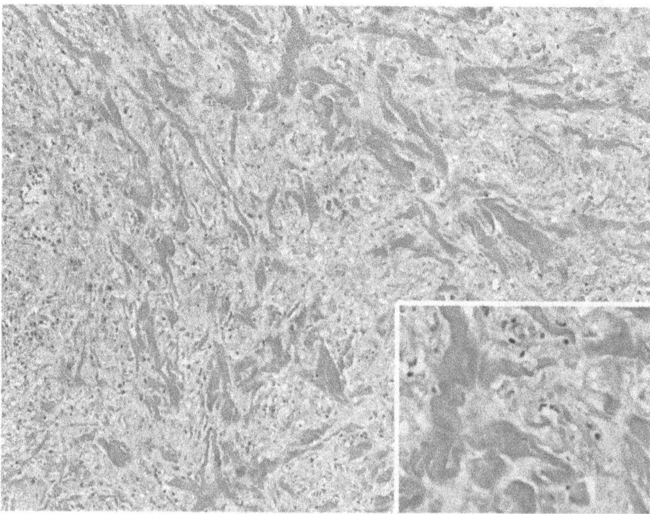

Figure 12 Pulmonary hyalinizing granuloma. The lesion is paucicellular with small amounts of lymphocytes and plasma cells and contains thick lamellar collagen bundles (inset). H&E stain, ×100; inset: ×400.

typical waxy, homogeneous appearance of amyloid, and usually stain positive with Congo red. Giant cells are frequently observed at the periphery of the nodular masses of amyloid, and phagocytosis of amyloid material may be noted. Clusters of plasma cells are often seen scattered within the lesions. Calcification and even ossification may be noted. This latter finding is not specific, however, and ossification may be observed to varying degrees within most of the fibrotic disorders described in this chapter.

Finally, one must consider neoplastic processes in the differential diagnosis of mature fibrosis within the lungs. For example, prominent sclerosis is frequently observed at the center of peripheral pulmonary adenocarcinomas, and many tumors metastatic to the lung may have a striking desmoplatic appearance, including some carcinomas, sarcomas, and lymphomas. Careful examination will disclose the neoplastic cells between the collagenous bundles, and use of immunohistochemical markers may assist in their identification.

V. Conclusion

In this chapter, we have sought to summarize the more common lesions presenting with mature fibrosis within the lungs. Every conceivable lesion associated with pulmonary fibrosis has not been covered in this review, and not all diseases follow the distribution pattern indicated in Figure 1. For example, sarcoidosis is sometimes more severe in the lower lung zones, and in rare cases, asbestosis is more severe in the upper zones. Nevertheless, careful attention to the distribution patterns and histologic features and familiarity with the clinical picture will permit the correct diagnosis in most cases.

References

1. Churg A. An inflation procedure for open lung biopsies. Am J Surg Pathol 1983; 7:69–71.
2. Wall CP, Gaensler EA, Carrington CB, et al. Comparison of transbronchial and open biopsies in chronic infiltrative lung diseases. Am Rev Respir Dis 1981; 123:280–285.
3. Katzenstein AL, Zisman DA, Litzky LA, et al. Usual interstitial pneumonia: histologic study of biopsy and explant specimens. Am J Surg Pathol 2002 (12):1567–1577.
4. Travis WD, Matsui K, Moss J, et al. Idiopathic nonspecific interstitial pneumonia: prognostic significance of cellular and fibrosing patterns: survival comparison with usual interstitial pneumonia and desquamative interstitial pneumonia. Am J Surg Pathol 2000; 24:19–33.
5. American Thoracic Society, European Respiratory Society. American Thoracic Society/ European Respiratory Society International Multidisciplinary Consensus Classification of the Idiopathic Interstitial Pneumonias. Am Rev Respir Crit Care Med 2002; 165:277–304.
6. Myers JL. Nonspecific interstitial pneumonia: pathologic features and clinical implications. Semin Diagn Pathol 2007; 24(3):183–187.
7. Leslie KO, Trahan S, Gruden J. Pulmonary pathology of the rheumatic diseases. Semin Respir Crit Care Med 2007; 28(4):369–378.
8. Hammar SP, Winterbauer RH, Bockus D, et al. Endothelial cell damage and tubuloreticular structures in interstitial lung disease associated with collagen vascular disease and viral pneumonia. Am Rev Respir Dis 1983; 127:77–84.
9. Sporn TA, Roggli VL. Asbestosis. In: Roggli VL, Oury TD, Sporn TA, eds. Pathology of Asbestos-Associated Diseases. 2nd ed. New York: Springer, 2004:71–103.
10. Roggli VL. Scanning electron microscopic analysis of mineral fiber content of lung tissue in the evaluation of diffuse pulmonary fibrosis. Scanning Microsc 1991; 5:71–83.

11. Travis WD, Colby TV, Koss MN, et al., eds. Occupational lung diseases and pneumoconiosies. In: Non-Neoplastic Disorders of the Lower Respiratory Tract. Atlas of Nontumor Pathology First Series Fascicle 2. Washington DC: American Registry of Pathology, 2002.
12. Honma K, Abraham JL, Chiyotani K, et al. Proposed criteria for mixed dust pneumoconiosis: definition, descriptions and guidelines for pathologic diagnosis and clinical correlation. Hum Pathol 2004; 35(12):1515–1523.
13. Churg A, Muller NL, Flint J, et al. Hypersenstivity pneumonitis. Am J Surg Pathol 2006; 30(2): 201–208.
14. Hargett CW, Sporn TA, Roggli VL, et al. Giant cell interstitial pneumonia associated with nitrofurantion. Lung 2006; 184(3):147–149.
15. Cooper JAD, White DA, Matthay RA. Drug-induced pulmonary disease. Part I: Cytotoxic drugs. Am Rev Respir Dis 1986; 133:321–340.
16. Cooper JAD, White DA, Matthay RA. Drug-induced pulmonary disease. Part II: Noncytotoxic drugs. Am Rev Respir Dis 1986; 133:488–505.
17. Rossi SE, Erasmus JJ, McAdams HP, et al. Pulmonary drug toxicity: radiologic and pathologic manifestations. Radiographics 2000; 20(5):1245–1259.
18. Tomashefski JF Jr. Pulmonary pathology of the acute respiratory distress syndrome. Clin Chest Med 2000; 21(3):435–466.
19. Pratt PC. Pathology of adult respiratory distress syndrome: implications regarding therapy. Semin Respir Med 1982; 4:79–85.
20. Collard HR, Moore BB, Flaherty KR, et al. Acute exacerbation of idiopathic pulmonary fibrosis. Am J Respir Crit Care Med 2007; 176:636–651.
21. Travis WD, Borok Z, Roum JH, et al. Pulmonary Langerhans cell granulomatosis (Histiocytosis X): a clinicopathologic study of 48 cases. Am J Surg Pathol 1993; 17:971–986.
22. Lie JT. Rheumatic connective tissue diseases. In: Dail DH, Hammar SP, eds. Pulmonary Pathology. 2nd ed. New York: Springer-Verlag, 1994:679–705.
23. McDonald JW, Roggli VL. Demonstration of silica particles in lung tissue by polarizing light microscopy. Arch Pathol Lab Med 1995; 119:242–246.
24. Kleinerman J, Green F, Laquer W, et al. Pathology standards for coal workers' pneumoconiosis. Arch Pathol Lab Med 1979; 103:375–431.
25. Green FHY, Vallyathan V. Coal workers' pneumoconiosis and pneumoconiosis due to other carboanceous dusts. In: Churg A, Green FHY, eds. Pathology of Occupational Lung Disease. 2nd ed. Baltimore, MD: Williams and Wilkins, 1988:89–154.
26. Pare JP, Cote G, Fraser RS. Long-term follow-up of drug abusers with intravenous talcosis. Am Rev Respir Dis 1989; 139:78–129.
27. Yousem S. Pulmonary apical cap: a distinctive but poorly recognized lesion in pulmonary surgical pathology. Am J Surg Pathol 2001; 25(5):679–683.
28. Oury TD. Benign asbestos-related pleural diseases. In: Roggli VL, Oury TD, Sporn TA, eds. Pathology of Asbestos-Associated Diseases. 2nd ed. New York: Springer, 2004:169–192.
29. Dail DH. Uncommon tumors. In: Dail DH, Hammar SP, eds. Pulmonary Pathology. 2nd ed. New York: Springer-Verlag, 1994:1279–1461.

6
Clinical and Radiologic Diagnosis of Interstitial Infiltrates

TALMADGE E. KING, JR.
Department of Medicine, University of California San Francisco,
San Francisco, California, U.S.A.

The diffuse parenchymal lung diseases (DPLDs), often collectively referred to as the interstitial lung diseases (ILDs), are a heterogeneous group of lung disorders that are classified together because of similar clinical, roentgenographic, physiologic, or pathologic manifestations. The most common causes of ILD are related to occupational and environmental exposures, especially to inorganic or organic dusts (Table 1). Sarcoidosis, idiopathic pulmonary fibrosis (IPF), and pulmonary fibrosis associated with connective tissue diseases (CTDs) are the most common ILDs of unknown etiology. The precise pathway(s) leading from injury to fibrosis is not known (1). However, the development of irreversible pulmonary scarring (fibrosis) to the alveolar wall, airways, or vasculature is the most feared outcome because it is progressive and irreversible. Consequently, management of patients with pulmonary fibrosis is problematic. Most treatments result in no improvement for the majority of patients and only partial or transient suppression of disease progression for the others (2).

A clinical diagnosis is not possible in many forms of ILD. Consequently, tissue examination, usually obtained by surgical lung biopsy, is critical to making or most often, confirming the diagnosis. This chapter will describe the clinical and radiologic approach to the differential diagnosis of DPLDs.

I. Clinical Presentation

Patients with ILD commonly come to medical attention because of the onset of progressive breathlessness with exertion (dyspnea) and/or a persistent, usually nonproductive cough (3). Other important symptoms and signs include hemoptysis, wheezing, and chest pain. Commonly, it is the identification of interstitial opacities on chest X ray that focuses the diagnostic approach toward one of the ILDs versus other pulmonary disorders [such as asthma or chronic obstructive pulmonary disease (COPD)].

Some patients present with pulmonary symptoms associated with another disease, such as a CTD. Importantly, clinical findings suggestive of a CTD (musculoskeletal pain, weakness, fatigue, fever, joint pains or swelling, photosensitivity, Raynaud's phenomenon, pleuritis, dry eyes, dry mouth) should be carefully elicited. The CTDs may be difficult to

Table 1 Etiologic Classification of Interstitial Lung Disease

I. Occupational and environmental exposures (partial list)
  Inorganic dust
    Silica, asbestos, hard metal dusts, beryllium
  Organic dusts (hypersensitivity pneumonitis or extrinsic allergic alveolitis)
    Thermophilic bacteria (e.g., *Micropolyspora faeni, Thermoactinomyces vulgaris, Thermoactinomyces sacchari*)
    Other bacteria (e.g., *Bacillus subtilis, B. sereus*)
    True fungi (e.g., *Aspergillus, Cryptostroma corticale, Aureobasidium pullulans*, Penicillin species)
    Animal Proteins (e.g., Bird Fancier's disease)
    Bacterial products (byssinosis)
    Chemical Sources,
      gases, fumes, vapors, aerosols
  Radiation
II. Drugs (partial list)
  Chemotherapeutic agents (carmustine, busulfan, bleomycin, methotrexate)
  Antibiotics (nitrofurantoin, sulfasalazine)
  Drug-induced lupus (diphenylhydantoin, procainamide)
  Gold salts
  Amiodarone
  Radiation
III. Connective tissue disease
  Systemic lupus erythematosus
  Rheumatoid arthritis
  Progressive systemic sclerosis
  Sjogren's syndrome
  Polymyositis and dermatomyositis
  Mixed connective tissue disease
  Ankylosing spondylitis
IV. Diseases of unknown etiology
  Sarcoidosis
  Vasculitides
    Wegener's granulomatosis
    Churg–Strauss syndrome
  Hemorrhagic syndromes
    Goodpasture's syndrome
    Idiopathic pulmonary hemosiderosis
  Pulmonary Langerhans cell histiocytosis (eosinophilic granuloma of the lung)
  Eosinophilic pneumonia (acute or chronic)
  Chronic gastric microaspiration
  Lymphangitic carcinomatosis
  Chronic pulmonary edema
  Chronic uremia
  Alveolar proteinosis
V. Idiopathic interstitial pneumonias
  Idiopathic pulmonary fibrosis
  Nonspecific interstitial pneumonia
  Cryptogenic organizing pneumonia
  Respiratory bronchiolitis/desquamative interstitial pneumonia
  Acute interstitial pneumonia
  Lymphocytic interstitial pneumonia
VI. Infections (Residue of active infection of any type)

rule out since the pulmonary manifestations occasionally precede the more typical systemic manifestations by months or years [particularly in rheumatoid arthritis (RA), systemic lupus erythematosus (SLE), and polymyositis/dermatomyositis (PM/DM)].

A. Dyspnea

A sense of shortness of breath, i.e., dyspnea, is a common complaint in patients with cardiac or pulmonary disease (4). In most instances, the patient has attributed the insidious onset of breathlessness with exertion to deconditioning, obesity, aging, or a recent upper respiratory tract illness. Some patients have so limited the amount of activity such that they do not "experience" any significant dyspnea. Frequently, a spouse or friend brings the problem to the patient's attention. Thus, the clinician must carefully inquire as to the level of activity the patient normally participates in, the frequency of exercise or exertion of any kind (especially walking stairs, doing housework, or carrying packages), the level of exertion that causes the sensation of breathlessness, and the length of time it takes for the patient to recover (4). Some patients, especially patients with sarcoidosis, silicosis, pulmonary Langerhans cell histiocytosis, may have extensive parenchymal lung disease on chest X ray without significant dyspnea, especially early in the course of their disease.

B. Cough

A dry cough may be particularly disturbing for patients with processes that involve the airways, such as sarcoidosis, organizing pneumonia, respiratory bronchiolitis (RB), pulmonary Langerhans cell histiocytosis, hypersensitivity pneumonitis, lipoid pneumonia, or lymphangitic carcinomatosis. A productive cough is unusual for most ILDs; however, a mucoid, salty-tasting sputum is sometimes reported with diffuse alveolar cell carcinoma.

C. Chest Pain

Clinically significant chest pain is uncommon in most ILDs. Pleuritic chest pain may occur in ILD associated with RA, SLE, mixed CTD, and some drug-induced disorders. Substernal chest pain or discomfort is common in sarcoidosis. Sudden worsening of dyspnea, especially if associated with pleural pain, may indicate a spontaneous pneumothorax. Spontaneous pneumothorax is a characteristic finding for pulmonary Langerhans cell histiocytosis, tuberous sclerosis, lymphangioleiomyomatosis, and neurofibromatosis.

D. Hemoptysis

Gross blood or blood-streaked sputum is rarely a presenting manifestation of ILD. It can be seen in the diffuse alveolar hemorrhage syndromes, lymphangioleiomyomatosis, tuberous sclerosis, pulmonary veno-occlusive disease, long-standing mitral valve disease, and granulomatous vasculitides. Occasionally, diffuse alveolar bleeding may be present without hemoptysis; the clinical manifestations of dyspnea, diffuse parenchymal opacities on chest X ray, and an iron deficiency anemia may be the presenting features. New onset of hemoptysis in a patient with known ILD should raise the possibility of a complicating malignancy.

E. Wheezing

Wheezing is an uncommon manifestation of ILD but has been described in cases of lymphangitic carcinomatosis, chronic eosinophilic pneumonia (CEP), Churg–Strauss syndrome, and RB.

II. Initial Evaluation

The initial evaluation should include a complete history and physical examination followed by laboratory testing that should include: routine blood tests, serologic studies, chest X ray, high-resolution computed tomography (HRCT), pulmonary function testing, and arterial blood gas analysis.

A. Past Medical History

Careful documentation of the past medical history is important in the initial assessment because the cause of the illness is often recognized from the patient's history. Key areas of focus include:

Age

The majority of patients with sarcoidosis, CTD-associated ILD, lymphangioleiomyomatosis, pulmonary Langerhans cell histiocytosis, inherited forms of ILD (familial IPF, Gaucher's disease, Hermansky-Pudlak syndrome) present between 20 to 40 years. Conversely, most patients with IPF are aged over 50 years.

Gender

Lymphangioleiomyomatosis and pulmonary involvement in tuberous sclerosis occurs exclusively in premenopausal women. In addition, lymphocytic interstitial pneumonitis (LIP), ILD in Hermansky-Pudlak syndrome, and the CTDs are more common in women; the exception is ILD in RA, which is more common in men. Because of occupational exposures, men are more likely to have pneumoconiosis. History of risk factors for acquired immune deficiency syndrome (AIDS) should be elicited from all patients with ILD.

Smoking History

A history of tobacco use is important since some diseases occur largely among current or former smokers (pulmonary Langerhans cell histiocytosis, desquamative interstitial pneumonitis, IPF, RB, and acute eosinophilic pneumonia) (5) or among never or former smokers (sarcoidosis and hypersensitivity pneumonitis) (6). Active smoking can lead to complications in some process such as Goodpasture's syndrome where pulmonary hemorrhage is far more frequent in current smokers.

Prior Medication Use

A detailed history of the medications taken by the patients is needed to exclude the possibility of drug-induced disease, including over-the-counter medications, oily nose drops, or petroleum products (7). Importantly, lung disease may occur weeks to years after the drug has been discontinued (for example, carmustine).

Family History

The family history is occasionally helpful since familial associations (with an autosomal-dominant pattern) have been identified in cases of IPF, sarcoidosis, tuberous sclerosis, and neurofibromatosis (8). An autosomal-recessive pattern of inheritance occurs in Niemann-Pick disease, Gaucher's disease, and Hermansky-Pudlak syndrome.

Occupational History

A strict chronologic listing of the patient's entire lifelong employment must be sought, including specific duties and known exposures to dusts, gases, and chemicals. The degree of exposure, duration, latency of exposure, and the use of protective devices should also be elicited.

Environmental Exposures

Review of the home and work environment, including that of spouse and children, is invaluable. Hypersensitivity pneumonitis, respiratory symptoms, fever, chills, and an abnormal chest roentgenogram are often temporally related to the workplace (farmer's lung) or to a hobby (pigeon breeder's disease). Symptoms may diminish or disappear after the patient leaves the exposure for several days; similarly, symptoms reappear on returning to the exposure. Thus, it is important to determine if the patient has had exposures to pets (especially any birds or feather products), air conditioners, humidifiers, hot tubs, evaporative cooling systems (e.g., swamp coolers), and water damage in the home or work environment. Family members may develop disease as a result of "passive" exposure to dusts, from the hobby, or occupation of another member of the family (for example, asbestosis and berylliosis).

Duration of Illness

The duration of illness prior to presentation and diagnosis may be helpful in narrowing the differential diagnosis. In the vast majority of ILDs, the symptoms and signs are chronic, i.e., lasting for months to years, (IPF, sarcoidosis, and pulmonary Langerhans cell histiocytosis). Acute presentations (days to weeks) are unusual and should suggest acute idiopathic interstitial pneumonia (IIP), acute eosinophilic pneumonia, hypersensitivity pneumonitis, or organizing pneumonia. These latter processes are often confused with atypical pneumonias since many have diffuse radiographic opacities, fever, or relapses of disease activity. Subacute presentations (weeks to months) may be seen in all ILDs but can suggest sarcoidosis, some drug-induced ILDs, the alveolar hemorrhage syndromes, cryptogenic organizing pneumonia, and the acute immunologic pneumonia that complicates either SLE or polymyositis.

III. Physical Examination

The physical examination is commonly not specific. It frequently reveals tachypnea, reduced chest expansion, and bibasilar end-inspiratory dry crackles.

Crackles or "velcro rales" are common in most forms of ILD, although they are less likely to be heard in the granulomatous lung diseases, especially sarcoidosis. Crackles may be present in the absence of radiographic abnormalities on the chest radiograph.

Inspiratory squeaks are scattered late-inspiratory high-pitched rhonchi that are frequently heard on chest examination in patients with bronchiolitis.

For cor pulmonale, the cardiac examination is usually normal except in the mid- or late stages of the disease when findings of pulmonary hypertension (i.e., augmented P2, right-sided lift, and S3 gallop) and cor pulmonale may become evident. Signs of pulmonary hypertension and cor pulmonale are generally secondary manifestations of advanced ILD, although they may be primary manifestations of a connective tissue disorder (e.g., progressive systemic sclerosis).

Cyanosis is uncommon and is usually a late manifestation indicative of advanced disease.

Clubbing of the digits, i.e., the distal part of the finger is enlarged compared with the proximal part, is common in some patients (IPF, asbestosis) and rare in others (sarcoidosis, hypersensitivity pneumonitis, histiocytosis X). In most patients, clubbing is a late manifestation suggesting advanced derangement of the lung.

Extrapulmonary physical findings and other manifestations may be helpful in narrowing the differential diagnosis (Table 2).

Table 2 Extrapulmonary Findings in the Interstitial Lung Diseases

Physical findings	Associated conditions
Systemic arterial hypertension	Connective tissue disease; neurofibromatosis; some diffuse alveolar hemorrhage syndromes
Skin changes:	
Erythema nodosum	Sarcoidosis; connective tissue disease; Behcet's syndrome, histoplasmosis, coccidioidomycosis
Maculopapular rash	Drug-induced; amyloidosis; lipoidosis; connective tissue disease; Gaucher's disease
Heliotrope rash	Dermatomyositis
Telangiectasia	Scleroderma
Raynaud's phenomena	Idiopathic pulmonary fibrosis; connective tissue disease (scleroderma)
Cutaneous vasculitis	Systemic vasculitides; connective tissue disease
Subcutaneous nodules	von Reckinghausen's disease; rheumatoid arthritis
café'-au-lait spots	Neurofibromatosis
Calcinosis	Dermatomyositis; scleroderma
Albinism	Hermansky-Pudlak syndrome
Eye changes:	
Uveitis	Sarcoidosis; Behcet's syndrome; ankylosing spondylitis
Scleritis	Systemic vasculitis; systemic lupus erythematosus; scleroderma; sarcoidosis
Keratoconjunctivitis sicca	Sjogren's syndrome
Salivary gland enlargement	Sarcoidosis, Sjogren's syndrome
Peripheral lymphadenopathy	Sarcoidosis; lymphangitic carcinomatosis; Sjogren's syndrome; lymphocytic interstitial pneumonia; lymphoma
Hepatosplenomegaly	Sarcoidosis; Pulmonary Langerhans cell histiocytosis; connective tissue disease; amyloidosis; lymphocytic interstitial pneumonia
Pericarditis	Radiation pneumonitis; connective tissue disease, systemic vasculitis

Table 2 Extrapulmonary Findings in the Interstitial Lung Diseases (*Continued*)

Physical findings	Associated conditions
Myositis/Muscle weakness	Connective tissue disease; drugs (L-tryptophan)
Arthritis	Sarcoidosis; connective tissue disease; systemic vasculitis
Diabetes insipidus	Sarcoidosis; Pulmonary Langerhans cell histiocytosis
Bone involvement	Sarcoidosis; Pulmonary Langerhans cell histiocytosis; lymphangitic carcinomatosis; lymphocytic interstitial pneumonia
Kidney involvement	
Renal mass	Lymphangioleiomyotosis, tuberous sclerosis
Glomerulonephritis	Systemic vasculitis, connective tissue disease; sarcoidosis
Nephrotic syndrome	Amyloidosis, drug-induced lung disease; systemic lupus erythematosus; sarcoidosis

Source: Adapted from Ref. 93.

IV. Role of the Laboratory and Other Studies

A. Routine Laboratory Evaluation

The initial laboratory evaluation should include biochemical tests to evaluate liver and renal function and hematologic tests to check for evidence of anemia, polycythemia or leukocytosis. Serologic studies should be obtained if clinically indicated by features suggestive of a CTD or vasculitis: sedimentation rate, antinuclear antibodies, rheumatoid factor, antineutrophil cytoplasmic antibodies, and antibasement membrane antibody. The routine laboratory evaluation is often not helpful (Table 3). An elevated erythrocyte sedimentation rate and hypergammaglobulinemia are commonly observed but are nondiagnostic. Elevation of the lactate dehydrogenase (LDH) may be noted but is a nonspecific finding common to pulmonary disorders (e.g., alveolar proteinosis, IPF). An increase in the angiotensin converting enzyme (ACE) level may be observed in sarcoidosis but is nonspecific as elevated ACE levels have been noted in several interstitial diseases including hypersensitivity pneumonitis. Antibodies to organic antigens (hypersensitivity panel) may be helpful in confirming exposure when hypersensitivity pneumonitis is suspected, although they are not diagnostic. The electrocardiogram is usually normal in the absence of pulmonary hypertension or concurrent cardiac disease.

B. Chest Imaging Studies

The diagnosis of ILD will often be suspected initially on the basis of an abnormal chest roentgenogram. A recent chest X ray should be obtained and it is also important to review all previous chest X rays to assess the rate of change in disease activity. Unfortunately, the chest roentgenogram may be normal in as many as 10% of patients with some forms of ILD, particularly patients with hypersensitivity pneumonitis. The physician should not ignore or incompletely evaluate a symptomatic patient with a normal chest X ray or an asymptomatic patient with radiographic evidence of ILD. Failure to completely evaluate such individuals often leads to progressive disease, which may be irreversible by the time the patient seeks additional medical attention.

Table 3 Laboratory Findings in the Interstitial Lung Diseases

Abnormality	Associated condition
Leukopenia	Sarcoidosis; connective tissue disease; lymphoma; drug-induced;
Eosinophilia	eosinophilic pneumonia; sarcoidosis; systemic vasculitis; drug induced (sulfa, methotrexate);
Thrombocytopenia	Sarcoidosis; connective tissue disease; drug induced; Gaucher's disease;
Hemolytic anemia	Connective tissue disease; sarcoidosis; lymphoma; drug induced
Normocytic anemia	Diffuse alveolar hemorrhage syndromes; connective tissue disease; lymphangitic carcinomatosis
Urinary sediment abnormalities	Connective tissue disease; systemic vasculitis; drug induced
Hypogammaglobulinemia	Lymphocytic interstitial pneumonitis
Hypergammaglobulinemia	Connective tissue disease; sarcoidosis; systemic vasculitis; lymphocytic interstitial pneumonia; lymphoma
Serum angiotensin-converting enzyme	Sarcoidosis; hypersensitivity pneumonitis; silicosis; Gaucher's disease
Antibasement membrane antibody	Goodpasture's syndrome
Antineutrophil cytoplasmic antibody	Wegener's granulomatosis, Churg–Strauss syndrome, microscopic polyangiitis
Serum precipitating antibodies	Hypersensitivity pneumonitis
Lymphocyte transformation test to specific antigens	Chronic beryllium disease, aluminum potroom workers disease, gold-induced pneumonitis

Source: Adapted from Ref. 93.

Chest X Ray

The most common radiographic abnormality is a reticular pattern; however, a nodular or mixed pattern of alveolar filling and increased interstitial markings is not unusual. Most ILDs have predilection for the lower lung zones. As the disease progresses, there is widespread infiltration associated with reductions in lung volume and the appearance of pulmonary hypertension. A subgroup of ILDs have predilection for the upper lung zones and often produce nodular opacities that result in upward contraction of the pulmonary hilus. With progression of the disease, small cystic structures appear representing fibrous replacement of the normal alveolar architecture and radiographic honeycombing. Table 4 outlines the likely diagnosis for certain radiographic patterns. Although the chest roentgenogram is useful in suggesting the presence of ILD, the correlation between the roentgenographic pattern and the stage of disease (clinical or histopathologic) is generally poor. Only the radiographic finding of honeycombing (small cystic spaces) correlates with pathologic findings and, when present, portends a poor prognosis.

Computed Tomography of the Chest

HRCT is well suited for evaluation of diffuse pulmonary parenchymal disease (9,10). Pattern recognition in diffuse lung disease is enhanced because HRCT avoids the problem of superimposition of structures and is exposure independent. It offers more accuracy than conventional chest X ray in distinguishing airspace from interstitial involvement (11–13).

Table 4 Helpful Radiographic Patterns in the Differential Diagnosis of Interstitial Lung Disease

- Airspace opacities
  - Pulmonary hemorrhage
  - Chronic or acute eosinophilic pneumonia
  - Organizing pneumonia
  - Alveolar proteinosis
- Reticular or linear opacities
  - Peripheral lung zone
    - Organizing pneumonia
    - Eosinophilic pneumonia
  - Upper zone predominance
    - Granulomatous disease
      - Sarcoidosis
      - Pulmonary Langerhans cell histiocytosis (Eosinophilic granuloma)
      - Chronic hypersensitivity pneumonitis
      - Chronic infectious diseases (e.g., tuberculosis, histoplasmosis)
    - Pneumoconiosis
      - Silicosis
      - Berylliosis
      - Coal miners' pneumoconiosis
      - Hard metal disease
    - Miscellaneous
      - Rheumatoid arthritis (necrobiotic nodular form)
      - Ankylosing spondylitis
      - Radiation fibrosis
      - Drug induced (amiodarone, gold)
  - Lower zone predominance
    - Idiopathic pulmonary fibrosis (usual interstitial pneumonia pattern)
    - Rheumatoid arthritis (associated with usual interstitial pneumonia)
- Asbestosis
- End-stage or honeycomb lung
  - Upper zone predominance
    - Sarcoidosis
    - Pulmonary Langerhans cell histiocytosis (eosinophilic granuloma)
    - Chronic hypersensitivity pneumonitis
    - Lymphangiomyomatosis
  - Lower zone predominance
    - Idiopathic pulmonary fibrosis (usual interstitial pneumonia pattern
    - Rheumatoid arthritis (associated with usual interstitial pneumonia)
    - Asbestosis
- Increased lung volumes
  - Lymphangiomyomatosis
  - Tuberous sclerosis
  - Sarcoidosis (stage 3)
  - Pulmonary Langerhans cell histiocytosis (chronic with cyst formation)
  - Neurofibromotosis
  - Chronic hypersensitivity pneumonitis
- Reticular or nodular opacities, increased lung volumes and bullous changes
  - Lymphangiomyomatosis
  - Tuberous sclerosis

(*Continued*)

Table 4 Helpful Radiographic Patterns in the Differential Diagnosis of Interstitial Lung Disease (*Continued*)

- Neurofibromatosis
- Chronic sarcoidosis
- Pulmonary Langerhans cell histiocytosis
- Chronic hypersensitivity pneumonia
- End-stage pulmonary involvement in microscopic polyangiitis
- Intravenous drug abuse (Ritalin)

Associated with pneumothorax
- Pulmonary Langerhans cell histiocytosis
- Lymphangiomyomatosis
- Tuberous sclerosis

Pleural involvement
- Asbestosis
- Connective tissue disorders
  1. Systemic lupus erythematosus
  2. Rheumatoid arthritis
  3. Scleroderma
  4. Mixed connective tissue disease
- Lymphangitic carcinomatosis
- Lymphangiomyomatosis (chylous effusion)
- Drug induced
  - Nitrofurantoin
- Sarcoidosis (lymphocytic effusion)
- Radiation pneumonitis (chronic with mediastinal lymphatic obstruction)

Hilar or mediastinal lymphadenopathy
- Sarcoidosis
- Lymphoma
- Kaposi's sarcoma
- Methotrexate-induced lung disease
- Lymphangitic carcinomatosis
- Berylliosis
- Amyloidosis
- Gaucher's disease
- Acute disseminated histoplasmosis or coccidioidomycosis

Eggshell calcification of lymph nodes
- Silicosis
- Sarcoidosis
- Radiation

Associated with Kerley B lines
- Lymphangitic carcinomatosis
- Chronic left ventricular failure
- Mitral valve disease
- Lymphoma
- Lymphangioleiomyomatosis
- Amyloidosis

Subcutaneous calcinosis
- Scleroderma (CREST)
- Dermatopolymyositis

Miliary pattern
- Sarcoidosis

Table 4 Helpful Radiographic Patterns in the Differential Diagnosis of Interstitial Lung Disease (*Continued*)

Silicosis
Hypersensitivity pneumonitis
Bronchiolitis obliterans
Infectious granulomatous disease (tuberculosis, histoplasmosis, coccidiomycosis)
Metastatic malignant disease
Hypernephroma
Adenocarcinoma of breast
Malignant melanoma
Fleeting or migratory infiltrates
Organizing pneumonia (idiopathic or radiation induced)
Simple pulmonary eosinophilia (Loffler's syndrome)
Hypersensitivity to drugs
Parasitic infections
Fungus-induced, especially allergic bronchopulmonary aspergillosis
Normal[a]
Hypersensitivity pneumonitis (common in population studies, rare in isolated chronic cases)
Sarcoidosis
Connective tissue disease
Bronchiolitis obliterans
IPF (especially early "cellular" stage)
Asbestosis
Lymphangioleiomyotosis

[a]The HRCT scan may be abnormal in many of these cases.
Source: Adapted from Ref. 94.

Also, earlier detection and confirmation of suspected diffuse lung disease, especially in the investigation of a symptomatic patient with a normal chest radiograph, is best achieved by HRCT. HRCT allows better assessment of the extent and distribution of disease. Coexisting disease, e.g., discern occult mediastinal adenopathy, carcinoma, or emphysema is often best recognized on CT scanning. Table 5 outlines the likely diagnosis for certain HRCT patterns.

Other Imaging Techniques

Several other techniques have not lived up to expectations and to date have no well-documented clinical role in the diagnosis, management, or prognosis of most diffuse lung processes. These include (14) magnetic resonance imaging, gallium 67 citrate scanning, positron emission tomography, and technetium 99m-diethylenetriamine penta-acetate (99mTc-DTPA) scanning.

C. Pulmonary Function Testing

Complete lung function testing (spirometry, lung volumes, diffusing capacity) and resting room air arterial blood gases should be obtained (15). Measurement of lung volumes and spirometry function testing are important tests in assessing the severity of lung involvement in patients with ILD (16). Also, the finding of an obstructive or restrictive pattern is useful in narrowing the number of possible diagnoses. Common diseases, such as COPD, anemia, heart failure, mycobacterial or fungal disease can mimic ILD. So they must be ruled out.

Table 5 Helpful HRCT Patterns in the Differential Diagnosis of Interstitial Lung Disease

- Normal
  - Hypersensitivity pneumonitis
  - Sarcoidosis
  - Bronchiolitis obliterans
  - Asbestosis
- Distribution of disease within the lung
  - Peripheral lung zone
    - Idiopathic pulmonary fibrosis
    - Asbestosis
    - Connective tissue disease
    - Organizing pneumonia
    - Eosinophilic pneumonia
- Central disease (bronchovascular thickening)
  - Sarcoidosis
  - Lymphangitic carcinoma
- Upper zone predominance
  - Granulomatous disease
    - Sarcoidosis
    - Pulmonary Langerhans cell histiocytosis (Eosinophilic granuloma)
    - Chronic hypersensitivity pneumonitis
    - Chronic infectious diseases (e.g., tuberculosis, histoplasmosis)
  - Pneumoconiosis
    - Silicosis
    - Berylliosis
    - Coal miners' pneumoconiosis
- Lower zone predominance
  - Idiopathic pulmonary fibrosis
  - Rheumatoid arthritis (associated with usual interstitial pneumonia)
  - Asbestosis
- Airspace opacities
  - Haze or ground-glass attenuation
  - Hypersensitivity pneumonitis
  - Desquamative interstitial pneumonia
  - Respiratory bronchiolitis associated interstitial lung disease
  - Drug toxicity
  - Pulmonary hemorrhage
  - Lung consolidation
  - Chronic or acute eosinophilic pneumonia
  - Organizing pneumonia
  - Aspiration pneumonitis and chronic microaspiration (e g., lipoid pneumonia)
  - Alveolar carcinoma
  - Lymphoma
  - Alveolar proteinosis
- Reticular opacities
  - Idiopathic pulmonary fibrosis
  - Asbestosis
  - Connective tissue disease
  - Hypersensitivity pneumonitis
- Nodules
  - Hypersensitivity pneumonitis
  - Respiratory bronchiolitis associated interstitial lung disease

Table 5 Helpful HRCT Patterns in the Differential Diagnosis of Interstitial Lung Disease (*Continued*)

Sarcoidosis
Pulmonary Langerhans cell histiocytosis
Silicosis
Coal worker's pneumoconiosis
Metastatic cancer
Isolated lung cysts
Pulmonary Langerhans cell histiocytosis
Lymphangiomyomatosis
Chronic PCP

Measurement of Spirometry and Lung Volume

Most of the interstitial disorders have a restrictive defect with reduced total lung capacity (TLC), residual capacity (FRC), and residual volume (RV). Flow rates are decreased [forced expiratory volume in one second (FEV_1) and forced vital capacity (FVC)], but this is related to the decreased lung volumes. The FEV_1/FVC ratio is usually normal or increased. Reductions in lung volumes increase as lung stiffness worsens with disease progression. Smoking history must be considered when interpreting the functional studies. A few disorders produce interstitial opacities on chest X ray and obstructive airflow limitation on lung function testing, e.g., sarcoidosis, lymphangioleiomyomatosis, hypersensitivity pneumonitis, tuberous sclerosis, and COPD with superimposed ILD.

Measurement of Diffusing Capacity

A reduction in the diffusing capacity for carbon monoxide (DL_{CO}) is a very common but nonspecific finding in ILDs. The decrease in DL_{CO} is due primarily to the extent of mismatching of ventilation and perfusion of the alveoli. Lung regions with reduced compliance due either to fibrosis or excessive cellularity may be poorly ventilated, but still be well perfused. The severity of the DL_{CO} reduction does not correlate well with disease stage. In some ILDs, there can be considerable reduction in lung volumes and/or severe hypoxemia but normal or only slight reduction in DL_{CO}, especially in sarcoidosis. The presence of moderate to severe reductions of DL_{CO} in the presence of normal lung volumes should suggest ILD with associated emphysema, pulmonary vascular disease, pulmonary Langerhans cell histiocytosis, or lymphangioleiomyomatosis.

Measurements of Arterial Blood Gas

The resting arterial blood gas may be normal or reveal hypoxemia (secondary to a mismatching of ventilation to perfusion) and respiratory alkalosis. CO_2 retention is rare and usually a manifestation of far-advanced end-stage disease. Importantly, a normal resting partial pressure of oxygen in arterial blood (PaO_2) (or normal O_2 saturation by oximetry) does not rule out significant hypoxemia during exercise or sleep. Further, although hypoxemia with exercise and sleep is very common, secondary erythrocytosis is rarely observed in uncomplicated ILD.

Because resting hypoxemia is not always evident and because severe exercise-induced hypoxemia may go undetected, it is important to perform exercise testing with serial measurement of arterial blood gases. Useful information regarding physiologic abnormalities and extent of disease include: arterial oxygen desaturation, a failure to decrease dead space appropriately with exercise [i.e., a high dead-space/tidal volume (V_D/V_T) ratio], and an excessive increase in respiratory rate with a lower than expected recruitment of tidal volume. There is increasing evidence that serial assessments of resting and exercise gas exchange are the best methods to identify disease activity and responsiveness to treatment, especially in IPF (17). Oximetry testing is not a reliable method to identify exercise-induced hypoxemia in patients with ILD.

D. Bronchoalveolar Lavage

In selected cases, bronchoalveolar lavage (BAL) cellular analysis studies may be useful to narrow the differential diagnostic possibilities between various types of ILD. BAL may help define the stage of disease and allow for the assessment of disease progression or response to therapy (18,19). However, the utility of BAL in the clinical assessment and management of ILD patients remains to be established (20,21). Table 6 shows the diagnostic value of BAL findings in some ILDs.

E. Screening for Common Comorbidities

Patients with DPLD (especially patients with IPF) have a high prevalence of several comorbidities: gastroesophageal reflux (GER) (22–25), pulmonary hypertension (26–28), and sleep-disordered breathing. Chronic progressive lung fibrosis may be related to GER and repeated microaspiration of gastric contents over long periods of time (29,30). Chronic microaspiration may be detected by different methods (tracheal penetration on barium swallow, radioactivity in the lung on scintigraphy, BAL finding of large numbers of

Table 6 Diagnostic Value of Bronchoalveolar Lavage in Interstitial Lung Disease

Condition	Lavage finding
Lymphangitic carcinomatosis, alveolar cell carcinoma, pulmonary lymphoma	Malignant cells
Diffuse alveolar bleeding	Hemosiderin-laden macrophages, red blood cells
Alveolar proteinosis	Lipoproteinaceous intra-alveolar material (periodic acid-Schiff stain)
Lipoid pneumonia	Fat globules in macrophages
Pulmonary Langerhans cell histiocytosis	Monoclonal antibody (T6) positive histiocytes Electron microscopy demonstrating Birbeck granule in lavaged macrophage (expensive and difficult to perform)
Asbestos-related pulmonary disease	Ferruginous bodies
Lipoidosis	Accumulation of specific lipopigment in alveolar macrophages
Berylliosis	+ Lymphocyte transformation test
Silicosis	Dust particles by polarized light microscopy
Wegener's granulomatosis	ANCA may be positive

Abbreviation: ANCA, antineutrophil cytoplasmic antibodies.
Source: Adapted from Ref. 94.

lipid-laden macrophages, or a foreign body reaction on lung biopsy) (31,32). Pulmonary hypertension is common in patients with advanced fibrotic lung disease and contributes to substantial morbidity and mortality (26–28). In subjects whose vital capacity (VC) is less than 50% of predicted or whose diffusing capacity (DL_{CO}) falls below 45% of predicted, pulmonary hypertension can be expected (33). Echocardiography is an inaccurate method in identifying pulmonary arterial hypertension (PAH) in this setting. Right heart catheterization is preferred in patients with ILD suspected to have clinically significant pulmonary hypertension. Sleep-disordered breathing is associated with chronic lung diseases. Patients with DPLD have been shown to have nocturnal desaturations and pulmonary hypertension (34). Subjects identified to be at risk for sleep apnea should be referred for nocturnal polysomnography.

F. The Role of Tissue Examination

Lung biopsy need not be performed in all patients with suspected ILD (35–37). However, following the initial evaluation, it is important to confirm the diagnosis and establish the stage of disease. This is often only possible following careful examination of adequate lung tissue.

In many instances, lung biopsy is indicated because it provides a specific diagnosis, especially in alveolar proteinosis, sarcoidosis, pulmonary Langerhans cell histiocytosis, RB, lymphangioleiomyomatosis, organizing pneumonia, veno-occlusive disease, and vasculitis limited to the lung. Lung biopsy is a useful method to assess disease activity. Other reasons for obtaining a lung biopsy includes the likelihood of excluding neoplastic and infectious processes that occasionally mimic chronic, progressive interstitial disease. Commonly, the lung biopsy may identify a more treatable process than originally suspected, particularly, chronic hypersensitivity pneumonitis, organizing pneumonia, RB-associated ILD (RB-ILD), or sarcoidosis. Clinicians need to achieve a definitive diagnosis to be most comfortable in proceeding with therapies, which may have serious side effects (38). Failure to secure a definitive diagnosis or to determine the stage of disease prior to the initiation of treatment can result in unnecessary anguish for the physician caring for the patient with ILD and may result in potentially avoidable morbidity for the patient. Often a definitive diagnosis avoids confusion and anxiety later in the clinical course if patient is "failing" therapy or suffering serious side effects of therapy.

Fiberoptic Bronchoscopy with Transbronchial Lung Biopsy

Fiberoptic bronchoscopy with transbronchial lung biopsy is often the initial procedure of choice, especially when sarcoidosis, lymphangitic carcinomatosis, eosinophilic pneumonia, Goodpasture's syndrome, or infection is suspected. If a specific diagnosis is not made by transbronchial biopsy then an open, or more commonly, a thoracoscopic lung biopsy is indicated.

Surgical Lung Biopsy

Open or thoracoscopic lung biopsy is the most definitive method to diagnose and stage the disease so that appropriate prognostic and therapeutic decisions can be made. Open lung biopsy via thoracotomy or video thoracoscopy is relatively safe procedures with little morbidity and less than 1% mortality. Currently, video-assisted thoracoscopic lung biopsy is the preferred method for obtaining multiple lung tissue samples for analysis. Relative contraindications to lung biopsy include: serious cardiovascular disease, roentgenographic evidence of diffuse end-stage disease, i.e., "honeycombing," severe pulmonary dysfunction, or other major operative risks (especially in the elderly population). Several technical issues have been resolved: (*i*) the thoracic surgeon should obtain adequate-sized biopsies from multiple sites, usually from two lobes of the lung; (*ii*) the site of the biopsy should be the edge of the grossly abnormal areas of the lung to include grossly normal lung parenchyma and avoid the radiologically or grossly palpable "worst" areas and not the tips of the lingula and right middle lobe; and (*iii*) size of the biopsy specimens must be deep, extending well into the subpleural lung parenchyma (~3 to 5 cm in greatest dimension) (39).

V. Major Histopathologic Patterns

Two major histopathologic patterns are found in patients with ILD: granulomatous process and interstitial pneumonitis. Important histopathologic patterns found in ILDs include: usual interstitial pneumonia (UIP), nonspecific interstitial pneumonia, diffuse alveolar damage, desquamative interstitial pneumonia (DIP), RB, LIP, giant cell interstitial pneumonia, and organizing pneumonia. Different pathologic findings exist in other rarer forms of ILD. For example, several diseases are characterized not by inflammation and fibrosis of the alveolar walls but rather by filling of the alveolar space with blood (diffuse alveolar hemorrhage), lipoproteinaceous fluid (alveolar proteinosis), malignant cells (alveolar cell carcinoma), or calcium microliths (alveolar microlithiasis). A hamartomatous proliferation of smooth muscle cells in the alveolar septa, around vessels and lymphatics, and in the pleura, without clearly evident alveolitis is seen in lymphangioleiomyomatosis. Amyloid fibrillary proteins are deposited in the alveolar walls, within the walls of small blood vessels, and in the alveolar capillary basement membrane in pulmonary amyloidosis; and in lymphangitic carcinomatosis, tumor cells obstruct both pulmonary lymphatics and muscular pulmonary arteries.

A. Granulomatous Lung Disease

The granulomatous process is characterized by an accumulation of T lymphocytes, macrophages, and epithelioid cells organized into discrete structures (granulomas) that result in derangement of normal tissue architecture. Patients with a granulomatous lung disease can progress to clinically significant pulmonary fibrosis. However, many of these patients remain free of severe impairment of lung function or even improve after treatment. When this lesion is found, the main differential diagnosis is between sarcoidosis and hypersensitivity pneumonitis (see chapter 16, "Clinical and Radiologic Diagnosis and Types of Granulomas," for more information).

B. Interstitial Pneumonias

Histopathologic evaluation has become the basis for the classification of the interstitial pneumonias, and it has been shown that the morphologic patterns provide important prognostic information that can guide therapy. In 2001, an American Thoracic Society

(ATS)/European Respiratory Society (ERS) consensus panel revised the classification schema to emphasize the importance of an integrated clinical, radiologic, and pathologic approach to the diagnosis of IIP (40). In addition, they concluded that the idiopathic interstitial pneumonias (IIP) comprised a number of clinicopathologic entities, which were sufficiently different from one another to be designated as separate disease entities (Tables 7 and 8).

The ATS/ERS classification combined the histopathologic pattern seen on lung biopsy with clinical and radiologic information to arrive at a final diagnosis (40). This approach allowed for the preservation of existing histopathologic and clinical terms while precisely defining the relationship between them. When the terms are same for the histopathologic pattern and the clinical diagnosis (e.g., DIP), it was recommended that the pathologist use the addendum "pattern" when referring to the appearance on lung biopsy (e.g., DIP pattern), reserving the initial term for the final diagnosis. The new "gold standard" for the diagnosis of IIP is a combination of "clinical-radiographic-pathologic" features arrived at by a dynamic, integrated process among clinicians, radiologists, and pathologists (when a surgical lung biopsy is available) (39–43). Importantly, lung biopsy is no longer considered the gold standard for the diagnosis but is one integral part of the diagnosis (44).

Usual Interstitial Pneumonia

Patients with the UIP lesion often have a devastating illness characterized by unrelenting progression to end-stage fibrosis and death, especially for the patients with IPF. The key histologic features of the UIP pattern are architectural destruction, fibrosis often with honeycombing, scattered fibroblastic foci, patchy distribution, and involvement of the periphery of the acinus or lobule (15,45). It has a heterogeneous appearance at low magnification, with alternating areas of normal lung, interstitial inflammation, fibrosis, and honeycomb change. Interstitial inflammation is usually mild to moderate, patchy, and consists of an alveolar septal infiltrate of lymphocytes, plasma cells, and histiocytes associated with hyperplasia of type II pneumocytes (15,45).

A UIP-like pattern can be seen in patients with connective tissue disorders (CTDs) [e.g., RA, SLE, progressive systemic sclerosis (PSS), mixed connective tissue disease (MCTD), DM], pneumoconioses (e.g., asbestosis, berylliosis, silicosis, hard metal pneumoconiosis), radiation injury, certain drug-induced lung diseases (e.g., nitrofurantoin), and chronic aspiration. Since there are other histopathologic features frequently present in these other syndromes, we reserve the term UIP for those patients in whom the lesion is idiopathic and not associated with another condition; i.e., for patients with IPF.

Nonspecific Interstitial Pneumonia

Nonspecific interstitial pneumonia (NSIP) is characterized by varying degrees of inflammation and fibrosis, with some forms being primarily inflammatory ("cellular NSIP") and others primarily fibrotic ("fibrotic NSIP") (46). Most investigators believe that cellular NSIP is the early stage of fibrotic NSIP. While NSIP may have significant fibrosis, it is usually of uniform temporality and fibroblastic foci, and, honeycombing, if present, are rare. Fibrotic NSIP can be difficult to distinguish from UIP even by expert pathologists. NSIP (not UIP) is most often found on lung biopsy in patients with CTD, and this pattern is identified in hypersensitivity pneumonitis and some cases of drug-induced lung disease.

Table 7 Clinical and Radiologic Features of the Idiopathic Interstitial Pneumonias

Clinical-radiographic-pathologic diagnosis	Idiopathic pulmonary fibrosis (IPF)	Nonspecific interstitial pneumonia (NSIP)	Cryptogenic organizing pneumonia (COP)	Acute interstital pneumonia (AIP)	Desquamative interstitial pneumonia (DIP) Respiratory bronchiolitis-associated interstitial lung disease (RB-ILD)	Lymphocytic interstitial pneumonia (LIP)
Duration of illness	Chronic (>12 mo)	Subacute to chronic (mo to yr)	Subacute (<3 mo)	Abrupt (1–2 wk)	Subacute (wk to mo); smoker	Chronic (>12 mo); women
Frequency of diagnosis	47–64%	14–36%	4–12%	Rare (<2%)	10–17%	Rare
HRCT	Peripheral, subpleural, basal predominance	Peripheral, subpleural, basal, symmetric	Subpleural or peribronchial	Diffuse, bilateral	DIP: Diffuse ground-glass opacity in the middle and lower lung zones	Diffuse
	Reticular opacities	Ground-glass attenuation	Patchy consolidation	Ground-glass opacities often with lobular sparing	RB-ILD: Bronchial wall thickening; Centrilobular nodules; Patchy ground-glass opacity	Centrilobular nodules,
	Honeycombing	Consolidation (uncommon)	Nodules			Ground-glass attenuation
	Traction bronchiectasis/ bronchiolectasis	Lower lobe volume loss				Septal and bronchovascular thickening
	Architectural distortion	Subpleural sparing may be seen				Thin-walled cysts

Abbreviation: HRCT, high-resolution computed tomography.
Source: Adapted from Ref. 39.

Table 8 Treatment and Prognosis of the Idiopathic Interstitial Pneumonias

Clinical-radiographic-pathologic diagnosis	Idiopathic pulmonary fibrosis (IPF)	Nonspecific interstitial pneumonia (NSIP)	Cryptogenic organizing pneumonia (COP)	Acute interstital pneumonia (AIP)	Desquamative interstitial pneumonia (DIP) Respiratory bronchiolitis-associated interstitial lung disease (RB-ILD)	Lymphocytic interstitial pneumonia (LIP)
Treatment	No effective treatment	Corticosteroid responsiveness	Corticosteroid responsiveness	No effective treatment	Smoking cessation Partially corticosteroid responsiveness	Corticosteroid responsiveness
Prognosis	50–80% mortality in 5 yr	Unclear; <10% mortality in 5 yr	Deaths rare	60% mortality in <6 mo	5% mortality in 5 yr	Not well defined

Source: Adapted from Ref. 39.

When lung tissue is obtained from multiple sites, an NSIP-like pattern is sometimes found in association with another histopathologic pattern, particularly UIP. To date, there has been no report documenting progression from NSIP to UIP (or vice versa) (38). As Katzenstein and coworkers have stated, for NSIP (a uniform process with minimal architectural destruction) to evolve into UIP (a nonuniform process with alternating zones of dense fibrosis, fibroblast foci, scant inflammation, normal lung, and honeycomb change), one would have to postulate that some of the involved areas in NSIP revert to normal while others progress to irreversible fibrosis and honeycomb change (47). One explanation for the coexistence of NSIP-like areas and UIP is that two different mechanisms of fibrosis are occurring. Conceivably, the initial injury in UIP could itself cause secondary inflammation and fibrosis that resemble NSIP, thus explaining the finding of NSIP-like areas in UIP (47). Importantly, in cases where UIP and NSIP coexist in the same lung specimen, the clinical behavior of the patient is most consistent with that of UIP, i.e., UIP injury is the dominant factor controlling prognosis and treatment responsiveness (48).

Respiratory Bronchiolitis

RB is an accurate histologic marker of cigarette smoking, and it may be found many years after smoking cessation (49). In RB, the changes are patchy at low magnification and have a bronchiolocentric distribution (15). Respiratory bronchioles, alveolar ducts, and peribronchiolar alveolar spaces contain clusters of dusty brown macrophages. The lightly pigmented cells have abundant cytoplasm, which contains finely granular golden brown particles. Intralumenal macrophages are accompanied by a patchy submucosal and peribronchiolar infiltrate of lymphocytes and histiocytes. Mild peribronchiolar fibrosis is also seen and expands contiguous alveolar septa, which are lined by hyperplastic type II cells and cuboidal bronchiolar-type epithelium. Centrilobular emphysema is common.

Desquamative Interstitial Pneumonia

DIP is characterized by diffuse involvement of the lung by numerous macrophage accumulations within most of the distal airspaces (15). The alveolar septa are thickened by a sparse inflammatory infiltrate that often includes plasma cells and occasional eosinophils, and they are lined by plump cuboidal pneumocytes. Lymphoid aggregates may be present.

The main feature that distinguishes DIP from RB is that DIP affects the lung in a uniform diffuse manner and lacks the bronchiolocentric distribution seen in RB (15). The intralumenal macrophages in DIP frequently contain dusty brown pigment identical to that seen in RB. Finely granular iron may be seen in the macrophage cytoplasm (50,51). Emphysema is often present. A semiquantitative histologic evaluation disclosed significantly more lymphoid follicles, interstitial fibrosis, and eosinophils in DIP compared with RB. Both RB and DIP may evolve into a pattern resembling fibrotic NSIP (51).

The DIP-like reaction in UIP is usually minimal and does not have the uniform involvement of lung parenchyma as seen in DIP. In addition, a DIP-like pattern can be seen in a number of other processes, usually to only a minor degree: pulmonary Langerhans cell histiocytosis, drug reactions (e.g., amiodarone), chronic alveolar hemorrhage, eosinophilic pneumonia, pneumoconioses (e.g., talcosis, hard metal disease, and asbestosis), obstructive pneumonias, and exogenous lipoid pneumonia.

Diffuse Alveolar Damage

Diffuse alveolar damage (DAD) is a relatively common histopathologic finding at autopsy, particularly in patients dying with adult respiratory distress syndrome (ARDS) and can result from a variety of causes (52). Infections and acute interstitial pneumonia (AIP) are the most common causes of DAD diagnosed by surgical lung biopsy (52). The histologic features of DAD include a diffuse distribution, uniform temporal appearance, and alveolar septal thickening due to organizing fibrosis and patchy or diffuse airspace organization (15). Hyaline membranes are characteristic lesions Thrombi are common in small- to medium-sized pulmonary arterioles. If the patient survives, the lungs may resolve to normal. The lungs may also progress to end-stage honeycomb fibrosis.

Organizing Pneumonia

The organizing pneumonia pattern is a patchy process characterized primarily by organizing pneumonia involving alveolar ducts and alveoli with or without bronchiolar intralumenal polyps (15). The connective tissue is all the same age. There is a mild associated interstitial inflammatory infiltrate, type II cell metaplasia, and an increase in alveolar macrophages, some of which may be foamy. There is relative preservation of background lung architecture.

Foci of organizing pneumonia [i.e., a bronchiolitis obliterans with organizing pneumonia (BOOP) pattern] are a nonspecific reaction to lung injury and can occur as a secondary finding adjacent to other pathologic processes or as a component of other primary pulmonary disorders (e.g., cryptococcosis, Wegener's granulomatosis, lymphoma, hypersensitivity pneumonitis, and eosinophilic pneumonia). Consequently, the clinician must carefully re-evaluate any patient found to have this histopathologic lesion to rule out these possibilities.

Lymphocytic Interstitial Pneumonitis

LIP is defined as a dense interstitial lymphoid infiltrate, including lymphocytes, plasma cells, and histiocytes with associated type II cell hyperplasia and a mild increase in alveolar macrophages (15). Lymphoid follicles, including follicles with germinal centers, are often present, usually in the distribution of pulmonary lymphatics.

VI. Clinical and Radiologic Manifestations of the Idiopathic Interstitial Pneumonias

The ATS/ERS consensus classification separates the IIPs into seven clinical-radiologic-pathologic entities (in order of relative frequency): IPF (frequency, ~47–64%), idiopathic NSIP (frequency, ~14–36%), RB-ILD/DIP (frequency, ~10–17%), cryptogenic organizing pneumonia (frequency, ~4–12%), AIP (frequency ~2%), and LIP (frequency ~2%) (53).

A. Idiopathic Pulmonary Fibrosis

IPF is one of the more commonly occurring ILDs of unknown etiology. IPF occurs worldwide and the majority of the patients reported are white. It mainly affects people aged

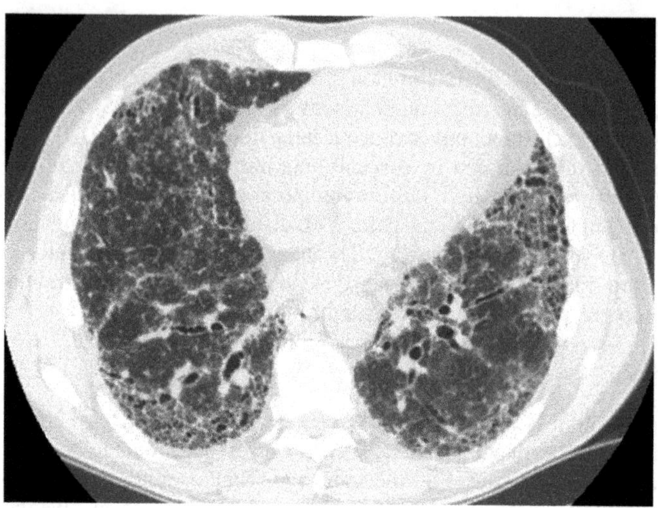

Figure 1 Idiopathic pulmonary fibrosis: CT manifestations. This HRCT scan shows honeycomb changes in the lower lung zones in a patient with UIP lesion on lung biopsy. *Abbreviations*: HRCT, high-resolution computed tomography; UIP, usual interstitial pneumonia.

over 50 years. The incidence of IPF is estimated at 6.8 cases per 100,000 and the prevalence is estimated to be 14.0 per 100,000 (54). Cigarette smoking has been identified as a risk factor for developing IPF.

The clinical manifestations of IPF include dyspnea on exertion, nonproductive cough, and "velcro"-type inspiratory crackles with or without digital clubbing noted on physical examination. The chest roentgenogram and HRCT typically reveal diffuse lower lung zone predominant interstitial opacities and honeycombing (Fig. 1). Pulmonary function tests often reveal restrictive impairment (decreased static lung volumes), reduced DL_{CO}, and arterial hypoxemia exaggerated or elicited by exercise. The confirmation of the diagnosis of IPF generally requires tissue obtained by surgical lung biopsy, and the UIP pattern is essential to confirm this diagnosis.

The clinical course is variable with a mean survival of four to six years after the time of diagnosis. Acute deterioration in IPF—that is an abrupt and unexpected worsening of the underlying lung disease—may occur secondary to infections, pulmonary embolism, pneumothorax, or heart failure. Often, however, there is no identifiable cause for the acute decline, and these episodes are called "acute exacerbations" of IPF (55). The impact of acute exacerbation on mortality was unclear, however, recent studies have suggested mortality rates from 20% to 86% (53,55). Patients with IPF continue to experience an inexorable progression to death, with lung transplantation being the only measure shown to prolong survival (2). Walter and colleagues summarized the management of IPF as follows (2): no specific drug treatment recommendations can be made; treatment of IPF with corticosteroids alone should not be considered a standard therapy; treatment of IPF with corticosteroids and cytotoxic agents is of unproven benefit and causes substantial morbidity; agents such as coumadin (56), *N*-acetylcysteine (57), pirfenidone (58), or bosentan (59) show promise, but there is insufficient evidence to recommend their general use;

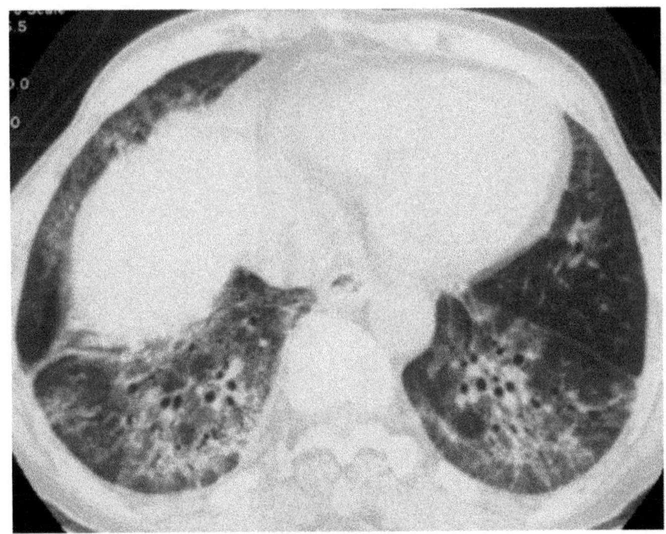

Figure 2 Nonspecific interstitial pneumonia (NSIP). This HRCT scan shows peripheral, basal, and symmetric ground-glass attenuation with associated subpleural sparing. *Abbreviation*: HRCT, high-resolution computed tomography.

efforts must be made to better understand and manage the acute exacerbations that seem to be a harbinger of death in patients with IPF; appropriate patients should receive pulmonary rehabilitation and oxygen therapy; and all suitable patients should be referred for lung transplant evaluation at the time of diagnosis.

B. Idiopathic NSIP

The existence of idiopathic NSIP remains controversial (38,60,61). A recent ATS workshop has proposed that idiopathic NSIP is a distinct clinical entity that occurs worldwide (62). It occurs mostly in middle-aged women who are never-smokers. The most common symptoms are dyspnea (96%) and cough (87%) and 69% had restrictive pulmonary function. By HRCT, the lower lung zones were predominantly involved in 92% of cases; 46% had a peripheral distribution; 47% were diffuse (Fig. 2) (62). Most showed a reticular pattern (87%) with traction bronchiectasis (82%) and volume loss (77%). Lung biopsies showed uniform thickening of alveolar walls with a spectrum of cellular to fibrosing patterns (62). The five-year survival was 82.3% (62). Kinder and coworkers have suggested that most patients diagnosed with idiopathic NSIP meet the case definition of undifferentiated CTD (63).

C. Respiratory Bronchiolitis-Associated ILD

RB-ILD is a distinct clinical syndrome found in current or former cigarette smokers (64). The clinical presentation resembles those with other ILDs like cough and breathlessness with exertion and crackles on chest examine. Routine laboratory studies are not helpful.

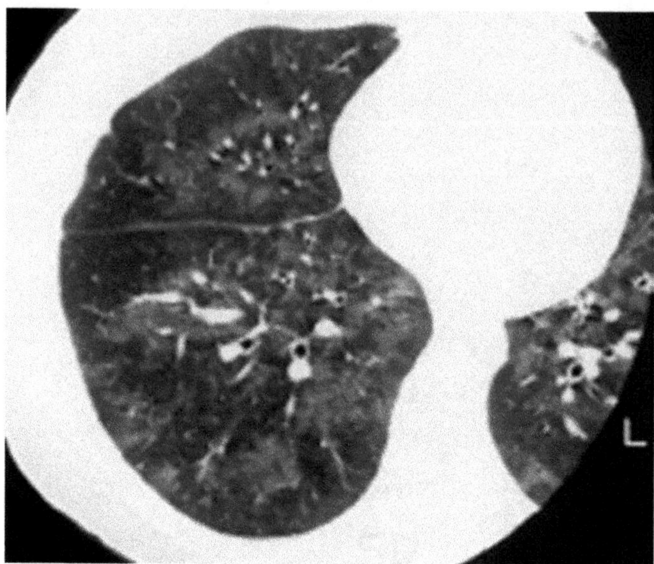

Figure 3 Respiratory bronchiolitis-associated ILD: CT manifestations. HRCT scan shows patchy, diffuse ground-glass opacification. *Abbreviations*: ILD, interstitial lung diseases; HRCT, high-resolution computed tomography.

Diffuse, fine reticular, or nodular interstitial opacities are found on chest radiograph usually with normal appearing lung volumes (50,65). Other reported features include: bronchial wall thickening; prominence of peribronchovascular interstitium; small, regular, and irregular opacities; and small peripheral ring shadows. HRCT scanning often reveals centrilobular nodules, ground-glass opacity, and air trapping (Fig. 3) (50,65). A mixed obstructive-restrictive pattern is common on lung function testing. An isolated increase in RV may be found. Arterial blood gases show mild hypoxemia. The clinical course and prognosis of RB is unknown. Smoking cessation is important in the resolution of these lesions. Prolonged survival is common in RB-ILD. However, symptomatic and physiologic improvement occurs in only a minority of patients, and neither smoking cessation nor immunosuppressive therapy is regularly associated with clinically significant benefit (66).

D. Desquamative Interstitial Pneumonia

DIP affects cigarette smokers in their fourth or fifth decades of life with most patients presenting with dyspnea. Lung function testing shows a restrictive pattern with reduced DL_{CO} and hypoxemia on blood gas analysis. The chest X ray shows less severe changes compared with IPF and may be normal in up to 20% of cases. The incidence of the clinicopathologic syndrome of DIP is quite rare (probably <3% of all ILD cases). In fact, many cases previously called DIP are cases of RB-ILD. Clinical recognition of DIP is important because the process is associated with a better prognosis (overall survival is about 70% after 10 years) and a better response to smoking cessation. Corticosteroid therapy appeared to be associated with modest clinical benefit but usually not with resolution of disease (67). Progressive disease with eventual death can occur in subjects with DIP, especially with continued cigarette smoking (67).

E. Acute Interstitial Pneumonia

AIP is a rare fulminant form of lung injury that presents acutely (days to weeks from onset of symptoms), usually in a previously healthy individual (52,68). Most patients are aged over 40 years (mean age 50 years, range 7–83 years). AIP is similar in presentation to the ARDS and probably corresponds to the subset of cases of idiopathic ARDS. The onset is usually abrupt, although a prodromal illness lasting usually 7 to 14 days before presentation is common. The clinical signs and symptoms were most often fever, cough, and shortness of breath. There is no sexual predilection. Routine laboratory studies are nonspecific and generally not helpful. Diffuse, bilateral, airspace opacification is seen on chest radiograph (69). CT scans show bilateral, patchy, symmetric areas of ground-glass attenuation (70). Bilateral areas of air space consolidation may also be present. A predominantly subpleural distribution may be seen. Mild honeycombing, usually involving less than 10% of the lung may be seen on CT examination. These radiographic findings are similar to those seen in ARDS. Most patients have moderate to severe hypoxemia and develop respiratory failure. Mechanical ventilation is often required. The diagnosis of AIP requires the presence of a clinical syndrome of idiopathic ARDS and pathologic confirmation of organizing DAD (71). Consequently, a surgical lung biopsy is required to confirm the diagnosis. The mortality from AIP is high (>60%) with the majority of patients dying within six months of presentation. However, those who recover usually do not have recurrence of the disease and most have substantial or complete recovery of lung function. It is not clear whether corticosteroid therapy is effective in AIP. The main treatment is supportive care.

F. Cryptogenic Organizing Pneumonia

Cryptogenic organizing pneumonitis (COP) (or idiopathic BOOP) is a specific clinicopathologic syndrome of unknown etiology (72). The disease onset occurs usually in the fifth and sixth decade and affects men and women equally. Almost three-fourths of the patients have their symptoms for less than two months and few have symptoms for greater than six months prior to diagnosis. A flu-like illness, characterized by cough, fever, malaise, fatigue, and weight loss herald the onset of COP in two-fifths of the patients. Inspiratory crackles are frequently present on chest examination. Routine laboratory studies are nonspecific. A leukocytosis without increase in eosinophils is seen in approximately half of the patients. The initial erythrocyte sedimentation rate (ESR) was frequently elevated in patients with COP. Pulmonary function is usually impaired with a restrictive defect being most common. Resting and exercise arterial hypoxemia is also common. The roentgenographic manifestations are quite distinctive. Bilateral, diffuse alveolar opacities in the presence of normal lung volume constituted the characteristic radiographic appearance in patients with COP (Fig. 4). A peripheral distribution of the opacities, very similar to that thought to be "virtually pathognomic" for CEP, is also seen in COP. Rarely, the alveolar opacities may be unilateral. Recurrent and migratory pulmonary opacities are common (73). Irregular linear or nodular interstitial infiltrates or honeycombing are rarely seen at presentation. HRCT scans of the lung reveal patchy airspace consolidation, ground-glass opacities, small nodular opacities, and bronchial wall thickening and dilation (74). These

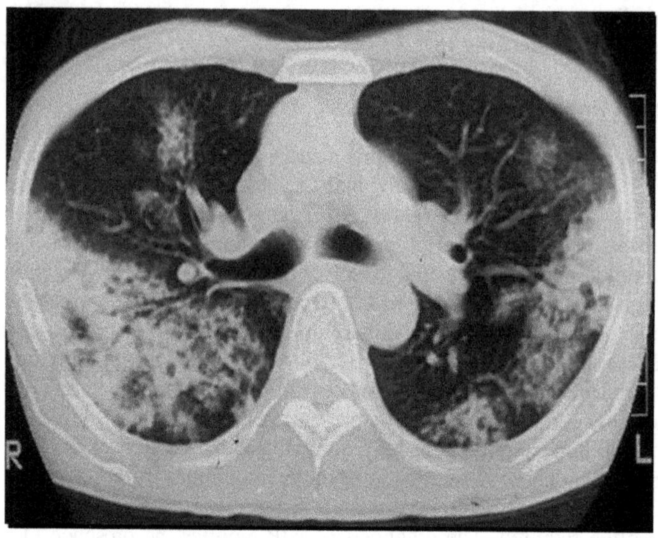

Figure 4 Cryptogenic Organizing Pneumonia (COP). HRCT scan shows patchy areas of consolidation. *Abbreviation*: HRCT, high-resolution computed tomography.

patchy opacities occur more frequently in the periphery of the lung and are often in the lower lung zone. The CT scan may reveal much more extensive disease then is expected by review of the plain chest X ray. Corticosteroid therapy was the most common treatment used in these patients. It results in clinical recovery in two-thirds of the patients (72,75).

G. Lymphocytic Interstitial Pneumonitis

LIP is a rare form of ILD in adults but is more common in the pediatric population (76). The cause of LIP is unknown. Up to three-fourths of patients with LIP will have a serum protein abnormality, most commonly the dysproteinemia, which is a polyclonal gammopathy, and, especially in children, hypogammaglobulinemia (77). Sjogren's syndrome (SS) is associated with one-fourth of reported cases of LIP and, as with other autoimmune or dysproteinemic states, the pulmonary disease may precede or follow the diagnosis of the underlying process. HIV-associated LIP may be the presenting problem in up to one half of children and infants infected with HIV (78). Cough and dyspnea, slowly progressive over months and in some cases years, are the most common presenting symptoms of LIP. Other symptoms include constitutional features such as weight loss, fevers, arthralgias, and pleuritic chest pain. Physical examination may reveal crackles on chest examine. Other findings, e.g., hepatosplenomegaly, arthritis, lymphadenopathy, etc., refer to the underlying disease state. Pulmonary function testing shows reduced lung volumes and diffusing capacity with preserved airflow. Marked hypoxemia may occur. BAL may reveal increased numbers of lymphocytes. LIP has a varied radiographic appearance. It can appear as a basilar linear interstitial opacities or as a nodular process. HRCT scanning of the chest is useful to better establish the extent of disease, define the hilar anatomy, and identify any pleural involvement. The natural history and prognosis of LIP is poorly understood.

Spontaneous resolution, resolution following treatment with corticosteroids or other immunosuppressive agents, progression to lymphoma, or development of pulmonary fibrosis with respiratory insufficiency are all potential outcomes. Corticosteroid therapy alone or in combination with other agents has been used to treat symptomatic patients with LIP although its efficacy has not been established in a controlled trial.

VII. Clinical and Radiologic Manifestations of Other Interstitial Pneumonias

A. Connective Tissue Disorders

ILD associated with CTD usually occurs after the CTD has been recognized. Occasionally, the ILD may precede the development of the characteristic systemic signs and symptoms of the particular CTD, especially RA or polymyositis. The most common form of pulmonary involvement is a chronic interstitial pattern characterized by NSIP on lung biopsy. However, determining the precise nature of lung involvement in most of the CTD is difficult because of the high incidence of lung disease caused by disease-associated complications of esophageal dysfunction (predisposing to aspiration and secondary infections), respiratory muscle weakness (atelectasis and secondary infections), therapeutic complications (opportunistic infections), and associated malignancies.

Progressive Systemic Sclerosis

PSS (scleroderma) is a systemic disease characterized by dermatologic changes (skin thickening, ulcerations), visceral microvascular abnormalities, and esophageal dysfunction. The incidence of ILD associated with PSS ranges from 14% to 90% in clinical studies and from 60% to 100% in autopsy studies. Pulmonary function tests usually reveal a restrictive pattern with reduced lung compliance and impaired diffusing capacity, often before any clinical or radiographic evidence of lung disease appears. Pulmonary vascular disease alone or in association with pulmonary fibrosis, pleuritis, recurrent aspiration pneumonitis, and bronchiolar carcinoma can also occur. The ILD and pulmonary hypertension associated with scleroderma are strikingly resistant to current modes of therapy (79–83).

Rheumatoid Arthritis

Although RA itself has a female predominance, pulmonary disease associated with RA is more common in men. Manifestations of RA in the lung include pleurisy with or without effusion, ILD (in up to 20% of cases), necrobiotic nodules (nonpneumoconiotic intrapulmonary rheumatoid nodules) with or without cavities, Caplan's syndrome (rheumatoid pneumoconiosis), pulmonary hypertension secondary to rheumatoid pulmonary vasculitis, bronchiolitis obliterans, BOPP, and upper airway obstruction due to arytenoid arthritis. Gold-induced pneumonitis may occur in RA patients treated with gold (84).

Systemic Lupus Erythematosus

SLE is a systemic disorder of unknown etiology characterized by immunologically mediated tissue damage, with a variable presentation. Multiple organ systems may be involved including renal, central nervous system, musculoskeletal, mucocutaneous, and others. Pleuritis with or without effusion is the most common pulmonary manifestation of SLE. Other lung manifestations include atelectasis, diaphragmatic dysfunction with loss of lung volumes, pulmonary vascular disease, pulmonary hemorrhage, uremic pulmonary edema, infectious pneumonia, bronchiolitis obliterans, and ILD.

Polymyositis/Dermatomyositis

ILD occurs in approximately 10% of patients with PM/DM, and the clinical features are similar to IPF. Less commonly, a rapidly progressive Hamman-Rich syndrome (DAD) may occur with respiratory failure. Diffuse reticular or nodular opacities with or without an alveolar component occur radiographically, with a predilection for the lung bases.

Sjogren's Syndrome

SS manifested by keratoconjunctivitis sicca, xerostomia, and recurrent swelling of the parotid gland may be associated with ILD (85). LIP, lymphoma, pseudolymphoma, and bronchiolitis and bronchiolitis obliterans are also associated with SS. Surgical lung biopsy is frequently required to discern a precise pulmonary diagnosis in SS. In the absence of controlled trials, corticosteroids have been used in the management of SS-associated ILD with some degree of clinical success.

B. Drug-Induced ILD

Many drugs are known to have the potential to induce diffuse interstitial opacities with associated symptoms of dyspnea and nonproductive cough. In most cases, the pathogenesis of this aberrant pulmonary response to a given drug is unknown, although a combination of direct toxic effects of the drug (or its metabolite) and indirect inflammatory and immunologic events are likely. This topic is too extensive to discuss thoroughly; several generalizations can be made: (*i*) the extent and severity of disease is usually dose related, (*ii*) many classes of drugs may cause disease, (*iii*) the onset of illness may be insidious over weeks to months or may be abrupt and fulminant, (*iv*) treatment always includes discontinuation of any possible offending drug and supportive care, (*v*) since the addition of corticosteroids is often ineffective the decision must be taken on the basis of available data for a given drug, and (*vi*) a syndrome of drug-induced lupus, manifested in the lung principally as pleural disease can be seen (particularly with procainamide and rarely quinidine).

C. Pneumoconioses

Silicosis

Silicosis is found in miners, sandblasters, glass manufacturers, quarry workers, stone dressers, foundry workers, and boiler scalers. Radiographically, silicosis appears as bilateral, multinodular, rounded densities predominantly in the upper lung zones. The radiographic changes usually occur before the clinical and functional abnormalities. Progression from simple to progressive massive fibrosis occurs in a minority of patients. Patients with silicosis are highly susceptible to infection by *Mycobacterium tuberculosis* and other atypical mycobacteria. Also, scleroderma and RA are unusually prevalent in silicosis. Laboratory findings in simple silicosis may include an increased sedimentation rate, immunoglobulins, immune complexes, antinuclear antibodies, and anti-immunoglobulin antibodies (rheumatoid factors). There is no known effective treatment at present for silicosis.

Asbestosis

Asbestos exposure is widespread because it is used extensively as an insulation material, fire retardant, and noise reduction agent in many public facilities. More than 90% of the asbestos used is chrysolite or white asbestos. Workers employed in the shipyard, automotive, insulation, cement, textile, and asbestos mining industries are at greatest risk. There is a long latent period between exposure and the development of lung diseases. In general, individuals who develop asbestos-induced disease will have markedly increased numbers of asbestos fibers in their lung compared to the general population. Smoking appears to facilitate the damaging effects of asbestos inhalation. It is important to distinguish evidence of asbestos exposure from asbestosis. Asbestosis is characterized by a history of exposure to asbestos and the presence of interstitial pulmonary fibrosis manifested by dyspnea, cough, and bibasilar inspiratory crackles with or without digital clubbing on examination. Bilateral pleural thickening along the lower or midthoracic walls, calcified pleural plaques on the parietal pleura and diaphragm, and hazy opacities composed of irregular or linear small opacities, especially in the lower lung zones, are the most common roentgenographic changes. Pulmonary function studies may reveal a restrictive pattern, and the DL_{CO} is often reduced. Asbestos-induced fibrosis of the visceral pleura can produce restrictive functional abnormalities. The clinical course of asbestosis is usually one of slow but progressive deterioration, and death is often a result of either respiratory compromise or cancer. The synergistic effect of cigarette smoking and asbestosis exposure on the development of lung cancer is well established, with 30% to 40% of patients with asbestosis developing lung cancer.

D. Pulmonary Langerhans Cell Histiocytosis (Eosinophilic Granuloma)

Pulmonary Langerhans cell histiocytosis of the lung is a rare, smoking-related diffuse lung disease that primarily afflicts young adults aged between 20 and 40 years (86–89). Pulmonary Langerhans cell histiocytosis occurs more commonly in men. The clinical presentation is variable, from an asymptomatic state (~16%) to a rapidly progressive condition. The most common clinical manifestations at presentation are cough, dyspnea, chest pain, weight loss, and fever. Pneumothorax occurs in about 25% of patients and is occasionally the first manifestation of the illness. Hemoptysis and diabetes insipidus are rare manifestations. The physical examination is usually normal. Routine laboratory studies are not helpful. The radiographic features vary depending on the stage of the disease (90). The combination of ill-defined or stellate nodules (2–10 mm in size), reticular or nodular opacities, upper zone cysts or honeycombing, preservation of lung volume, and costophrenic angle sparing are felt to be highly specific for pulmonary Langerhans cell histiocytosis (Fig. 5) (91). However, the differentiation of pulmonary Langerhans cell histiocytosis from other fibrosing lung diseases by chest radiographic features alone can be

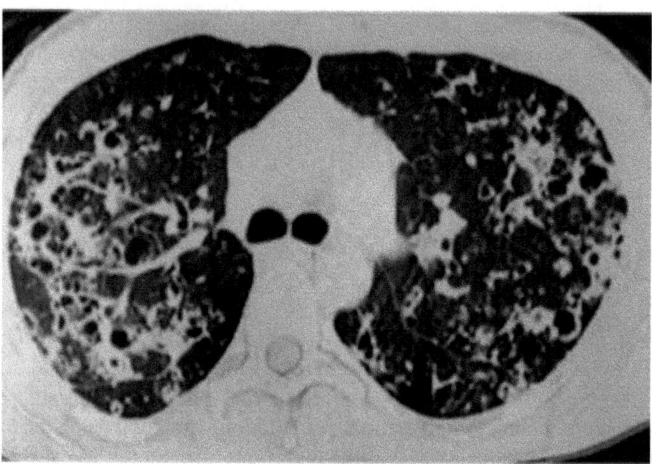

Figure 5 Pulmonary Langerhans cell histiocytosis. HRCT lung scan in this patient shows the combination of nodules and thin- and thick-walled cysts in the upper lung zones. *Abbreviation*: HRCT, high-resolution computed tomography.

difficult. HRCT lung scanning that reveals the combination of nodules and thin-walled cysts is virtually diagnostic of Pulmonary Langerhans cell histiocytosis. Physiologically, the most prominent and frequent pulmonary function abnormality reported is a markedly reduced DL_{CO}, though varying degrees of restrictive disease, airflow limitation, and diminished exercise capacity are described (92). Discontinuance of smoking is the key treatment, resulting in clinical improvement in 33% of the subjects. Most patients with pulmonary Langerhans cell histiocytosis suffer persistent or progressive disease. Death due to respiratory failure occurs in approximately 10% of patients.

E. Eosinophilic Pneumonia

CEP is often a fulminant illness characterized by fever, night sweats, weight loss, and progressive breathlessness and asthma (accompany or precede the illness in 50% of cases). Acute idiopathic eosinophilic pneumonia is a cause of acute respiratory failure. The etiology is unknown but an inhaled antigen is suspected. These entities are discussed in chapter 11 "Clinical Diagnosis of Pulmonary Eosinophilia."

VIII. Summary

The ILDs are a diverse group of pulmonary disorders with overlapping clinical, radiographic, physiologic, and histopathologic characteristics. The clinical history is the most valuable factor in the assessment of patients with parenchymal lung disease. Velcro crackles are commonly present on auscultation of the chest, and restriction is the most frequent finding in pulmonary function testing. Widening of the alveolar-arterial oxygen gradient is a sensitive indicator of physiologic impairment, which may detect early disease.

Thin-section HRCT is the most valuable and informative chest imaging technique. BAL allows the sampling and characterization of the types of cells and mediators within the alveolar space but is not necessarily representative of the processes within the interstitium. Lastly, histopathologic examination of lung tissue remains a key feature in confirming the diagnosis and assessment of severity in many ILDs.

Management of most ILDs is difficult, and different approaches are taken depending on the specific entity. Regardless of etiology, end-stage fibrosis is irreversible and untreatable. An extensive and aggressive early diagnostic evaluation, even in patients with relatively few symptoms, is recommended. Patients with evidence of functional impairment, signs of progression, or evidence of active disease should be treated, if no contraindications to therapy exist. Cases in which an inciting agent can be identified, cessation of exposure is the principal therapeutic intervention. Smoking cessation is a key treatment in many ILDs. Many of the patients with ILD are elderly, consequently, the decision to treat them with immunosuppressive drugs should not be taken lightly, as the toxicity and side effects of these medications can be substantial. Lung transplantation is an increasing treatment for end-stage disease.

References

1. Selman M, King TE Jr., Pardo A. Idiopathic pulmonary fibrosis: prevailing and evolving hypotheses about its pathogenesis and implications for therapy. Ann Intern Med 2001; 134:136–151.
2. Walter N, Collard HR, King TE Jr. Current perspectives on the treatment of idiopathic pulmonary fibrosis. Proc Am Thorac Soc 2006; 3(4):330–338.
3. King TE Jr. Interstitial lung diseases: general approaches. In: Parsons PE, Heffner JE, eds. Pulmonary and Respiratory Therapy Secrets. Philadelphia, PA: Handley & Belfus, Inc., 1997:231–242.
4. Schwartzstein RM. Approach to the patient with dyspnea. In: Rose BD, ed. UpToDate. Wellesley, MA: UpToDate, 2007.
5. Shorr AF, Scoville SL, Cersovsky SB, et al. Acute eosinophilic pneumonia among US military personnel deployed in or near iraq. JAMA 2004; 292(24):2997–3005.
6. Ryu JH, Colby TV, Hartman TE, et al. Smoking-related interstitial lung diseases: a concise review. Eur Respir J 2001; 17(1):122–132.
7. Franquet T, Giménez A, Rosón N, et al. Aspiration diseases: findings, pitfalls, and differential diagnosis. Radiographics 2000; 20(3):673–685.
8. Rosas IO, Ren P, Avila NA, et al. Early interstitial lung disease in familial pulmonary fibrosis. Am J Respir Crit Care Med 2007; 176(7):698–705.
9. Lynch DA, Travis WD, Muller NL, et al. Idiopathic interstitial pneumonias: CT features. Radiology 2005; 236(1):10–21.
10. Gotway MB, Freemer MM, King TE Jr. Challenges in pulmonary fibrosis 1: use of high resolution CT scanning of the lung for the evaluation of patients with idiopathic interstitial pneumonias. Thorax 2007; 62(6):546–553.
11. Raghu G, Mageto YN, Lockhart D, et al. The accuracy of the clinical diagnosis of new-onset idiopathic pulmonary fibrosis and other interstitial lung disease: a prospective study. Chest 1999; 116(5):1168–1174.
12. Hunninghake GW, Lynch DA, Galvin JR, et al. Radiologic findings are strongly associated with a pathologic diagnosis of usual interstitial pneumonia. Chest 2003; 124(4):1215–1223.
13. Aziz ZA, Wells AU, Hansell DM, et al. HRCT diagnosis of diffuse parenchymal lung disease: inter-observer variation. Thorax 2004; 59(6):506–511.

14. Singh S, Wells AU, Du Bois RM. Other imaging techniques for idiopathic interstitial pneumonias. In: Lynch JP III, ed. Idiopathic Pulmonary Fibrosis. New York, NY: Marcel Dekker, Inc., 2004:237–252.
15. American Thoracic Society/European Respiratory Society International Multidisciplinary Consensus Classification of the Idiopathic Interstitial Pneumonias. Am J Respir Crit Care Med 2002; 165:277–304.
16. Jegal Y, Kim DS, Shim TS, et al. Physiology is a stronger predictor of survival than pathology in fibrotic interstitial pneumonia. Am J Respir Crit Care Med 2005; 171(6):639–644.
17. King TE Jr., Tooze JA, Schwarz MI, et al. Predicting survival in idiopathic pulmonary fibrosis. Scoring system and survival model. Am J Respir Crit Care Med 2001; 164:1171–1181.
18. King TE Jr. Role of bronchoalveolar lavage in the diagnosis of interstitial lung disease. In: Rose BD, ed. UpToDate Wellesley, MA: UpToDate, 2007.
19. Kinder BW, Brown KK, Schwarz MI, et al. Baseline bronchoalveolar lavage neutrophilia predicts early mortality in idiopathic pulmonary fibrosis. Chest 2008; 133(1):226–232.
20. Klech H, Pohl W. Technical recommendations and guidelines for bronchoalveolar lavage (BAL). Eur Respir J 1989; 2:561–585.
21. King TE Jr. Interstitial lung disease. In: Feinsilver SH, Fein AM, eds. Textbook of Bronchoscopy. Baltimore, MD: Williams & Wilkins, 1995:185–220.
22. Sweet MP, Hoopes C, Golden J, et al. Prevalence of delayed gastric emptying and gastroesophageal reflux in patients with end-stage lung disease. Ann Thorac Surg 2006; 82(4):1570.
23. Raghu G, Freudenberger TD, Yang S, et al. High prevalence of abnormal acid gastro-oesophageal reflux in idiopathic pulmonary fibrosis. Eur Respir J 2006; 27(1):136–142.
24. Tobin RW, Pope CE II, Pellegrini CA, et al. Increased prevalence of gastroesophageal reflux in patients with idiopathic pulmonary fibrosis. Am J Respir Crit Care Med 1998; 158(6): 1804–1808.
25. Sweet MP, Patti MG, Leard LE, et al. Gastroesophageal reflux in patients with idiopathic pulmonary fibrosis referred for lung transplantation. J Thorac Cardiovasc Surg 2007; 133(4): 1078–1084.
26. Arcasoy SM, Christie JD, Ferrari VA, et al. Echocardiographic assessment of pulmonary hypertension in patients with advanced lung disease. Am J Respir Crit Care Med 2003; 167(5): 735–740.
27. Ghofrani HA, Wiedemann R, Rose F, et al. Sildenafil for treatment of lung fibrosis and pulmonary hypertension: a randomised controlled trial. Lancet 2002; 360(9337):895–900.
28. Nadrous HF, Pellikka PA, Krowka MJ, et al. Pulmonary hypertension in patients with idiopathic pulmonary fibrosis. Chest 2005; 128(4):2393–2399.
29. Mays EE, Dubois JJ, Hamilton GB. Pulmonary fibrosis associated with tracheobronchial aspiration. Chest 1976; 69:512–515.
30. Bandla HP, Davis SH, Hopkins NE. Lipoid pneumonia: a silent complication of mineral oil aspiration. Pediatrics 1999; 103(2):E19.
31. Corwin RW, Irwin RS. The lipid-laden alveolar macrophage as a marker of aspiration in parenchymal lung disease. Am Rev Respir Dis 1985; 132:576–581.
32. Marom EM, McAdams HP, Erasmus JJ, et al. The many faces of pulmonary aspiration. AJR Am J Roentgenol 1999; 172(1):121–128.
33. Campbell EJ, Harris B. Idiopathic pulmonary fibrosis (clinical conference). Arch Intern Med 1981; 141:771–774.
34. Bye PT, Issa F, Berthon-Jones M, et al. Studies of oxygenation during sleep in patients with interstitial lung disease. Am Rev Respir Dis 1984; 129:27–32.
35. King TE Jr. The role of lung biopsy in the diagnosis of interstitial lung disease. In: Rose BD, ed. UpToDate. Wellesley, MA: UpToDate, 2004.
36. Glaspole IN, Wells AU, du Bois RM. Lung biopsy in diffuse parenchymal lung disease. Monaldi Arch Chest Dis 2001; 56(3):225–232.

37. Collard HR, King TE Jr. Lung biopsy in patients with usual interstitial pneumonia. Eur Respir J 2001; 18(5):895–898.
38. du Bois R, King TE Jr. Challenges in pulmonary fibrosis 5: the NSIP/UIP debate. Thorax 2007; 62(11):1008–1012.
39. King TE Jr. Clinical advances in the diagnosis and therapy of the interstitial lung diseases. Am J Respir Crit Care Med 2005; 172(3):268–279.
40. Travis WD, King TE Jr., Bateman ED, et al. American thoracic society/european respiratory society international multidisciplinary consensus classification of the idiopathic interstitial pneumonias. Am J Respir Crit Care Med 2002; 165:277–304.
41. British thoracic society. The diagnosis, assessment and treatment of diffuse parenchymal lung disease in adults. Thorax 1999; 54(suppl 1):S1–S28.
42. Hunninghake G, Zimmerman MB, Schwartz DA, et al. Utility of lung biopsy for the diagnosis of idiopathic pulmonary fibrosis. Am J Respir Crit Care Med 2001; 164:193–196.
43. Flaherty KR, King TE Jr., Raghu G, et al. Idiopathic interstitial pneumonia: what is the effect of a multidisciplinary approach to diagnosis? Am J Respir Crit Care Med 2004; 170(8):904–910.
44. Wells AU. Histopathologic diagnosis in diffuse lung disease: an ailing gold standard. Am J Respir Crit Care Med 2004; 170(8):828–829.
45. American Thoracic Society. Idiopathic pulmonary fibrosis: diagnosis and treatment. International consensus statement. American Thoracic Society (ATS), and the European Respiratory Society (ERS). Am J Respir Crit Care Med 2000; 161:646–664.
46. Katzenstein AL, Fiorelli RF. Nonspecific interstitial pneumonia/fibrosis. Histologic features and clinical significance. Am J Surg Pathol 1994; 18(2):136–147.
47. Katzenstein AL, Zisman DA, Litzky LA, et al. Usual interstitial pneumonia: histologic study of biopsy and explant specimens. Am J Surg Pathol 2002; 26(12):1567–1577.
48. Flaherty KR, Travis WD, Colby TV, et al. Histopathologic variability in usual and nonspecific interstitial pneumonias. Am J Respir Crit Care Med 2001; 164(9):1722–1727.
49. Fraig M, Shreesha U, Savici D, et al. Respiratory bronchiolitis: a clinicopathologic study in current smokers, ex-smokers, and never-smokers. Am J Surg Pathol 2002; 26(5):647–653.
50. Vassallo R, Jensen EA, Colby TV, et al. The overlap between respiratory bronchiolitis and desquamative interstitial pneumonia in pulmonary Langerhans cell histiocytosis: high-resolution CT, histologic, and functional correlations. Chest 2003; 124(4):1199–1205.
51. Craig PJ, Wells AU, Doffman S, et al. Desquamative interstitial pneumonia, respiratory bronchiolitis and their relationship to smoking. Histopathology 2004; 45(3):275–282.
52. Parambil JG, Myers JL, Aubry M-C, et al. Causes and prognosis of diffuse alveolar damage diagnosed on surgical lung biopsy. Chest 2007; 132(1):50–57.
53. Kim DS, Collard HR, King TE Jr. Classification and natural history of the idiopathic interstitial pneumonias. Proc Am Thorac Soc 2006; 3(4):285–292.
54. Raghu G, Weycker D, Edelsberg J, et al. Incidence and prevalence of idiopathic pulmonary fibrosis. Am J Respir Crit Care Med 2006; 174(7):810–816.
55. Collard HR, Moore BB, Flaherty KR, et al. Acute exacerbations of idiopathic pulmonary fibrosis. Am J Respir Crit Care Med 2007; 176(7):636–643.
56. Kubo H, Nakayama K, Yanai M, et al. Anticoagulant therapy for idiopathic pulmonary fibrosis. Chest 2005; 128(3):1475–1482.
57. Demedts M, Behr J, Buhl R, et al. High-dose acetylcysteine in idiopathic pulmonary fibrosis. N Engl J Med 2005; 353(21):2229–2242.
58. Azuma A, Nukiwa T, Tsuboi E, et al. Double-blind, placebo-controlled trial of pirfenidone in patients with idiopathic pulmonary fibrosis. Am J Respir Crit Care Med 2005; 171(9):1040–1047.
59. King TE Jr., Behr J, Brown KK, et al. BUILD-1: a randomized placebo-controlled trial of bosentan in idiopathic pulmonary fibrosis. Am J Respir Crit Care Med 2008; 177(1):75–81.
60. Myers JL. NSIP, UIP, and the ABCs of idiopathic interstitial pneumonias. Eur Respir J 1998; 12 (5):1003–1004.

61. Maher TM, Wells AU, Laurent GJ. Idiopathic pulmonary fibrosis: multiple causes and multiple mechanisms? Eur Respir J 2007; 30(5):835–839.
62. Travis WD, Hunninghake G, King TE Jr., et al. Idiopathic nonspecific interstitial pneumonia: report of an ATS workshop. Am J Respir Crit Care Med (in press).
63. Kinder BW, Collard HR, Koth L, et al. Idiopathic nonspecific interstitial pneumonia: lung manifestation of undifferentiated connective tissue disease? Am J Respir Crit Care Med 2007; 176(7):691–697.
64. King TE Jr. Respiratory bronchiolitis-associated interstitial lung disease. Clin Chest Med 1993; 14:693–698.
65. Park JS, Brown KK, Tuder RM, et al. Respiratory bronchiolitis associated interstitial lung disease: radiologic features with clinical and pathologic correlation. J Comput Assist Tomogr 2002; 26:13–20.
66. Portnoy J, Veraldi KL, Schwarz MI, et al. Respiratory bronchiolitis-interstitial lung disease: long-term outcome. Chest 2007; 131(3):664–671.
67. Ryu JH, Myers JL, Capizzi SA, et al. Desquamative interstitial pneumonia and respiratory bronchiolitis-associated interstitial lung disease. Chest 2005; 127(1):178–184.
68. Olson J, Colby TV, Elliott CG. Hamman-rich syndrome revisited. Mayo Clin Proc 1990; 65(12): 1538–1548.
69. Primack SL, Hartman TE, Ikezoe J, et al. Acute interstitial pneumonia: radiographic and CT findings in nine patients. Radiology 1993; 188(3):817–820.
70. Johkoh T, Muller NL, Taniguchi H, et al. Acute interstitial pneumonia: thin-section CT findings in 36 patients. Radiology 1999; 211(3):859–863.
71. Askin FB. Acute interstitial pneumonia: histopathologic patterns of acute lung injury and the hamman-rich syndrome revisited. Radiology 1993; 188(3):620–621.
72. King TE Jr., Mortenson RL. Cryptogenic organizing pneumonia. The North American experience. Chest 1992; 102:8S–13S.
73. King TE Jr. BOOP: an important cause of migratory pulmonary infiltrates? Euro Respir J 1995; 8:193–195.
74. Nishimura K, Itoh H. High-resolution computed tomographic features of bronchiolitis obliterans organizing pneumonia. Chest 1992; 102:26S–31S.
75. Cordier JF. Cryptogenic organizing pneumonitis. Clinics Chest Med 1993; 14:677–692.
76. Pitt J. Lymphocytic interstitial pneumonia. Pediatr Clin North Am 1991; 38:89–95.
77. Popa V. Lymphocytic interstitial pneumonia of common variable immunodeficiency. Ann Allergy 1988; 60:203–206.
78. Travis WD, Fox CH, Devaney KO, et al. Lymphoid pneumonitis in 50 adult patients infected with the human immunodeficiency virus: lymphocytic interstitial pneumonitis versus nonspecific interstitial pneumonitis. Hum Pathol 1992; 23:529–541.
79. Tashkin DP, Elashoff R, Clements PJ, et al. Cyclophosphamide versus placebo in scleroderma lung disease. N Engl J Med 2006; 354(25):2655–2666.
80. Ahmadi-Simab K, Hellmich B, Gross WL. Bosentan for severe pulmonary arterial hypertension related to systemic sclerosis with interstitial lung disease. Eur J Clin Invest 2006 36(suppl 3):44–48.
81. Benan M, Hande I, Gul O. The natural course of progressive systemic sclerosis patients with interstitial lung involvement. Clin Rheumatol 2007; 26(3):349–354.
82. Berezne A, Valeyre D, Ranque B, et al. Interstitial lung disease associated with systemic sclerosis: what is the evidence for efficacy of cyclophosphamide? Ann N Y Acad Sci 2007; 1110: 271–284.
83. Tashkin DP, Elashoff R, Clements PJ, et al. Effects of 1-year treatment with cyclophosphamide on outcomes at 2 years in scleroderma lung disease. Am J Respir Crit Care Med 2007; 176 (10):1026–1034.
84. Tomioka H, King TE Jr. Gold-induced pulmonary disease: clinical features, outcome, and differentiation from rheumatoid lung disease. Am J Respir Crit Care Med 1997; 155:1011–1020.

85. Deheinzelin D, Capelozzi VL, Kairalla RA, et al. Interstitial lung disease in primary Sjögren's syndrome. Clinico-pathological evaluation and response to treatment. Am J Respir Crit Care Med 1996; 154:794–799.
86. Travis WD, Borok Z, Roum JH, et al. Pulmonary Langerhans cell granulomatosis (histiocytosis X). A clinicopathologic study of 48 cases. Am J Surg Pathol 1993; 17:971–986.
87. Vassallo R, Ryu JH, Schroeder DR, et al. Clinical outcomes of pulmonary Langerhans'-cell histiocytosis in adults. N Engl J Med 2002; 346(7):484–490.
88. Crausman RS, King TE Jr. Primary pulmonary histiocytosis X in the adult: clincal features, diagnosis, and treatment. In: Rose B, ed. UpToDate. Wellesley, MA: UpToDate, 2004.
89. Caminati A, Harari S. Smoking-related interstitial pneumonias and pulmonary Langerhans cell histiocytosis. Proc Am Thorac Soc 2006; 3(4):299–306.
90. Kulwiec EL, Lynch DA, Aguayo S, et al. Imaging of pulmonary histiocytosis X. Radiographics 1992; 12:515–526.
91. Lacronique J, Roth C, Battesti J-P, et al. Chest radiological features of pulmonary histiocytosis X: a report based on 50 adult cases. Thorax 1982; 37:104–109.
92. Crausman RS, Jennings CA, Tuder R, et al. Pulmonary histiocytosis X: pulmonary function and exercise pathophysiology. Am J Respir Crit Care Med 1996; 153:426–435.
93. Schwarz MI, King TE Jr., Cherniack RM. General principles and diagnostic approach to the interstitial lung diseases. In: Murray JF, Nadel JA, eds. Textbook of Respiratory Medicine. 2nd ed. Philadelphia, PA: W.B. Saunders, 1994:1803–1826.
94. King TE Jr. Approach to the patient with interstitial lung disease. In: Kelley W, ed. Textbook of Internal Medicine. 3rd ed. Philadelphia, PA: L. B. Lippincott, 1997:1954–1962.

7
Predominantly Immature Interstitial and Intra-alveolar Fibrosis

EUNHEE S. YI
Mayo Clinic, Rochester, Minnesota, U.S.A.

I. Introduction

Immature fibrosis is characterized histologically by fibroblastic proliferation in a background of edematous stroma with little or no collagen deposition. Immature fibrosis in the lung usually occurs as a component of acute lung injury pattern in various clinicopathological conditions but it can also be seen as a feature of chronic processes such as usual interstitial pneumonia (UIP). Fibroblastic proliferation comprising immature fibrosis is potentially reversible and has been shown to be completely resolved on clinical and pathological follow-up in human diseases as well as in animal models of fibrosis (1). The Masson body, an intraluminal or intra-alveolar bud of immature fibrotic tissue, is composed of fibroblasts and myofibroblasts. Previous ultrastructural studies have shown that Masson bodies not only progress to obliterate the alveolar spaces but also may incorporate into the alveolar septa (2). Immature fibrosis can be localized to either intra-alveolar/intraluminal or interstitial spaces but is usually seen to some degree in both compartments. Diagnostic approaches to the cases with immature fibrosis as a major or minor component would be stepwise processes: first, confirm the presence of immature fibrosis and differentiate from proliferation of other types of cells; second, recognize the major pattern of immature fibrosis; third, examine the presence of associated changes in the background; finally, identify the specific clinical disorder(s) manifesting as diffuse alveolar damage (DAD) or bronchiolitis obliterans organizing pneumonia (BOOP).

II. Acute Lung Injury Pattern: Prototype of Predominantly Immature Fibrosis

The concept of acute lung injury pattern was introduced by Katzenstein and Askin to acknowledge the stereotypical response of the lung to a wide range of acute pulmonary insults (3). Organizing DAD and BOOP are the two major histological findings of acute lung injury presenting as temporally uniform fibroblastic proliferation. Typically, DAD and BOOP are readily distinguishable histologically and they also follow quite distinct clinical courses: acute and fulminate with poor prognosis in DAD, subacute and less catastrophic with favorable outcome in BOOP. Histological changes of DAD generally correlate with clinical manifestations of acute or adult respiratory distress syndrome (ARDS). When the features of DAD and BOOP coexist in a biopsy, acute lung injury would be a useful term for such cases. These cases usually follow the clinical course of ARDS as in DAD. In small biopsies, distinction of DAD and BOOP may be difficult. Such cases can also be diagnosed as acute lung injury and clinical radiological correlation would be helpful.

Liebow has asserted that the word "diffuse" in DAD refers to all parts of the alveolus (i.e., epithelium, endothelium, and interstitial stroma), but not necessarily indicates diffuse involvement of most alveoli in the lung. Thus, diffuse involvement of the lung is not required for the diagnosis of DAD and some DAD cases show only "focal" involvement affecting a limited region of the lung. However, typical DAD cases show widespread involvement of the lung and manifest as two phases: acute and organizing. Acute or exudative phase occurs within a week after the onset of symptoms and is characterized by diffuse interstitial, intra-alveolar, and septal edema and hyaline membranes along the walls of alveolar ducts and distal alveolar spaces. A later organizing stage of DAD usually, but not always, follows the earlier exudative stage, appearing one to two weeks after clinical onset, and is dominated by exuberant immature interstitial fibrosis. Diffuse type II pneumocyte hyperplasia along the markedly thickened alveolar septa is another prominent feature in the organizing stage of DAD (Fig. 1). Arterial fibrin thrombi are commonly seen in cases of DAD or in cases showing mixed findings of DAD and BOOP. However, fibrin thrombi are generally not present in pure BOOP cases. Immunohistochemical and ultrastructural studies have demonstrated mural incorporation of intra-alveolar exudates and remnants of hyaline membranes between the denuded alveolar septal basement membrane and proliferating type II cells, suggesting a pathogenic relationship between intra-alveolar and interstitial fibrosis (4).

A clinicopathological study on acute fibrinous and organizing pneumonia (AFOP) was first reported by Beasley et al. in 2002 (5). In contrast to the hyaline membrane

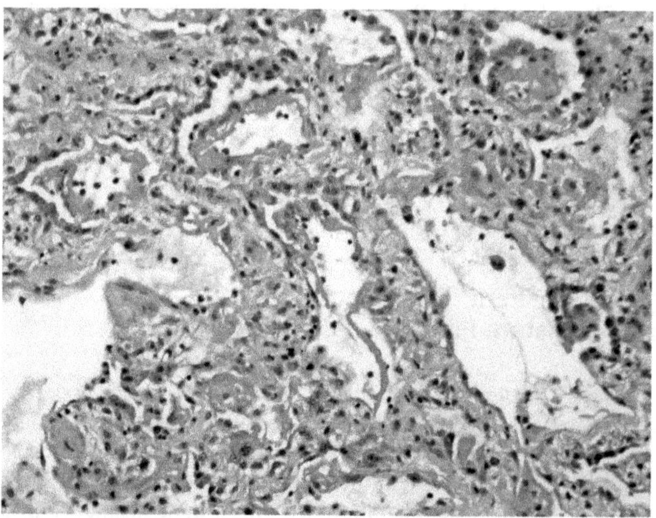

Figure 1 DAD in early organizing stage. Remnants of hyaline membranes are incorporating into the septal fibroblastic proliferation. A marked type II pneumocyte hyperplasia is present (H&E, 200×). *Abbreviations*: DAD, diffuse alveolar damage; H&E, hematoxylin and eosin.

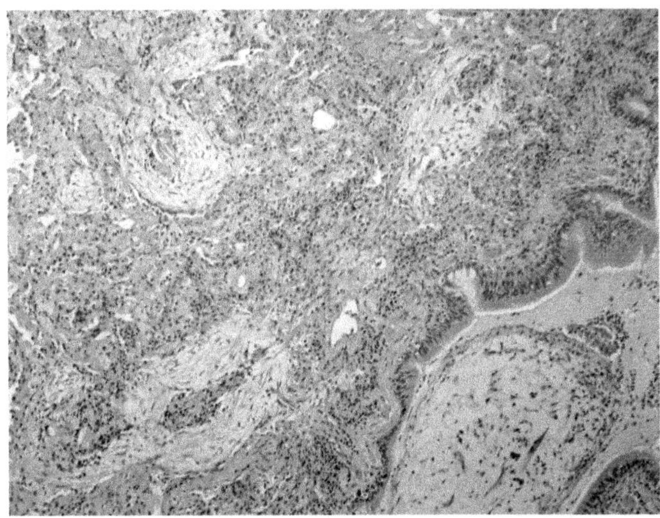

Figure 2 BOOP. Fibromyxoid plugs filling the bronchiolar lumens and alveolar spaces (H&E, 100×). *Abbreviations*: BOOP, bronchiolitis obliterans organizing pneumonia; H&E, hematoxylin and eosin.

formation in acute DAD, alveolar fibrinous exudates in AFOP form rounded plugs within the alveolar spaces showing variable degrees of organization. Alveolar septal fibroblastic proliferation is not prominent in AFOP, if any. Many AFOP cases clinically manifested as acute lung injury with a similar mortality rate to DAD, suggesting that AFOP might be a histological variant of DAD (5). However, some cases follow a subacute clinical course, which suggests that some AFOP cases may represent an early form of BOOP.

The histological hallmark of BOOP is polypoid fibromyxoid tissue plugging the bronchiolar lumens, alveolar ducts, and distal airspaces, frequently forming a continuous, elongated, or serpiginous mass (Fig. 2). BOOP is a common nonspecific histological pattern in reaction to a number of injuries including infections, toxic inhalants, drugs, radiation, collagen vascular diseases, and aspiration, to name a few. Fibroblastic plugs in organizing pneumonia (OP) may contain mixed inflammatory cells including some giant cells and food particles in cases with aspiration (Figs. 3 and 4). It is frequently seen at the edge of granulomas, necrosis, tumors, abscesses, and vasculitis. Rarely, malignant cell nests may be entrapped within the intra-alveolar fibrotic tissue (Fig. 5). BOOP can be a minor component of some respiratory illnesses including hypersensitivity pneumonitis (HP), nonspecific interstitial pneumonia (NSIP), eosinophilic pneumonia (EP), and Langerhans cells histiocytosis (LCH). Idiopathic BOOP without any associated underlying condition has been well recognized as a clinicopathological entity since the report by Epler in 1985 (6).

The consensus statement by American Thoracic Society (ATS)/European Respiratory Society (ERS) used the term cryptogenic organizing pneumonia (COP) for idiopathic BOOP cases (7). It also has recommended the term "organizing pneumonia" in lieu of BOOP to describe the histological pattern (7). However, this chapter used the term BOOP throughout since BOOP has been well understood as generic descriptive term encompassing the cases with variable proportions of bronchiolitis obliterans (BO) and OP. Cases showing

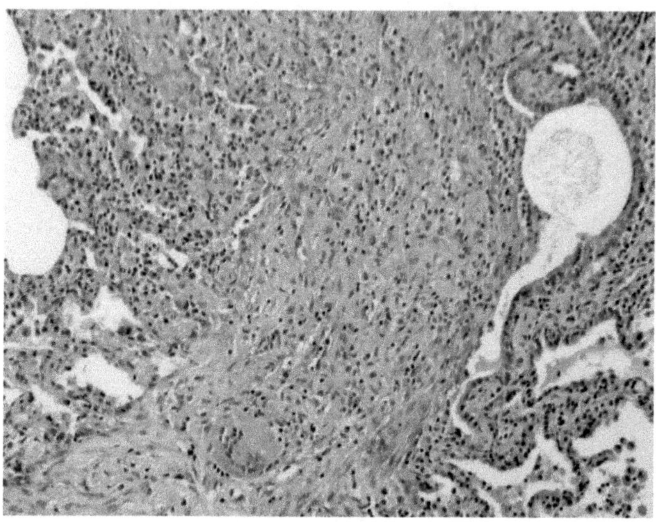

Figure 3 HP case associated with pet birds at home showing mixed inflammatory cells within the intra-alveolar Masson bodies. A few giant cells are also noted. (H&E, 200×). *Abbreviations*: HP, hypersensitivity pneumonitis; H&E, hematoxylin and eosin.

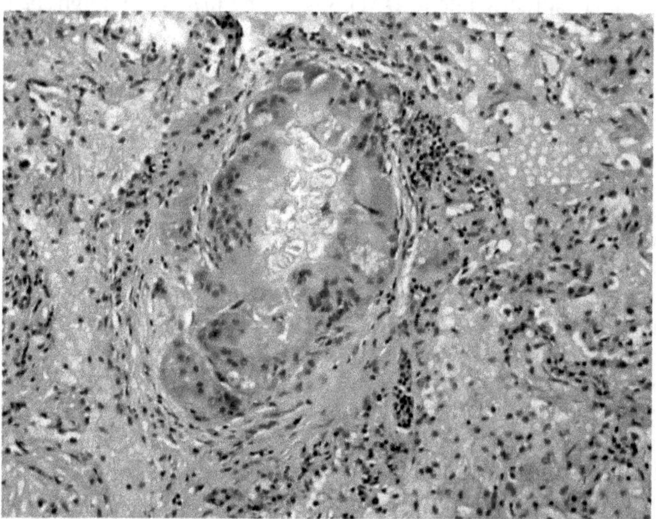

Figure 4 Vegetable matter within the intra-alveolar fibrous plug in OP secondary to chronic aspiration (H&E, 200×). *Abbreviations*: OP, organizing pneumonia; H&E, hematoxylin and eosin.

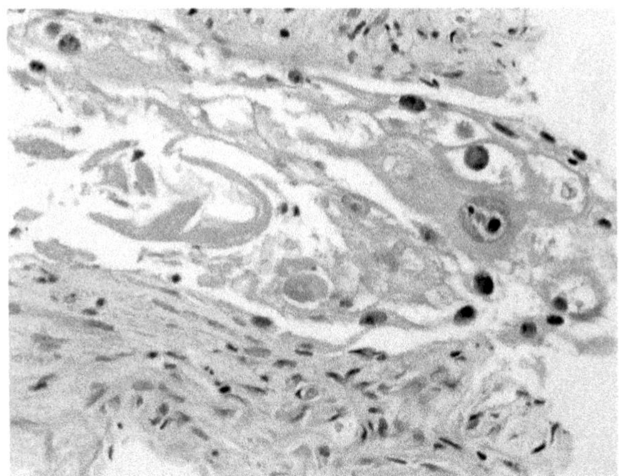

Figure 5 BOOP reaction is common in the lung tissue adjacent to tumor masses but malignant cells may be present within the BOOP area as shown. Squamous carcinoma cell nests entrapped within the fibrous plug (H&E, 200×). *Abbreviations*: BOOP, bronchiolitis obliterans organizing pneumonia; H&E, hematoxylin and eosin.

fibromyxoid plugs only in the alveolar spaces without significant bronchiolar plugging are not uncommon. On the other hand, isolated BO without histological evidence of alveolar involvement in the biopsy is a rare finding and probably represents an inadequate sampling. Thus, it could be appropriate to diagnose such cases as BOOP. However, examples of pure BO have been described and were reported to follow an unfavorable clinical course as compared to typical BOOP (8). Also, it is important to distinguish it from "obliterative bronchiolitis" (OB), which refers to a bronchiololar disease showing peribronchiolar fibrosis with luminal narrowing (9). This entity is better designated as "constrictive bronchiolitis" to avoid confusion. OB is clinically associated with BO syndrome. Pertinent issues in the diagnosis of OB are not included in the following discussion; the reader is referred to other chapters concerning small airway diseases and transplant-related pathology. BOOP may present as a discrete nodular lesion on imaging study and the patients may undergo needle biopsy or wedge resection. In such cases, it is still important to exclude the possibility of neoplasm in the vicinity.

III. Chronic Interstitial Disease with Immature Fibrosis

UIP shows temporally heterogeneous patchy interstitial fibrosis with scattered dome-shaped fibroblast foci over dense collagen deposition (Fig. 6). Some UIP cases may show very exuberant fibroblast foci, which could mimic acute lung injury. The clinical and prognostic significance of prominent fibroblast foci in UIP is not entirely clear but previous studies have suggested that the prominence of fibroblastic foci as an adverse prognostic parameter (10,11). Many methods of quantitative analysis of fibroblastic foci in UIP have been reported as well (10–13).

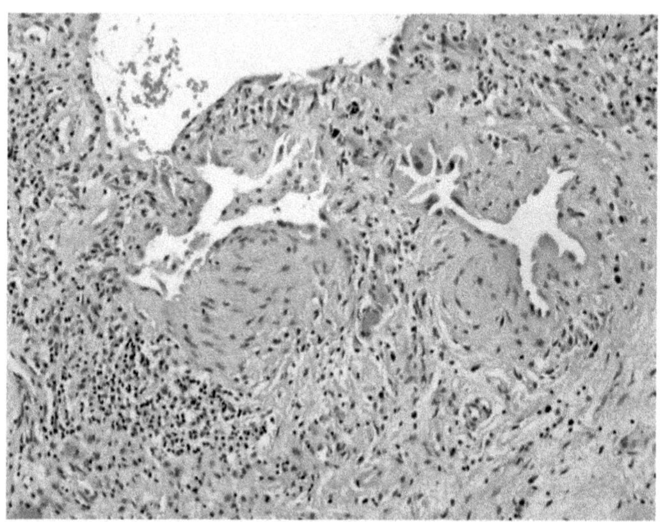

Figure 6 Dome-shaped fibroblastic foci over collagen fibrosis and architectural distortion in UIP (H&E, 200×). *Abbreviations*: UIP, usual interstitial pneumonia; H&E, hematoxylin and eosin.

It is also important to note that full-blown acute lung injury can be superimposed on UIP. Infectious etiology needs to be carefully searched in such cases. If there is no clinically or histologically apparent infection or other detectable cause, a possibility of acute exacerbation of UIP can be considered (14). The clinical criteria have been proposed by Kondoh et al. and Akira et al. (14,15): (1) acute worsening of dyspnea within 1 month of presentation, (2) new pulmonary infiltrates on chest radiography or CT scan, (3) deterioration in pulmonary function measurements or gas exchange, and (4) absence of an identifiable cause including infections or cardiovascular disease. Less commonly, other types of chronic interstitial lung diseases including fibrosing NSIP and chronic HP may have superimposed acute lung injury with acute exacerbation of the disease clinically (16). Three microscopic patterns of acute lung injury were seen in UIP and other forms of fibrotic interstitial pneumonias: DAD, OP, and a pattern of numerous very large fibroblastic foci superimposed on underlying fibrosis (16). Thus, it is imperative to examine the presence of underlying chronic abnormalities in the lung biopsies showing acute lung injury.

IV. Differential Diagnoses

Recognition of the general histopathological patterns of DAD and BOOP is the first step in interpretation of the biopsies showing predominantly immature fibrosis. Although classifying the dominant injury pattern as DAD or OP is generally not a problem in thoracoscopic or open-lung biopsies, it may be difficult in transbronchial biopsies. The histological distribution of fibrosis and radiological pattern of infiltrates tend to be diffuse in DAD but somewhat patchy in BOOP. Type II pneumocyte hyperplasia is more prominent in DAD and is an essential feature in the organizing stage of this pattern. Collections of foamy macrophages comprise endogenous lipid pneumonia and are frequently seen in BOOP due to the clinical or subclinical obstruction of small airways. Overlapping features of DAD and BOOP can be seen and the term of acute lung injury would be appropriate to indicate such cases.

Temporal uniformity of immature fibrosis and a paucity of collagen deposition in DAD and BOOP are important distinguishing features from UIP. UIP shows predominantly collagen fibrosis and minor interstitial foci of fibroblastic proliferation in the background of normal or distorted underlying lung architectures. Movat's pentachrome stain or combined elastic and trichrome stains are helpful in localizing the major site of injury, assessing the degree of collagen fibrosis, and identifying the presence of vasculitis. Appropriate histochemical or immunohistochemical stains for infectious agents are needed if clinical suspicion for infection is high and biopsies show marked acute and chronic inflammation or granulomas.

Proliferating fibroblasts are immunopositive for vimentin and sometimes for smooth muscle actin antibodies, indicating myofibroblastic differentiation, but they are generally negative for desmin. Immunohistochemical stains, though usually not necessary, can be useful in differentiating immature smooth muscle proliferation in lymphangioleimyomatosis (LAM), which is additionally positive for desmin, HMB-45, and melanoma-associated antigen recognized by T cells 1 (MART1) in addition to vimentin and smooth muscle actin. CD1a and S100 protein stains help to detect Langerhans cell collections in LCH cases. In small biopsies, inflammatory myofibroblastic tumor (IMT), also known as inflammatory pseudotumor and plasma cell granuloma, may mimic BOOP. IMT shows a spectrum of fibroblastic and myofibroblastic cellular proliferations that contain variable amount of inflammatory cells including plasma cells, lymphocytes, macrophages, and occasional eosinophils. IMT typically presents as a solitary, well-demarcated and lobulated mass on radiological study, which replaces the underlying lung tissue, in contrast to BOOP that has preserved underlying alveolar architecture (Fig. 7). In small biopsies, distinction can be difficult. Besides, IMT may show BOOP reaction at the periphery. A subset of IMT cases, especially in patients younger than 30 years of age, show strong anaplastic lymphoma

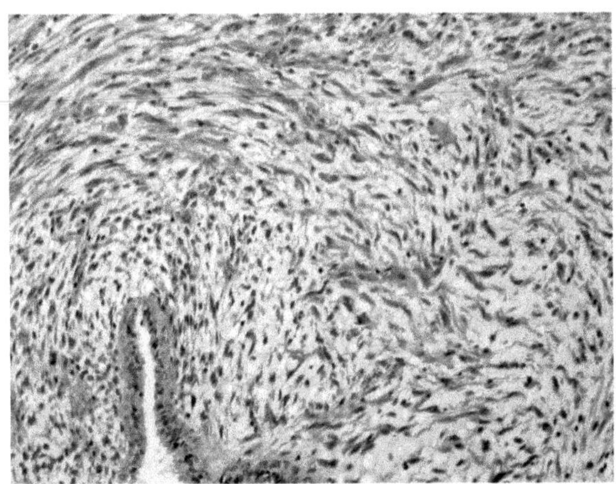

Figure 7 IMT. Myofibroblastic proliferation obliterating the underlying lung parenchyma (H&E, 200×). *Abbreviations*: IMT, inflammatory myofibroblastic tumor; H&E, hematoxylin and eosin.

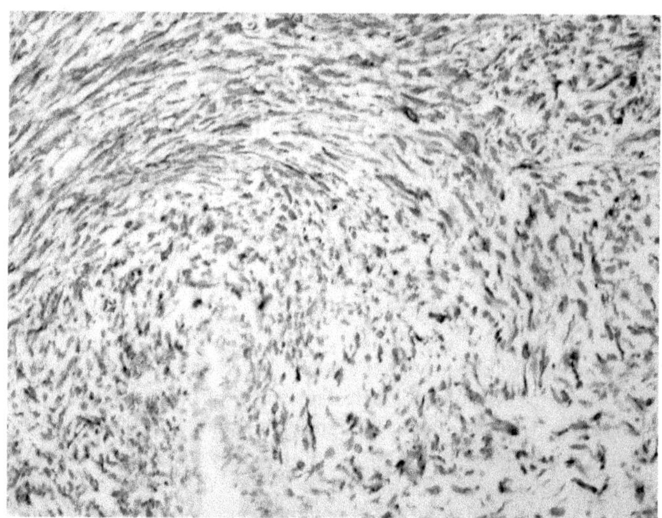

Figure 8 Diffuse positivity for ALK-1 immunostain is virtually pathognomonic for IMT in young patients with chromosomal translocation involving 2p23 (anti-ALK-1, 200×). *Abbreviations*: ALK-1, anaplastic lymphoma kinase 1; IMT, inflammatory myofibroblastic tumor.

kinase 1 (ALK-1) positivity, which would be also helpful (Fig. 8). An algorithm for histopathological differential diagnosis of immature fibrosis is summarized in Tables 1 and 2.

A wide variety of pulmonary and systemic diseases may produce the changes of DAD or BOOP. For cases in which the specific etiology cannot be identified after careful pathological and clinical evaluation, a diagnosis of idiopathic DAD or idiopathic BOOP is warranted. Idiopathic DAD [also known as acute interstitial pneumonia (AIP), Hamman-Rich

Table 1 Diagnostic Approach in Biopsies with Immature Fibrosis[a]

Predominantly Immature fibrosis:

1. Differential diagnosis with other conditions mimicking immature fibrosis e.g. LAM (HMB45/MART1/desmin +), LCH (CD1a/S100 +), IMT (ALK1 +)
2. Location of immature fibrosis
   - Interstitial: DAD
   - Intraluminal: BOOP
3. Evaluation of possible underlying chronic interstitial pneumonia e.g. acute exacerbation of UIP

Immature fibrosis as a minor component

1. Assess the pattern of chronic fibrosing pneumonia, e.g. UIP

[a]Checklist for underlying conditions: Infectious agents, granulomas, degree and pattern of inflammatory responses, tumors, abscesses, vasculitis, bronchial epithelial necrosis or metaplasia, clinical history of various therapies (drugs, radiation, transplantation, oxygen) and other events.

Abbreviations: LAM, lymphangioleimyomatosis; HMB45, human melanoma black 45; MART1, melanoma-associated antigen recognized by T cells 1; +, positive; LCH, Langerhans cells histiocytosis; IMT, inflammatory myofibroblastic tumor; ALK-1, anaplastic lymphoma kinase 1; UIP, usual interstitial pneumonia; DAD, diffuse alveolar damage; BOOP, bronchiolitis obliterans organizing pneumonia.

Table 2 Histopathological Differential Diagnosis

DAD	BOOP	UIP
Fibroblastic proliferation		
Interstitial/diffuse	Intraluminal/patchy	Interstitial/variegated
Temporally uniform	Temporally uniform	Temporally heterogeneous
Type II cell hyperplasia		
Diffuse, linear	Scattered, less conspicuous	Variable
Remnants of hyaline membranes and microthrombi		
Often present	Absent	Absent
Intra-alveolar foamy macrophage collection		
Rare	Common	Rare

Abbreviations: DAD, diffuse alveolar damage; BOOP, bronchiolitis obliterans organizing pneumonia; UIP, usual interstitial pneumonia.

disease, or accelerated interstitial pneumonitis] is a rapidly progressive, often fatal condition occurring in a previously healthy person and produces histological changes of organizing DAD (17). Idiopathic BOOP undergoes a less catastrophic course than AIP, although the onset of illness in idiopathic BOOP is still relatively acute as compared with NSIP and UIP (6). The prognosis of idiopathic BOOP is regarded as excellent, with complete recovery within weeks or months in many cases after the treatment with glucocorticoids or antibiotics or sometimes even without therapy (6). OP may present as a nodule, which results in a local resection (18). Focal OP may mimic lung cancer on radiological examination with positive contrast-enhancement CT scan and PET scan (18). Most cases of focal OP are cryptogenic and infection is identified in a minority of cases (18).

The major causes of DAD listed in Table 3 usually induce diffuse bilateral lung involvement, but some insults such as radiation injury may cause a localized reaction. Changes of BOOP may present as the primary pulmonary parenchymal abnormality

Table 3 Causes and Conditions Associated with Diffuse Alveolar Damage

1. Idiopathic	AIP, Hamman-Rich disease
2. Infectious agents	Viruses, mycoplasma, any organisms causing severe infection
3. Inhalants	Oxygen, nitrogen dioxide (silo-filler's lung), other noxious gases and fumes
4. Drugs and ingestants	Chemotherapeutic agents (bleomycin, cytoxan, methotrexate, etc.), narcotic drugs (heroin), paraquat, and others
5. Sepsis and shock of any cause	
6. Aspiration	Gastric contents, near-drowning (fresh or salt water)
7. Radiation	Thoracic irradiation for lung, mediastinal, or breast cancers
8. Miscellaneous	Trauma (pulmonary or extrapulmonary), pancreatitis, uremia, high altitude, preservation injury or severe acute rejection of lung allograft, and others

Abbreviation: AIP, acute interstitial pneumonia.

Table 4 Conditions Showing BOOP as Major (Primary) or Minor (Secondary) Component of Histological Lung Injury Pattern

A. Primary BOOP
1. Idiopathic (idiopathic BOOP)
2. Organizing infections (bacterial, viral, mycoplasmal)
3. Collagen vascular diseases (rheumatoid arthritis, SLE, dermatomyositis, etc.)
4. Drugs (bleomycin, amiodarone, gold, etc.)
5. Toxic inhalants (silo-filler's lung)

B. Secondary BOOP
1. Periphery of mass or nodular lesions (tumors, granulomas, abscesses, infarcts, Wegener's granulomatosis)
2. Distal to proximal bronchial obstruction (tumors, foreign bodies)
3. Component of inflammatory lung disorders (chronic EP, HP, eosinophilic granuloma)
4. Adjacent to any severe lung disorders

Abbreviations: BOOP, bronchiolitis obliterans organizing pneumonia; SLE, systemic lupus erythematosus; EP, eosinophilic pneumonia; HP, hypersensitivity pneumonitis.

associated with a causative etiology. BOOP may occur as a secondary reaction at the periphery of a mass or nodular lesion (neoplasms, abscesses, infarcts, Wegener's granulomatosis, etc.) or as a minor component of other significant inflammatory lesions such as hypersensitivity pneumonia and chronic EP. The primary and secondary causes of BOOP are summarized in Table 4. Diagnostic problems in relatively common conditions that often present as DAD and/or BOOP on histopathological examination are discussed briefly in the following section.

V. Pulmonary Disorders Commonly Presenting as DAD or BOOP

A. Infectious Pneumonia

Recognition of the common lung injury patterns by different microorganisms may be useful in narrowing down the differential diagnosis, although specific histopathological diagnosis of infectious pneumonia requires special histochemical and immunostains, typical cytopathic changes for some viruses, or microbiological cultures. Virus, especially cytomegalovirus (CMV) or herpes simplex virus (HSV), in immunocompromised hosts may be the most frequently encountered etiology among infectious agents for the changes of DAD. DAD, caused by viral pneumonia, usually accompanies diffuse interstitial and perivascular infiltrates of chronic inflammatory cells and sometimes shows marked reactive and metaplastic changes in the bronchiolar epithelium, with or without viral inclusions. Organizing bacterial, mycoplasmal, and *Legionella* pneumonia usually show the pattern of BOOP rather than DAD. Dr. Liebow had postulated that viral pneumonia superimposed by bacterial pneumonia is a common cause of BOOP (unpublished communication). Necrotizing granulomatous inflammation is predominant in fungal and mycobacterial pneumonia; it may show a pattern of BOOP at the periphery of the granulomas as a secondary change. Secondary BOOP is frequently seen in the lung parenchyma adjacent to the abscesses or suppurative inflammation caused by pulmonary actinomycosis and nocardiosis. *Pneumocystis carinii* pneumonia rarely causes the changes of DAD in severely immunocompromised hosts.

B. Collagen Vascular Diseases

Histopathological changes in the lungs associated with the specific types of collagen vascular diseases vary greatly, as do clinical manifestations. DAD with or without active vasculitis and hemorrhage can be seen in systemic lupus erythematosus (SLE). BOOP is another frequent pattern in SLE as well as in rheumatoid arthritis. Rheumatoid arthritis may also show follicular bronchiolitis, vascular changes, and rheumatoid nodules. Scleroderma tends to present as pulmonary hypertension with a collagen type of chronic interstitial fibrosis rather than immature fibrosis. Lymphocytic interstitial pneumonia is characteristic of Sjögren's syndrome, but features of BOOP can also be seen. UlP-like reaction has been described in most collagen vascular diseases as a late manifestation of pulmonary involvement.

C. Drug-Induced Pulmonary Diseases

Correlation with a history of drug therapy is crucial in the interpretation of any biopsies showing DAD or BOOP, since many commonly used drugs may cause these pulmonary reactions (19,20). Pulmonary reaction to drugs may be dose-related toxicity or idiosyncratic phenomena. A toxic pulmonary reaction histologically manifests as DAD in most cases, and cytotoxic chemotherapeutic agents have most frequently been implicated as causes of drug-induced pulmonary toxicity. Bleomycin, one of the best-characterized pulmonary toxic agents, causes dose- and time-dependent alveolar damage similar to that of organizing DAD in humans and animal models and may result in irreversible fibrosis, especially when administered in high doses or combined with thoracic irradiation (21). Nonspecific but supportive findings for cytotoxic drug reactions include marked cytological atypia in alveolar lining cells and unusual intranuclear tubular structures within type II cells on electron microscopy (19). Histological features associated with idiosyncratic and allergic reaction to drugs include BOOP, OB, and EP, to name a few (20). Temporal eligibility, responses to rechallenge and dechallenge, known histopathological patterns of specific drugs, and exclusion of other causes are important factors for identifying pulmonary drug reactions.

D. Oxygen Toxicity

A high concentration of inspired oxygen is one of the most common causes of DAD among hospitalized patients receiving mechanical ventilation. Underlying lung diseases, often present in individuals requiring mechanical ventilation, may complicate histopathological changes of DAD. Bronchopulmonary dysplasia (BPD) is a complex structural and physiological alteration of the neonatal lungs, similar but not identical to DAD in adults. BPD was first identified in premature infants with hyaline membrane diseases who were treated with high concentrations of inspired oxygen. Subsequent studies have shown that mechanical ventilation alone with, or occasionally without, high oxygen concentrations can induce the development of BPD, suggesting BPD as a variant of DAD associated with oxygen toxicity and barotrauma in neonates and infants. Necrosis of bronchiolar epithelium and fibromyxoid plugging of small airways, simulating the features of BOOP, are frequently seen in acute and subacute stages of BPD.

E. Changes in Allograft Lungs

DAD in allograft lungs may represent a severe infectious pneumonia (especially viral), perioperative (reperfusion/ischemic, preservation) lung injury, or severe acute cellular rejection (grade A4). In grade A4 acute rejection, there are diffuse perivascular, interstitial, and airspace infiltrates of mononuclear cells as well as prominent alveolar pneumocyte damage associated with intra-alveolar necrotic cells, macrophages, hyaline membranes, hemorrhage, and neutrophils (22). The above changes may be accompanied by parenchymal necrosis, infarction, or necrotizing vasculitis (22). Posttransplantation acute lung injury (preservation injury) manifests histologically as DAD relatively early in the course after transplantation, not necessarily causing full-blown clinical ARDS. DAD in preservation injury may accompany scattered intra-alveolar neutrophils and acute bronchiolitis, in contrast to the prominent perivascular and interstitial mononuclear cell infiltrates in severe acute rejection (22).

BOOP-like reaction in the allograft lungs have been reported to be associated with infection, ischemic injury, and acute rejection (23). A recent study reported changes of BOOP in 17 out of 163 allograft lungs, including transbronchial biopsies, open-lung biopsies, and autopsies between 2 and 43 months (mean, 8.5 months) after transplantation (24). The BOOP pattern in allograft lungs was most often associated with acute rejection (23,24) and has been suggested as a possible predictor of the later development of OB, an irreversible outcome of chronic rejection (24).

VI. Summary

Immature interstitial and intra-alveolar fibrosis usually parallels ongoing acute and subacute lung damage and is a potentially reversible process. Organizing DAD and BOOP represent the major stereotypical pulmonary reaction patterns of predominantly immature fibrosis in response to variety of lung injuries. Fibroblastic proliferation is mainly localized to alveolar septa in DAD as opposed to intraluminal spaces in BOOP. Idiopathic cases of DAD and BOOP show distinctive clinicopathological manifestations despite an apparently similar pathogenesis and some overlapping pathological features. Acute lung injury may be superimposed on chronic interstitial lung diseases especially UIP. Identification of underlying conditions and etiologies for DAD and BOOP requires thorough examination of associated histopathological changes in the background and careful correlation with clinical and radiological findings.

References

1. Yi ES, Lee H, Yin S, et al. Platelet-derived growth factor causes pulmonary cell proliferation and collagen deposition in vivo. Am J Pathol 1996; 149:539–548.
2. Myers JL, Katzenstein ALA. Ultrastructural evidence of alveolar epithelial injury in idiopathic bronchiolitis obliterans–organizing pneumonia. Am J Pathol 1988; 132:102–109.
3. Kazenstein ALA, Askin FB. Acute lung injury patterns: diffuse alveolar damage, acute interstitial pneumonia, bronchiolitis obliterans–organizing pneumonia. In: Kazenstein ALA, Askin FB, eds. Surgical Pathology of Non-neoplastic Lung Diseases. Philadelphia: Saunders, 1990:9–57.

4. Fukuda Y, Ishizaki M, Masuda Y, et al. The role of intraalveolar fibrosis in the process of pulmonary structural remodeling in patients with diffuse alveolar damage. Am J Pathol 1987; 126:171–182.
5. Beasley MB, Franks TJ, Galvin JR, et al. Acute fibrinous and organizing pneumonia. A histologic pattern of lung injury and possible variant of diffuse alveolar damage. Arch Pathol Lab Med 2002; 126:1064–1070.
6. Epler GR, Colby TV, Mcleod TC, et al. Bronchiolitis obliterans–organizing pneumonia. N Engl J Med 1985; 312:152–158.
7. American Thoracic Society/European Respiratory Society International Multidisciplinary Consensus Classification Of The Idiopathic Interstitial Pneumonias, . This joint statement of the American Thoracic Society (ATS), and the European Respiratory Society (ERS) was adopted by the ATS board of directors, June 2001 and by the ERS Executive Committee, June 2001. Am J Respir Crit Care Med 2002; 165:277–304.
8. Guerry-Force ML, Muller NL, Wright JL, et al. A comparison of bronchiolitis obliterans–organizing pneumonia, usual interstitial pneumonia, and small airway disease. Am Rev Respir Dis 1987; 135:705–712.
9. Glanville A, Baldwin J, Burke C, et al. Obliterative bronchiolitis after hear-lung transplantation: apparent arrest by augmented immunosuppression. Ann Intern Med 1987; 107:300–304.
10. King TE, Schwartz MI, Brown K, et al. Idiopathic pulmonary fibrosis: relationship between histopathologic features and mortality. Am J Respir Crit Care Med 2001; 164:1025–1032.
11. Nicholson AG, Fulford LG, Colby TV, et al. The relationship between individual histologic features and disease progression in idiopathic pulmonary fibrosis. Am J Respir Crit Care Med 2002; 166:173–177.
12. Cherniack RM, Colby TV, Flint A, et al. Quantitative assessment of lung pathology in idiopathic pulmonary fibrosis: the BAL Cooperative Group Steering Committee. Am Rev Respir Dis 1001; 144:892–900.
13. Enomoto NE, Takafumi S, Kato M, et al. Quantitative analysis of fibroblastic foci in usual interstitial pneumonia. Chest 2006; 130:22–29.
14. Kondoh Y, Taniguchi H, Kawabata Y, et al. Acute exacerbation in idiopathic pulmonary fibrosis. Analysis of clinical and pathologic findings in three cases. Chest 1993; 103:1808–1812.
15. Akira M, Hamada H, Sakatani M, et al. CT findings during phase of accelerated deterioration in patients with idiopathic pulmonary fibrosis. AJR Am J Roentgenol 1997; 168:79–83.
16. Churg A, Muller NL, Silva IS, et al. Acute exacerbation (acute lung injury of unknown cause) in UIP and other forms of fibrotic interstitial pneumonias. Am J Surg Pathol 2007; 31:277–284.
17. Olson J, Colby TV. Hamman-Rich syndrome revisited. Mayo Clin Proc 1990; 65:1538–1548.
18. Maldonado F, Daniels CE, Hoffman EA, et al. Focal organizing pneumonia on surgical lung biopsy. Causes, clinicoradiologic features, and outcomes. Chest 2007; 132:1579–1583.
19. Cooper J, White D, Matthay R. Drag-induced pulmonary disease: Part 1. Cytotoxic drugs. Am Rev Respir Dis 1986; 133:321–340.
20. Cooper J, White D, Matthay R. Drug-induced pulmonary disease. Part 2: Noncytotoxic drugs. Am Rev Respir Dis 1986; 133:488–505.
21. Yi ES, Williams S, Malicki DM, et al. Keratinocyte growth factor ameliorates radiation and bleomycin-induced lung injury and mortality. Am J Pathol 1996; 149:1963–1970.
22. Yousem SA, Berry GJ, Cagle PT, et al. Revision of the 1990 working formulation for the classification of pulmonary allograft rejection: Lung Rejection Study Group. J Heart Lung Transplant 1996; 15:1–15.
23. Yousem SA, Steven RD, Griffith BP. Interstitial and airspace granulation tissue reactions in lung transplant recipients. Am J Surg Pathol 1992; 16:877–884.
24. Chaparro C, Chamberlain D, Maurer J, et al. Bronchiolitis obliterans organizing pneumonia (BOOP) in lung transplant recipients. Chest 1996; 110:1150–1154.

8
Intra-alveolar Exudates and Infiltrates

MARY BETH BEASLEY
Mount Sinai Medical Center, New York, New York, U.S.A.

I. Introduction

Intra-alveolar infiltrates are frequently encountered, either as the primary pathologic process or as secondary reactions in the setting of other pulmonary parenchymal diseases. Such infiltrates may be relatively acellular and consist of eosinophilic material or fibrin, or they may be cellular, usually consisting of inflammatory cells, macrophages or fibroblastic proliferations. The focus of this chapter will be to address the pulmonary disorders in which intra-alveolar infiltrates are the primary pathologic process. Those in which an associated interstitial process is also a component or are otherwise included in another chapter will be covered elsewhere as indicated.

II. Pulmonary Edema

Pulmonary edema is usually secondary to a passive increase in pulmonary venous pressure, but may also result from a direct insult to the alveolar capillaries. Histologically, edema is characterized by the intra-alveolar accumulation of finely granular eosinophilic material (Fig. 1). Vascular congestion is frequently present and mild interstitial widening may also been seen. The eosinophilic material lacks the coarse granularity, large granules, and cholesterol clefts seen in alveolar proteinosis. Similarly, edema fluid lacks the foamy vacuolated appearance of the exudates seen in association with Pneumocystis infection.

III. Pulmonary Alveolar Proteinosis

Pulmonary alveolar proteinosis (PAP) is a rare disorder characterized by the accumulation of proteinaceous, surfactant-like material within the alveolar spaces. The mechanism has been largely unknown but was previously thought to be secondary to a defect in surfactant clearance either by macrophages or lymphatics. More recent research has demonstrated that defective function of granulocyte macrophage colony stimulating factor (GM-CSF) is involved in the development of this disorder, and autoantibodies to GM-CSF have been demonstrated in patients with PAP, suggesting that PAP may in fact be autoimmune in origin (1). PAP may be idiopathic but may also occur in the setting of immunodeficiency or underlying malignancies, especially lymphoproliferative disorders. PAP may also occur in the setting of massive exposure to silica producing so-called "silicoproteinosis." Coexisting

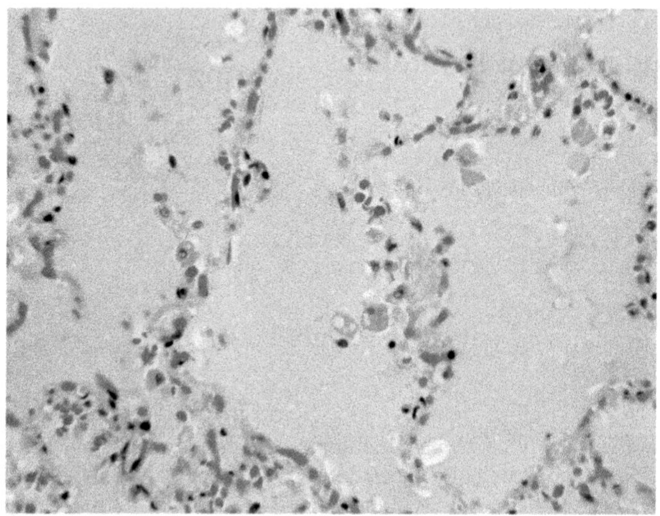

Figure 1 Pulmonary edema is characterized by finely granular, eosinophilic material within alveolar spaces (H&E, 200×). *Abbreviation*: H&E, hematoxylin and eosin.

infection with Nocardia may also occur (2). Rarely, PAP may occur as a complication of lung transplantation (3).

PAP is characterized histologically by the accumulation of coarsely granular eosinophilic material comprising protein and lipid. Large granules and cholesterol clefts may be observed, which help distinguish PAP from pulmonary edema (Fig. 2). The surrounding alveolar septa are relatively unremarkable. The material is characteristically PAS positive (2).

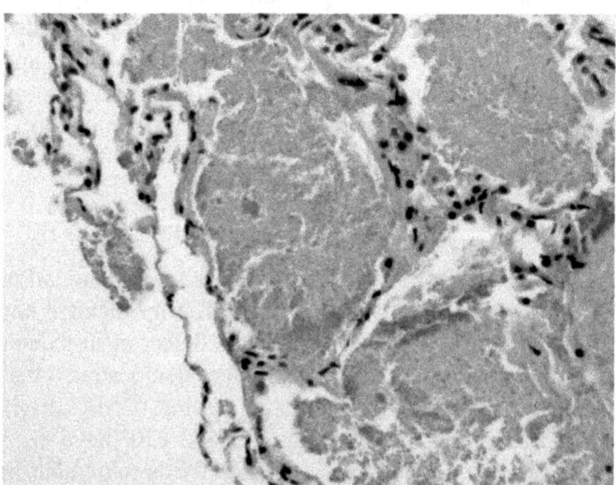

Figure 2 Pulmonary alveolar proteinosis is characterized by coarsely granular proteinaceous material that may contain larger granules (H&E, 200×). *Abbreviation*: H&E, hematoxylin and eosin.

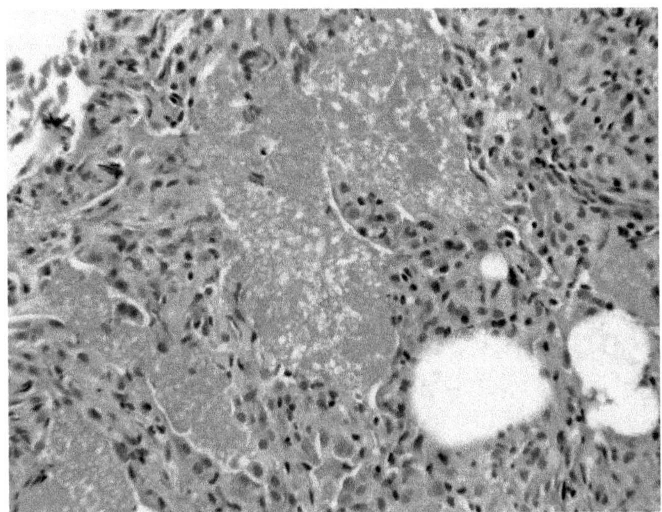

Figure 3 Pneumocystis pneumonia is classically characterized by frothy vacuolated intra-alveolar exudates (H&E 200×). *Abbreviation*: H&E, hematoxylin and eosin.

IV. *Pneumocystis jiroveci* Pneumonia

Pneumocystis jiroveci (formerly *carinii*) classically produces a pneumonia characterized by the intra-alveolar accumulation of frothy eosinophilic intra-alveolar exudates. Chronic inflammation is present to varying degrees in the interstitium, but is generally mild in degree. The intra-alveolar material has a vacuolated appearance secondary to the presence of organisms (Fig. 3). GMS stains readily identify the organisms that are roughly five microns in diameter and may have a central dark region (Fig. 4). While this histologic pattern is the most typical produced by pneumocystis infection, the organisms may produce a wide range of findings, including interstitial accumulation of the exudates, a nonspecific interstitial pneumonia pattern, or relatively minimal histologic change (4,5).

V. Acute Fibrinous and Organizing Pneumonia

Acute fibrinous and organizing pneumonia (AFOP) is a relatively recently described pattern of acute lung injury characterized by the presence of intra-alveolar fibrin balls (Fig. 5). Varying degrees of associated organizing fibroblastic tissue may be present, which often retain a central fibrin core. The alveolar septa contain mild-to-moderate chronic inflammatory cell infiltrates. Classic hyaline membranes are not present and significant eosinophils or neutrophils are not seen. As intra-alveolar fibrin may occur as a secondary reaction adjacent to an unrelated process such as a necrotizing granuloma, or may be found focally in cases otherwise showing typical features of diffuse alveolar damage (DAD), a diagnosis of AFOP should be restricted to cases in which large biopsy specimen has been obtained. At

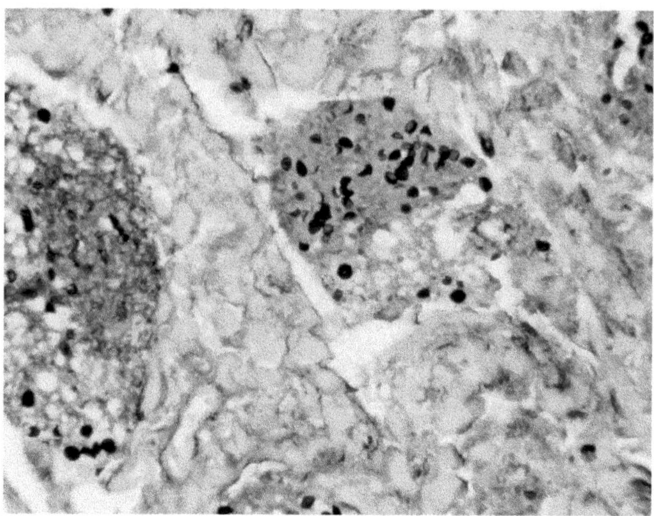

Figure 4 Pneumocystis pneumonia: numerous pneumocystis organisms are present within the alveolar exudates (GMS, 200×). *Abbreviation*: GMS, Grocott Methenamine Silver.

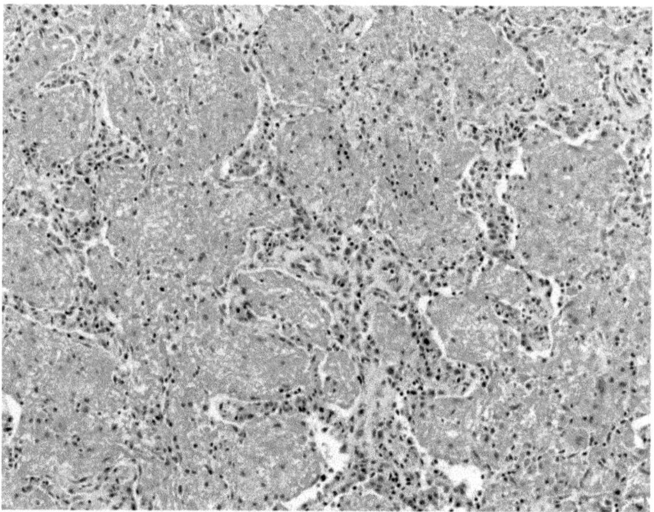

Figure 5 Acute fibrinous and organizing pneumonia is characterized by organizing balls of intra-alveolar fibrin without associated hyaline membrane formation or significant eosinophils (H&E, 100×). *Abbreviation*: H&E, hematoxylin and eosin.

present, AFOP appears to most likely represent a histologic variant of DAD, with most cases of AFOP having a similar clinical course and outcome. However, a significant number of patients experienced an indolent clinical course with eventual recovery. Clinically, AFOP appears to be associated with a wide spectrum of underlying etiologies or may be idiopathic, similar to other forms of acute lung injury (6).

The differential diagnosis of AFOP primarily includes eosinophilic pneumonia, organizing pneumonia and DAD. Eosinophilic pneumonia may greatly resemble AFOP as prominent intra-alveolar fibrin may be present; however, macrophages and prominent eosinophils are not features of AFOP. Eosinophils disappear very quickly following initiation of steroid therapy and therefore it may be difficult to separate partially treated eosinophilic pneumonia from AFOP on histologic grounds in patients who have received steroids prior to biopsy. The clinical finding of peripheral blood eosinophilia, typical of eosionophilic pneumonia, has not been documented thus far in AFOP and may be an important discriminating point. Organizing pneumonia is characterized by intra-alveolar plugs of organizing fibroblastic tissue, but does not exhibit the prominent fibrin present in AFOP. Additionally, the organizing fibroblastic tissue seen in some cases of AFOP often retains a central fibrin core. Organizing fibrin may be observed in DAD, but the finding of typical hyaline membranes separates DAD from AFOP (6).

VI. Eosinophilic Pneumonia

Eosinophilic pneumonia is characterized by varying amounts of intra-alveolar fibrin and macrophages admixed with large numbers of eosinophils. Eosinophilic pneumonia has overlapping histologic features with AFOP which are discussed above. Eosinophilic pneumonia is discussed in detail in chapter 10.

VII. Organizing Pneumonia

Organizing pneumonia is characterized by intra-alveolar organizing fibroblastic tissue, which is patchy and bronchiolocentric in distribution. The interstitium contains relatively sparse chronic inflammation. The distinction between organizing pneumonia and AFOP is discussed above and organizing pneumonia is discussed in detail in chapter 7.

VIII. Acute Bronchopneumonia/Lobar Pneumonia

Acute pneumonia is characterized by the accumulation of neutrophils within alveolar spaces and bronchiolar lumens (Fig. 6). When the distribution is patchy and centered around bronchioles, the term *bronchopneumonia* is used. Although infrequently seen today, lobar pneumonia is characterized by confluent filling of alveolar spaces with neutrophils, classically involving essentially an entire lobe. Most cases of acute pneumonia are caused by bacteria, and while the histologic findings may provide clues to the causative organism, correlation with culture results is required for definitive identification. Acute pneumonia may result in abscess formation or an associated empyema. The finding of associated giant cells should prompt a search for aspirated material which typically may be observable as vegetable material or skeletal muscle fragments (7,8).

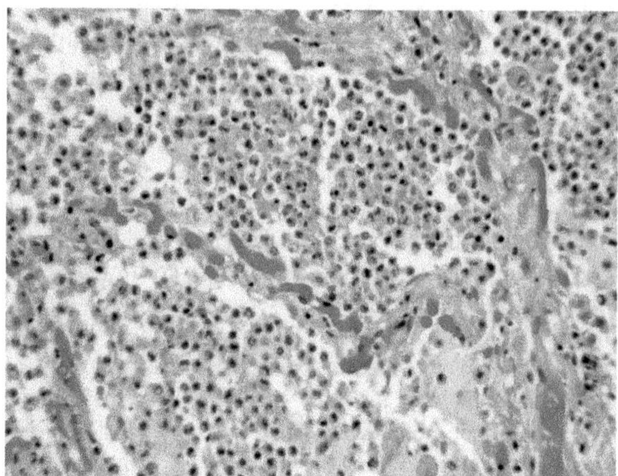

Figure 6 Acute pneumonia is characterized by the accumulation of neutrophils within the alveolar spaces and bronchiolar lumens (H&E, 100×). *Abbreviation*: H&E, hematoxylin and eosin.

IX. Endogenous Lipid Pneumonia/Obstructive Pneumonia

Pneumonia secondary to obstruction typically contains abundant finely vacuolated macrophages (Fig. 7). An associated acute pneumonia may be present to varying degrees. The lipid material in this situation is due to impaired clearance of cellular breakdown products that are phagocytized by macrophages. Finely vacuolated lipid macrophages may be present to some degree in association with any type of small-airway obstruction; however, the presence of this finding to a significant extent should prompt a search for an obstructing endobronchial lesion (8).

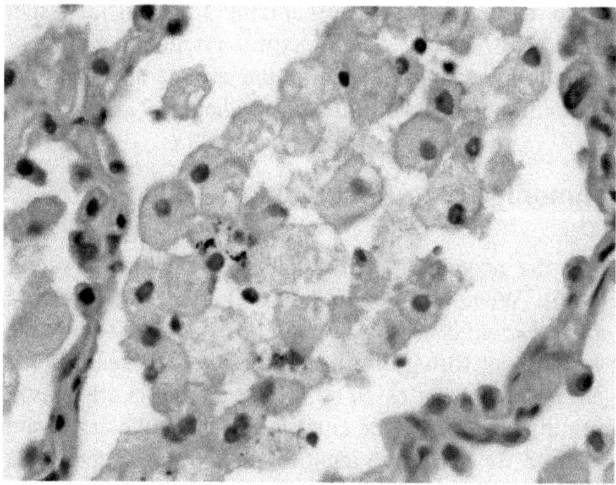

Figure 7 Endogenous lipid pneumonia is characterized by the accumulation of macrophages containing relatively uniform small lipid vacuoles. This process is typically a secondary reaction to airway obstruction (H&E, 400×). *Abbreviation*: H&E, hematoxylin and eosin.

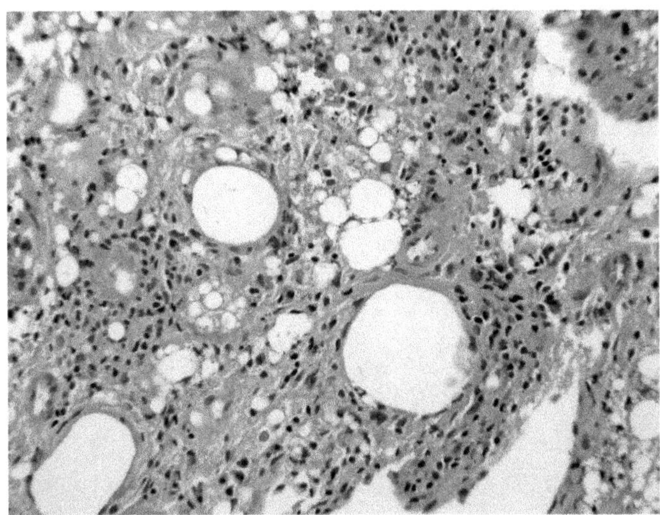

Figure 8 Exogenous lipid pneumonia is characterized by large, variably sized lipid vacuoles surrounded by varying degrees of fibrosis and foreign body giant cell reaction (H&E, 200×). *Abbreviation*: H&E, hematoxylin and eosin.

X. Exogenous Lipid Pneumonia

Exogenous lipid pneumonia is characterized by large variably shaped lipid vacuoles, which are usually associated with a foreign body type giant cell reaction (Fig. 8). Exogenous lipid pneumonia, as the name implies, occurs secondary to the aspiration of oily materials. The process begins within the alveoli, but over time the aspirated lipid elicits a fibrotic reaction that may form a mass lesion. Necrosis may also be present. The finding of giant cells and necrosis may cause confusion with a granulomatous process, but the giant cells in exogenous lipid pneumonia are found surrounding the lipid material, which may be present only as clear spaces. True granulomas composed of epithelioid histiocytes are not seen (8,9).

XI. Respiratory Bronchiolitis/Desquamative Interstitial Pneumonia

Respiratory bronchiolitis is characterized by the accumulation of macrophages within alveolar spaces and bronchiolar lumens. The macrophages contain finely granular brown pigment that may be positive with iron stains (Fig. 9). Bronchiolar metaplasia of adjacent alveolar spaces and associated small-airway remodeling may be variably present. The accumulation of pigmented macrophages may be found in transbronchial biopsies from almost every patient who smokes and may or may not be of clinical significance. However, in the setting of symptomatic lung disease in which respiratory bronchiolitis is the only finding on wedge biopsy, the term respiratory bronchiolitis interstitial lung disease (RB-ILD) is appropriate (10). Desquamative interstitial pneumonia (DIP), in comparison, is characterized by the relatively diffuse accumulation of intra-alveolar pigmented macrophages (Fig. 10). DIP and RB-ILD are thought to represent a spectrum of cigarette

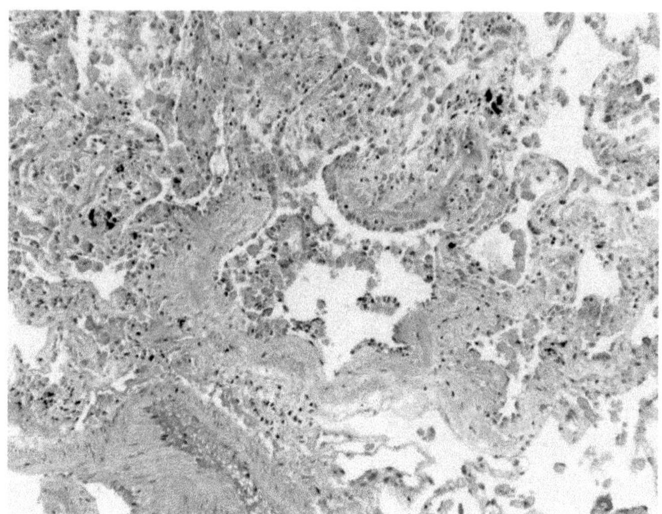

Figure 9 Respiratory bronchiolitis is characterized by the accumulation of macrophages containing finely granular brown pigment in the small airways and immediately adjacent alveolar spaces (H&E, 100×). *Abbreviation*: H&E, hematoxylin and eosin.

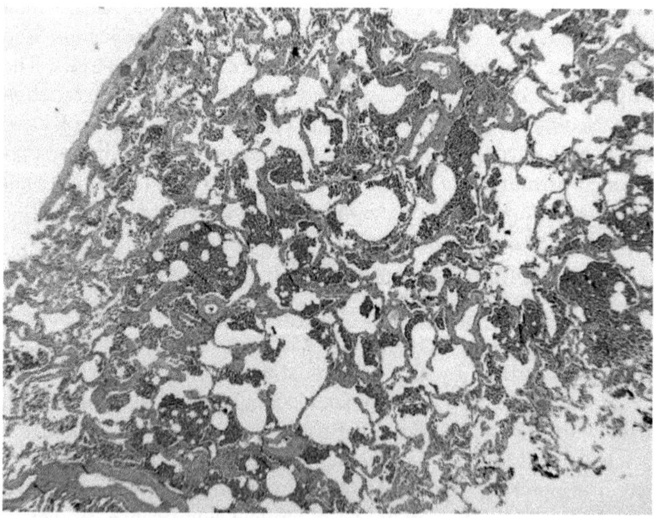

Figure 10 Desquamative interstitial pneumonia is characterized by the relatively diffuse accumulation of macrophages containing finely granular brown pigment (H&E, 50×). *Abbreviation*: H&E, hematoxylin and eosin.

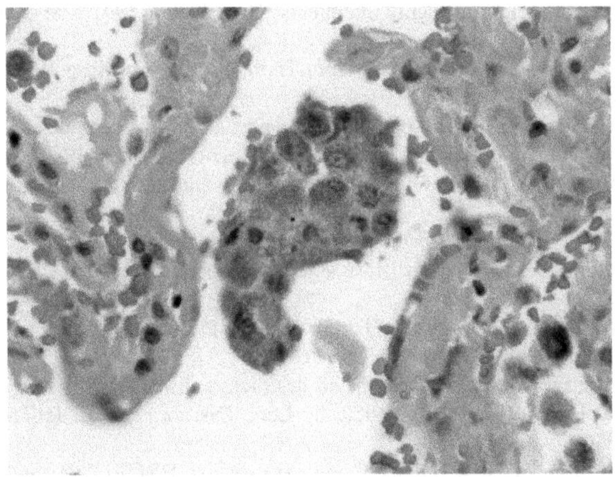

Figure 11 Alveolar hemorrhage is characterized by macrophages containing coarse hemosiderin, in contrast to the finely granular pigment seen in respiratory bronchiolitis or DIP (H&E, 200×). *Abbreviation*: H&E, hematoxylin and eosin.

smoking–associated interstitial lung disease, although some cases of DIP do occasionally occur in the absence of a smoking history (11–13). The background lung in both disorders is relatively unremarkable, particularly in RB-ILD. DIP may have associated interstitial chronic inflammation or some minimal fibrosis, but the macrophages remain the dominant finding. As accumulation of macrophages (so-called "DIP-like reaction") may occur in association with most interstitial lung disease, the presence of significant fibrosis should prompt consideration of other interstitial lung diseases such as usual interstitial pneumonia, the fibrosing subtype of nonspecific interstitial pneumonia or pulmonary Langerhans cell histiocytosis (11,14).

XII. Alveolar Hemorrhage

Alveolar hemorrhage is characterized by the accumulation of macrophages containing coarse refractile hemosiderin granules (Fig. 11), in contrast to the finely granular pigment seen in respiratory bronchiolitis. Such macrophages may be seen to some degree in association with cardiac failure, but in the situation of a lung biopsy in a patient with hemoptysis, they are usually the hallmark of a pulmonary hemorrhage syndrome, often in association with capillaritis or large vessel vasculitis. These disorders are discussed in detail in chapter 13.

References

1. Bonfield TL, Russell D, Burgess S, et al. Autoantibodies against granulocyte macrophage colony-stimulating factor are diagnostic for pulmonary alveolar proteinosis. Am J Respir Cell Mol Biol 2002; 27(4):481–486.
2. Goldstein LS, Kavuru MS, Curtis-McCarthy P, et al. Pulmonary alveolar proteinosis: clinical features and outcomes. Chest 1998; 114(5):1357–1362.

3. Yousem SA. Alveolar lipoproteinosis in lung allograft recipients. Hum Pathol 1997; 28(12): 1383–1386.
4. Travis WD. Surgical pathology of pulmonary infections. Semin Thorac Cardiovasc Surg 1995; 7(2):62–69.
5. Travis WD, Pittaluga S, Lipschik GY, et al. Atypical pathologic manifestations of Pneumocystis carinii pneumonia in the acquired immune deficiency syndrome. Review of 123 lung biopsies from 76 patients with emphasis on cysts, vascular invasion, vasculitis, and granulomas. Am J Surg Pathol 1990; 14(7):615–625.
6. Beasley MB, Franks TJ, Galvin JR, et al. Acute fibrinous and organizing pneumonia: a histological pattern of lung injury and possible variant of diffuse alveolar damage. Arch Pathol Lab Med 2002; 126(9):1064–1070.
7. Winn W, Chandler F. Bacterial Infections. In: Dail DH, Hammar SP, ed. Pulmonary Pathology. 2nd ed. New York: Springer-Verlag, 1994:255–330.
8. Katzenstein AL. Miscellaneous: nonspecific inflammatory and destructive disease of the lung. Katzenstein and Askin's Surgical Pathology of Non-neoplastic Lung Disease. 3rd ed. Philadelphia: W.B. Saunders Co., 1997:417–441.
9. Laurent F, Philippe JC, Vergier B, et al. Exogenous lipoid pneumonia: HRCT, MR, and pathologic findings. Eur Radiol 1999; 9(6):1190–1196.
10. Myers JL, Veal CF Jr., Shin MS, et al. Respiratory bronchiolitis causing interstitial lung disease. A clinicopathologic study of six cases. Am Rev Respir Dis 1987; 135(4):880–884.
11. Aubry MC, Wright JL, Myers JL. The pathology of smoking-related lung diseases. Clin Chest Med 2000; 21(1):11–35, vii.
12. Craig PJ, Wells AU, Doffman S, et al. Desquamative interstitial pneumonia, respiratory bronchiolitis and their relationship to smoking. Histopathology 2004; 45(3):275–282.
13. Yousem SA, Colby TV, Gaensler EA. Respiratory bronchiolitis-associated interstitial lung disease and its relationship to desquamative interstitial pneumonia. Mayo Clin Proc 1989; 64(11):1373–1380.
14. Travis WD, Matsui K, Moss J, et al. Idiopathic nonspecific interstitial pneumonia: prognostic significance of cellular and fibrosing patterns: survival comparison with usual interstitial pneumonia and desquamative interstitial pneumonia. Am J Surg Pathol 2000; 24(1):19–33.

9
Clinical Diagnosis of Intra-alveolar Infiltrates and Exudates

LESLIE H. ZIMMERMAN
Veterans Administration Medical Center, San Francisco, California, U.S.A.

I. Introduction

Alveolar filling processes represent a wide variety of infectious, inflammatory, and idiopathic diseases. A specific approach starts with clues from the history, physical examination, and chest radiograph. Intra-alveolar processes (i.e., alveoli filled with blood, water, lipoproteinaceous material, or inflammatory cells with or without infectious organisms) typically have acinar filling patterns with or without air bronchograms on chest radiographs. For a specific diagnosis, additional studies such as sputum examination, examination of pleural fluid (if present), blood studies, plain and/or computed tomographic (CT) radiography, pulmonary function tests, bronchoscopy, or lung biopsy may be necessary. In some cases, an empirical therapeutic trial is appropriate and, when successful, will strengthen a presumptive diagnosis (Table 1).

II. Bacterial Pneumonia

Mycoplasma pneumoniae, *Streptococcus pneumoniae*, *Chlamydophila pneumoniae*, *Legionella*, and *Haemophilus influenzae* are the most common pathogens of community-acquired bacterial pneumonia in immunocompetent adults without coexistent medical illnesses (1). The rate of pneumonia increases with in patients with immunocompromise, structural lung disease, exposure to and colonization with organisms and a variety of other factors. The risk of pneumococcal pneumonia increases with age, smoking, asthma, COPD, alcoholism, asplenia, and B-cell defects. Bacterial pneumonia is more common in patients with HIV infection and the incidence increases as HIV immunosuppression progresses. *S. pneumoniae* is the most commonly isolated bacterial pathogen in this population. Patients with poor dental hygiene and alcoholism are at increased risk for infection from oral anaerobes; sites of pneumonias and cavities in these patients are typically in gravity-dependent portions of the lung. In addition to anaerobic infection, cavitation can also occur with *Staphylococcus aureus* or gram-negative bacteria. Bronchogenic cancer, particularly squamous cell carcinoma, can also cavitate and should be considered in patients with poor radiographic resolution despite appropriate antibiotics. Recently hospitalized patients or nursing home residents are at increased risk for gram-negative bacilli and *S. aureus* pneumonia. *S. aureus* pneumonia also occurs more commonly in patients with intravenous

Table 1 Intra-alveolar Infiltrates and Exudates

Diagnosis	History and physical	Chest radiograph	Sputum examination	Laboratory, pulmonary function, and other supportive tests
Bacterial pneumonia	Acute onset, fever, dyspnea, cough with purulent sputum, rales, egophony; if pleural effusion, dullness to percussion	Lobar and lobular distribution; pleural effusion may be present	Purulent, microscopically may have predominant organism	Elevated WBC with left shift
Atypical infectious pneumonia	Acute to subacute onset, fever, dyspnea, cough may be nonproductive, rales	Typically lobular or interstitial infiltrates; pleural effusion less common than usual bacterial	Scant, microscopically often no predominant organism	WBC variable; positive serology for influenza, *Legionella*, etc.; decreased diffusion capacity for carbon monoxide in *Pneumocystis jirovecii* pneumonia
Pulmonary edema (cardiogenic)	Dyspnea, PND, orthopnea, history of cardiac disease, may have cough, crackles, JVD, S_3, peripheral edema	Usually bilateral and symmetrical, cardiomegaly, Kerley B lines, pleural effusions (small to moderate)	Variable in amount, low protein content	Elevated B-type natriuretic peptide or poor contractility or diastolic dysfunction by echocardiography
Alveolar hemorrhage	Dyspnea, cough, hemoptysis (may be delayed or even absent, despite significant alveolar hemorrhage) Pallor if anemic, lung exam variable	Typically widespread distribution; acutely, acinar pattern, then interstitial	Bloody, without purulence	Active hemorrhage usually associated with fall in hemoglobin; diffusion capacity for carbon monoxide elevated in acute setting; if pulmonary-renal syndrome, abnormal U/A or elevated BUN, creatinine. Positive serology for specific diseases

Eosinophilic pneumonia	Dyspnea (usually mild in chronic), cough, lung exam normal, or with rales or wheezes	Peripheral lung zones without lobar distribution; may be transitory and/or migratory	Occasionally, mucoid sputum	Acute EP: elevated serum eosinophils rare on presentation. Chronic EP: elevated serum eosinophils in most
Exogenous lipoid pneumonia	Dyspnea, risk factors for aspiration, use of mineral oil, or other oily substances; occasional industrial aerosolized exposures; lung exam variable, poor gag reflex in those at risk for aspiration	Distribution in dependent portions of upper and lower lobes	Scant, but may have lipid-laden macrophages	Nonspecific
Exogenous lipoid pneumonia	Dyspnea, risk factors for aspiration, use of mineral oil, or other oily substances; occasional industrial aerosolized exposures; lung exam variable, poor gag reflex in those at risk for aspiration	Distribution in dependent portions of upper and lower lobes	Scant, but may have lipid-laden macrophages	Nonspecific
Diffuse alveolar damage	Acute onset after inciting insult, marked dyspnea; risk factors for ARDS, crackles	Usually diffuse on plain chest films, CT scan; patchy bilateral involvement	Scant, but with high protein content	Severe hypoxemia; stiff, noncompliant lungs, PCWP <18 if pulmonary artery catheter present

(*Continued*)

Table 1 Intra-alveolar Infiltrates and Exudates (*Continued*)

Diagnosis	History and physical	Chest radiograph	Sputum examination	Laboratory, pulmonary function, and other supportive tests
Alveolar proteinosis	Most with gradual onset of dyspnea, nonproductive cough; low-grade fever, weight loss, and clubbing in some; crackles or lack of breath sounds	Typically bilateral and symmetrical; tends to spare costophrenic angles. Lack of air bronchograms. "Crazy paving" on CT	Occasionally productive of thick, chunky, or gummy consistency	Elevated serum lactate dehydrogenase in 50%; hypoxemia common, though may only be seen during exercise in some
COP	Dyspnea, waxing/waning flu-like symptoms	Bilateral, patchy, peripheral infiltrates; CT scan with "ground-glass" infiltrates	Scant	Nonspecific
Desquamative interstitial pneumonia	Dyspnea, nonproductive cough	Bilateral infiltrates; CT scan may have peribronchovascular cysts	Scant	Nonspecific

Abbreviations: PND, paroxysonal nocturnal dyspnea; JVD, jugular venous distension; PCWP, pulmonary capillary wedge pressure; BUN, blood urea nitrogen; U/A, urinalysis; ARDS, acute respiratory distress syndrome.

drug use and recent influenza infection. Patients with structural lung disease are at increased risk for pneumonia with gram-negative bacteria, including *Pseudomonas aeruginosa. M. pneumoniae*, *C. pneumoniae*, and respiratory viral infections, especially influenza virus, are also common causes of community-acquired pneumonia and sometimes referred to as "atypical" pneumonia because of the propensity for a more gradual onset, a nonproductive cough, and extrapulmonary symptoms such as headache, mylagias, fatigue. In contrast to *M. pneumoniae* infection that occurs most commonly in younger patients, pneumonia due to *C. pneumoniae* is more common in the elderly and has been the etiological agent in of outbreaks in nursing home–acquired pneumonia.

A. Differential Diagnosis of Bacterial Pneumonia

Radiographic patterns (2) of bacterial pneumonia can be classified as lobar, lobular (bronchopneumonia), or interstitial. Lobar pneumonia is typically from a bacterial infection, particularly *S. pneumoniae* and *Klebsiella pneumoniae*, and reflects rapid production of edema fluid that spreads from acinus to acinus. Larger bronchi often remain patent and correlate to the air bronchograms seen on radiographs. *S. aureus* and most gram-negative bacteria more commonly cause lobular or bronchopneumonia. With these pathogens, infection and inflammation are predominant around airways. Radiographs typically have a poorly defined, patchy appearance with peribronchial thickening. With more severe disease, multilobe patchy consolidation occurs. An interstitial pattern in which edema and infiltrate are centered in the alveolar septa, surrounding small airways, and vessels is typical for mycoplasma (as well as viral and *Pneumocystis jiroveci* infection). Infection with *C. pneumoniae* can have a variety of radiographic appearances, including alveolar opacities, interstitial infiltrates, or mixed pattern.

In the majority of patients, empirical therapy based on patient presentation and underlying comorbid illnesses is appropriate. Risks factors for tuberculosis and immunocompromise, specifically HIV infection, should always be sought. Therapy can be guided by an adequate gram stain of sputum if a predominant organism is present. A positive pleural fluid or blood culture is definitive for the specific organism and can help tailor empirical antibiotics. The need for tissue confirmation of bacterial infection is rare but occasionally warranted. Thoracoscopic or open lung biopsy is sometimes performed in severely ill patients with respiratory failure who do not respond to empirical antibiotics. Alternatively, bronchoscopic lavage is sometimes useful to rule out alternative infectious or inflammatory etiologies in patients responding poorly to empirical antibiotics. Bronchoscopic lavage and/or protected brush specimens via bronchoscopy are also employed for the diagnosis of ventilator-associated pneumonia as clinical and radiographic features are nonspecific. A lobar pneumonia with slow resolution or a recurrent lobar pneumonia in the same lung segment should prompt consideration of airway inspection for endobronchial tumor or foreign body.

For patients who do undergo biopsy, usually because of a poor clinical response to antibiotics, transbronchial, thoracoscopic, or open lung biopsy specimens should be divided into samples for microbiology and pathology at the time of the procedure. Pathological specimens of bacterial pneumonia reveal alveoli filled with neutrophils, macrophages, and edema; obviously the specimen should be examined specifically for bacteria, fungi, and mycobacteria with appropriate stains. Necrosis is less common in pneumococcal pneumonia and more often seen in *S. aureus*, gram-negative rod, and anaerobic pneumonias.

Alveoli filled with a foamy exudate should be stained for *P. jiroveci* pneumonia. The presence of food particles suggests aspiration. Because infections can trigger acute respiratory distress syndrome (ARDS), the presence of hyaline membranes suggests the additional complication of diffuse alveolar damage (DAD) associated with ARDS. Although the distinction between neutrophils and eosinophils seems intuitively obvious, the cellular infiltrate should be specifically examined for eosinophils. A significant number of eosinophils in the exudate suggest a primary eosinophilic pneumonia or possibly a secondary drug reaction complicating the treatment of the pneumonia.

III. Eosinophilic Pneumonias: Acute and Chronic

Eosinophilic pneumonias will be covered in more depth in chapters 10 and 11. Acute (3) and chronic eosinophilic pneumonias are rare disorders marked by eosinophilic lung parenchymal infiltration, which may be accompanied by excess eosinophils in the peripheral blood. Eosinophilic pneumonias are associated with helminthic, bacterial, and fungal infections, including allergic bronchopulmonary aspergillosis, drug reactions, toxin and dust exposure, connective tissue diseases, vasculitides, Hodgkin's disease, sarcoidosis, systemic hypereosinophilic syndrome, Churg-Strauss syndrome, and other forms of bronchocentric granulomatosis. One-third of acute eosinophilic pneumonias are idiopathic. The distinction between acute and chronic forms, based on clinical presentation and course, may be arbitrary or valid. Acute forms tend to be more common in men, while chronic forms are more common in women. In acute eosinophilic pneumonia, patients may present with fever, dyspnea, cough, chest pain; many progress to acute hypoxemic respiratory failure. The physical examination typically reveals crackles. Eosinophilia in peripheral blood is unusual on presentation, however most patients, but not all, have some elevation during in their clinical course. Chest radiographs typically have bilateral airspace or bilateral mixed airspace and interstitial opacities. CT scans reveal the bilateral airspace opacification; many will have small effusions. By definition, patients with acute eosinophilic pneumonia have >25% eosinophils on bronchoalveolar lavage or eosinophilic pneumonia on biopsy. In chronic eosinophilic pneumonia (4), patients usually have an insidious onset over weeks to months of fevers, dyspnea, nonproductive or mucoid-productive cough, malaise, weight loss, and chest pain. Asthma or atopy is present in more than half. Physical examination may reveal crackles or wheezes. Mild-to-moderate elevation of eosinophils in the peripheral blood is typical, usually higher than in the acute variety. Radiographically, the classic pattern in chronic eosinophilic pneumonia of migratory, dense, bilateral, peripheral infiltrates occurs in only 25% of patients; however, the infiltrate(s) are peripheral (the outer two-thirds of the lung field) in most patients. CT scans are often better at revealing the peripheral nature of the infiltrates. Peripheral blood eosinophilia is quite common. Eosinophilia recovered by bronchoalveolar lavage (>25% of recovered cells), as with acute eosinophilic pneumonia, correlates well with the presence of lung eosinophils.

A. Differential Diagnosis of Eosinophilic Pneumonia

Secondary causes should be considered in any eosinophilic pneumonia, especially drug reactions and parasitic infections. If eosinophils are not specifically sought in the tissue specimen, other inflammatory pneumonias may be erroneously diagnosed, such as acute interstitial pneumonia, DAD, desquamative interstitial pneumonia (DIP), or cryptogenic organizing pneumonia; the number of tissue eosinophils should distinguish the eosinophilic pneumonias. Although some forms of interstitial lung disease, such as idiopathic pulmonary fibrosis may have increased eosinophils recovered on bronchoalveolar lavage, the percentage of eosinophils in the total cell count is usually <10%. There should be particular attention to examination of transbronchial biopsies for eosinophils, as the process can be patchy. In the healing or recovery phase of eosinophilic pneumonias, the number of tissue eosinophils may decline rapidly and an alveolar infiltrate of mostly macrophages may be left, erroneously suggesting a DIP. Allergic bronchopulmonary aspergillosis, Churg-Strauss syndrome, and even occasionally asthma may have parenchymal infiltrates with eosinophils. Allergic bronchopulmonary aspergillosis is associated with central airway saccular bronchiectasis, elevated IgE levels, precipitating antibodies to *Aspergillus*, and an immediate-type skin reaction. Specimens that reveal bronchiectasis, bronchocentric granulomatosis, or fungal stain/cultures suggesting *Aspergillus* should raise suspicion for this disease. Churg-Strauss syndrome, also called allergic granulomatosis and angiitis, is a rare, acute to subacute, often systemic illness associated with asthma. As in the case of acute and chronic eosinophilic pneumonias, the lung parenchyma is infiltrated with eosinophils. However, the findings of a necrotizing granulomatous vasculitis suggests Churg-Strauss syndrome. Some pulmonary infections, especially tuberculosis and coccidioidomycosis, can have significant lung tissue eosinophilia; consideration of these infections should be included in the clinical history. Of note, acute and chronic eosinophilic pneumonias typically respond rapidly to glucocorticoid therapy; such a response supports this diagnosis.

IV. Pulmonary Alveolar Proteinosis

Pulmonary alveolar proteinosis (PAP), also referred to as alveolar lipoproteinosis, alveolar phospholipidosis, and pulmonary alveolar phospholipoproteinosis, is a rare lung disorder characterized by alveolar accumulation of an acellular, amorphous, insoluble surfactant derived lipoproteinaceous material (5). Primary or idiopathic PAP is the most common form of this lung disease and accounts for 90% of reported cases. The pathogenesis of idiopathic PAP is uncertain, but it may be an autoimmune disorder due to circulating anti-granulocyte macrophage colony–stimulating factor (GM-CSF) antibodies that cause a relative deficiency of GM-CSF (6,7). This in turn leads to impaired processing of surfactant by alveolar macrophages. Secondary PAP has been associated with hematological malignancies, especially myeloid leukemias, immunodeficiency disorders, infection with *P. jiroveci*, and acute dust and fume exposure, especially silica (typically in sandblasters). The average age of presentation is between 30 and 50 and there is a 2:1 male to female predominance. Most patients have a gradual onset of dyspnea and nonproductive cough, though some may report production of thick, gummy phlegm. Low-grade fevers, pleuritic chest pain, scant hemoptysis, and weight loss may be present. Physical examination may reveal crackles or lack of breath sounds in densely consolidated lung segments. Hypoxemia is common, which worsens with exercise. Pulmonary function testing shows a restrictive defect with decreased diffusion capacity for carbon monoxide. Chest radiographs typically show bilateral mid to low symmetrical alveolar infiltrates that spare costophrenic angles. Air bronchograms are not usually seen. High-resolution CT scans show ground-glass opacification in polygonal shapes representing the secondary pulmonary lobule; this leads

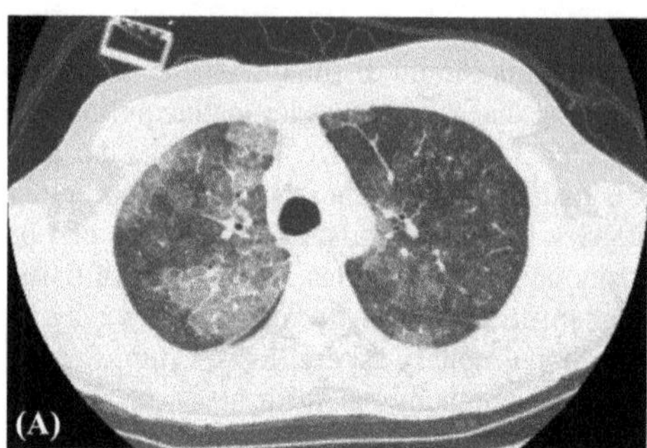

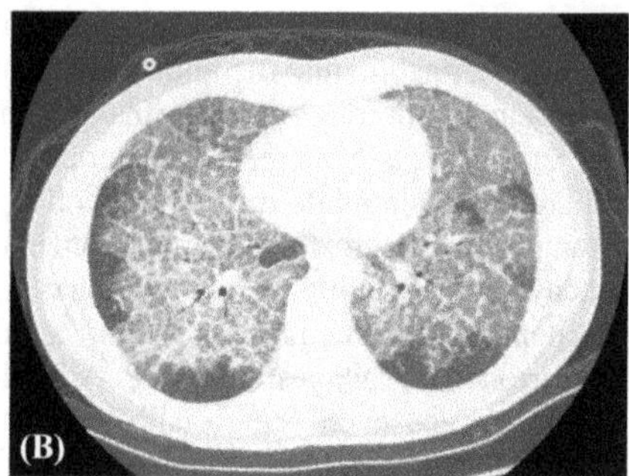

Figure 1 (**A and B**) Pulmonary alveolar proteinosis. High-resolution CT scans reveal the ground-glass opacification in a "crazy paving" pattern and thickened intra- and interlobular septa characteristic of PAP. *Source*: Radiographs courtesy of Brett Elicker, MD.

to the characteristic "crazy paving" pattern (8). While a "crazy paving" pattern is classic for PAP, it can also be seen in *P. jirovecii* pneumonia, bronchioloalveolar carcinoma, sarcoidosis, nonspecific interstitial pneumonia, organizing pneumonia, exogenous lipoid pneumonia, adult respiratory distress syndrome, and pulmonary hemorrhage syndromes. In addition to the "crazy paving" pattern of PAP, there is also superimposed thickening of the intra- and interlobular septa (see Fig. 1A and B). In long-standing cases, fibrosis may occur and an interstitial or reticulonodular pattern may be seen. Bronchoalveolar lavage material is turbid, opaque, and opalescent, with a tan, dense sediment. Under light microscopy, the sediment contains large amounts of acellular eosinophilic material with "foamy" macrophages, which are engorged with periodic acid-Schiff (PAS)-positive material. Transbronchial or open lung biopsy confirms the diagnosis, with the characteristic PAS-positive acellular eosinophilic material that fills the alveoli and terminal bronchioles. Except when pulmonary fibrosis has occurred, the alveolar architecture is usually well preserved. A typical presentation, classic HRCT findings, and characteristic findings on bronchoalveolar lavage or transbronchial biopsy obviate the need for open or thoracoscopic biopsy in most patients. Electron microscopic demonstrating phospholipid lamellar bodies in alveolar airspaces, alveolar macrophages, and type II cells confirms the diagnosis in difficult cases. Therapy in symptomatic patients is unique and consists of whole lung lavage with sterile saline; the efficacy of lavage is due to the mechanical removal of Intra-alveolar phospholipids.

A. Different Diagnosis of PAP

On biopsy, alveoli and terminal bronchioles are filled with large amounts of an acellular eosinophilic PAS-positive material. This material has a granular pink appearance with darker pink clumps and slit-like cholesterol clefts. Alveolar macrophages are "foamy" or vacuolated (filled with ingested lipoproteinaceous material), giant, and poorly mobile. Inflammation and fibrosis have been detected in some cases, but there is generally preservation of parenchymal architecture. The finding of PAP on biopsy should lead to consideration of secondary causes, including infection, inhaled inorganic dusts, underlying immunosuppression, or hematological malignancy. *P. jirovecii* infection is characterized by foamy eosinophilic alveolar material containing cysts, trophozoites, and macrophages. In some cases of *P. jirovecii* pneumonia, the extracellular material has PAP-like lamellar structures evident by electron microscopy. *P. jirovecii* infection can not only mimic PAP histologically but can also trigger a PAP reaction, so lavage material should be examined for this organism. Because patients with PAP appear to be prone to pulmonary infections from *Nocardia*, mycobacterial species, and fungi, lavage material should also be cultured for these organisms. Pulmonary edema from cardiogenic or noncardiogenic causes produces pink, homogenous, edema-filled alveoli but not the granular appearance or the slit-like clefts of PAP. Mucin-producing well-differentiated bronchoalveolar cell carcinoma can also be mistaken for PAP; the alveolar exudate from both processes can stain positively with the PAS reagent. Close inspection of cellular detail can help to differentiate these two diseases.

V. Lipoid Pneumonia

Aspiration of lipid material may cause asymptomatic radiographic abnormalities or an acute, subacute, or chronic clinical pneumonia (9). Patients typically have risk factors for aspiration or are otherwise healthy people with exposures to aerosols of oily substances, as in workplace exposures or from oil-based nose drops. Symptomatic patients may have fever, weight loss, cough, dyspnea, and hypoxemia. Physical examination reveals crackles in some. Radiographic imaging most frequently shows bilateral alveolar consolidation or ground-glass opacification but can also show nodules, masses, or a reticulonodular pattern. Locations in dependent portions of the lungs are typical. The characteristic CT finding (10) is lung consolidation with areas of hypodensity as assessed by Hounsfield units corresponding to the low density of accumulated fat (see Fig. 2A and B). Once inhaled, alveolar macrophages ingest the oil, fill the alveoli, and an acute and chronic pneumonitis can result. Alveolar macrophages transport the oil to the interlobular septa, which can lead to localized granulomas and pulmonary fibrosis. When the diagnosis is suspected on clinical grounds, sputum cytology with lipid-laden macrophages supports the diagnosis.

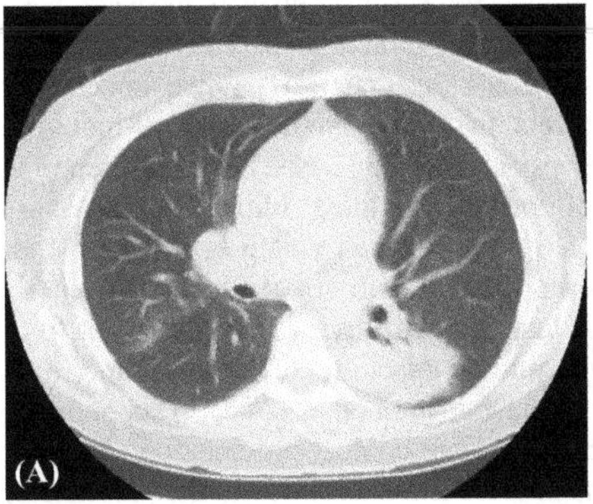

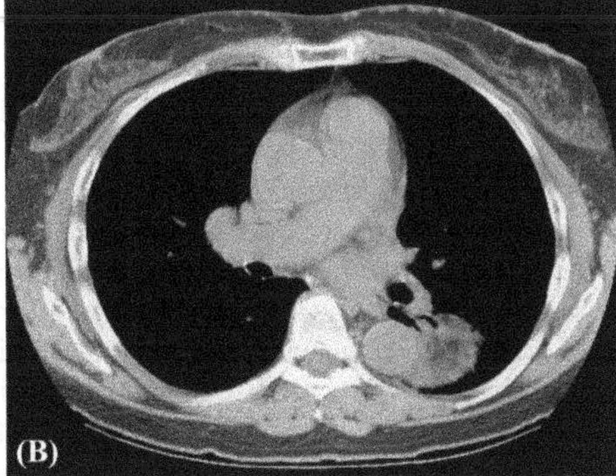

Figure 2 (**A and B**) Lipoid pneumonia. Image 1 (CT scan—lung windows) reveals a localized left lower lobe process. In Image 2 (CT scan—mediastinal windows), areas of low attenuation with in the process suggests a lipoid pneumonia. *Source*: Radiographs courtesy of Brett Elicker, MD.

Bronchoscopic lavage may show visible fat globules on the surface of the recovered fluid. Cytology from lavage reveals lipid-laden macrophages that stain for fat with Sudan black, Sudan red, or oil red O. Multinucleated giant cells with cytoplasmic lipid droplets may also be present. Biopsy specimens may reveal patchy areas of chronic inflammation and scarring. Treatment is the avoidance of the aspirated material, although there have been reports of additional improvement with glucocorticoid therapy.

A. Differential Diagnosis of Lipoid Pneumonia

In contrast to the foamy, finely stippled macrophages filled with endogenous lipid, as seen behind obstructed airways distal to endobronchial tumors or as in cryptogenic organizing pneumonitis (COP), macrophages from exogenous aspirated lipid have large, coalesced vacuoles. In addition, there are large, extracellular lipid vacuoles in lipoid pneumonia that would be unusual in COP or distal to obstructed airways. In patients with aspiration of a variety of substances, undigested food particles and a granulomatous reaction with scarring and fibrosis may be present. Close inspection of biopsy material for food substances will help distinguish aspiration from other granulomatous inflammatory pneumonias.

VI. Alveolar Hemorrhage

Alveolar hemorrhage (11) will be covered in more depth in chapters 13 and 14. Etiologies include capillaritis (e.g., Wegener's granulomatosis, microscopic polyangitis), collagen vascular diseases (e.g., systemic lupus erythematosus, scleroderma, rheumatoid arthritis, mixed connective tissue disease), Goodpasture's syndrome, crack cocaine use, idiopathic pulmonary hemosiderosis, and nonpulmonary processes such as mitral stenosis and systemic coagulopathies. In any of these disorders, hemoptysis can be mild to life threatening or even absent, despite extensive alveolar hemorrhage. Anemia is common and primarily due to pulmonary blood loss. Patients may also have dyspnea, cough, fatigue, and, if there is renal involvement, hematuria, proteinuria, and renal insufficiency. With vasculitides, joint pains and skin rashes may be present. In Goodpasture's syndrome (12), circulating antiglomerular basement membrane antibodies can be detected in over 90% of patients and appear to have specificity of greater than 95%. An elevated level of antiglomerular basement membrane antibodies in the appropriate clinical setting establishes the diagnosis. When uncertainty exists or if there is delay in obtaining antibody levels, tissue may be obtained for immunofluorescent staining. The kidney is the preferred biopsy site, as lung tissue has higher reported false-positive and false-negative rates of immunofluorescent staining. Idiopathic pulmonary hemosiderosis is a rare disease that tends to occur in children and young adults; its pathogenesis is unknown and specific antibodies or serum markers are not available. Wegener's granulomatosis is a systemic vasculitis of small and medium arteries characterized by a necrotizing granulomatous process especially involving the upper and lower respiratory tract and the kidneys. The presence of antineutrophil cytoplasmic antibodies (ANCA) supports the diagnosis of Wegener's granulomatosis with the appropriate clinical presentation. Alveolar hemorrhage in the setting of systemic lupus erythematosus is associated with the presence of serum antinuclear antibodies and reduced serum complement levels.

Radiographically, patients with alveolar hemorrhage have nonspecific patchy or diffuse perihilar alveolar infiltrates. Several days after a bout of alveolar hemorrhage, a reticulonodular pattern may emerge; it is thought to reflect clearance of hemoglobin by macrophages into lymphatics and the interstitium. After repeated bouts of hemorrhage, interstitial fibrosis may be seen. Pulmonary function testing may reveal an elevated diffusion capacity for carbon monoxide consistent with recent alveolar hemorrhage, but most patients are too dyspneic to perform the test. Occasionally, significant pulmonary hemorrhage occurs without apparent hemoptysis. Bronchoscopy suggests alveolar hemorrhage if the recovered lavage material is or becomes increasingly bloody during the lavage. Lavage typically reveals hemosiderin-laden macrophages; this is a nonspecific finding occurring in any type of bleeding in the lung. Therapy includes supportive care and treatment directed at the underlying process.

A. Differential Diagnosis of Alveolar Hemorrhage

With any form of alveolar hemorrhage, there are alveolar red blood cells and hemosiderin-laden macrophages. Repeated hemorrhage into the lung can lead to fibrosis, which may potentially be confused with a primary fibrotic lung process. Conversely, any acute inflammatory lung disease may be accompanied by some degree of alveolar hemorrhage. The presence of hyaline membranes suggests ARDS/DAD as the primary lung process. Wegener's granulomatosis, microscopic polyangiitis, and collagen vascular diseases are associated with pulmonary vasculitis. Serological markers in the appropriate clinical setting can help narrow the differential diagnosis among these diseases. Idiopathic pulmonary hemosiderosis, DAD from ARDS, and mitral stenosis should not show evidence of capillaritis. Of note, idiopathic pulmonary hemosiderosis is a disease confined to the lung; evidence of other organ involvement argues against this disease.

VII. Cryptogenic Organizing Pneumonitis

COP (13) is a clinical pathological entity characterized by a subacute respiratory illness with plugs of loose granulation tissue in distal airways with an associated organizing pneumonitis. COP is the idiopathic form of bronchiolitis obliterans organizing pneumonia (BOOP), the most common form of BOOP. Rarely, secondary BOOP has been associated with viral, *Legionella*, and mycoplasmal infections, toxic fume exposure, HIV infection, connective tissue diseases, radiation therapy, myelodysplastic syndrome, and various drugs. Patients with COP typically present in their 40s to 50s with a subacute flu-like illness with fatigue, fever, nonproductive cough, weight loss, and dyspnea on exertion. COP may be suspected in an adult patient with a prolonged viral-like respiratory illness that does not respond to antibiotics. Physical examination reveals inspiratory crackles in most. Chest radiographs typically show bilateral, patchy, often peripheral, alveolar infiltrates. Infiltrates may be dense or partially opaque with a ground-glass appearance. Infiltrates may resolve spontaneously and reappear in different lung segments ("fleeting" or "migratory" infiltrates). High-resolution CT scans also reveal the patchy, dense, or ground-glass alveolar infiltrates. Although nondiagnostic, CT scanning may distinguish the process from interstitial pulmonary fibrosis, which typically shows radiographic evidence of subpleural fibrosis, and can direct the pulmonologist or surgeon to optimal sites for biopsy. Lung biopsy is recommended because of the wide clinical differential diagnosis and the prolonged glucocorticoid therapy required in most cases. Transbronchial biopsy may be diagnostic if a piece of tissue of sufficient size is obtained that contains all the elements of the lesion. However, most cases will require either thoracoscopic or open lung biopsy. Diagnosis is made by finding the characteristic pathology in the appropriate clinical setting. Over two-third of treated patients respond to corticosteroids; symptomatic relief can be rapid, over days to weeks.

A. Differential Diagnosis of Cryptogenic Organizing Pneumonia

Although idiopathic COP is the most common form of BOOP, secondary causes (listed above) should be considered. The finding of a coincident infectious pathogen, a clinical history of underlying connective tissue disorder, or recent toxin exposure suggests a secondary form. Because the diagnosis of COP pathologically requires a specimen that exhibits both the tufts of granulation tissue in the airways and the pneumonitis, small specimens or samples that are on the periphery of involvement of the patchy process may exhibit only part of the entire lesion. A biopsy specimen that contains only the airway lesion may be confused with a primary bronchiolitis; a specimen that contains only alveoli may be confused with other idiopathic inflammatory pneumonias.

VIII. Diffuse Alveolar Damage

ARDS is a clinical, physiological, and radiographic syndrome characterized by alveolar capillary membrane injury with increased vascular permeability. It is the severe form of acute lung injury. It is defined (14,15) by three features: bilateral infiltrates, hypoxemia with a ratio of the partial pressure of arterial oxygen to the fraction of inspired oxygen of $\leq$200 mmHg, and no evidence of an elevated left atrial pressure. Sepsis, aspiration, pneumonia, burns, massive blood transfusion, and trauma are the most common precipitants of ARDS, but dozens of other local and systemic insults have been associated with acute lung injury. Despite numerous possible triggers, patients typically present with a history of a preceding noxious event, followed by rapid and progressive hypoxemia, development of stiff, noncompliant lungs, and diffuse pulmonary infiltrates over the course of hours to days. There are no clinical or laboratory findings specific for the diagnosis of ARDS; however, an acute lung injury score, based on the extent of the physiological and radiographic derangements, is used to quantify the degree of injury (Fig. 3) (16).

Radiographs are nonspecific but usually reveal bilateral alveolar and interstitial infiltrates; CT scans are also nonspecific but show the patchy nature of the infiltrates, not usually appreciated on plain chest radiographs. There is often dense consolidation in areas of dependent lung (see Fig. 4). Therapy is directed at minimizing additional trauma from the ventilator by using a low tidal volume strategy, in addition to supportive care of a critically ill patient. A large randomized trial (17) did not find a mortality benefit with the use of methylprednisolone for persistent ARDS.

A. Differential Diagnosis of DAD

ARDS with DAD initially has widespread alveolar and interstitial edema and hemorrhage, loss of type I alveolar epithelial cells, type II cell hyperplasia, and respiratory bronchiolar and alveolar hyaline membranes. After this exudative stage, a proliferative or organizing stage ensues, marked by fibrin organization, type II cell proliferation, an inflammatory

Acute Lung Injury Score

Chest Radiograph Score		
No alveolar consolidation		0
Alveolar consolidation confined to 1 quadrant		1
Alveolar consolidation confined to 2 quadrants		2
Alveolar consolidation confined to 3 quadrants		3
Alveolar consolidation in all 4 quadrants		4
Hypoxemia Score		
PaO_2/FIO_2	≥ 300	0
PaO_2/FIO_2	225-299	1
PaO_2/FIO_2	175-224	2
PaO_2/FIO_2	100-174	3
PaO_2/FIO_2	<100	4
PEEP (if ventilated)		
	≥ 5 cm H_2O	0
	6-8 cm H_2O	1
	9-11 cm H_2O	2
	12-14 cm H_2O	3
	≥ 15 cm H_2O	4
Respiratory Compliance (if ventilated)		
	≥ 80 ml/cm H_2O	0
	60-79 ml/cm H_2O	1
	40-59 ml/cm H_2O	2
	20-39 ml/cm H_2O	3
	≤19 ml/cm H_2O	4

Final score: divide sum by number of components used

Mild to moderate lung injury:	.1-2.5
Severe lung injury:	> 2.5

Adapted with permission from: Murray JF, Matthay MA, Luce JM, Flick MR. An expanded definition of the adult respiratory distress syndrome. Amer Rev Respir Dis 1988;138:720-723.

Figure 3 Acute lung injury score.

infiltrate with fibroblasts, edema resorption, and thickening of the alveolar septa. Most patients who survive the medical illness precipitating ARDS recover significant lung function, but occasionally significant fibrosis of the parenchyma can lead to permanent physiological and pulmonary function abnormalities. Biopsy is occasionally warranted in patients in whom the diagnosis is not straightforward or in whom infectious agents have not been satisfactorily excluded. Because of the acuity in onset, ARDS may appear clinically similar to acute interstitial pneumonia, though the time course from onset to respiratory compromise is usually much shorter in ARDS. Diffuse alveolar hemorrhage can present with rapid respiratory failure without hemoptysis, although typically laboratories reveal a drop in hemoglobin. If the patient is intubated, blood may be more evident in the endotracheal tube; progressively bloodier return with bronchoalveolar lavage should also raise the possibility of diffuse alveolar hemorrhage. Evidence of hyaline membranes on biopsy would strongly favor ARDS/DAD rather than acute interstitial pneumonia or acute hemorrhage. Numerous eosinophils should prompt consideration of an acute eosinophilic pneumonia. Severe pneumonia can precipitate acute respiratory failure with or without secondary ARDS. The distinction between severe pneumonia with or without ARDS may

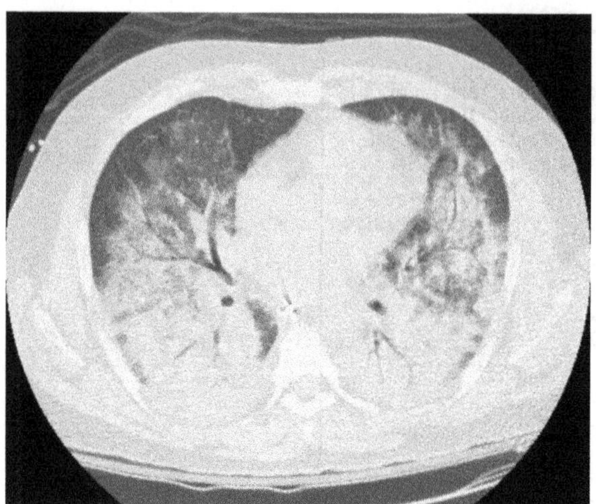

Figure 4 ARDS. CT scan reveals the patchy nature of ARDS and the increased density of the infiltrates in the dependent portions of the lungs. *Source*: Radiographs courtesy of Brett Elicker, MD.

be difficult and not always clinically necessary, as patients with clinical pneumonia with or without ARDS often receive the same supportive care in addition to antibiotics for the pneumonia. If ARDS is a possibility, a lung-protective strategy (18) with low tidal volume ventilation in those patients who require mechanical ventilation should be considered. Cardiogenic pulmonary edema is often difficult to distinguish clinically and radiographically from ARDS. An elevated B-type natriuretic peptide or poor contractility by echocardiography favors cardiogenic pulmonary edema (19). Although pulmonary artery catheter–guided management of fluid status has not been shown to decrease mortality in patients with ARDS (20), the finding of an elevated pulmonary capillary wedge pressure supports that there is some degree of cardiogenic pulmonary edema.

IX. Desquamative Interstitial Pneumonia

DIP is a rare idiopathic inflammatory lung disease that typically affects middle-aged smokers with 2:1 male to female predominance. The term *desquamative* describes the abundance of alveolar macrophages, originally thought to represent desquamating type II cells. In general, patients with DIP present with a subacute (weeks to months) illness with dyspnea and nonproductive cough; clubbing occurs in 20%. Plain chest radiographs may have bilateral airspace opacification or can be fairly normal in a minority; however, high-resolution CT scans (21,22) reveal patchy or diffuse ground-glass, basilar, and peripheral predominant opacification, occasionally with peribronchovascular cysts. Honeycombing is unusual. These radiographic findings are not distinguishable from other acute inflammatory lung diseases such as hypersensitivity pneumonitis and nonspecific interstitial pneumonia. As with most undiagnosed inflammatory lung processes, CT scans can direct clinicians to appropriate biopsy sites, avoiding areas of honeycombing. Transbronchial biopsies usually provide insufficient material for diagnosis. Therapy consists of smoking abstinence and glucocorticoids.

A. Different Diagnosis of DIP

In DIP, there is prominent thickening of alveolar walls with inflammatory cells, including plasma cells and occasional eosinophils and a marked accumulation of large numbers of alveolar macrophages. The macrophages may contain a dusty brown pigment. The process appears temporally uniform. DIP is very similar to smoking-related respiratory bronchiolitis. The macrophages tend to be more alveolar in DIP, while more centered around peribronchiolar areas in smoking-related respiratory bronchiolitis, and the CT scan typically has a more diffuse ground-glass involvement with DIP, but these entities have a great deal of clinical and pathological overlap. DIP lacks granulomas found in hypersensitivity pneumonitis and sarcoidosis. As compared to DAD, DIP lacks the hyaline membranes of DAD. Subpleural honeycombing or traction bronchiectasis on high-resolution CT or these pathological findings along with spatial and temporal heterogeneity and fibroblastic foci support the diagnosis of usual interstitial pneumonia process rather than DIP.

References

1. Campbell GD. Overview of community-acquired pneumonia: prognosis and clinical features. Med Clin North Am 1994; 78:1035–1048.
2. Tarver RD, Teague SD, Heitkamp DE, et al. Radiology of community-acquired pneumonia. Rad Clin North Am 2005; 43:497–512.
3. Philit F, Etienne-Mastroïanni B, Parrot A, et al. Idiopathic acute eosinophilic pneumonia: a study of 22 patients. Am J Respir Crit Care Med 2002; 166:1235–1239.
4. Marchand E, Reynaud-Gaubert M, Lauque D, et al. Idiopathic chronic eosinophilic pneumonia: a clinical and follow-up study of 62 cases. Medicine 1998; 77:299–312.
5. Seymour JF, Presneill JJ. Pulmonary alveolar proteinosis: progress in the first 44 years. Am J Respir Crit Care Med 2002; 166:215–235.
6. Venkateshiah SB, Yan TD, Bonfield TL, et al. An open-label trial of granulocyte macrophage colony stimulating factor therapy for moderate symptomatic pulmonary alveolar proteinosis. Chest 2006; 130:227–237.
7. Tazawa R, Hamano E, Arai T, et al. Granulocyte-macrophage colony–stimulating factor and lung immunity in pulmonary alveolar proteinosis. Am J Respir Crit Care Med 2005; 171: 1142–1149.
8. Rossi SE, Erasmus JJ, Volpacchio M, et al. Crazy-Paving pattern at thin-section CT of the lungs: radiologic-pathologic overview. Radiographics 2003; 23:1509–1519.
9. Gondouin A, Manzoni Ph, Ranfaing E, et al. Exogenous lipid pneumonia: a retrospective multicentre study of 44 cases in France. Eur Respir J 1996; 9:1463–1469.
10. Gaerte SC, Meyer CA, Winer-Muram HT, et al. Fat-containing lesions of the chest. Radiographics 2002; 22:S61–S78.
11. Green RJ, Ruoss SJ, Kraft SA, et al. Pulmonary capillaritis and alveolar hemorrhage. Update on diagnosis and management. Chest 1996; 110:1305–1316.
12. Hudson BG, Tryggvason K, Sundaramoorthy M, et al. Alport's syndrome, Goodpasture's syndrome, and type IV collagen. N Engl J Med 2003; 348:2543–2556.
13. Epler EG. Bronchiolitis obliterans organizing pneumonia. Arch Intern Med 2001; 161:158.
14. Murray JF, Matthay MA, Luce JM, et al. An expanded definition of the adult respiratory distress syndrome. Am Rev Respir Dis 1988; 138:720–723.
15. Leaver SK, Evans TW. BMJ Acute respiratory distress syndrome. BMJ 2007; 335:389–394.
16. Cherniak RM, Colby TV, Flint A, et al. Correlation of structure and function in idiopathic pulmonary fibrosis. Am J Respir Crit Care Med 1995; 151:1180–1188.

17. The National Heart, Lung, and Blood Institute Acute Respiratory Distress Syndrome (ARDS) Clinical Trials Network. Efficacy and safety of corticosteroids for persistent acute respiratory distress syndrome. N Engl J Med 2006; 354:1671–1684.
18. Acute Respiratory Distress Syndrome Network. Ventilation with lower tidal volumes as compared with traditional tidal volumes for acute lung injury and the acute respiratory distress syndrome. N Engl J Med 2000; 342:1301–1308.
19. McCullough PA, Nowak RM, McCord J, et al. B-type natriuretic peptide and clinical judgment in emergency diagnosis of heart failure: analysis from breathing not properly (BNP) multinational study. Circulation 2002; 106:416–422.
20. The National Heart, Lung, and Blood Institute Acute Respiratory Distress Syndrome (ARDS) Clinical Trials Network. Pulmonary-artery versus central venous catheter to guide treatment of acute lung injury. N Engl J Med 2006; 354:2213–2224.
21. Lynch DA, Travis WD, Muller NL, et al. Idiopathic interstitial pneumonias: CT features. Radiology 2005; 236:10–21.
22. Gruden JF, Webb WR. CT findings in proved case of respiratory bronchiolitis. Am J Respir 1993; 161:44–46.

10
Pulmonary Eosinophilia

DONALD G. GUINEE, JR.
Virginia Mason Medical Center, Seattle, Washington, U.S.A.

I. General Pathologic Approach to Eosinophilic Pulmonary Infiltrates

II. Eosinophilic Pneumonia Pattern (Without Other Patterns)

- Simple eosinophilic pneumonia
- Chronic eosinophilic pneumonia
- Tropical pulmonary eosinophilia

III. Acute Eosinophilic Pneumonia Pattern

- Acute eosinophilic pneumonia

IV. Eosinophilic Pneumonia Combined with Other Patterns

- Allergic bronchopulmonary aspergillosis
  - Eosinophilic pneumonia—diffuse
  - Mucoid impaction—bronchiolocentric (see below)
  - Bronchocentric granulomatosis—bronchiolocentric
- Churg-Strauss syndrome (also a multifocal or focal infiltrate—see below)
  - Eosinophilic pneumonia
  - Necrotizing angiitis
  - Necrotizing granulomas
- Infection

V. Multifocal or Focal Eosinophilic Infiltrates

A. Bronchiolocentric Distribution

- Pulmonary Langerhans cell histiocytosis
- Asthma
- Non-eosinophilic Asthma
- Eosinophilic bronchitis

- Mucoid impaction (either idiopathic or allergic bronchopulmonary aspergillosis)
- Bronchocentric granulomatosis (either idiopathic or allergic bronchopulmonary aspergillosis)

B. Angiocentric Distribution

- Churg-Strauss syndrome
- Wegener's granulomatosis

C. Lymphatic Distribution

- Hodgkin's disease

D. Pleural Distribution

- Reactive eosinophilic pleuritis

VI. Extremely Rare Disorders

- Hypereosinophilic syndrome

I. General Pathologic Approach to Eosinophilic Pulmonary Infiltrates

Eosinophils are a major component of many pulmonary diseases. Eosinophils may be the predominate cell type, as in eosinophilic pneumonia, or part of a mixed cellular infiltrate that varies in both composition and quantity such as in Hodgkin's disease or pulmonary Langerhans cell histiocytosis.

Eosinophilic pulmonary infiltrates, like other pulmonary infiltrates, may be distinguished through consideration of the distribution and the cytologic features of the cellular infiltrate (1). Eosinophilic infiltrates may either be "diffuse," "multifocal," or "focal." A diffuse infiltrate involves either a lobe or part of a lobe diffusely (i.e., eosinophilic pneumonia) whereas multifocal or focal processes show areas of relatively normal pulmonary parenchyma alternating with areas of diseased lung (i.e., pulmonary Langerhans cell histiocytosis). Diffuse processes may involve predominately airspaces, the interstitium, or both (i.e., eosinophilic pneumonia). Multifocal processes, on the other hand, are often centered around bronchioles (bronchiolocentric, i.e., pulmonary Langerhans cell histiocytosis), lymphatics, blood vessels (angiocentric, i.e., Churg-Strauss syndrome), the pleura (pleural and subpleural, i.e., reactive eosinophilic pleuritis) or are entirely random (1). The cytologic features are also important in the diagnosis of an infiltrate, especially in combination with the pattern of infiltration. For example, the diagnosis of Hodgkin's disease relies on recognition of the classic Reed-Sternberg cell or its variants. This approach to eosinophilic pulmonary infiltrates is listed above.

A pathologic diagnosis may sometimes be diagnostic of a distinct clinical entity (i.e., pulmonary Langerhans cell histiocytosis), but more often describes a pattern that has a variety of clinical etiologies (i.e., eosinophilic pneumonia). In this case, correlation with clinical history is helpful in allowing a more specific clinical diagnosis and the institution of appropriate therapy. A comment in the pathologic report listing the clinical possibilities may also be helpful.

II. Eosinophilic Pneumonia Pattern

Histologic Features

Major Features

- Diffuse process involving airspaces and interstitium
- Numerous eosinophils and/or macrophages within alveoli
- Interstitial infiltrate with eosinophils, lymphocytes, and plasma cells (Fig. 1A–D)

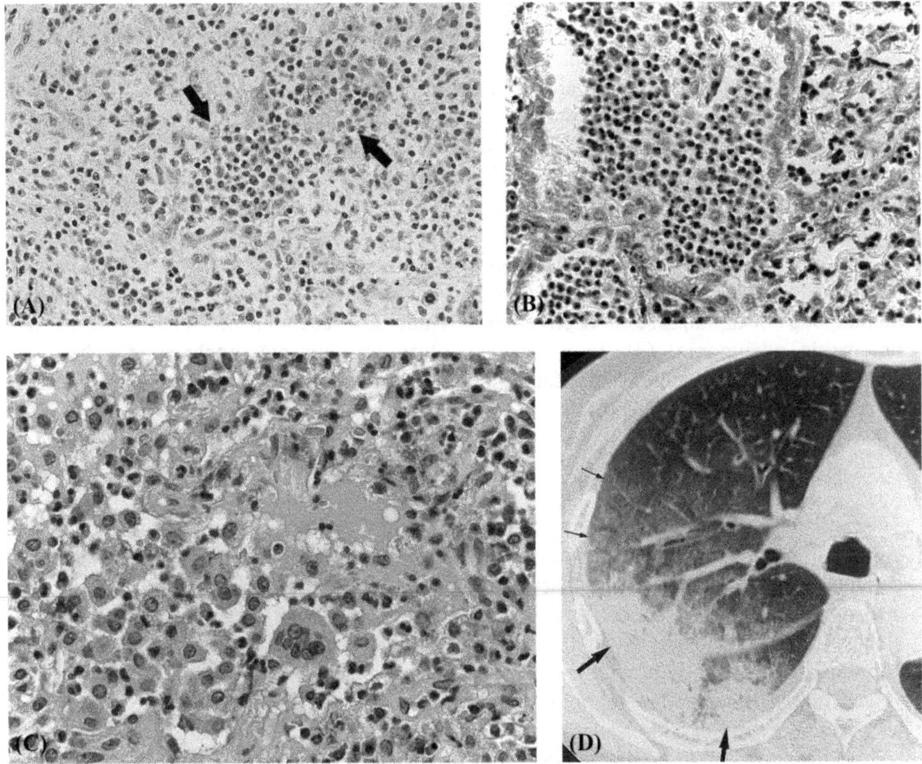

Figure 1 (**A**) Eosinophilic pneumonia. There are numerous eosinophils within alveolar air spaces (*arrows*) as well as an interstitial infiltrate consisting of eosinophils and mononuclear cells. (**B**) Eosinophilic pneumonia (Giemsa stain). Higher power view highlighting eosinophils within alveolar space. (**C**) Eosinophilic pneumonia. In this example of eosinophilic pneumonia, there are collections of both eosinophils and macrophages within alveolar airspaces. Occasional multinucleated giant cells are present. In some cases of eosinophilic pneumonia, histiocytes may be the predominant cell type. (**D**) Chronic eosinophilic pneumonia. High-resolution CT scan at level of carina shows extensive peripheral airspace consolidation (*large arrows*) as well as areas of ground-glass attenuation (*small arrows*). *Source*: From Ref. 25.

Minor Features (present in some cases)

- Rare scattered multinucleated giant cells or granulomas
- Eosinophilic microabscesses
- Scattered neutrophils
- Non-necrotizing small vessel vasculitis with eosinophils and lymphocytes
- Intraluminal buds of organizing connective tissue (foci of organizing pneumonia pattern)
- Eosinophilic granules and/or Charcot-Leyden crystals within macrophages

The major pathologic pattern associated with a diffuse eosinophilic pulmonary infiltrate is eosinophilic pneumonia. The pattern of eosinophilic pneumonia is characterized by collections of eosinophils and macrophages within alveolar air spaces admixed with fibrin and proteinaceous debris (Fig. 1A and B) (2–8). Admixed histiocytes may often contain eosinophilic granules and even Charcot-Leyden crystals. Occasionally, rare scattered multinucleated giant cells are present (Fig. 1C). Scattered lymphocytes and plasma cells may also be present within alveoli, but are usually overshadowed by the predominance of eosinophils and macrophages. In some cases, there are eosinophilic microabscesses consisting of necrotic eosinophils and debris surrounded by a poorly formed palisaded rim of epithelioid histiocytes. Occasionally, there may be scattered neutrophils. The interstitium is also involved, and is expanded by an infiltrate consisting of eosinophils, lymphocytes, and plasma cells. A non-necrotizing small vessel vasculitis consisting of eosinophils and lymphocytes is a common, but not prominent feature. Additional, but variable features, include buds of organizing connective tissue within air spaces (bronchiolitis obliterans and organizing pneumonia) (3). In some cases, intra-alveolar macrophages may be more prominent than eosinophils. This feature may reflect the duration of the lesion or its course of resolution with treatment (6).

Differential Diagnosis

The pathologic differential diagnosis of eosinophilic pneumonia (Table 1) includes acute eosinophilic pneumonia, desquamative interstitial pneumonia (DIP), and pulmonary Langerhans cell histiocytosis (pulmonary eosinophilic granuloma). Eosininophilic pneumonia is distinguished from "acute" eosinophilic pneumonia by the absence of superimposed changes of DAD (see below) (9,10). Like eosinophilic pneumonia, DIP consists of a diffuse pulmonary infiltrate with prominent collections of macrophages within alveolar spaces (11). Usually, however, eosinophilic pneumonia can be distinguished by the presence, at least in some areas, of prominent aggregates of eosinophils. Pulmonary Langerhans cell histiocytosis also often contains aggregates of eosinophils and macrophages. Unlike eosinophilic pneumonia, however, pulmonary Langerhans cell histiocytosis is a multifocal, patchy process with a bronchiolocentric distribution. The lesion characteristically effaces the underlying pulmonary parenchyma. Identification of collections of Langerhans cells is

Table 1 Pathologic Differential Diagnosis of Eosinophilic Pneumonia Pattern

I.	Acute eosinophilic pneumonia pattern
II.	Desquamative interstitial pneumonia pattern
III.	Pulmonary Langerhans cell histiocytosis (pulmonary eosinophilic granuloma)

required to make this diagnosis and also helps to further distinguish it from eosinophilic pneumonia (12,13). One should also remember that areas of eosinophilic pneumonia may be either part of, or the predominate response to, an infectious agent such as coccidiomycosis, atypical mycobacteria, and others (14–21). One should always search for features more typical of infection such as prominent necrotizing granulomatous inflammation. In some cases special stains may identify a microorganism.

Ancillary Techniques

In the right clinical setting, the diagnosis of eosinophilic pneumonia may sometimes be supported by ancillary techniques such as bronchoalveolar lavage (BAL). While eosinophils in BAL fluid may sometimes be increased in interstitial lung disease, this increase is usually below 10%. A finding of 20% or greater eosinophils within BAL is almost always associated with an eosinophilic alveolitis (22).

Clinical Syndromes Manifested by Eosinophilic Pneumonia

Eosinophilic pneumonia is best regarded as a histologic pattern, which may be present in a variety of clinical conditions. For this reason, I prefer the term "eosinophilic pneumonia" as a diagnosis, followed by a comment listing the possible clinical syndromes and their etiologies. Clinical syndromes associated with eosinophilic pneumonia may be further subdivided according to whether eosinophilic pneumonia is the only finding or whether eosinophilic pneumonia most often occurs in association with other histologic patterns.

Eosinophilic pneumonia is often the only finding in the clinical syndromes of simple eosinophilic pneumonia (Löffler's syndrome), chronic eosinophilic pneumonia, and tropical pulmonary eosinophilia (Table 2). Separation of these entities requires detailed knowledge of the clinical presentation and course.

Simple eosinophilic pneumonia (Löffler's syndrome) consists of a self-limited illness characterized by mild respiratory symptoms and fever associated with transient pulmonary infiltrates on chest x-ray and peripheral blood eosinophilia (23,24). High-resolution CT scan shows transient, peripheral areas of ground-glass opacity and/or consolidation, or nodules, preferentially involving the mid- and upper-lung fields (24,25). This syndrome is often associated with ascaris infection (2,3), and is thought to be due to passage of larva through the lung. Although usually self-limited, this disorder will also respond well to corticosteroids.

Chronic eosinophilic pneumonia is a rare illness characterized by severe dyspnea, high fever, peripheral blood eosinophilia, and peripheral pulmonary infiltrates on chest x-ray. In about half of the cases, the infiltrates have a characteristic appearance referred to as the "photographic negative of pulmonary edema." High-resolution CT scan typically shows peripherally located, often subpleural, patchy, areas of consolidation, predominantly

Table 2 Clinical Syndromes Manifested by Eosinophilic Pneumonia (with Eosinophilic Pneumonia as the Sole Histologic Manifestation)

I. Simple eosinophilic pneumonia (Löffler's syndrome)
II. Chronic eosinophilic pneumonia
III. Tropical pulmonary eosinophilia

Table 3 Causes of Eosinophilic Pneumonia

I.	Idiopathic
II.	Fungal colonization of airways (allergic bronchopulmonary aspergillosis)
III.	Infection
IV.	Fungal (i.e., coccidiomycosis)
V.	Parasitic (i.e., ascaris, filaria, strongyloides)
VI.	Drugs (i.e., penicillin, nitrofurantoin)
VII.	Toxic inhalation (i.e., nickel carbonyl vapor)

in the mid- to upper-lung fields (Fig. 1D) (24,25). The majority of patients are middle-aged females (female to male ratio 2:1), although males may also be affected. About half of patients have asthma. The cause is unknown in many cases, although hypersensitivity reactions to drugs may show identical histologic features. These patients will have a dramatic response to corticosteroid therapy (4,5,7,26,27).

Tropical pulmonary eosinophilia is a clinical syndrome common in the tropics characterized by intense eosinophilia in the peripheral blood, accompanied by a paroxysmal, nonproductive cough, wheezing and peripheral adenopathy. This disease is believed, in most instances to be a manifestation of filariasis (*Wucheria bancrofti*), although microfilaria are usually not identified in the peripheral blood (28). Occasional cases appear to be manifestations of helminthic infections (i.e., ascariasis) or other parasites such as Strongyloidiasis (29). In these cases, identification of characteristic ova or larva in stool may be helpful in identifying an etiology. Pathologically, the histologic pattern evolves from an eosinophilic bronchopneumonia to a mixed nodular granulomatous infiltrate with fibrosis (30).

While eosinophilic pneumonia is associated with separate clinical syndromes, the etiologic agents behind these syndromes are varied and overlapping (Table 3). Löffler's pneumonia is most often due to underlying ascaris infection, although it may occur from other causes (i.e., hypersensitivity drug reactions) as well. Chronic eosinophilic pneumonia is often idiopathic, but has been associated with asthma, hypersensitivity reactions to drugs (i.e., penicillin), parasites, fungi (especially coccidiodes), and inhalation of nickel carbonyl vapor. Tropical pulmonary eosinophilia is most often a manifestation of filariasis (*Wucheria bancrofti*), but may be associated with helminthic infections, or other parasites. Regardless of the clinical syndrome, therefore, a specific etiology should be sought in all cases by obtaining a detailed history of drug use, stool analysis for ova cysts and parasites, and examination of sputum and histologic sections for fungi and other microorganisms.

Eosinophilic pneumonia is often a focal component of Churg-Strauss syndrome and allergic bronchopulmonary aspergillosis (21,31–37). In these cases, the identification of additional histopathologic features allows their diagnosis. Occasionally, however, eosinophilic pneumonia may be the most prominent or only finding. In this case, clinicopathologic correlation is essential.

Churg-Strauss syndrome often has areas of eosinophilic pneumonia, but in addition may also have necrotizing granulomas and a necrotizing vasculitis affecting small- and medium-sized vessels (see below) (32–35). Clinical history is extremely helpful in this regard as eosinophilic pneumonia may be the only histologic finding in patients with limited biopsies or early disease (35).

III. Acute Eosinophilic Pneumonia Pattern

Histologic Features

Major Features

- Interstitial and intra-alveolar infiltrate of eosinophils
- Superimposed changes of acute and organizing DAD including:
  - Hyaline membranes
  - Interstitial edema
  - Variable degrees of interstitial and organizing pneumonia (Fig. 2A and B)

Minor Features

- Type II pneumocyte hyperplasia
- Perivascular mixed eosinophilic inflammation without necrosis
- Occasional mucus plugging

Acute eosinophilic pneumonia is a histologic pattern characterized by a combination of eosinophilic pneumonia with superimposed changes of acute and organizing DAD. Biopsies show interstitial and intra-alveolar infiltrates of eosinophils. There are associated hyaline membranes, edematous thickened alveolar septa, and varying degrees of interstitial and intra-alveolar organization by loose fibromyxoid connective tissue (Fig. 2A) (9).

Differential Diagnosis

The pathologic differential diagnosis of acute eosinophilic pneumonia includes more typical patterns of DAD and eosinophilic pneumonia. DAD can be excluded by the absence of a significant eosinophilic infiltrate. Likewise, a typical pattern of eosinophilic pneumonia

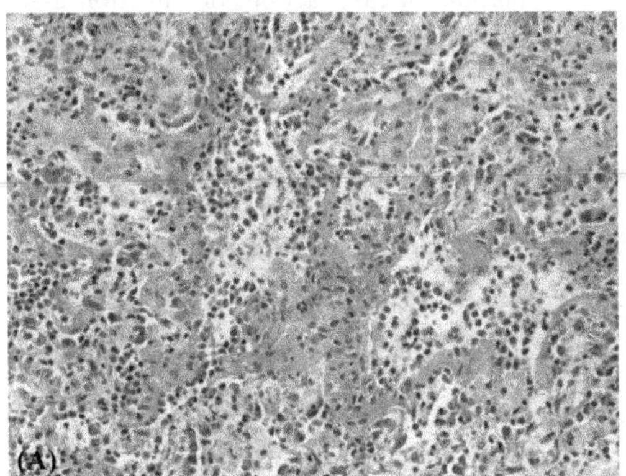

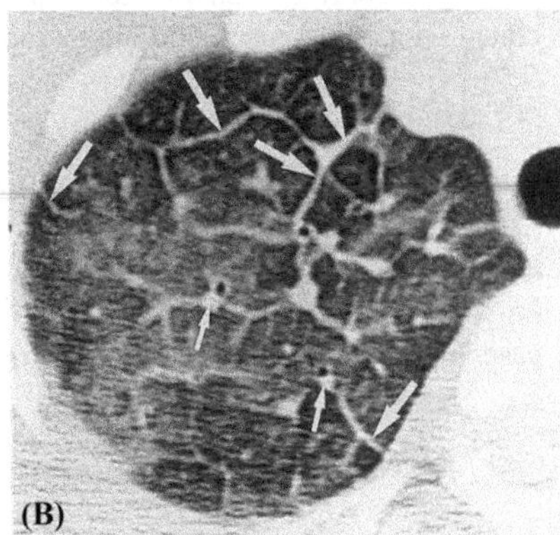

Figure 2 **(A)** Acute eosinophilic pneumonia. Medium power view shows hyaline membranes lining alveolar septa. There is a background infiltrate of eosinophils within alveoli and adjacent septa. **(B)** Acute eosinophilic pneumonia. High-resolution CT scan at apex shows areas of ground-glass attenuation, thickened interlobular septa (*large arrows*) and peripheral thickened bronchovascular bundles (*small arrows*). *Source*: From Ref. 25.

lacks hyaline membranes, type II pneumocyte hyperplasia, and interstitial and organizing fibrosis (9).

Clinical Features

Clinically, acute eosinophilic pneumonia is characterized by the development of acute respiratory failure in young, previously healthy adults. Patients are not asthmatic and are nonsmokers. Initial symptoms include cough, dyspnea, fever, pleuritic chest pain, and myalgias. Respiratory failure usually occurs rapidly within one week from the onset of symptoms. Eosinophilia (>25%) is present on bronchioloalveolar lavage, and in the right clinical setting, may be used to support the diagnosis. In contrast to chronic eosinophilic pneumonia, peripheral blood eosinophilia is absent in the majority of cases (10,38–42).

Radiographic Features

High-resolution CT scan shows patchy areas of ground-glass attenuation accompanied by interlobular septal thickening and sometimes by consolidation or poorly defined nodules (Fig. 2B) (24,25).

Pathogenesis

In addition to idiopathic cases, both the clinical syndrome and the histologic pattern of acute eosinophilic pneumonia may have a variety of secondary causes. Possible etiologies include toxic inhalation and hypersensitivity reactions to pharmaceutical agents. Similar to simple pulmonary eosinophilia and chronic eosinophilic pneumonia, acute eosinophilic pneumonia may also be associated with underlying infection.

With regard to toxic inhalation, one intriguing observation is that in many patients, acute eosinophilic pneumonia appears to follow the recent initiation of cigarette smoking (42–45). Reported agents of toxic inhalation, pharmaceutical reaction, or infection associated with acute eosinophilic pneumonia are listed in Table 4.

Prognosis and Treatment

Recognition of the histologic pattern of acute eosinophilic pneumonia is important because of its prompt response to therapy. Patients respond rapidly to therapy with corticosteroids and do not relapse (10,38,39,42). As noted above, however, secondary causes such as infection, drug reactions, or toxic inhalation should always be excluded as therapy in these cases will be directed toward the offending agent.

IV. Eosinophilic Pneumonia Combined with Other Patterns

Eosinophilic pneumonia may be combined with other histopathologic patterns in allergic bronchopulmonary aspergillosis, Churg-Strauss syndrome, or infection. For example, while eosinophilic pneumonia in allergic bronchopulmonary aspergillosis may present pathologically as a diffuse infiltrate, more often eosinophilic pneumonia is a focal component of a limited spectrum of histologic patterns, which includes bronchocentric granulomatosis and mucoid impaction. Eosinophilic pneumonia, either diffuse or multifocal, may also be a

Table 4 Secondary Causes of Acute Eosinophilic Pneumonia

I. Idiopathic

II. Toxic Inhalation
- a. Recent initiation of cigarette smoking (42–45)
- b. Nickel dust (174)
- c. Exposure to World Trade Center dust (175).
- d. Heroin smoking (176)
- e. Acetylene (177)
- f. Scotchguard (178)
- g. Smoke from fireworks (179)

III. Drug reactions
- a. Trazodone (180)
- b. Ranitidine (181)
- c. Progesterone (182)
- d. Tendinap (183)
- e. Clomipramine and sertaline (184)
- f. Calcium stearate (additive agent for oral antihistamine) (185)
- g. GM-CSF (186)
- h. Pentamidine isethiocyanate (187)

IV. Infection
- a. HIV and AIDS (188,189)
- b. *Trichosporon terrestre* (190)
- c. Intravesicle BCG (191)
- d. Aspergillosis (21)
- e. Toxocariasis (20)

Abbreviations: GM-CSF, granulocyte macrophage colony stimulating factor; BCG, Bacillus Calmette-Guérin.

primary or focal pulmonary manifestation of active infection by mycobacteria (15,18), parasites such as filiaria (30), fungi such as *Coccidioides immitis* (14) or *Schizophyllum commune* (46), or unusual bacteria (17,47).

Allergic Bronchopulmonary Aspergillosis

General Features

Allergic bronchopulmonary aspergillosis is a clinical syndrome thought to result from a hypersensitivity reaction to chronic colonization of airways by Aspergillus. The disorder is characterized clinically by fever, radiographic infiltrates, peripheral blood eosinophilia, and immediate cutaneous reactivity to antigens of Aspergillus. Allergic bronchopulmonary aspergillosis most commonly affects patients who seem to have an underlying disorder with clearance of mucus and is therefore most common in patients with underlying asthma or cystic fibrosis (48–50). Pathologically, allergic bronchopulmonary aspergillosis is characterized by variable combinations of one or more of three distinctive types of major reaction patterns. These reaction patterns include areas of eosinophilic pneumonia, mucoid impaction of the bronchi and/or bronchocentric granulomatosis (36,37,51). Eosinophilic pneumonia as a reaction pattern has been previously discussed (see above). Mucoid impaction of the bronchi and bronchocentric granulomatosis may occur either in association with allergic bronchopulmonary aspergillosis or independently and are described below.

Radiographic Features

Radiologic findings in allergic bronchopulmonary aspergillosis correspond to the extent of these reaction patterns. Accordingly thin-section CT scans show variable combinations of ground-glass attenuation, mucus plugs and bronchiectasis, and centrilobular nodules or masses (Fig. 3A) (24,25).

Mucoid Impaction of the Bronchi

Histologic Features

Major Features

- Distention of bronchi by "allergic mucin"
- Rare fragments of noninvasive fungal hyphae may be identified within centers of inspissated mucus (Fig. 3B)

Minor Features

- Ulceration of bronchial wall
- Thinned bronchial wall
- Peribronchial chronic inflammation with scattered eosinophils
- Squamous and goblet cell metaplasia of bronchial mucosa

Mucoid impaction is characterized grossly by distention of bronchi and bronchioles by firm, rubbery, yellow to gray, plugs of inspissated mucin (36,51–53). Histologically, the inspissated mucus often contains concentric layers of pale pink to basophilic mucus with viable and disintegrating eosinophils admixed with sloughed epithelial cells, Charcot-Leyden crystals, and granular debris (Fig. 3B). "Allergic mucin" is a term used to describe this appearance. Within the "allergic mucin" rare noninvasive fungal hyphae, morphologically consistent with Aspergillus, are sometimes but not always, present (36). The surrounding bronchial wall is often thinned with an intramural and/or peribronchial chronic inflammatory infiltrate admixed with eosinophils. The bronchial mucosa may be ulcerated, or show prominent goblet cell or squamous metaplasia. Mucoid impaction may be present in conditions other than allergic bronchopulmonary aspergillosis such as chronic bronchitis or cystic fibrosis. However, in these conditions, the mucin is more often composed of degenerating neutrophils rather than eosinophils and lacks the concentric layering distinctive of "allergic mucin" (36).

Ancillary Techniques

Endobronchial biopsy may aid in the diagnosis of mucoid impaction associated with allergic bronchopulmonary aspergillosis. Aubry et al. (54) reported that a combination of

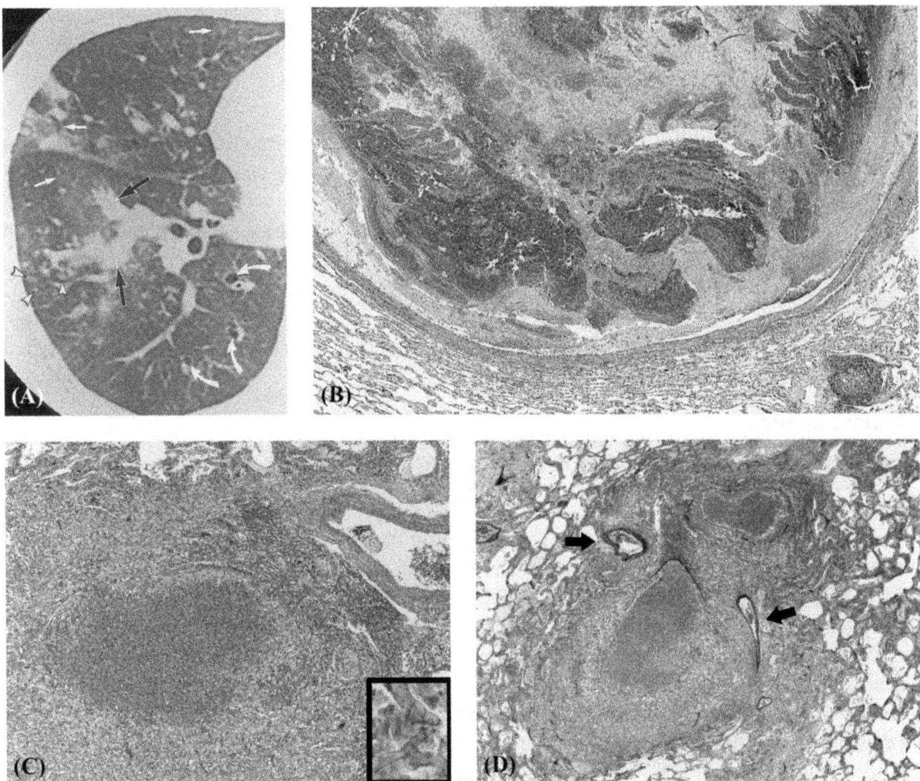

Figure 3 **(A)** Allergic bronchopulmonary aspergillosis. High-resolution CT scan shows areas of mucus plugging (*black arrows*), ground-glass attenuation (*straight white arrows*), centrilobular nodules (*arrowheads*), bronchial wall thickening and bronchiectasis (*curved arrows*). These features generally correspond to pathologic features of mucoid impaction, eosinophilic pneumonia, bronchocentric granulomatosis, and bronchiectasis. **(B)** Mucoid impaction. A markedly dilated bronchiole is distended by thick mucus. **(C)** Bronchocentric granulomatosis. The wall of a bronchiole has been almost completely replaced by granulomatous inflammation. A small portion of bronchial mucosa remains. The center of the bronchiole consists of necrotic debris. The identification of fungal hyphae by special stain within the center of these areas of necrotic debris (*inset*) confirms the diagnosis of allergic bronchopulmonary aspergillosis. **(D)** Bronchocentric granulomatosis (Movat pentachrome stain). The key to the recognition of bronchocentric granulomatosis is the presence of this lesion next to a pulmonary arteriole (*arrows*). The distribution of lesions can be highlighted, as in this case, on special stains for elastic tissue. *Source*: From Ref. 25.

allergic mucin and fungal hyphae within bronchial biopsy specimens prompted consideration of allergic bronchopulmonary aspergillosis in five patients in which the disease was originally not suspected. Bronchoscopy confirmed the presence of mucoid impaction in all three patients (54).

Bronchocentric Granulomatosis

Histologic Features

Major Features

- Replacement of bronchi/bronchioles by necrotizing granulomatous inflammation
- Affected bronchioles have thick walls and central "caseous" or mucopurulent necrosis
- Degenerated noninvasive fragments of fungal hyphae may be identified within centers of the granulomas
- Parenchymal granulomas typical of invasive fungal or mycobacterial infections are not present
- Besides hyphal fragments, other organisms (i.e., mycobacteria) are not identified (Fig. 3C and D)

Minor Features

- Exudative bronchiolitis may be present
- Chronic bronchiolitis may be present

Bronchocentric granulomatosis refers to an unusual histologic pattern of pulmonary disease characterized by either the partial or total replacement of bronchi or bronchioles by necrotizing granulomatous inflammation (51,55,56). Grossly, involved bronchi and bronchioles have thick walls and contain central "caseous" or sometimes mucopurulent necrosis. Histologically, there is replacement of bronchiolar epithelium by epithelioid histiocytes and occasional giant cells, sometimes in a palisaded array. In cases where there is complete replacement of bronchi and bronchioles, this pattern may be identified only by noting the presence of the granulomas adjacent to pulmonary arteries and arterioles (Fig. 3C and D). An elastic tissue stain may be helpful in confirming this impression by demonstrating remnants of the bronchiolar elastic lamina (Fig. 3D). Secondary involvement of adjacent pulmonary arteries by chronic inflammation is a common, but not prominent feature. Within the lumen of the affected airways, there is cellular debris admixed with degenerated eosinophils, neutrophils, and red blood cells. As in mucoid impaction, degenerated noninvasive hyphal fragments of Aspergillus may be identified (Fig. 3C). Although difficult to find in occasional cases, when found, the presence of degenerated hyphae are essentially diagnostic of allergic bronchopulmonary aspergillosis (36,51,55).

Other histologic features commonly present in bronchocentric granulomatosis include a distinctive "exudative bronchiolitis" and a chronic bronchiolitis. These pathologic features are often present in those airways not involved by granulomatous inflammation. "Exudative bronchiolitis" refers to the presence of necrotic debris admixed with disintegrating eosinophils and/or neutrophils within bronchiolar lumens. This material is histologically identical to the necrotizing centers of the granulomas and probably represents passive extension of the exudates in bronchiolar lumens distal to the granulomatous inflammation. Chronic bronchiolitis is also probably a secondary phenomenon, and is characterized by marked infiltration of bronchiolar walls by lymphocytes and plasma cells (36).

Like mucoid impaction, and eosinophilic pneumonia, bronchocentric granulomatosis is not always associated with allergic bronchopulmonary aspergillosis, and may be a histologic feature of other disorders. Approximately half of the patients have bronchocentric granulomatosis that is unassociated with asthma, peripheral eosinophilia, associated mucoid impaction, or eosinophilic pneumonia. The failure to identify fungal hyphae in this subset of patients, suggests that their pathogenesis is distinct from allergic bronchopulmonary aspergillosis. A pattern of bronchocentric granulomatosis may also be present as the primary histologic manifestation of infection by various agents including *Mycobacterium tuberculosis*, histoplasma, blastomycosis, mycoplasma pneumonia, and even influenza A virus (57–59). In cases with an infectious etiology, however, there are usually extrabronchial granulomas. Special stains to exclude infection should always be performed (55,57) in any case considered to show bronchocentric granulomatosis to exclude this possibility. If infection is carefully excluded, cases of idiopathic bronchocentric granulomatosis may respond to steroid therapy (55).

While allergic bronchopulmonary aspergillosis describes the clinical syndrome resulting from hypersensitivity to Aspergillus, similar clinical symptoms and pathologic findings may occur from other fungi as well, including candida, curvularia, geotrichum, and others (60). In this case, the generic term allergic bronchopulmonary fungal disease is appropriate.

V. Multifocal or Focal Eosinophilic Infiltrates

Disorders with focal or multifocal eosinophilic components include pulmonary Langerhans cell histiocytosis, asthma, eosinophilic bronchitis, Churg-Strauss syndrome, Wegener's granulomatosis, Hodgkin's disease, and reactive eosinophilic pleuritis. These disorders may be bronchiolocentric (pulmonary Langerhans cell histiocytosis, asthma, eosinophilic bronchitis), angiocentric (Churg-Strauss syndrome), distributed along lymphatic routes (Hodgkin's disease), or random.

A. Bronchiolocentric Distribution

Pulmonary Langerhans Cell Histiocytosis (Pulmonary Eosinophilic Granuloma)

Histologic Features

Major Features

- Bronchiolocentric distribution
- Discrete symmetric stellate nodules of varying cellularity
- Younger lesions are cellular, older lesions may be entirely fibrotic
- Lesions of different age coexist within the same biopsy
- There may be central cavitation and cyst formation
- Nodules are composed of varying numbers of Langerhans cells, histiocytes, lymphocytes, and fibroblasts
- Immunohistochemical staining for S100, CD1a, and/or langerin helps to confirm Langerhans cells (Fig. 4A–D).

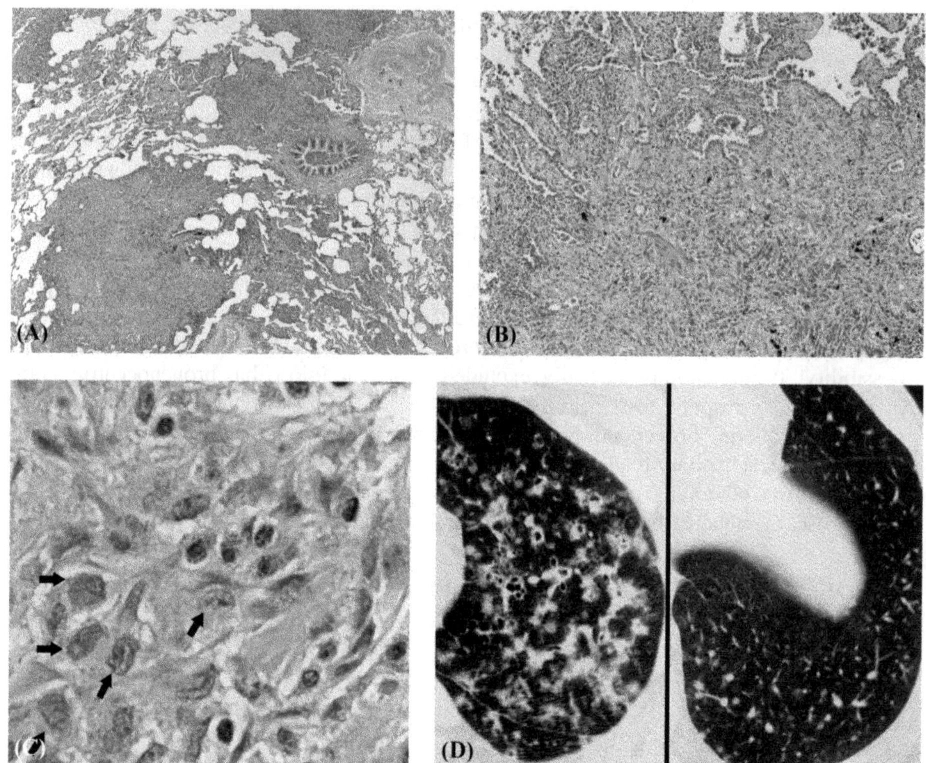

Figure 4 **(A)** Pulmonary Langerhans cell histiocytosis (pulmonary eosinophilic granuloma). Low power view shows irregular nodules with a bronchiolocentric distribution. **(B)** Pulmonary Langerhans cell histiocytosis (pulmonary eosinophilic granuloma). Intermediate power view shows the stellate character of the nodule's border. Within the nodules, aggregates of Langerhans cells are present admixed with histiocytes, lymphocytes and eosinophils (Fig. 4C). **(C)** Pulmonary Langerhans cell histiocytosis (pulmonary eosinophilic granuloma). In this high power field, numerous Langerhans cells are identified by their irregular convoluted nuclei (*arrows*). Also present are scattered eosinophils within the background. **(D)** Pulmonary Langerhans cell histiocytosis. Composite of high-resolution CT scans (lung windows) shows irregular nodules and thick-walled cysts in the superior lung (*left image*) with relative sparing of the lung bases (*right image*). *Source*: From Ref. 75.

Minor Features

- Intraluminal buds of organizing connective tissue (organizing pneumonia pattern) may be present within airspaces at the periphery
- There may be prominent collections of macrophages in alveoli adjacent to nodules ("pseudo DIP-like reaction")
- Focal areas of honeycombing may be present in areas of dense fibrosis

Pulmonary Langerhans cell histiocytosis is characterized by a multifocal infiltrate with a bronchiolocentric distribution. The histologic appearance of the infiltrate varies with the age of the lesions. Low power examination usually shows discrete symmetric stellate nodules with varying degrees of cellularity and fibrosis (Fig. 4A and B). Sometimes there is central cavitation and cyst formation. Early lesions of pulmonary Langerhans cell histiocytosis are cellular and consist of variable numbers of Langerhans cells admixed with eosinophils, lymphocytes, histiocytes, giant cells, and fibroblasts. The number of Langerhans cells, as well as eosinophils, varies from lesion to lesion. Some lesions may contain predominantly eosinophils and lymphocytes, whereas other lesions may consist predominantly of Langerhans cells. As lesions evolve, fibrosis replaces much of the cellular infiltrate. Dense fibrosis may be associated with honeycombing, a feature that is prominent in rare individuals with progressive disease (12,13,61,62).

The identification of Langerhans cells is key to the diagnosis in both early, cellular, or old fibrotic lesions. Langerhans cells have pale eosinophilic cytoplasm, irregular or convoluted oval nuclei, and indistinct cell borders. In well-prepared sections, they may be easily distinguished from histiocytes (Fig. 4C). Histiocytes are usually intra-alveolar rather than interstitial, have distinct rather than indistinct cell borders, and dense rather than pale eosinophilic cytoplasm.

While the bronchiolocentric distribution and appearance of lesions at low power may suggest pulmonary Langerhans cell histiocytosis, Langerhans cells may be difficult to find, especially in older lesions. In problematic cases, their demonstration may require examination of multiple levels. Immunohistochemical staining for S100 and CD1a may also be helpful in confirming their identity (63–65). In addition to S100 and CD1a, langerin, a Langerhans cell-specific lectin that initiates Birbeck granule formation, has also been shown to be expressed preferentially in this disorder (66). Caution is necessary interpreting these stains, however, as other types of interstitial lung disease may show a mild increase in scattered Langerhans cells. Nonetheless, identification of significant aggregates of these cells is consistent with pulmonary Langerhans cell histiocytosis. In the past, electron microscopy was also helpful for demonstration of Birbeck granules but is usually not necessary in current samples (12,62–65).

In an open lung biopsy, lesions of different activity are usually present so that cellular lesions coexist with stellate fibrotic scars. In alveoli adjacent to the scars there are often prominent collections of macrophages (DIP-like reaction). Collections of Langerhans cells, however, are most often found within the interstitial nodules.

Ancillary Techniques

Ancillary techniques such as transbronchial biopsy and BAL may sometimes be helpful in the diagnosis of pulmonary Langerhans cell histiocytosis. While most transbronchial biopsies in pulmonary Langerhans cell histiocytosis are nondiagnostic, in occasional cases, diagnostic lesions will be sampled and obviate the need for an open lung biopsy (12). An increased number of Langerhans cells in BAL has also been suggested as a diagnostic feature. Langerhans cells are less than 1% in normal BAL fluid and increased in patients with pulmonary Langerhans cell histiocytosis (67). A cutoff of 5% CD1-positive cells has been proposed as diagnostically useful in diagnosis (68,69). However, this finding is not entirely specific and should be correlated with other clinical and radiographic features as slightly increased Langerhans cells in BAL fluid can occur in patients with other interstitial lung disorders (68–70) and in healthy smokers without interstitial lung diseases (68,71).

Radiographic Features

Radiographically, pulmonary Langerhans cell histiocytosis is characterized by a diffuse bilateral upper to midzonal reticulonodular radiographic appearance with frequent cavitation and sparing of the costophrenic angles. High-resolution CT scans show diffuse lung involvement with thin-walled cysts and nodules in a peribronchiolar distribution (Fig. 4D) (72–75). The lung disease may progress to honeycomb fibrosis.

Clinical Features

Pulmonary Langerhans cell histiocytosis (pulmonary eosinophilic granuloma) is caused by the uncontrolled proliferation of Langerhans cells within the lungs. Langerhans cells are a particular type of antigen presenting dendritic cell distributed widely in normal tissues including the skin, lymph nodes, and lung. In the lung, the dendritic processes of Langerhans cells form a continuous network associated with the epithelium lining airways (76,77).

Langerhans cells are also the proliferative cells in a spectrum of clinicopathologic syndromes in children (eosinophilic granuloma of bone, Letterer-Siwe disease, Hand-Schüller-Christian disease) collectively referred to as Histiocytosis-X. In contrast to Langerhans cell histiocytosis occurring in children, pulmonary Langerhans cell histiocytosis has a distinctly different clinical presentation with different prognostic and therapeutic implications.

Pulmonary Langerhans cell histiocytosis virtually always appears in adult smokers and is usually restricted to the lung (12,13,61). Affected patients most commonly present in the third and fourth decades of life (12,61). Up to 25% of patients may be asymptomatic at diagnosis. The most common presenting symptoms are nonproductive cough, dyspnea on exertion, chest pain, dizziness, weight loss, and spontaneous pneumothorax (61). A restrictive pattern of pulmonary function testing is often present. Extrapulmonary involvement, such as bone lesions or diabetes insipidus, occurs in about 10% to 15% of cases (12,61).

Although rare, atypical presentations of pulmonary Langerhans cell histiocytosis can occur and include isolated nodules, isolated endobronchial or endotracheal disease, focal alveolar consolidation, pleural effusion, and mediastinal adenopathy (76,78–81). The diagnosis of pulmonary Langerhans cell histiocytosis is often strongly suspected on clinical and radiologic grounds; however, a lung biopsy may be needed for definitive diagnosis.

While disease is localized to the lung in most patients, 10% to 15% of patients will have limited involvement of other organs such as bone, lymph node, or anterior pituitary (diabetes insipidus). The pathologic manifestations in the lung in these patients are similar to the pathologic features observed in patients with exclusive pulmonary disease (12,61). Pulmonary involvement in severe disseminated disease affecting children, however, such as Letterer-Siwe disease, is manifested by relatively more cellular, monomorphous interstitial infiltrates of Langerhans cells with correspondingly less fibrosis (13).

Differential Diagnosis

The differential diagnosis of pulmonary Langerhans cell histiocytosis includes the usual interstitial pneumonia (UIP) pattern, respiratory bronchiolitis, desquamative interstitial pneumonitis, eosinophilic pneumonia, pulmonary involvement by Erdheim-Chester disease, and reactive eosinophilic pleuritis. Distinction of late forms of pulmonary Langerhans cell histiocytosis from a UIP pattern may be difficult. Helpful clues include the subpleural and paraseptal distribution of scarring with fibroblast foci in UIP in contrast to the irregular stellate bronchiolocentric nodules of pulmonary Langerhans cell histiocytosis. While individual Langerhans cells may be present in fibrotic lung diseases when studied by immunohistochemistry or electron microscopy, clusters of Langerhans cells are absent (12,13).

Pulmonary Langerhans cell histiocytosis may also be confused with respiratory bronchiolitis and DIP. Although collections of macrophages may be identified within alveolar spaces around lesions of pulmonary Langerhans cell histiocytosis, the presence of discrete cellular nodules or stellate scars is not a feature of either respiratory bronchiolitis or DIP. Clusters of Langerhans cells are also not identified within these conditions. Eosinophilic pneumonia is likewise distinguished from Langerhans cell histiocytosis by the absence of nodules or stellate scars, and the absence of collections of Langerhans cells.

Reactive eosinophilic pleuritis is a nonspecific reaction consisting of a proliferation of histiocytes, and mesothelial cells admixed with eosinophils involving the pleural surface (82). Occasional cases may show associated vascular and perivascular infiltration of small to medium-sized muscular pulmonary arterioles and pulmonary veins by eosinophils (83). Unlike pulmonary Langerhans cell histiocytosis, however, these cases lack parenchymal nodules or scars containing collections of Langerhans cells. Since pulmonary Langerhans cell histiocytosis may involve the pleura, and may itself evoke reactive eosinophilic pleuritis, immunohistochemical stains marking Langerhans cells (S100, CD1a, and/or langerin) may be helpful to confirm or exclude diagnostic collections of Langerhans cells (12,13,63–66).

Erdheim-Chester disease is a rare non-Langerhans cell histiocytosis that typically presents as symmetrical sclerosis involving the diaphyseal aspects of long bones. Extra-osseous lesions may be present. Lesions of Erdheim-Chester diseases typically consist of a proliferation of large histiocytes with abundant pale staining eosinophilic to foamy cytoplasm associated with a variable lymphoplasmacytic infiltrate and fibrosis (84). In Erdheim-Chester disease, histiocytes may stain variably positively for S100, but in contrast to Langerhans cells, lack staining for CD1a (84).

Pathogenesis

The almost exclusive occurrence of pulmonary Langerhans cell histiocytosis in smokers and its peribronchiolocentric distribution pathologically suggests that cigarette smoking is fundamental to the development of this disease. In support of this hypothesis, increased numbers of Langerhans cells are present in the BAL fluid of smokers (71,85). Cytokines such as granulocyte macrophage colony stimulating factor (GM-CSF) and others also appear to be important (86–88).

Yousem et al. recently examined cases of pulmonary Langerhans cell histiocytosis using the X-linked polymorphic human androgen receptor assay (HUMARA) locus to assess clonality in female patients with one or more discrete LCH cell nodules in open lung biopsies (89). They found 7 (29%) were clonal and 17 (71%) were non-clonal. Of the six cases with multiple discrete nodules, three (50%) showed a non-clonal Langerhans cell population. They speculated that in most cases, pulmonary Langerhans cell histiocytosis appears to be primarily a reactive process in which lesions are non-clonal. In this way it is distinct from the systemic or multifocal Langerhans cell disorders in children most of which are clonal (86). Nonetheless, in approximately 30% of cases of pulmonary Langerhans cell histiocytosis, nonlethal, nonmalignant clonal evolution of LCH cells may arise in the setting of Langerhans cell hyperplasia.

Prognosis and Treatment

Most patients spontaneously recover and have a good prognosis. There is some evidence that pulmonary Langerhans cell histiocytosis may sometimes resolve if patients stop smoking (90). However, a significant percentage develops chronic pulmonary dysfunction, and progressive pulmonary fibrosis can lead to death in a small subset of cases (12,61). Treatment for patients with progressive disease is varied and includes corticosteroids and cytotoxic agents (76). Overall median survival is 12.5 years, which is significantly worse than expected for matched controls (91). Lung transplant has also been used successfully in some patients (92).

Asthma

Histologic Features

Major Features

- Bronchiolocentric distribution
- Bronchial walls permeated by mixed inflammatory infiltrate with prominent eosinophils
- Hyperplastic bronchial/bronchiolar smooth muscle (two to three times normal)
- Goblet cell metaplasia of bronchial/bronchiolar epithelium
- Thick mucus plugs may be present within bronchial lumens
- Basement membrane thickening (up to twice normal) (Fig. 5A and B)

Minor Features

- Slight increase in size of submucosal seromucinous glands

The pathologic features of asthma are largely extrapolated from studies of patients dying of status asthmaticus. These results have been largely confirmed by recent studies of bronchial biopsies and BAL fluid in patients with less severe disease (93–98) At autopsy, the lungs are overexpanded with occasional alternating areas of atelectasis. Thick mucous

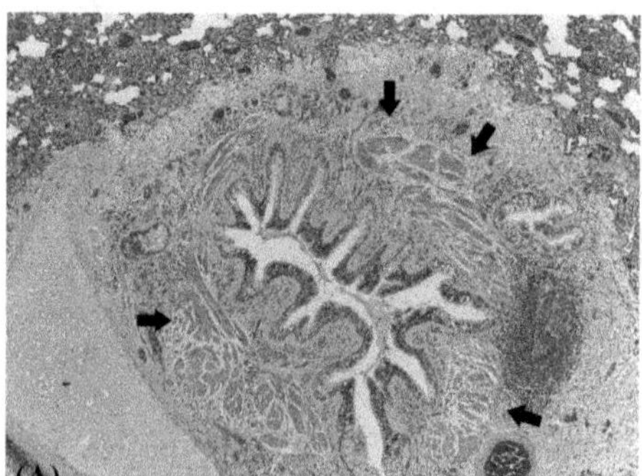

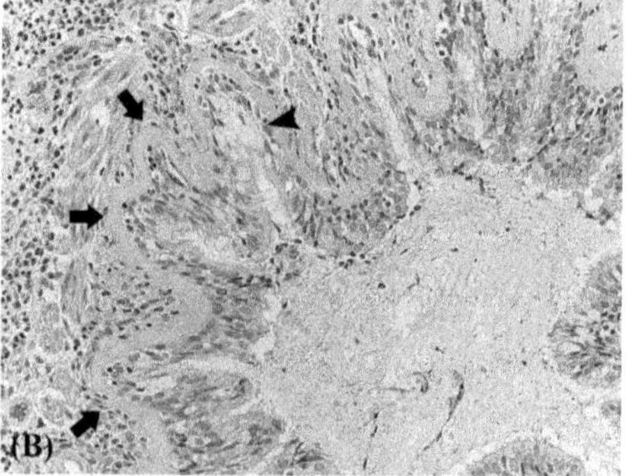

Figure 5 **(A)** Asthma. A small bronchus shows striking smooth muscle hyperplasia (*arrows*). **(B)** Asthma. At higher power, there is thickening of the basement membrane (*arrows*), a marked submucosal infiltrate of eosinophils and prominent goblet cell metaplasia (*arrowhead*).

plugs are often present in bronchi and bronchioles. Severely affected patients may have areas of saccular bronchiectasis, most commonly in the upper lobes (99,100).

Histologic abnormalities are predominantly within bronchi and bronchioles reflecting bronchial and bronchiolocentric distribution of asthma. Bronchi and bronchioles show hyperplasia of smooth muscle (2 to 3 times normal thickness) and marked thickening of the basement membrane (up to twice normal) (Fig. 5A and B). Bronchial walls are permeated by a mixed inflammatory infiltrate consisting of eosinophils, lymphocytes, plasma cells, and sometimes neutrophils. Eosinophils are usually prominent and an important histologic feature of asthma (100).

Another prominent histologic feature of asthma is a striking hyperplasia of goblet cells (Fig. 5B). Goblet cells comprise approximately 5% to 10% of surface epithelial cells in normal bronchi, the remainder consisting predominantly of ciliated cells and Clara cells. The percentage of goblet cells decreases in smaller bronchi, and goblet cells are normally absent in bronchioles. In asthma, however, the percentage of goblet cells is markedly increased in large airways and goblet cells are often prominent in bronchioles. In large airways, there may be a slight increase in size of submucosal seromucinous glands, and a slight increase in percentage of mucous cells compared to normal subjects (100–102).

Within the lumen of bronchi and bronchioles, mucous plugs consist of large amounts of mucus, detached fragments of epithelium (Creola bodies) admixed with eosinophils and Charcot-Leyden crystals. The detached fragments of epithelium frequently result in focal areas of denuded bronchial mucosa with only a basal layer of cells present (99).

The main differential diagnosis of asthma is chronic bronchitis. Chronic bronchitis and asthma both show hyperplasia of goblet cells, thickening of the basement membrane and a peri-/intrabronchial inflammatory infiltrate. Other histologic features, however, usually allow their separation. The smooth muscle hyperplasia and prominent eosinophils observed in asthma are not a feature of chronic bronchitis. The increase in submucosal glands is also greater in chronic bronchitis than asthma (101,102).

Since asthma is associated with other diseases such as Churg-Strauss syndrome, allergic bronchopulmonary aspergillosis, and eosinophilic pneumonia, biopsies from asthmatic patients should be correlated with clinical impression. Besides documenting asthmatic changes, biopsies should be examined for other histopathologic features suggesting associated diseases such as a necrotizing vasculitis in Churg-Strauss syndrome, or mucoid impaction with hyphal fragments in allergic bronchopulmonary aspergillosis (103).

Clinical Features

Asthma is characterized by increased irritability of the tracheobronchial tree with acute, episodic paroxysmal narrowing of airways, which may reverse spontaneously or as a result of treatment. Asthmatic attacks are manifested clinically by cough, wheezing, and feelings of suffocation. Asthma has been subdivided clinically into atopic and nonatopic forms. In this context, "atopy" refers to a genetic predisposition to develop a hypersensitivity type I reaction to certain antigens (i.e., pollen). Asthma has also been classified according to the provoking agent (i.e., exercise induced asthma) (104–106).

Pathogenesis

The pathogenesis of asthma is complex but involves airway inflammation by TH2 lymphocytes, cytokines including IL-4 and IL-13, leukotrienes C4, D4, and E4, and eotaxins

(107–110). One recent intriguing observation comes from a detailed comparison of a series of endobronchial biopsies from patients with eosinophilic bronchitis (see below) and patients with asthma. This study showed markedly increased mast cells within bronchial smooth muscle compared to either patients with eosinophilic bronchitis or normal controls. This interesting finding suggests that the presence of intramuscular mast cells may underlie bronchoconstriction in asthma and its lack thereof in eosinophilic bronchitis (106,111).

Treatment

Treatment of asthma consists of relief of symptoms through bronchodilators and long-term suppression of airway inflammation. Bronchodilaters generally include long-acting β_2 agonists such as terbutaline or albuterol. Inhaled and systemic corticosteroids and leukotriene antagonists such as montelukast are helpful in suppressing airway inflammation (107,112). More recently, bronchial thermoplasty has been advocated as efficacious in the treatment of severe refractory asthma (113,114).

Non-eosinophilic Asthma

Non-eosinophilic asthma refers to a recently described but poorly understood subset of patients with asthma. In contrast to more typical asthmatic patients, eosinophilia is absent on assessment of common fluid or tissue samples including BAL, induced sputa, or endobronchial biopsies. In addition, studies show an increase in neutrophilia in some, but not all of these patients. Furthermore, unlike conventional findings in asthma, tissue samples from patients with non-eosinophilic asthma show no increase in basement membrane thickness. These findings suggest that non-eosinophilic asthma refers to a distinct subset of asthma whose etiology, pathogenesis, and treatment are different than conventional eosinophilic asthma (115–120).

In contrast to eosinophilic asthma, which is usually precipitated by atopic (extrinsic) factors, asthmatic attacks and exacerbations in patients with non-eosinophilic asthma occur predominantly in response to non-atopic (intrinsic) factors. These factors include viruses, endotoxin, particulates, and NO_2/ozone particulates among others (119,121). Treatment of patients with non-eosinophilic asthma with corticosteroid agents has been less effective than in patients with the more conventional eosinophilic asthma (116,117,122). The finding of neutrophils within the submucosa in some patients with sudden onset asthma or "sudden asphyxic" asthma has suggested that this type of clinical presentation may represent a form of non-eosinophilic asthma (123). Likewise, neutrophilia has been observed as a dominant inflammatory response in tracheal aspirates and bronchial lavage of patients with acute severe asthma and status asthmaticus suggesting a role in these presentations as well (124,125).

Eosinophilic Bronchitis

Eosinophilic bronchitis is another recently described entity consisting of patients who have a pattern of airway eosinophilia and inflammation typical of asthma yet whose only symptom is chronic cough. Unlike patients with asthma, wheezing, or dyspnea is not prominent and tests of airway responsiveness are normal. Morphologic studies are few, but patients identified with eosinophilic bronchitis show pathologic features on endobronchial biopsy otherwise typical of asthma including submucosal and intraepithelial eosinophilia and commensurate thickening of the basement membrane. A similar pattern of eosinophilia is likewise present on assessment of BAL and induced sputa (126–132). As noted above, in comparison to patients with asthma, patients with eosinophilic bronchitis as well as normal control lack mast cells within bronchial smooth muscle—a finding that suggests a role for the intramuscular localization of mast cells in the airway hyperreactivity and bronchoconstriction of asthma (111).

Mucoid Impaction (see page 190)

Bronchocentric Granulomatosis (see page 192)

B. Angiocentric Distribution

Churg-Strauss Syndrome

Histologic Features

Early Prevasculitic Phase

Major features

- Areas of eosinophilic pneumonia

Vasculitic Phase

Major features

- Necrotizing vasculitis of medium and small pulmonary arteries and veins
- Associated multinucleated giant cells within vessel wall
- Dense subintimal and perivascular infiltrate of eosinophils within affected vessels
- Extravascular granulomas with central necrotic eosinophils ("Churg-Strauss granulomas")
- Areas of eosinophilic pneumonia
- Non-necrotizing vasculitis preferentially affecting walls of veins and venules (Fig. 6A–C)

Minor features

- Extravascular granulomas may involve the bronchial wall.

Postvasculitic Phase

Major features

- Healed vasculitis
    - Scarring of vessel walls
    - Organized thromboemboli
- Eosinophils may be scant or few

In classic descriptions based on series of autopsies, pulmonary involvement by Churg-Strauss syndrome consists of a multifocal/focal infiltrate with several distinctive features including areas of eosinophilic pneumonia, extravascular granulomas with central areas of eosinophilic necrosis, and a necrotizing "giant cell" vasculitis. Areas of eosinophilic pneumonia consist of aggregates of eosinophils and histiocytes within airspaces

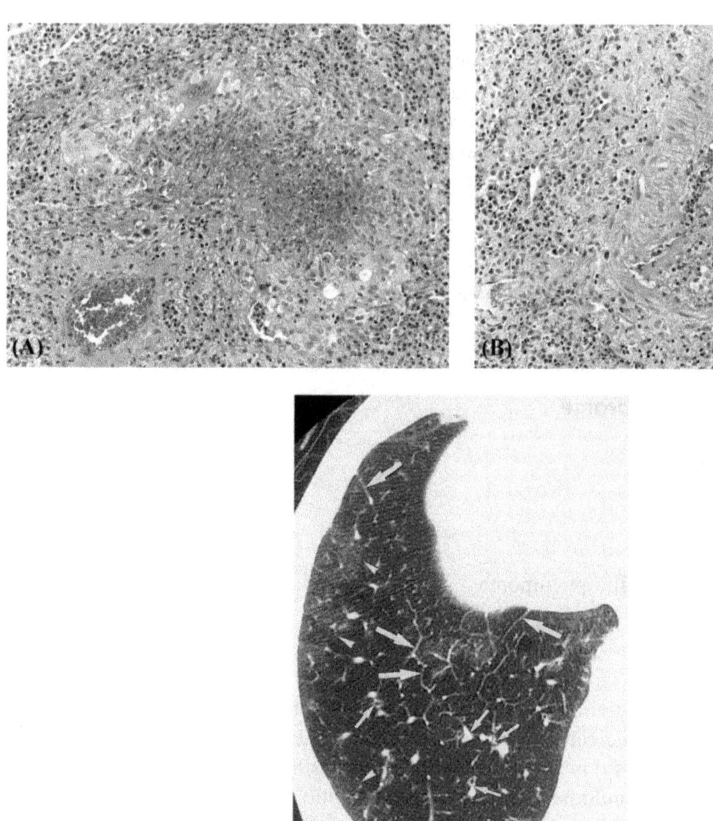

Figure 6 (**A**) Churg-Strauss syndrome. Allergic granuloma consisting of a circumscribed collection of epithelioid histiocytes surrounding central eosinophilic necrosis. (**B**) Churg-Strauss syndrome. There is segmental permeation of the vessel intima and wall by epithelioid histiocytes and eosinophils. (**C**) Churg-Strauss syndrome. High-resolution CT scan shows diffusely thickened interlobular septa (*large arrows*), thickened bronchovascular bundles (*small arrows*) and areas of peripheral ground-glass accentuation (*arrowheads*). From Ref. 25.

accompanied by an interstitial eosinophilic infiltrate. There may be associated eosinophilic microabscesses (32,133–135).

Extravascular granulomas (termed Churg-Strauss granulomas) are distinctive and show central areas of necrotic eosinophils surrounded by a rim of epithelioid histiocytes and giant cells (Fig. 6A). In some cases, there may also be focal involvement of bronchioles by granulomatous inflammation (133,134). As with necrotizing vasculitis, granulomas are not always present in Churg-Strauss disease and their absence should not exclude the diagnosis if other clinical and pathologic features are present (35).

The vasculitis in Churg-Strauss has classically been described as necrotizing, involving the walls of small arteries, arterioles, veins, and venules. The vasculitis is manifested by fibrinoid necrosis of the vascular wall associated with infiltration of the media by multinucleated giant cells, and a dense subintimal and perivascular infiltrate of eosinophils. An elastic stain will show fragmentation of the internal and external elastic lamina (33,34,133). Recent studies have shown that necrotizing vasculitis may not be present on many lung biopsy specimens. In many cases of otherwise classic disease, the only vasculitis present is non-necrotizing, consisting of eosinophilic infiltrates without necrosis or fibrin often within the walls of small veins or venules. This non-necrotizing eosinophilic vasculitis is a common feature in lung biopsies with this disorder and consistent with diagnosis of Churg-Strauss disease even if a true necrotizing vasculitis is not identified (Fig. 6B) (35).

Churg has emphasized that the natural history in many cases of Churg-Strauss disease includes an early prevasculitic stage in which the predominant manifestation is tissue eosinophilia. In the lung, this takes the form of areas of eosinophilic pneumonia (without vasculitis or granulomas). In the appropriate clinical setting, recognition of this pattern as consistent with Churg-Strauss syndrome is important as response to therapy is better than in the later vasculitic phase.

A postvasculitic phase may also be present in successfully treated patients. Biopsies from these patients show evidence of a healed vasculitis. The healed vasculitis is recognizable by segmental scarring of the vessel wall associated with organized thromboemboli. Eosinophils may be scant or absent (35).

Differential Diagnosis

The differential diagnosis of pulmonary involvement by Churg-Strauss syndrome includes polyarteritis nodosa, Wegener's granulomatosis with prominent tissue eosinophilia, and eosinophilic pneumonia (33,136). Involvement of the lung by classic polyarteritis nodosa (PAN) is rare. When it does occur, involvement usually consists of segmental involvement of bronchial arteries. The arteritis in PAN is usually neutrophilic rather than eosinophilic and lacks the granulomatous features present in Churg-Strauss syndrome. Finally, while asthma may occur in PAN, it is much rarer than in Churg-Strauss syndrome (32,137).

Wegener's granulomatosis may also be confused with Churg-Strauss syndrome. Wegener's granulomatosis, like Churg-Strauss syndrome, is a systemic vasculitis characterized by a necrotizing vasculitis and necrotizing granulomatous inflammation. Most cases can be distinguished histologically by the absence of asthmatic features and the lack of a prominent eosinophilic infiltrate in Wegener's granulomatosis. In addition, the granulomas in Churg-Strauss syndrome ("Churg-Strauss granulomas") have eosinophilic necrosis, whereas neutrophilic necrosis is more typical of the granulomas in Wegener's granulomatosis (35). Nonetheless, rare cases of Wegener's granulomatosis may have a preponderance of eosinophils (138). In this case, clinical features help to separate the diseases. Churg-Strauss syndrome occurs predominantly in patients with asthma, whereas asthma occurs only rarely in Wegener's granulomatosis. Peripheral blood eosinophilia is likewise rare in Wegener's granulomatosis but a prominent feature in Churg-Strauss syndrome (138,139). Other helpful clinical features include the distribution and location of lesions on physical examination and radiographic studies.

In laboratory tests, serum of patients with Wegener's granulomatosis and Churg-Strauss syndrome may have antineutrophil cytoplasmic antibodies (ANCA). However, in Churg-Strauss syndrome, antimyeloperoxidase antibodies (P-ANCA) are common, whereas antiproteinase 3 antibodies (C-ANCA) are more typical of Wegener's granulomatosis (140,141). Eosinophilic pneumonia may also be confused with Churg-Strauss syndrome.

While Churg-Strauss syndrome frequently contains areas of eosinophilic pneumonia, the presence of an associated prominent necrotizing vasculitis in some cases and the clinical presentation as a systemic vasculitis usually allows its separation (33). Nonetheless, Churg has suggested that some cases diagnosed as chronic eosinophilic pneumonia may actually represent the early prevasculitic phase of Churg-Strauss syndrome.

Clinical Features

Churg-Strauss syndrome is a systemic vasculitis that closely resembles polyarteritis nodosa. It is distinguished from this condition by the presence of (1) asthma, (2) peripheral eosinophilia, and (3) pulmonary involvement in up to half of all patients (32,133–135). Other involved sites include the skin, gastrointestinal tract, heart, brain, and kidney.

Radiographic Features

Radiographic features are not specific, but in the right clinical setting may be helpful and obviate the need for biopsy. Thin-section CT scan characteristically shows patchy areas of consolidation, ground-glass opacities, centrilobular nodules, thickening of interlobular septa, and bronchial wall thickening and bronchiectasis (Fig. 6C) (24,25).

Pathogenesis

The pathogenesis of Churg-Strauss syndrome is not well understood. Original studies postulated a role for immune complexes based on increased serum IgE levels and immune complexes containing IgE. More recent studies have noted the presence of ANCA in a significant minority (38%) of patients most of which are antimyeloperoxidase. Based on these findings, some authors have suggested that Churg-Strauss syndrome is heterogeneous with distinct clinical phenotypes (ANCA-positive and -negative) reflecting different underlying pathogenetic mechanisms. This suggestion is bolstered by the observation that the clinical manifestations of ANCA-positive patients tend to be dominated by vasculitic complications (alveolar hemorrhage, necrotizing glomerulonephritis, purpura, and/or mononeuritis multiplex) while those of ANCA-negative patients are dominated by the effects of eosinophilic tissue infiltration (eosinophilic pneumonia, cardiomyopathy, mono-/polyneuropathy, eosinophilic gastritis/enteritis) (142,143).

Prognosis and Treatment

Most patients (greater than 80%) respond well to corticosteroids. Other immunosuppressants may be added in severe or recalcitrant cases (142).

C. Lymphatic Distribution

Primary Pulmonary Hodgkin's Disease

Histologic Features

Major Features

- Single or multiple nodules are present that tend to have a lymphatic distribution along bronchovascular bundles, septa, and the pleura

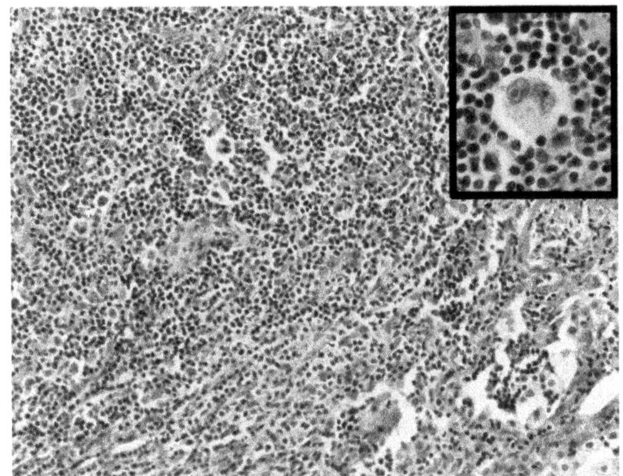

Figure 7 Pulmonary Hodgkin's disease. A nodule with mixed lymphoid infiltrate contains scattered Reed-Sternberg cells and their variants. Inset shows a higher power view of a classic Reed-Sternberg cell.

- The nodules consist of varying numbers of lymphocytes, plasma cells, eosinophils, and Reed-Sternberg cells or their variants
- Eosinophils are often prominent (Fig. 7)

Minor Features

- Eosinophilic microabascesses may occur
- Necrosis is common and may have a geographic pattern
- There may be granulomatous inflammation surrounding areas of necrosis
- Secondary areas of obstructive or acute bronchopneumonia may occur

Primary pulmonary Hodgkin's disease usually presents with a single or multiple nodules tending to have a lymphatic distribution along bronchovascular bundles, septa, and pleura. The nodules consist of varying numbers of lymphocytes, plasma cells, eosinophils, and Reed-Sternberg cells or their variants (Fig. 7). Eosinophils are often prominent, and eosinophilic microabscesses may also occur. Necrosis is common within the centers of nodules and may have a geographic pattern. The cytologic composition and constituent cells are similar to Hodgkin's disease in lymph nodes. Approximately two-thirds of cases are classified as nodular sclerosing Hodgkin's disease, and one-third are classified as mixed cellularity (144).

Other histopathologic features identified in primary pulmonary Hodgkin's disease include granulomatous inflammation surrounding areas of necrosis, involvement of the bronchial wall with destruction of cartilage plates and bronchial smooth muscle, involvement of the pleura, and permeation of arteries and veins by the infiltrate at sites separate from the main nodule. Secondary inflammatory changes consist of areas of obstructive or acute bronchopneumonia (144).

Differential Diagnosis

The differential diagnosis of primary pulmonary Hodgkin's disease includes Non-Hodgkin's lymphoma, lymphomatoid granulomatosis, Wegener's granulomatosis, granulomatous infections, and pulmonary Langerhans cell histiocytosis. Non-Hodgkin's lymphoma may involve the lungs as single or multiple nodules and appear similar histologically to primary pulmonary Hodgkin's disease. Use of immunohistochemical stains for Reed-Sternberg cells including CD30, CD15, and stains for B- and T-cell lymphomas including CD20, CD45, and CD45RO are often helpful in making this distinction (145). Lymphomatoid granulomatosis may be difficult to distinguish from Hodgkin's disease. The atypical cells in lymphomatoid granulomatosis, however, unlike Reed-Sternberg cells will stain positively for B-cell markers in most cases (146). Although Wegener's granulomatosis and Hodgkin's disease may have areas of geographic necrosis, vascular involvement, granulomatous inflammation, and prominent numbers of eosinophils, Wegener's granulomatosis lacks Reed-Sternberg cells required for diagnosis of Hodgkin's disease. The absence of nasopharyngeal and renal involvement, and absence of serum C-ANCA also help to exclude Wegener's granulomatosis (139). While granulomatous infections may accompany Hodgkin's disease, those cases unassociated with Hodgkin's disease will lack Reed-Sternberg cells. The etiologic organism may also be identified on special stains or culture. While the nodules of pulmonary Langerhans cell histiocytosis may superficially resemble primary pulmonary Hodgkin's disease, the Langerhans cells of pulmonary Langerhans cell histiocytosis may be separated from Reed-Sternberg cells by their distinctive morphology, and positive staining for S100, langerin, and CD1a (12,13,63–66).

Clinical Features

While secondary involvement of the lung is common occurring in up to half of all patients with Hodgkin's disease (144,147), primary pulmonary Hodgkin's disease is rare. The diagnosis of primary pulmonary Hodgkin's disease requires adherence to three criteria: (1) typical histologic and immunohistochemical features of Hodgkin's disease, (2) restriction of the findings to the lung without evidence of involvement by hilar lymph nodes, and (3) adequate clinical or pathologic exclusion of Hodgkin's disease at other sites (144).

In primary pulmonary Hodgkin's disease, the most common presenting symptoms are cough, fever, and weight loss. Females are affected more often than males (2:1). There is a bimodal age distribution with a peak incidence between 20 to 30 years and 60 to 80 years (144,147,148).

Radiographic Features

Radiographically, almost all patients have either a solitary mass or multiple nodules. Some nodules may show central cavitation (144,148). Occasional cases may have bilateral reticulonodular infiltrates or localized pneumonic consolidation. Peripheral or mediastinal adenopathy is not identified.

Pathogenesis

The pathogenesis of primary pulmonary Hodgkin's disease is uncertain but may reflect initial development in bronchus associated lymphoid tissue or an intrapulmonary lymph node (144).

Prognosis and Treatment

Primary pulmonary Hodgkin's disease tends to have a variable prognosis. Radin reported two-year survival of approximately 50% of patients (148). Adverse prognostic factors include multilobar or bilateral involvement, cavitary disease, pleural involvement and type B symptoms. Treatment is variable and consists of combinations of chemotherapy and radiation therapy (148).

D. Pleural Distribution

Reactive Eosinophilic Pleuritis

Histologic Features

Major Features

- Pleural inflammatory infiltrate consisting of eosinophils, reactive mesothelial cells, histiocytes, lymphocytes, and giant cells (Fig. 8A and B)

Minor Features

- Adjacent lung may show focal non-necrotizing eosinophilic infiltrates within small vessels

Reactive eosinophilic pleuritis is a fairly common pleural reaction to pneumothorax identified in the tissues of patients undergoing pleurectomy and/or excision of blebs. Histologically, this condition is manifested by a pleural inflammatory infiltrate consisting of numerous eosinophils, reactive mesothelial cells, histiocytes, lymphocytes, and occasional giant cells (Fig. 8A and B) (82,149). In some patients there may be associated focal

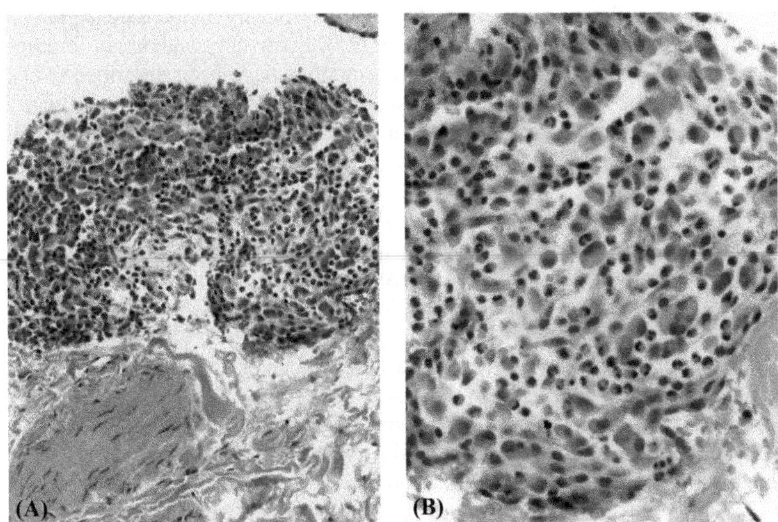

Figure 8 **(A)** Reactive eosinophilic pleuritis. The pleura is thickened by an inflammatory infiltrate. The adjacent lung showed fibrobullous disease. **(B)** Reactive eosinophilic pleuritis. The inflammatory infiltrate consists of numerous eosinophils admixed with histiocytes, some of which are multinucleated. This lesion is distinguished from pulmonary Langerhans cell histiocytosis by the absence of characteristic Langerhans cells.

non-necrotizing vascular and perivascular eosinophilic infiltrates within the adjacent pulmonary parenchyma (83). While the histologic features may superficially resemble pulmonary Langerhans cell histiocytosis, and pulmonary Langerhans cell histiocytosis may involve the pleura, reactive eosinophilic pleuritis lacks collections of Langerhans cells. Parenchymal nodules containing Langerhans cells are also present in Langerhans cell histiocytosis but not in reactive eosinophilic pleuritis. In equivocal cases, immunohistochemical stains for Langerhans cells (S100, CD1a, and langerin) can help in the differential diagnosis (63–66).

VI. Extremely Rare Disorders

Hypereosinophilic Syndrome

Histologic Features

- Interstitial eosinophilic infiltrate
- There may be areas of pulmonary parenchymal necrosis
- The histologic appearance may be similar to Churg-Strauss syndrome

Hypereosinophilic syndrome is an extremely rare disorder characterized by persistent marked eosinophilia in the peripheral blood (>1500 eosinophils/mm^3), no known causes for eosinophilia, and signs of multiple organ involvement. Patients commonly present with weakness and fatigue, cough, dyspnea, myalgia or angioedema, rash, fever, or rhinitis. Pulmonary involvement is common, occurring in up to 40% of patients (150–152). High-resolution CT findings in pulmonary involvement consist of patchy areas of consolidaton or nodules variably accompanied by pleural effusion (25). Pulmonary pathologic findings are not well documented. Interstitial infiltrates of eosinophils have been described (151). An isolated report describes eosinophilic infiltration and cuffing of small pulmonary arteries (153). Likewise there is a case report of a patient with pulmonary parenchymal necrosis and infarction (154) as well as another case with features similar to Churg-Strauss syndrome (151).

New findings have greatly increased our understanding of hypereosinophilic syndrome. Recent studies have shown that imatinib mesylate (Gleevec, Novartis®) is an effective treatment for this disorder and causes remission in many patients (155–162). Most patients who respond have a novel fusion tyrosine kinase FIP1L1-PDGFR-α. This protein is generated as the result of an 800 kb deletion on chromosome 4q12, which leads to the fusion of the newly discovered gene FIP1L1 to the kinase domain of the platelet-derived growth factor receptor alpha (PDGFR-α) (163,164). The fusion protein is inhibited by imatinib in vitro, thus likely accounting for the response of these patients clinically. This form of the disease is termed the "myeloproliferative form" (165,166).

In a second group of patients, the disorder appears to have a different pathogenesis unrelated to FIP1L1-PDGFR-α. These cases are instead associated with the elaboration of IL-5 by expansion of an aberrant clone of CD3−, CD4+ T cells (166–170). Preliminary results of ongoing trials with anti–IL-5 antibodies have resulted in clinical improvement and sustained reduction in blood eosinophil counts in some patients (165,166,171–173).

References

1. Colby TV, Lombard C, Yousem SA, et al. Approach to lung biopsies. In: Atlas of Pulmonary Surgical Pathology. 1st ed. Philadelphia: W.B. Saunders Company; 1991:1–45.
2. Crofton JW, Livingstone JL, Oswald NC, et al. Pulmonary eosinophilia. Thorax 1952; 7(1):1–35.
3. Liebow AA, Carrington CB. The eosinophilic pneumonias. Medicine 1969; 48:251–285.
4. Jederlinic PJ, Sicilian L, Gaensler EA. Chronic eosinophilic pneumonia. A report of 19 cases and a review of the literature. Medicine 1988; 67:154–162.
5. Carrington CB, Addington WW, Goff AM, et al. Chronic eosinophilic pneumonia. N Engl J Med 1969; 280:787–798.
6. Colby TV, Carrington CB. Interstitial lung disease. In: Thurlbeck WM, Churg AM, eds. Pathology of the Lung. 2 ed. New York: Thieme Medical Publishers, Inc.; 1995:589–737.
7. Hayakawa H, Sato A, Toyoshima M, et al. A clinical study of idiopathic eosinophilic pneumonia. Chest 1994; 105(5):1462–1466.
8. Cottin V, Cordier JF. Eosinophilic pneumonias. Allergy 2005; 60(7):841–857.
9. Tazelaar HD, Linz LJ, Colby TV, et al. Acute eosinophilic pneumonia: histopathologic findings in nine patients. Am J Respir Crit Care Med 1997; 155(1):296–302.
10. Allen J. Acute eosinophilic pneumonia. Semin Respir Crit Care Med 2006; 27(2):142–147.
11. Katzenstein AL, Askin FB. Surgical pathology of non-neoplastic lung disease. 4th ed. Philadelphia: Saunders Elsevier; 2006.
12. Travis WD, Borok Z, Roum JH, et al. Pulmonary Langerhans cell granulomatosis (Histiocytosis X). A clinicopathologic study of 48 cases. Am J Surg Pathol 1993; 17:971–986.
13. Colby TV, Lombard C. Histiocytosis X in the lung. Hum Pathol 1983; 14:847–856.
14. Lombard CM, Tazelaar HD, Krasne DL. Pulmonary eosinophilia in coccidioidal infections. Chest 1987; 91:734–736.
15. Wright JL, Pare PD, Hammond M, et al. Eosinophilic pneumonia and atypical mycobacterial infection. Am Rev Respir Dis 1983; 127:497–499.
16. Keslin MH, McCoy EL, McCusker JJ, et al. Corynebacterium pseudotuberculosis. A new cause of infectious and eosinophilic pneumonia. Am J Med 1979; 67:228–231.
17. Butland RJA, Coulson IH. Pulmonary eosinophilia associated with cutaneous larva migrans. Thorax 1985; 40:76–77.
18. Vijayan V-K, Reetha A-M, Jawahar MS, et al. Pulmonary eosinophilia in pulmonary tuberculosis. Chest 1992; 101:1708–1709.
19. Dines DE. Chronic eosinophilic pneumonia: a roentgenographic diagnosis. Mayo Clin Proc 1978; 53(2):129–130.
20. Roig J, Romeu J, Rivera C, et al. Acute eosinophilic pneumonia due to toxocariasis with bronchoalveolar lavage findings. Chest 1992; 102:294–296.
21. Ricker DH, Taylor SR, Gartner JC Jr., et al. Fatal pulmonary aspergillosis presenting as acute eosinophilic pneumonia in a previously healthy child. Chest 1991; 100:875–877.
22. Pesci A, Bertorelli G, Manganelli P, et al. Bronchoalveolar lavage in chronic eosinophilic pneumonia. Analysis of six cases in comparison with other interstitial lung diseases. Respiration 1988; 54 (suppl):16–22.
23. Allen JN, Davis WB. Eosinophilic lung diseases. Am J Respir Crit Care Med 1994; 150(5 pt 1): 1423–1438.
24. Jeong YJ, Kim KI, Seo IJ, et al. Eosinophilic lung diseases: a clinical, radiologic, and pathologic overview. Radiographics 2007; 27(3):617–637; discussion 37–39.
25. Johkoh T, Muller NL, Akira M, et al. Eosinophilic lung diseases: diagnostic accuracy of thin-section CT in 111 patients. Radiology 2000; 216(3):773–780.
26. Marchand E, Cordier JF. Idiopathic chronic eosinophilic pneumonia. Semin Respir Crit Care Med 2006; 27(2):134–141.

27. Marchand E, Reynaud-Gaubert M, Lauque D, et al. Idiopathic chronic eosinophilic pneumonia. A clinical and follow-up study of 62 cases. The Groupe d'Etudes et de Recherche sur les Maladies "Orphelines" Pulmonaires (GERM"O"P). Medicine 1998; 77(5):299–312.
28. Gopinathan VP. Tropical pulmonary eosinophilia. A clinical study. Med J Aust 1983; 1:69–72.
29. Enright T, Chua S, Lim DT. Pulmonary eosinophilic syndromes. Ann Allergy 1989; 62(4):277–283.
30. Neva FA, Ottesen EA. Current concepts in parasitology. Tropical (filarial) eosinophilia. N Engl J Med 1978; 298:1129–1131.
31. Warnock ML, Fennessy J, Rippon J. Chronic eosinophilic pneumonia, a manifestation of allergic aspergillosis. Am J Clin Pathol 1974; 62:73–81.
32. Chumbley LC, Harrison EG, DeRemee RA. Allergic granulomatosis and angiitis (Churg-Strauss syndrome). Report and analysis of 30 cases. Mayo Clin Proc 1977; 52:477–484.
33. Koss MN, Antonovych T, Hochholzer L. Allergic granulomatosis (Churg-Strauss syndrome). Pulmonary and renal morphologic findings. Am J Surg Pathol 1981; 5:21–28.
34. Churg J. Churg-Strauss syndrome. In: Thurlbeck WM, Churg AM, eds. Pathology of the lung. 2nd ed. New York: Thieme Medical Publishers, Inc.; 1995:425–436.
35. Churg A. Recent advances in the diagnosis of Churg-Strauss syndrome. Mod Pathol 2001; 14(12):1284–1293.
36. Bosken CH, Myers JL, Greenberger PA, et al. Pathologic features of allergic bronchopulmonary aspergillosis. Am J Surg Pathol 1988; 12(3):216–222.
37. Zander DS. Allergic bronchopulmonary aspergillosis: an overview. Arch Pathol Lab Med 2005; 129(7):924–928.
38. Allen JN, Pacht ER, Gadek JE, et al. Acute eosinophilic pneumonia as a reversible cause of noninfectious respiratory failure. N Engl J Med 1989; 321(9):569–574.
39. Pope-Harman AL, Davis WB, Allen ED, et al. Acute eosinophilic pneumonia. A summary of 15 cases and review of the literature. Medicine 1996; 75(6):334–342.
40. King MA, Pope-Harman AL, Allen JN, et al. Acute eosinophilic pneumonia: radiologic and clinical features. Radiology 1997; 203(3):715–719.
41. Badesch DB, King TE Jr., Schwarz MI. Acute eosinophilic pneumonia: a hypersensitivity phenomenon? Am Rev Respir Dis 1989; 139(1):249–252.
42. Philit F, Etienne-Mastroianni B, Parrot A, et al. Idiopathic acute eosinophilic pneumonia: a study of 22 patients. Am J Respir Crit Care Med 2002; 166(9):1235–1239.
43. Shintani H, Fujimura M, Ishiura Y, et al. A case of cigarette smoking-induced acute eosinophilic pneumonia showing tolerance. Chest 2000; 117(1):277–279.
44. Shintani H, Fujimura M, Yasui M, et al. Acute eosinophilic pneumonia caused by cigarette smoking. Internal medicine (Tokyo, Japan) 2000; 39(1):66–68.
45. Taki R, Sawada M, Isogai S, et al. A possible role of cigarette smoking in the pathogenesis of acute eosinophilic pneumonia (abstr). Am J Respir Crit Care Med 1996; 153:A271.
46. Kawayama T, Fujiki R, Rikimaru T, et al. Chronic eosinophilic pneumonia associated with Schizophyllum commune. Respirology 2003; 8(4):529–531.
47. Elsom KA, Ingelfinger FJ. Eosinophilia and pneumonitis in chronic brucellosis; a report of two cases. Ann Intern Med 1942; 16:995–1002.
48. Wardlaw A, Geddes DM. Allergic bronchopulmonary aspergillosis: a review. J R Soc Med 1992; 85:747–751.
49. Ricketti AJ, Greenberger PA, Mintzer RA, et al. Allergic bronchopulmonary aspergillosis. Chest 1984; 86:773–778.
50. Virnig C, Bush RK. Allergic bronchopulmonary aspergillosis: a US perspective. Curr Opin Pulm Med 2007; 13(1):67–71.
51. Katzenstein AL, Liebow AA, Friedman PJ. Bronchocentric granulomatosis, mucoid impaction, and hypersensitivity reactions to fungi. Am Rev Respir Dis 1975; 111:497–537.
52. Shaw RR. Mucoid impaction of the bronchi. J Thorac Surg 1951; 22:149–163.

53. Urschel HC Jr., Paulson DL, Shaw RR. Mucoid impaction of the bronchi. Ann Thorac Surg 1966; 2:1–16.
54. Aubry MC, Fraser R. The role of bronchial biopsy and washing in the diagnosis of allergic bronchopulmonary aspergillosis. Mod Pathol 1998; 11(7):607–611.
55. Koss MN, Robinson RG, Hochholzer L. Bronchocentric granulomatosis. Hum Pathol 1981; 12:632–638.
56. Liebow AA. Pulmonary angiitis and granulomatosis. Am Rev Respir Dis 1973; 108:1–18.
57. Myers JL, Katzenstein A-LA. Granulomatous infection mimicking bronchocentric granulomatosis. Am J Surg Pathol 1986; 10:317–322.
58. van der Klooster JM, Nurmohamed LA, van Kaam NA. Bronchocentric granulomatosis associated with influenza-A virus infection. Respiration 2004; 71(4):412–416.
59. Keijzer A, Daniels JM, Slieker WA, et al. [Bronchocentric granulomatosis and mycoplasmal pneumonia]. Ned Tijdschr Geneeskd 2004; 148(7):332–336.
60. Travis WD, Kwon Chung KJ, Kleiner DE, et al. Unusual aspects of allergic bronchopulmonary fungal disease: report of two cases due to Curvularia organisms associated with allergic fungal sinusitis. Hum Pathol 1991; 22:1240–1248.
61. Friedman PJ, Liebow AA, Sokoloff J. Eosinophilic granuloma of lung. Clinical aspects of primary pulmonary histiocytosis in the adult. Medicine 1981; 60:385–396.
62. Fukuda Y, Basset F, Soler P, et al. Intraluminal fibrosis and elastic fiber degradation lead to lung remodeling in pulmonary Langerhans cell granulomatosis (histiocytosis X). Am J Pathol 1990; 137(2):415–424.
63. Flint A, Lloyd RV, Colby TV, et al. Pulmonary histiocytosis X. Immunoperoxidase staining for HLA-DR antigen and S100 protein. Arch Pathol Lab Med 1986; 110:930–933.
64. Webber D, Tron V, Askin F, et al. S-100 staining in the diagnosis of eosinophilic granuloma of lung. Am J Clin Pathol 1985; 84:447–453.
65. Krenacs L, Tiszalvicz L, Krenacs T, et al. Immunohistochemical detection of CD1A antigen in formalin-fixed and paraffin-embedded tissue sections with monoclonal antibody 010. J Pathol 1993; 171(2):99–104.
66. Sholl LM, Hornick JL, Pinkus JL, et al. Immunohistochemical analysis of langerin in langerhans cell histiocytosis and pulmonary inflammatory and infectious diseases. Am J Surg Pathol 2007; 31(6):947–952.
67. Chollet S, Soler P, Dournovo P, et al. Diagnosis of pulmonary histiocytosis X by immunodetection of Langerhans cells in bronchoalveolar lavage fluid. Am J Pathol 1984; 115(2):225–232.
68. Xaubet A, Agusti C, Picado C, et al. Bronchoalveolar lavage analysis with anti-T6 monoclonal antibody in the evaluation of diffuse lung diseases. Respiration 1989; 56:161–166.
69. Auerswald U, Barth J, Magnussen H. Value of CD-1-positive cells in bronchoalveolar lavage fluid for the diagnosis of pulmonary histiocytosis X. Lung 1991; 169(6):305–309.
70. Sledziewska J, Roginska E, Oblakowski P, et al. [Usefulness of CD1 expression on surfaces of cells in bronchoalveolar fluid for diagnosis of histiocytosis X—our experience]. Pneumonol Alergol Pol 1999; 67(7–8):311–317.
71. Casolaro MA, Bernaudin JF, Saltini C, et al. Accumulation of Langerhans' cells on the epithelial surface of the lower respiratory tract in normal subjects in association with cigarette smoking. Am Rev Respir Dis 1988; 137(2):406–411.
72. Brauner MW, Grenier P, Tijani K, et al. Pulmonary Langerhans cell histiocytosis: evolution of lesions on CT scans. Radiology 1997; 204(2):497–502.
73. Brauner MW, Grenier P, Mouelhi MM, et al. Pulmonary histiocytosis X: evaluation with high-resolution CT. Radiology 1989; 172(1):255–258.
74. Moore ADA, Godwin JD, Muller NL, et al. Pulmonary histiocytosis X: Comparison of radiographic and CT findings. Radiology 1989; 172:249–254.
75. Abbott GF, Rosado-de-Christenson ML, Franks TJ, et al. From the archives of the AFIP: pulmonary Langerhans cell histiocytosis. Radiographics 2004; 24(3):821–841.
76. Tazi A. Adult pulmonary Langerhans' cell histiocytosis. Eur Respir J 2006; 27(6):1272–1285.

77. Schon-Hegrad MA, Oliver J, McMenamin PG, et al. Studies on the density, distribution, and surface phenotype of intraepithelial class II major histocompatibility complex antigen (Ia)-bearing dendritic cells (DC) in the conducting airways. J Exp Med 1991; 173(6):1345–1356.
78. Khoor A, Myers JL, Tazelaar HD, et al. Pulmonary Langerhans cell histiocytosis presenting as a solitary nodule. Mayo Clinic Proc 2001; 76(2):209–211.
79. O'Donnell AE, Tsou E, Awh C, et al. Endobronchial eosinophilic granuloma: a rare cause of total lung atelectasis. Am Rev Respir Dis 1987; 136(6):1478–1480.
80. Loukides S, Karameris A, Lachanis S, et al. Eosinophilic granuloma of the lung presenting as an endobronchial mass. Monaldi archives for chest disease = Archivio Monaldi per le malattie del torace/Fondazione clinica del lavoro, IRCCS [and] Istituto di clinica tisiologica e malattie apparato respiratorio, Universita di Napoli, Secondo ateneo 2000; 55(3):208–209.
81. Fridlender ZG, Glazer M, Amir G, et al. Obstructing tracheal pulmonary Langerhans cell histiocytosis. Chest 2005; 128(2):1057–1058.
82. Askin FB, McCann BG, Kuhn C. Reactive eosinophilic pleuritis. A lesion to be distinguished from pulmonary eosinophilic granuloma. Arch Pathol Lab Med 1977; 101:187–192.
83. Luna E, Tomashefski JF, Brown D, et al. Reactive eosinophilic pulmonary vascular infiltration in patients with spontaneous pneumothorax. Am J Surg Pathol 1994; 18:195–199.
84. Rush WL, Andriko JA, Galateau-Salle F, et al. Pulmonary pathology of Erdheim-Chester disease. Mod Pathol 2000; 13(7):747–754.
85. Soler P, Moreau A, Basset F, et al. Cigarette smoking-induced changes in the number and differentiated state of pulmonary dendritic cells/Langerhans cells. Am Rev Respir Dis 1989; 139(5):1112–1117.
86. Vassallo R, Ryu JH. Pulmonary Langerhans' cell histiocytosis. Clin Chest Med 2004; 25(3): 561–571, vii.
87. de Graaf JH, Tamminga RY, Dam-Meiring A, et al. The presence of cytokines in Langerhans' cell histiocytosis. J Pathol 1996; 180(4):400–406.
88. Asakura S, Colby TV, Limper AH. Tissue localization of transforming growth factor-beta1 in pulmonary eosinophilic granuloma. Am J Respir Crit Care Med 1996; 154(5):1525–1530.
89. Yousem SA, Colby TV, Chen YY, et al. Pulmonary Langerhans' cell histiocytosis: molecular analysis of clonality. Am J Surg Pathol 2001; 25(5):630–636.
90. Mogulkoc N, Veral A, Bishop PW, et al. Pulmonary Langerhans' cell histiocytosis: radiologic resolution following smoking cessation. Chest 1999; 115(5):1452–1455.
91. Vassallo R, Ryu JH, Schroeder DR, et al. Clinical outcomes of pulmonary Langerhans'-cell histiocytosis in adults. N Engl J Med 2002; 346(7):484–490.
92. Dauriat G, Mal H, Thabut G, et al. Lung transplantation for pulmonary Langerhans' cell histiocytosis: a multicenter analysis. Transplantation 2006; 81(5):746–750.
93. Beasley R, Roche WR, Roberts JA, et al. Cellular events in the bronchi in mild asthma and after bronchial provocation. Am Rev Respir Dis 1989; 139(3):806–817.
94. Beasley R, Burgess C, Crane J, et al. Pathology of asthma and its clinical implications. J Allergy Clin Immunol 1993; 92(1 pt 2):148–154.
95. Bradley BL, Azzawi M, Jacobson M, et al. Eosinophils, T-lymphocytes, mast cells, neutrophils, and macrophages in bronchial biopsy specimens from atopic subjects with asthma: comparison with biopsy specimens from atopic subjects without asthma and normal control subjects and relationship to bronchial hyperresponsiveness. J Allergy Clin Immunol 1991; 88(4):661–674.
96. Djukanovic R, Wilson JW, Britten KM, et al. Quantitation of mast cells and eosinophils in the bronchial mucosa of symptomatic atopic asthmatics and healthy control subjects using immunohistochemistry. Am Rev Respir Dis 1990; 142(4):863–871.
97. Kay AB. Pathology of mild, severe, and fatal asthma. Am J Respir Crit Care Med 1996; 154 (2 pt 2):S66–S69.
98. Bourdin A, Neveu D, Vachier I, et al. Specificity of basement membrane thickening in severe asthma. J Allergy Clin Immunol 2007; 119(6):1367–1374.
99. Thurlbeck WM. Chronic airflow obstruction. In: Thurlbeck WM, Churg AM, eds. Pathology of the lung. 2nd ed. New York: Thieme Medical Publishers; 1995:739–825.

100. Dunnill MS. The pathology of asthma, with special reference to changes in the bronchial mucosa. J Clin Pathol 1960; 13:27–33.
101. Takizawa T, Thurlbeck WM. Muscle and mucous gland size in the major bronchi of patients with chronic bronchitis, asthma, and asthmatic bronchitis. Am Rev Respir Dis 1971; 104:331–336.
102. Pratt PC. Emphysema and chronic airways disease. In: Dail DH, Hammar SP, eds. Pulmonary Pathology. 2nd ed. New York: Springer-Verlag; 1994:847–865.
103. Colby TV, Lombard C, Yousem SA, et al. Airway and obstructive diseases. In: Atlas of pulmonary pathology. 1st ed. Philadelphia: W.B. Saunders Company; 1991:205–226.
104. Expert Panel Report 2: Guidelines for the Diagnosis and Management of Asthma. In: National Institutes of Health, National Heart, Lung, and Blood Institute publication # 97-4051. Bethesda, MD; 1997:1–153.
105. Novak N, Bieber T. Allergic and nonallergic forms of atopic diseases. J Allergy Clin Immunol 2003; 112(2):252–262.
106. Wardlaw AJ, Brightling CE, Green R, et al. New insights into the relationship between airway inflammation and asthma. Clin Sci (Lond) 2002; 103(2):201–211.
107. Busse WW, Lemanske RF Jr. Asthma. N Engl J Med 2001; 344(5):350–362.
108. Hamid Q, Azzawi M, Ying S, et al. Interleukin-5 mRNA in mucosal bronchial biopsies from asthmatic subjects. Int Arch Allergy Appl Immunol 1991; 94(1–4):169–170.
109. Brightling CE, Symon FA, Birring SS, et al. TH2 cytokine expression in bronchoalveolar lavage fluid T lymphocytes and bronchial submucosa is a feature of asthma and eosinophilic bronchitis. J Allergy Clin Immunol 2002; 110(6):899–905.
110. Azzawi M, Bradley B, Jeffery PK, et al. Identification of activated T lymphocytes and eosinophils in bronchial biopsies in stable atopic asthma. Am Rev Respir Dis 1990; 142(6 pt 1): 1407–1413.
111. Brightling CE, Bradding P, Symon FA, et al. Mast-cell infiltration of airway smooth muscle in asthma. N Engl J Med 2002; 346(22):1699–1705.
112. Drazen JM, Israel E, O'Byrne PM. Treatment of asthma with drugs modifying the leukotriene pathway. N Engl J Med 1999; 340(3):197–206.
113. Cox G, Miller JD, McWilliams A, et al. Bronchial thermoplasty for asthma. Am J Respir Crit Care Med 2006; 173(9):965–969.
114. Cox G, Thomson NC, Rubin AS, et al. Asthma control during the year after bronchial thermoplasty. N Engl J Med 2007; 356(13):1327–1337.
115. Wenzel SE, Schwartz LB, Langmack EL, et al. Evidence that severe asthma can be divided pathologically into two inflammatory subtypes with distinct physiologic and clinical characteristics. Am J Respir Crit Care Med 1999; 160(3):1001–1008.
116. Pavord ID, Brightling CE, Woltmann G, et al. Non-eosinophilic corticosteroid unresponsive asthma. Lancet 1999; 353(9171):2213–2214.
117. Douwes J, Gibson P, Pekkanen J, et al. Non-eosinophilic asthma: importance and possible mechanisms. Thorax 2002; 57(7):643–648.
118. Haldar P, Pavord ID. Noneosinophilic asthma: a distinct clinical and pathologic phenotype. J Allergy Clin Immunol 2007; 119(5):1043–1052; quiz 53–54.
119. Green RH, Brightling CE, Bradding P. The reclassification of asthma based on subphenotypes. Curr Opin Allergy Clin Immunol 2007; 7(1):43–50.
120. Gibson PG, Simpson JL, Saltos N. Heterogeneity of airway inflammation in persistent asthma: evidence of neutrophilic inflammation and increased sputum interleukin-8. Chest 2001; 119(5): 1329–1336.
121. Green RH, Brightling CE, Woltmann G, et al. Analysis of induced sputum in adults with asthma: identification of subgroup with isolated sputum neutrophilia and poor response to inhaled corticosteroids. Thorax 2002; 57(10):875–879.
122. Berry M, Morgan A, Shaw DE, et al. Pathological features and inhaled corticosteroid response of eosinophilic and non-eosinophilic asthma. Thorax 2007; 62(12):1043–1049.

123. Sur S, Crotty TB, Kephart GM, et al. Sudden-onset fatal asthma. A distinct entity with few eosinophils and relatively more neutrophils in the airway submucosa? Am Rev Respir Dis 1993; 148(3):713–719.
124. Lamblin C, Gosset P, Tillie-Leblond I, et al. Bronchial neutrophilia in patients with noninfectious status asthmaticus. Am J Respir Crit Care Med 1998; 157(2):394–402.
125. Ordonez CL, Shaughnessy TE, Matthay MA, et al. Increased neutrophil numbers and IL-8 levels in airway secretions in acute severe asthma: clinical and biologic significance. Am J Respir Crit Care Med 2000; 161(4 pt 1):1185–1190.
126. Gibson PG, Dolovich J, Denburg J, et al. Chronic cough: eosinophilic bronchitis without asthma. Lancet 1989; 1(8651):1346–1348.
127. Gibson PG, Fujimura M, Niimi A. Eosinophilic bronchitis: clinical manifestations and implications for treatment. Thorax 2002; 57(2):178–182.
128. Birring SS, Berry M, Brightling CE, et al. Eosinophilic bronchitis: clinical features, management and pathogenesis. Am J Respir Med 2003; 2(2):169–173.
129. Brightling CE, Pavord ID. Eosinophilic bronchitis: an important cause of prolonged cough. Ann Med 2000; 32(7):446–451.
130. Brightling CE, Pavord ID. Eosinophilic bronchitis—what is it and why is it important? Clin Exp Allergy 2000; 30(1):4–6.
131. Brightling CE. Chronic cough due to nonasthmatic eosinophilic bronchitis: ACCP evidence-based clinical practice guidelines. Chest 2006; 129(1 suppl):116S–121S.
132. Scott KA, Wardlaw AJ. Eosinophilic airway disorders. Semin Respir Crit Care Med 2006; 27(2):128–133.
133. Churg J, Strauss L. Allergic granulomatosis, allergic angiitis, and periarteritis nodosa. Am J Pathol 1951; 27:277–301.
134. Churg A. Pulmonary angiitis and granulomatosis revisited. Hum Pathol 1983; 14:868–883.
135. Lie JT. The classification of vasculitis and a reappraisal of allergic granulomatosis and angiitis (Churg-Strauss syndrome). Mt Sinai J Med 1986; 53:429–439.
136. Katzenstein A-LA, Askin FB. Pulmonary vasculitis. In: Surgical Pathology of Non-neoplastic lung disease. 4th ed. Philadelphia: Elsevier Saunders; 2006:217–236.
137. Matsumoto T, Homma S, Okada M, et al. The lung in polyarteritis nodosa: a pathologic study of 10 cases. Hum Pathol 1993; 24:717–724.
138. Yousem SA, Lombard CM. The eosinophilic variant of Wegener's granulomatosis. Hum Pathol 1988; 19:682–688.
139. Travis WD, Hoffman GS, Leavitt RY, et al. Surgical pathology of the lung in Wegener's granulomatosis. Review of 87 open lung biopsies from 67 patients. Am J Surg Pathol 1991; 15:315–333.
140. Fienberg R, Mark EJ, Goodman M, et al. Correlation of antineutrophil cytoplasmic antibodies with the extrarenal histopathology of Wegener's (pathergic) granulomatosis and related forms of vasculitis. Hum Pathol 1993; 24:160–168.
141. Tervaert JWC, Goldschmeding R, Elema JD, et al. Antimyeloperoxidase antibodies in the Churg-Strauss syndrome. Thorax 1991; 46:70–71.
142. Pagnoux C, Guilpain P, Guillevin L. Churg-Strauss syndrome. Curr Opin Rheumatol 2007; 19(1):25–32.
143. Kallenberg CG. Churg-Strauss syndrome: just one disease entity? Arthritis and rheumatism 2005; 52(9):2589–2593.
144. Yousem SA, Weiss LM, Colby TV. Primary pulmonary Hodgkin's disease. Cancer 1986; 57:1217–1224.
145. Chittal SM, Caveriviere P, Schwarting R, et al. Monoclonal antibodies in the diagnosis of Hodgkin's disease. The search for a rational panel. Am J Surg Pathol 1988; 12:9–21.
146. Guinee D Jr., Jaffe E, Kingma D, et al. Pulmonary lymphomatoid granulomatosis. Evidence for a proliferation of Epstein-Barr virus infected B-lymphocytes with a prominent T-cell component and vasculitis. Am J Surg Pathol 1994; 18:753–764.

147. Colby TV, Hoppe RT, Warnke RA. Hodgkin's disease at autopsy: 1972–1977. Cancer 1981; 47:1852–1862.
148. Radin AI. Primary pulmonary Hodgkin's disease. Cancer 1990; 65:550–563.
149. McDonnell TJ, Crouch EC, Gonzalez JG. Reactive eosinophilic pleuritis. A sequela of pnemothorax in pulmonary eosinophilic granuloma. Am J Clin Pathol 1989; 91:107–111.
150. Weller PF, Bubley GJ. The idiopathic hypereosinophilic syndrome. Blood 1994; 83(10): 2759–2779.
151. Chusid MJ, Dale DC, West BC, et al. The hypereosinophilic syndrome. Medicine 1975; 54:1–27.
152. Fauci AS, Harley JB, Roberts WC, et al. NIH conference. The idiopathic hypereosinophilic syndrome. Clinical, pathophysiologic, and therapeutic considerations. Ann Intern Med 1982; 97(1):78–92.
153. Hill R, Wang NS, Berry G. Hypereosinophilic syndrome with pulmonary vascular involvement. Angiology 1984; 35(4):238–244.
154. Suenaga N, Hayashi F, Miyauhi N, et al. [A case of hypereosinophilic syndrome associated with pulmonary infarction and hepatic vein obstruction (Budd-Chiari syndrome)]. Nihon Kyobu Shikkan Gakkai Zasshi 1991; 29(2):239–244.
155. Frickhofen N, Marker-Hermann E, Reiter A, et al. Complete molecular remission of chronic eosinophilic leukemia complicated by CNS disease after targeted therapy with imatinib. Ann Hematol 2004; 83(7):477–480.
156. Muller AM, Martens UM, Hofmann SC, et al. Imatinib mesylate as a novel treatment option for hypereosinophilic syndrome: two case reports and a comprehensive review of the literature. Ann Hematol 2006; 85(1):1–16.
157. Apperley JF, Gardembas M, Melo JV, et al. Response to imatinib mesylate in patients with chronic myeloproliferative diseases with rearrangements of the platelet-derived growth factor receptor beta. N Engl J Med 2002; 347(7):481–487.
158. Ault P, Cortes J, Koller C, et al. Response of idiopathic hypereosinophilic syndrome to treatment with imatinib mesylate. Leuk Res 2002; 26(9):881–884.
159. Cortes J, Ault P, Koller C, et al. Efficacy of imatinib mesylate in the treatment of idiopathic hypereosinophilic syndrome. Blood 2003; 101(12):4714–4716.
160. Gleich GJ, Leiferman KM, Pardanani A, et al. Treatment of hypereosinophilic syndrome with imatinib mesilate. Lancet 2002; 359(9317):1577–1578.
161. Pardanani A, Reeder T, Porrata LF, et al. Imatinib therapy for hypereosinophilic syndrome and other eosinophilic disorders. Blood 2003; 101(9):3391–3397.
162. Schaller JL, Burkland GA. Case report: rapid and complete control of idiopathic hypereosinophilia with imatinib mesylate. MedGenMed 2001; 3(5):9.
163. Gotlib J, Cools J, Malone JM IIIrd, et al. The FIP1L1-PDGFR alpha fusion tyrosine kinase in hypereosinophilic syndrome and chronic eosinophilic leukemia: implications for diagnosis, classification, and management. Blood 2004; 103(8):2879–2891.
164. Cools J, DeAngelo DJ, Gotlib J, et al. A tyrosine kinase created by fusion of the PDGFRA and FIP1L1 genes as a therapeutic target of imatinib in idiopathic hypereosinophilic syndrome. N Engl J Med 2003; 348(13):1201–1214.
165. Gleich GJ, Leiferman KM. The hypereosinophilic syndromes: still more heterogeneity. Curr Opin Immunol 2005; 17(6):679–684.
166. Roufosse F, Goldman M, Cogan E. Hypereosinophilic syndrome: lymphoproliferative and myeloproliferative variants. Semin Respir Crit Care Med 2006; 27(2):158–1570.
167. Roufosse F, Cogan E, Goldman M. Recent advances in pathogenesis and management of hypereosinophilic syndromes. Allergy 2004; 59(7):673–689.
168. Roufosse F, Schandene L, Sibille C, et al. Clonal Th2 lymphocytes in patients with the idiopathic hypereosinophilic syndrome. Br J Haematol 2000; 109(3):540–548.
169. Simon HU, Plotz SG, Dummer R, et al. Abnormal clones of T cells producing interleukin-5 in idiopathic eosinophilia. N Engl J Med 1999; 341(15):1112–1120.

170. Bank I, Amariglio N, Reshef A, et al. The hypereosinophilic syndrome associated with CD4+CD3- helper type 2 (Th2) lymphocytes. Leuk Lymphoma 2001; 42(1–2):123–133.
171. Klion AD, Law MA, Noel P, et al. Safety and efficacy of the monoclonal anti-interleukin-5 antibody SCH55700 in the treatment of patients with hypereosinophilic syndrome. Blood 2004; 103(8):2939–2941.
172. Garrett JK, Jameson SC, Thomson B, et al. Anti-interleukin-5 (mepolizumab) therapy for hypereosinophilic syndromes. J Allergy Clin Immunol 2004; 113(1):115–119.
173. Plotz SG, Simon HU, Darsow U, et al. Use of an anti-interleukin-5 antibody in the hypereosinophilic syndrome with eosinophilic dermatitis. N Engl J Med 2003; 349(24):2334–2339.
174. Toyoshima M, Sato A, Taniguchi M, et al. A case of eosinophilic pneumonia caused by inhalation of nickel dusts. Nihon Kyobu Shikkan Gakkai Zasshi 1994; 32(5):480–484.
175. Rom WN, Weiden M, Garcia R, et al. Acute eosinophilic pneumonia in a New York City firefighter exposed to World Trade Center dust. Am J Respir Crit Care Med 2002; 166(6): 797–800.
176. Brander PE, Tukiainen P. Acute eosinophilic pneumonia in a heroin smoker. Eur Respir J 1993; 6(5):750–752.
177. Takamizawa A, Amari T, Kubo K. [A case of acute eosinophilic pneumonia induced by inhalation of acetylene]. Nihon Kokyuki Gakkai zasshi (J Jpn Respir Soc) 2000; 38(12): 947–951.
178. Kelly KJ, Ruffing R. Acute eosinophilic pneumonia following intentional inhalation of Scotchguard. Ann Allergy 1993; 71(4):358–361.
179. Hirai K, Yamazaki Y, Okada K, et al. Acute eosinophilic pneumonia associated with smoke from fireworks. Intern Med (Tokyo, Japan) 2000; 39(5):401–403.
180. Salerno SM, Strong JS, Roth BJ, et al. Eosinophilic pneumonia and respiratory failure associated with a trazodone overdose. Am J Respir Crit Care Med 1995; 152(6 pt 1):2170–2172.
181. Andreu V, Bataller R, Caballeria J, et al. Acute eosinophilic pneumonia associated with ranitidine. J Clin Gastroenterol 1996; 23(2):160–162.
182. Bouckaert Y, Robert F, Englert Y, et al. Acute eosinophilic pneumonia associated with intramuscular administration of progesterone as luteal phase support after IVF: case report. Hum Reprod 2004; 19(8):1806–1810.
183. Martinez BM, Domingo P. Acute eosinophilic pneumonia associated with tenidap. BMJ 1997; 314(7077):349.
184. Barnes MT, Bascunana J, Garcia B, et al. Acute eosinophilic pneumonia associated with antidepressant agents. Pharm World Sci 1999; 21(5):241–242.
185. Kurai J, Chikumi H, Kodani M, et al. Acute eosinophilic pneumonia caused by calcium stearate, an additive agent for an oral antihistaminic medication. Internal medicine (Tokyo, Japan) 2006; 45(17):1011–1016.
186. Seebach J, Speich R, Fehr J, et al. GM-CSF-induced acute eosinophilic pneumonia. Br J Haematol 1995; 90(4):963–965.
187. Dupon M, Malou M, Rogues AM, et al. Acute eosinophilic pneumonia induced by inhaled pentamidine isethionate. BMJ 1993; 306(6870):109.
188. Mayo J, Collazos J, Martinez E, et al. Acute eosinophilic pneumonia in a patient infected with the human immunodeficiency virus. Tuber Lung Dis 1995; 76(1):77–79.
189. Glazer CS, Cohen LB, Schwarz MI. Acute eosinophilic pneumonia in AIDS. Chest 2001; 120(5):1732–1735.
190. Miyazaki E, Sugisaki K, Shigenaga T, et al. A case of acute eosinophilic pneumonia caused by inhalation of Trichosporon terrestre. Am J Respir Crit Care Med 1995; 151(2 pt 1):541–543.
191. Orikasa K, Namima T, Ota S, et al. Acute eosinophilic pneumonia associated with intravesical bacillus Calmette-Guerin therapy of carcinoma in situ of the bladder. Int J Urol 2003; 10(11):622–624.

11
Clinical Diagnosis of Pulmonary Eosinophilia

LISA KOPAS and ZEENAT SAFDAR
Baylor College of Medicine, Houston, Texas, U.S.A.

I. Introduction

Eosinophilic pneumonias are a diverse group of disorders that demonstrate blood and/or tissue eosinophilia and pulmonary infiltrates. Sir William Osler first described this entity in 1895 and then Löffler described transient pulmonary infiltrates in 1932 (1). In 1952, William Reeder and Ben Goodrich coined the term "Pulmonary Infiltration with Eosinophilia" or the PIE syndrome (2). This nomenclature was proposed to group together the previously individually named syndromes including Löffler's syndrome, allergic bronchopneumonia, and cases associated with periarteritis nodosa. Crofton et al. in the same year redefined the classification under the general term of pulmonary eosinophilia (3). He proposed a classification of simple pulmonary eosinophilia (Löffler's syndrome), prolonged pulmonary eosinophilia, pulmonary eosinophilia with asthma, tropical pulmonary eosinophilia, and polyarteritis nodosa. It is helpful to classify pulmonary eosinophilic syndromes as shown in Table 1 to aid in diagnosis and treatment of this diverse group of disorders. A list of secondary causes of pulmonary eosinophilia is given in Table 2.

II. Idiopathic Eosinophilic Pneumonias

A. Acute Eosinophilic Pneumonia

Acute eosinophilic pneumonia (AEP) is the most recently described of the eosinophilic pneumonias. In 1989, Allen et al. and Badesch et al. described a distinct entity of rapidly progressive eosinophilic pneumonias (4,5). The clinical presentation was similar to acute lung injury (ALI), but presence of pulmonary eosinophilia distinguished it from ALI. King et al. proposed that the diagnosis of AEP be made in a patient with a febrile illness for one to five days, severe hypoxemia ($PaO_2 < 60$ mmHg), marked elevation of eosinophils in bronchoalveolar lavage (BAL) fluid, and nonspecific pulmonary infiltrates (6).

The etiology of AEP is not currently known, although it may be related to antigenic stimulation or a hypersensitivity reaction (5). Cigarette smoking and occupational exposures have been theorized to be offending agents (6,7). Males are more commonly affected and the patients tend to be younger than in chronic eosinophilic pneumonia (CEP) (8). Histologically, AEP is defined by diffuse alveolar damage with interstitial and alveolar eosinophilia (9). BAL is sufficient to make the diagnosis in the absence of infection. Open lung biopsy is not required or recommended for a definitive diagnosis. Several

Table 1 Eosinophilic Pneumonias

Idiopathic
Acute eosinophilic pneumonia
Chronic eosinophilic pneumonia
Eosinophilic pneumonia caused by parasites and fungi
Löffler's syndrome
Tropical pulmonary eosinophilia
Allergic bronchopulmonary aspergillosis
Eosinophilic pneumonia caused by drugs, toxins, and radiation therapy
Drug- and toxin-related eosinophilic pneumonias
Radiation therapy–related eosinophilic pneumonias
Vasculitic eosinophilic pneumonia
Churg-Strauss syndrome

Table 2 Partial List of Secondary Causes of Pulmonary Eosinophilia

Infection
Histoplasmosis
Coccidiomycosis
Mycobacterial
Brucellosis
Collagen vascular disease
Rheumatoid arthritis
Sjogren's syndrome
Malignancy
Lung carcinoma
Lymphoma
Acute eosinophilic pneumonia
Sézary syndrome with lung involvement
Transplantation
Graft vs. host disease
Lung allograft rejection
Others
Hypersensitivity pneumonitis
Hypereosinophilic syndrome
Idiopathic pulmonary fibrosis
Sarcoidosis
Cryptogenic organizing pneumonia
Psittacosis
Farmer's lung

inflammatory markers and chemokines/cytokines have been found to be elevated in this disorder such as IL-5 (10), sADAM8, and sVCAM and as well as serum surfactant proteins (11,12).

Patients with AEP have eosinophils that are equal to or greater than 25% in the bronchoalveolar lavage fluid (BALF) without significant peripheral eosinophilia (8). Lack of peripheral eosinophilia distinguishes it from CEP. Radiographically, AEP may present as diffuse bilateral ground glass, micronodular infiltrates, or localized infiltrates (8). Pleural effusions (usually bilateral) are commonly found (6).

The mainstay treatment of nearly all eosinophilic pneumonias is systemic corticosteroids. In AEP, methylprednisolone is typically given parenterally at a dose of up to 125 mg every six hours. This may be switched to prednisone as patients are able to tolerate oral therapy. However, no standard with regard to optimum length of treatment has been clearly defined. Two- to 12-week courses have not shown a difference in efficacy (13). Relapses after treatment are extremely unusual and there have been reports of spontaneous improvement without any treatment (7).

B. Chronic Eosinophilic Pneumonia

CEP is another type of idiopathic eosinophilic pneumonia initially described in 1960 and later clinically defined by Carrington in 1969. He described nine cases of CEP in women, all of whom presented with fevers, night sweats, weight loss, and dyspnea (14).

The etiology of CEP is not understood and is thought to be related to an unknown trigger. IL-5, which is elevated in BALF from CEP patients, is thought to be the major mediator along with other chemokines such as RANTES acting on the Th2 cell to cause eosinophil migration to the lung (15,16). On biopsy, large amounts of eosinophils are found in the alveoli, lymphocytes, plasma cells, and polymorphonuclear neutrophils are also seen (17). Lack of distal airway intraluminal organization distinguishes CEP from cryptogenic organizing pneumonia (18). Lung biopsy is not required to make the diagnosis, and BAL is sufficient to confirm diagnosis. A BAL fluid cell count of >40% eosinophils can be diagnostic of CEP in the absence of infection (19).

The clinical presentation consists of a subacute illness spanning over several weeks to months. Common symptoms are high fevers, night sweats, weight loss, and dyspnea. There is a female to male predominance of about 2:1 (20,21). When compared with AEP, the patients with CEP are generally older with peak incidence at age 40 to 50, though patients of varied ages ranging from 18 to 80 have been reported (20). There has been some disagreement on the history of asthma and atopy in the literature. In the original report by Carrington, a history of both asthma and allergic rhinitis was seen in majority of cases.

Hypoxia is generally mild but there has been a report of significant respiratory failure in a patient with CEP (17). Peripheral eosinophilia is generally present, though not required for diagnosis, and erythrocyte sedimentation rate is usually elevated (21). Chest radiographs show infiltrates that are located at lung periphery without lobar or segmental demarcation. This has been called the "photographic negative of pulmonary edema" (14,22). In a minority of cases reported by Gaensler and Carrington, the peripheral infiltrate surrounded the lung, but was more commonly present in the upper or lateral locations. Patients often develop asthmatic symptoms and an obstructive pattern on pulmonary function testing occurring concomitantly with CEP or after its resolution (14,21).

In CEP, rapid improvement in symptoms and complete resolution of infiltrates after treatment with corticosteroids often occur (14,22). Oral prednisone 20 to 40 mg daily have been shown to be effective. Clinical improvement can be within a few hours, while infiltrates resolve in a few days to weeks (14,22). Spontaneous resolution without steroid treatment has also been reported. Some patients have been found to relapse after completing steroid treatment. Usually the infiltrates recur in the same location and distribution as the first episode, and this may indicate sensitization of previously affected sections of the lungs (21,22). Although the overall prognosis in this disease is good, patients who have recurrences may be on steroids off and on for years (21). In a minority of those who relapse, fibrosis with honeycombing has been reported (14,22).

III. Eosinophilic Pneumonias Caused by Parasites and Fungi

A. Löeffler's Syndrome

Löffler's syndrome, also known as simple pulmonary eosinophilia, was first described in 1932 by a Swiss physician Wilhelm Löffler (1). Löffler reported four cases of pulmonary infiltrations with eosinophilia. Symptoms were mild and chest radiograph showed fleeting variable infiltrates that lasted up to 6 to 12 days (3). At that time the etiology of this syndrome was unknown. By 1958, *Ascaris lumbricoides* (a roundworm) infection was noted in patients with Löffler's syndrome (23), and in 1968, a form of Löffler's syndrome was described in Saudi Arabia because of ascaris larva (24). List of parasites causing pulmonary eosinophilia is given in Table 3.

Ascaris infection is the most common cause of Löffler's syndrome worldwide. Other common causes are *Ancylostoma duodenale* and *Necator americanus* (hookworms). Poor, minority groups, immunosuppressed, and those in institutions are more commonly infected.

During *Ascaris* infection, eggs are ingested and hatch into larvae. The pulmonary manifestations are thought to be a hypersensitivity reaction to larval migration through the lung tissue (25).

The clinical presentation is mild with nonproductive cough, substernal pleuritic chest pain, low-grade fever, and rarely, hemoptysis. Rales and wheezing are noted on physical exam. Eosinophil count is elevated except in HIV positive patients where it may be normal. Transient, migratory pulmonary infiltrates that clear spontaneously are the hallmarks of the syndrome (24,25). Sputum contains eosinophils and Charcot-Leyden crystals. At the time of the syndrome, the stool may not contain eggs (25) as the hypersensitivity reaction happens early in infestation.

Pathologically, eosinophils and fibrin are found within bronchioles as well as interstitial pneumonitis with thickened septa. Larvae are seen within bronchioles, bronchi, and alveoli. Intraalveolar hemorrhage is also possible (25).

Treatment consists of mebendazole 100 mg twice daily for three days or 500 mg once. Pyrantel pamoate, albendazole, and ivermectin are also effective therapy. Ivermectin though is only partially effective for hookworms.

Strongyloides stercoralis can also cause a form of Löffler's syndrome similar to that caused by *Ascaris*. *Strongyloides* is found commonly in the tropics and in the southeastern United States. Infection is through percutaneous penetration after contact with soil. *Strongyloides* is able to reproduce within the human host that can cause a chronic infection. The life cycle of this nematode consists of larvae migrating from the site of penetration either skin or gut, then migrating to the lungs via the blood. The parasites then climb

Table 3 Parasites Causing Pulmonary Eosinophilia

Western world	India/Southeast Asia	Other
Strongyloides	*Wuchereria bancrofti*	*Schistosoma*
Ascaris	*Brugia malayi*	*Clonorchis sinensis*
Toxacara	–	Opisthorchiasis
Ancylostoma	–	*Trichinella spiralis*
Paragonimus westermani	–	*Echinococcus granulosus*
–	–	*Dirofilaria immitis*

through the bronchial tree to the oropharynx where they are swallowed and travel to the small bowel to reproduce.

Diagnosis of *Strongyloides* is difficult given low concentration in the stool. In endemic areas, elevated eosinophilic count with high IgE is sufficient to make the diagnosis. Treatment consists of thiabendazole 25 mg/kg two times daily for two days (25).

B. Tropical Pulmonary Eosinophilia

Since the early 20th century, cases of eosinophilia associated with lung manifestations in the tropics have been reported. In 1950, the term tropical pulmonary eosinophila (TPE) was coined by Ball, which is used today. In the early 1960s, it was hypothesized that TPE is cause by a filarial infection (26); however, it took 25 years of investigation to definitively identify the inciting organism.

Less than 1% of patients infected with lymphatic filariae develop TPE (27). TPE has been reported in India, Sri Lanka, Southeast Asia, Africa, West Indies, and China. It has been noted that TPE is more likely to be found in Indians even when the endemic area is outside the country of India (28).

The microfilariae implicated in TPE are *Wuchereria bancrofti* and *Brugia malayi* (29,30). The microfilariae must develop in an insect vector in order to be transmitted to another host (27). The adult worms reproduce forming microfilariae that circulate in the blood. These microfilariae are opsonized by antifilarial antibodies in the lymphatic system and cleared in the pulmonary vasculature. TPE is the result of heightened immune responses to filarial antigens in certain people, such as those who do not live in the endemic areas (27).

In 1963, Donohugh delineated the criteria for diagnosis of TPE that consisted of major criteria: pulmonary symptoms of nocturnal dry cough and dyspnea, peripheral eosinophilia of over 2000/mL, positive filarial complement-fixation test, and response to treatment of diethylcarbamazine (28). Minor criteria included presence in an endemic area, male, crepitations or rhonchi on exam, a chest radiograph showing miliary pattern, elevated sedimentation rate and symptoms of malaise, weight loss, fatigue, and anorexia (28). IgE levels are generally elevated (31). The characteristic chest radiograph demonstrates increased linear markings, hilar enlargement, and miliary pattern (32). Airway obstruction is the main abnormality on pulmonary function testing (33).

On biopsy, nodules consist of large numbers of eosinophils that aggregate around fragments of microfilaria. These microfilariae are small in number and easily missed under routine microscopic examination (34).

Currently recommended treatment is diethylcarbamazine 6 to 12 mg/kg (25). Length of treatment varies but 7 to 10 days has been shown to be effective (27).

C. Allergic Bronchopulmonary Aspergillosis

Hinson et al. in 1952 described allergic bronchopulmonary aspergillosis (ABPA) in three patients (35). In 1930s positivity to skin tests for *Aspergillus* was recorded in up to 20% of asthmatics. The fungus *Aspergillus* is ubiquitous in the environment. *Aspergillus fumigatus* is the most common species infecting humans. ABPA is a hypersensitivity reaction to *Aspergillus* and is not a manifestation of the infection itself. ABPA occurs in non-immunocompromised host in contrast to invasive aspergillosis that occurs in

Table 4 Diagnostic Criteria for Allergic Bronchopulmonary Aspergillosis

Asthma or cystic fibrosis[a]
Immediate cutaneous reaction to *A. fumigatus*[a]
Peripheral eosinophilia
Chest radiograph infiltrates
Central bronchiectasis
Total IgE (>1000 ng/mL)[a]
Elevated serum *A. fumigatus*–specific IgE or IgE[a]
Precipitating antibodies to *A. fumigatus*
Positive sputum culture for *Aspergillus*
History of brown plug expectoration
Arthus reactivity to *Aspergillus*[a]

[a]The essential criteria for diagnosis.

immunocompromised patients (36). Most patients who develop ABPA have a predisposing condition such as asthma or cystic fibrosis (CF) (37,38).

Pathogenesis of ABPA is not entirely clear. In patients with ABPA, several host factors may be associated with an increased susceptibility to developing ABPA. HLA-DR2 gene expression, increased CF transmembrane conductance regulator gene mutations IL-10, and surface protein A have been shown to play a role in the pathogenesis (39–42). These predisposing genetic abnormalities may allow sensitization to *Aspergillus* antigens. The immunological pathway of sensitization involves activation of Th2 cells with release of IL-5 and eosinophilic infiltration (37,43).

ABPA is estimated to occur in 1% to 2% of asthmatics and up to 10% of patients with CF. The diagnostic criteria for ABPA is given in Table 4 (44). The stages and the treatment at each stage are outlined in Table 5 (45).

In CF, diagnosis can be more difficult because several of the criteria required for ABPA are manifestations of CF disease (38). The Cystic Fibrosis Foundation recommends the following criteria to diagnose ABPA: clinical deterioration, immediate hypersensitivity to *A. fumigatus*, total IgE >1000 kUI/L, precipitating antibodies to *A. fumigatus*, and abnormal chest radiograph including unexplained new change in radiograph (46). Patients should only be treated with steroids; however, if there is a high fungal burden or locally invasive disease, the preferred antifungal therapy is voriconazole (47).

Table 5 Stages and Treatment of ABPA

Stage	Description	IgE	Treatment
I	Acute: upper or middle lobe infiltrate	Markedly elevated	Prednisone 0.5 mg/kg for 2 wk then taper
II	Remission: no infiltrate	Normal or elevated	None
III	Exacerbation: upper or middle lobe infiltrate	Markedly elevated	Prednisone taper
IV	Steroid-dependent asthma	Normal or elevated	Chronic low dose steroids
V	End stage: fibrotic changes	Normal	Unclear efficacy of steroids

Abbreviation: ABPA, allergic bronchopulmonary aspergillosis.

Table 6 Partial List of Drugs Associated with Eosinophilic Pneumonias

Class or drug	Cases in literature	Classic drug in class
Antidepressant/antipsychotic	7	Amitriptyline
Antibiotic	>25	Minocycline/nitrofurantoin, PCN
ACE inhibitor	4	Captopril
NSAIDS	23	Sulfasalazine
Chemotherapeutic agent	6	Bleomycin
Cholesterol-lowering agent	2	Simvastatin
Antimalarial	3	Maloprim
Antiseizure	3	Carbemazapine, dilantin
Miscellaneous	Multiple	Amiodarone
	1	Glafenine, progesterone, BCG, aminoglutethiamide, ranitidine, isotretinoin, acetaminophen, cromoglycate, gold salts

Source: From Refs. 48–62.

IV. Eosinophilic Pneumonias Caused by Drugs, Toxins, and Radiation Therapy

A. Drug- and Toxin-Related Eosinophilic Pneumonia

Eosinophilic pneumonia can be directly related to the ingestion of drugs and toxins. This association has been known since 1969, and as the number of prescribed medications grows, the number of drugs causing eosinophilic pneumonia grows as well. There are more than 100 known agents causing this syndrome. Nonsteroidal anti-inflammatory medications and antibiotics are commonly implicated (Table 6). The website PNEUMOTOX ON LINE (www.pneumotox.com) maintains a comprehensive and current list of drug-related lung diseases.

The clinical presentation is mild with complaints of cough, fever, and dyspnea. Pulmonary infiltrates are present on chest radiograph. Diagnosis is made by BAL with elevated eosinophil on cell count (>25%). Peripheral eosinophilia is also usually present. Pathology is nonspecific and shows eosinophilic infiltration in the lung parenchyma and alveolar spaces.

Eosinophilic pneumonia related to toxins is similar to drug-related disease. Some toxins such as cigarette smoke are causal agents implicated in a severe form of eosinophilic pneumonia known as AEP (63).

B. Radiation-Related Eosinophilic Pneumonia

Radiation therapy causes a variety of diseases in lungs including acute and chronic pneumonitis, fibrosis, and cryptogenic organizing pneumonia. There are rare reports of eosinophilic pneumonia due to radiation therapy and these cases responded well to steroid therapy (63,64).

V. Vasculitic Eosinophilic Pneumonia

A. Churg-Strauss Syndrome

In 1951, Churg and Strauss described a syndrome in 13 patients who had asthma, fever, sinusitis, hypereosinophilia, and pulmonary and extrapulmonary involvement (65). Autopsy showed extravascular granulomatous nodules and periarteritis nodosa. This syndrome was termed Churg-Struass syndrome (CSS) after the two pathologists who initially described it. CSS is predominantly an adult disease. Most patients have a history of asthma, allergic rhinitis, nasal polyp, and sinusitis (66). In recent reports, use of leukotriene receptor antagonists has been implicated as inciting agents (67,68).

Clinical diagnostic criterion outlined by Lanham et al. includes three criteria (69):

1. Asthma
2. Peak peripheral blood eosinophil counts in excess of 1.5×10^9/L
3. Systemic vasculitis involving two or more extrapulmonary organs

According to the American College of Rheumatology, the diagnostic criteria for classification of CSS include asthma, eosinophilia >10% on differential blood count and a history of allergy other than asthma or drug sensitivity (70). Symptoms included weight loss, abdominal pain, joint pain (migratory arthritis), allergic rhinitis, subcutaneous nodules, and mononeuritis monoplex (71). Three phases of the syndrome have been described (69): a prodromal phase in which allergic manifestations predominate, a second phase in which eosinophilia and eosinophilic infiltration occur, and a third phase of vasculitic changes that may occur up to 30 years after the onset of asthma (69). Interestingly, approximately 50% of cases have regression of their asthma symptoms with the onset of vasculitis (69). Although upper respiratory and pulmonary disease is the hallmark of CSS, many other organs can be affected (Table 7). Laboratory abnormalities include elevated erythrocyte sedimentation rates, leukocytosis, eosinophilia, positive rheumatoid factor, anemia, thrombocytosis, proteinuria, hematuria, depressed complement levels, immune complexes, cryoglobulins, elevated IgE levels, and positive perinuclear ANCA (66,69,72). The average time of death from onset of signs and symptoms of vasculitis is 4.6 years (55). The most common cause of death is by cardiac involvement (66).

Pathologically, the typical necrotizing granulomas and necrotizing vasculitis of small arteries and veins are seen which are similar to those of polyarteritis nodosa (71). What sets

Table 7 Systemic Features in CSS

System involved	Manifestation	Frequency (%)
Cardiovascular	Heart failure	25
	Hypertension	38–75
Gastrointestinal	Abdominal pain	14–44
	Diarrhea	31
	GI bleed	25
Renal	Mild kidney disease	30–88
	Nephrotic syndrome	19
	Renal failure	3–6
Cutaneous	Subcutaneous nodules	13–53
	Purpura/petechiae	37–56
	Erythema/urticaria	56
Musculoskeletal	Arthritis	20–69
	Myalgias	69
Nervous system	Mononeuritis multiplex	63–75
	Central nervous system	25

Abbreviation: CSS, Churg-Struass syndrome.
Source: From Refs. 65,69,71.

CSS apart according to Fauci in his review on vasculitides is the high occurrence of lesions in the pulmonary vasculature, involvement of both small- and medium-sized arteries/arterioles and veins/venules, intravascular and extravascular lesions, presence of eosinophilia in the tissue, and the associated clinical picture (72).

Most patients respond well to treatment with corticosteroids. Treatment in the vasculitic phase generally requires high dose steroids such as prednisolone 40 to 60 mg for several weeks. The general practice is to taper steroids based on clinical improvement. Often in cases with mononeuritis multiplex, steroid therapy must be prolonged.

References

1. Löffler W. Zur Differential der Lungenifiltrierungen: II. Uber fluchtige succedan Infiltrate (mit Eosinophile). Beitr Klin Tuberk 1932; 79:368.
2. Reeder W, Goodrich B. Pulmonary infiltration with eosinophilia (PIE syndrome). Ann Intern Med 1952; 36:1217–1240.
3. Crofton JW, Livingstone JL, Oswald NC, et al. Pulmonary eosinophilia. Thorax 1952; 7:1–35.
4. Allen JN, Pacht ER, Gadek JE, et al. Acute eosinophilic pneumonia as a reversible cause of noninfectious respiratory failure. N Engl J Med 1989; 321:569–574.
5. Badesch DB, King TE Jr., Schwarz MI. Acute eosinophilic pneumonia: a hypersensitivity phenomenon? Am Rev Respir Dis 1989; 139:249–252.
6. King MA, Pope-Harman AL, Allen JN, et al. Acute eosinophilic pneumonia: radiologic and clinical features. Radiology 1997; 203:715–719.
7. Philit F, Etienne-Mastroianni B, Parrot A, et al. Idiopathic acute eosinophilic pneumonia: a study of 22 patients. Am J Respir Crit Care Med 2002; 166:1235–1239.
8. Hayakawa H, Sato A, Toyoshima M, et al. A clinical study of idiopathic eosinophilic pneumonia. Chest 1994; 105:1462–1466.
9. Tazelaar HD, Linz LJ, Colby TV, et al. Acute eosinophilic pneumonia: histopathologic findings in nine patients. Am J Respir Crit Care Med 1997; 155:296–302.
10. Okubo Y, Horie S, Hachiya T, et al. Predominant implication of IL-5 in acute eosinophilic pneumonia: comparison with chronic eosinophilic pneumonia. Int Arch Allergy Immunol 1998; 116:76–80.
11. Fujii M, Tanaka H, Kameda M, et al. Elevated serum surfactant protein A and D in a case of acute eosinophilic pneumonia. Intern Med 2004; 43:423–426.
12. Matsuno O, Miyazaki E, Nureki S, et al. Elevated soluble ADAM8 in bronchoalveolar lavage fluid in patients with eosinophilic pneumonia. Int Arch Allergy Immunol 2007; 142:285–290.
13. Pope-Harman AL, Davis WB, Allen ED, et al. Acute eosinophilic pneumonia. A summary of 15 cases and review of the literature. Medicine (Baltimore) 1996; 75:334–342.
14. Carrington CB, Addington WW, Goff AM, et al. Chronic eosinophilic pneumonia. N Engl J Med 1969; 280:787–798.
15. Kita H, Sur S, Hunt LW, et al. Cytokine production at the site of disease in chronic eosinophilic pneumonitis. Am J Respir Crit Care Med 1996; 153:1437–1441.
16. Miyazaki E, Nureki S, Fukami T, et al. Elevated levels of thymus- and activation-regulated chemokine in bronchoalveolar lavage fluid from patients with eosinophilic pneumonia. Am J Respir Crit Care Med 2002; 165:1125–1131.
17. Libby DM, Murphy TF, Edwards A, et al. Chronic eosinophilic pneumonia: an unusual cause of acute respiratory failure. Am Rev Respir Dis 1980; 122:497–500.
18. Olopade CO, Crotty TB, Douglas WW, et al. Chronic eosinophilic pneumonia and idiopathic bronchiolitis obliterans organizing pneumonia: comparison of eosinophil number and degranulation by immunofluorescence staining for eosinophil-derived major basic protein. Mayo Clin Proc 1995; 70:137–142.
19. Cottin V, Cordier JF. Eosinophilic pneumonias. Allergy 2005; 60:841–857.

20. Alam M, Burki NK. Chronic eosinophilic pneumonia: a review. South Med J 2007; 100:49–53.
21. Pearson DL, Rosenow EC III. Chronic eosinophilic pneumonia (Carrington's): a follow-up study. Mayo Clin Proc 1978; 53:73–78.
22. Gaensler EA, Carrington CB. Peripheral opacities in chronic eosinophilic pneumonia: the photographic negative of pulmonary edema. AJR Am J Roentgenol 1977; 128:1–13.
23. Beaver PC, Danaraj TJ. Pulmonary ascariasis resembling eosinophilic lung; autopsy report with description of larvae in the bronchioles. Am J Trop Med Hyg 1958; 7:100–111.
24. Gelpi AP, Mustafa A. Ascaris pneumonia. Am J Med 1968; 44:377–389.
25. Chitkara RK, Krishna G. Parasitic pulmonary eosinophilia. Semin Respir Crit Care Med 2006; 27:171–184.
26. Ball JD. Tropical pulmonary eosinophilia. Trans R Soc Trop Med Hyg 1950; 44:237–258.
27. Ong RK, Doyle RL. Tropical pulmonary eosinophilia. Chest 1998; 113:1673–1679.
28. Donohugh DL. Tropical eosinophilia. An etiologic inquiry. N Engl J Med 1963; 269:1357–1364.
29. Beaver PC. Filariasis without microfilaremia. Am J Trop Med Hyg 1970; 19:181–189.
30. Joshi VV. Eosinophilic reactions in the lung. N Engl J Med 1969; 281:50–51.
31. Spry CJ, Kumaraswami V. Tropical eosinophilia. Semin Hematol 1982; 19:107–115.
32. Herlinger H. Pulmonary changes in tropical eosinophilia. Br J Radiol 1963; 36:889–901.
33. Nesarajah MS. Pulmonary function in tropical eosinophilia. Thorax 1972; 27:185–187.
34. Joe LK. Occult filariasis: its relationship with tropical pulmonary eosinophilia. Am J Trop Med Hyg 1962; 11:646–651.
35. Hinson KF, Moon AJ, Plummer NS. Broncho-pulmonary aspergillosis; a review and a report of eight new cases. Thorax 1952; 7:317–333.
36. Safdar A, Papadopoulos EB, Young JW. Breakthrough Scedosporium apiospermum (Pseudallescheria boydii) brain abscess during therapy for invasive pulmonary aspergillosis following high-risk allogeneic hematopoietic stem cell transplantation. Scedosporiasis and recent advances in antifungal therapy. Transpl Infect Dis 2002; 4:212–217.
37. Gibson PG. Allergic bronchopulmonary aspergillosis. Semin Respir Crit Care Med 2006; 27:185–191.
38. Laufer P, Fink JN, Bruns WT, et al. Allergic bronchopulmonary aspergillosis in cystic fibrosis. J Allergy Clin Immunol 1984; 73:44–48.
39. Brouard J, Knauer N, Boelle PY, et al. Influence of interleukin-10 on Aspergillus fumigatus infection in patients with cystic fibrosis. J Infect Dis 2005; 191:1988–1991.
40. Chauhan B, Santiago L, Hutcheson PS, et al. Evidence for the involvement of two different MHC class II regions in susceptibility or protection in allergic bronchopulmonary aspergillosis. J Allergy Clin Immunol 2000; 106:723–729.
41. Marchand E, Verellen-Dumoulin C, Mairesse M, et al. Frequency of cystic fibrosis transmembrane conductance regulator gene mutations and 5T allele in patients with allergic bronchopulmonary aspergillosis. Chest 2001; 119:762–767.
42. Saxena S, Madan T, Shah A, et al. Association of polymorphisms in the collagen region of SP-A2 with increased levels of total IgE antibodies and eosinophilia in patients with allergic bronchopulmonary aspergillosis. J Allergy Clin Immunol 2003; 111:1001–1007.
43. Skov M, Poulsen LK, Koch C. Increased antigen-specific Th-2 response in allergic bronchopulmonary aspergillosis (ABPA) in patients with cystic fibrosis. Pediatr Pulmonol 1999; 27:74–79.
44. Rosenberg M, Patterson R, Mintzer R, et al. Clinical and immunologic criteria for the diagnosis of allergic bronchopulmonary aspergillosis. Ann Intern Med 1977; 86:405–414.
45. Patterson R, Greenberger PA, Radin RC, et al. Allergic bronchopulmonary aspergillosis: staging as an aid to management. Ann Intern Med 1982; 96:286–291.
46. Tillie-Leblond I, Tonnel AB. Allergic bronchopulmonary aspergillosis. Allergy 2005; 60:1004–1013.
47. Herbrecht R, Denning DW, Patterson TF, et al. Voriconazole versus amphotericin B for primary therapy of invasive aspergillosis. N Engl J Med 2002; 347:408–415.

48. Bouckaert Y, Robert F, Englert Y, et al. Acute eosinophilic pneumonia associated with intramuscular administration of progesterone as luteal phase support after IVF: case report. Hum Reprod 2004; 19:1806–1810.
49. Espeleta VJ, Moore WH, Kane PB, et al. Eosinophilic pneumonia due to duloxetine. Chest 2007; 131:901–903.
50. Hakoda Y, Aoshima M, Kinoshita M, et al. [A case of eosinophilic pneumonia possibly associated with 5-aminosalicylic acid (5-ASA)]. Nihon Kokyuki Gakkai Zasshi 2004; 42:404–409.
51. Ho D, Tashkin DP, Bein ME, et al. Pulmonary infiltrates with eosinophilia associated with tetracycline. Chest 1979; 76:33–36.
52. Kaur J, Khandpur S, Seith A, et al. Dapsone-induced eosinophilic pneumonitis in a leprosy patient. Indian J Lepr 2005; 77:267–271.
53. Michael JR, Rudin ML. Acute pulmonary disease caused by phenytoin. Ann Intern Med 1981; 95:452–454.
54. Nader DA, Schillaci RF. Pulmonary infiltrates with eosinophilia due to naproxen. Chest 1983; 83:280–282.
55. Oddo M, Liaudet L, Lepori M, et al. Relapsing acute respiratory failure induced by minocycline. Chest 2003; 123:2146–2148.
56. Ohnishi H, Abe M, Yokoyama A, et al. Clarithromycin-induced eosinophilic pneumonia. Intern Med 2004; 43:231–235.
57. Orikasa K, Namima T, Ota S, et al. Acute eosinophilic pneumonia associated with intravesical bacillus Calmette-Guerin therapy of carcinoma in situ of the bladder. Int J Urol 2003; 10: 622–624.
58. Perez C, Errazuriz I, Brockmann P, et al. [Eosinophilic pneumonia caused by mesalazine. Report of one case]. Rev Med Chil 2003; 131:81–84.
59. Sato S, Watanabe K, Ishida T, et al. [Amiodarone-induced pneumonitis associated with marked eosinophilia in BALF]. Nippon Naika Gakkai Zasshi 2006; 95:356–358.
60. Slesnick TC, Mott AR, Fraser CD Jr., et al. Captopril-induced pulmonary infiltrates with eosinophilia in an infant with congenital heart disease. Pediatr Cardiol 2005; 26:690–693.
61. Wang KK, Bowyer BA, Fleming CR, et al. Pulmonary infiltrates and eosinophilia associated with sulfasalazine. Mayo Clin Proc 1984; 59:343–346.
62. Yoshioka S, Mukae H, Ishii H, et al. [A case of drug-induced pneumonia possibly associated with simvastatin]. Nihon Kokyuki Gakkai Zasshi 2005; 43:600–604.
63. Solomon J, Schwarz M. Drug-, toxin-, and radiation therapy-induced eosinophilic pneumonia. Semin Respir Crit Care Med 2006; 27:192–197.
64. Cottin V, Frognier R, Monnot H, et al. Chronic eosinophilic pneumonia after radiation therapy for breast cancer. Eur Respir J 2004; 23:9–13.
65. Churg J, Strauss L. Allergic granulomatosis, allergic angiitis, and periarteritis nodosa. Am J Pathol 1951; 27:277–301.
66. Katzenstein AL. Diagnostic features and differential diagnosis of Churg-Strauss syndrome in the lung. A review. Am J Clin Pathol 2000; 114:767–772.
67. Cuchacovich R, Justiniano M, Espinoza LR. Churg-Strauss syndrome associated with leukotriene receptor antagonists (LTRA). Clin Rheumatol 2007; 26:1769–1771.
68. Oberndorfer S, Beate U, Sabine U, et al. Churg Strauss syndrome during treatment of bronchial asthma with a leucotriene receptor antagonist presenting with polyneuropathy. Neurologia 2004; 19:134–138.
69. Lanham JG, Elkon KB, Pusey CD, et al. Systemic vasculitis with asthma and eosinophilia: a clinical approach to the Churg-Strauss syndrome. Medicine (Baltimore) 1984; 63:65–81.
70. Masi AT, Hunder GG, Lie JT, et al. The American College of Rheumatology 1990 criteria for the classification of Churg-Strauss syndrome (allergic granulomatosis and angiitis). Arthritis Rheum 1990; 33:1094–1100.
71. Chumbley LC, Harrison EG Jr., DeRemee RA. Allergic granulomatosis and angiitis (Churg-Strauss syndrome). Report and analysis of 30 cases. Mayo Clin Proc 1977; 52:477–484.
72. Fauci AS. Vasculitis. J Allergy Clin Immunol 1983; 72:211–223.

12
Small Airway Lesions

CHIH-WEI WANG
Chang Gung Memorial Hospital, Taoyuan, Taiwan

JOHN R. MUHM, THOMAS V. COLBY, and KEVIN O. LESLIE
Mayo Clinic Arizona, Scottsdale, Arizona, U.S.A.

I. Introduction

A diverse group of pathologic conditions involve the small airways compartment (terminal bronchiole to alveolar duct). Airway diameters in this distal region are typically less than 1 mm. Pathology of the small airways can present as the main lesion of a pulmonary disease or occur as a secondary manifestation related to primary pathology in adjacent parenchymal (or even large airway) disease. In practice, lesions in the small airways can be classified into several pathologic patterns, which are somewhat descriptive (Table 1) (1,2). After these basic pathologic patterns are recognized, further refinement of the differential diagnosis can be achieved with the aid of clinical, functional, and radiologic correlation.

Noncontrast chest CT with 3-mm reconstructed images is the preferred radiologic technique for the study of airway disease such as bronchiectasis, bronchiolectasis, acute bronchiolitis, and constrictive bronchiolitis. Viewing reformatted coronal and sagittal images, with slices as thin as 0.6 mm, on a dedicated workstation is also helpful.

In normal lungs studied with chest CT, bronchi are visible in the medial two-thirds of the lungs. The normal bronchus has thin, smooth walls, and its lumen tapers gradually toward the chest wall. The normal bronchi in the outer third of the lungs, less than 1 mm in diameter, are too small to be seen with chest CT. The segmental bronchi and bronchioles are accompanied by a pulmonary artery branch, and the airway and its artery have identical diameters. In the periphery of the lungs, each bronchiole and its accompanying pulmonary arteriole are located in the center of a secondary pulmonary lobule. The secondary pulmonary lobule, the smallest portion of the lung that is surrounded by a connective tissue septum, is polyhedral in shape and is 1.5 to 3 cm in diameter. Since the peripheral bronchiole and its accompanying pulmonary arteriole are in the center of the secondary pulmonary lobule, abnormalities of the bronchiole or pulmonary arteriole can produce abnormalities that are visible with CT and are called "centrilobular nodules."

Bronchiectasis and bronchiolectasis, the permanent dilatation of bronchi and bronchioles, are well depicted with chest CT (3,4). Bronchiectasis is identified by abnormal dilatation of a bronchus, by bronchial-wall thickening, by lack of tapering of its lumen, and by irregularity of the shape of the bronchial lumen. It is helpful to compare the diameter of

Table 1 Pathologic Patterns of Small Airway Lesions

Asthmatic-type changes
Chronic bronchitis/emphysema-associated small airway changes
Cellular bronchiolitis (acute, chronic, acute and chronic, with or without fibrosis)
Subtypes: follicular bronchiolitis, diffuse panbronchiolitis
Respiratory bronchiolitis
Bronchiolitis obliterans with intraluminal polyps
Constrictive bronchiolitis
Mineral dustassociated airways disease
Peribronchiolar metaplasia
Bronchiolocentric nodules

Source: From Refs. 1,2.

a bronchus with the diameter of its accompanying artery to determine if the bronchus is dilated. The lumen of the abnormal bronchus may be air-filled or filled with a mucus plug or pus. When large airway disease is visible on CT, the lung biopsy (always taken from the periphery of the lung) will often have histopathologic abnormalities. The reverse is not always true. The patient with small airway disease may have little in the way of CT-visible abnormalities of the large airways.

Bronchiolectasis is diagnosed by the visualization of bronchioles in the outer half of the lung. The abnormal bronchiole may be air filled, thick walled, dilated, and nontapering. It may also appear as a sharply marginated solid, tubular, branching structure due to plugging of the bronchiole by pus or mucus. When seen on end, the abnormal bronchiole can be seen as a sharply marginated centrilobular dot in the secondary pulmonary lobule (5). Extensive bronchiolectasis, when accompanied by bronchiolar impaction with mucus or pus, can have the "tree-in-bud" appearance when seen in profile. When seen in cross section, extensive bronchiolectasis with bronchiolar impaction has an irregularly branching pattern, resembling a child's jack.

Bronchiectasis and bronchiolectasis are commonly the result of infection, typically occurring early in life. Infections occurring later in life, such as those occurring in immunocompromised patients (e.g., HIV-positive patients) and in older patients (e.g., Nocardia or Mycobacterium avium-intracellulare), can also cause bronchiectasis and bronchiolectasis. Other causes of bronchiectasis and bronchiolectasis are allergic bronchopulmonary aspergillus (occurring in asthmatic patients) and conditions that compromise the lung's normal defense mechanisms, such as cystic fibrosis, abnormal ciliary motility, immune deficiency, and bronchial wall cartilage abnormalities (Williams-Campbell syndrome).

Acute and subacute inflammation of the bronchioles can be seen with chest CT as fluffy centrilobular nodules. Acute bronchiolitis can be caused by acute viral, bacterial, or mycobacterial infections, aspiration, hypersensitivity pneumonitis, respiratory bronchiolitis due to smoking, and toxic gas inhalation.

Constrictive bronchiolitis is a chronic condition due to fibrotic narrowing or obliteration of the bronchiole, causing air trapping in the secondary pulmonary lobule (6). In this condition, chest CT shows decreased density in the affected secondary pulmonary lobules due to decreased perfusion of the underventilated secondary lobules. This finding can be accentuated by expiratory images. The abnormal secondary pulmonary lobules are usually interspersed with normally aerated secondary pulmonary lobules, giving the "mosaic perfusion" appearance. Less frequently, constrictive bronchiolitis can be widespread, resulting in large areas of lung with decreased density, as in the Swyer-James syndrome. Constrictive bronchiolitis can be due to infection, especially early in life, toxic gas inhalation, including cigarette smoke, hypersensitivity pneumonitis, lung and bone marrow transplants, drugs such as amiodarone and penicillamine, and connective tissue diseases such as rheumatoid arthritis.

The radiographic distribution of small airway disease can give clues to its etiology. Bronchiectasis and/or bronchiolectasis localized to a segment or a lobe is usually due to previous infection, whereas widespread bronchiectasis or bronchiolectasis suggests conditions that compromise the lungs' normal defense mechanisms, such as cystic fibrosis or ciliary dyskinesia, or inflammatory injury to the airways resulting from autoimmune or drug reactions. Central bronchiectasis without peripheral bronchiectasis suggests allergic bronchopulmonary aspergillus due to asthma.

The appearance of the centrilobular nodules, tree-in-bud appearance, or the irregularly branching pattern resembling a child's jack can suggest the chronicity of the disease causing the airway abnormalities. A fluffy appearance of these findings suggests an acute or subacute condition such as infection, aspiration, hypersensitivity pneumonitis, or respiratory bronchiolitis. A sharply marginated appearance of these findings suggests a chronic condition such as bronchiolectasis.

II. General Histopathologic Types of Small Airway Pathology

Asthmatic-type changes in the airways include mucous stasis, bronchiolar epithelial sloughing, luminal and mural infiltrate of eosinophils and eosinophil debris, submucosal edema, smooth muscle hypertrophy, goblet-cell metaplasia and hyperplasia, basement membrane thickening, and, in bronchi, bronchial gland hypertrophy (7,8). Submucosal lymphocytic infiltrates are also common in this setting. These changes are typically more prominent in proximal small bronchi than in the bronchioles. Some asthmatic-type histopathologic changes may be reversible and therefore may be absent in patients with treated or inactive asthma, or in patients between asthmatic attacks.

Chronic bronchitis and emphysema (chronic obstructive pulmonary disease)-associated small airway changes are usually not dramatic but include some degree of chronic inflammation of the walls of bronchioles, respiratory bronchiolitis (see below), mild fibrosis of the bronchiolar wall, mucous stasis with some dilatation or distortion of the luminal shape, and loss of radial attachments (9,10).

Cellular bronchiolitis is a descriptive histologic term that refers to inflammatory infiltrates of the bronchioles, which may or may not be associated with other bronchiolar changes, such as fibrosis or peribronchiolar metaplasia, described below (1,11). The inflammatory infiltrate may be acute (acute bronchiolitis), chronic (chronic bronchiolitis), or mixed with both acute and chronic inflammation (acute and chronic bronchiolitis). Conditions associated with various forms of cellular bronchiolitis are discussed later.

Two distinctive subtypes of cellular bronchiolitis include follicular bronchiolitis (FB) (12) and diffuse panbronchiolitis (DPB) (13). In FB, there is a dramatic proliferation of lymphoid follicles with germinal centers along the airways accompanied by some chronic inflammatory infiltrate of the epithelium. FB is thought to be due to hyperplasia of mucosa-associated lymphoid tissue along the airways in response to chronic antigenic stimulation. DPB is a distinctive disease entity with characteristic clinical, radiologic, and pathologic features (14–17). Pathologically, there is an acute or chronic cellular bronchiolitis with interstitial accumulation of foam cells, most prominent in and around respiratory bronchioles, producing gross and microscopic bronchiolocentric nodules. The interstitial foam cells are a characteristic feature helpful in separating DPB from other forms of small airway pathology.

Respiratory bronchiolitis describes the cellular reaction seen in and around respiratory bronchioles that is almost exclusively associated with cigarette smoking (18,19). The characteristic changes of respiratory bronchiolitis include (*i*) smoker's macrophages in the lumens of respiratory bronchioles and the surrounding alveolar spaces, (*ii*) mild chronic bronchiolitis with variable extension into surrounding alveolar parenchyma, and (*iii*) minimal peribronchiolar fibrosis. The macrophages of respiratory bronchiolitis are commonly referred to as "smoker's macrophages" and are characterized by the presence of tan-brown cytoplasmic pigment accentuated by fine black punctuate dots and flecks. These cells may show variable positivity with iron stains. Respiratory bronchiolitis is frequently seen in the lung specimens of smokers, and sometimes this may be an incidental finding. Whenever respiratory bronchiolitis is identified in a lung specimen, a careful search for other more significant pathology is warranted. When respiratory bronchiolitis occurs as the only pathologic finding in a surgical lung biopsy, consideration for respiratory bronchiolitis-associated interstitial lung disease is warranted (see later discussion).

The term bronchiolitis obliterans with intraluminal polyps was originally used for a reparative reaction seen in bronchioles accompanied by intraluminal polypoid plugs of loose fibroblastic tissue (1,9,11,20). It usually occurs in combination with similar organizing tissue plugs in the alveolar ducts and alveolar spaces (organizing pneumonia). These two histologic manifestations have been collectively referred to as bronchiolitis obliterans organizing pneumonia (BOOP), although in most casesthe organizing pneumonia component tends to predominate. Organizing pneumonia pattern is an alternative and more "transparent" descriptive term for BOOP, and this has been suggested as a preferable nomenclature by a recent American Thoracic Society/European Respiratory Society (ATS/ERS) consensus on classification of idiopathic interstitial pneumonias (21). BOOP/organizing pneumonia pattern is a common reparative reaction seen in a number of clinical settings, as discussed below. Idiopathic BOOP/cryptogenic organizing pneumonia is the appropriate term when no underlying etiology is found (20,21).

The pathologic findings seen in constrictive bronchiolitis include varying degrees of mucus stasis, submucosal scarring, bronchiolar smooth muscle hypertrophy, adventitial scarring, and cellular infiltrates of bronchioles. These changes lead to narrowed bronchiolar lumens and obstructive pulmonary functional deficits. Sometimes, complete luminal obliteration by an acellular scar can occur and is best visualized with the trichrome stain for collagen. Obliterative bronchiolitis and bronchiolitis obliterans are synonyms of constrictive bronchiolitis but these terms are easily confused with BOOP (9,11). While BOOP/organizing pneumonia pattern is usually a reversible process with excellent prognosis, constrictive bronchiolitis is usually irreversible with guarded outcome. Clinically, BOOP presents as a restrictive disorder, while constrictive bronchiolitis is generally associated with airflow obstruction. Constrictive bronchiolitis can occur as a late complication of

Table 2 Causes of Constrictive Bronchiolitis

Healed infections (especially adenovirus)
Healed fume or toxin exposures
As a minor component of chronic bronchitis/emphysema
Distal to bronchiectasis (regardless of cause)
Collagen vascular diseases, especially rheumatoid arthritis
Following bone marrow, lung, or heart-lung transplantation
Drug reactions
Inflammatory bowel disease–associated
Diffuse idiopathic pulmonary neuroendocrine cell hyperplasia/carcinoid/tumorlets (23)
As a complication of asthma or cellular bronchiolitis
Idiopathic

Source: From Ref. 2.

various kinds of bronchiolar injuries, although idiopathic cases do occur (22). Causes of constrictive bronchiolitis are listed in Table 2 (2).

Mineral dust associated airway disease is a term applied to pathologic changes involving bronchioles and, more commonly, alveolar ducts following inhalation of a variety of mineral dusts such as asbestos, iron oxide, aluminum oxide, silica, silicate, and coal (9). There is mild thickening and fibrosis of walls of alveolar ducts with usually little inflammation. Dust-laden macrophages and/or free dust deposition are seen around the bronchioles and alveolar ducts. Mineral dust airways disease is more of pneumoconiosis than a bronchiolitis.

Peribronchiolar metaplasia (bronchiolarization) presents as metaplastic bronchiolar epithelium involving alveoli immediately surrounding the bronchiole. Mild mural thickening and fibrosis of the alveolar walls may also be seen. This phenomenon is presumably postinflammatory in origin and thus may be a component of other forms of bronchiolitis such as cellular bronchiolitis, respiratory bronchiolitis, and constrictive bronchiolitis (1,24). Occasionally, peribronchiolar metaplasia is the sole pathologic lesion, which manifests as infiltrative ILD (25).

Bronchiolocentric nodules are a heterogeneous group of conditions in which one sees bronchiolocentric aggregates of cells, granulomatous inflammation, and/or fibrosis, grossly or under low-power magnification (2,24). Such nodular small airway disease may overlap with groups listed in Table 1, but recognizing this pattern may be helpful in the initial differential diagnoses. Lesions that may produce bronchiolocentric nodules at low-power magnification are listed in Table 3.

III. Histopathology of Small Airway Lesions and Their Differential Diagnosis

In assessing bronchiolar pathology, it is critical to know whether the changes under examination represent part of a diffuse process or simply a localized inflammatory reaction (e.g., changes related to localized bronchiectasis). In the latter instance, the changes may be dramatic yet not as significant as when there is widespread but less conspicuous bronchiolar damage. Clinical and CT correlation is invaluable in this setting.

Table 3 Lesions Associated with Bronchiolocentric Nodules

Primarily Inflammatory
Cellular bronchiolitis—including follicular bronchiolitis and diffuse panbronchiolitis
Hypersensitivity pneumonitis/Extrinsic allergic alveolitis
Respiratory bronchiolitis (see above)
Inflammatory and fibrotic
Bronchiolitis obliterans organizing pneumonia/Organizing pneumonia
Pulmonary Langerhans cell histiocytosis
Pneumoconioses
Granulomatous conditions—sarcoidosis, infections, bronchocentric granulomatosis, bronchocentric Wegener granulomatosis.
Miscellaneous
Diffuse idiopathic pulmonary neuroendocrine cell hyperplasia/carcinoid/tumorlets
Lymphangitic and interstitial infiltrating neoplasms involving peribronchiolar lymphatic regions

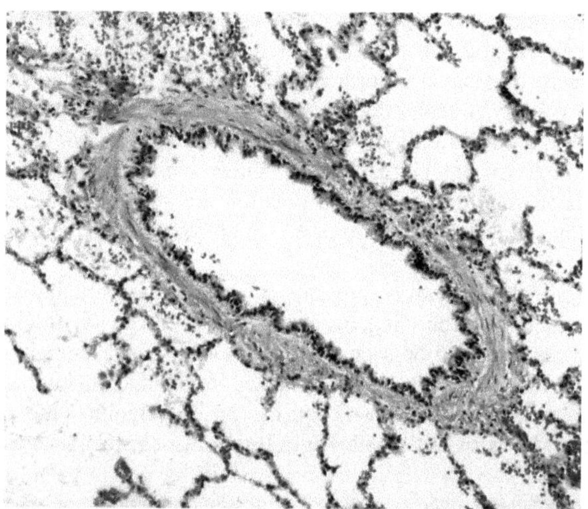

Figure 1 Normal bronchiole. The normal bronchiole has an easily identifiable lumen and variably enfolded columnar to cuboidal epithelium overlying an inconspicuous lamina propria, giving this structure the appearance of epithelium superimposed directly on the underlying smooth muscle wall. The surrounding alveolar septa appear to interface abruptly with the smooth muscle, despite a delicate connective tissue adventitia at this intersection.

The following is a compilation of individual histologic lesions and the clinical conditions that should be considered when these are encountered. For comparison, a normal bronchiole is included (Fig. 1).

1. Acute bronchiolitis (acute inflammation is usually luminal in location; with or without epithelial necrosis and sloughing) (Fig. 2).

    Infections—bacterial and viral; if there is epithelial necrosis, look for viral inclusions

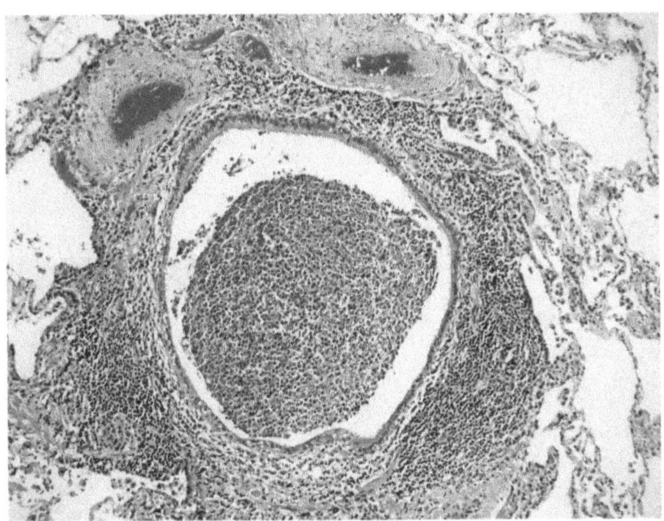

Figure 2 Acute and chronic bronchiolitis. Dense chronic inflammation in the bronchiolar wall with acute luminal inflammation constitutes acute and chronic bronchiolitis. There may or may not be visible epithelial injury, depending on the etiology. (From a case of bronchiolitis associated with inflammatory bowel disease.)

Acute fume/toxic exposure
Acute aspiration (look for foreign material)
Wegener granulomatosis (rare)
Part of a localized reaction/acute bronchopneumonia

2. Acute and chronic bronchiolitis (acute luminal inflammation with mural chronic inflammation; with or without epithelial necrosis, reparative bronchiolar epithelium or changes of constrictive bronchiolitis; may have associated or secondary organizing pneumonia) (Fig. 2).

CT differential diagnosis of tree-in-bud pattern

Centrilobular nodules, tree-in-bud, jacks—acute/subacute disease (fluffy) (Fig. 3)
Infection
Aspiration pneumonia
Hypersensitivity pneumonitis
Respiratory bronchiolitis
Toxic gas inhalation

Centrilobular nodules, tree-in-bud, jacks—chronic disease (well defined)

Bronchiectasis
Bronchiolectasis

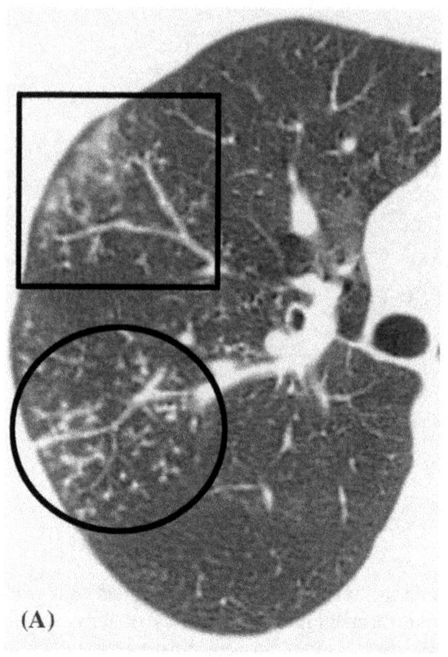

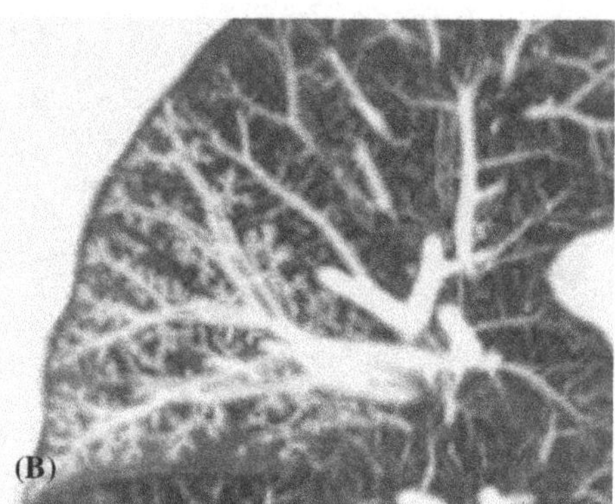

Figure 3 Tree-in-bud CT pattern of acute/subacute and chronic airway infection. (**A**) Axial 3-mm reconstructed image of right upper lobe shows fluffy centrilobular nodules at the end of dilated bronchioles in the anterior portion of the right upper lobe due to acute/subacute airway infection (*black square*). The posterior portion of the right upper lobe shows sharply marginated dilated bronchioles and sharply marginated centrilobular nodules due to chronic airway infection (*black circle*). (**B**) Coronal 10-mm reformatted maximum intensity projection (MIP) of right upper lobe shows sharply marginated dilated bronchioles and sharply marginated centrilobular nodules due to chronic airway infection.

Histopathologic differential diagnosis of acute and chronic bronchiolitis

- Infections—bacterial, viral, mycoplasmal
- Distal to bronchiectasis (regardless of the cause of bronchiectasis)
- Allergic reactions (asthma, hypersensitivity pneumonitis)
- Inflammatory bowel disease–related airway disease
- Diffuse panbronchiolitis
- Bronchocentric granulomatosis
- Collagen vascular disease manifesting in the lung
- Aspiration—giant cells and foreign material may be apparent
- Posttransplantation
- Wegener granulomatosis—giant cells and microabscesses may be found
- Idiopathic
- Part of a localized inflammatory reaction

Comment: Acute and chronic bronchiolitis may be associated with obstructive, restrictive, or mixed obstructive/restrictive pulmonary physiology and also may be associated with radiographic infiltrates (which may be nodular in character).

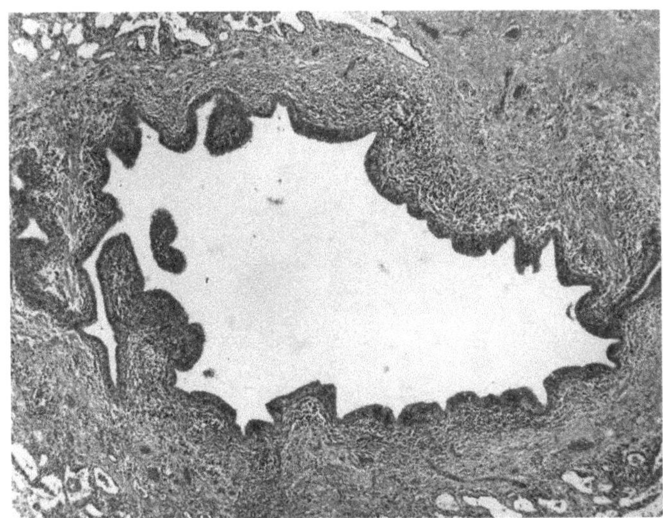

Figure 4 Chronic bronchiolitis in bronchiectasis. In this case of bronchiectasis, the bronchiolar lumen is irregularly dilated with chronic inflammatory infiltrate in the wall.

Morphologic changes of constrictive bronchiolitis may be an accompanied feature. Reactive lymphoid follicles may be present.

3. Chronic bronchiolitis (chronic inflammation of bronchioles, mural in distribution, with or without associated germinal centers or changes of constrictive bronchiolitis) (Figs. 4 to 7).

   Histopathologic differential diagnosis of chronic bronchiolitis

   - Distal to bronchiectasis (regardless of the cause of bronchiectasis)
   - Collagen vascular diseases
   - Inflammatory bowel disease
   - Allergic reactions (asthma, hypersensitivity pneumonitis)
   - Posttransplantation
   - Lymphoproliferative disease
   - Diffuse panbronchiolitis
   - Chronic aspiration—giant cells and foreign material may be present
   - Langerhans cell histiocytosis
   - Idiopathic
   - Part of a localized inflammatory reaction [e.g., middle lobe syndrome (MLS)]

   Comment: Acute and chronic bronchiolitis and chronic bronchiolitis often overlap. Cases of chronic bronchiolitis with prominent germinal centers are termed follicular bronchiolitis (Fig. 5). The presence of follicular bronchiolitis raises the possibility of congenital and acquired immunodeficiency syndromes

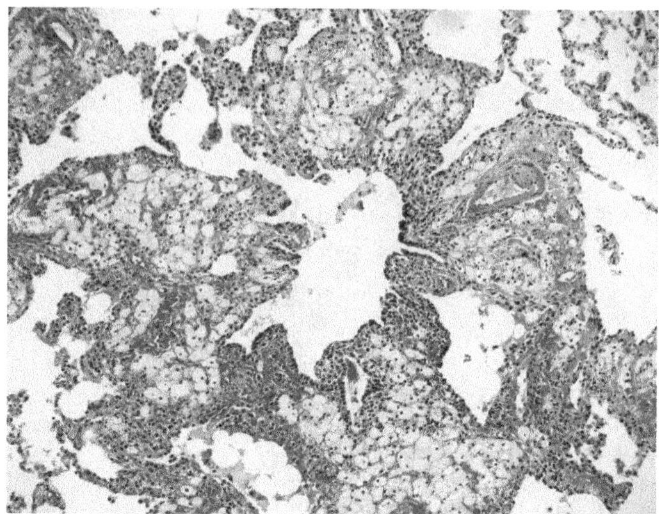

Figure 5 Diffuse panbronchiolitis. The respiratory bronchiole shows chronic inflammation with a characteristic foam-cell infiltrate in the surrounding alveolar interstitium and airspaces. The lesion is concentrated around the terminal bronchiole with relative sparing of the lung parenchyma. Secondary acute inflammation may also be seen.

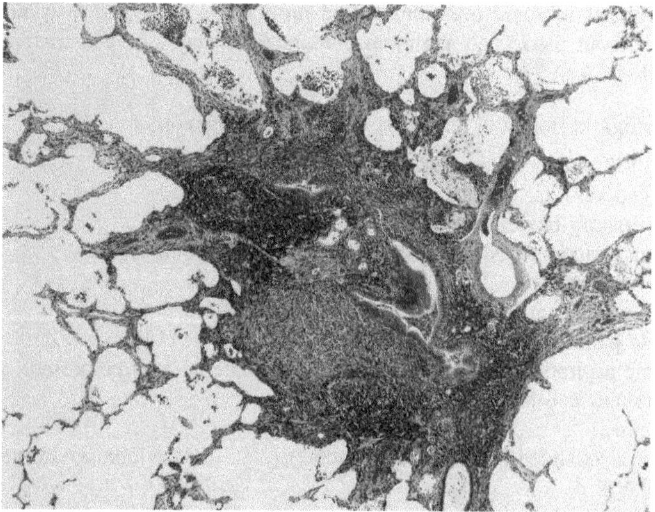

Figure 6 Follicular bronchiolitis. Reactive lymphoid follicles surrounding the bronchiole are seen. The bronchiolar lumen is distorted. From a case of follicular bronchiolitis associated with rheumatoid arthritis.

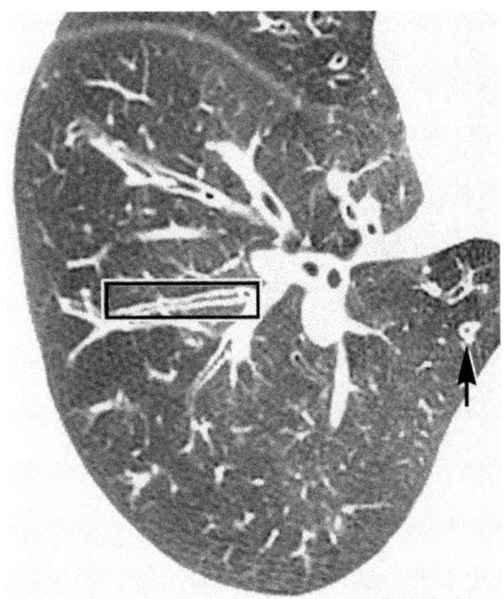

Figure 7 Bronchiolectasis on CT. Thickened bronchiolar walls and slightly enlarged luminal diameters seen en face (*white box*) and on end (*black arrow*).

(including HIV infection and acquired immunoglobulin deficiencies), collagen vascular disease (especially rheumatoid arthritis), systemic hypersensitivity reactions, lymphoproliferative disease (including lymphocytic interstitial pneumonia/diffuse lymphoid hyperplasia), diffuse panbronchiolitis, as a reaction distal to bronchiectasis, and as a local inflammatory reaction (especially MLS of the lingula or right middle lobe) (26).

4. Bronchiolar necrosis (mucosal necrosis and sloughing with or without mural necrosis) (Fig. 8).

   Histopathologic differential diagnosis for bronchiolar necrosis

   Infections—bacterial and viral (especially adenovirus, influenza, herpes virus), bronchocentric fungal infections
   Toxic fume exposure
   Bronchocentric granulomatosis
   Wegener granulomatosis

5. Respiratory bronchiolitis includes (*i*) smoker's macrophages in the lumens of respiratory bronchioles and the surrounding alveolar spaces, (*ii*) mild chronic bronchiolitis with variable extension into surrounding alveolar parenchyma, and (*iii*) minimal peribronchiolar fibrosis (Fig. 9).

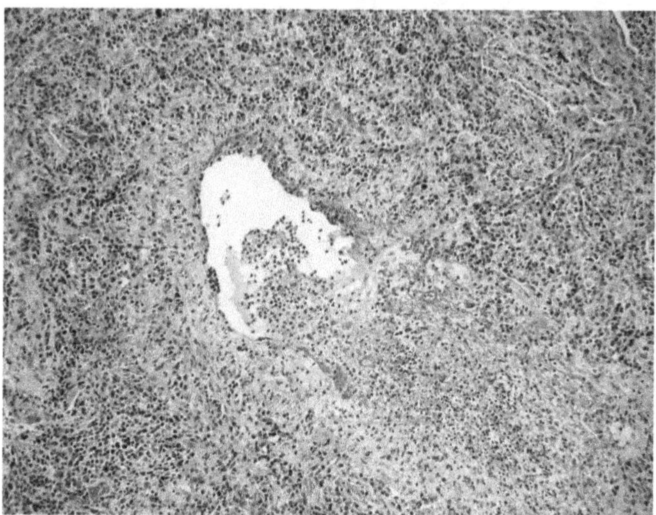

Figure 8 Bronchiolar necrosis. In this case of bronchocentric granulomatosis, the bronchial wall is partially necrotic and replaced by granulomatous inflammation.

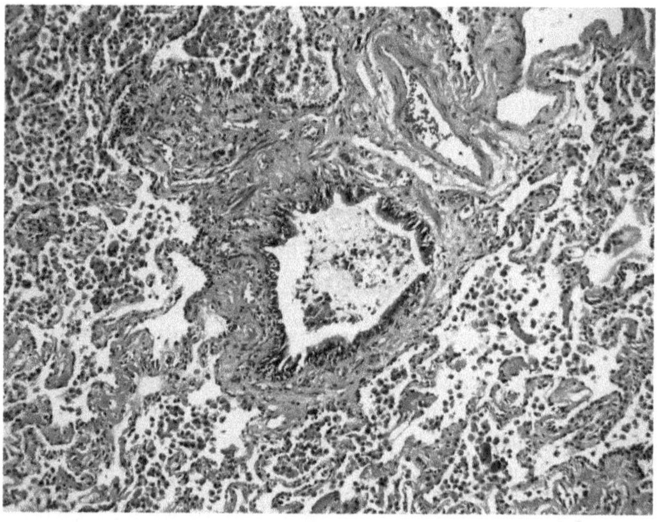

Figure 9 Respiratory bronchiolitis. The characteristic small airways lesion of respiratory bronchiolitis consists of thickened and mildly fibrotic respiratory bronchioles with pigmented macrophages within the bronchiolar lumen and adjacent alveolar spaces. Mucostasis is also present. The iron stain may show fine positivity in the macrophages.

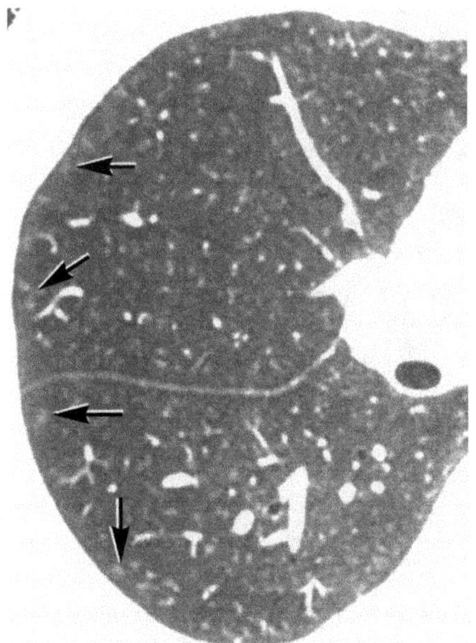

Figure 10 Respiratory bronchiolitis. There are numerous fluffy centrilobular nodules (*arrows*) in the right upper lobe and right lower lobe due to chronic bronchiolar inflammation and peribronchiolar macrophage accumulation in alveolar spaces.

Histopathologic differential diagnosis of respiratory bronchiolitis

- Cigarette smokers
- Respiratory bronchiolitis-ILD/desquamative interstitial pneumonia (DIP) (see comment)
- Langerhans cell histiocytosis (see comment)

Comment: Respiratory bronchiolitis-interstitial lung disease/desquamative interstitial pneumonia (RB-ILD/DIP) is a spectrum of smoking-related ILD (21). It is diagnosed when respiratory bronchiolitis is the sole pathologic finding and there are clinical and radiologic evidences of diffuse ILD (Fig. 10). Langerhans cell histiocytosis commonly occurs in a background of respiratory bronchiolitis (27). Therefore, the possibility of concurrent Langerhans cell histiocytosis should be evaluated when encountering cases of respiratory bronchiolitis.

6. Peribronchiolar metaplasia (bronchiolarization) (Fig. 11).

Histopathologic differential diagnosis for peribronchiolar metaplasia

- Healed bronchiolitis (regardless of the cause)
- Distal to bronchiectasis (regardless of the cause)
- Associated with various causes of interstitial fibrosis
- Chronic hypersensitivity pneumonitis (Fig. 12)
- As a component of constrictive bronchiolitis
- Idiopathic (may be associated with evidence of ILD)

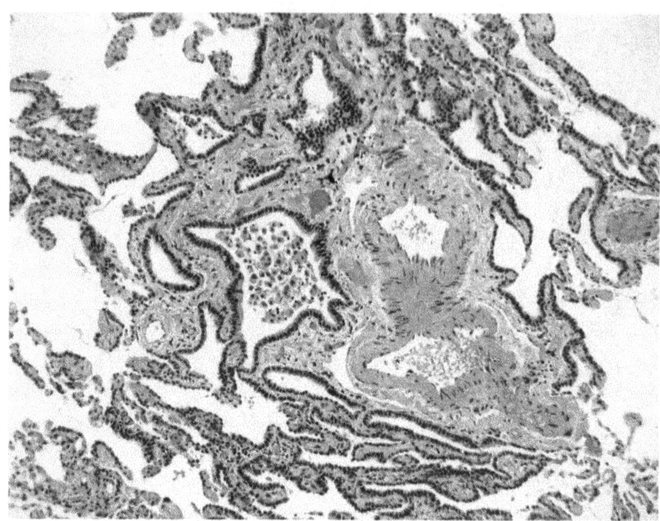

Figure 11 Peribronchiolar metaplasia (bronchiolization). It is characterized by thickening of the bronchiolar wall with extension of cuboidal or low columnar epithelium from the respiratory bronchiole to adjacent alveolar ducts and alveoli. A few mucin and some histiocytes are seen within the bronchiolar lumen. There is usually some degree of interstitial fibrosis in the affected alveoli. (From a case of hypersensitivity pneumonitis.)

7. Alveolar duct fibrosis and dust deposition—mineral dust associated airway disease.

   Histopathologic differential diagnosis for alveolar duct fibrosis with dust deposition

   Mineral dust exposure
   Cigarette smoking

   Comment: Heavy smokers may also have anthracotic pigment deposited along respiratory bronchioles and alveolar ducts, but this condition is usually considerably less prominent and involves less fibrosis than in patients with significant occupational dust exposure.

8. Mucostasis/luminal histiocytes in bronchioles (stasis of mucus and/or histiocytes within the lumen of bronchioles, which often show irregular shapes and distorted lumens) (Fig. 13).

   Histopathologic differential diagnosis for mucostasis

   Chronic bronchitis/emphysema
   Respiratory bronchiolitis
   Asthma (including status asthmaticus)
   Mucoid impaction/allergic bronchopulmonary aspergillosis (28)
   Constrictive bronchiolitis
   Distal to bronchiectasis
   As part of a local inflammatory process (e.g., MLS)

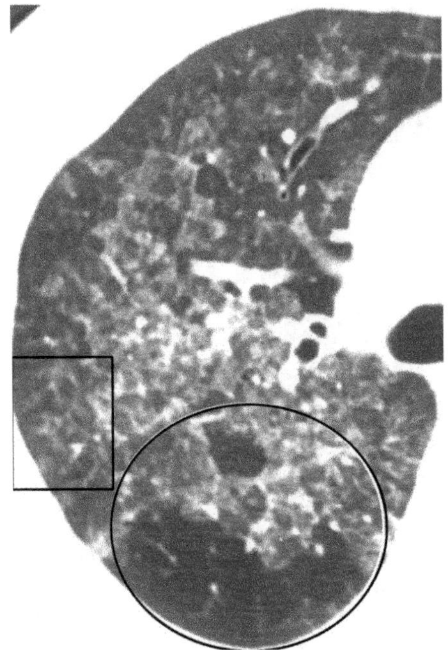

Figure 12 Chronic hypersensitivity pneumonitis. Numerous fluffy centrilobular nodules (*black rectangle*) representing acute/subacute bronchiolitis and areas of constrictive bronchiolitis (*black circle*) mosaic perfusion can be seen.

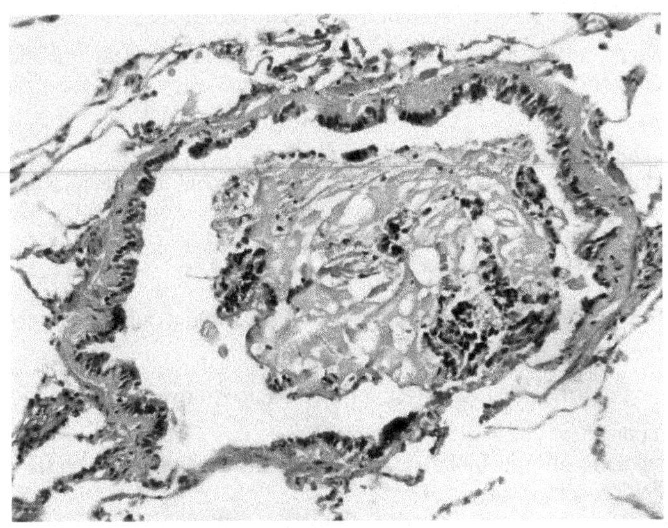

Figure 13 Mucostasis. There is mucus stasis with sloughed epithelium in an airway. The bronchiolar wall shows mild fibrosis. (From a case of chronic asthma.)

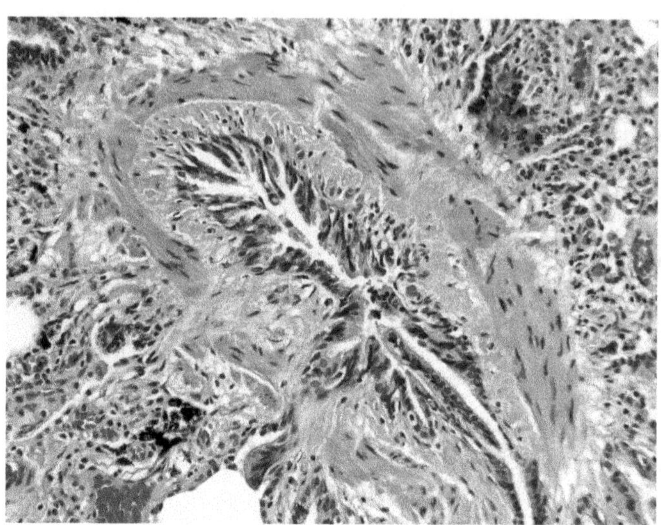

Figure 14 Bronchiolar fibrosis. The bronchiole shows feature of constrictive bronchiolitis with submucosal fibrosis, bronchiolar smooth muscle hypertrophy, and adventitial scarring, leading to a narrowed bronchiolar lumen. (From a case of constrictive bronchiolitis associated with chronic asthma.)

9. Bronchiolar smooth muscle hypertrophy (usually best appreciated subjectively at low-power magnification; there is considerably normal variation; may be accentuated at lobar tips) (Fig. 14).

   Histopathologic differential diagnosis for bronchiolar smooth muscle hypertrophy

   Asthma
   A component of constrictive bronchiolitis
   A component of bronchiolar scarring and peribronchiolar metaplasia
   Associated with fibrotic lung disease
   Part of a localized inflammatory process
   A focal incidental finding

10. Bronchiolar fibrosis (adventitial, submucosal, with or without muscle hypertrophy or peribronchiolar metaplasia) (Figs. 14–16).

    Histopathologic differential diagnosis for bronchiolar fibrosis

    A component of constrictive bronchiolitis
    A component of bronchiolar scarring and peribronchiolar metaplasia
    Distal to bronchiectasis
    Associated with chronic interstitial fibrosis
    Part of a localized inflammatory process (e.g., MLS)

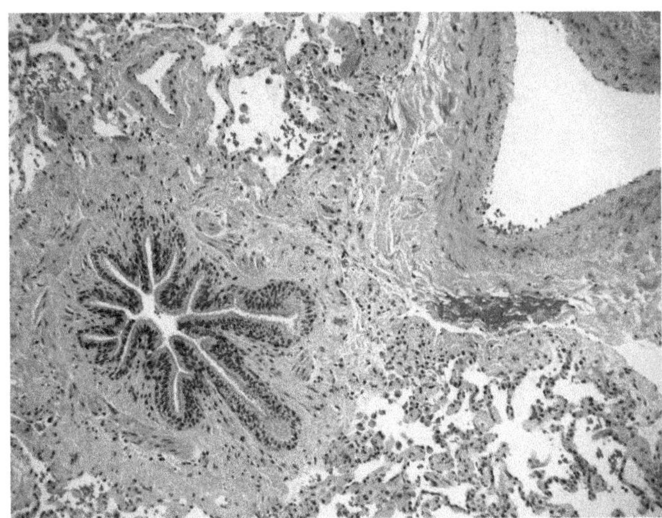

Figure 15 Bronchiolar fibrosis. In this case of constrictive bronchiolitis, the bronchiole shows dense submucosal and advential fibrosis. The bronchiolar lumen is marked narrowed in comparison with the accompanying pulmonary artery.

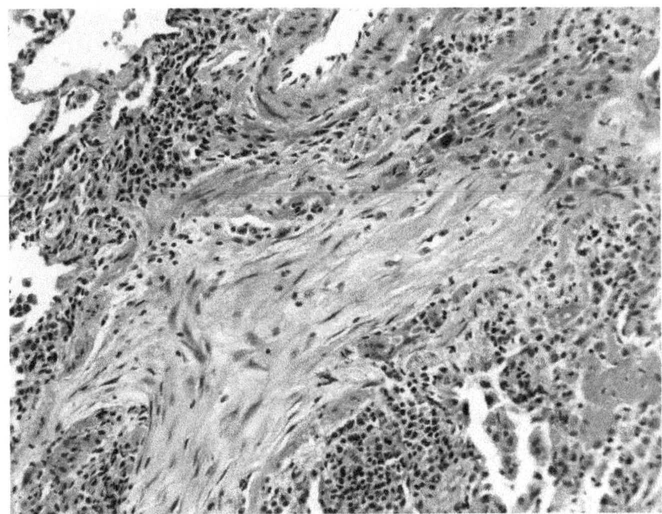

Figure 16 Bronchiolar fibrosis with complete luminal obliteration. The lumen is entirely replaced by fibrous tissue, which is surrounded by remnants of bronchiolar smooth muscle.

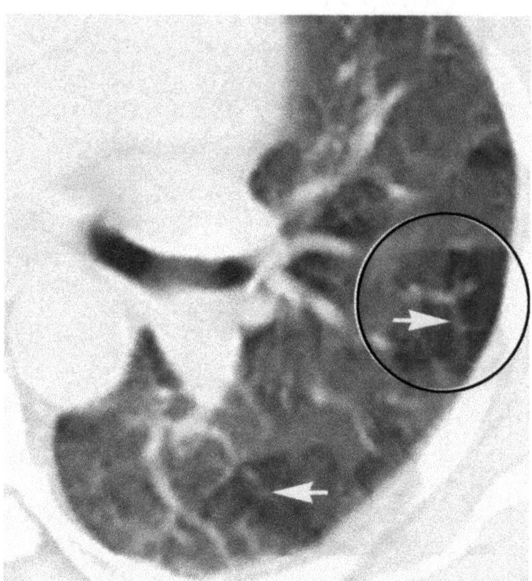

Figure 17 Constrictive bronchiolitis. There are numerous lucent (*blacker*) 1.5- to 3.5-cm well-circumscribed polyhedral areas (*circled area*) scattered around the periphery of the left lower lobe representing secondary pulmonary lobules involved by constrictive bronchiolitis. The constrictive bronchiolitis has caused hypoventilation of the involved secondary pulmonary lobules. The hypoventilated lobules have become hypoxic, resulting in shunting of pulmonary arterial flow away from the hypoxic hypoventilated lobules. The involved lobules are blacker than the surrounding normally ventilated lobules because they contain less blood than the normal lobules. Notice that the pulmonary arterioles in the affected lobules are smaller than those in the normally perfused lobules (*arrows*).

11. Irregular bronchiolar shapes/bronchiolectasis (Figs. 4–6, 11, 13–15).

    Chronic bronchitis/emphysema
    A component of constrictive bronchiolitis
    Distal to bronchiectasis
    Diffuse panbronchiolitis
    Associated with chronic interstitial fibrosis
    As part of a localized inflammatory process (e.g., MLS)

12. Decreased bronchiolar size (in comparison to the accompanying artery, which is usually about the same size as the bronchiole in cross-sectional view) (Figs. 14–17).

    Constrictive bronchiolitis
    Healed neonatal respiratory distress syndrome/bronchopulmonary Dysplasia

13. Bronchiolitis obliterans with intraluminal polyps/BOOP/organizing pneumonia pattern (Fig. 18) (2).

    Histopathologic differential diagnosis for bronchiolitis obliterans with intraluminal polyps

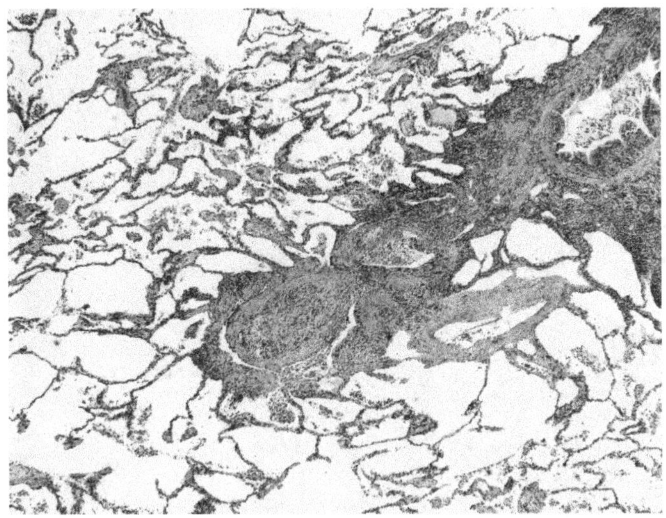

Figure 18 Bronchiolitis obliterans with intraluminal polyps. The bronchiole shows mild chronic inflammation in the wall (chronic bronchiolitis) and an intraluminal polypoid plug of loose fibroblastic tissue (bronchiolitis obliterans with intraluminal polyps). Similar organizing tissue plugs also occur in the alveolar ducts and alveolar spaces (organizing pneumonia). This whole feature is termed as bronchiolitis obliterans organizing pneumonia/organizing pneumonia pattern.

- Organizing diffuse alveolar damage
- Organizing infections
- Organization distal to obstruction
- Organizing aspiration pneumonia
- Drug reactions, fume, or toxic exposures (in the phase of organization)
- Collagen vascular diseases
- Hypersensitivity pneumonitis
- Chronic eosinophilic pneumonia
- As a secondary reaction in patients with chronic bronchiolitis or diffuse panbronchiolitis
- As an idiopathic process that is either localized or more widespread (idiopathic BOOP/cryptogenic organizing pneumonia)
- As a part of a reparative reaction around some other processes such as Wegener granulomatosis, infarcts, abscesses, necrotic tumors

14. Granulomatous bronchiolitis (with or without necrosis and/or giant cells) (Fig. 19).

    Histopathologic differential diagnosis for granulomatous bronchiolitis

    - Infections—fungal, mycobacterial (including atypical mycobacterial)
    - Sarcoidosis
    - Hypersensitivity pneumonitis
    - Bronchocentric granulomatosis

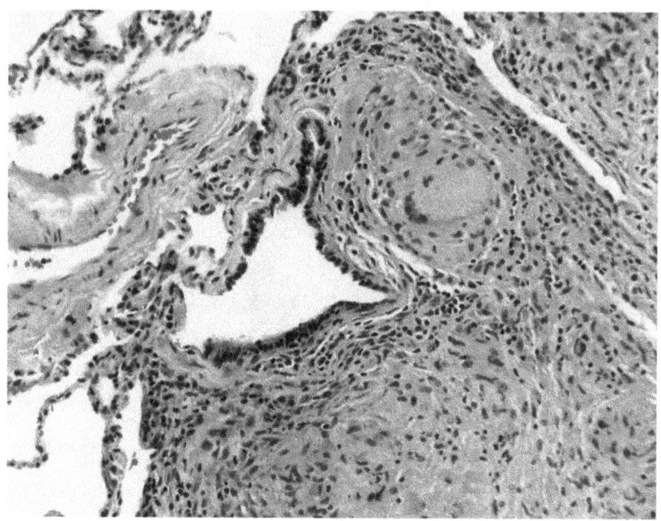

Figure 19 Granulomatous bronchiolitis. The bronchiole is surrounded by confluent nonnecrotizing granulomas. (From a case of sarcoidosis.)

Wegener granulomatosis
Aspiration—foreign material may be present
Hard-metal disease/cobalt pneumoconiosis/giant cell interstitial pneumonia—intra-alveolar giant cells in a peribronchiolar distribution

References

1. Epler GR, ed. Diseases of the Bronchioles. New York: Raven Press, 1994.
2. Colby TV. Bronchial disorders. In: Travis WD, Colby TV, Koss MN, et al., eds. Atlas of Nontumor Pathology, fascicle 2. Non-neoplastic Disorders of the Lower Respiratory Tract. Washington, DC: American Registry of Pathology and the Armed Forces Institute of Pathology, 2002:351–380.
3. Grenier P, Cordeau MP, Beigelman C. High-resolution computed tomography of the airways. J. Thorac Imaging 1993; 8:213–229.
4. Gruden JF, Webb WR, Warnock M. Centrilobular opacities in the lung on high-resolution CT: diagnostic considerations and pathologic correlation. AJR Am J Roentgenol 1994; 162:569–574.
5. Collins J, Blankenbaker D, Stern EJ. CT Patterns of bronchiolar disease: what is "tree-in bud"? AJR Am J Roentgenol 1998; 171:365–370.
6. Müller NL, Miller RR. Diseases of the bronchioles: CT and histopathologic findings. Radiology 1995; 196:3–12.
7. Dunnill MS. The pathology of asthma with special reference to changes in the bronchial mucosa. J Clin Pathol 1960; 13:27–33.
8. Hogg JC. Asthma as a bronchiolitis. Semin Respir Med 1992; 13:114–118.
9. Wright JL, Cagle P, Churg A, et al. Diseases of the small airways. Am Rev Respir Dis 1992; 146:240–262.
10. Colby TV. Bronchiolitis. Pathologic considerations. Semin Respir Med 1992; 13:119–133.

11. Colby TV, Myers JL. Clinical and histologic spectrum of bronchiolitis obliterans including bronchiolitis obliterans organizing pneumonia. Semin Respir Med 1992; 13:119–133.
12. Yousem S, Colby TV, Carrington CB. Follicular bronchiolitis. Hum Pathol 1985; 16:700–706.
13. Kitaichi M, Nishimura K, Izumi T. Diffuse panbronchiolitis. In: Sharma OP, ed. Lung Disease in the Tropics. New York: Marcel Dekker, 1991:479–509.
14. Yamanaka A, Saiki S, Tamura S, et al. Problems in chronic obstructive bronchial disease, with special reference to diffuse panbronchiolitis. Naika 1969; 23:442–451.
15. Homma H, Yamanaka A, Tanimoto S, et al. Diffuse panbronchiolitis: a disease of the transitional zone of the lung. Chest 1983; 83:63–69.
16. Randhawa P, Hoagland MH, Yousem SA. Diffuse panbronchiolitis in North America. Report of three cases and review of the literature. Am J Surg Pathol 1991; 15:43–47.
17. Poletti V, Casoni G, Chilosi M, et al. Diffuse panbronchiolitis. Eur Respir J 2006; 28:862–871.
18. Niewoehner D, Kleinerman J, Rice D. Pathological changes in the peripheral airways of young cigarette smokers. N Engl J Med 1974; 291:755–758.
19. Myers J, Veal C Jr., Shin M, et al. Respiratory bronchiolitis causing interstitial lung disease: a clinicopathologic study of six cases. Am Rev Respir Dis 1987; 135:880–884.
20. Cordier JF. Cryptogenic organising pneumonia. Eur Respir J 2006; 28:422–446.
21. Travis WD, King TE Jr., Bateman ED, et al. ATS/ERS international multidisciplinary consensus classification of idiopathic interstitial pneumonia. Am J Respir Crit Care Med 2002; 165: 277–304.
22. King TE Jr. Bronchiolitis. In: Schwartz MI, King TE Jr., eds. Interstitial Lung Disease, 3rd ed. London: BC Decker, 1998:645–684.
23. Aguayo SM, Miller YE, Waldron JA, et al. Idiopathic diffuse hyperplasia of pulmonary neuroendocrine cells and airway disease. N Engl J Med 1992; 327:1285–1288.
24. Colby TV, Lombard CL, Yousem SA, et al. Atlas of Pulmonary Surgical Pathology. Philadelphia: Saunders, 1991.
25. Fukuoka J, Franks TJ, Colby TV. Peribronchiolar metaplasia: a common histologic lesion in diffuse lung disease and a rare cause of interstitial lung disease: clinicopathologic features of 15 cases. Am J Surg Pathol 2005; 29:948–954.
26. Kwon KY, Myers JL, Swensen SJ. Middle lobe syndrome: a clinicopathological study of 21 patients. Hum Pathol 1995; 26:302–307.
27. Tazi A. Adult pulmonary Langerhans' cell histiocytosis. Eur Respir J 2006; 27:1272–1285.
28. Bosken CH, Myers JL, Greenberger PA, et al. Pathologic features of allergic bronchopulmonary aspergillosis. Am J Surg Pathol 1988; 12:216–222.

13
Pulmonary Hemorrhage

ANDRAS KHOOR
Mayo Clinic, Jacksonville, Florida, U.S.A.

HENRY D. TAZELAAR
Mayo Clinic, Scottsdale, Arizona, U.S.A.

I. Introduction

Hemorrhage into the pulmonary parenchyma is a common histologic finding. It may be acute in the form of extravasated red blood cells or remote in the form of hemosiderin. It may be focal or diffusely involve the entire lung. It may have dramatic clinical manifestations in a variety of conditions and may be a clinically insignificant incidental finding in others. Knowledge of the clinical history is essential in determining which of these applies to a particular patient.

In a biopsy specimen, it is often difficult to determine whether the presence of red blood cells in alveolar spaces represents true pulmonary hemorrhage or an artifact of the procedure. This type of artifact is actually more common than true hemorrhage and can be seen in transbronchial as well as surgical lung biopsies and, interestingly, it is seen more frequently in biopsies obtained by video-assisted thoracoscopy than traditional thoracotomy (1,2). In general, acute pulmonary hemorrhage should not be diagnosed in the absence of an appropriate clinical history. Histologic features that suggest artifactual extravasation of red blood cells include absence of hemosiderin and fibrin. When hemosiderin-laden macrophages are seen, the recognition that pulmonary hemorrhage has taken place is relatively straightforward.

Hemosiderin, the hallmark of old hemorrhage, should be differentiated from other types of pigment, which may be present in the lung. Hemosiderin is dark brown to gold and coarsely granular. Smoker's pigment is usually light brown. It can form relatively quickly (as early as 24–48 hours) (3). In contrast to hemosiderin, smoker's pigment is less coarse, finely dispersed, or "dusty" (Figs. 1 and 2). It may also be associated with small flecks of carbonaceous material. Both pigments are readily identifiable with iron stains, such as Prussian blue. However, hemosiderin stains darker blue and forms more distinct granules. Formalin pigment is another dark brown to black granular material (Fig. 3), which may be present in the lung. As opposed to hemosiderin and smoker's pigment, it is birefringent and is easily identifiable under polarized light (Fig. 4). If there is any question, formalin pigment can be removed from histologic sections with a mixture of acetone, hydrogen peroxide, and ammonium hydroxide. Anthracotic pigment is a black granular pigment that consists mainly of carbon. Although anthracotic pigment is not birefringent, it is often associated with needle-shaped birefringent silicates.

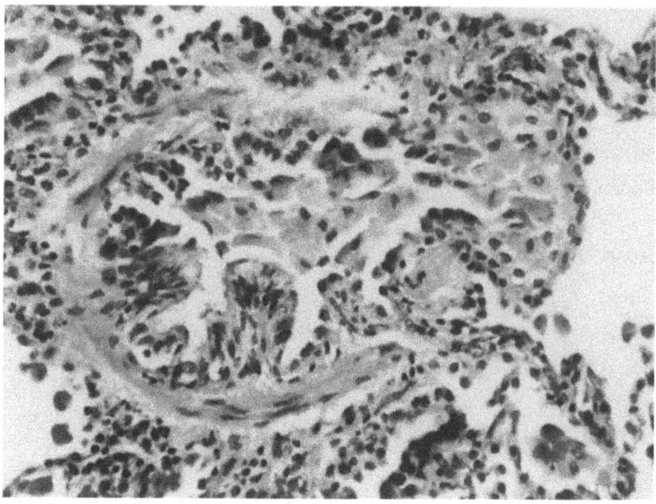

Figure 1 Respiratory (smoker's) bronchiolitis. There is an accumulation of alveolar macrophages in a respiratory bronchiole. The macrophages spill over into the surrounding alveoli.

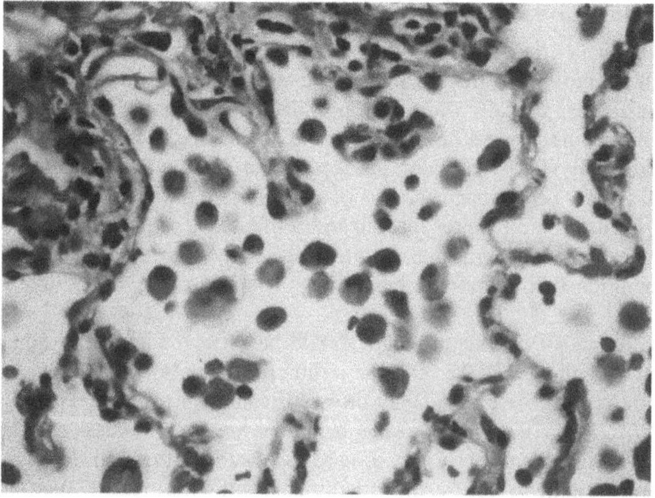

Figure 2 Respiratory (smoker's) bronchiolitis. The alveolar macrophages contain finely granular brown "smoker's" pigment.

II. Localized Hemorrhage

Once intra-alveolar blood has been judged to be pathologic hemorrhage, it is helpful to know whether the hemorrhage is focal or diffuse. The most common causes of pulmonary

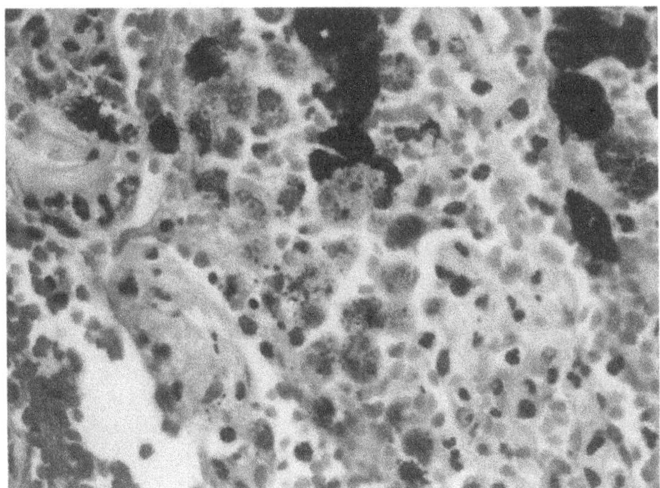

Figure 3 Formalin pigment. It appears as a brown-black, granular material.

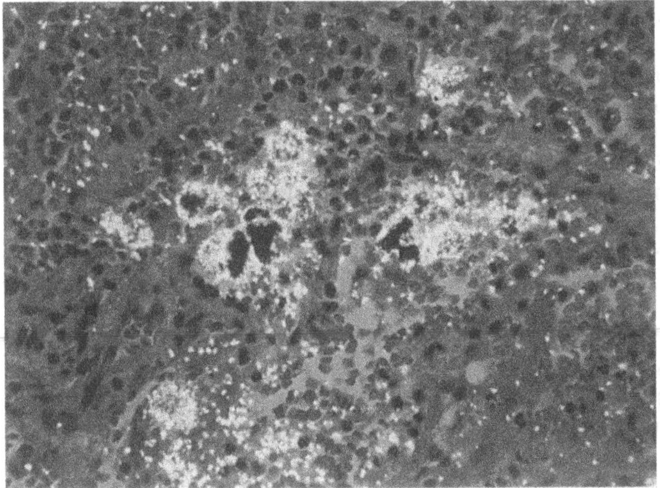

Figure 4 Formalin pigment. Under polarized light, it is birefringent.

hemorrhage are focal (Table 1). In some of these conditions, the bronchial as opposed to the pulmonary circulation is the source of the bleeding. Most patients with focal pulmonary hemorrhage can be successfully treated conservatively. However, in some situations, a resection may be indicated.

Chronic bronchitis due to cigarette smoking is a major cause of hemoptysis. In a prospective analysis of 184 cases, the main causes of hemoptysis were bronchiectasis

Table 1 Causes of Localized Hemorrhage

Chronic and acute bronchitis
Bronchiectasis
Arteriovenous malformation
Dieulafoy disease (superficial submucosal bronchial artery)
Broncholithiasis
Foreign body
Aspiration
Pulmonary infarction
Infection, including abscess and mycetoma
Endometriosis
Neoplasms
Miscellaneous
Transbronchial biopsy in pulmonary amyloidosis
Transbronchial biopsy during mechanical ventilation
Thoracic injury
Aspiration of maternal blood
Congenital cystic adenomatoid malformation
Cystic fibrosis

(26%), chronic bronchitis (23%), acute bronchitis (15%), and lung cancer (13%) (4). However, patients with chronic bronchitis very rarely undergo surgery or biopsy and, therefore, pathologists are occasionally called upon to make this clinicopathologic correlation. In some cases, however, the etiology of focal hemorrhage may not be apparent on pathologic examination. If the history suggests that the hemorrhage is confined to a specific lobe and a lobectomy has been performed, resulting in "cure," the hemorrhage is most likely secondary to chronic bronchitis, even though a definite bleeding site may be difficult to identify. The presence of findings associated with chronic bronchitis and the lack of other histologic changes may suggest the diagnosis.

Bronchiectasis is most often the result of chronic infection and predisposing conditions include airway obstruction (tumors, foreign bodies, mucous plugs, etc.), cystic fibrosis, Kartagener's syndrome, and immune deficiency. Noninfectious bronchiectasis may be associated with connective tissue and inflammatory bowel diseases. Due to the inflammation being frequently associated with bronchiectasis, ulceration of the mucosa may lead to brisk hemoptysis and hemorrhage. Demonstration of the site of bleeding in the rare instance when a lobectomy may be performed in this setting may require examination of the entire affected large airway.

Arteriovenous malformations are vascular anomalies characterized by an abnormal communication between arteries and veins. They are commonly associated with hereditary hemorrhagic telangiectasia or Rendu-Osler-Weber syndrome (5). Arteriovenous malformations are usually diagnosed radiographically, and the pathologist's role is to confirm the diagnosis. Microscopically, they are composed of enlarged, anastomosing blood vessels with irregular mural thickening (Fig. 5). They are quite uncommon, however.

Dieulofoy disease refers to bleeding from mucosal erosion over a superficial submucosal bronchial artery. A recent study identified this abnormality in almost half of patients with a clinical diagnosis of cryptogenic hemoptysis (6).

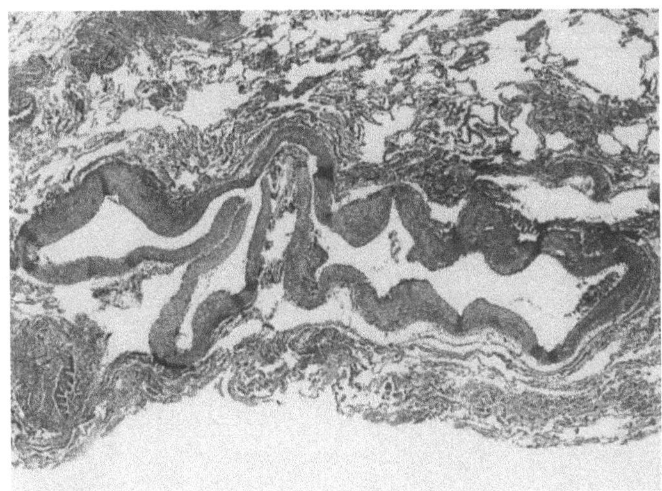

Figure 5 Arteriovenous malformation. There are large, anastomosing, thick-walled vessels.

III. Diffuse Alveolar Hemorrhage

Diffuse alveolar hemorrhage is caused by a heterogeneous group of disorders (Table 2) (7–34). Their unifying feature is their clinical and radiographic presentation, which usually comprises the triad of hemoptysis, anemia, and alveolar filling opacities on imaging. Assessment of patients with diffuse alveolar hemorrhage includes a search for the presence of serologic abnormalities [anti-glomerular basement membrane antibody, antinuclear

Table 2 Causes of Diffuse Alveolar Hemorrhage

Goodpasture's syndrome
Idiopathic vasculitides
Wegener's granulomatosis
Microscopic polyangiitis
Churg-Strauss syndrome
Behcet's disease
Henoch-Schonlein purpura
Essential mixed cryoglobulinemia
Isolated pulmonary capillaritis
Mixed cryoglobulinemia
Connective tissue diseases
Systemic lupus erythematosus
Rheumatoid arthritis
Scleroderma/Systemic sclerosis
Mixed connective tissue disease
Polymyositis
Antiphospholipid antibody syndromes
Ehlers-Danlos syndrome

(Continued)

Table 2 Causes of Diffuse Alveolar Hemorrhage (*Continued*)

Idiopathic glomerulonephritis
With immune complexes
Without immune complexes
Idiopathic pulmonary hemosiderosis
Chemical and drug related
Anticoagulants
Bevacizumab
Cocaine
D-penicillamine
Enoxaparin
Lymphangiogram associated
Paraquat
Propylthiouracil
Rituximab
Sirolimus
Streptokinase
Trimellitic anhydride
Warfarin
Infections
SARS
Leptospirosis
Influenza
Neoplasms
Metastatic angiosarcoma
Choriocarcinoma
Miscellaneous
Autoimmune hemolytic anemia
Bone marrow transplantation
Exercise
High-altitude pulmonary edema
Fat embolism
IgA nephropathy
Malignant hypertension
Silicone embolism
Strangulation
Unclassified pulmonary-renal syndromes

Abbreviations: SARS, severe acute respiratory syndrome; IgA, immunoglobulin A.

antibodies (ANAs), antineutrophil cytoplasmic antibody (ANCA), and immune complexes] and renal abnormalities. In a clinicopathologic study of 34 patients with biopsy-confirmed diffuse pulmonary hemorrhage, Travis et al. encountered the following causes (15): Wegener's granulomatosis (WG) (11 cases), Goodpasture's syndrome (4 cases), idiopathic pulmonary hemosiderosis (IPH) (4 cases), microscopic polyangiitis (3 cases), systemic lupus erythematosus (SLE) (2 cases), rheumatoid arthritis (RA) (2 cases), idiopathic glomerulonephritis (2 cases), immunoglobulin A (IgA) nephropathy (1 case), and unclassified pulmonary-renal syndrome (5 cases).

Diffuse alveolar hemorrhage is defined by the presence of blood in alveolar spaces, which is similar regardless of etiology, but this may be accompanied by other features (see

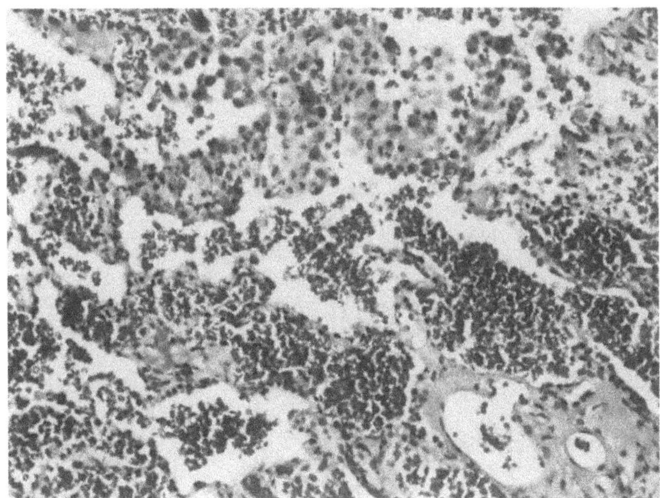

Figure 6 Diffuse alveolar hemorrhage. There are intra-alveolar red blood cells and hemosiderin-laden macrophages.

below), some of which are helpful in limiting the diagnostic possibilities (35). Hemorrhage is manifest by the presence of red blood cells, fibrin, and hemosiderin-laden macrophages in the airspaces (Fig. 6). The alveolar walls may show evidence of acute lung injury in the form of hyaline membranes and reactive type II cells. Foci of organization may be prominent (Fig. 7). The degree of organization can be so prominent as to suggest the diagnosis of cryptogenic organizing pneumonia. Recognition of the presence of abundant

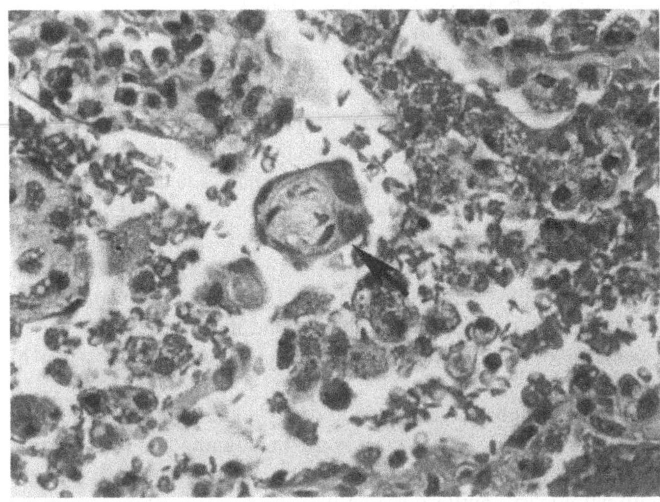

Figure 7 Diffuse alveolar hemorrhage. A focus of organization is present (*arrow*).

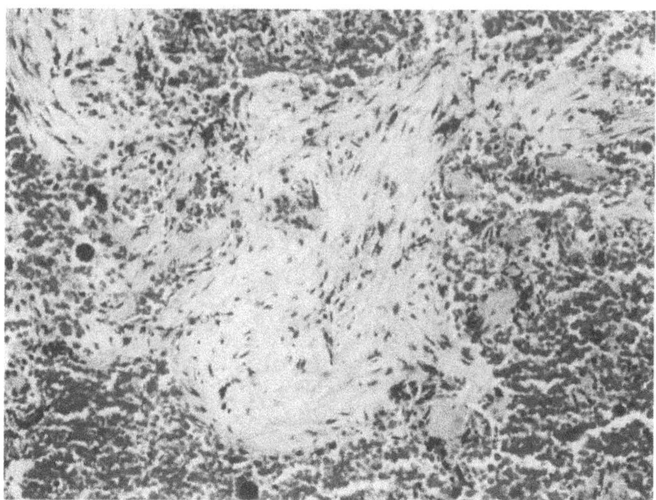

Figure 8 Organizing hemorrhage. In addition to the extravasated red blood cells, connective tissue plugs and hemosiderin-laden macrophages are present within airspaces.

hemosiderin-laden macrophages in the plugs of granulation tissue may suggest the diagnosis of organizing hemorrhage (Fig. 8).

Subclassification of diffuse alveolar hemorrhage cannot be done on morphologic grounds alone, with the exception of typical cases of WG. Electron microscopy is rarely useful. Immunofluorescent microscopic studies may be helpful and, therefore, some authors suggest that a portion of the lung biopsy should always be frozen for these studies. Determining which disease a patient has, however, usually requires a synthesis of the clinical information, ancillary laboratory tests, and biopsy findings.

Damage to endothelial cells is of course at the root of pulmonary hemorrhage and, therefore, one may see evidence of damage to vessels in cases of diffuse alveolar hemorrhage. Vasculitis and necrosis can involve any size or type of vessel in the pulmonary vasculature, and vasculitis in the lung has an appearance similar to that occurring in other organs. Because of its anatomy, however, damage to the capillaries (capillaritis) is a form of vascular injury of special interest in the lung. Histologically, capillaritis is characterized by the presence of neutrophils within the alveolar septa (Figs 9–11). Karyorrhectic debris, thrombosis, and capillary wall necrosis can occasionally be observed. If the capillary wall injury leads to accumulation of neutrophils in the airspaces, differentiation of capillaritis from acute pneumonia may be difficult. Features that may still suggest an alveolar hemorrhage syndrome over a hemorrhagic pneumonia are the clinical history, the presence of focally necrotic alveolar walls associated with early organization, and the presence of hemosiderin-laden macrophages.

Pulmonary capillaritis usually signals the presence of an underlying systemic vasculitis or connective tissue disease (36,37). However, it is not pathognomonic of a specific disorder and has been reported with virtually any of the diffuse alveolar hemorrhage syndromes (15,38). Patients with pulmonary capillaritis usually present with bilateral infiltrates on chest radiographs and can be acutely ill with diffuse alveolar hemorrhage that may be life

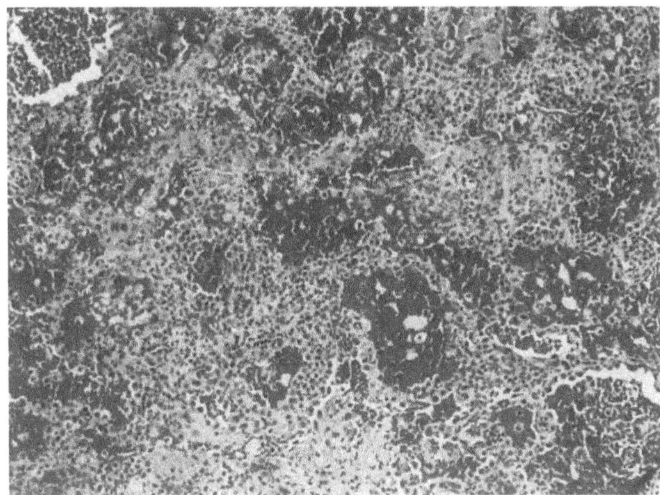

Figure 9 Capillaritis. The alveolar septa are highlighted by a neutrophilic infiltrate. Alveolar hemorrhage is also seen.

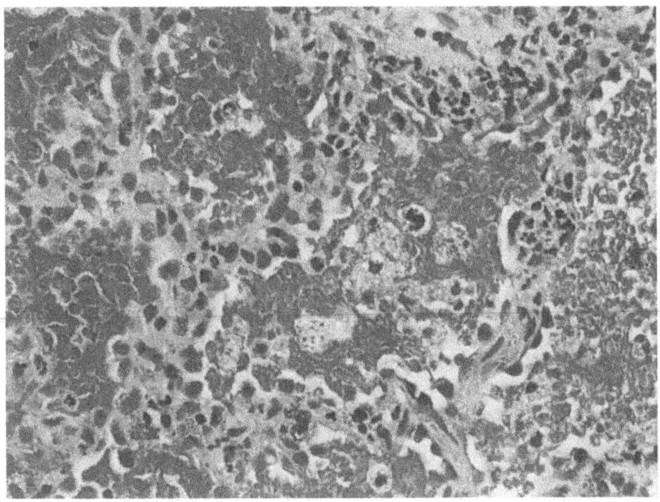

Figure 10 Capillaritis. The alveolar septa contain clusters of neutrophils and are lined by hyperplastic type II cells.

threatening (36). Among patients with WG, for example, patients who present with diffuse pulmonary hemorrhage have the highest acute mortality. Therapy depends on diagnosis of the underlying disease that gave rise to the capillaritis. Since many of the disorders leading to capillaritis are treated by immunosuppression with corticosteroids and cyclophosphamide or azathioprine, infection must be excluded early in the course of therapy.

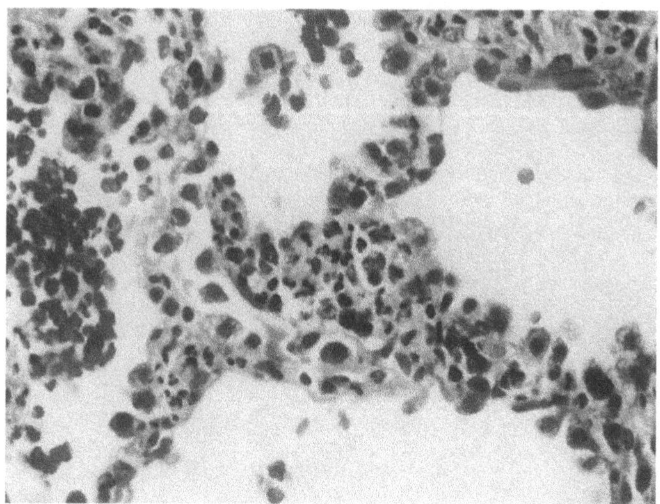

Figure 11 Capillaritis. Numerous neutrophils are present in capillary walls. The airspaces contain a large number of red blood cells, but only occasional neutrophils.

A. Goodpasture's Syndrome

Goodpasture's syndrome or antibasement membrane antibody (ABMA) disease typically occurs in young men, but can affect both sexes and all ages. The diagnostic requirements include the presence of alveolar hemorrhage, crescentic glomerulonephritis, and the presence of ABMA (39). ABMA is detectable in the serum in at least 95% of the patients. The diagnosis can usually be confirmed by a renal biopsy showing the characteristic linear pattern of immunofluorescence for IgG.

Lung biopsy is usually not necessary for the diagnosis of Goodpasture's syndrome. In some cases, however, it may be done if WG is also in the differential diagnosis. The dominant pathologic finding is usually alveolar hemorrhage (40). Hyaline membranes, edematous thickening of alveolar walls, and capillaritis may also be seen. By immunofluorescent microscopy, linear deposition of IgG can be demonstrated along the basement membrane of the alveolar capillaries (Fig. 12) (41).

B. Idiopathic Vasculitides

The two idiopathic vasculitides that most commonly cause diffuse alveolar hemorrhage are WG and microscopic polyangiitis. Secondary vasculitides leading to alveolar hemorrhage include connective tissue diseases, discussed below.

ANCAs are useful serologic markers for systemic vasculitides (42–48). Two major patterns of reactivity are seen when the indirect fluorescent antibody technique is used: diffuse cytoplasmic staining (c-ANCA) and perinuclear staining (p-ANCA) (49). The c-ANCA pattern is caused by antibodies to proteinase 3, whereas the p-ANCA pattern has several reactivities including myeloperoxidase, cathepsin G, and neutrophil elastase (50). The sensitivity of c-ANCA for active WG is greater than 90% in patients with active

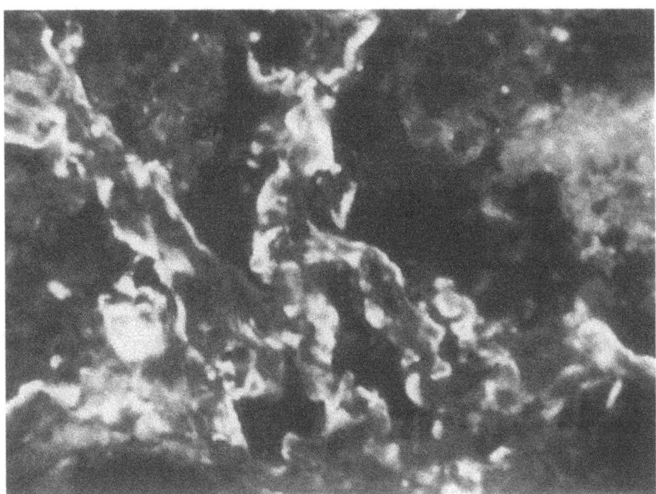

Figure 12 Goodpasture's syndrome. There is linear deposition of IgG along capillary basement membranes, as seen by immunofluorescent microscopy. *Abbreviation*: IgG, immunoglobulin G.

multiorgan disease. c-ANCA reactivity has been described in approximately 50% of patients with microscopic polyangiitis. The specificity of c-ANCA for WG and microscopic polyangiitis is greater than 98%. Reactivity for p-ANCA occurs in a wide range of diseases (51). Antibodies to myeloperoxidase have been found in patients with microscopic polyangiitis, polyarteritis nodosa, WG, idiopathic crescentic glomerulonephritis, SLE, mixed connective tissue disease (MCTD), and Churg-Strauss syndrome (52,53). Additional information on the sensitivity and specificity of these tests and their utility in diagnosis of patients can be found in a consensus statement (54). Subclinical alveolar bleeding as detected by the presence of iron-positive macrophages in bronchoalveolar lavage fluid is a common finding in ANCA-associated vasculitis (55).

Wegener's Granulomatosis

WG is a clinicopathologic syndrome characterized by necrotizing granulomatous vasculitis of the upper and lower respiratory tract and focal segmental glomerulonephritis. The vasculitis may also involve the eyes, joints, skin, nervous system, and heart. WG most often affects middle-aged adults. Affected men outnumber women by a ratio of 2:1. It rarely occurs in children.

The three major histologic manifestations of WG include parenchymal necrosis, vasculitis, and a mixed inflammatory infiltrate with scattered individual giant cells (Figs. 13 and 14) (56,57). If at least two of these three major histologic criteria are present, the lung biopsy may be considered compatible with WG. Although the histopathologic features of WG are usually distinctive enough to suggest the diagnosis on hematoxylin- and eosin-stained sections, special stains should always be performed to rule out an infectious etiology. Rarely, alveolar hemorrhage and capillaritis are the only pathologic findings (58–61). Alveolar hemorrhage is one of the minor manifestations of WG and is present in

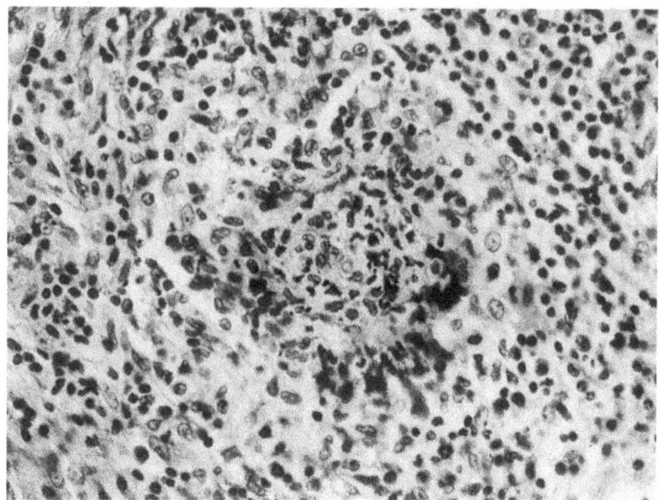

Figure 13 Wegener's granulomatosis. Neutrophils form a microabscess in the background of a mixed inflammatory infiltrate.

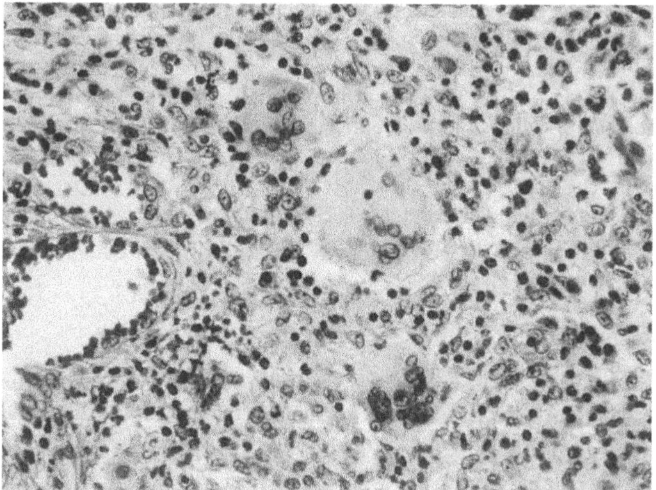

Figure 14 Wegener's granulomatosis. Individual giant cells are present.

approximately half of the cases. It is usually found at the periphery of typical nodules of WG. If alveolar hemorrhage and capillaritis are the dominant features, WG cannot be separated from other alveolar hemorrhage syndromes on histologic grounds alone, although, the presence of even a few giant cells in this setting would favor a diagnosis of WG over the other possibilities. The differentiation of WG from microscopic polyangiitis can be especially difficult.

Microscopic Polyangiitis

Microscopic polyangiitis is characterized by focal segmental glomerulonephritis and a small vessel vasculitis that predominantly affects the skin and musculoskeletal system. It is thought to be a variant of polyarteritis nodosa, but grossly visible aneurysms are not seen. Unlike classic polyarteritis nodosa, patients with microscopic polyangiitis commonly have pulmonary involvement (62).

The lung reveals intra-alveolar hemorrhage, small vessel vasculitis with fibrinoid necrosis, and hemosiderin-laden macrophages. Nonspecific pulmonary fibrosis may be present. No medium-sized vessel involvement, granulomatous inflammation, or bronchiolar obliteration are seen. Immunofluorescent studies of the lung show minimal or no reactivity.

C. Connective Tissue Diseases

Connective tissue diseases are immunologically mediated musculoskeletal disorders. Their diagnostic criteria include the presence of various autoantibodies including ANAs and rheumatoid factor (RF).

Systemic Lupus Erythematosus

SLE is a multisystem disease. ANAs are commonly found in the serum. The first symptoms usually occur between the second and fourth decades of life. The female-male ratio in this age group is 9:1. The female predominance is less striking in children and elderly patients. While lupus occurs in all races, it is more common in blacks than in whites.

Pulmonary hemorrhage is a rare, but severe complication of SLE (63). Acute alveolar hemorrhage in SLE usually occurs as a pulmonary-renal syndrome. In most cases, the lungs show "bland" alveolar hemorrhage with little or no inflammation (64). However, small vessel vasculitis characterized by acute necrotizing inflammation of capillaries, arterioles, and small muscular arteries can also occur (65). Immunofluorescent and electron microscopic studies demonstrate immune complexes in approximately half of the cases. Other histologic manifestations of SLE in the lung include chronic interstitial pneumonia, interstitial fibrosis, diffuse alveolar damage, pulmonary hypertension, and pleuritis.

Rheumatoid Arthritis

RA is a chronic inflammatory disorder characterized by nonsuppurative arthritis and frequent involvement of other organs. Although a positive RF is observed in 80% of the patients, it is not considered specific for RA. RA affects 1% to 2% of the U.S. population and the female-male ratio is 3:1. Men, however, are more commonly affected by pulmonary complications. Although pulmonary involvement is more common in patients with active disease, the respiratory findings may precede the onset of skeletal symptoms. Recurrent alveolar hemorrhage, hemosiderosis, and vasculitis are rare manifestations of RA in the lung (66). The vasculitis may be granulomatous (67). There are no other histologic features, which can be used to separate pulmonary hemorrhage in this setting from other diffuse pulmonary hemorrhage syndromes.

Scleroderma

Scleroderma (progressive systemic sclerosis) is characterized by microvascular abnormalities and excessive deposition of collagen and other matrix proteins in the skin and internal organs. Limited scleroderma consists of calcinosis, Raynaud phenomenon, esophageal dysfunction, sclerodactyly and teleangiectasia (CREST syndrome). Women are affected four times more often than men. The disease generally appears in the third or fourth decade of life.

Hemoptysis due to endobronchial teleangiectasias has been described in patients with scleroderma. Pulmonary veno-occlusive disease is rarely associated with scleroderma, but may become the source of chronic hemorrhage.

Mixed Connective Tissue Disease

MCTD demonstrates overlapping features of several rheumatic diseases and high titers of a specific antibody to an extractable nuclear antigen (ENA). The majority of patients are women, and the average age at the time of presentation is 37 years.

Pulmonary hemorrhage is a rare but life-threatening complication of MCTD (68,69). Other pleuropulmonary manifestations include interstitial lung disease, pulmonary hypertension, and pleural effusion.

D. Idiopathic Pulmonary Hemosiderosis

IPH is a diagnosis of exclusion (70–72). It occurs most frequently in children (73). Patients with IPH develop pulmonary hemorrhage without any systemic manifestations or renal disease. No ABMA can be detected in the serum or in a renal biopsy. Some patients diagnosed initially as having IPH may develop manifestations of another diffuse alveolar hemorrhage syndrome later. IPH has been described in association with celiac disease.

Microscopically, numerous hemosiderin-laden macrophages are seen. These lungs lack any evidence of capillaritis or acute injury, but appear relatively quiescent. Recurrent alveolar hemorrhage may lead to interstitial fibrosis.

IV. Iron Deposition Without Significant Acute Hemorrhage

Some diseases are commonly associated with hemosiderosis but are infrequently seen with acute alveolar hemorrhage (Table 3). Lesions that present with hemosiderosis should be separated from smoking-related changes including respiratory bronchiolitis, respiratory

Table 3 Causes of Pulmonary Iron Deposition Without Significant Acute Hemorrhage

Chronic passive congestion
Desquamative interstitial pneumonia
Lymphangioleiomyomatosis
Pulmonary Langerhans Cell Histiocytosis
Pulmonary veno-occlusive disease
Respiratory bronchiolitis
Respiratory bronchiolitis–associated interstitial lung disease

bronchiolitis–associated interstitial lung disease, eosinophilic granuloma, and desquamative interstitial pneumonia. Respiratory bronchiolitis is a common incidental finding in lung biopsy specimens of cigarette smokers characterized by accumulations of pigment-laden macrophages in and around terminal and respiratory bronchioles. In contrast to hemosiderin, smoker's pigment is indistinct and finely dispersed. Respiratory bronchiolitis is sometimes accompanied by mild interstitial fibrosis and chronic inflammation. This usually incidental finding can occasionally be the sole pathologic feature present in patients with signs and symptoms of interstitial lung disease and is referred to as respiratory bronchiolitis–associated interstitial lung disease (74). Respiratory bronchiolitis can also be associated with pulmonary Langerhans cell histiocytosis (eosinophilic granuloma, histiocytosis X). Desquamative interstitial pneumonia is characterized by diffuse interstitial fibrosis and chronic interstitial pneumonia associated with uniform filling of airspaces by smoker's pigment containing macrophages.

Lymphangioleiomyomatosis presents almost exclusively in women. However, rare cases have been described in men with and without tuberous sclerosis (75,76) Lymphangioleiomyomatosis may show patchy foci of old hemorrhage adjacent to pulmonary veins. Additionally, the characteristic parenchymal airspace enlargement and HMB-45-positive immature smooth muscle cells are also seen. The pulmonary lesions in patients with tuberous sclerosis are pathologically identical to lymphangioleiomyomatosis.

In pulmonary veno-occlusive disease, the accumulation of hemosiderin-filled alveolar macrophages is associated with interstitial edema and fibrosis. The diagnostic changes are in the small veins and include intimal fibrosis and the presence of recanalized thrombi.

Chronic passive congestion is another common incidental finding in histologic specimens of the lung. It is characterized by the presence of numerous hemosiderin-laden macrophages or "heart failure cells" (Fig. 15). When there is extensive hemosiderosis, mild

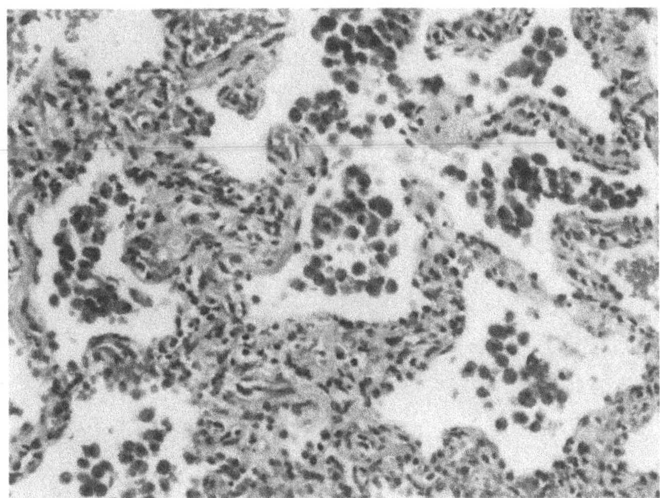

Figure 15 Chronic passive congestion. Numerous hemosiderin-laden macrophages are present in the airspaces.

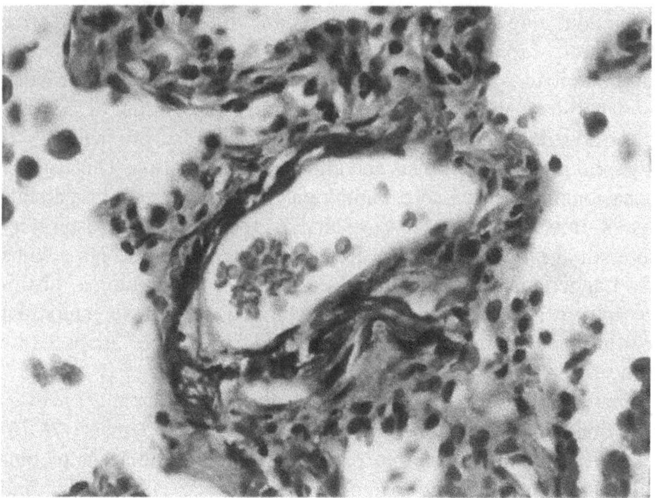

Figure 16 Chronic passive congestion. An elastic vessel shows encrustation by iron.

interstitial fibrosis may be seen. As an extremely rare complication, fatal pulmonary hemorrhage can occur in patients with mitral stenosis and congenital heart disease.

Occasionally, hemosiderosis becomes so great that the elastic tissues in the walls of vessels (usually pulmonary veins) become encrusted with iron. This has been called "endogenous pneumoconiosis," although the term "mineralizing elastosis" is probably a better moniker (Figs. 16 and 17). When observed, elastic fibers frequently appear black or deep purple and careful observation may reveal the presence of occasional giant cells.

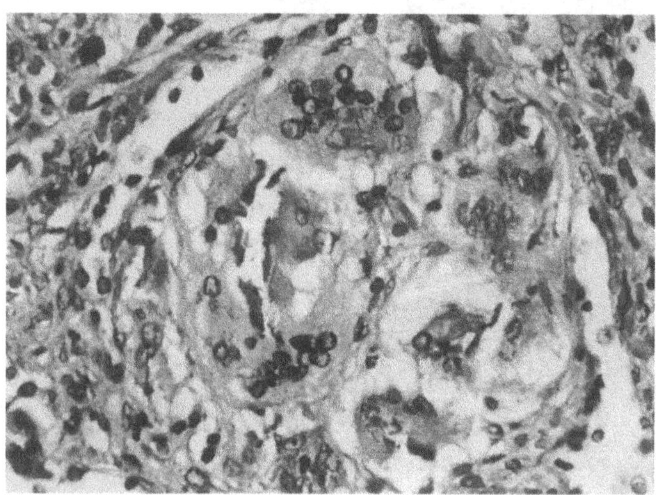

Figure 17 Chronic passive congestion. Multinucleated giant cells engulf elastic fibers.

Sometimes the fibers actually calcify. The finding of mineralizing elastosis indicates that there has been chronic hemorrhage. It is most commonly observed in the setting of chronic passive congestion, veno-occlusive disease, or disease with pulmonary outflow obstruction such as sclerosing mediastinitis.

References

1. Kadokura M, Colby TV, Myers JL, et al. Pathologic comparison of video-assisted thoracic surgical lung biopsy with traditional open lung biopsy. J Thorac Cardiovasc Surg 1995; 109:494–498.
2. Colby TV, Fukuoka J, Ewaskow SP, et al. Pathologic approach to pulmonary hemorrhage. Ann Diagn Pathol 2001; 5:309–319.
3. Vanezis P. Interpreting bruises at necropsy. J Clin Pathol 2001; 54:348–355.
4. Tsoumakidou M, Chrysofakis G, Tsiligianni I, et al. A prospective analysis of 184 hemoptysis cases: diagnostic impact of chest X-ray, computed tomography, bronchoscopy. Respiration 2006; 73:808–814.
5. Cottin V, Chinet T, Lavole A, et al. Pulmonary arteriovenous malformations in hereditary hemorrhagic telangiectasia: a series of 126 patients. Medicine (Baltimore) 2007; 86:1–17.
6. Savale L, Parrot A, Khalil A, et al. Cryptogenic hemoptysis: from a benign to a life-threatening pathologic vascular condition. Am J Respir Crit Care Med 2007; 175:1181–1185.
7. De Lassence A, Fleury-Feith J, Escudier E, et al. Alveolar hemorrhage. Diagnostic criteria and results in 194 immunocompromised hosts. Am J Respir Crit Care Med 1995; 151:157–163.
8. Lai FM, Li EK, Suen MW, et al. Pulmonary hemorrhage. A fatal manifestation in IgA nephropathy. Arch Pathol Lab Med 1994; 118:542–546.
9. Leatherman JW. Immune alveolar hemorrhage. Chest 1987; 91:891–897.
10. Leatherman JW, Davies SF, Hoidal JR. Alveolar hemorrhage syndromes: diffuse microvascular lung hemorrhage in immune and idiopathic disorders. Medicine (Baltimore) 1984; 63:343–361.
11. Matsumoto T, Homma S, Okada M, et al. The lung in polyarteritis nodosa: a pathologic study of 10 cases. Hum Pathol 1993; 24:717–724.
12. Moss M, Neff TA, Colby TV, et al. Diffuse alveolar hemorrhage due to antibasement membrane antibody disease appearing with a polyglandular autoimmune syndrome. Chest 1994; 105:296–298.
13. Schmidt-Wolf I, Schwerdtfeger R, Schwella N, et al. Diffuse pulmonary alveolar hemorrhage after allogeneic bone marrow transplantation. Ann Hematol 1993; 67:139–141.
14. Schwarz MI, Sutarik JM, Nick JA, et al. Pulmonary capillaritis and diffuse alveolar hemorrhage. A primary manifestation of polymyositis. Am J Respir Crit Care Med 1995; 151:2037–2040.
15. Travis WD, Colby TV, Lombard C, et al. A clinicopathologic study of 34 cases of diffuse pulmonary hemorrhage with lung biopsy confirmation. Am J Surg Pathol 1990; 14:1112–1125.
16. Dhillon SS, Singh D, Doe N, et al. Diffuse alveolar hemorrhage and pulmonary capillaritis due to propylthiouracil. Chest 1999; 116:1485–1488.
17. Colby TV. Pulmonary pathology in patients with systemic autoimmune diseases. Clin Chest Med 1998; 19:587–612, vii (review).
18. Grissom CK, Albertine KH, Elstad MR. Alveolar haemorrhage in a case of high altitude pulmonary oedema. Thorax 2000; 55:167–169.
19. Hida K, Wada J, Odawara M, et al. Malignant hypertension with a rare complication of pulmonary alveolar hemorrhage. Am J Nephrol 2000; 20:64–67.
20. Lewis ID, DeFor T, Weisdorf DJ. Increasing incidence of diffuse alveolar hemorrhage following allogeneic bone marrow transplantation: cryptic etiology and uncertain therapy. Bone Marrow Transplant 2000; 26:539–543.
21. Rossi SE, Erasmus JJ, McAdams HP, et al. Pulmonary drug toxicity: radiologic and pathologic manifestations. Radiographics 2000; 20:1245–1259.
22. Delmonte C, Capelozzi VL. Morphologic determinants of asphyxia in lungs: a semiquantitative study in forensic autopsies. Am J Forensic Med Pathol 2001; 22:139–149.

23. Droma Y, Hanaoka M, Hotta J, et al. Pathological features of the lung in fatal high altitude pulmonary edema occurring at moderate altitude in Japan. High Alt Med Biol 2001; 2:515–523.
24. Morelon E, Stern M, Israel-Biet D, et al. Characteristics of sirolimus-associated interstitial pneumonitis in renal transplant patients. Transplantation 2001; 72:787–790.
25. Specks U. Diffuse alveolar hemorrhage syndromes. Curr Opin Rheumatol 2001; 13:12–17.
26. Alexandrescu DT, Dutcher JP, O'Boyle K, et al. Fatal intra-alveolar hemorrhage after rituximab in a patient with non-Hodgkin lymphoma. Leuk Lymphoma 2004; 45:2321–2325.
27. Erdogan D, Kocaman O, Oflaz H, et al. Alveolar hemorrhage associated with warfarin therapy: a case report and literature review. Int J Cardiovasc Imaging 2004; 20:155–159.
28. Nadrous HF, Yu AC, Specks U, et al. Pulmonary involvement in Henoch-Schonlein purpura. Mayo Clin Proc 2004; 79:1151–1157.
29. Vlahakis NE, Rickman OB, Morgenthaler T. Sirolimus-associated diffuse alveolar hemorrhage. Mayo Clin Proc 2004; 79:541–545.
30. Roychowdhury M, Pambuccian SE, Aslan DL et al. Pulmonary complications after bone marrow transplantation: an autopsy study from a large transplantation center. Arch Pathol Lab Med 2005; 129:366–371.
31. Schmid A, Tzur A, Leshko L, et al. Silicone embolism syndrome: a case report, review of the literature, and comparison with fat embolism syndrome. Chest 2005; 127:2276–2281.
32. Sharma S, Nadrous HF, Peters SG, et al. Pulmonary complications in adult blood and marrow transplant recipients: autopsy findings. Chest 2005; 128:1385–1392.
33. Guarner J, Paddock CD, Shieh WJ, et al. Histopathologic and immunohistochemical features of fatal influenza virus infection in children during the 2003–2004 season. Clin Infect Dis 2006; 43: 132–140.
34. Hadjiangelis NP, Harkin TJ. Propylthiouracil-related diffuse alveolar hemorrhage with negative serologies and without capillaritis. Respir Med 2007; 101:865–867.
35. Leslie KO, Gruden JF, Parish JM, et al. Transbronchial biopsy interpretation in the patient with diffuse parenchymal lung disease. Arch Pathol Lab Med 2007; 131:407–423.
36. Franks TJ, Koss MN. Pulmonary capillaritis. Curr Opin Pulm Med 2000; 6:430–435.
37. Sinico RA, Di Toma L, Maggiore U, et al. Prevalence and clinical significance of antineutrophil cytoplasmic antibodies in Churg-Strauss syndrome. Arthritis Rheum 2005; 52:2926–2935.
38. Mark EJ, Ramirez JF. Pulmonary capillaritis and hemorrhage in patients with systemic vasculitis. Arch Pathol Lab Med 1985; 109:413–418.
39. Lazor R, Bigay-Game L, Cottin V, et al. Alveolar hemorrhage in anti-basement membrane antibody disease: a series of 28 cases. Medicine (Baltimore) 2007; 86:181–193.
40. Lombard CM, Colby TV, Elliott CG. Surgical pathology of the lung in anti-basement membrane antibody-associated Goodpasture's syndrome. Hum Pathol 1989; 20:445–451.
41. Magro CM, Morrison C, Pope-Harman A, et al. Direct and indirect immunofluorescence as a diagnostic adjunct in the interpretation of nonneoplastic medical lung disease. Am J Clin Pathol 2003; 119:279–289.
42. Bosch X, Lopez-Soto A, Mirapeix E, et al. Antineutrophil cytoplasmic autoantibody-associated alveolar capillaritis in patients presenting with pulmonary hemorrhage. Arch Pathol Lab Med 1994; 118:517–522.
43. Fienberg R, Mark EJ, Goodman M, et al. Correlation of antineutrophil cytoplasmic antibodies with the extrarenal histopathology of Wegener's (pathergic) granulomatosis and related forms of vasculitis. Hum Pathol 1993; 24:160–168.
44. Rao JK, Allen NB, Feussner JR, et al. A prospective study of antineutrophil cytoplasmic antibody (c-ANCA) and clinical criteria in diagnosing Wegener's granulomatosis. Lancet 1995; 346: 926–931.
45. Ritter JH. Anti-neutrophil cytoplasmic autoantibodies and patterns of pulmonary disease. A spectrum of pathologic findings. Am J Clin Pathol 1995; 104:1–2.

46. Ding Y, Wang H, Shen H, et al. The clinical pathology of severe acute respiratory syndrome (SARS): a report from China. J Pathol 2003; 200:282–289.
47. Lang ZW, Zhang LJ, Zhang SJ, et al. A clinicopathological study of three cases of severe acute respiratory syndrome (SARS). Pathology 2003; 35:526–531.
48. Luks AM, Lakshminarayanan S, Hirschmann JV. Leptospirosis presenting as diffuse alveolar hemorrhage: case report and literature review. Chest 2003; 123:639–643.
49. Gross WL, Schmitt WH, Csernok E. Antineutrophil cytoplasmic autoantibody-associated diseases: a rheumatologist's perspective. Am J Kidney Dis 1991; 18:175–179.
50. Jennette JC, Falk RJ. The coming of age of serologic testing for anti-neutrophil cytoplasmic autoantibodies. Mayo Clin Proc 1994; 69:908–910.
51. Gal AA, Velasquez A. Antineutrophil cytoplasmic autoantibody in the absence of Wegener's granulomatosis or microscopic polyangiitis: implications for the surgical pathologist. Mod Pathol 2002; 15:197–204.
52. Gaudin PB, Askin FB, Falk RJ, et al. The pathologic spectrum of pulmonary lesions in patients with anti-neutrophil cytoplasmic autoantibodies specific for anti-proteinase 3 and anti-myeloperoxidase. Am J Clin Pathol 1995; 104:7–16.
53. Kitaura K, Miyagawa T, Asano K, et al. Mixed connective tissue disease associated with MPO-ANCA-positive polyangiitis. Intern Med 2006; 45:1177–1182.
54. Savige J, Dimech W, Fritzler M, et al. Addendum to the International Consensus Statement on testing and reporting of antineutrophil cytoplasmic antibodies. Quality control guidelines, comments, and recommendations for testing in other autoimmune diseases. Am J Clin Pathol 2003; 120:312–318.
55. Schnabel A, Reuter M, Csernok E, et al. Subclinical alveolar bleeding in pulmonary vasculitides: correlation with indices of disease activity. Eur Respir J 1999; 14:118–124.
56. Mark EJ, Matsubara O, Tan-Liu NS, et al. The pulmonary biopsy in the early diagnosis of Wegener's (pathergic) granulomatosis: a study based on 35 open lung biopsies. Hum Pathol 1988; 19:1065–1071.
57. Travis WD, Hoffman GS, Leavitt RY, et al. Surgical pathology of the lung in Wegener's granulomatosis. Review of 87 open lung biopsies from 67 patients. Am J Surg Pathol 1991; 15: 315–333.
58. Bax J, Gooszen HC, Hoorntje SJ. Acute fulminating alveolar hemorrhage as presenting symptom in Wegener's granulomatosis. Anticytoplasmatic antibodies as a diagnostic tool. Eur J Respir Dis 1987; 71:202–205.
59. Myers JL, Katzenstein AL. Wegener's granulomatosis presenting with massive pulmonary hemorrhage and capillaritis. Am J Surg Pathol 1987; 11:895–898.
60. Stokes TC, McCann BG, Rees RT, et al. Acute fulminating intrapulmonary haemorrhage in Wegener's granulomatosis. Thorax 1982; 37:315–316.
61. Travis WD, Carpenter HA, Lie JT. Diffuse pulmonary hemorrhage. An uncommon manifestation of Wegener's granulomatosis. Am J Surg Pathol 1987; 11:702–708.
62. Lauque D, Cadranel J, Lazor R, et al. Microscopic polyangiitis with alveolar hemorrhage. A study of 29 cases and review of the literature. Groupe d'Etudes et de Recherche sur les Maladies "Orphelines" Pulmonaires (GERM"O"P). Medicine (Baltimore) 2000; 79:222–233.
63. Lee JG, Joo KW, Chung WK, et al. Diffuse alveolar hemorrhage in lupus nephritis. Clin Nephrol 2001; 55:282–288.
64. Hughson MD, He Z, Henegar J, et al. Alveolar hemorrhage and renal microangiopathy in systemic lupus erythematosus. Arch Pathol Lab Med 2001; 125:475–483.
65. Myers JL, Katzenstein AA. Microangiitis in lupus-induced pulmonary hemorrhage. Am J Clin Pathol 1986; 85:552–556.
66. Yousem SA, Colby TV, Carrington CB. Lung biopsy in rheumatoid arthritis. Am Rev Respir Dis 1985; 131:770–777.

67. Hakala M, Paakko P, Huhti E, et al. Open lung biopsy of patients with rheumatoid arthritis. Clin Rheumatol 1990; 9:452–460.
68. Sanchez-Guerrero J, Cesarman G, Alarcon-Segovia D. Massive pulmonary hemorrhage in mixed connective tissue diseases. J Rheumatol 1989; 16:1132–1134.
69. Horiki T, Fuyuno G, Ishii M, et al. Fatal alveolar hemorrhage in a patient with mixed connective tissue disease presenting polymyositis features. Intern Med 1998; 37:554–560.
70. Cutz E. Idiopathic pulmonary hemosiderosis and related disorders in infancy and childhood. Perspect Pediatr Pathol 1987; 11:47–81.
71. Milman N, Pedersen FM. Idiopathic pulmonary haemosiderosis. Epidemiology, pathogenic aspects and diagnosis. Respir Med 1998; 92:902–907.
72. Cohen S. Idiopathic pulmonary hemosiderosis. Am J Med Sci 1999; 317:67–74.
73. Ioachimescu OC, Sieber S, Kotch A. Idiopathic pulmonary haemosiderosis revisited. Eur Respir J 2004; 24:162–170.
74. Myers JL, Veal CF Jr., Shin MS, et al. Respiratory bronchiolitis causing interstitial lung disease. A clinicopathologic study of six cases. Am Rev Respir Dis 1987; 135:880–884.
75. Schiavina M, Di Scioscio V, Contini P, et al. Pulmonary lymphangioleiomyomatosis in a karyotypically normal man without tuberous sclerosis complex. Am J Respir Crit Care Med 2007; 176:96–98.
76. Aubry MC, Myers JL, Ryu JH, et al. Pulmonary lymphangioleiomyomatosis in a man. Am J Respir Crit Care Med 2000; 162:749–752.

14
Clinical Diagnosis of Pulmonary Hemorrhage

HARALD SAUTHOFF and JOHN G. HAY
New York University School of Medicine, New York, New York, U.S.A.

I. Introduction

Diffuse alveolar hemorrhage is an uncommon condition with protean causes. The clinical presentation can range from acute and life-threatening hemorrhage, which may or may not be associated with obvious hemoptysis, to a much more chronic and indolent condition characterized by dyspnea and anemia. Furthermore, the pulmonary disease may or may not be associated with disease in other organ systems. The diagnosis is therefore sometimes inapparent and has many masquerades. Pulmonary hemorrhage may be clinically manifested in three predominant clinical patterns:

1. Massive alveolar hemorrhage sometimes with substantial hemoptysis
2. Recurrent hemorrhage and usually hemoptysis with pulmonary infiltrates
3. Progressive dyspnea and pulmonary infiltrates and anemia that may be associated with hemoptysis

II. Is There Alveolar Hemorrhage?

A presentation of dyspnea, with or without hemoptysis, and bilateral alveolar infiltrates should always prompt the consideration of alveolar hemorrhage. It is critical to keep the diagnosis in mind, as even massive alveolar hemorrhage can present without hemoptysis.

When hemoptysis is substantial the diagnosis of bleeding into the respiratory tract is not difficult. The difficulty lies in determining the site and cause of the bleeding. Alveolar hemorrhage is usually bilateral and the chest radiogram typically reveals an alveolar filling pattern in both lung fields. History and chest radiogram may identify chronic bronchial disease that could lead to massive hemoptysis, in particular bronchiectasis and bronchogenic tumor. Bleeding from a localized lesion can lead to diffuse aspiration of blood. If there is any doubt, a chest CT and a bronchoscopy will be helpful to identify a focal site of bleeding. In the case of alveolar hemorrhage, sequential bronchoalveolar lavage will show progressive hemorrhagic return. In contrast, aspirated blood will be cleared with sequential lavage.

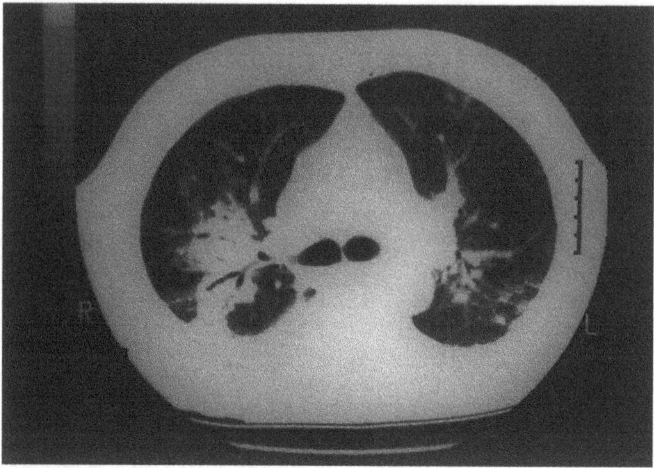

Figure 1 CT scan with features of an alveolar filling pattern in a young man with diffuse alveolar hemorrhage in association with a connective tissue disease and diffuse alveolar damage.

When alveolar hemorrhage is substantial without hemoptysis the diagnosis can be confused with pulmonary edema. Indications are a drop in hematocrit and echocardiographic findings that are inconsistent with congestive heart failure or valvular disease.

When alveolar hemorrhage is not massive and infiltrates are being investigated, helpful clues are hemosiderin staining of macrophages obtained at bronchoalveolar lavage or on biopsy. The carbon monoxide diffusing capacity (DLCO) is increased when there is blood within the alveoli, and although not a useful initial diagnostic test, this test can be useful in the sequential follow up of patients with new infiltrates.

A. Imaging

The chest radiograph most commonly shows nonspecific bilateral diffuse alveolar infiltrates. However, asymmetrical or even focal consolidations are not unusual. When the chest radiogram is normal, a chest CT may reveal areas of ground glass attenuation. In the presence of an abnormal chest radiograph, the CT is likely to reveal alveolar consolidation, which is not specific for any disease process (1) (Fig. 1).

III. What is the Specific Etiology?

A classification of diffuse pulmonary hemorrhage with the focus on the clinical presentation is given in Table 1. It should be understood that certain conditions, particularly systemic lupus and the connective tissue diseases fit into more than one group. The following questions direct the investigation toward the eventual diagnosis, and a diagnostic algorithm is outlined in Table 2.

Table 1 Clinical Classification of Diffuse Alveolar Hemorrhage

1. In association with exposure to toxic agents
   - Illicit drugs
     - Crack cocaine
     - Marijuana contaminated with paraquat
   - Occupational exposure
     - Trimetallic anhydride
   - Therapeutic agents
     - Propylthiouracil
     - Penicillamine
     - Nitrofurantoin
     - Sirolimus
     - Surfactant therapy
     - Thrombolytics
     - Clopidogrel and glycoprotein IIb/IIIa receptor blocker
2. In association with pulmonary hypertension/venous obstruction
   - Mitral stenosis
   - Pulmonary veno-occlusive disease
   - Lymphangioleiomyomatosis
   - Tuberous sclerosis
   - Pulmonary capillary hemangiomatosis
3. In association with renal disease
   - Not associated with a pulmonary capillaritis
     - Anti-GBM antibody disease
   - Associated with a pulmonary capillaritis
     - ANCA positive
     - WG
     - Microscopic polyangiitis
     - Churg-Straus syndrome
   - Immune complexes present
     - Behcet's syndrome
     - Henoch-Schönlein purpura
     - Mixed cryoglobulinemia
     - IgA nephropathy
4. In association with isolated pulmonary capillaritis
5. In association with a connective tissue disease
   - SLE
   - Scleroderma
   - Rheumatoid arthritis
   - Mixed connective tissue disease
   - Relapsing polychondritis
   - Antiphospholipid antibody syndrome
6. In association with bone marrow transplantation
   - Graft versus host
   - Total body irradiation
   - Chemotherapy
   - Pulmonary infection
7. In association with diffuse alveolar damage
8. Idiopathic pulmonary hemosiderosis

Abbreviation: GBM, glomerular basement membrane; SLE, systemic lupus erythematosis; ANCA, anti-neutrophil cytoplasmic antibodies; WG, Wegener's granulomatosis; IgA, Immunoglobin A.

Table 2 Diagnosis of Alveolar Hemorrhage

Confirm alveolar hemorrhage
(hemoptysis, fall in hemoglobin, increase in DLCO with new infiltrates, bronchoscopy, alveolar lavage, lung biopsy)
↓
History of exposure to toxic agents?
↓
Clinical signs of pulmonary hypertension or mitral stenosis?
(echocardiogram, PFTs, chest CT, lung biopsy)

↙	↓	↘
Renal disease? (creatinine, urinary sediment, renal biopsy)		**Clinical signs of connective tissue disease?**
Serum antibodies? Anti-glomerular basement Antineutrophil cytoplasmic Antinuclear		Serum antibodies? Antineutrophil cytoplasmic Antinuclear

Isolated pulmonary capillaritis?
(lung biopsy)
↓
Diffuse alveolar damage?
↓
Idiopathic pulmonary hemosiderosis?
(lung biopsy)

Abbreviations: DLCO, carbon monoxide diffusing capacity; PFT, pulmonary function test; GBM, glomerular basement membrane.

1. Has the patient been exposed to potentially toxic agents?
2. Is there evidence of pulmonary hypertension/vascular disease?
3. Is there evidence of renal disease?
   a. without systemic vasculitis.
   b. with systemic vasculitis.
4. Is there evidence for isolated pulmonary capillaritis?
5. Is there evidence of a connective tissue disease?
6. Has the patient had a recent bone marrow transplant?
7. Could there be diffuse alveolar damage?
8. Could this be idiopathic pulmonary hemosiderosis?

A. Has the Patient Been Exposed to Potentially Toxic Agents?

The first step is a careful review of the history for evidence of possible exposure to potential causative agents. This includes illicit drug use, occupational exposure, and medical treatment.

Massive hemoptysis has been associated with smoking of alkaloidal cocaine ("crack"), and evidence of alveolar hemorrhage is seen in 30% of individuals who die suddenly from cocaine overdose (2,3). The clinical presentation is usually one of fever, hypoxemia, hemoptysis, and respiratory failure with diffuse alveolar infiltrates seen on chest radiograms. Paraquat ingestion leads to diffuse alveolar damage and alveolar hemorrhage, and the smoking of marijuana contaminated with paraquat has lead to alveolar hemorrhage.

Inhalation of trimetallic anhydride, which is used in the manufacture of resins and plastics, can lead to pulmonary infiltrates and anemia resulting from alveolar hemorrhage. This is usually associated with a hemolytic anemia, and antibodies to trimetallic anhydride conjugated to albumin and red blood cells can be detected. Recovery is usually spontaneous when exposure is stopped (4).

Therapeutic drugs are an important cause of pulmonary hemorrhage. Multiple reports have related alveolar hemorrhage to propylthiouracil, mostly but not always with pulmonary capillaritis (5–8). Therapy with d-penicillamine can cause alveolar hemorrhage and glomerulonephritis (9). Nitrofurantoin (10–12) and the immunosuppressant drug sirolimus have also been associated with alveolar hemorrhage (13,14). There is also a risk of pulmonary hemorrhage with surfactant therapy in respiratory distress syndrome (15).

The increasing use of thrombolytics, platelet inhibitors such as clopidogrel and glycoprotein IIb/IIIa receptor blocker, used often in combination in the management of acute coronary syndrome, has led to multiple reports of alveolar hemorrhage (16,17). Patients commonly present with dyspnea, hemoptysis, hypoxemia, new pulmonary infiltrates, and a drop in the hematocrit. The diagnosis can be confused with cardiogenic pulmonary edema and may have a fatal outcome (18–20).

B. Is There Evidence of Pulmonary Hypertension/Vascular Disease?

The clinical examination should carefully try to detect evidence of pulmonary hypertension that may be associated with mitral stenosis or be more suggestive of pulmonary hypertension and cor pulmonale.

Mitral Stenosis

Mitral stenosis can lead to massive hemoptysis from rupture of anastomotic bronchial varicosities secondary to chronically raised left atrial pressure, or recurrent small hemoptysis can lead to organization and interstitial fibrosis (21). The underlying cardiac disease may not have been previously recognized. If there is doubt, an echocardiogram should be performed.

Occlusion of Pulmonary Venules

Pulmonary veno-occlusive disease is a rare cause of pulmonary hypertension that presents with dyspnea and syncope secondary to postcapillary obstruction of pulmonary capillaries. Occult alveolar hemorrhage may be a more common feature of this disease than previously recognized (22). The chest radiograph will usually show evidence of pulmonary hypertension and Kerley's B lines may be visible. Alveolar infiltrates may be superimposed when alveolar hemorrhage occurs.

Lymphangioleiomyomatosis is also associated with obstruction to pulmonary venules and may be associated with alveolar hemorrhage. This disease is limited to premenopausal women and is associated with airflow obstruction. Similar manifestations are associated with tuberous sclerosis in both males and females.

Pulmonary capillary hemangiomatosis is a rare condition that may be familial and is associated with proliferation of pulmonary capillaries and obstruction of pulmonary veins, leading to alveolar hemorrhage that can be severe.

In these conditions, CT scans, respiratory function tests, and frequent open lung biopsy establish the diagnosis.

C. Is There Evidence of Renal Disease?

Evidence of renal disease should be carefully sought after, as glomerulonephritis may precede or follow alveolar hemorrhage. Examination of urine for the presence of blood and protein and of urinary sediment for red cell casts to suggest glomerulonephritis is essential. Blood levels of creatinine and urea should also be measured. If renal disease is found, the next step is to determine the cause. Renal disease in association with alveolar hemorrhage falls into two main groups:

1. Anti–glomerular basement membrane (anti-GBM) antibody disease, which is also called Goodpasture's syndrome
2. A vasculitis involving glomeruli and pulmonary capillaries

Anti-GBM Disease (Goodpasture's Syndrome)

Anti-GBM antibody disease is an autoimmune disorder causing glomerulonephritis and alveolar hemorrhage. The combination of glomerulonephritis and alveolar hemorrhage is the most common presentation (60–80%), although glomerulonephritis may occur alone (20–40%), but alveolar hemorrhage alone is unusual (10%). The disease may follow a fulminant course with rapidly progressive renal failure, which, without therapy, is usually fatal. The presentation of the renal disease is nonspecific, and hemoptysis is frequently associated with the alveolar hemorrhage. Young men (second through fifth decade) are most commonly affected, and associated clinical findings are not present.

The tissue injury is mediated by antibodies that bind the carboxy terminal NC1 domain of the alpha 3 chain of type IV collagen in glomerular and alveolar basement membranes (23). The diagnosis can be established by detection of these antibodies in circulation (24). Smoking (25), infection (26), or organic solvents may possibly expose the antigen, and in genetically predisposed individuals (27) stimulate an autoimmune response (28,29).

The diagnosis can therefore be made on the basis of detection of anti-GBM antibodies in the serum, most commonly by enzyme-linked immunoabsorbent assay (ELISA). However, serum antibody testing is not always completely reliable. A renal biopsy will confirm the diagnosis by the detection of linear immunoglobulin along the GBM by immunofluorescence. Light microscopy most commonly shows crescentic glomerulonephritis, and the degree of crescentic involvement has import prognostic implications. A renal biopsy is preferable to a lung biopsy but the same findings of basement membrane linear immunostaining will be seen.

Early diagnosis and treatment is critical to prevent end-stage renal disease and death. The anti-GBM antibodies and other inflammatory mediators are removed by plasmapheresis. In addition, the production of new antibodies is suppressed by the administration of corticosteroids and cyclophosphamide (30).

Vasculitis Involving Glomeruli and Pulmonary Capillaries

Several disease entities can lead to glomerulonephritis and pulmonary capillaritis. Features of the history and physical examination may direct the clinician to the correct diagnosis, but the typical features of these diseases may not be present in the acute presentation associated with alveolar hemorrhage (Table 3).

Serological tests, in particular serum antineutrophil cytoplasmic antibodies (ANCA) can be of great value. The diseases under consideration that can cause pulmonary and glomerular capillaritis can therefore be divided into those associated with various antibodies and immune complexes.

Vasculitis Associated with ANCA

The ANCA-associated small-vessel vasculitides include Wegener's granulomatosis (WG), microscopic polyangiitis (MPA) and Churg-Strauss syndrome (CSS) (31). Two patterns of staining can be detected by indirect immunofluoresence, cytoplasmic staining (c-ANCA) and perinuclear staining (p-ANCA). c-ANCA is associated with antibodies to anti-proteinase-3 (APR-3), whereas p-ANCA is associated with antibodies to myeloperoxidase (AMPo). c-ANCA has a high sensitivity and specificity for WG and, in the right clinical setting, may be of great diagnostic value. p-ANCA is relatively common in MPA and CSS but lacks sufficient sensitivity and specificity. When ANCA-associated vasculitides presents with alveolar hemorrhage, pulmonary capillaritis is generally found on lung biopsy. In addition, granulomas may be seen in WG.

WG is the most common ANCA-associated vasculitis. The typical triad of upper airway disease, lower respiratory tract disease, and glomerulonephritis may not always be present, especially at first presentation. The disease can present with massive pulmonary hemorrhage, and may be difficult to diagnose both clinically due to the absence of associated features and on lung biopsy due to the absence of granulomas (32,33). The presence of sinusitis or nodular and cavitating pulmonary infiltrates would be supportive evidence in conjunction with positive c-ANCA testing. In active systemic disease, a positive c-ANCA test is found in 85% to 95%. In organ-limited disease, the sensitivity is only 60% to 65%. The specificity of c-ANCA testing is high (approximately 90%) (31,34). However, as with any test, the pretest probability is critical for the interpretation of a positive or negative result. In a patient with typical clinical features, a positive c-ANCA may have a sufficient positive predictive value that a biopsy can be deferred.

Microscopic polyangiitis often presents with constitutional symptoms, followed by renal diseases, characterized by a rapidly progressive glomerulonephritis. The lungs are affected in approximately 30% of cases (35), and diffuse alveolar hemorrhage is the most common pulmonary manifestation. The musculoskeletal and peripheral nervous systems are frequently involved, as is the skin and gastrointestinal mucosa. p-ANCA testing is positive in 50% to 75% and c-ANCA can be positive in 10% to 30% of patients (31,34).

Table 3 Clinical Features and Antibody Studies of Various Syndromes Associated with Diffuse Alveolar Hemorrhage

	Clinical features			Antibody studies					
Syndrome	Renal disease	Skin vasculitis	Arthritis	ABMA	ANA	p-ANCA	c-ANCA	anti-DNA	Complement
Anti-GBM disease	+	–	–	+	–	–	–	–	N
WG	+	+	+	–	+/–	+	++	–	N
Microscopic polyangiitis	+	+	+	–	+/–	++	+	–	N
SLE	+	+	+	–	+	+/–	–	++	L
Behcet's syndrome	+	+	+	–	+/–	–	–	–	N
Henoch-Schönlein purpura	+	+	+	–	–	–	–	–	N
Mixed cryoglobulinemia	+	+	+	–	+/–	–	–	–	N/L
IgA nephropathy	+	–		–		–	–	–	N
Scleroderma	+/–	+	+	–	+/–	–	–	–	N
Rheumatoid arthritis	+/–	+	+	–	+/–	–	–	–	N
Mixed connective tissue disease	+/–	+	+	–	+/–	–	–	–	N
Antiphospholipid antibody syndrome	–	–	–	–	–	–	–	–	N
IPH	–	–	–	–	–	–	–	–	N
Pauci-immune pulmonary capillaritis	–	–	–	–	–	–	–	–	N

Abbreviations: ABMA, antibasement membrane antibodies; ANA, antinuclear antibodies; GBM, glomerular basement membrane; WG, Wegener's granulomatosis; ANCA, antineutrophil cytoplasmic antibodies; IgA, Immunoglobin A; IPH, idiopathic pulmonary hemosiderosis; N, normal; L, low.

Churg-Strauss syndrome commonly presents in three phases with long-standing asthma preceding a hypereosinophilic phase that is ultimately followed by a necrotizing systemic vasculitis. Cutaneous and neurological manifestations are common. Cardiac and gastrointestinal complications, as well as status asthmaticus can be life threatening. Pulmonary hemorrhage and glomerulonephritis are less common than with the other small-vessel vasculitides. Typical laboratory findings are marked eosinophilia and elevated immunoglobulin E (IgE) levels. p-ANCA is positive in 44% to 66% of patients with active disease, c-ANCA positivity, however, is uncommon (36).

Vasculitis Associated with Immune Complexes

Behcet's syndrome is a chronic relapsing multisystem illness characterized by oral and genital ulceration, cutaneous vasculitis, arthritis, glomerulonephritis, and meningoencepalitis. Pulmonary hemorrhage can result from small-vessel vasculitis, large-vessel vasculitis with arterial aneurysms that can erode into bronchi and pulmonary artery occlusion associated with pulmonary infarction.

Henoch-Schönlein purpura presents with a palpable purpuric rash and glomerulonephritis. The joints and gastrointestinal tract are frequently involved. Pulmonary capillaritis and alveolar hemorrhage is however rare (37).

Mixed cryoglobulinemia is a systemic vasculitis associated with purpura, arthritis, hepatitis, and glomerulonephritis in which diffuse alveolar hemorrhage has been described.

Immunoglobulin A (IgA) nephropathy, either symptomatic or as a cause of renal failure, can lead to fatal alveolar hemorrhage associated with a pulmonary capillaritis (38).

D. Is There an Isolated Pauci-immune Pulmonary Capillaritis?

Isolated (or idiopathic) pauci-immune pulmonary capillaritis, although most often ANCA negative, is considered to be an organ specific subtype of MPA. The disease is characterized by pulmonary capillaritis with alveolar hemorrhage in the absence of systemic vasculitis. It was the most common diagnosis in a series of 29 cases of biopsy-proven pulmonary capillaritis. No pathological evidence of a systemic vasculitis was found nor did evidence of a vasculitis appear over 43 months of follow up (39).

E. Is There Evidence of a Connective Tissue Disease?

Systemic lupus erythematosis (SLE), scleroderma, rheumatoid arthritis, and mixed connective tissue disease, have all been described associated with alveolar hemorrhage usually in the presence of vasculitis and renal disease. Of these conditions, SLE most commonly is associated with alveolar hemorrhage. Alveolar hemorrhage is an unusual presenting feature of SLE, and thus occurs in an individual with established disease and is often life threatening. The differential diagnosis therefore involves excluding other forms of lung disease in particular lupus pneumonitis or infection from alveolar hemorrhage. Other clinical features of lupus are apparent, and anti-DNA antibody is present in the serum and complement levels decreased. The mortality is high in pulmonary hemorrhage associated with systemic lupus. Treatment with high-dose steroids and cyclophosphamide has been of modest value, and plasmapheresis may result in radiographic and clinical improvement (40,41).

In an unusual occurrence scleroderma (42), rheumatoid arthritis, relapsing polychondritis, or mixed connective tissue disease can be associated with alveolar hemorrhage (43).

The antiphospholipid antibody syndrome is a disorder associated with hypercoagulability, thrombocytopenia, and thromboembolic phenomena. Pulmonary hemorrhage due to pulmonary capillaritis with evidence of perivascular immune complex deposition without systemic lupus erythematosus has been described (44).

F. Bone Marrow Transplantation

Bone marrow transplantation has been associated with a clinical syndrome characterized by progressive dyspnea, hypoxia, cough, and diffuse consolidation on chest radiograph. Bronchoalveolar lavage confirms the diagnosis of alveolar hemorrhage (34). The radiographic abnormalities of the diffuse alveolar hemorrhage are nonspecific and usually precede the clinical diagnosis. The clinical course after hemorrhage is short, often resulting in death (45).

The pulmonary hemorrhage may occur at the time of white cell recovery and be a feature of graft versus host disease but is also associated with preparation for transplantation, either with total body irradiation or chemotherapy using busulphan (46,47).

G. Diffuse Alveolar Damage

Diffuse alveolar damage can lead to injury of the alveolar-capillary interface with leakage of red cells into the alveolar spaces and sometimes hemoptysis. Some of the more common processes associated with diffuse alveolar damage include sepsis, trauma, aspiration of gastric content, pancreatitis, pulmonary infections, blood transfusions, and drugs.

H. Idiopathic Pulmonary Hemosiderosis

The diagnosis of idiopathic pulmonary hemosiderosis requires the exclusion of known causes of diffuse alveolar hemorrhage. There is no associated vasculitis, connective tissue disease, or renal disease. Circulating autoantibodies are not detected although IgA levels may be elevated and a case with circulating immune complexes has been described (48).

This condition usually occurs in children and young adults, predominately young men, but can also present later in life. The presentation may be with acute and massive alveolar hemorrhage, recurrent hemoptysis, or progressive dyspnea with clinical features similar to idiopathic pulmonary fibrosis (49). The finger clubbing and basal crackles of the chronic disease are associated with iron deficiency and anemia, and on occasions the anemia may precede the lung disease. In childhood cases, hepatosplenomegaly may also be found. A chest radiograph of the acute presentation is likely to show an alveolar filling pattern. This may resolve or progress to a reticular infiltrate and diffuse nonconfluent shadows that may persist. In childhood cases, hilar and mediastinal adenopathy may be found. Idiopathic pulmonary hemosiderosis has been described in association with gluten intolerance and small bowel villous atrophy (50), and in some instances, a gluten free diet may improve outcome (51). Overall, the prognosis of this disease is considered to be poor, but long-term survival has been reported (49,52). Steroids or immunosuppressive therapy with azathioprine or cyclophosphamide may be beneficial (53).

References

1. Primack SL, Miller RR, Muller NL. Diffuse pulmonary hemorrhage: clinical, pathologic, and imaging features. AJR Am J Roentgenol 1995; 164(2):295–300 (review).
2. Forrester J, Steele A, Waldron J, et al. Crack lung: an acute pulmonary syndrome with a spectrum of clinical and histopathologic findings. Am Rev Respir Dis 1990; 142:462–467.
3. Haim D, Lippmann M, Goldberg S, et al. The pulmonary complications of crack cocaine. Chest 1995; 107:233–240.
4. Ahmad D, Morgan WK, Patterson R, et al. Pulmonary haemorrhage and haemolytic anaemia due to trimellitic. Lancet 1979; 2(8138):328–330.
5. Dhillon SS, Singh D, Doe N, et al. Diffuse alveolar hemorrhage and pulmonary capillaritis due to propylthiouracil. Chest 1999; 116(5):1485–1488.
6. Hadjiangelis NP, Harkin TJ. Propylthiouracil-related diffuse alveolar hemorrhage with negative serologies and without capillaritis. Respir Med 2007; 101(4):865–867.
7. Pirot AL, Goldsmith D, Pascasio J, et al. Pulmonary capillaritis with hemorrhage due to propylthiouracil therapy in a child. Pediatr Pulmonol 2005; 39(1):88–92.
8. Yamauchi K, Sata M, Machiya J, et al. Antineutrophil cytoplasmic antibody positive alveolar haemorrhage during propylthiouracil therapy for hyperthyroidism. Respirology 2003; 8(4): 532–535.
9. Zitnik RJ, Cooper JA Jr. Pulmonary disease due to antirheumatic agents. Clin Chest Med 1990; 11(1):139–150 (review).
10. Averbuch SD, Yungbluth P. Fatal pulmonary hemorrhage due to nitrofurantoin. Arch Intern Med 1980; 140(2):271–273.
11. Bucknall CE, Adamson MR, Banham SW. Non fatal pulmonary haemorrhage associated with nitrofurantoin. Thorax 1987; 42(6):475–476.
12. Meyer MM, Meyer RJ. Nitrofurantoin-induced pulmonary hemorrhage in a renal transplant recipient receiving immunosuppressive therapy: case report and review of the literature. J Urol 1994; 152(3):938–940.
13. Khalife WI, Kogoj P, Kar B. Sirolimus-induced alveolar hemorrhage. J Heart Lung Transplant 2007; 26(6):652–657.
14. Vlahakis NE, Rickman OB, Morgenthaler T. Sirolimus-associated diffuse alveolar hemorrhage. Mayo Clin Proc 2004; 79(4):541–545.
15. Raju TN, Langenberg P. Pulmonary hemorrhage and exogenous surfactant therapy: a meta-analysis. J Pediatr 1993; 123(4):603–610 (comments).
16. Kilaru PK, Schweiger MJ, Kozman HA, et al. Diffuse alveolar hemorrhage after clopidogrel use. J Invasive Cardiol 2001; 13(7):535–537.
17. Khanlou H, Tsiodras S, Eiger G, et al. Fatal alveolar hemorrhage and Abciximab (ReoPro) therapy for acute myocardial infarction. Cathet Cardiovasc Diagn 1998; 44(3):313–316.
18. Awadh N, Ronco JJ, Bernstein V, et al. Spontaneous pulmonary hemorrhage after thrombolytic therapy for acute myocardial infarction. Chest 1994; 106(5):1622–1624 (review).
19. Brown DL, MacIsaac AI, Topol EJ. Pulmonary hemorrhage after intracoronary stent placement. J Am Coll Cardiol 1994; 24(1):91–94.
20. Kok LC, Sugihara J, Druger G. First case report of spontaneous pulmonary hemorrhage following heparin therapy in acute myocardial infarction. Hawaii Med J 1996; 55(5):83–84.
21. Cortese DA. Pulmonary function in mitral stenosis. Mayo Clin Proc 1978; 53(5):321–326.
22. Rabiller A, Jais X, Hamid A, et al. Occult alveolar haemorrhage in pulmonary veno-occlusive disease. Eur Respir J 2006; 27(1):108–113.
23. Hudson BG, Kalluri R, Gunwar S, et al. Molecular characteristics of the Goodpasture autoantigen. Kidney Int 1993; 43(1):135–139 (review).
24. Kalluri R, Melendez E, Rumpf KW, et al. Specificity of circulating and tissue-bound autoantibodies in Goodpasture syndrome. Proc Assoc Am Physicians 1996; 108(2):134–139.

25. Donaghy M, Rees AJ. Cigarette smoking and lung haemorrhage in glomerulonephritis caused by autoantibodies to glomerular basement membrane. Lancet 1983; 2(8364):1390–1393.
26. Rees AJ, Lockwood CM, Peters DK. Enhanced allergic tissue injury in Goodpasture's syndrome by intercurrent bacterial infection. Br Med J 1977; 2(6089):723–726.
27. Rees AJ, Peters DK, Amos N, et al. The influence of HLA-linked genes on the severity of anti-GBM antibody-mediated nephritis. Kidney Int 1984; 26(4):445–450.
28. Kalluri R, Gattone VHn, Noelken ME, et al. The alpha 3 chain of type IV collagen induces autoimmune Goodpasture syndrome. Proc Natl Acad Sci U S A 1994; 91(13):6201–6205.
29. Kelly PT, Haponik EF. Goodpasture syndrome: molecular and clinical advances. Medicine (Baltimore) 1994; 73(4):171–185 (review).
30. Levy JB, Turner AN, Rees AJ, et al. Long-term outcome of anti-glomerular basement membrane antibody disease treated with plasma exchange and immunosuppression. Ann Intern Med 2001; 134(11):1033–1042.
31. Bosch X, Guilabert A, Font J. Antineutrophil cytoplasmic antibodies. Lancet 2006; 368(9533): 404–418.
32. Myers JL, Katzenstein AL. Wegener's granulomatosis presenting with massive pulmonary hemorrhage and capillaritis. Am J Surg Pathol 1987; 11(11):895–898.
33. Travis WD, Carpenter HA, Lie JT. Diffuse pulmonary hemorrhage. An uncommon manifestation of Wegener's granulomatosis. Am J Surg Pathol 1987; 11(9):702–708.
34. Brown KK. Pulmonary vasculitis. Proc Am Thorac Soc 2006; 3(1):48–57.
35. Savage CO, Winearls CG, Evans DJ, et al. Microscopic polyarteritis: presentation, pathology and prognosis. Q J Med 1985; 56(220):467–483.
36. Conron M, Beynon HL. Churg-Strauss syndrome. Thorax 2000; 55(10):870–877.
37. Wright WK, Krous HF, Griswold WR, et al. Pulmonary vasculitis with hemorrhage in anaphylactoid purpura. Pediatr Pulmonol 1994; 17(4):269–271.
38. Lai FM, Li EK, Suen MW, et al. Pulmonary hemorrhage. A fatal manifestation in IgA nephropathy. Arch Pathol Lab Med 1994; 118(5):542–546.
39. Jennings CA, King TE Jr., Tuder R, et al. Diffuse alveolar hemorrhage with underlying isolated, pauciimmune pulmonary capillaritis. Am J Respir Crit Care Med 1997; 155(3):1101–1109.
40. Erickson RW, Franklin WA, Emlen W. Treatment of hemorrhagic lupus pneumonitis with plasmapheresis. [Semin Arthritis Rheum 1994; 24(2):114–123 (review).
41. Badsha H, Teh CL, Kong KO, et al. Pulmonary hemorrhage in systemic lupus erythematosus. Semin Arthritis Rheum 2004; 33(6):414–421.
42. Griffin MT, Robb JD, Martin JR. Diffuse alveolar haemorrhage associated with progressive systemic sclerosis. Thorax 1990; 45(11):903–904.
43. Leatherman JW, Sibley RK, Davies SF. Diffuse intrapulmonary hemorrhage and glomerulonephritis unrelated to anti-glomerular basement membrane antibody. Am J Med 1982; 72(3): 401–410.
44. Crausman RS, Achenbach GA, Pluss WT, et al. Pulmonary capillaritis and alveolar hemorrhage associated with the antiphospholipid antibody syndrome. J Rheumatol 1995; 22(3):554–556.
45. Witte RJ, Gurney JW, Robbins RA, et al. Diffuse pulmonary alveolar hemorrhage after bone marrow transplantation: radiographic findings in 39 patients. AJR Am J Roentgenol 1991; 157(3):461–464.
46. Wojno KJ, Vogelsang GB, Beschorner WE, et al. Pulmonary hemorrhage as a cause of death in allogeneic bone marrow recipients with severe acute graft-versus-host disease. Transplantation 1994; 57(1):88–92.
47. Majhail NS, Parks K, Defor TE, et al. Diffuse alveolar hemorrhage and infection-associated alveolar hemorrhage following hematopoietic stem cell transplantation: related and high-risk clinical syndromes. Biol Blood Marrow Transplant 2006; 12(10):1038–1046.
48. Louie S, Russell LA, Richeson RBd, et al. Circulating immune complexes with pulmonary hemorrhage during pregnancy in idiopathic pulmonary hemosiderosis. Chest 1993; 104(6): 1907–1909.

49. Soergel K, Sommers S. Idiopathic pulmonary hemosiderosis and related syndromes. Am J Med 1962; 32:499–511.
50. Wright PH, Menzies IS, Pounder RE, et al. Adult idiopathic pulmonary haemosiderosis and coeliac disease. Q J Med 1981; 50(197):95–102.
51. Pacheco A, Casanova C, Fogue L, et al. Long-term clinical follow-up of adult idiopathic pulmonary hemosiderosis and celiac disease. Chest 1991; 99(6):1525–1526.
52. Le Clainche L, Le Bourgeois M, Fauroux B, et al. Long-term outcome of idiopathic pulmonary hemosiderosis in children. Medicine (Baltimore) 2000; 79(5):318–326.
53. Colombo JL, Stolz SM. Treatment of life-threatening primary pulmonary hemosiderosis with cyclophosphamide. Chest 1992; 102(3):959–960.

15
Granulomas and Granulomatous Inflammation

HELMUT H. POPPER
Institute of Pathology, Medical University of Graz, Graz, Austria

I. Introduction

The name granuloma is derived from the Latin word granulum, which means grain. The Greek suffix "-oma" is used to designate a nodular swelling. Therefore, granuloma is a nodular, well-circumscribed lesion. With the invention of microscopy, this term has been extended to a small nodular aggregate of cells. Over the decades, the definition has undergone different interpretations. Some use the term granuloma, strictly, when there is a well-circumscribed lesion in an otherwise uninvolved organ, whereas others also designate a more loose aggregate of inflammatory cells as granuloma (1).

We will use the word granuloma and granulomatous in a wider sense, and therefore will include, for example, loose nodular aggregates of histiocytes as granulomatous inflammation. An argument for doing so can be found in the process of granuloma formation itself. If we use the classical epithelioid cell granuloma as a model, we can encounter different stages of granuloma formation. First, we see a loose aggregation of macrophages, histiocytes, lymphocytes, and even neutrophils (Fig. 1). This is followed by the cytokine-induced transformation of macrophages into epithelioid and foreign body giant cells, of which the latter can differentiate into Langhans giant cells (2,3). During each step in granuloma formation, the granuloma becomes more compact, and the margins are better circumscribed. However, in other diseases like extrinsic allergic alveolitis (EAA) (hypersensitivity pneumonitis), the epithelioid cell granulomas are less well delineated and tend to be more loosely arranged. Also a spillover of lymphocytes into adjacent alveolar septa is seen (Fig. 2) (4). As they age, epithelioid cell granulomas may undergo fibrosis and hyalinization (Fig. 3). A similar process can be seen in anthracosilicosis: Early on a loose aggregate of histiocytes can be seen (Fig. 4), followed by the development of foreign body granulomas with giant cells (Fig. 5) and then formation of the well-known hyalinized granulomas (Fig. 6). At this stage, everyone will call this a granuloma, however, even the early aggregates are centered on blood vessels and lymphatics, with minimal extension into surrounding alveolar walls. We, therefore, will also call these aggregates granulomas.

In the following paragraphs we will follow the routine path of diagnosing granulomatous diseases. We first recognize granulomatous inflammation in a tissue specimen. The next step is to describe the cellular and structural elements on the basis of H&E stains. This will provide a differential diagnosis, which then will force us to employ special stains for a final diagnosis. Immunohistochemical stains and molecular biological investigations

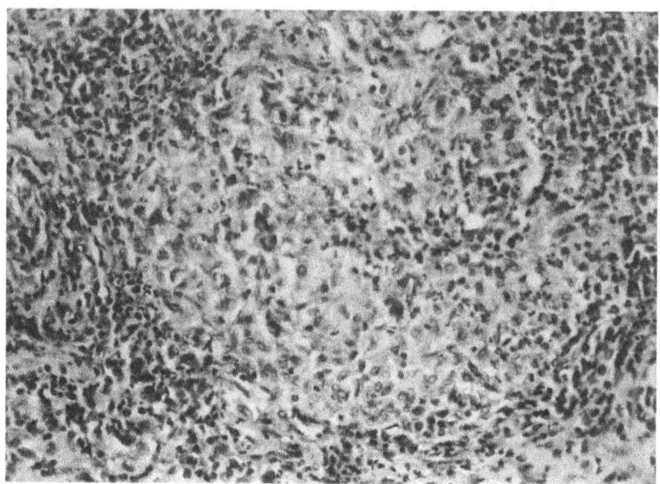

Figure 1 Early epithelioid cell granuloma. Note neutrophilic granulocytes in the center and histiocytes/macrophages at the outer layer of the granuloma (tuberculosis).

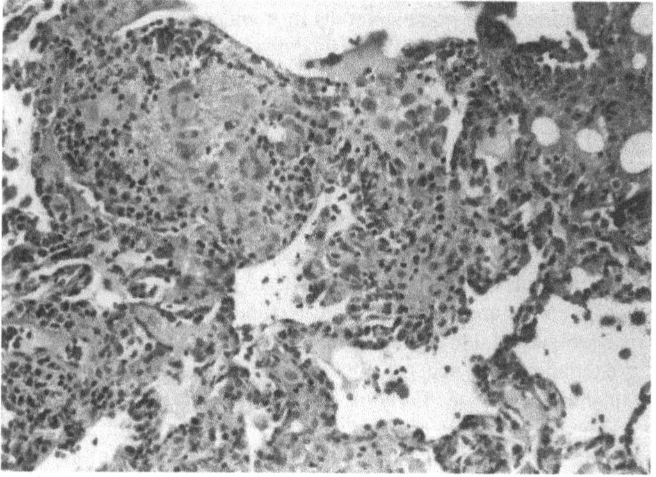

Figure 2 Extrinsic allergic alveolitis with epithelioid cell granuloma. Note the spillover of lymphocytes into adjacent alveolar walls.

will be mentioned, where needed to confirm the diagnosis. Otherwise, tests that are unnecessary for diagnostic purposes will not be discussed, although they might be utilized for scientific research studies. Citations will be at a minimum. For a complete reference list, the reader is referred to standard textbooks on pulmonary pathology and electronic databases.

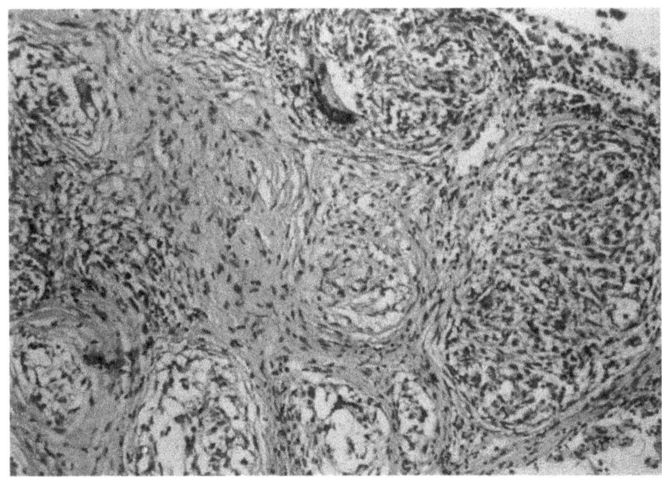

Figure 3 Epithelioid cell granulomas with fibrosis in sarcoidosis. Note that unlike in tuberculosis, fibrosis starts from the outer layers of the granulomas.

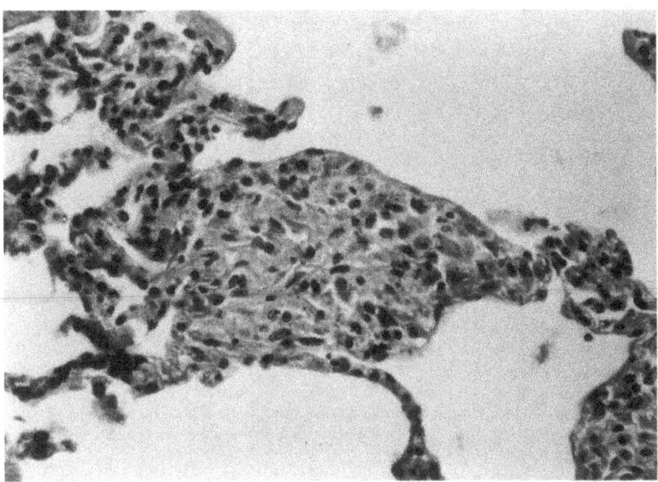

Figure 4 Histiocytic granulomas as an early event in silicosis/anthracosilicosis.

II. The Epithelioid Cell Granuloma

The epithelioid cell granuloma is composed of epithelioid cells, a specialized secretory macrophage (Fig. 7A), multinucleated giant cells, either foreign body or Langhans cells

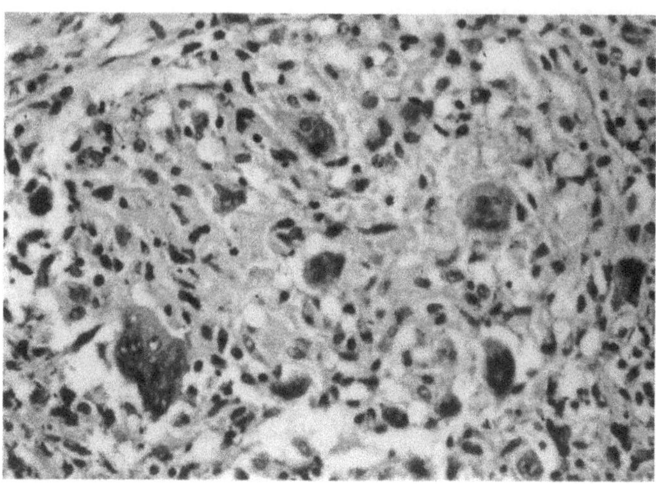

Figure 5 Developing anthracosilicotic granuloma with foreign body giant cells.

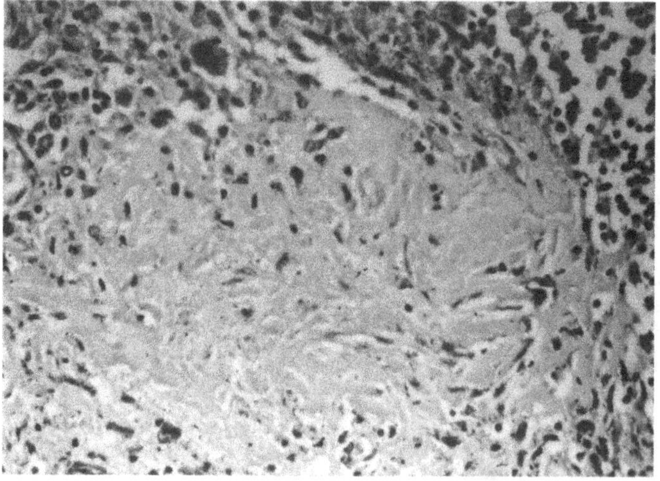

Figure 6 Hyalinized granuloma: the late stage of granuloma formation in silicosis/anthracosilicosis.

(Fig. 7B, C), specialized for phagocytosis of nondigestible and insoluble material (3–5), and lymphocytes. Lymphocytes might be numerous or scarce, which is often related to the age of the granuloma. Most important is to examine the center and edges of the granuloma: Is there central necrosis or not, and, is there a spillover of lymphocytes into the surrounding alveolar walls or not?

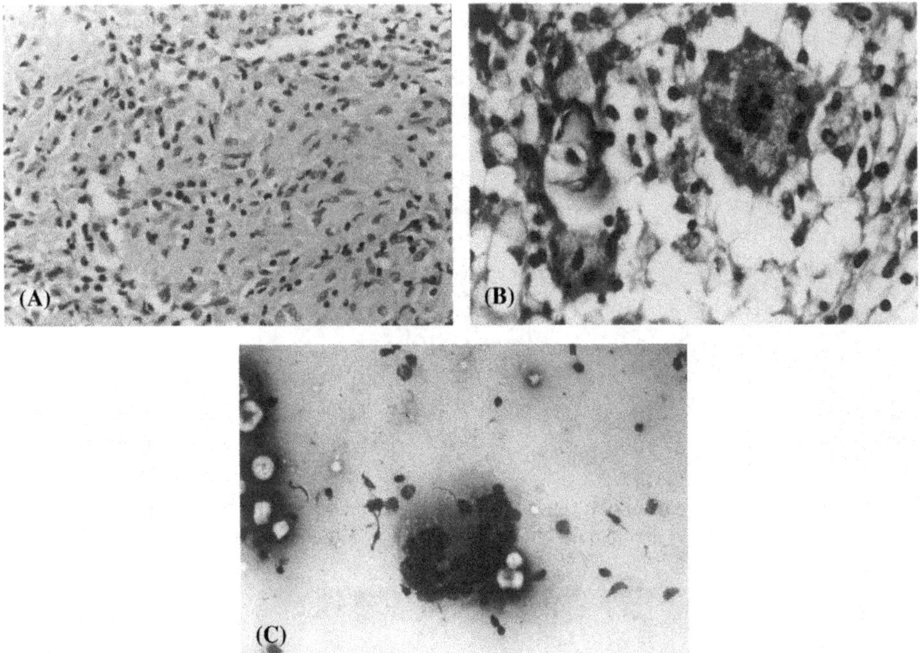

Figure 7 (**A**) Epithelioid cells, (**B**) foreign body giant cell in transition to Langhans cell, and (**C**) Langhans giant cell are all elements of sarcoid granulomas; the nuclei of epithelioid cells are often twisted, the chromatin is finely distributed, and the cell membranes are indistinct (**A**). Note a conchoid body in the left giant cell in **B**. Langhans cells are sometimes seen in cytology specimen, where the huge amount of nuclei can be appreciated (**C**).

A. The Necrotizing Epithelioid Cell Granuloma

As the term indicates, necrosis is observed in the center of the necrotizing epithelioid cell granuloma (Fig. 8) (6). Small necrobiotic foci or few apoptotic cells are not regarded as necrosis and may be encountered in nonnecrotizing epithelioid cell granulomas as well (see below). The necrosis either stains eosinophilic with minimal amounts of nuclear debris or may contain large amounts of nuclear debris that is finely granular and stains blue-violet with hematoxylin. In early necrosis, neutrophils can be found. The term "caseous necrosis" is often used to describe the necrosis; however, it should be remembered that this term was coined to describe a type of necrosis seen on gross examination: Caseous necrosis is a term for macroscopic necrosis characterized by a yellowish color and soft, cheese-like consistency (Fig. 9).

Having found at least one necrotizing epithelioid cell granuloma in a tissue specimen, the following infectious diseases enter the differential diagnosis: tuberculosis, mycobacteriosis, histoplasmosis, cryptococcosis, blastomycosis, coccidiomycosis, paracoccidiomycosis, and other rare mycotic and bacterial diseases.

To further investigate these infections, special stains are necessary (Table 1). First, an AFB (acid fast bacillus) stain [either auramine-rhodamine fluorescence (7) or Ziehl-Nelson

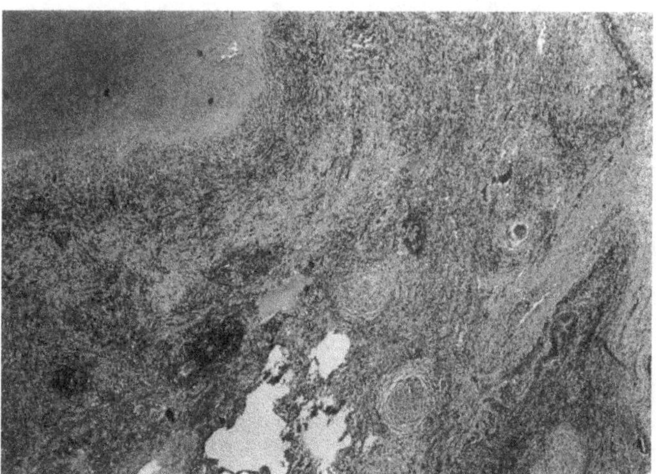

Figure 8 Necrotizing epithelioid cell granuloma (*left upper corner*); in addition, small non-necrotizing epithelioid cell granulomas are seen (*lower right corner*) (tuberculosis).

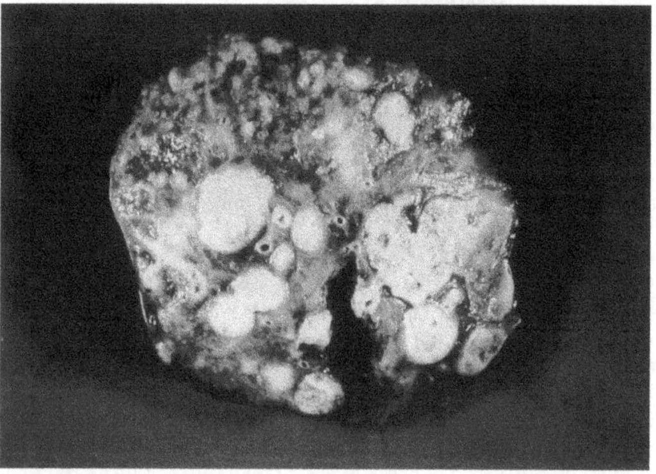

Figure 9 Caseous necrosis in tuberculosis: the macroscopic appearance of a case of acino-nodous tuberculosis. Involvement of bronchi and blood vessels can even be seen macroscopically.

stain], a GMS (methenamine-silver impregnation according to Grocott) stain, and a PAS (periodic acid–Schiff) stain should be done simultaneously. We prefer the auramin-rhodamine stain, because in paucibacillary tuberculosis the few mycobacteria cannot be missed: They are orange fluorescent in a black background. On the basis of these findings, a differential diagnosis of tuberculosis or mycobacteriosis can be made in AFB-positive cases (Fig. 10A). It should be noted that mycobacteria can also be silver impregnated by the GMS

Table 1 Differential Diagnosis of Necrotizing (Caseous) Epithelioid Cell Granulomas

Epithelioid cell granulomas with necrosis	→ Auramine-rhodamine fluorescence-positive (Ziehl-Neelsen stain, PCR-positive, paucibacillary cases)	→ Tuberculosis or mycobacteriosis, differentiate by PCR or culture
	→ Auramine-rhodamine fluorescence-negative (Ziehl-Neelsen stain, PCR-negative), Grocott stain or PAS-positive	→ Different mycoses (histoplasmosis, cryptococcosis, sporotrichosis, and other rare fungi); differentiate by morphology and staining behavior (PAS, mucicarmine, Grocott) and by culture
	→ Auramine-rhodamine fluorescence-negative (Ziehl-Neelsen stain, PCR-negative), PAS-negative, Grocott or other silver impregnation stain (Gomori, Warthin-Starry)–positive	→ Syphilis (typical long, corkscrew organisms; also positive serology); can also be confirmed immunohistochemically using specific antibodies

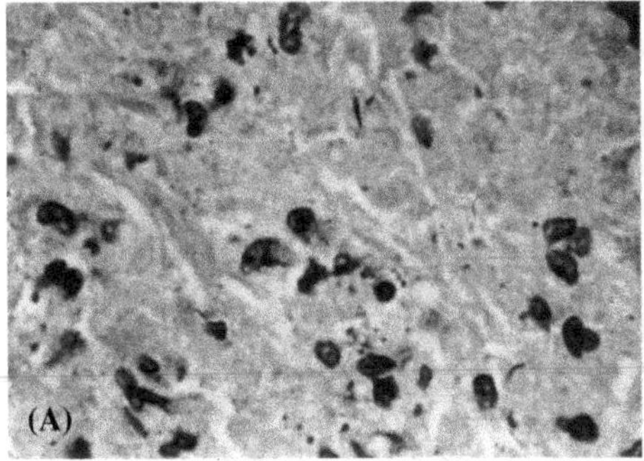

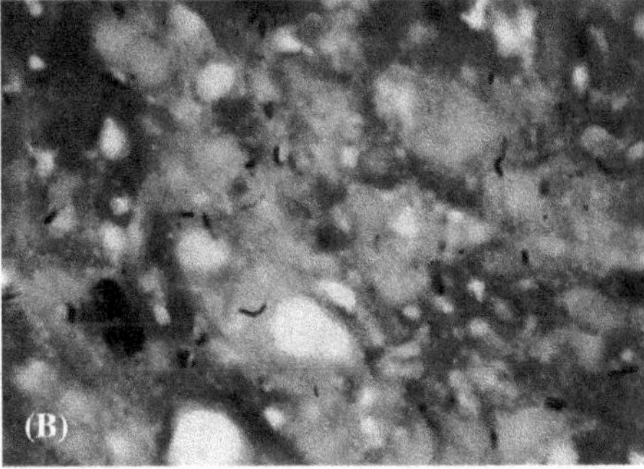

Figure 10 Demonstration of *M. tuberculosis* by (**A**) acid-fast stain and (**B**) silver impregnation.

stain (Fig. 10B). In an otherwise immunocompetent patient, and based on clinical information, most cases can be signed out as consistent with tuberculosis. In immunosuppressed patients and in patients having acquired immunodeficiency syndrome (AIDS), the diagnosis of a mycobacteriosis (a disease caused by members of the Mycobacteriaceae other than tuberculosis complex) should enter our differential diagnosis. The nontuberculous mycobacteria are sometimes described as having a shorter and thicker appearance on AFB stain; however, this should always be proven by polymerase chain reaction (PCR) and microbiologic culture. It should be noted that *Mycobacterium fortuitum* is similarly long and slender like *M. tuberculosis*. A PCR-based characterization is recommended, because a culture of some mycobacteria, for example, *M. avium*, can be very time consuming (up to 11 weeks), whereas a PCR result can be reported within two days. We prefer a PCR for the mycobacterial chaperonin (65 kDa antigen coding gene), and for specific insertion sequences, unique for different mycobacteria (8,9). The insertion sequence IS 6110, for example, can be used to demonstrate DNA of *M. tuberculosis*, *M. bovis*, *M. africanum*, and BCG—all members of the *M. tuberculosis* complex.

Mycosis

A negative AFB stain and positive GMS stain is found in different mycoses. However, it should be noted that epithelioid cell granulomas are not always found in these mycoses. A granulomatous reaction is usually a sign of a competent immune system. In immunosuppressed patients, often a nonspecific inflammatory reaction is seen (10,11). Whereas central necrosis is quite common in histoplasmosis and blastomycosis, it is rare in the other fungal diseases (12).

On the basis of the different forms of cysts and sporozoites and with the aid of additional stains, the following mycoses can be differentiated (a PCR procedure for several of these fungi is also available).

Histoplasmosis

Histoplasma capsulatum is a yeast-like uninucleate organism, 2 to 4 μm in diameter. It reproduces by budding. The organisms are usually found within macrophages and histiocytes, but also in necrotic debris. Capsules of *Histoplasma* can be stained by GMS (Fig. 11A) and PAS, leaving the center unstained. With Giemsa the nucleus is stained, leaving the capsule more or less unstained.

The African variant is *H. duboisii*, which is larger than *H. capsulatum*. Lung lesions in African histoplasmosis are less frequent than with the North American form. Epithelioid cell granulomas are seen in both; however, necrotizing granulomas are more frequent in *H. capsulatum*–induced lesions (Fig. 11B). *Leishmania* species might be mistaken for *Histoplasma*; however, these former organisms can be differentiated by their kinetoplasts (Giemsa) and their PAS-negative cell wall. In addition, *Leishmania* infection in the lungs does not induce a granulomatous reaction.

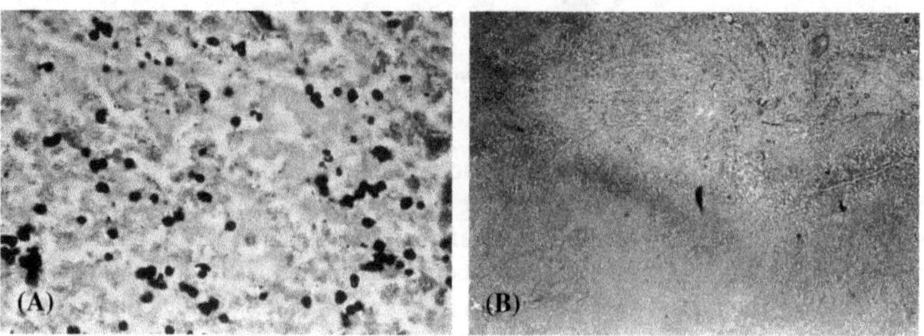

Figure 11 (**A**) *Histoplasma capsulatum* demonstrated by GMS. Note that only few *Histoplasma* show the cup-like shape (*middle right*). (**B**) *H. capsulatum* can cause large necrotizing epithelioid cell granulomas very much like tuberculosis.

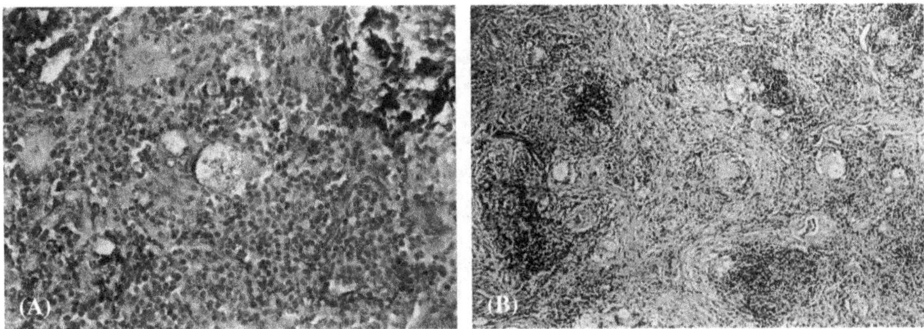

Figure 12 (**A**) *Cryptococcus neoformans* with cyst rupture (**B**) within Langhans giant cells). In **A** the capsule and the sporozoites are stained, whereas in **B** central portions of the organisms are stained by H&E. *Abbreviation*: H&E, haematoxylin and eosin.

Cryptococcosis

Cryptococcus neoformans is distributed worldwide. The organisms are 4 to 7 μm in diameter; their cell walls can be stained by H&E; and the mucinous capsule is usually unstained. Mucicarmine or PAS stains are helpful in highlighting the capsule. The organisms reproduce by budding. Variably sized (small and/or large) yeast-like organisms are found adjacent to each other. Buds may be small or large and show prominent fragmentation, which distinguishes them from *Histoplasma* and *Blastomyces* (Fig. 12A). The organisms are usually found within Langhans giant cells (Fig. 12B), but may also be found lying free within necrosis.

Blastomycosis

Blastomyces dermatitidis is found in North America and Africa. It is a thick-walled, round, 8 to 15 μm measuring organism, which reproduces by budding. The buds are numerous and are broad-based, attached to the parent yeast. The fungus has many nuclei, which distinguishes it from *Cryptococcus*, *Coccidioides*, and *Paracoccidioides*. GMS stains the entire yeast, and the capsule can be highlighted by PAS or mucicarmine stains (Fig. 13). *Blastomyces* regularly induces a granulomatous reaction; however, the necrosis is not of the classical caseous type and contains cellular debris and many neutrophils.

Coccidio- and Paracoccidiomycosis

Coccidioides immitis is found in southern parts of North America, and Central and South America. It is characterized by large sporangia, 30 to 60 μmin diameter; the endospores are each 1 to 5 μm. They can be identified in H&E-stained sections; however, they are also stained by GMS and PAS. The sporangia can be found within giant cells or free within necrosis. *Paracoccidioides brasiliensis*—found in South America—is characterized by multiple buds growing out of one organism. The single fungus is 5 to 15 μm in diameter, but with budding may approach 20 to 40 μm. The fungus is uninucleate, and the buds are of varying size and shape. The organisms can be demonstrated by H&E, PAS, and GMS stains (Fig. 14).

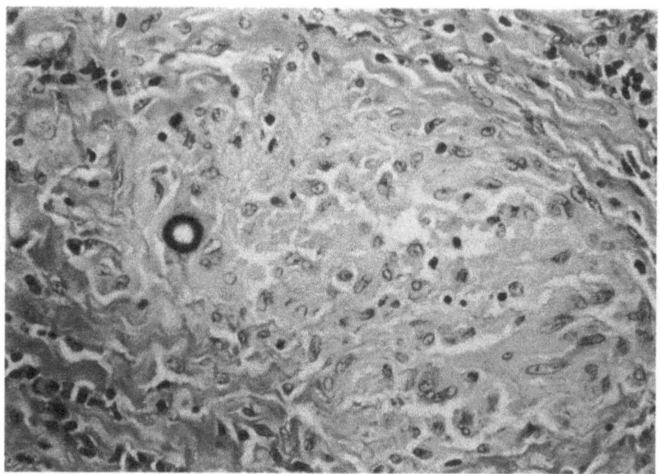

Figure 13 Mucicarmine stained capsule of *Coccidioides immitis* in an epithelioid cell granuloma.

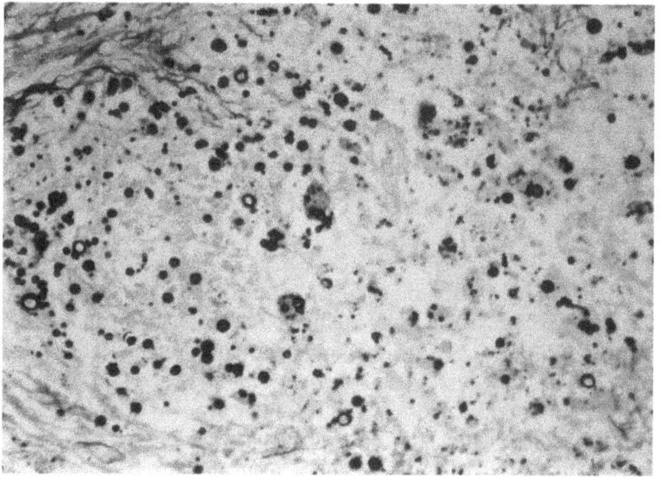

Figure 14 *Paracoccidioides brasiliensis* organisms in an epithelioid cell granuloma, stained by GMS; note the irregular budding of the organisms and the formation of large aggregates. *Abbreviation*: GMS, Grocott's methenamine silver stain.

Other Rare Mycoses

Other fungi causing deep mycosis rarely induce epithelioid cell granulomas. In most instances organisms, like *Aspergillus*, *Candida*, and others, cause a localized mycetoma, or a diffuse invasive mycosis, or an allergic reaction (allergic bronchopulmonary aspergillosis/mycosis, see later). The reason that organisms like *Aspergillus* sometimes induce a necrotizing epithelioid cell granulomatous inflammation (Fig. 15) is largely unknown.

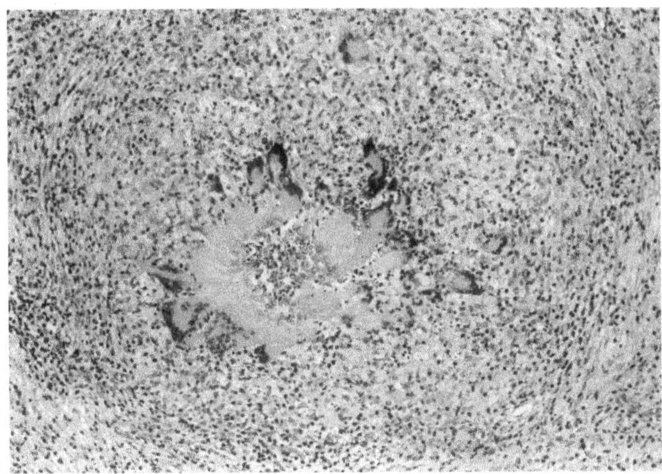

Figure 15 Necrotizing granulomatous aspergillosis. In the center the mycelia can be seen in addition to necrotic debris; the fungi are surrounded by epithelioid and Langhans giant cells; however, there is also a granulocytic and lymphocytic infiltrate.

Rare Bacterial Diseases

Treponema pallidum, the causative agent of syphilitic gumma, still exists, although rare in Western countries. The primary infection sites are the external genitalia, where a granulomatous and ulcerating inflammation is found. After bacteremia, the organisms can enter the lungs. Inflammation is characterized by necrotizing epithelioid cell granulomas, similar to tuberculosis, but also numerous neutrophilic granulocytes are seen (Fig. 16). The name gumma, used for these granulomas, is derived from their macroscopic appearance: The central necrosis is not caseous as in tuberculosis, but has a gum-like consistency, hence the name (*gummi arabicum*). The *Treponema* organisms can be stained by silver impregnation (modified Warthin-Starry stain) or immunohistochemically by specific antibodies.

B. The Nonnecrotizing Epithelioid Cell Granuloma

These granulomas are characterized by the absence of central necrosis, however, necrobiotic foci can occur (6). It is very important to look for vasculitis: Cases of epithelioid cell granulomatosis with foci of neutrophilic, eosinophilic, or lymphocytic vasculitis should be excluded from this group. However, granulomatous vasculitis showing epithelioid cell granulomas in the walls of different-sized blood vessels are not infrequently encountered in all variants of epithelioid cell granulomatosis.

Having found nonnecrotizing epithelioid cell granulomas without granulocytic or lymphocytic vasculitis in the tissue specimen, the following diseases enter the differential diagnosis: tuberculosis, mycobacteriosis, histoplasmosis, cryptococcosis, blastomycosis, coccidiomycosis, paracoccidiomycosis, sarcoidosis, necrotizing sarcoid granulomatosis (NSG), EAA, berylliosis, sarcoid-like reaction, rheumatoid arthritis, and Crohn's disease (Table 2).

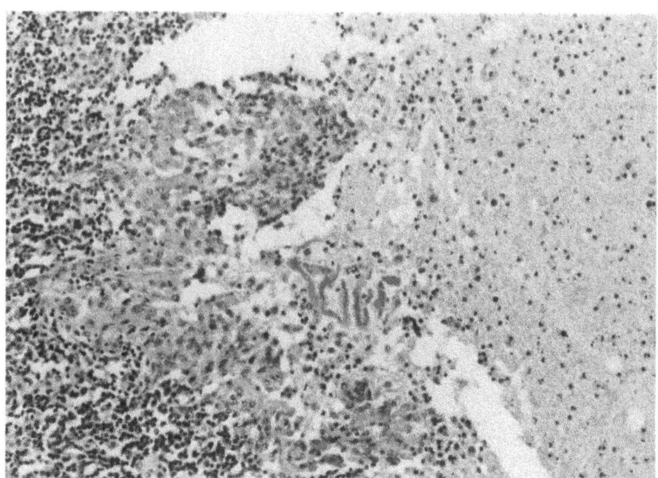

Figure 16 Epithelioid cell granuloma with central necrosis in a case of *Treponema pallidum* infection; note the inflammatory reaction is similar to tuberculosis, however unusual numbers of neutrophils are seen within the necrosis. *Source*: Courtesy of Drs. Woeckel and Morresi/Hauf, Gauting.

We will not discuss tuberculosis, mycobacteriosis, and the different mycoses, because the necessary information has been provided in the previous section. For the diagnosis of an infection, the same special stains are necessary and the same morphologic characteristics of the organisms observed. The reason why mycobacteria sometimes cause a nonnecrotizing epithelioid cell granuloma and sometimes cause caseous necrosis usually is related to the virulence of the organism and the immunocompetence of the host (Table 3) (6).

Sarcoidosis

Sarcoidosis is an epithelioid cell granulomatosis for which no etiology is known. The diagnosis requires the exclusion of infectious organisms. The granulomas are most frequently found along bronchovascular bundles and very often obstruct lymphatics. High-resolution computerized tomography (HRCT) scans are very useful to highlight this distribution pattern. Usually, alveolar septa adjacent to the granulomas are devoid of inflammatory infiltrates, so the granulomas are conspicuous within otherwise normal peripheral lung tissue. This is especially apparent in transbronchial biopsies, where some of the pieces of tissue are negative for granulomas and a few pieces of tissue contain granulomas. A granulomatous vasculitis pattern can be seen in some cases (Fig. 17). Some intracellular materials were previously regarded as specific for sarcoidosis (for example, asteroid bodies, Schaumann bodies, and conchoid bodies) (Fig. 18A, B); however, these structures can be seen in granulomas of diverse etiology and are not specific for the diagnosis of sarcoidosis (13). Oxalate, carbonate, and pyrophosphate crystals can be found in sarcoidosis granulomas, sometimes combined with calcium as a component of Schaumann bodies: however, they are also not specific for a diagnosis of sarcoidosis (Fig. 19A, B) (14). Bilateral, symmetric lymph node swelling in the hilum, induced by granulomatous lymphadenitis, and a

Table 2 Differential Diagnosis of Nonnecrotizing Sarcoid Granulomas

Epithelioid cell granulomas without necrosis	→ Auramine/rhodamine fluorescence-positive (Ziehl-Neelsen stain, PCR positive)	→ Tuberculosis or mycobacteriosis, differentiate by PCR or culture
	→ Auramine/rhodamine fluorescence-negative (Ziehl-Neelsen stain, PCR-negative), Grocott stain or PAS-positive	→ Mycosis (cryptococcosis, blastomycosis, paracoccidiomycosis, sporotrichosis, and other rare fungi), differentiate by morphology and staining behavior (PAS, mucicarmine, Grocott) and by culture
	→ Auramine/rhodamine fluorescence-negative (Ziehl-Neelsen stain, PCR-negative), Grocott stain or PAS-negative	→ Sarcoidosis, beryllosis (differentiate by lymphocyte transformation test, exposure anamnesis, element analysis); both show a T-H-lymphocyte dominated alveolitis in BAL
	→ Auramine/rhodamine fluorescence-negative (Ziehl-Neelsen stain, PCR-negative), Grocott stain or PAS-negative, in the vicinity of a pulmonary tumor	→ Epitheloid cell reaction along draining lymphatics and in lymph nodes; usually induced by different cytokines derived from tumor necrosis and surrounding inflammation
Epithelioid cell granulomatous vasculitis and ischemic parenchymal necrosis	→ Auramine/rhodamine fluorescence-negative (Ziehl-Neelsen stain, PCR-negative), Grocott stain or PAS-negative	→ Necrotizing sarcoid granulomatosis/vasculitis, a variant of nodular sarcoidosis
Combined with lymphocytic interstitial pneumonia	→ Auramine/rhodamine fluorescence-negative (Ziehl-Neelsen stain, PCR-negative), Grocott stain or PAS-negative	→ Hypersensitivity pneumonia (Ts lymphocyte predominance in BAL, exposure anamnesis)

(Continued)

Table 2 Differential Diagnosis of Nonnecrotizing Sarcoid Granulomas (*Continued*)

Additional pallisading histiocytic granulomas	→	Auramine/rhodamine fluorescence-negative (Ziehl-Neelsen stain, PCR-negative), Grocott stain or PAS-negative	→	Rheumatoid arthritis with lung involvement
Combined with eosinophilic or neutrophilic necrotizing bronchiolitis and palisading histiocytic granulomas	→	Auramine/rhodamine fluorescence-negative (Ziehl-Neelsen stain, PCR-negative), Grocott stain or PAS-positive—usually remnants of fungi	→	Bronchocentric granulomatosis as a manifestation of allergic bronchopulmonary aspergillosis
Combined with neutrophilic or eosinophilic vasculitis (small and medium-sized blood vessels, with or without ischemic necroses)	→	Auramine/rhodamine fluorescence-negative (Ziehl-Neelsen stain, PCR-negative), Grocott stain or PAS-negative	→	Wegener's granulomatosis (positive ANCA test)

Table 3 Influence of the Virulence of *Mycobacterium tuberculosis* and the Immune Status of the Patient on the Morphological Presentation of Tuberculosis

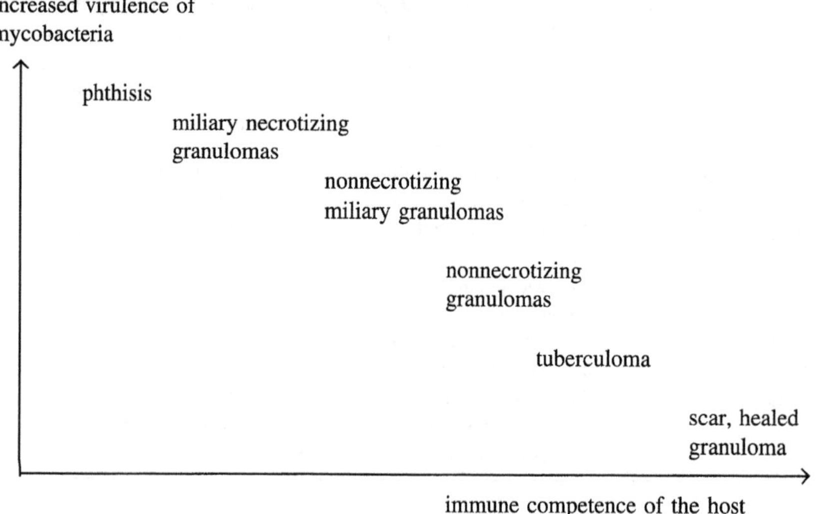

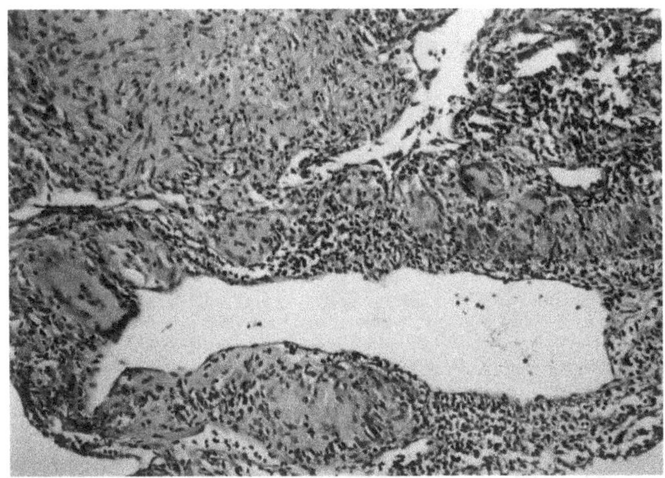

Figure 17 Granulomatous vasculitis in sarcoidosis with many epithelioid cell granulomas and giant cells.

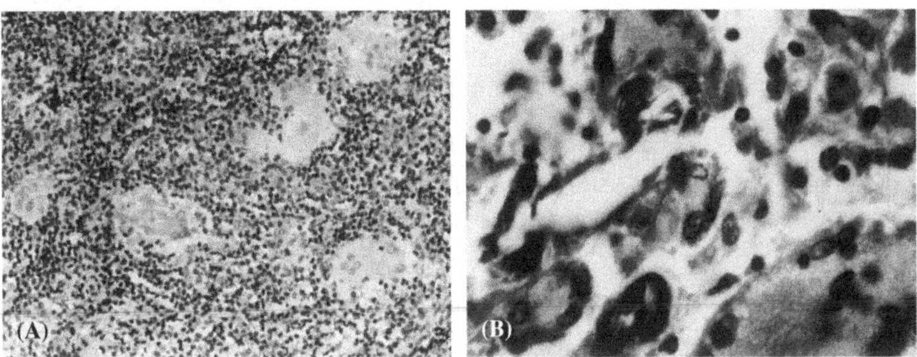

Figure 18 (**A**) Two asteroid bodies in Langhans giant cells stained by H&E in a case of sarcoid reaction in a hilar lymph node due to bronchogenic carcinoma. (**B**) Schaumann and conchoid bodies in Langhans cells also containing a crystalline structure in a case of sarcoidosis. The fragmentation of the bodies is due to a sectioning artifact.

T-helper lymphocyte–dominated alveolitis in the bronchoalveolar lavage (BAL) may supplement the histologic diagnosis of sarcoidosis. PCR for nonspecific mycobacteria is useless in the workup of the granulomas, because mycobacterial DNA can be found in up to one-third of sarcoidosis cases (9). However, a specific and positive PCR for *M. tuberculosis* rules out sarcoidosis, since it is only nontuberculous mycobacterial DNA or RNA that has been described in sarcoidosis. Therefore, the diagnosis of sarcoidosis is based on the exclusion of infectious organisms in epithelioid cell granulomas and on clinical data.

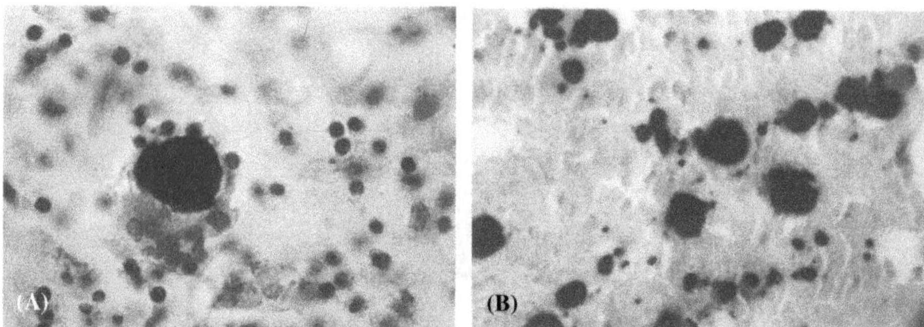

Figure 19 Some bodies are positive for iron (**A**, Prussian blue reaction), most bodies are positive for calcium (**B**, Alizarin red reaction).

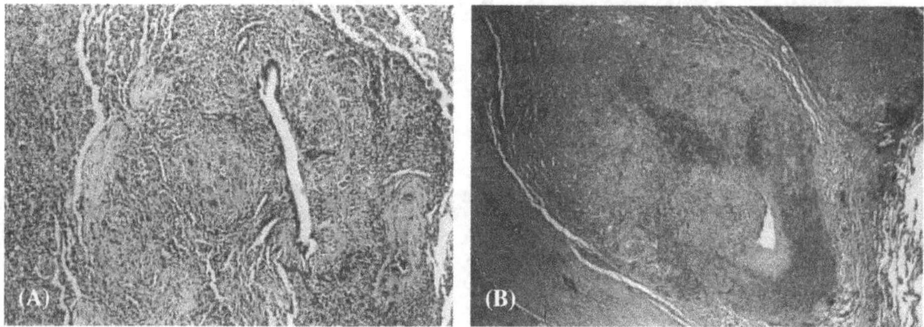

Figure 20 (**A**) Confluent (nodular) epithelioid cell granulomas in necrotizing sarcoid angiitis/granulomatosis with a bronchocentric arrangement and involvement of a pulmonary artery (vasculitis) (*right lower corner*). (**B**) Large ischemic necrosis in another area due to vasculitis.

Necrotizing Sarcoid Granulomatosis (NSG)

Noncaseating epithelioid cell granulomas are observed in NSG. The distribution of the granulomas is similar to sarcoidosis with a dominant involvement of the bronchovascular bundle (Fig. 20A). In addition, there is vasculitis and parenchymal necrosis, usually an ischemic type of necrosis (Fig. 20A, B) (15). The granulomas can be confluent, forming large nodules, usually with a prominent lymphocytic rim. Originally, the disease was thought to involve only the lungs; however, subsequent reports have demonstrated that NSG can be a systemic disease with multiple organ involvement (16). Some of the histologic features are mixtures of features of sarcoidosis and Wegener's granulomatosis (WG), namely vasculitis, nodular aggregates of granulomas, and necrosis. It may be difficult to separate NSG from nodular sarcoidosis, because granulomatous vasculitis and nodular aggregates of granulomas do occur in the latter. In addition, granulomatous vasculitis is not uncommonly found in sarcoidosis. One of these tissue reactions that is uncommon in sarcoidosis is necrosis. NSG may represent a variant of nodular sarcoidosis. Mycobacterial DNA has not been found in NSG (unpublished observation).

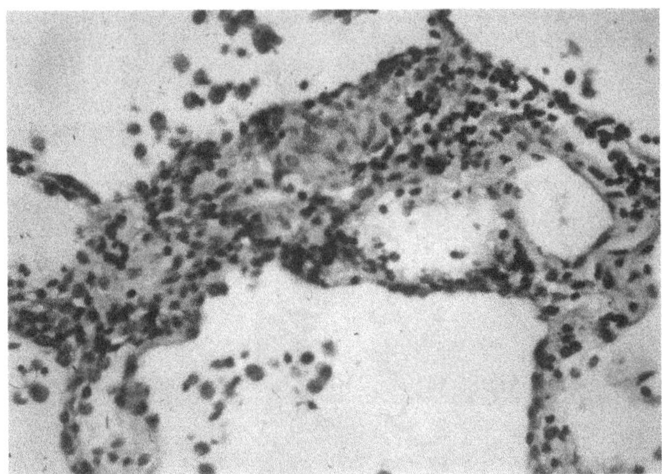

Figure 21 Minute epithelioid cell granuloma in extrinsic allergic alveolitis, a rare finding in transbronchial biopsies.

Extrinsic Allergic Alveolitis (Hypersensitivity Pneumonitis)

This is a granulomatous lung disease induced by an allergic reaction against different fungi, plant pollens, and also animal proteins. In open lung biopsies, epithelioid cell granulomas are frequently seen in EAA (Fig. 2), whereas they are quite rare in transbronchial biopsies (Fig. 21). This might be a disease-specific distribution phenomenon: Whereas granulomas in sarcoidosis are easily found in the bronchial mucosa, in EAA the granulomas are more frequent in the periphery of the lung, most probably caused by the deposition of immune complexes. As in sarcoidosis, all special stains for infectious organisms are negative. In contrast to sarcoidosis, the granulomas in EAA are more loosely organized and usually have a broader rim of lymphocytes with the lymphocytes spilling over into the adjacent alveolar septa (Fig. 2). In active disease, there may be an interstitial pneumonia composed of lymphocytic interstitial infiltrates with or without lymphoid follicle hyperplasia (Fig. 22) (4). The BAL specimen may be very helpful. In EAA there is a lymphocytic alveolitis with a predominance of $CD8^+$-T lymphocytes. The CD4/CD8 ratio should be less than 0.8 (17). However, it should be mentioned that a few rare exceptions to this rule have been reported, and there is also a time effect: With antigen restriction so that the patient is not exposed to the antigen, the CD4/CD8 ratio normalizes within a week (unpublished observations).

Berylliosis

Berylliosis is another allergic epithelioid cell granulomatosis. The granulomas tend to be larger than in EAA or sarcoidosis; however, it might be impossible to differentiate them from those of sarcoidosis on morphologic grounds alone (Fig. 23). The granuloma itself is histologically identical to the granuloma in sarcoidosis (18). As in sarcoidosis, no infectious organisms can be demonstrated in the granulomas. No large series of BAL has been reported for berylliosis so far. However, from experimental data, a predominance of

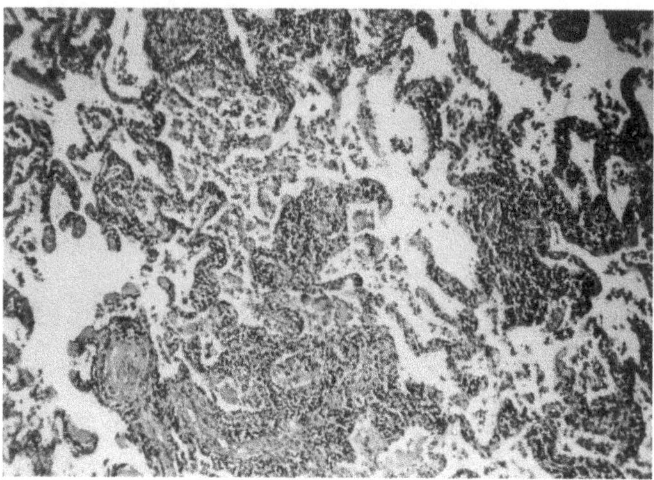

Figure 22 Lymphocytic interstitial pneumonia is quite common in active extrinsic allergic alveolitis.

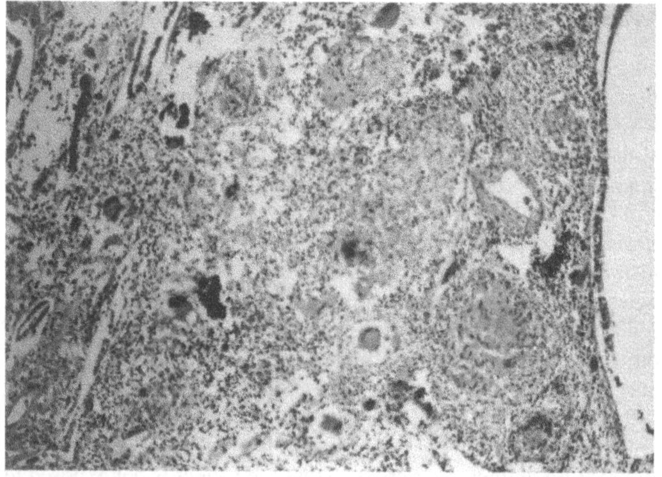

Figure 23 Epithelioid cell granulomas in berylliosis, on morphologic ground alone, indistinguishable from sarcoidosis.

T-helper lymphocytes has been reported, making BAL a potentially useless tool for the differentiation of berylliosis and sarcoidosis (18). For diagnosis, a lymphocyte transformation test is usually recommended, and an exposure anamnesis is necessary to suggest berylliosis (19). By electron microscopy and energy-dispersive X-ray analysis (EDXA), beryllium oxide may be demonstrated in the granulomas. However, it should be remembered that in routinely processed specimens the beryllium oxide might be leached out from

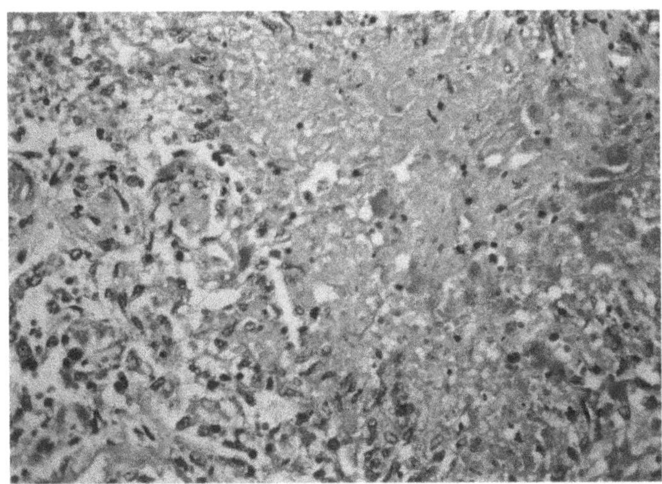

Figure 24 Pallisading epithelioid cell and histiocytic granuloma with necrotic center in seropositive rheumatoid arthritis with lung involvement; sometimes remnants of collagen within the necrosis might help establishing the correct diagnosis.

the tissue by the solvents used for fixation, dehydration, and embedding. The same is true for a laser-assisted mass spectrophotometric analysis (LAMA) using formalin-fixed tissue.

Another rare occupational allergic granulomatous reaction against metal compounds was reported for zirconium. Zirconium dust can induce nonnecrotizing epithelioid cell granulomas, similar to beryllium oxide following a similar mechanism (20).

Rheumatoid Arthritis

In cases of a negative AFB, GMS, and PAS stains, one should think of rheumatoid arthritis involving the lung and/or pleura. Although in the majority of cases of rheumatoid arthritis lung involvement is usually associated with one of the variants of interstitial pneumonia (21), sometimes a granulomatous reaction can be found. This might take the form of a classic rheumatoid nodule with palisading histiocytes (Fig. 24) or an epithelioid cell granuloma without central necrosis (Fig. 25A), associated most often with seropositivity (22). In our experience, both types of granulomas are found side by side. For confirmation, immunohistochemical stains for immunoglobulins and complement components can be used. It should be mentioned that rare cases of coincident rheumatoid arthritis and tuberculosis do exist; therefore, mycobacteria should be excluded in these epithelioid cell granulomas.

Crohn's Disease

Lung involvement in chronic inflammatory bowels diseases was first reported in 1990 (23). Since the first description, numerous reports have been published demonstrating epithelioid cell granulomas in the bronchial and bronchiolar mucosa of patients with Crohn's disease (24–27). Most often, these are loosely formed granulomas with ill-defined borders, rarely

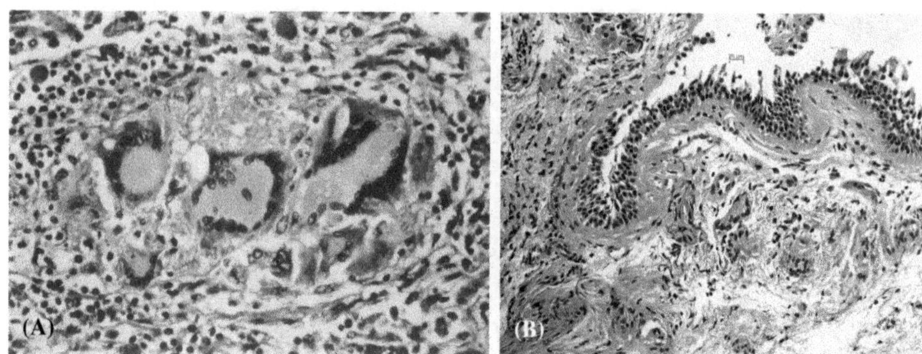

Figure 25 (**A**) Few epithelioid cells and many Langhans giant cells form this epithelioid cell granuloma in the same case of rheumatoid arthritis with extensive lung involvement. (**B**) Loosely scattered epithelioid and giant cells within the bronchial mucosa in Crohn's disease.

with necrobiotic centers (Fig. 25B). In addition, interstitial pneumonias of various patterns have been described in these patients; however, most often these are related to sulfasalazine treatment of Crohn's disease (28).

Sarcoid-Like Reaction in the Setting of a Lung Tumor

Not infrequently we see an epithelioid cell granulomatous inflammation in the lung and hilar lymph nodes in the setting of a bronchial carcinoma. The granulomas are indistinguishable from sarcoidosis granulomas and, therefore, a careful examination of all available data is necessary to separate this reaction from sarcoidosis. First, clinical information should favor a reaction to a lung tumor. Second, there should be no radiologic features favoring sarcoidosis. If we are dealing with lymph nodes excised during mediastinoscopy, we usually end up with a differential diagnosis of epithelioid cell granulomatous lymphadenitis, sarcoidosis versus sarcoid-like reaction.

III. Epithelioid Cell Granuloma Combined with Vasculitis

The diagnostic hallmark of this group of diseases is a granulocytic vasculitis, either neutrophils or eosinophils (Table 2; Fig. 26). In addition, nonnecrotizing epithelioid cell granulomas are found—sometimes many, sometimes few (Fig. 27). It is important to diagnose vasculitis in areas apart from the granulomas to avoid secondary vasculitis commonly seen in infectious diseases. Vasculitis can induce large areas of ischemic necrosis (Fig. 28). Lymphocytes, plasma cells, and histiocytes/macrophages can be seen in small numbers. First of all, infectious organisms should be ruled out by AFB, GMS, and PAS stains (29). If infections are ruled out by appropriate studies such as special stains and cultures, a diagnosis of WG can be made when these histologic features are present. A positive ANCA test can help in confirming the diagnosis (30). However, the diagnosis of WG should never be based on ANCA serology alone (31–33).

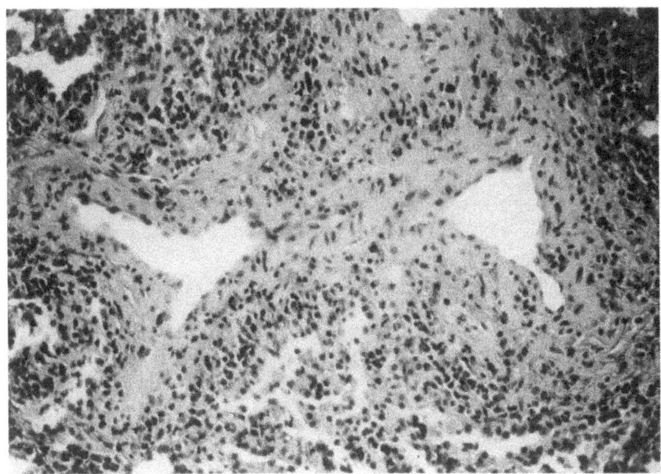

Figure 26 Granulocytic vasculitis in a case of Wegener's disease.

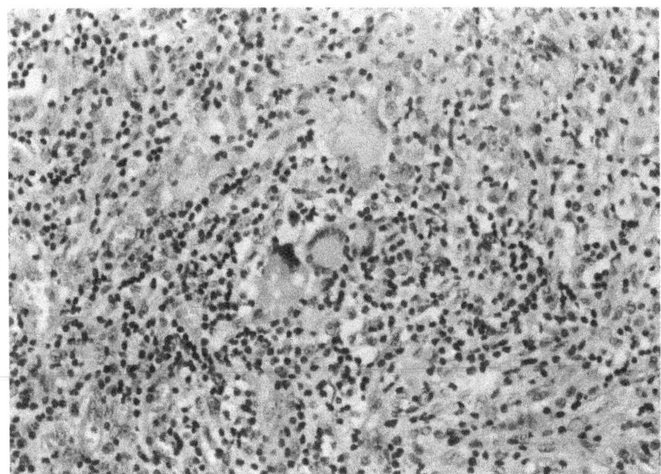

Figure 27 Epithelioid cell granulomas in Wegener's disease are usually loosely arranged.

IV. Epithelioid Cell and Palisading Histiocytic Granulomas with Necrotizing Bronchiolitis

The hallmark of so-called bronchocentric granulomatosis is a necrotizing bronchiolitis with peribronchiolar extension of the inflammatory infiltrates. Necrotic debris can be seen in the lumina. Epithelioid cell granulomas and/or palisading histiocytic granulomas are found

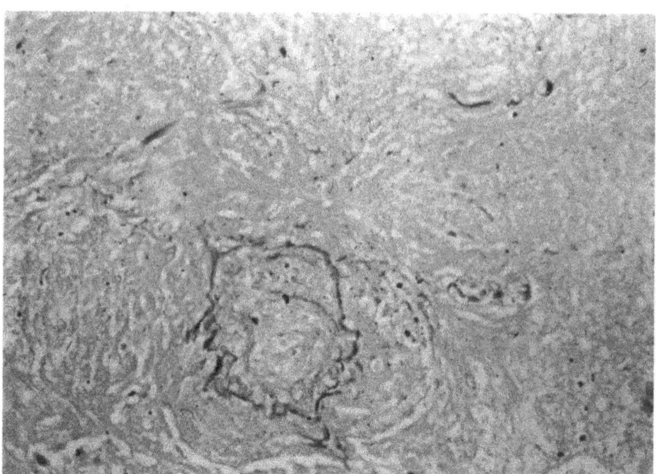

Figure 28 Ischemic necrosis of a large lung area. Remnants of a blood vessel are highlighted by an Elastic van Gieson stain.

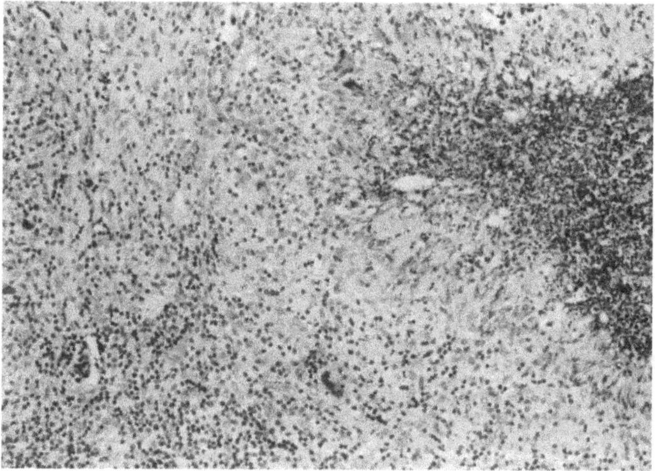

Figure 29 Pallisading histiocytic and epithelioid cell granulomas in a case of necrotizing bronchocentric granulomatosis due to allergic bronchopulmonary aspergillosis.

within the bronchiolar walls (Fig. 29). In addition, there is usually a dense infiltrate of eosinophils or neutrophils. AFB stains should always be performed to exclude mycobacteria, which not uncommonly induce a bronchocentric granulomatous inflammation (especially in the setting of a neutrophilic infiltrate) (6,34,35). If infection is ruled out by appropriate studies, a diagnosis of a bronchocentric granulomatosis as a morphologic variant of allergic bronchopulmonary mycosis/aspergillosis (ABPA) can be made (36). In my experience, it is often necessary to perform serial sections to demonstrate the *Aspergillus* in these cases. Therefore, a negative GMS or PAS reaction in a few sections does not exclude bronchocentric granulomatosis. The clinical information about positive allergy tests may be helpful. Combinations of type 1 and 4 immune reactions can be seen in this form of ABPA (36). In rare cases, bronchocentric necrotizing granulomatosis might also be seen in the setting of WG (37). Therefore, ANCA tests can be helpful in this difficult differential diagnosis.

V. The Histiocytic Granuloma

This type of granuloma is defined by a more or less circumscribed aggregate of histiocytes. In addition, other cells may be found, for example, macrophages, foreign body giant cells, lymphocytes, plasma cells, and occasionally neutrophils. There may be central necrosis and palisading of the histiocytes or no necrosis at all. Histiocytes may have a foamy cytoplasm or may contain pigment and/or an inorganic crystalline material (Table 4). Special stains are required to arrive at a definite diagnosis.

A. Histiocytic Granuloma Without Palisading

In AFB-positive cases, the tentative diagnosis of a mycobacteriosis can be made, which should be confirmed by culture and/or PCR. In immunosuppressed and AIDS patients, *M. tuberculosis* can sometimes induce this type of reaction (6,35,38). Fungal infection should be investigated by a GMS and PAS stain. Some rare bacterial infections, usually intracytoplasmic bacteria like *Chlamydia* and *Afipia* species, or Whipple's disease can induce this type of reaction. A PAS stain will show the intracytoplasmic bacteria. In special geographic regions of the world the induction of histiocytic granulomas by *M. leprae* should also be considered (39). If AFB, GMS, and PAS are all negative, silicosis or anthracosilicosis should be considered. The histiocytes should be examined under polarized light (Fig. 30). White birefringent crystals, usually 7 to 14 μm in length, establish the diagnosis of early silicosis or anthracosilicosis (if there is an additional intra- and extracellular accumulation of anthracotic pigment (see section Silicosis and Anthracosilicosis).

B. Histiocytic Granuloma with Palisading

"Palisading" means that the histiocytes are arranged around central necrosis with their nuclei perpendicular to the necrotic center (Fig. 31). Mycobacterial and fungal infection have to be excluded by AFB and GMS stains. In cases with PAS-positive granules, actinomycosis can be present; therefore a Gram stain should be performed, which will show the thin blue filaments of *Actinomyces* species. Most of these patients will also present with actinomycosis of the paranasal sinuses. If other, usually gram-positive, bacteria are encountered, the diagnosis of a botryomycosis or bacterial pseudomycosis can be made (40).

If all special stains are negative, the diagnosis of rheumatoid arthritis involving the lung can be considered. To confirm the diagnosis, immunohistochemical stains for immunoglobulins G and M and complement components C5-9 complex can be done, which should be positive in the necrosis and the adjacent area. It should be mentioned that within the necrosis remnants of destroyed collagen fibers are often seen, which can be highlighted under polarized light.

Table 4 Differential Diagnosis of Histiocytic Granulomas with and Without Palisading

Histiocytic granulomas with or without palisading, with or without central necrosis	→ Auramine/rhodamine fluorescence-positive (Ziehl-Neelsen stain, PCR-negative), Grocott stain or PAS-negative	→ Mycobacterioses, differentiate by culture or PCR, in immunosuppressed patients
With palisading and necrosis	→ Auramine/rhodamine fluorescence-negative (Ziehl-Neelsen stain, PCR negative), Grocott stain, gram- or PAS-positive	→ Actinomycosis or botryomycosis, differentiate by Gram stain
With palisading and necrotizing bronchiolitis	→ Auramine/rhodamine fluorescence-negative (Ziehl-Neelsen stain, PCR-negative), Grocott and PAS-positive	→ Bronchocentric granulomatosis in the setting of allergic bronchopulmonary aspergillosis/mycosis
Usually with fibrinoid necrosis	→ Auramine/rhodamine fluorescence-negative (Ziehl-Neelsen stain, PCR-negative), Grocott stain, gram- or PAS negative	→ Rheumatoid arthritis
Loose histiocytic granulomas without palisading, with birefringent crystals with or without anthracotic pigment	→ Auramine/rhodamine fluorescence-negative (Ziehl-Neelsen stain, PCR-negative), Grocott stain, gram– or PAS-negative, birefringent crystals corresponding to silicates	→ Early silicotic or anthracosilicotic granulomas

VI. Eosinophilic Granulomas

An accumulation of eosinophils together with histiocytes, Langerhans cells, and, in specific cases, also giant cells of the foreign body and Langhans type characterize eosinophilic granulomas. In transbronchial biopsies, it might not be possible to discern between an eosinophilic granuloma and an eosinophilic pneumonia (41). Therefore, the knowledge of

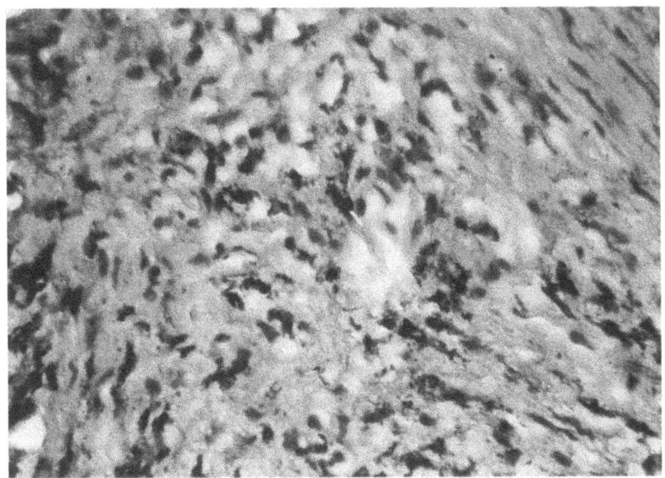

Figure 30 Histiocytic granuloma under semipolarized light: in the center a silicium oxide needle can be seen; the macrophages/histiocytes contain anthracotic pigment, in this case of anthracosilicosis.

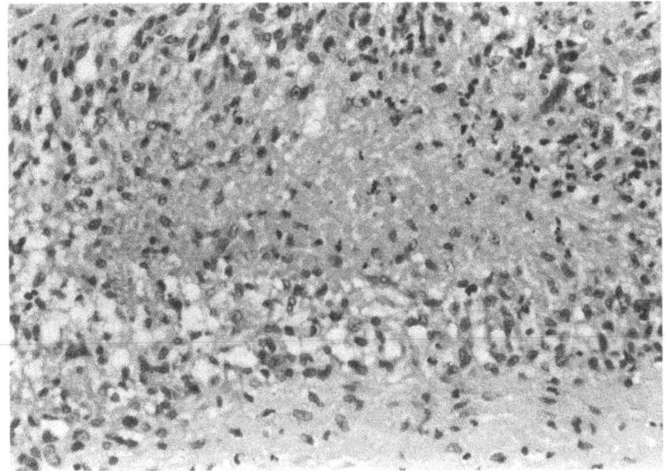

Figure 31 Histiocytic and foam cell granulomas in bronchocentric necrotizing granulomatosis in a case of actinomycosis; in another area the causing organisms could be found forming the well-known PAS-positive granules.

the HRCT scan is necessary. A vasculitis might or might not be encountered. If there is a doubt about the type of granulocytes, eosinophils can be efficiently stained by Congo red, which will highlight the specific eosinophilic granules. Cases of eosinophilic pneumonia associated with granulomas will not be discussed in this chapter. Depending on the cellular composition, three different entities enter our differential diagnosis (Table 5).

Table 5 Differential Diagnosis of Eosinophilic Granulomas

Eosinophilic granulomas	→ Along bronchioles with or without necroses, with proliferating Langerhans cells	→ Histiocytosis X, confirm by CD1a and S100 stains and by CDla positive Langerhans cells >6% in BAL
	→ With or without necroses, with foreign-body and Langerhans giant cells	→ Often multiple sections required to detect parasites or parasitic eggs/larvae; differentiate by morphology and exact (geographic) exposure anamnesis
With bronchocentric necrosis and histiocytes	→ Auramine/rhodamine fluorescence negative (Ziehl-Neelsen stain, PCR negative), Grocott stain or PAS positive—usually remnants of fungi	→ Bronchocentric granulomatosis as a manifestation of allergic bronchopulmonary aspergillosis

A. Histiocytosis X (Langerhans Cell Granulomatosis)

This disease is usually found in young and middle-aged patients with a history of cigarette smoking (42). In histiocytosis X, the pattern is a bronchiolocentric granulomatous inflammation with necrosis of the bronchiolar mucosa, which is replaced by granulomas composed of eosinophils, histiocytes and macrophages, and Langerhans cells (Fig. 32). In early lesions, the Langerhans cells might be obscured by the dense eosinophilic infiltrate, whereas in matured lesions they can be discerned easily (Fig. 33). Langerhans as well as dendritic cells belong to the antigen-presenting cells of the body and are characterized by oval nuclei with finely distributed euchromatin and an inconspicuous cytoplasm and cell membrane. They can be highlighted by immunohistochemical stains with S100 protein antibodies, but more specifically by CD1a or Langerin antibodies (Fig. 34). In BAL of patients with histiocytosis X, the Langerhans cells are quite numerous, whereas in other conditions they are rarely seen. In our experience, more than 6% Langerhans cells in BAL fluid are suspicious for histiocytosis X and more than 10% are diagnostic for histiocytosis X. In old scarred cases, a definitive histologic diagnosis of histiocytosis X may be impossible.

B. Bronchocentric Granulomatosis

This type of bronchocentric granulomatous inflammation requires the demonstration of fungi or remnants of fungi and a clinical history of an allergic reaction. The features have already been described in the previous section.

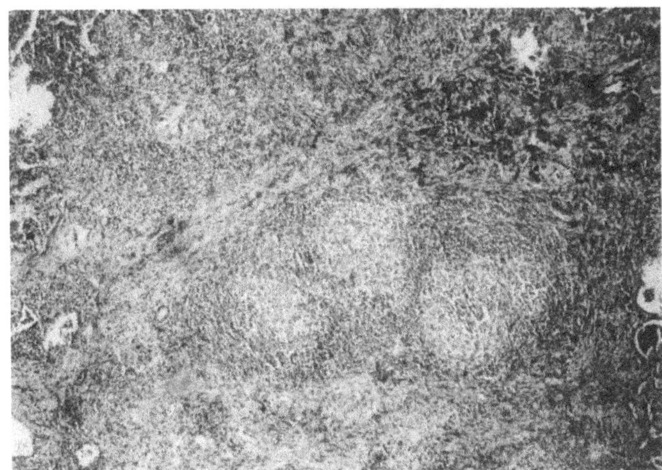

Figure 32 Low-power view of an eosinophilic bronchiolocentric granuloma in a case of histiocytosis X; the bronchioles are all destroyed in this area.

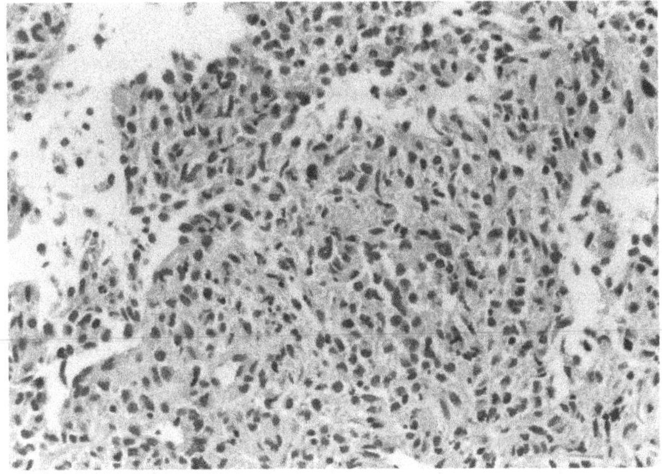

Figure 33 Langerhans cells in histiocytosis X; more advanced stage of granuloma formation with numerous Langerhans cells.

C. Parasitic Granulomas

Parasitic granulomas are composed of numerous eosinophils, together with histiocytes, macrophages, and giant cells (43,44). The outer wall of the granuloma, especially, may be entirely composed of eosinophils, whereas, toward the center, foreign body giant cells with numerous eosinophils prevail. The distribution can be of a bronchocentric or a

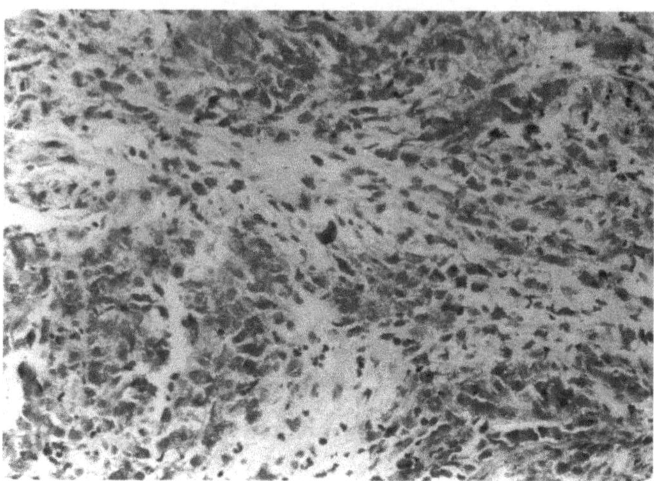

Figure 34 Langerhans cells in histiocytosis X highlighted by an immunohistochemical stain for CD1a.

vasculocentric pattern, depending on the route by which the parasites have entered the lung. It is often necessary to perform multiple sections to detect the parasite; therefore, ample tissue is required (Fig. 35A–C). An open lung biopsy is preferred for this diagnosis. A GMS stain in many instances will assist in the search for the parasites, because the egg and parasite membranes very often can be silver impregnated. The parasites or their eggs may be hidden very deep in the center of the granuloma. Some of the parasites can be identified on morphologic grounds and information about the geographic region where they may have been acquired. However, I recommend contacting specialists for a definite identification, especially when dealing with worm eggs (45).

VII. Foreign Body Granulomas

Histiocytes, macrophages, and foreign body giant cells characterize these granulomas. There will always be a few granulocytes and/or lymphocytes in the surrounding area. The giant cells may show inclusions and foreign material in their cytoplasm, which can be seen by light microscopy in H&E-stained sections or under polarized light (Table 6).

A. Drug or Medical Device Induced

Some common drugs like corticosteroids might induce a foreign body granulomatous reaction. Very often the giant cells contain negative imprints of cholesterol crystals (Fig. 36). In addition to giant cells, macrophages can be seen, sometimes with foamy cytoplasm. Characteristically, the foreign body granulomas are centered around small blood vessels. The mechanism is not known, but interference with surfactant metabolism

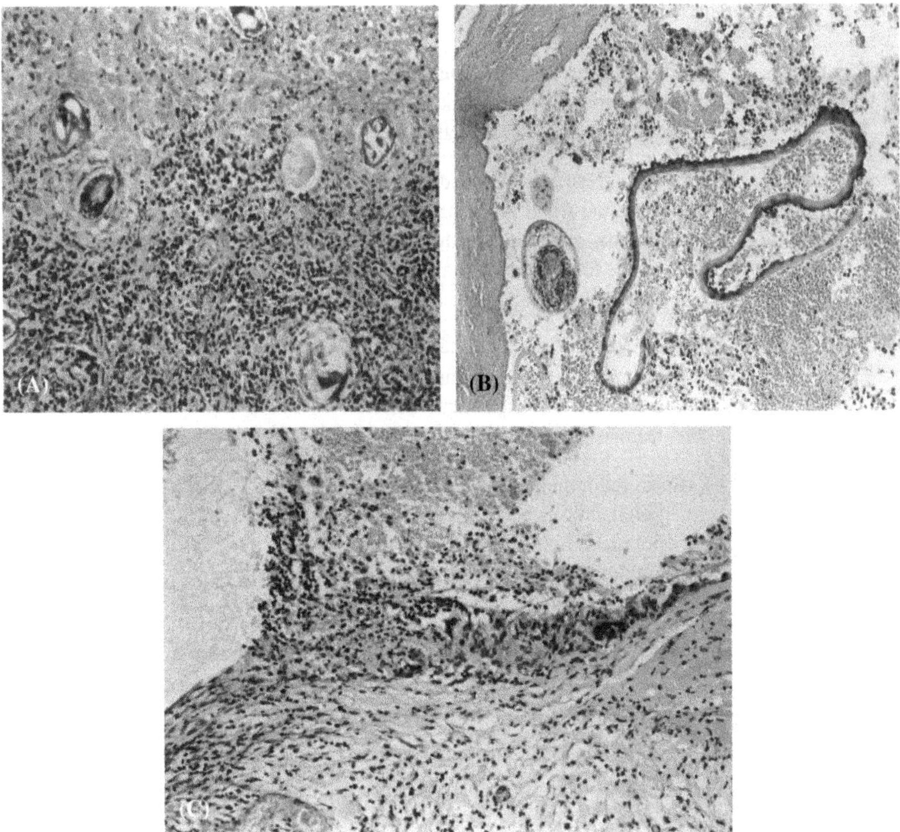

Figure 35 (**A**) Eosinophilic granulomas with parasites in a case of *Paragonimus brasiliensis* infection, and (**B**) in a case of *Echinococcus* infection, (**C**) note the granulomatous reaction with epithelioid and Langhans cells and numerous eosinophils.

is suspected. The diagnosis is based on the exclusion of other causes and a clinical history of drug medication.

A very similar reaction has been found in patients undergoing dialysis. In these cases, cellulose from the dialysis membranes is liberated and embolizes to the lungs, causing a vasculocentric foreign body granulomatous reaction (Fig. 37).

B. In Intravenous Drug Abusers

The characteristic features are talcum crystals, which can be polarized, in foreign body giant cells and a vasculocentric arrangement of the granulomas. There can be obstruction of the small blood vessels and focal bleeding. The disease is caused by intravenous injection of narcotic drugs used as a replacement for heroin. These drugs contain talcum as the

Table 6 Differential Diagnosis of Foreign-Body Granulomas

Foreign-body granulomas	→ Within alveolar walls, and strictly in and around small pulmonary blood vessels, cholesterol clefts	→ Drug-induced, often seen in corticoid-treated patients
	→ Within alveolar walls, and strictly in and around small pulmonary blood vessels, polarizing membranous material, sometimes typical cellulose structure, or polarizing talcum crystals	→ Material from dialysis membranes, or talcum granulomas in intravenous drug abusers
	→ With or without foamy macrophages, cellulose or animal tissue derived from vegetables or meat	→ Aspirated material (food)
	→ Eosin red homogeneous material, Kongored stain positive, green under polarized light, positive for A- or P-amyloid, often associated with calcification and bone formation	→ Nodular amyloidosis
	→ With multiple phagocytosed alveoliths lying in alveolar walls and free in aveoli	→ Pulmonary microlithiasis
	→ Usually combined with histiocytic infiltrates or loose histiocytic granulomas, with/without central hyalinosis, with positively polarizing needle-like crystals, and anthracotic pigment	→ Early silicosis and anthracosilicosis

binding material. Talcum becomes trapped in the pulmonary capillaries and venules and induces foreign body granulomatous inflammation (Fig. 38).

C. Inhaled Material and Food Aspiration

Many types of particulate matter can induce a granulomatous reaction, usually of foreign body type (46–48). With food aspiration, all variants of food can potentially be found in the developing foreign body granulomas: Vegetables can be diagnosed under polarized light because the cellulose backbone of the plants is resistant to degradation and is birefringent. Aspirated animal-derived food can be diagnosed by remnants of skeletal muscle tissue or sheets of cells such as liver cells (Fig. 39). Normally, the nuclei are no longer visible, but the cytoplasm is preserved. Very often, well-preserved food remnants can be found in the

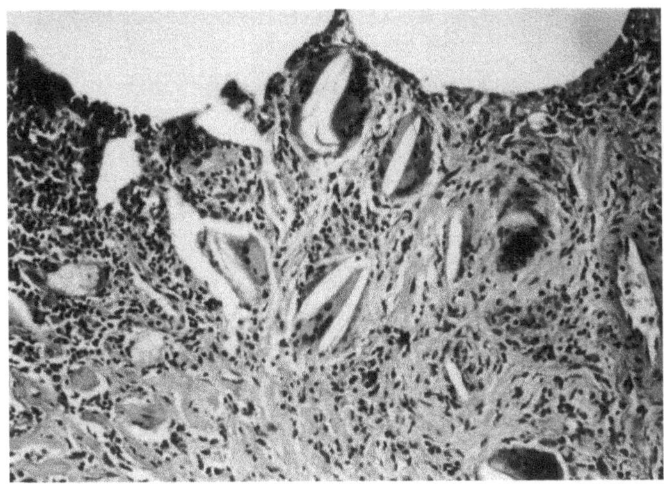

Figure 36 Drug-induced foreign body granulomas in a case of high dose corticosteroid treatment. The granuloma is composed of foreign body giant cells, lymphocytes, and granulocytes; the former contain many imprints of cholesterol crystals, which have been dissolved during tissue preparation.

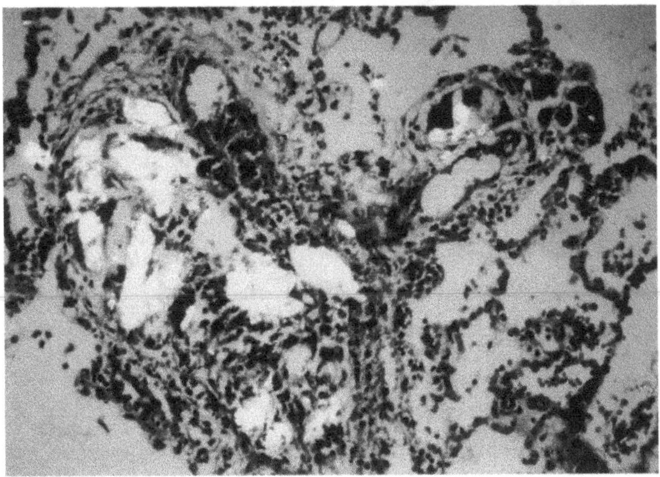

Figure 37 Foreign body granuloma in the alveolar wall, centered around blood vessels; the giant cells contain birefringent material (seen under semipolarized light) which turned out to be cellulose, derived from a dialysis membrane.

centers of the granulomas, surrounded by the giant cells. The diagnosis of aspirated bone remnants, usually from chicken, can sometimes be difficult, because the inspissated bone fragments might be mistaken for an ossification of the bronchial cartilage. Therefore, a careful search for foreign body giant cells is essential.

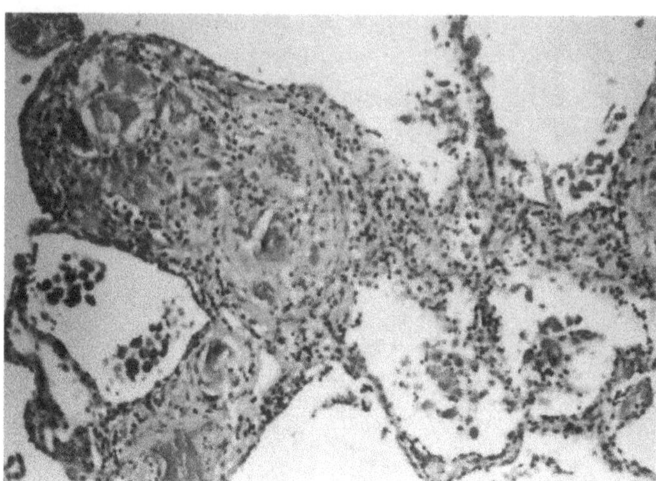

Figure 38 Foreign body granuloma in an intravenous drug abuser; the birefringent material turned out to be talcum.

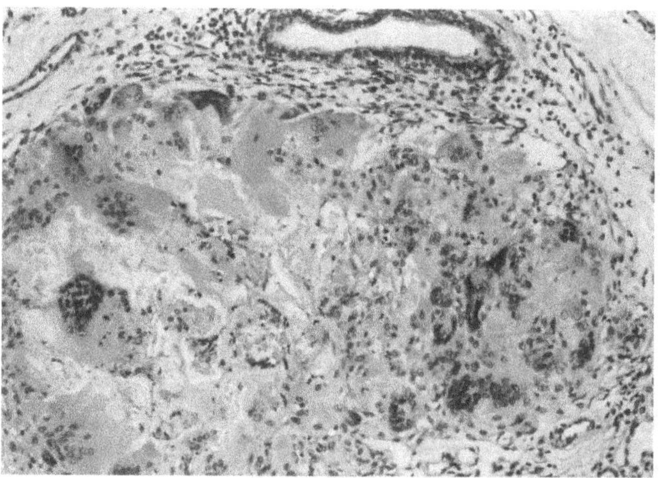

Figure 39 Foreign body granuloma in a case of food aspiration. Many foreign body giant cells form a rather large granuloma; in between them remnants of the food can be seen.

D. Nodular Amyloidosis

Amyloid deposition can occur as either a diffuse or a nodular pattern in the lung. Only nodular amyloidosis poses some problems in the differential diagnosis of granulomas because of a usually prominent foreign body granulomatous reaction (49). The foreign body

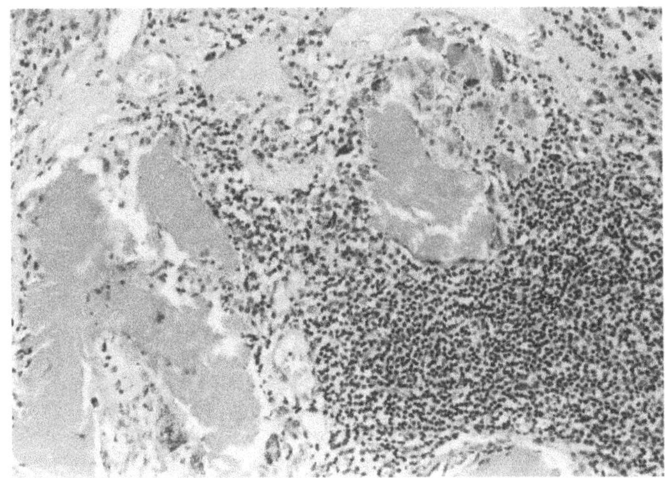

Figure 40 Foreign body granulomas in a case of nodular amyloidosis of the lung; deposited amyloid is in part phagocytosed by foreign body giant cells.

reaction surrounds the deposited amyloid. The granulomas tend to be large and often confluent, depending on the amount of amyloid deposited. In addition, other metaplastic changes can be seen such as bone formation. The tentative diagnosis is made on H&E section (Fig. 40), because the characteristic eosinophilic acellular material is typical, and, together with the foreign body reaction, is unique to amyloidosis. A positive Congo red stain examined under polarized light will confirm the diagnosis, as well as immunohistochemical stains for the different amyloid proteins.

E. Pulmonary Microlithiasis

In this condition, many large and small granules can be found, surrounded by foreign body giant cells, sometimes forming granulomas. These granules show a concentric lamellar structure and contain different minerals, among them calcium carbonate and calcium pyrophosphates. Some of the granules may lie free in the alveoli, but most of them are within the alveolar walls. A few granules encountered in biopsies and in BAL are nonspecific, and they should be discerned from alveoliths, which are not lamellated. They are either phagocytosed by giant cells or may lie free in the alveoli. However, if they are numerous and elicit a foreign body granulomatous reaction (Fig. 41), pulmonary microlithiasis can be diagnosed (50).

VIII. Hyalinizing Granulomas

The characteristic feature of hyalinizing granulomas is their sharp delineation and their acellular centers. Under polarized light, the typical features of collagen fibers are seen. Two diseases enter our differential diagnosis (Table 7).

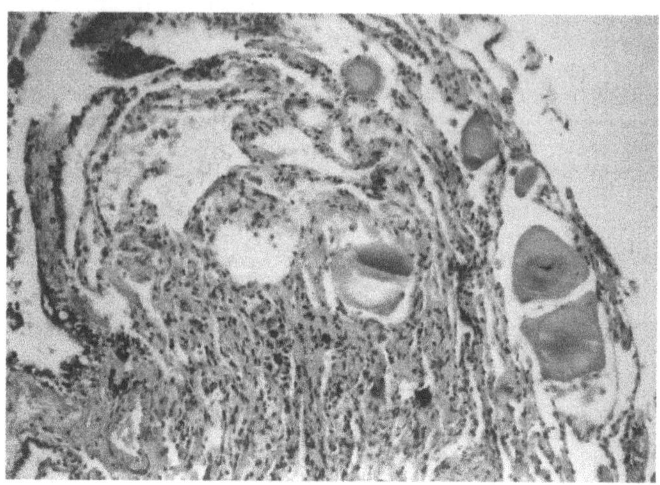

Figure 41 Pulmonary microlithiasis; in this area the few foreign body giant cells are obscured, however, many granules in the alveoli and one in the alveolar wall are seen.

Table 7 Differential Diagnosis of Hyalinizing Granulomas

Hyalinizing Granulomas	→ Loose histiocytic granulomas without palisading, with birefringent crystals with or without anthracotic pigment; sometimes puriform necrosis in the center	→	Silicotic or anthracosilicotic nodules
	→ Hyalinized granulomas, often confluent, simulating silicosis nodules; without crystals, with predominantly plasmocytic infiltrates around the granulomas, negative for all infectious organisms	→	Hyalinizing granulomatosis of lung and mediastinum

A. Silicosis and Anthracosilicosis

Hyalinized granulomas, sometimes confluent, are the characteristic features of silicosis and anthracosilicosis. The centers might be homogeneous or might show necrosis. In the later case, cholesterol can be found in these centers. In early silicotic nodules, a foreign body granulomatous reaction can be seen in the periphery. Later on, the rim of the granuloma is composed of macrophages, which are stuffed with anthracotic pigment and crystalline material (Fig. 5). A few lymphocytes can be found too. The diagnosis is confirmed by examination under polarized light: white birefringent needles of silicium oxides are seen, usually 7 to 15 μm long (Fig. 30). Although rare, in the presence of central necrosis one should be aware of the combination of silicosis and tuberculosis and silicosis and

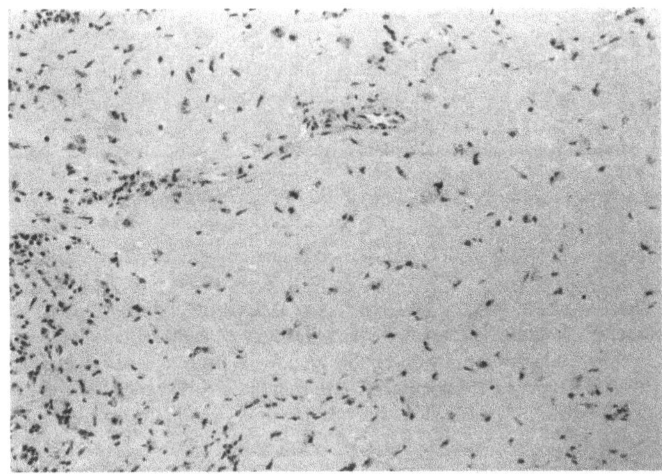

Figure 42 Hyalinizing granuloma in the lungs of a young boy suffering from hyalinizing granulomatosis of lung and mediastinum.

rheumatoid arthritis (51). Therefore, AFB and GMS stains should be performed and the clinical report should be studied carefully.

B. Hyalinizing Granulomatosis of Lung, Pleura, and Mediastinum

In cases where AFB and GMS are negative and no epithelioid cells or birefringent material are found, the diagnosis of hyalinizing granulomatosis of the lung should be considered (52). Usually a dense lymphocytic and plasmocytic infiltration is seen at the rim of the hyalinized nodules, but also within the nodule (Fig. 42). Most patients are either children or patients in their second decade of life.

References

1. Muns G, West WW, Gurney J, et al. Non-sarcoid granulomatous disease with involvement of the lungs. Sarcoidosis 1995; 12:99–110.
2. Flynn JL, Goldstein MM, Chan J, et al. Tumor necrosis factor-alpha is required in the protective immune response against Mycobacterium tuberculosis in mice. Immunity 1995; 2:561–572.
3. McNally AK, Anderson JM. Interleukin-4 induces foreign body giant cells from human monocytes/macrophages. Differential lymphokine regulation of macrophage fusion leads to morphological variants of multinucleated giant cells. Am J Pathol 1995; 147:1487–1499.
4. Sharma OP, Fujimura N. Hypersensitivity pneumonitis: a noninfectious granulomatosis. Semin Respir Infect 1995; 10:96–106.
5. Enelow RI, Sullivan GW, Carper HT, et al. Induction of multinucleated giant cell formation from in vitro culture of human monocytes with interleukin-3 and interferon-gamma: comparison with other stimulating factors. Am J Respir Cell Mol Biol 1992; 6:57–62.
6. Ridley DS, Ridley MJ. Rationale for the histological spectrum of tuberculosis. A basis for classification. Pathology 1987; 19:186–192.

7. Wöckel W. Auramine fluorescence for acid fast bacilli in formalin-fixed, paraffin-embedded tissues. Am J Clin Pathol 1995; 103:667.
8. Popper HH, Winter E, Höfler G. DNA of Mycobacterium tuberculosis in formalin fixed and paraffin embedded tissue in tuberculosis and sarcoidosis detected by PCR. Am J Clin Pathol 1994; 101:738–741.
9. Popper HH, Klemen H, Höfler G, et al. Presence of mycobacterial DNA in sarcoidosis. Hum Pathol 1997; 28(7):796–800.
10. McAdams HP, Rosado-de-Christenson ML, Templeton PA, et al. Thoracic mycoses from opportunistic fungi: radiologic-pathologic correlation. Radiographics 1995; 15:271–286.
11. White DA. Pulmonary infection in the immunocompromised patient. Semin Thorac Cardiovasc Surg 1995; 7:78–87.
12. Binford H, Dooley JR. Deep mycoses. In: Binford CH, Connor DH, eds. Pathology of Tropical and Extraordinary Diseases. Washington, DC: Armed Forces Institute of Pathology, 1976:565ff.
13. Katzenstein AL, Askin FB. Systemic diseases involving the lung. In: Katzenstein AL, Askin FB, eds. Surgical Pathology of non-neoplastic Lung Disease. Philadelphia, PA: Saunders, 1990:235.
14. Visscher D, Churg A, Katzenstein AL. Significance of crystalline inclusions in lung granulomas. Mod Pathol 1988; 1:415–419.
15. Liebow AA. The J. Burns Amberson Lecture: pulmonary angiitis and granulomatosis. Am Rev Respir Dis 1973; 108:1–18 (review).
16. Churg A. Pulmonary angiitis and granulomatosis revisited. Hum Pathol 1978; 89:660.
17. Popper HH, Pongratz M. Aussage- und Einsatzmöglichkeiten der bronchioloalveolären Lavage kombiniert mit transbronchialer Lungenbiopsie (Findings and relevance of bronchoalveolar lavage combined with transbronchial biopsy). Wien Klin Wochenschr 1987; 99:848–855.
18. Votto JJ, Barton RW, Gionfriddo MA, et al. A model of pulmonary granulomata induced by beryllium sulfate in the rat. Sarcoidosis 1987; 4:71–76.
19. Kreiss K, Wasserman S, Mroz MM, et al. Beryllium disease screening in the ceramics industry. Blood lymphocyte test performance and exposure-disease relations. J Occup Med 1993; 35:267–274.
20. Romeo L, Cazzadori A, Bontempini L, et al. Interstitial lung granulomas as a possible consequence of exposure to zirconium dust. Med Lav 1994; 85:219–222.
21. Hakala M, Paakko P, Huhti E, et al. Open lung biopsy of patients with rheumatoid arthritis. Clin Rheumatol 1990; 9:452–460.
22. Fellbaum C, Domej W, Popper H. Rheumatoid arthritis with extensive lung lesions. Thorax 1989; 44:70–71.
23. Puntis JW, Tarlow MJ, Raafat F, et al. Crohn's disease of the lung. Arch Dis Child 1990; 65: 1270–1271.
24. Camus P, Piard F, Ashcroft T, et al. The lung in inflammatory bowel disease. Medicine 1993; 72: 151–183.
25. Freeman HJ, Davis JE, Prest ME, et al. Granulomatous bronchiolitis with necrobiotic pulmonary nodules in Crohn's disease. Can J Gastroenterol 2004; 18:687–690.
26. Vandenplas O, Casel S, Delos M, et al. Granulomatous bronchiolitis associated with Crohn's disease. Am J Respir Crit Care Med 1998; 158:1676–1679.
27. Wallaert B, Colombel JF, Tonnel AB, et al. Evidence of lymphocyte alveolitis in Crohn's disease. Chest 1985; 87:363–367.
28. Yaffe BH, Korelitz BI. Sulfasalazine pneumonitis. Am J Gastroenterol 1983; 78:493–494.
29. Hammar SP. Granulomatous vasculitis. Semin Respir Infect 1995; 10:107–120.
30. Fienberg R, Mark EJ, Goodman M, et al. Correlation of antineutrophil cytoplasmic antibodies with the extrarenal histopathology of Wegener's (pathergic) granulomatosis and related forms of vasculitis. Hum Pathol 1993; 24:160–168.
31. Davenport A, Lock RJ, Wallington TB. Clinical relevance of testing for antineutrophil cytoplasm antibodies (ANCA) with a standard indirect immunofluorescence ANCA test in patients with upper or lower respiratory tract symptoms. Thorax 1994; 49:213–217.

32. Gaudin PB, Askin FB, Falk RJ, et al. The pathologic spectrum of pulmonary lesions in patients with anti-neutrophil cytoplasmic autoantibodies specific for anti-proteinase 3 and anti-myeloperoxidase. Am J Clin Pathol 1995; 104:7–16.
33. Wöckel W, Haussinger K, Weis R, et al. Anticytoplasmic antibodies (cANCA) in syphilitic nodules of the lung. Dtsch Med Wochenschr 1996; 121:617–621.
34. Myers JL, Katzenstein AL. Granulomatous infection mimicking bronchocentric granulomatosis. Am J Surg Pathol 1986; 10:317–322.
35. Farhi DC, Mason UG III, Horsburgh CR Jr. Pathologic findings in disseminated Mycobacterium avium-intracellulare infection. A report of 11 cases. Am J Clin Pathol 1986; 85:67–72.
36. Kauffman HF, Tomee JF, van der Werf TS, et al. Review of fungus-induced asthmatic reactions. Am J Respir Crit Care Med 1995; 151:2109–2115.
37. Yousem SA. Bronchocentric injury in Wegener's granulomatosis: a report of five cases. Hum Pathol 1991; 22:535–540.
38. Klatt EC, Jensen DF, Meyer PR. Pathology of Mycobacterium avium-intracellulare infection in acquired immunodeficiency syndrome. Hum Pathol 1987; 18:709–714.
39. Silva CL, Foss NT. Inflammation induced by a glycolipid fraction from Mycobacterium leprae. Braz J Med Biol Res 1989; 22:327–339.
40. Katapadi K, Pujol F, Vuletin JC, et al. Pulmonary botryomycosis in a patient with AIDS. Chest 1996; 109:276–278.
41. Housini I, Tomashefski JF Jr., Cohen A, et al. Transbronchial biopsy in patients with pulmonary eosinophilic granuloma. Comparison with findings on open lung biopsy. Arch Pathol Lab Med 1994; 118:523–530.
42. Youkeles LH, Grizzanti JN, Liao Z, et al. Decreased tobacco-glycoprotein-induced lymphocyte proliferation in vitro in pulmonary eosinophilic granuloma. Am J Respir Crit Care Med 1995; 151:145–150.
43. Piergili Fioretti D, Moretti A, Mughetti L, et al. Eosinophilia, granuloma formation, migratory behaviour of second stage larvae in murine Toxocara canis infection. Effect of the inoculum size. Parassitologia 1989; 31:153–166.
44. Botros SS, Hassanein HI, Hassan SI, et al. Immunoregulatory potential of exogenous Schistosoma mansoni soluble egg antigen in a model of experimental schistosomiasis—I. Regulation of granuloma formation in vivo. Int J Immunopharmacol 1995; 17:291–302.
45. Sharma OP, Maheshwari A. Lung diseases in the tropics. Part 1: Tropical granulomatous disorders of the lung: diagnosis and management. Tuber Lung Dis 1993; 74:295–304.
46. Annobil SH, Morad NA, Khurana P, et al. Reaction of human lungs to aspirated animal fat (ghee): a clinicopathological study. Virchows Arch 1995; 426:301–305.
47. Henderson RF, Driscoll KE, Harkema JR, et al. A comparison of the inflammatory response of the lung to inhaled versus instilled particles in F344 rats. Fundam Appl Toxicol 1995; 24:183–197.
48. Sakamoto O, Saita N, Yamasaki H, et al. Pulmonary granulomatosis caused by aspirated green tea. Chest 1994; 106:308–309.
49. Hui AN, Koss MN, Hochholzer L, et al. Amyloidosis presenting in the lower respiratory tract. Clinicopathologic, radiologic, immunohistochemical, and histochemical studies on 48 cases. Arch Pathol Lab Med 1986; 110:212.
50. Ravines HT. Pulmonary alveolar microlithiasis: report of nine cases with familial incidence in seven of the nine cases among three families. Am J Clin Pathol 1969; 52:767.
51. Gough J. Pathology of rheumatoid pneumoconiosis. Beitr Silikoseforsch 1965; 6(suppl):307.
52. Yousem SA, Hochholzer L. Pulmonary hyalinizing granuloma. Am J Clin Pathol 1987; 87:1–6.

16
Clinical and Radiological Diagnosis and Causes of Pulmonary Granulomas

OM P. SHARMA
Keck School of Medicine, Los Angeles, California, U.S.A.

I. Introduction

Granuloma is an immunological battleground where a series of complex inflammatory events determine the success of an offending agent or survival of the host. A cascade of interacting extracellular signaling proteins orchestrates the trafficking of immune cells that stage the formation of granuloma. Combining with relevant receptors on the neighboring cells, cytokine regulate expression of adhesion molecules on the vascular endothelium. This interaction in turn favors activation of effector cells and modulates local survival and proliferation of immune cells. If the inciting agent(s) is subdued, the inflammatory response generally resolves. The persistence of the causative agent and/or imbalance of mechanisms that remove inflammatory cells and their byproducts may lead to perpetuation of the granulomatous reaction (1).

The classification of respiratory granulomas is based on the synthesis of evidence based on the clinical features enhanced by histological, microbiological, radiological, and immunological changes. Often radiologists suspect the presence of granulomatous reaction, but it is a pathologist who recognizes histological features. Diagnosis is then completed by a clinician who collates and links clinical, radiological, and histological information. Many pulmonary granulomatous illnesses occur worldwide and are well known; others are endemic in certain areas and only partially identified; still others are rare and barely understood. The causative agents of these disorders range from intracellular organisms (bacteria, mycobacteria, viruses, fungi) to complicated metazoans (helminthes), inanimate substances (metals, chemical agents), and organic antigens (Table 1) (2).

II. History and Physical Examination

A. Location

Tuberculosis and sarcoidosis are the two common causes of pulmonary granulomas in the world. Tuberculosis is particularly rampant in India, Southeast Asia, and Africa; whereas, sarcoidosis has assumed an increasing importance in the United States, Japan, and the European Continent. In Egypt and North Africa schistosomiasis is added to the diagnostic list. Granulomas of visceral leishmaniasis are seen in inhabitants of eastern India and the Mediterranean littorals, while those in association with helminthic infestations should be considered in residents of almost every developing country. Coccidioidomycosis is endemic

Table 1 Some of the Known Causes of Pulmonary Granulomatous Diseases

Infectious agents	
Bacteria	*Brucella abortus*
	Francisella tularensis
	Yersinia
Mycobacteria	*Mycobcaterium tuberculosis*
	M. kansasii
	M. avium
	M. leprae
	M. marinum
Spirochetes	*Treponema pallidum*
	T. carateum
Protozoa	*Toxoplasma gondii*
	Leishmania donovanii
Metazoa	*Schistoma*
	Toxocara
Fungi	*Coccidiodes immitis*
	Histoplasma capsulatum
	Cryptococcus neoformans
Animal and plant proteins	Thermophilic actinomycetes
	Pigeon proteins
	Moldy cork fungus
	Moldy compost
	Moldy sugarcane
	Pituitary snuff
Drugs	Dilantin
	Methotrexate
	Talc
	Bacillus Calmette-Guerin
	Mineral oil
	Phenyl butazone
Chemicals	Beryllium
	Zirconium
	Hard metal
	Silicon

in California; whereas, histoplasmosis is the frequent culprit in the mid-western United States. Behcet's disease is common in Turkey, China, Japan, and Korea (3).

B. Occupational History

In the practice of pulmonary diseases, the occupational history is extremely helpful; ironically, it is often poorly obtained. It is a wise rule to secure the occupational history in a chronological order, from the time the patient left school and obtained his or her first job (part-time or full-time) since certain substances may continue to exert their effects long after the patient has discontinued contact with the particular agent. Asbestos and beryllium are excellent examples of such a delayed response.

Brucellosis is an occupational hazard of veterinary surgeons, laboratory personnel, and abattoir workers. Farmer's lung disease is caused by inhalation of antigenic products of thermophilic actinomycetes (*Micropolyspora faeni*). In Farmer's lung and other hypersensitivity pneumonitides, the causative agent is not detectable on a tissue specimen, but a positive history of exposure is of diagnostic value (Table 2) since it leads one to estimate levels of circulating precipitin antibodies against an appropriate offending antigen. Chronic beryllium disease continues to be hazardous because the metal is being used increasingly in a variety of industries, especially ceramics and metallurgy.

C. Hobbies and Reacreational Activities

Pigeon breeder's lung, parakeet lung, mushroom picker's lung, saxophone player's lung, and many others are acquired while the individual indulges in an apparently harmless pursuit of pleasure. Intravenous drug abuse involving an injection of talc-containing drugs intended for oral use is a known cause of granulomatous inflammation in the lung. Granulomas due to *Coccidioides immitis* may occur in individuals active in unearthing anthropological relics, rock hunting, and digging for bottles in the desert; whereas, spelunkers are at risk for developing histoplasmosis.

D. Family History

If more than one family member suffers from the same granulomatous disease, then the answer might be in the home environment. Poor housing with associated overcrowding increases the risk of infection or reinfection if one of the members has tuberculosis. Leprosy has long been considered to occur only after exposure to a human case, the most important mode of spread of *Mycobacterium leprae* being droplets from the sneezes of a leprosy patient with heavily infected nasal mucosa.

E. Physical Examination

Sarcoidosis, tuberculosis, coccidioidomycosis, histoplasmosis, brucellosis, leishmaniasis, and vasculitides are multisystem disorders with specific manifestations. The patient should be examined for ocular and dermatological lesions, joint involvement, peripheral lymphadenopathy, enlarged spleen, and neurological features. Remittent fever with enlarged liver and spleen in a chronically ill patient suggests leishmaniasis, malaria, and brucellosis. Diagnosis of sarcoidosis rests not only on the obtainment of positive histological findings, but also on the exclusion of diseases that produce sarcoid granulomas.

III. Chest Radiography and HRCT Imaging

An ability to recognize a few typical radiographic patterns goes a long way in evaluating patient with granulomatous lung disease (Table 3). In pulmonary tuberculosis, the characteristic features include unilateral hilar adenopathy, military infiltration, and upper lobe disease with or without cavity. In sarcoidosis bilateral hilar adenopathy occurs in more than 50% of the patients (Fig. 1). In lymphoma and Hodgkin's disease, mediastinal adenopathy is common; hilar adenopathy is less frequent (Fig. 2). Roentgenographic findings in beryllium disease are nonspecific; in early stage, there may be a generalized haziness or a ground-glass appearance throughout both lungs. As the disease progresses, however, bronchial markings and reticulation may appear primarily in the upper lung regions with emphysematous changes in the bases.

Table 2 Chest Radiographic Patterns of Common Pulmonary Granulomatosis

Features	TB	Sarcoidosis	HP	CBD	WG	Lymphoma	Fungi
Hilar adenopathy	Unilateral	Bilateral	Absent	Rare, bilateral	Absent	Uni- or bilateral	Unilateral
Lung infiltrate	Unilateral, upper lobes	Middle and lower lung fields	Diffuse, upper lobes	Diffuse	Patchy	Uncommon	Common
Cavity formation	Common	Rare	Absent	Absent	Common	Rare	Common
Mediastinal adenopathy	Unusual	May occur	Absent	Absent	Absent	Common	May occur
Pleural effusion	Common	Unusual	Absent	Absent	Rare	May occur	May occur
Large nodules	Rare	May occur	Absent	Absent	Common	Common	Common
Small nodules/ miliary	Common	May occur	May occur	May occur	Rare	Rare	Common

Abbreviations: TB, tuberculosis; HP, hypersensitivity pneumonitis; CBD, chronic beryllium disease; WG, Wegener's granulomatosis.

Table 3 Histological Appearance of Common Pulmonary Granulomas

Features	TB	Sarcoidosis	HP	Fungi	Leprosy	Brucellosis	WG
Caseation	Present	Absent	Absent	Absent	Present	Absent	Absent
Necrosis	Present	Rare	Absent	Present	Present	May be present	Present
Inclusion bodies	Present	Present	Rare	Rare	Rare	Rare	Rare
Alveolitis	Absent	Present	Present	Rare	Absent	Absent	Absent
Vasculitis	Rare	Present	Absent	Rare	Absent	Absent	Present
Bronchiolitis	Absent	Rare	Common	Absent	Absent	Absent	Absent

Abbreviations: TB, tuberculosis; HP, hypersensitivity pneumonitis; WG, Wegener's granulomatosis.

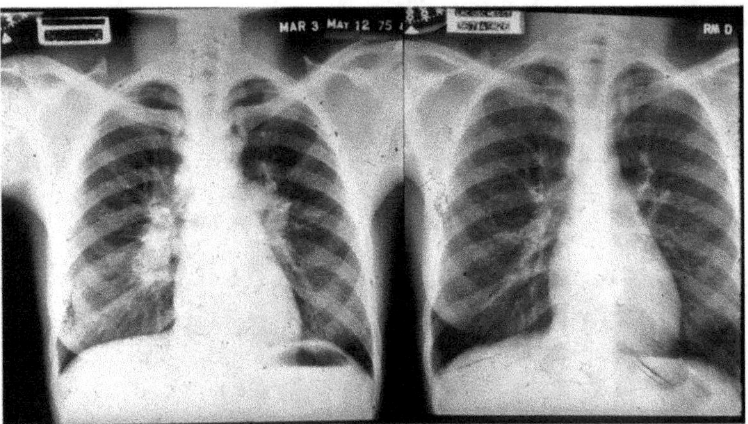

Figure 1 Posteroanterior view of the chest showing bilateral hilar adenopathy (*left*) in a patient with sarcoidosis. Hilar adenopathy subsided (*right*) after six months without treatment.

Chest radiographs are of limited value in patients with granulomatous lung disease. CT and high-resolution computerized tomography (HRCT) are more sensitive in detecting extent and severity of acute and chronic granulomatous lung disease. HRCT has also been used to assess the response to therapy. In most patients with sarcoidosis the main HRCT abnormality is parenchymal and subpleural nodules along with 'bronchovascular beading' (Fig. 3); whereas ground-glass opacity with nodules and a mosaic pattern are seen in hypersensitivity pneumonitis (4).

IV. Skin Tests

Tuberculin, histoplasmin, and coccidioidin skin tests have important roles. There are no skin tests for hypersensitivity pneumonitis, talc granulomatosis, Whipple's disease, and inorganic dust exposures. The Kveim-Siltzbach test is helpful in differentiating sarcoidosis from all other granulomatous disorders, but validated antigen is generally not available.

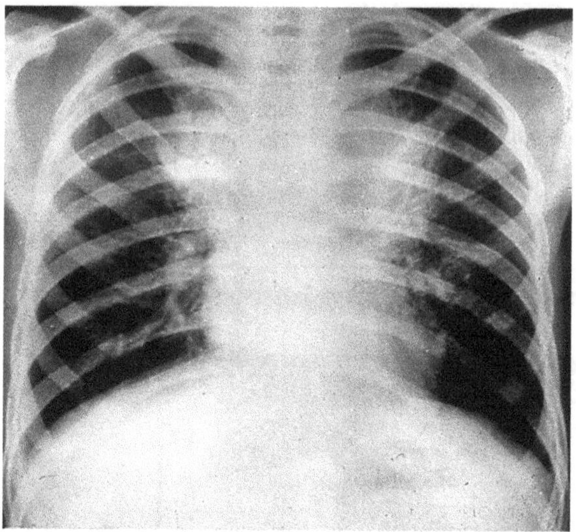

Figure 2 Mediastinal adenopathy in a patient with Hodgkin's disease.

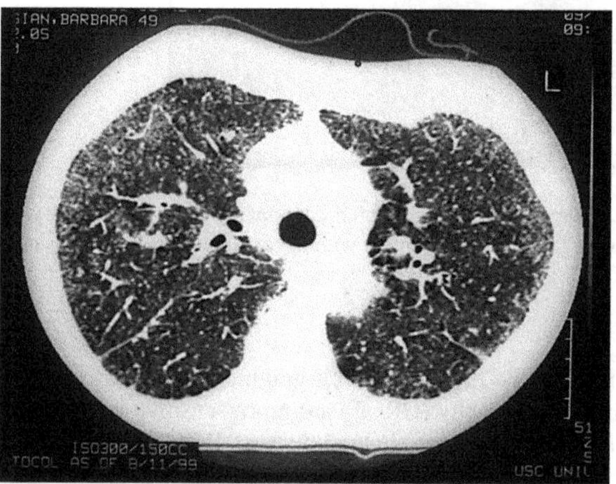

Figure 3 High-resolution computerized tomography (HRCT) showing parenchymal and pleural nodules with nodularity of bronchovascular bundles in a patient with sarcoidosis.

V. Laboratory Tests

Serum angiotensin converting enzyme (ACE) is helpful in supporting the diagnosis of sarcoidosis and monitoring its course and response to treatment. The serum level of ACE reflects the granuloma load; it is elevated in up to 80% of patients with sarcoidosis. SACE level falls with resolution of granulomas and are useful in monitoring the course of the disease. SACE levels are also elevated in other disease. Nevertheless elevated SACE levels associated with hypercalcemia strongly suggest sarcoidosis. This combination is rare in Hodgkin's disease and military tuberculosis. Both agglutinating and complement fixation antibody titers are used to diagnose brucellosis. Serological titers are important in the diagnosis of brucellosis because the organism is fastidious and requires special culture media for optimal growth. The abnormal laboratory finding helpful in diagnosing schistosomal infestation include peripheral eosinophilia and increased serum globulins, especially IgG. The sedimentation rate, C-reactive protein, and antineutrophil cytoplasmic antibody (ANCA) levels may be elevated in granulomas associated with vasculitides. There are two types of ANCA. The cytoplasmic-antineutrophil cytoplasmic antibody (C-ANCA) is specific for Wegener's granulomatosis or necrotizing granulomatous vasculitis. The test often obviates the need for an open lung biopsy. A negative C-ANCA, however does not exclude Wegener's granulomatosis. The perinuclear antineutrophil cytoplasmic antibody (P-ANCA) is nonspecific and present in many autoimmune diseases; however, P-ANCA with specificity against myeloperoxidase is closely associated with microscopic polyangitis affecting small vessels. Lymphocyte transformation test is helpful in diagnosing chronic berylliosis (5).

VI. Important Granulomatous Diseases

A. Mycobacterial Diseases

Tuberculosis

There are more documented tuberculosis cases in the world today than have ever been recorded before. Furthermore, bacterial resistance to single and multiple drugs has become a major health problem. The tuberculosis granulomas are typically necrotic, but in military tuberculosis noncaseating granulomas are common. Hypercalcemia and elevated serum angiotensin converting levels may occur in military tuberculosis. Acid-fast stains and culture of body fluids or tissue biopsy specimens are needed to confirm the diagnosis. Many laboratories use a fluorescent microscope for examination but standard microscopy is much faster because the slide can be scanned at a lower magnification.

Leprosy

This chronic infectious disease is caused by *Mycobacterium leprae*, an organism that has high infectivity, low pathogenicity, and preference for growth in cool, moist areas of the body. The disease is endemic in most of the tropical and warm temperate countries of the world including Southeast Asia, Africa, and South America. In tuberculoid leprosy, granulomas have little or no caseation and the bacilli are scant or altogether absent and can not be cultured or transmitted to usual laboratory animals. Elevated SACE levels may occur in patients with leprosy. Leprosy may mimic other diseases that involve skin and peripheral nerves. The diagnosis is established by clinical evidence of the disease and biopsy. The lepromin skin test is positive in tuberculoid leprosy and negative in lepromatous leprosy.

B. Non-mycobacterial Bacterial Diseases

Brucellosis

A zoonotic infection, brucellosis is caused by bacteria of the genus Brucella. It is an acute or chronic illness that manifests principally by chills, relapses of fever, weakness, body aches, and pains. In the United States, brucellosis is rare and largely an occupational hazard of slaughterhouse workers and veterinarians. It is common in the Far East, Kuwait, Saudi Arabia, and other Persian Gulf countries, South America, Mexico, and the Mediterranean region. The disease can be caused by any of the four species, each usually confined to its major animal host: *B. melitensis* (goat), *B. suis* (hogs), *B. abortus* (cattle), and *B. cannis* (dogs). Granulomas are small and poorly formed. Diagnosis depends on occupational history, clinical features, and serological evidence. A single titer of 1:160 or higher, or a fourfold or greater rise in titers in specimens drawn one to four weeks apart indicates recent infection (6).

Tularemia

Francisella (Pasturella) *tularensis*, a gram-negative coccobacillus, is spread by contact with infected animals or by insect vectors such as ticks. Tularemia, an occupational hazard of sheep herders, trappers, and butchers may present in different ways depending upon the site of inoculation. The common features are skin ulcers, regional lymphadenopathy, and systemic febrile illness. Septicemic tularemia causes military microabscesses in the liver, spleen, and lungs. Healed abscesses form granulomas and fibrosis. Because the organism is fastidious, serological tests are usually necessary for diagnosing tularemia.

C. Fungal Diseases

Histoplasmosis

This granulomatous infection, acquired by inhalation, has been reported from Africa, Asia, Mexico, and South America. In the United States, the midwestern section of the country is an area of the high endemicity.

Histoplasmosis may resemble sarcoidosis and tuberculosis clinically, histologically, and radiologically. Histoplasma granulomas tend to be round and solitary; if multiple, there is usually one dominant lesion. Serum complement fixation, immunodiffusion, and radioimmunoassay may be needed for accurately diagnosing histoplasmosis.

Coccidioidomycosis

Coccidioidomycosis is endemic in the southwestern United States, northern Mexico, and certain parts of central and South America. One-third of the patients develop primary infection after an incubation period of one to three weeks. About two-thirds of infected patients are asymptomatic. Primary coccidioidomycosis is associated with a flu-like illness, fever, chills, erythema nodosum, malaise, and night sweats. Chest X-ray films may show hilar adenopathy, pulmonary infiltrates, and pleural effusion. About 0.5% of patients develop disseminated disease with involvement of meninges, brain, bone, joints, and skin. Serological tests, fungal culture, and demonstration of coccidioidin spherules in the tissue are useful in establishing the diagnosis of coccidioidomycosis (7).

Cryptococcosis

Cryptococcosis is a systemic mycosis caused by the encapsulated yeast-like fungus *Cryptococcus neoformans* and *Cryptococcus neoformans var. gattii*. In immunocompetent

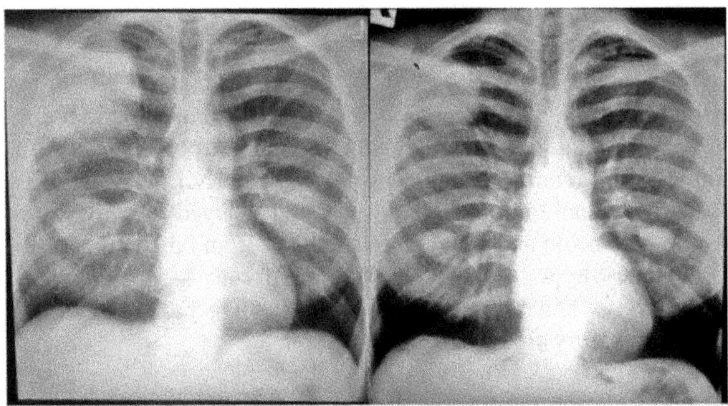

Figure 4 Posteroanterior chest radiograph showing large masses (*left*) in a patient with pulmonary cryptococcosis. The disease responded (*right*) to amphotericin-B therapy.

individuals the infection is usually asymptomatic. Chest radiographs usually single or multiple nodules or masses (Fig. 4). Diagnosis is made by sputum culture or on specimens obtained by bronchial lavage or by histological examination of transbronchial, open or percutaneous lung biopsy specimens. It is essential to exclude meningeal disease in patients with pulmonary cryptococcosis.

D. Parasitic Diseases

Protozoa

Leishmaniasis

Visceral leishmaniasis (kala-azar) has a long incubation period and a chronic course with remittent fever, leucopenia, anemia, and enlarged spleen and liver. The Mediterranean type is prevalent in the Mediterranean and Red Sea littorals, Sudan, Asian Russia, and Arabia; whereas, the Indian type is prevalent in parts of India and Burma bordering the Bay of Bengal. The parasite *Leishmania donovanii* is found in the form of Donovan bodies in the cytoplasm of reticuloendothelial cells or free in the blood plasma. Pulmonary involvement takes the form of bronchitis or bronchopneumonia. Serum IgG is increased. In Africa and other tropical countries, kala-azar is emerging as an important opportunistic infection in patients with acquired immunodeficiency syndrome (AIDS). A diagnostic assay for visceral leishmaniasis using monoclonal antibodies has recently been developed.

Metazoa

Helminthes are common in almost all developing countries. Migration of an helminth through the lung may induce a foreign type reaction with granuloma formation. Nematodes that cause pulmonary granuloma include *Ascaris lumbricoides*, *Toxocara canis*, and *Capillaria aerophila*. Eosinophils may be absent at the onset of the respiratory symptoms, particularly in immunosuppressed hosts. The absence of ova and parasites in stool samples compound the diagnostic dilemma.

Trematodes

Schistosomiasis

Schistoma mansoni has wide geographical distribution in Africa, the Eastern Mediterranean, South America, and the West Indies. The adult female worm deposits eggs in the tissues and induce granulomatous inflammation and fibrosis; particularly in the intestines, liver, and lungs. The *S. mansoni* granuloma is a T-cell-mediated delayed-type hypersensitivity response. Pulmonary hypertension and cor-pulmonale result from obstruction of the vasculature and arteritis. Pulmonary hypertension is less common with *S. japonicum* and *S. hematobium* infections. Diagnosis and assessment of morbidity are based on clinical features, stool egg count, and laboratory findings.

E. Granulomas of Unknown Origin

Sarcoidosis

Sarcoidosis is a multisystem granuloma that has no known cause. The disease has a worldwide distribution, although it is less frequently diagnosed in tropical Africa, India, and Southeast Asia. The frequency of sarcoidosis in the central mountainous district of Japan and the Scandinavian countries is high. It commonly affects young adults and most frequently with bilateral hilar adenopathy, pulmonary infiltration, and skin and eye lesions (Fig. 5). It can involve almost any organ and give rise to many easily recognizable clinical syndromes. Immunological features include depression of peripheral delayed-type hypersensitivity, hyperactivity of T lymphocytes at the site of granuloma formation, and elevated immunoglobulins. Alveolar macrophages from sarcoidosis patients are HLA-DR/D5 positive, can present a variety of antigens to autologous blood T cells, can spontaneously secrete interleukin-1(IL-1) immune interferon, and fibronectin and display C3b and Fc membrane receptors. The diagnosis depends on the evidence of multisystem involvement, typical chest

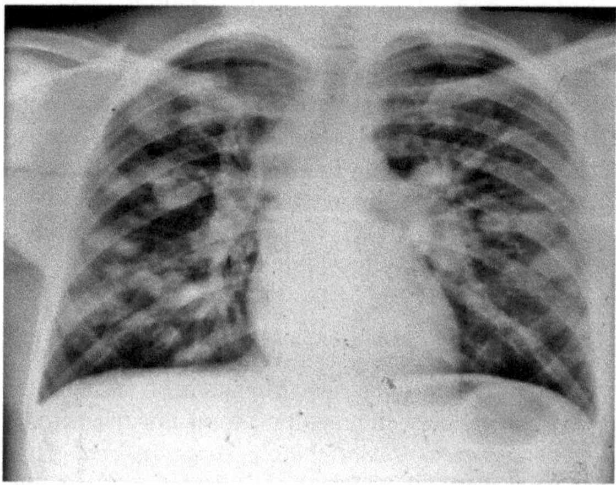

Figure 5 Posteroanterior view of the chest in a patient with sarcoidosis showing hilar and paratracheal adenopathy and pulmonary nodules.

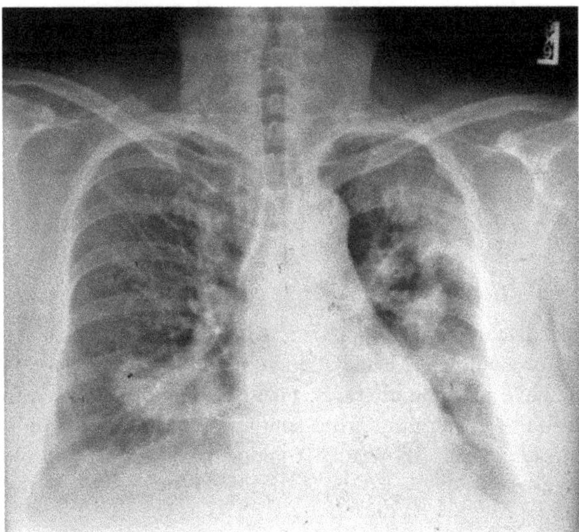

Figure 6 Posteroanterior view of the chest in a 45-year old man with Wegener's granulomatosis showing nodular lung infiltrates.

roentgenographic picture and the presence of noncaseating granulomas in tissue specimens. Elevated ACE levels support the diagnosis (8).

Wegener's Granulomatosis

Wegener's granulomatosis is an organ-specific necrotizing vasculitis involving principally the lungs, upper respiratory tract, and kidneys. The presentation may be generalized with involvement of the nose, sinuses, upper airways, lungs, and kidneys, or it may be limited only to the lungs (Fig. 6). Common presenting symptoms include nasal crusting and bleeding. Pulmonary symptoms include cough, hemoptysis, and chest pain. Renal symptoms, when present, appear after the onset of respiratory symptoms. Low-grade fever, weight loss, and malaise are common in the presence of respiratory symptoms. C-ANCA is almost always elevated in the patients with classical triad of upper airways, lungs, and kidney disease. Many of the patients with mild disease respond to treatment with trimethiprin-sulfamethoxazole; it is therefore possible that the causative agent for the disease may as yet be an unidentified infectious agent.

Pulmonary Allergic Granulomatosis

This relatively rarely diagnosed syndrome consists of asthma, eosinophilia, and vascular lesions similar to the type seen in polyarteritis nodosa. The chest radiographic picture is nonspecific, consisting of transient patchy infiltrates, multiple nodules with or without cavitation, and diffuse interstitial pattern. The cause of the illness is not known. Diagnosis is based on a history of asthma, the presence of eosinophilia and elevated serum IgE, and histological picture of necrotizing vasculitis with tissue eosinophilia, and extravascular granulomas.

Lymphomatoid Granulomatosis

It is characterized by pulmonary reticulo-infiltrates that are angiocentric and angiodestructive. Pulmonary symptoms of cough, dyspnea, and chest pain are common. Constitutional symptoms, skin lesions, and neurological involvement are frequent. Chest X-ray films show bilateral nodular infiltrates that are frequently peripheral and may be mistaken for metastatic tumors. Approximately 10% of pulmonary disease initially diagnosed as lymphomatoid granulomatosis (LG) eventually develop malignant lymphoma.

Bronchocentric Granulomatosis

This is a necrotizing granulomatous disease of the lungs in which the granulomas are centered principally on bronchi and bronchioles. Most patients with this disease have a history of chronic asthmas and some have multiple allergies. Positive skin tests and serum precipitins to Aspergillus, and isolation of Aspergillus from sputum cultures from several patients have been observed. Chest radiographs show involvement of single or multiple lobes with unilateral or bilateral disease.

Whipple's Disease

Whipple's disease is a rare multisystem disease, caused by infection with bacterium *Tropheryma whippelii*. The clinical picture varies greatly: patients can present with arthralgia or with cardiac, pulmonary, endocrine, ocular, neurological, psychiatric, and skin manifestations. Sarcoid-like granulomas have been described in various organs. Diagnostic tests include staining with periodic acid-Schiff (PAS), electron microscopy, immunohistochemistry, and polymerase chain reaction (9,10).

Multicentric Reticulohistiocytosis

Multicentric reticulohistiocytosis (MRH) is characterized by inflltration of multinucleated giant cells and histiocytes into various tissues. The typical clinical picture consists of papular skin nodules and destructive arthritis. The disease usually occurs in the fourth decade and affects women three times more often than men, predominantly Caucasian women. About one-third of the patients may have an associated malignant lymphoma. MRH consists of multinucleated giant cells and histiocytes with eosinophilic PAS-positive cytoplasm. It can spontaneously resolve or it may progress to severe arthritis (11).

F. Granulomas Caused by Organic Antigens

Hypersensitivity Pneumonitis

This group of pulmonary disorders includes several diseases. They all seem to be initiated by inhalation of organic dust, leading to chronic alveolar inflammation, granulomas formation and fibrosis. Hypersensitivity pneumonitis should be suspected when a person is exposed to organic antigens and complains of malaise, fatigue, dyspnea, cough. Wheezing is usually absent. If not detected early and further exposure to the causative agent is permitted, the symptoms continue, and become very severe in some cases. A chest X-ray film may show diffuse reticulonodular infiltrate or honeycombing. Lung-function impairment is usually of restrictive type; however, airway obstruction is not unusual. Diagnosis is supported by a positive precipitin test (12).

G. Granulomas Caused by Inorganic Granulomas

Berylliosis

The inhalation of beryllium dusts, salts, or fumes is associated with two types pulmonary disease; an acute chemical pneumonitis caused by short exposures to high concentrations and a chronic interstitial granulomatous disease caused by lower concentrations over long periods of time. Modern use of beryllium is found in the nuclear, electronics and aerospace industries. Because of the widespread use of beryllium and its salt in industry, the incidence of chronic, dermal, and pulmonary disease has increased. The chest X-ray may show a mottled appearance in both lungs, occasionally with bilateral hilar adenopathy. Chronic interstitial pneumonitis and noncaseating granulomas are seen in the lung biopsy specimens. The diagnosis depends on the history of exposure to beryllium, positive lymphocyte transformation tests, presence of beryllium in tissues and body fluids, and granulomas in tissue biopsies.

H. Drug-Induced Granulomas

The drugs that cause granulomatous reaction in the body are disodium chromoglycate, magnesium trisilicate, methotrexate, Bacillus Calmette-Guerin (BCG), aspirated oil, and chronic vaseline when used to the nose (13).

VII. Conclusion

The definitive diagnosis of the cause of pulmonary granulomatous disease requires a complete occupational and clinical history, physical examination, recognition of typical and atypical radiographic features, and appropriate serological and immunological tests. A tissue biopsy is needed to establish the diagnosis in difficult cases.

References

1. Agostini C, Semenzato G. Biology and immunology of granuloma. In: James DG, Zumla A, eds. The Granulomatous Disorders. Cambridge, UK: Cambridge University Press, 1999:3–16.
2. James D, Williams J. Classification of granulomatous disorders: a clinico-pathological synthesis. In: James DG, Zumla A, eds. The Granulomatous Disorders. Cambridge, UK: Cambridge University Press, 1999:17–27.
3. Zumla A, James D. Granulomatous infections: an overview. In: James DG, Zumla A, eds. The Granulomatous Disorders. Cambridge, UK: Cambridge University Press, 1999:103–121.
4. Richenberg J, Bomanji J. Imaging of granulomatous disorders. In: James D, Zumla A, eds. The Granulomatous Disorders. Cambridge, UK: Cambridge University Press, 1999:28–55.
5. Infante P, Newman L. Beryllium exposure and chronic beryllium disease. Lancet 2004; 363:415–416.
6. Lulu A, Araj G. Pulmonary complications of Brucellosis. In: Sharma O, ed. Lung Diseases in the Tropics. New York: Marcel Dekker, Inc., 1991:157–176.
7. Hage C, Sarosi G. Endemic Mycosis. In: Sharma O, ed. Tropical Lung Disease. 2nd ed. New York: Taylor and Francis Group, 2006:397–430.
8. Sharma OP. Sarcoidosis. London: Butterworths Inc., 1984:1–174.
9. Dzirlo L, Hubner M, Muller C, et al. A mimic of sarcoidosis. Lancet 2007; 369:1832.
10. Fenollar F, Puechal X, Raoult D. Whipple's disease. N Engl J Med 2007; 356:55–66.

11. Chauhan A, Mikulik Z, Hackshaw K, et al. Multicentric reticulohistiocytosis with positive anticyclic citrullinated antibodies. J Natl Med Assoc 2007; 99:678–680.
12. Rose C. Hypersensitivity pneumonitis. In: Mason R, Broaddus V, Murray J, et al., eds. Murray and Nadel's Textbook of Respiratory Medicine. 4th ed. Philadelphia: Elsevier Saunders, 2005: 1783–1799.
13. Limper A. Drug-induced pulmonary disease. In: Mason R, Broaddus V, Murray J, et al., eds. Murray and Nadel's Textbook of Respiratory Medicine. 4th ed. Philadelphia: Elsevier Saunders, 2005:1888–1912.

17
Enlarged Airspaces

ANNA E. SIENKO
The Methodist Hospital, Houston, Texas, U.S.A.

I. Introduction

Differential diagnosis of enlarged airspaces is relatively short and includes enlarged airspaces as part of a specific underlying pathological process or because of artifact. There are only few entities in adults where true enlarged airspaces are present on histological examination and include emphysema, lymphangioleiomyomatosis (LAM) and "honeycombing" due to end-stage lung disease fibrosis (Table 1).

II. Artifacts

The most common artifact is due to overinflation of resection or wedge biopsy specimens creating large airspaces (1). No destruction of alveolar walls is seen, which is characteristic of emphysema and histologically represented by short segments of detached fragmented alveolar septa.

Empty fat-like spaces or "bubble" artifacts are seen in the alveoli most often in biopsy specimens (transbronchial and wedge resection) and are due to crushing of the specimen and hemorrhage. Tissue processing leaves the bubble spaces on the tissue section slides, which can mimic exogenous lipoid pneumonia at first glance (Fig. 1). However, true lipoid pneumonia is accompanied by numerous intra-alveolar foamy macrophages, chronic interstitial inflammation, foreign body–type giant cell reaction, and a variable amount of fibrosis (2).

III. Emphysema

Emphysema is defined as permanent abnormal enlargement of airspaces distal to the terminal bronchioles with destruction of the alveolar walls without fibrosis. Emphysema is classified according to which portion of the acinus is affected (1,3).

Panacinar emphysema by definition involves the entire acinus equally and characteristically the lower lobes. Alpha-1-antitrypsin deficiency is most often associated with panacinar emphysema and is the form of emphysema seen in IV drug abusers (1,4,5).

Centrilobular (proximal acinar) emphysema involves the central or proximal portion of the bronchiole with emphysematous change limited to the bronchiole and surrounding airspace. The distal acini are not involved. Centrilobular emphysema is most often the form

Table 1 Comparison of True Enlarged Airspaces

True enlarged airspace	Features
Emphysema (panlobular, centrilobular, distal)	Damaged disrupted alveolar septa
LAM	Airspace surrounded by proliferation of spindle cells forming aggregates and nodules
Honeycombing	Background of surrounding lung parenchyma with fibrosis, chronic inflammation; no normal alveolated lung present

Abbreviation: LAM, lymphangioleiomyomatosis.

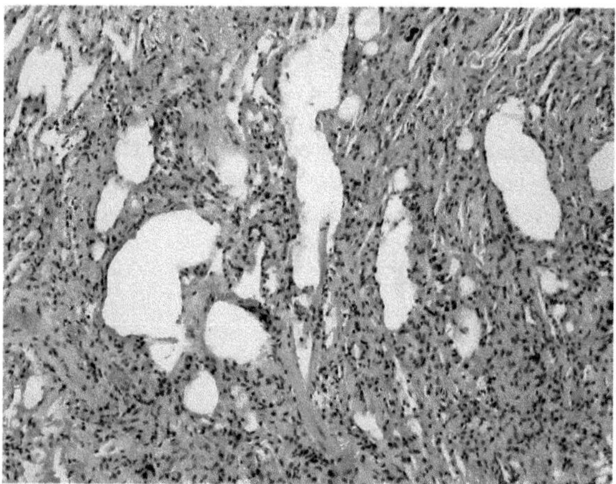

Figure 1 Pseudolipoid artifact. Transbronchial biopsy showing artifactual parenchymal condensation and "pseudolipoid" enlarged airspaces. (H&E, 10×).

associated with cigarette smoking and involves the upper lobes predominately (Figs. 2 and 3). Histological features similar to centrilobular emphysema can be seen secondary to dust exposure. The changes are usually focal and the result of mineral dusts such as coal dust, asbestos, hematite ore, and slate dust. Features of pigmentation, fibrosis, and distortion of the bronchioles can be seen within adjacent enlarged airspaces (4,6,7).

Distal acinar emphysema (paraseptal) involves the acinus distal portion including subpleural areas and along the intralobular septae. Pulmonary function is not greatly affected in distal acinar emphysema; however, there is increased risk for spontaneous pneumothorax and the formation of bullae (7).

IV. Other

Bullae are airspaces composed of thick fibrous walls in the visceral pleura that may extend to focally involve the subpleura or underlying lung parenchyma. Bullae by definition are usually larger than 1.0 cm in size and can be associated with emphysema regardless of type

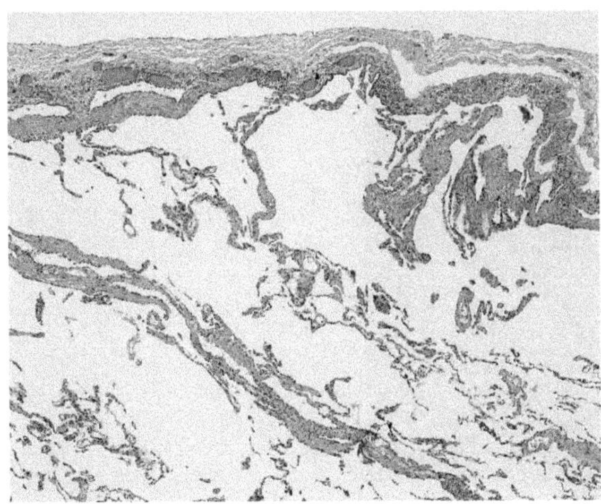

Figure 2 Emphysema. Variably sized enlarged air spaces with disrupted and fragmented alveolar septa. No increased fibrosis is present. (H&E, 4×). *Source*: Courtesy of Dr. Timothy Allen University of Texas Health Science Center Tyler, Tyler, Texas, U.S.A.

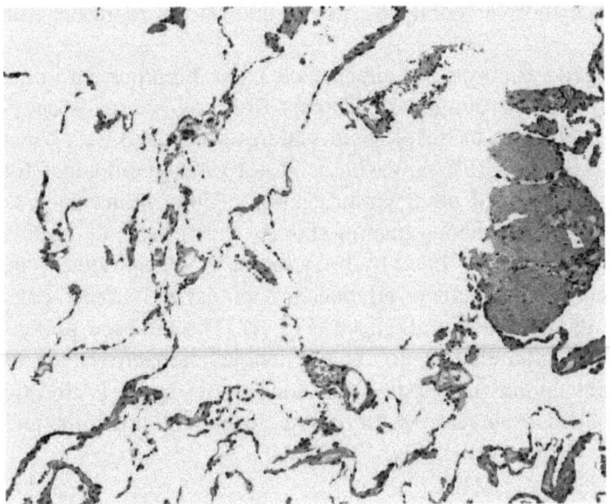

Figure 3 Emphysema. Loose fragments and segments of alveolar septa indicating destruction. (H&E, 10×). *Source*: Courtesy of Dr. Timothy Allen University of Texas Health Science Center Tyler, Tyler, Texas, U.S.A.

or uncommonly in normal lung. Giant bullous emphysema or vanishing lung syndrome refers to the occasional cases seen in distant acinar emphysema of prominent bilateral bullae with compression of adjacent lung parenchyma (4,6,7).

Parenchymal scars may have emphysema-like surrounding enlarged airspaces. The airspaces have also been termed scar emphysema, traction, or irregular emphysema. These

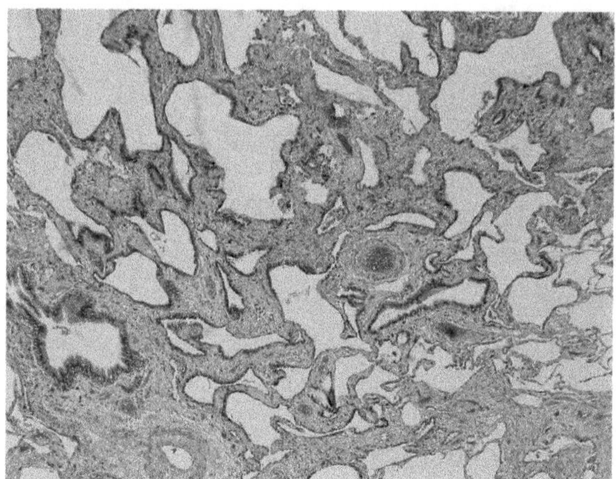

Figure 4 Honeycombing. Low-power view showing various sized enlarged airspaces with surrounding fibrotic lung parenchyma. (H&E, 4×).

enlarged air spaces, however, do not show alveolar destruction and do not represent true emphysema (1,7).

Honeycombing seen as enlarged variably sized airspaces is most often present in the background of end-stage lung disease and pulmonary fibrosis from any cause. Honeycombing can be seen as one of the spectrum of histological features associated with usual interstitial pneumonia or fibrosis (UIP or UIF); however, it is not pathognomonical for either. Honeycombing can be seen because of other varied causes of lung injury such as healing infarcts, resolving infections, spontaneous pneumothorax, aspirations, or trauma (8,9). Histologically, the honeycomb airspace is lined by bronchiolar type/respiratory type of epithelium consisting of columnar ciliated cells or attenuated cuboidal to flattened cells that can show metaplastic change to squamous epithelium (Fig. 4). The airspace lumens may be filled with mucinous material, inflammatory debris, pigment laden macrophages, or foamy macrophages. The lung parenchyma surrounding the honeycomb space is fibrotic with complete loss of normal alveolated architecture with foci of chronic inflammation and blood vessels with hypertrophy of vascular walls (Fig. 5) (8,9).

V. Lymphangioleiomyomatosis

LAM is a rare pulmonary disorder affecting predominately females of reproductive age. The lungs show cystic, enlarged airspaces with characteristic proliferation of smooth muscle fibers around or in the immediate adjacent lung parenchyma surrounding the enlarged airspace (Fig. 6). The LAM smooth muscle fibers are round or spindle shaped with moderate amounts of eosinophilic cytoplasm and are arranged in a disorderly fashion as nodules and aggregates around the airspace (Fig. 7). LAM cells stain with "usual" smooth muscle markers such as smooth muscle actin, desmin, and vimentin but unlike smooth

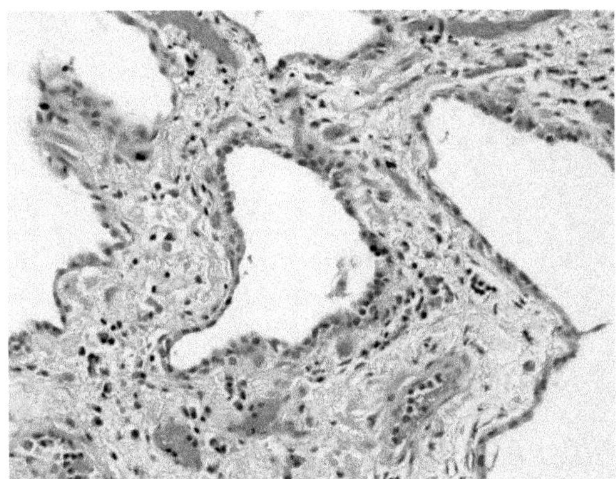

Figure 5 Honeycombing. High-power view of "honeycomb" airspace lined by metaplastic epithelium and surrounding expanded fibrotic interstitium with chronic inflammation. (H&E, 10×).

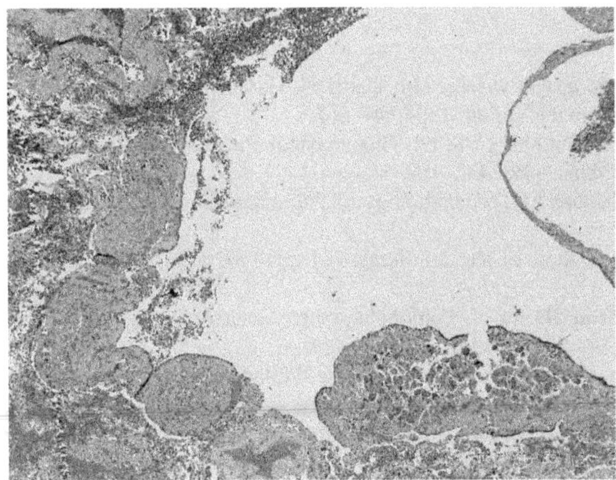

Figure 6 LAM. Low power of enlarged airspace with peripheral proliferation of spindle cells surrounding the airspace. (H&E, 4×). *Abbreviation*: LAM, lymphangioleiomyomatosis.

muscle fibers also stain with HMB-45, and estrogen and progesterone receptors (10). Variable mitosis and features of cytological atypia may be present.

The LAM cells can infiltrate blood vessels, airway walls, and lymphatics resulting in pulmonary hemorrhage with accumulations of hemosiderin-laden macrophages, chylous effusions, and pneumothorax. LAM can be associated with tuberous sclerosis (TSC); however, most patients with LAM do not have TSC. Progression of LAM is common with most patients eventually requiring lung transplantation that offers the only "cure" (11).

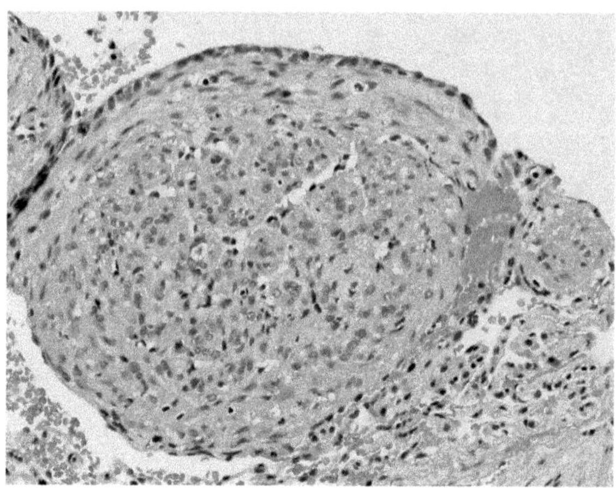

Figure 7 LAM. High power of LAM nodule composed of spindled cells underlying a layer of cuboidal to columnar pneumocytes. (H&E, 20×). *Abbreviation*: LAM, lymphangioleiomyomatosis.

References

1. Pratt PC. Emphysema and chronic airway disease. In: Dail DH, Hammer SP, eds. Pulmonary Pathology. 2nd ed. New York: Springer-Verlag, 1994:847–865.
2. Colby TV, Yousem SA. Lung. In: Sternberg SS, ed. Histology for Pathologists. 2nd ed. New York: Lippincott Williams & Wilkins, 1997:433–458.
3. Sononya RE. Emphysema. In: Saldana MJ, ed. Pathology of Pulmonary Disease. Philadelphia: Lippincott, 1994:275–286.
4. Wright JL, Cagle P, Churg A, et al. State of the art: diseases of small air ways. Am Rev Respir Dis 1991; 146:240–262.
5. Schmidt RA, Glenny RW, Godwin JD, et al. Panlobular emphysema in young intravenous Ritalin abusers. Am Rev Respir Dis 1991; 143:649.
6. Thurlbeck WM. Chronic Airflow Obstruction in Lung Disease. Philadelphia: Saunders, 1976.
7. Katzenstein, ALA. II. Miscellaneous nonspecific inflammatory and destructive diseases. In: Katzenstein, ALA, ed. Katzenstein & Askin's Surgical Pathology of Non-Neoplastic Lung Disease. Vol 13, 4th ed. Major Problems in Pathology Series. Philadelphia: Saunders Elsevier, 2006:445–475.
8. Cagle PT. Usual or non-specific interstitial pneumonia, interstitial fibrosis and the honeycomb lung. In: Saldana MJ, ed. Pathology of Pulmonary Disease. Philadelphia: Lippincott, 1994:325–339.
9. Katzenstein ALA. Idiopathic interstitial pneumonia: Chapter 3. In: Katzenstein ALA, ed. Katzenstein & Askin's Surgical Pathology of Non-Neoplastic Lung Disease. Vol 13, 4th ed. Major Problems in Pathology Series. Philadelphia: Saunders Elsevier, 2006:51–84.
10. Goncharova EA, Krymskaya VP. Pulmonary lymphangioleiomyomatosis (LAM): progress and current challenges. J Cell Biochem 2007; Epub ahead of print].
11. Pechet TT, Meyers BF, et al. Lung transplantation for lymphangioleiomyomatosis. J Heart Lung Transplant 2004; 23:301–308.

18
Pulmonary Vascular Lesions

JOHN C. ENGLISH
Vancouver General Hospital and The University of British Columbia,
Vancouver, British Columbia, Canada

I. Normal Microscopic Anatomy of the Pulmonary Vascular System

Many pathological lesions of the pulmonary vascular system are subtle and only focally present; therefore, familiarity with the normal anatomical disposition and microscopic features of pulmonary blood vessels is vital in order to make an accurate diagnosis. Careful fixation and appropriate selection of tissue stains provide the best starting point. Ideally, pneumonectomy and lobectomy specimens are inflated with formalin through the bronchi. Thoracoscopic or open lung wedge biopsies are carefully expanded with fixative by transalveolar needle inflation. Uncontrolled or excessively pressurized direct vascular perfusion may unnaturally overdistend vessels and is generally not recommended (1). Large specimens must be sampled liberally, given the focality of some lesions, and all tissue in a wedge biopsy should be submitted. The standard hematoxylin and eosin (H&E) stain is useful (and optimal) for general purposes, and use of an elastic stain (e.g., Verhoff-van Gieson or Movat pentachrome) is necessary for thorough tissue examination.

A. The Pulmonary Arterial System

The internal diameter of the pulmonary trunk approximates that of the aorta; however, the media is 60% thinner, with a more irregular arrangement of the elastic laminae. The pulmonary arterial branching pattern is not precisely dichotomous as it extends distally aside the airway within the bronchovascular sheath; there are approximately 17 orders of branching with supernumerary vessels periodically given off (2). The arteries branch slightly before the airway accounting for the frequent observation of two arterial profiles adjacent to one airway. The thinner pulmonary arterial/arteriolar wall (Fig. 1) reflects the low-pressure resident in the pulmonary circuit. As such, distinction from veins is difficult for the inexperienced observer. An anatomical classification of the pulmonary vasculature is given in Table 1. The basis for classification of these vessels originated with the work of Brenner (2).

B. Pulmonary Veins

Intra-acinar venules empty into the veins of the secondary lobular (interlobular) septae; a single vein drains each lobule (1). Pulmonary veins have no valves. Distinctive age-related intimal sclerosis affects acinar venules ubiquitously; inexperienced observers may mistakenly take these changes for hypertensive arterial remodeling.

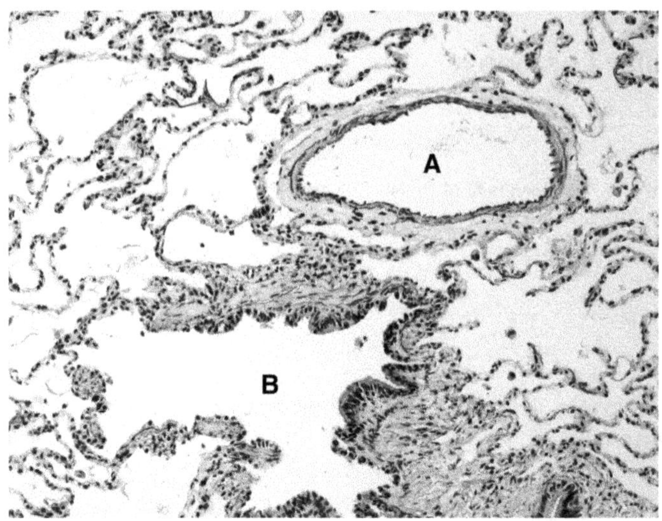

Figure 1 Normal pulmonary artery and vein. The pulmonary artery (**A**) diameter is similar to that of the accompanying bronchiole (**B**). The arterial tunica media is approximately 5% of the external diameter (external elastica to external elastica). Movat pentachrome stain.

II. Abnormal Connections (Congenital Malformations of the Pulmonary Vascular Tree)

Pulmonary vascular pathology as a result of congenital disease may manifest as a diffuse spectrum of changes involving large and small arterial and/or venous vessels. These are presented in Table 2.

III. Thickened Pulmonary Vasculature

A. Intimal Thickening

Age-Related Changes

With advancing age, and independently of pulmonary hypertension, eccentric patches of intimal fibrosis develop, which are morphologically suggestive of organizing thrombosis. The thickenings are consistent with the concept of focal intima hyperplasia as an adaptation to flow irregularities, particularly when present at bifurcations. These patches or plaques may reach thicknesses of 8% to 20% of the vessel's internal diameter (18). In elastic pulmonary arteries, shallow atheromas may be identified, sometimes as far distally as the lobar arteries; these may be the sequelae of the focal unfolding of vessels, producing local flow irregularities and inciting an inflammatory response along the lines of the "response-to-injury" hypothesis.

A commonly observed age-related change of the pulmonary venules and smaller veins is hyaline intimal sclerosis. This alteration is ubiquitous and should not necessarily be

Table 1 Anatomical Features of the Pulmonary Vasculature

Vessel type	Example	Accompanying airway or structure	Size limits	Composition
Elastic pulmonary artery	Pulmonary trunk, lobar, segmental arteries	Main bronchus, lobar, segmental, subsegmental bronchi	>500 or >1000 μm outside diameter (O.D.)	• Elastic laminae arranged concentrically, enclosing smooth muscle cells, collagen, and acid mucopolysaccharide ground substance • Elastic thick at birth, becomes more discontinuous with adulthood • Elastic/muscle layers more concentric in intrapulmonary arteries • No. of laminae 16–20 in large (>5000 μm diameter) vessels; 3–4 in smaller (500–1000 μm) vessels • Thick internal elastic lamina • Well-defined external elastic lamina only appears in the smallest elastic arteries • Vasa vasorum supply media
Musculo-elastic pulmonary arteries (some group these with elastic pulmonary arteries)	Segmental/subsegmental arteries (transitional)	Segmental, subsegmental bronchi	500–1000 μm O.D.	• Elastic laminae become discontinuous, gradually disappear • Retention of internal and external elastic laminae

(Continued)

Table 1 Anatomical Features of the Pulmonary Vasculature (*Continued*)

Vessel type	Example	Accompanying airway or structure	Size limits	Composition
Muscular pulmonary arteries	Subsegmental, intra-acinar vessels	Subsegmental bronchi terminal and respiratory bronchioles, alveolar ducts	50–1000 μm	• Muscular media, rare elastic fibers (especially proximally, elastic fibers with branching) • Medial thickness ~5% of O.D. • Distinct internal and external elastic laminae • Vasa vasorum (in adventitia) only in large muscular branches • Intima consists of endothelial layer and basement membrane only, resting on internal elastic lamina • Adventitia of variable thickness: thicker than media in larger muscular arteries; thinner than media in smaller branches
Arterioles	Intra-acinar vessels	Respiratory bronchioles, alveolar ducts, alveolar walls	15–150 μm	• Initial segments have distinct internal and external elastic laminae enclosing a complete muscle layer; muscle becomes discontinuous in vessels of ~70 μm diameter (respiratory bronchiolar level) • Smallest arterioles have only single elastic lamina
Venules	Intra-acinar vessels	As for arterioles	<100 μm	• Venule structure indistinct from arterioles (endothelial lining on single elastic lamina; negligible or absent adventitia) • Size increases as vessels reach periphery of acinus
Veins	Interlobular vessels	Interlobular septae	>100 μm	• Medial smooth muscle bundles divided by irregular elastic laminae • Adventitia contains collagen, elastic fibers, and often longitudinally oriented smooth muscle • No distinct external elastic lamina; media tends to “blend” with adventitia • Venous valves not present

Table 2 Abnormal Connections (Congenital Malformations of the Pulmonary Vascular Tree)

Abnormality	Comment	References
I. Pulmonary trunk		
A. Congenital idiopathic dilation of the pulmonary trunk	Simple dilation restricted to the pulmonary trunk, probably reflecting a developmental defect in the absence of chronic pulmonary disease, cardiac shunts, valve gradients, or chronic arterial disease such as syphilis or significant atherosclerosis. Some cases demonstrate cystic medial degeneration histologically. Generally benign, although dissection has been reported	3,4
B. Congenital stenosis of the pulmonary trunk	Supravalvular—thickening of the tunica media	5
	Bifurcation—("coarctation of the pulmonary artery")	
C. Pulmonary atresia	Possible association with tetralogy of Fallot/distal pulmonary stenoses	4
D. Persistent truncus arteriosus	Failure of partitioning of aorta from pulmonary trunk leaves single vessel exiting from ventricle. Associated with ventricular septal defect, pulmonary hypertension, other congenital defects	6
E. Aorticopulmonary septal defect (aorticopulmonary window)	Focal absence of the truncoconal septum. Associations include pulmonary hypertension, patent ductus arteriosus, and coarctation of the aorta	7
F. Anomalous origin of the coronary arteries from the pulmonary trunk	Typically left coronary arising from the pulmonary trunk producing severe postnatal left ventricular ischemia; anastomotic right coronary perfusion with retrograde flow into the pulmonary trunk results in pulmonary hypertension	1
II. Pulmonary arterial branches		
A. Anomalous origin of the pulmonary arteries		
1. "Crossed pulmonary arteries"	Right pulmonary artery arises below and to the left of the left pulmonary artery and crosses behind it and the aorta as it courses toward the right lung	
2. "Vascular sling"	The left pulmonary artery arises from the right pulmonary artery and crosses posterior to the trachea and anterior to the esophagus as it courses toward the right lung, often compressing the right bronchus. Tetralogy of Fallot is a recognized association	4
3. Origin from the aorta or its branches	(*i*) Origin of a pulmonary artery (usually the right) from the ascending aorta; the residual pulmonary trunk continues as the contralateral pulmonary artery; (*ii*) one or both arteries arise from the aortic arch or innominate artery; distal stenoses may coexist; (*iii*) sequestration of a lobe or portion thereof, with blood supply derived from the thoracic or abdominal aorta	4

(*Continued*)

Table 2 Abnormal Connections (Congenital Malformations of the Pulmonary Vascular Tree) (*Continued*)

Abnormality	Comment	References
B. Absent right or left pulmonary artery	Affected lung is supplied by an anomalous systemic connection. Associations include patent ductus arteriosus (absent right artery) and tetralogy of Fallot (absent left artery)	
C. Pulmonary stenosis/atresia	Stenoses: anatomical types include (*i*) localized stenosis with poststenotic segmental dilation, (*ii*) segmental stenosis, (*iii*) diffuse tubular hypoplasia, (*iv*) multiple peripheral pulmonary arterial stenoses. Intimal hyperplasia with medial thickening identified pathologically. Part of the spectrum of Alagille syndrome.	8,9,10
	Atresia: focal or diffuse changes seen in peripheral pulmonary arteries; if diffuse, the pulmonary trunk can be involved and associated with tetralogy of Fallot	
D. Misaligned pulmonary vessels (alveolar capillary dysplasia)	Seen as anatomical juxtaposition of pulmonary arteries and veins within the bronchovascular bundle and lobular parenchyma; arteries demonstrate medial thickening; parenchymal abnormalities are typically present and include a variably severe reduction in the capillary bed. Neonatal hypertension may be fatal if the condition is manifest in its complete form	11,12
III. Disorders of the pulmonary veins		
A. Anomalous pulmonary venous connection	Pulmonary venous circulation is anatomically diverted to the right atrium. Multiple variations are recognized: (*i*) most usually, a common chamber receives venous drainage and subsequently connects with the left innominate vein. Obstruction of this conduit occurs due to compression between the bronchus and left pulmonary artery. Other cardiac and extracardiac connections also occur. (*ii*) Subdiaphragmatic connection to the ductus venosus, portal or left gastric vein with attendant atrial septal defect or patent foramen ovale; pulmonary hypertension and right ventricular hypertrophy reflect obstructive hemodynamics. (*iii*) Partial anomalous drainage, typically from the right side through the superior vena cava. Associations include asplenia/polysplenia syndromes, sinus venosus atrial septal defect and the "scimitar syndrome", the latter named for the characteristic curvilinear roentgenographic density produced by the right lower lobe vein as it joins the vena cava; dextroposition of the heart forms part of this complex.	4,13

B. Cor triatrium	Presence of an accessory atrial chamber receiving the pulmonary outflow. The opening between this chamber and the left ventricle is related to the degree of pulmonary hypertension	
C. Congenital pulmonary venous stenosis	Focal segmental or diffuse tubular hypoplastic forms are recognized. The junction with the left atrium is particularly affected but peripheral stenoses may be present. Pathological changes include intimal fibrous thickening, fibrous cords, medial/intimal fibromuscular proliferation, and adventitial fibrosis. Pulmonary hypertension is a potential complication; atrial septal defect is the most commonly recognized cardiac anomaly	4,14
IV. Pulmonary arteriovenous aneurysm (PAA); pulmonary arteriovenous malformation (PAVM)	Abnormal communications between the pulmonary artery and vein. The pathological spectrum ranges from multiple telangiectatic lesions to single, large aneurysm-like structures. There is a strong association with hereditary hemorrhagic telangiectasia (HHT, Osler-Webber-Rendu disease). Pulmonary hypertension is uncommon (also see sect. VI)	15,16,17

Table 3 Clinical Classification of Pulmonary Hypertension (PH) ("Venice Classification", 2003)

- I. Pulmonary arterial hypertension (PAH)
  - A. Idiopathic pulmonary arterial hypertension (IPAH)
  - B. Familial pulmonary arterial hypertensions (FPAH)
  - C. Pulmonary arterial hypertension associated with other diseases (APAH)
    1. Collagen vascular diseases
    2. Congenital systemic-to-pulmonary shunts
    3. Portal hypertension
    4. HIV infection
    5. Drugs and toxins
    6. Other conditions
       - a. Thyroid disease
       - b. Glycogen storage disorders
       - c. Gaucher disease
       - d. Hereditary hemorrhagic telangiectasia
       - e. Hemoglobinopathies
       - f. Myeloproliferative disorders
       - g. Splenectomy
  - D. With significant venous or capillary involvement
    1. Pulmonary veno-occlusive disease (PVOD)
    2. Pulmonary capillary hemangiomatosis (PCH)
  - E. Persistent pulmonary hypertension of the newborn
- II. PH associated with left-sided heart disease
  - A. Atrial or ventricular heart disease
  - B. Valvular heart disease
- III. PH associated with (chronic) pulmonary disease and/or hypoxia
  - A. Chronic obstructive lung disease (COPD)
  - B. Interstitial lung disease (ILD)
  - C. Sleep-disordered breathing
  - D. Alveolar hypoventilation disorders
  - E. Chronic high altitude exposure
  - F. Neonatal lung disease
  - G. Alveolar-capillary dysplasia
  - H. Other
- IV. PH secondary to chronic thrombotic or embolic disease (CTEPH)
  - A. Thromboembolic obstruction of proximal pulmonary arteries
  - B. Thromboembolic obstruction of distal pulmonary arteries
  - C. Non-thrombotic pulmonary embolism
    1. Tumour
    2. Parasites
    3. Foreign material
- V. PH from miscellaneous causes
  - A. Sarcoidosis
  - B. Pulmonary Langerhans cell histiocytosis (PLCH)
  - C. Lymphangiomatosis
  - D. External vascular compression (adenopathy, neoplasm, fibrosing mediastinitis)

Abbreviation: PH, pulmonary hypertension.
Source: Modified from Ref. 20.

construed as a sign of pulmonary hypertension. Recognition of the vessel as venous rather than arterial usually obviates the potential for misinterpretation.

Lesions Identified in Pulmonary Arterial Hypertension

Many of the manifestations of vascular thickening (intimal, medial, and adventitial) are related to pulmonary arterial hypertension (PAH), a condition generally defined by resting mean pulmonary arterial pressure >25 mmHg (19). A contemporary clinical classification of PAH is presented in Table 3 (20).

Cellular Intimal Proliferation

This lesion is recognizable as layers of myofibroblasts and smooth muscle cells inserted between the internal elastic lamina and the endothelial layer, the orientation of which is often recognizably radial rather than circumferential. Vessels in the size range of 100 to 150 μm are most commonly involved (17). These are classified as Heath-Edwards grade 2.

Concentric Laminar Intimal Fibrosis

Following their migration into the intima, many medial smooth muscle cells convert into myofibroblasts and elaborate matrix consisting of collagen and proteoglycans, which becomes distributed to form a typical "onionskin" or lamellar appearance with slender spindle cells arranged circumferentially within the fibrous, often hyalinized matrix (Fig. 2). A later stage of the process involves production of elastic fibrils within the intima and thickening or reduplication of the elastic lamina. Any of these features is considered to be grade 3 in the Heath-Edwards classification.

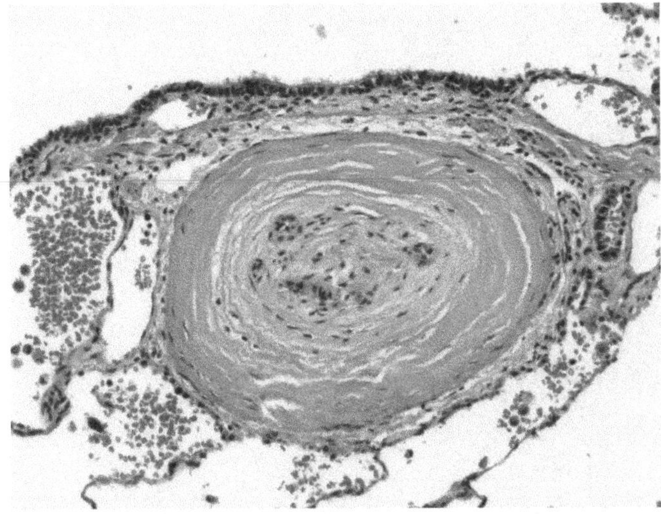

Figure 2 Concentric laminar intimal fibrosis. The normal arterial intima is replaced by a lamellar fibroproliferative process imparting the classical "onionskin" appearance. Small residual endothelialized lumens can be visualized in the center. The tunica media is thinned. A bronchiolar wall is identified adjacent to the artery. H&E stain.

Plexiform Lesion

Although the plexiform lesion is the characteristic lesion of plexogenic pulmonary arteriopathy, its presence is not required for the diagnosis (21). It has been designated as Heath-Edwards grade 4. Plexiform lesions are most commonly associated with primary pulmonary hypertension and pulmonary hypertension associated with portal hypertension and congenital cardiac left-to-right shunts. There is a tendency for the lesions to arise from perpendicular side branches of preacinar supernumerary pulmonary arteries in pulmonary hypertension secondary to congenital heart disease but to have an intra-acinar location in primary pulmonary hypertension (22). Their presence signifies severe pulmonary hypertension, but the distribution is often highly variable and multiple tissue blocks or serial sections may be required to demonstrate them.

In its classical form, the lesion consists of an intraluminal proliferation of vascular channels formed by connective tissue septa. The spaces may appear slit-like, with the septa containing smooth muscle, myofibroblasts, and fibrillary cells (23), imparting a "glomeruloid" appearance (Fig. 3). Fibrin is sometimes noted within the channel lumens in early lesions. The cells lining the vascular channels have a plump appearance and stain positively for factor VIII antigen by immunohistochemistry (17), but they differ from normal endothelial cells in that they have no basement membrane, pinocytotic vesicles, or Weibel-Palade bodies (23). The appearance of the plexiform lesion may change, presumably as a function of age, manifest by thickened septa formed by deposition of collagen and elastin as well as by infiltrating smooth muscle cells, although the overall appearance is generally less cellular than the younger lesions. The vascular channels may enlarge and assume a more rounded contour, making differentiation from the recanalized lesions of

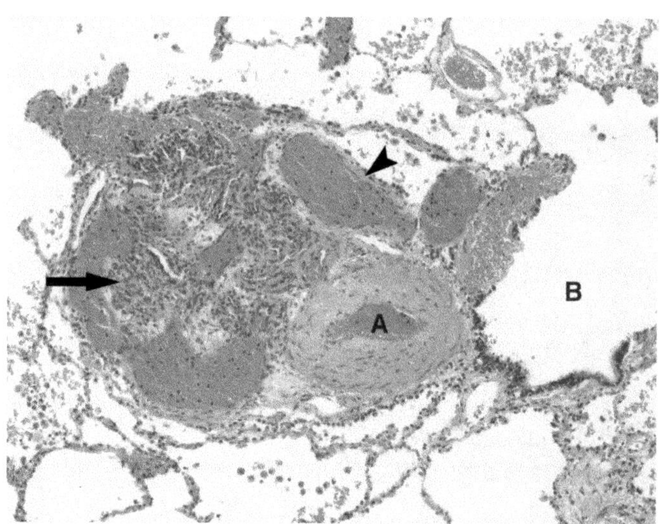

Figure 3 Plexiform and dilation lesion. Vague nodules composed of spindle cells that define slit-like channels (*arrow*) impart a "glomeruloid" appearance to this plexiform lesion. The parent pulmonary artery (**A**) demonstrates severe medial hypertrophy. Surrounding the cellular tufts is a collar of widened vessels that signifies the dilation lesion; (**B**) Bronchiole. H&E stain.

thrombotic/thromboembolic vasculopathy (see below) difficult. The septa may eventually be transformed into purely fibrotic or elastotic structures of variable thickness.

Dilation Lesion

Several types of arterial dilation lesions are recognized. One form is a component of the plexiform lesion, being the aneurysmally dilated segment that surrounds the proliferative tuft of endothelium-lined channels (Fig. 3). In this case, dilation is probably the result of weakening of the arterial wall secondary to fibrinoid degeneration. According to Heath (21), these changes antedate the cellular form of the plexiform lesion. Deposition of fibrinoid substances may, in fact, initiate the vasoformative processes characteristic of the plexiform lesion. In referring to this specific form of dilation, Heath-Edwards grade 4 is appropriate. With time and maturation of the intraluminal cellular tuft, the surrounding wall may become thinner, with virtual loss of the muscular media, and expansile, giving rise to the term *vein-like branches* (23). These dilated vessels may also continue distally as a form of poststenotic dilation; when clustered together, they are termed "angiomatoid lesions" (21). Similar dilated vessels may form proximal to a thickened arterial segment and surround it, probably forming a bypass channel around the obstructing artery. These vessels are prone to rupture and are responsible for focal hemorrhages and hemosiderin deposits in the lung (21). The term *cavernous lesion* has also been used to describe certain forms of dilation lesions and it may represent an intermediate stage between the vein-like branches and the angiomatoid lesion. All of these latter forms of dilation lesions are categorized as Heath-Edwards grade 5.

Eccentric Intimal Fibrosis

This lesion, while often associated with pulmonary hypertensive states, is not part of the Heath-Edwards grading system. Its presence is assumed to reflect healed thrombi, although whether the thrombi are of embolic or of in situ origin cannot be determined from this appearance.

Pulmonary Atherosclerosis

The lesions of pulmonary arterial atherosclerosis appear the same as those in the systemic circulation, demonstrating a lipid core with overlying fibrous cap. The reduced plaque thickness and the paucity of lesions are most likely a product of lower pulmonary circulatory pressure. Although the presence of atherosclerosis is not an absolute indicator of the presence of PAH, it is almost universal in cases with PAH from either congenital or acquired causes (24). It is possible that in older individuals there occurs an unfolding of the pulmonary artery trunk and proximal large elastic vessels, resulting in flow abnormalities that predispose to focal atheroma formation. If atheromas are identified in segmental or smaller vessels, however, other changes of PAH should be sought.

Transplant Vasculopathy

The vasculature of the transplanted lung may demonstrate thickening, presumably as a form of chronic rejection, analogous to the same process described in the coronary arteries of transplanted hearts. The change in elastic and muscular arteries is manifest as a concentric

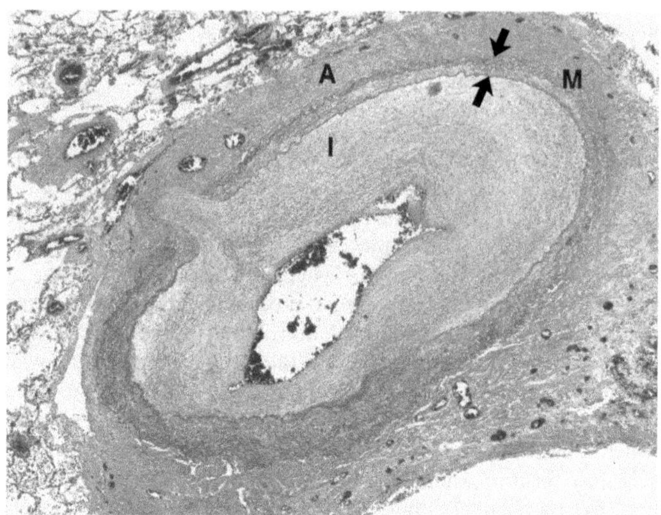

Figure 4 Transplant arteriopathy. Concentric fibrointimal proliferation with luminal encroachment is characteristic of transplant arteriopathy. The relatively narrow width of the tunica media (M) is demonstrated by the arrows. I represents tunica intima and A tunica adventitia. H&E stain.

fibrointimal proliferation (Fig. 4), occasionally with associated medial muscular hypertrophy (25). In veins and small venules, the lesion is usually concentric intimal sclerosis (26).

B. Thickening of the Arterial Media

Age-Related Changes

The media of muscular arteries is affected little with age (27), with changes essentially limited to irregular thickness of the muscle coat and coarsening of the elastic laminae. In older individuals, the arterioles may demonstrate concentric fibrosis, which may progress to complete hyalinization.

Lesions Identified in Pulmonary Arterial Hypertension

Medial Hypertrophy/Muscularization of the Pulmonary Arterioles

This lesion is assigned grade 1 in the Heath-Edwards scheme. It is also the most commonly identified lesion in pulmonary hypertension (27) and not restricted to pulmonary hypertension of any etiology. It is formed by an increase in the size and numbers of smooth muscle cells in the tunica media. The degree of medial hypertrophy is roughly proportional to physiological values (28) with values greater than 15% of the external diameter signifying severe hypertrophy (Fig. 5) (29).

Muscular transformation of arterioles represents the earliest histologically demonstrable lesion of pulmonary hypertension (30). Normally, the smooth muscle coat is completely dispersed by the time the vessel diameter is reduced to 70 to 100 μm, but in

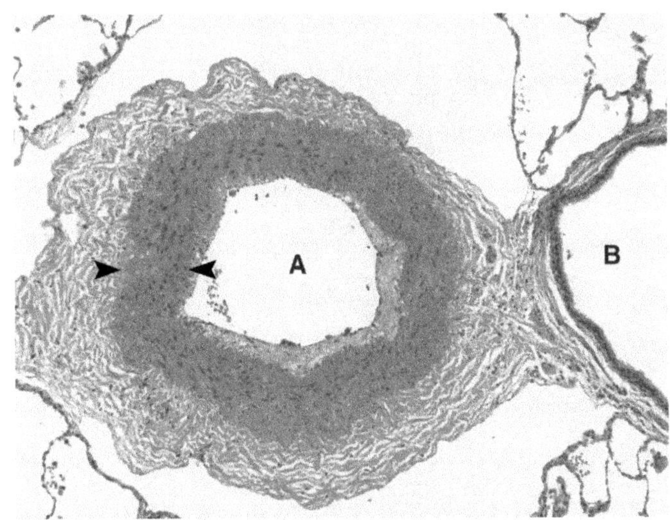

Figure 5 Arterial medial hyperplasia. The tunica media is enclosed between the internal and external elastic lamellae (*arrowheads*) and the ratio of its thickness (internal–external elastica on one side) to the outside diameter (external–external elastica) is approximately 18%, signifying severe hypertrophy (>15%). There is minimal intimal thickening. (**A**) Represents arterial lumen; (**B**) Bronchiole. H&E stain.

pulmonary hypertension, this muscular layer may extend to arterioles 20 to 30 μm in diameter and is enclosed by both an internal and external elastic lamina (17).

Fibrinoid Necrosis/Vasculitis

These changes primarily involve the media, although other components of the vessel wall may be involved. The spectrum of changes includes insudation of fibrinoid substances through the intimal layer into the media and degenerative changes of the medial smooth muscle cells, progressing in some cases to frank necrosis and classical necrotizing arteritis with a neutrophilic inflammatory infiltrate (Fig. 6) (1). Some cases may show the effects of healing with granulation tissue and/or granulomas in the vessel walls (31). The areas affected are usually focal and segmental (27). The fibrinoid change is recognizable as an area of relative acellularity where smooth muscle cells are replaced by bright eosinophilic material, the appearance of which may be enhanced by special stains for fibrin (Martius scarlet blue; acid picro-Mallory). Portions of the arterial wall are swollen by these deposits. Any of the above microscopic changes are associated with significant pulmonary hypertension.

Necrotizing arteritis is an uncommonly encountered lesion. In the Heath-Edwards classification scheme, this lesion is grade 6. Its position reflects earlier thinking that these changes represented the final step in the arterial response to increasing pressures. We now recognize that focal fibrinoid necrosis and arterial dilation may be precursors to formation of the plexiform lesion. This fact has stimulated some authors to question the validity of the grading system; however, as Heath points out (21), the full spectrum of necrotizing arteritis must be distinguished from focal fibrinoid degeneration, commonly identified as the antecedent lesion of plexiform changes.

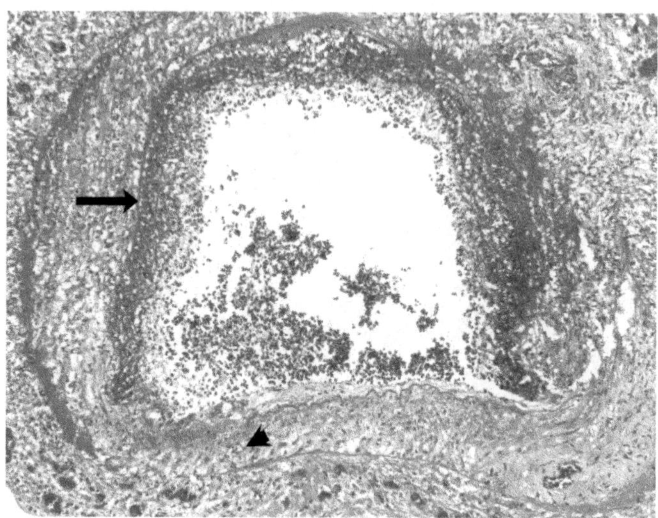

Figure 6 Fibrinous necrosis/necrotizing arteritis. Transmural inflammation with mural destruction, thrombosis, and deposition of fibrinoid material (*arrow*) characterize advanced changes of PAH in a child with congenital heart disease-related PAH. The arrowhead indicates disruption of the internal and external elastic laminae. H&E stain. *Abbreviation*: PAH, pulmonary arterial hypertension. *Source*: Case courtesy of Dr. Glen Taylor.

Deposition of Substances

Amyloidosis

Amyloid appears as a light eosinophilic, waxy, nonfibrillar amorphous deposit on routine H&E stains. It is classically demonstrated by the Congo red method, in which the substance displays characteristic apple-green birefringence on polarization. Ultrastructural examination reveals the diagnostic arrangement of a felt-work of nonbranching 7- to 10-nm fibrils. Amyloid may be present in the lung as diffuse or focal/nodular deposits related to a variety of clinical syndromes (32). Vascular deposits tend to be concentrated in the tunica media (Fig. 7) causing thickening and a rigid appearance with arterial luminal narrowing and likely impede normal physiological dilation/constriction. Although amyloid deposits in the lung may be significant, the cardiac and renal involvement typically determine prognosis (32,33).

Iron and Calcium Deposits ("Endogenous Pneumoconiosis," "Mineralizing Pulmonary Elastosis")

Impregnation of vascular elastica with iron and calcium salts is identified in many cases of recurrent pulmonary hemorrhage, especially idiopathic pulmonary hemosiderosis, pulmonary veno-occlusive disease (PVOD), and rarely, chronic venous congestion from heart failure (34). Both vascular and interstitial elastic fibers are transformed into blue-gray or amber structures as seen by routine light microscopy (34). The iron component stains

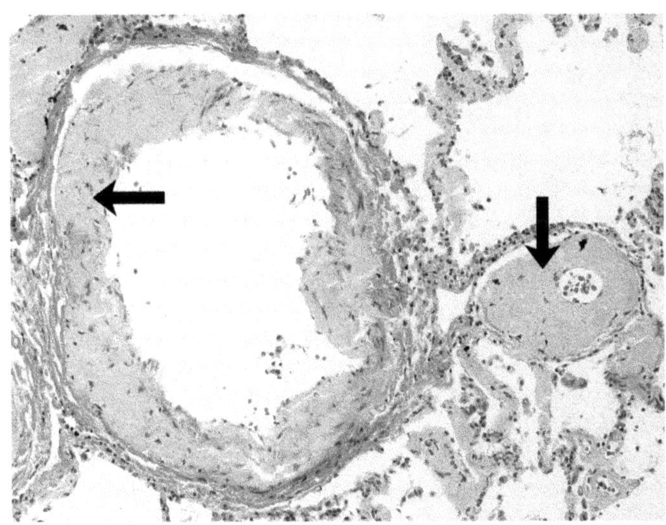

Figure 7 Amyloidosis. Pale, waxy, amorphous eosinophilic amyloid has become insudated within the tunica media (*arrows*) of a pulmonary artery and an adjacent small vessel. H&E stain.

positively with the Prussian blue method, while the calcium moiety will be revealed with either alizarin red or von Kossa techniques. Vascular involvement is more common in metastatic calcification (soft tissue calcium deposition in previously normal sites) versus dystrophic calcification (calcium deposition in pathologically altered soft tissues).

Metabolic Inclusions

In Fabry's disease, accumulated ceramide trihexoside, as a result of α-galactosidase deficiency, deposits in large and small pulmonary vessels. In muscular arteries, a characteristic bubbly appearance is produced by clear vesicles (present in the vascular smooth muscle cells) separated by the elastic lamellae (35). The lipid material stains positively with the Luxol fast blue method in paraffin sections or Sudan Black in frozen sections. Electron microscopy reveals the characteristic lamellar structure ("zebra bodies") of the inclusions. The significance of vascular involvement in the lung is uncertain; most clinical concerns are directed at obstructive airway disease (36).

C. Adventitial Thickening/Fibrosis

Direct contiguity of the adventitial layer with the surrounding pulmonary interstitium predisposes it to nonselective fibrous thickening as part of any of the spectrum of interstitial inflammatory/fibrosing diseases. Adventitial thickening has been mentioned in the context of bronchopulmonary dysplasia (37), persistent pulmonary hypertension of the newborn (38), pulmonary hypertension secondary to congenital heart disease (39), primary pulmonary hypertension (40), collagen vascular disease (Fig. 8), and pulmonary venous hypertension from mitral stenosis. In the latter instance, fibrous proliferation may result from persistent edema (41). Recent studies have identified a pivotal role of the adventitial fibroblast in vascular remodeling (42).

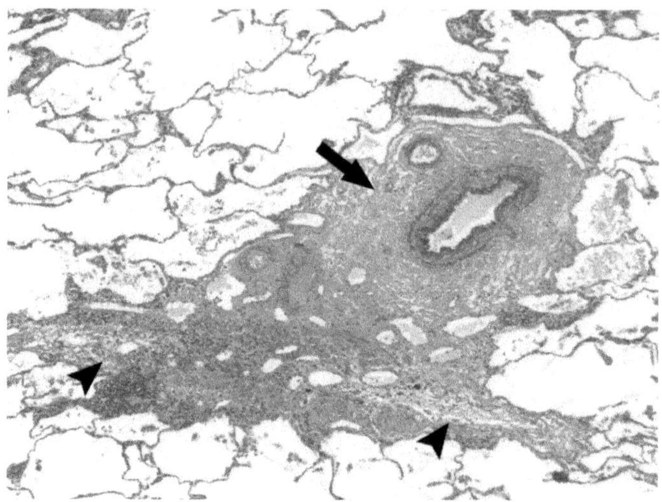

Figure 8 Adventitial thickening. A collar of dense, sclerotic collagen is seen expanding the periarterial adventitia (*arrow*) in this patient with rheumatoid arthritis-related pulmonary disease. The arrowheads define a linear scar that represents associated obliterative bronchiolitis. H&E stain.

Sarcoidosis is a nonnecrotizing granulomatous disorder of unknown etiology that, while not specifically thought of as a disease of the vascular adventitia, causes extensive thickening of that region by virtue of involvement of active granulomas as well as the characteristic fibrosis of healed lesions (43). Granulomas also infiltrate and disrupt the vascular media and intimal layers, causing stenosis or obliteration of the lumen. Healed lesions may be identified by discontinuities of the elastic laminae, a hallmark of vasculitis from many causes.

IV. Intraluminal Substances/Obstruction

A. Arterial Thrombus

Arterial thrombi are typically examined in two situations: as acute thrombi/thromboemboli in the setting of pulmonary infarction or sudden death and as subacute/chronic luminal obstructions in the context of pulmonary hypertension. The current classification of pulmonary hypertension contains separate definitions for obstruction of either proximal or distal pulmonary arteries (20).

Acute Thrombi/Thromboemboli

Barring recent lung/mediastinal trauma (including surgical intervention), thrombi identified within the pulmonary trunk and the lobar and segmental arteries are most commonly due to embolization from deep veins in the leg or pelvis (44). A V- or Y-shaped structure reflects origin within a venous confluence. Grossly, they are firm, rubbery, granular or dry masses that are lighter in color than a postmortem clot. They do not usually conform exactly to the receiving vessel, and if acute, will not adhere strongly to the vessel walls. Distinction of pulmonary thromboemboli from postmortem clots is often problematic. In general, postmortem clots conform more closely to the vessel walls. The classic gross appearance is of a yellow layer consisting of fibrin and platelets ("chicken fat" layer) distinctly partitioned from the deeper burgundy red mass of erythrocytes ("currant jelly" layer). In a true thrombus, the cut surface demonstrates alternating "lines of Zahn." Microscopically, there is a characteristic pattern of alternating layers of fibrin and platelets with erythrocytes and leukocytes. In the acute stage there is minimal neovascular/fibroblastic organization of the thrombus, although the periphery of an embolus may demonstrate such changes as derived from its relationship with the parent vein in which it was initially formed. Differences in the patient's coagulation status, microvascular environment, blood flow, and parenchymal disease may result in a variety of appearances of either postmortem clots or recent thrombi/thromboemboli.

Pulmonary Infarction

Pulmonary emboli are identified in 5% to 28% of autopsy cases (45) and are equally distributed in upper and lower lobes of the lung. Approximately 30% are associated with pulmonary infarction, and these generally favor the lower lobes. The majority of infarcts occur as a result of thromboemboli usually less than 3 mm in diameter (45,46) and in individuals with concomitant cardiorespiratory compromise (47). The average size of an infarct is 3 cm (17). It is usually triangular in shape with the apex defined by at least two pleural surfaces; thus, many occur in areas such as the costophrenic angles. Grossly, the acute infarct is hemorrhagic, typically with an overlying fibrinous pleuritis, but with organization/resolution the lesion becomes gray or tan and contracted, reflecting fibroelastic scarification. Microscopically, the earliest stages of the lesion demonstrate capillary engorgement, generalized vascular thrombosis, hemorrhage, and necrosis. Infarcts are not usually associated with excessive tissue neutrophilia, and the presence of same should suggest a septic embolic etiology. Organization is manifest as progressive granulation tissue remodeling from the periphery inwards. The late or healed infarct consists of extensive fibroelastic scarification. Lesions that are less developed are termed "incomplete" infarcts (48).

Uncertainties still exist in the pathogenesis of pulmonary infarcts but theories generally incorporate the role of dual blood supplies and hemodynamic autoregulatory capacity in the distal (peripheral) lung parenchyma (45,46) combined with venous outflow stasis in the setting of cardiac failure.

Large Vessel Thrombosis

From the current clinical perspective, a large (arterial) vessel is one that is accessible to surgical thromboendarterectomy for treatment of chronic thromboembolic pulmonary hypertension (CTEPH) and includes main, lobar, and, at best, proximal segmental arteries (49); this is also reflected in the contemporary classification of PAH (20) where the less anatomically precise term "proximal" is used. In subacute and chronic cases, progressive organization of the thrombus/thromboembolus will be found, manifested by influx from the periphery of small, primitive vascular channels, fibroblasts, and mononuclear cells. The process of organization results in fragmentation and erosion of the base of attachment of the

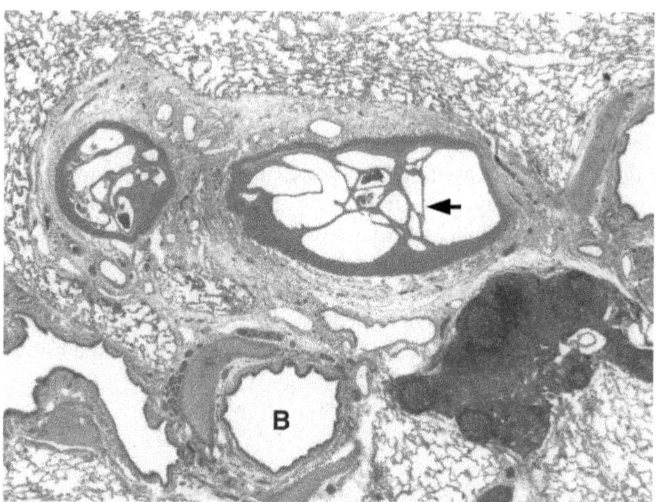

Figure 9 Chronic thromboembolic pulmonary hypertension (proximal). Attenuated fibrous strands (*arrow*) traversing an arterial lumen characterize the "webs" of a recanalized pulmonary arterial thrombus. Although this patient had thrombotic disease that preferentially involved the proximal arterial vasculature, smaller vessels were also involved. (**B**) Represents bronchiole. H&E stain.

embolus to the underlying arterial wall, leading to the formation of channels ("recanalization") through which some blood flow may return. Fibroelastic tissue becomes deposited in greater amounts, converting the thrombus into septa that traverse all or part of the arterial lumen (Fig. 9) (17). In the larger arteries, these are grossly recognizable in lung dissections as fibrous web or bands. Complete occlusion of large arteries by an organized thrombus is uncommon (50).

Small Vessel Thrombosis

In the clinical context of pulmonary hypertension, the term "small vessel" is likely to refer to the distal vascular bed inasmuch as lesions in this compartment may mandate medical rather than surgical therapy (51), even if proximal, large vessel thrombosis is present. In seminal investigations characterizing small vessel pathology in CTEPH (52), morphometric evaluation was conducted on vessels in the range of 25 to 100 μm, which essentially signifies intra-acinar vessels. The phases of organization are the same as thrombi/thromboemboli in larger vessels. The residual lesions may assume either an eccentric intimal plaque, if the thrombus remains sessile during organization, or totally occupy the lumen with a collagen matrix containing the rounded punched-out profiles of recanalizing vascular channels (Fig. 10). The latter feature is termed the "colander lesion" and the pattern of a series of rigid-appearing luminal spaces with rounded or curvilinear contours contrasts with the slit-like sinusoidal profiles and increased cellularity characteristic of plexiform lesions.

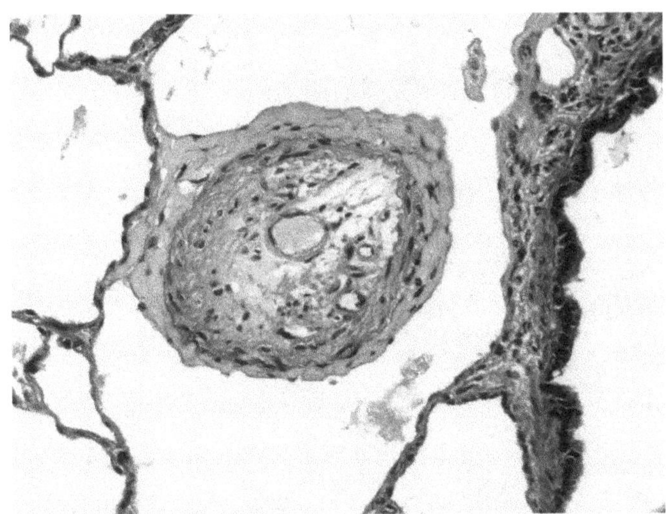

Figure 10 Chronic thromboembolic pulmonary hypertension (colander lesion). The lumen of this artery is virtually occluded by a hypocellular intimal plaque. The multiple small lumens signifying thrombus recanalization, characterize the "colander lesion." The rounded, "punched-out" profiles of these channels are distinguished from the slit-like spaces of a plexiform lesion. Movat pentachrome stain.

B. Venous Thrombosis/Pulmonary Veno-Occlusive Disease

PVOD [occasionally referred to as pulmonary occlusive venopathy, POV (53)] is an uncommon cause of pulmonary hypertension. Many cases are idiopathic but some demonstrate associations with chemotherapeutic treatment, oral contraceptives, viral infection, bone marrow transplantation, cardiomyopathy (54), and connective tissue disease (55). The lumens of intralobular or septal veins of varying sizes are plugged with fibrous tissue of either loose edematous or older sclerotic collagen, sometimes partitioned by septae characterizing the process of recanalization (Fig. 11). Recently formed thrombi are uncommon. Pulmonary veins may demonstrate medial thickening/arterialization (56) and adventitial fibrosis (57). Associated parenchymal changes include capillary engorgement, alveolar hemorrhage, hemosiderosis, and interstitial fibrosis, changes also identified in pulmonary capillary hemangiomatosis (PCH) (see below), a condition that shares a number of features with PVOD (58). Pulmonary arterial medial hypertrophy and intimal hyperplasia, but not plexiform lesions, are identified with frequency (58).

C. Foreign Material Emboli

Intravenous Illicit Drug Use

Foreign body embolism and granulomatosis secondary to intravenous injection of aqueous suspensions of insoluble binding agents in oral tablets is the most common vascular manifestation of intravenous drug use (59,60). Talc or hydrated magnesium silicate, (5- to 15-μm needle/plate-like aggregates) (Fig. 12), cornstarch (8- to 12-μm round/polyhedral bodies), and microcrystalline cellulose (25- to 200-μm rod/needle-like particles) (60,61) are

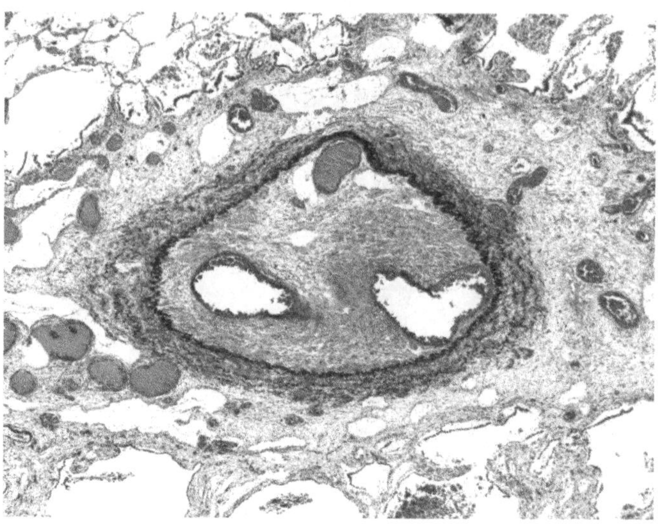

Figure 11 Pulmonary veno-occlusive disease. The lumen of an interlobular septal vein contains a recanalized intimal plaque, which, in this instance, is sclerotic and suggests a long-standing lesion. Dilated venules, capillaries, and lymphatic channels surround this obstruction. The adjacent parenchyma demonstrates interstitial fibrosis, a sequelae of PVOD. Movat pentachrome stain.

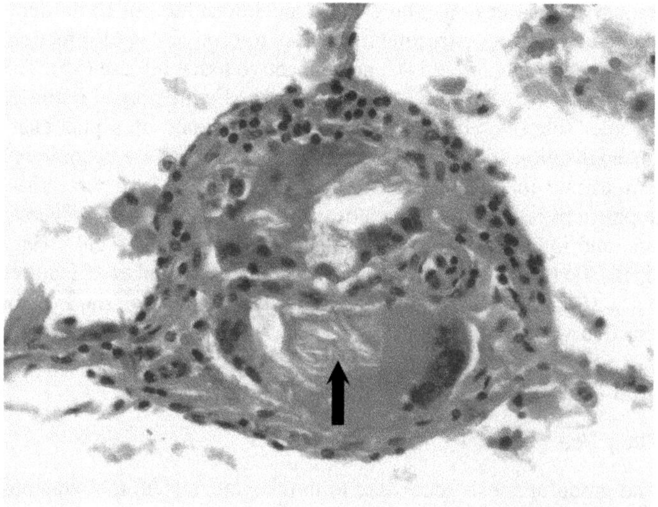

Figure 12 Intravascular talc embolization. This interstitial but extravascular foreign body granuloma sits at the confluence of three alveolar septae. Several multinucleated histiocytic giant cells contain the clear, slightly refractile plate-like aggregates of talc (*arrow*). H&E stain.

the common substances observed in these settings, although other filler substances may be observed in addition to cotton fibers (used in filtering suspensions) and hair (implanted from injection sites). Most of these particulates have characteristic birefringent properties on polarization microscopy (60). Intraluminal material with thrombosis signifies recent injection, but the substances tend to be extruded into the perivascular interstitium where they are embraced by multinucleated histiocytic giant cells. Cornstarch deposits may dissipate over time secondary to digestion (62). Interstitial fibrosis, panacinar emphysema (63), and a spectrum of thromboembolic vascular remodeling changes (64) can be observed. Pulmonary hypertension is a rare complication, possibly linked to progressive loss of the vascular bed with a decrease in diffusing capacity (65).

Iatrogenically Derived Substances

Invasive cardiovascular procedures may be associated with the embolization and impaction of cotton wool or gauze fibers within pulmonary vessels (66,67). Silicone antifoaming agents used in oxygenators for cardiopulmonary bypass procedures have been associated with capillary dispersion of clear, refractile (but nonbirefringent) particles in the lung and other organs (68). Materials such as polyvinyl alcohol beads and Gelfoam selectively injected into the bronchial arterial circulation in order to embolize bleeding neoplasms or other lesions may be encountered in subsequently resected specimens. These substances may have a variety of appearances in tissue sections since they may be altered by tissue processing. They are not always birefringent under polarized light.

D. Cellular Emboli/Impaction

Tumor Embolus

The most common malignancies that generate pulmonary tumor emboli are adenocarcinomas of the breast, stomach, lung, liver, prostate, and pancreas (69,70). The intravascular manifestations include pure cellular aggregates, malignant cells admixed with thrombus, or thrombus alone. The spectrum of tumor emboli, microangiopathic hemolytic anemia, and disseminated intravascular coagulation is termed "thrombotic microangiopathy" (Fig. 13) (71). Pulmonary hypertension and right heart failure may result from a combination of luminal obstruction and vascular remodeling (69), the latter including features of intimal and medial hyperplasia and fibrinoid necrosis (72,73). The diagnosis is usually made at autopsy.

Amniotic Fluid Embolus

Amniotic fluid components include epithelial squames, lanugo hairs, lipid, mucus, meconium, and bile, and its dissemination into the maternal circulation is a rare complication of pregnancy, therapeutic abortion, and cesarean section (74,75). The clinical syndrome consists of cardiovascular collapse and pulmonary edema, likely a result of anaphylactic shock reaction to fetal antigens. The gross features consist of the nonspecific findings of patchy edema, atelectasis, pulmonary hyperinflation, and evidence of disseminated intravascular coagulation (DIC) (74). The embolized material may be identified on routine sections as intralumenal stacked plate-like aggregates or thin linear structures (squames) or flocculent material (mucin) (Fig. 14). Additional histochemical and immunohistochemical techniques may highlight their presence (74).

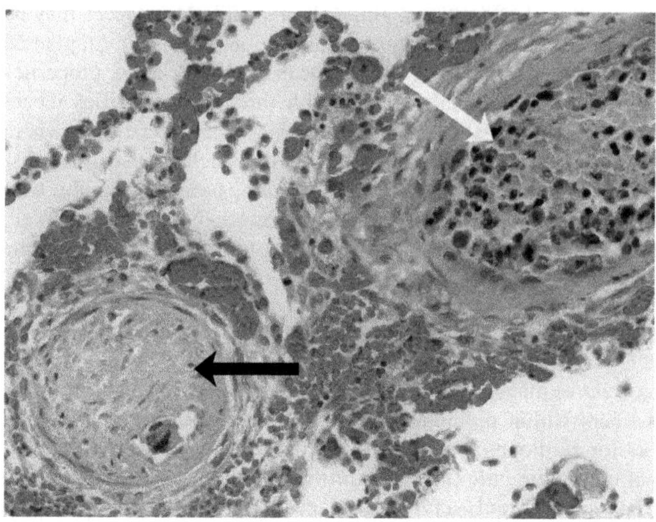

Figure 13 Intravascular tumor embolization. Two arterial profiles (presumably the same vessel) are seen in cross-section. In one (*white arrow*), the lumen is blocked by a necrotic tumor embolus (adenocarcinoma). In the other arterial section, the lumen is nearly obliterated by a fibroproliferative intimal plaque (*black arrow*), a manifestation of microangiopathic vascular remodeling. H&E stain.

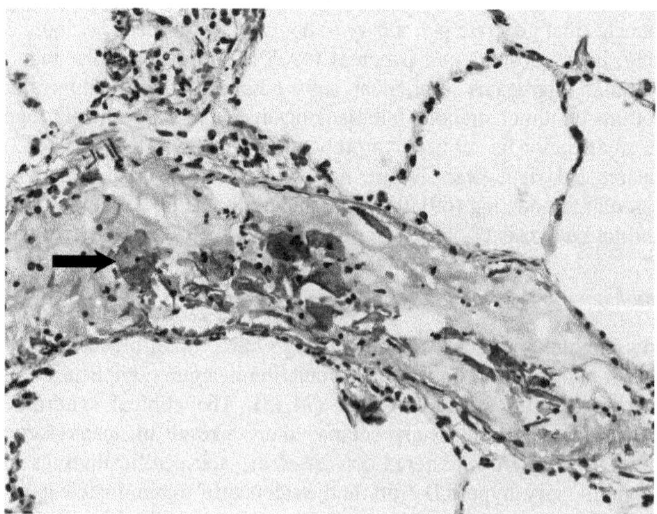

Figure 14 Amniotic fluid embolus. This intra-acinar artery is dilated by a plug of loose, myxoid amniotic fluid (Alcian blue–positive material) within which are suspended several flattened epithelial squames (*arrow*). Movat pentachrome stain.

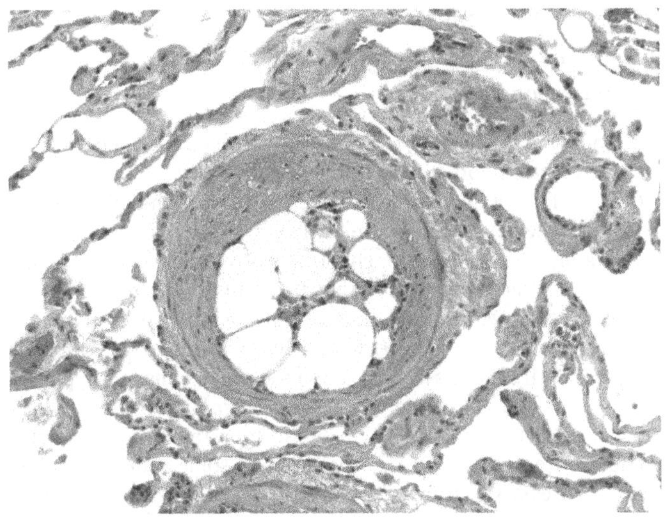

Figure 15 Fat/bone marrow embolus. Commonly identified at autopsy, bone marrow emboli are seen as cohesive cellular aggregates that define clear fat vacuoles by attenuated cellular processes that somewhat resemble the webs of recanalized thrombi. On higher magnification, immature myeloid/erythroid precursor cells and megakaryocytes may be identified. H&E stain.

Fat/Bone Marrow Embolus

Fragments of bone marrow and fat are often liberated at the time of traumatic injury, surgery, or chest compressions during resuscitation and may become lodged in the pulmonary arterial or capillary circulation. Marrow particulates are recognizable as cellular aggregates incorporating small clear spaces (Fig. 15) representing the lipid vacuoles of adipocytes; hematopoietic precursor cells may be clearly identified. These are usually incidental findings unless associated with the fat embolism syndrome, which presents as adult respiratory distress syndrome/diffuse alveolar damage, central nervous system abnormalities, and a petechial rash (75). Intravascular lipid may be difficult to diagnose due to the clearing effect of organic solvents used in tissue processing, but a clue to its existence is the rigid expansion of the lumen of small vessels and capillaries, without any obvious luminal content. Fat can be demonstrated in frozen section by the oil red O method or by postfixation en bloc with osmium tetroxide (76).

Parasitic Vascular Emboli

Chronic pulmonary infestation with *Schistosoma* ova (typically *S. mansoni*) may result in pulmonary hypertension and cor pulmonale (77). The arterial change is typically an endarteritis obliterans, but the spectrum of vascular histopathology includes intra- and perivascular (tuberculoid) granulomas, intimal hyperplasia, medial hypertrophy, vascular fibrosis, and angiomatoid lesions (1).

V. Proliferative Vascular Disease

A. Pulmonary Capillary Hemangiomatosis/ Pulmonary Microvasculopathy

PCH is a rare cause of pulmonary hypertension and it is still a matter of debate as to whether PCH is a low-grade neoplasm or a reactive vascular proliferation reflecting uncontrolled angiogenesis (53,78). Patchy, lobular-based areas of congestion with a spongy character are seen grossly (79). The characteristic microscopic pattern is one of proliferating and engorged capillaries extending throughout alveolar walls (Fig. 16) and investing themselves within interlobular septae and within the walls of airways and pulmonary veins, in the latter instance sometimes to a degree that compromises the venous lumen. Acute hemorrhage, hemosiderin-laden alveolar macrophages and interstitial fibrosis may be a sequelae of rupture of these fragile vessels. Concomitant arterial changes typically include intimal hyperplasia and medial hypertrophy, but plexiform/dilation lesions are characteristically absent. Pulmonary capillary hemangiomatosis/pulmonary microvasculopathy changes are noted so frequently in cases of PVOD that some authors feel they are both components of a certain disease spectrum (53). Similar vasculopathic features may be identified in cases of mitral valve stenosis or as incidental findings at autopsy without other evidence of pulmonary hypertension (80).

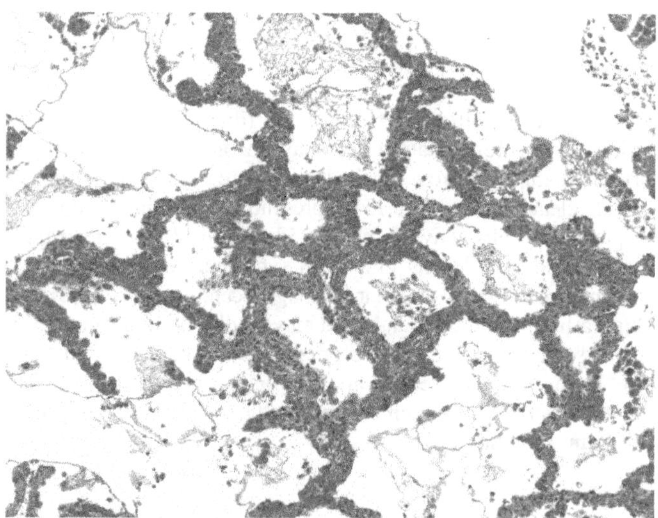

Figure 16 Pulmonary capillary hemangiomatosis. Although the normal septal architecture is retained, each alveolar septum is diffusely thickened by a proliferation of capillary vessels with an apparent increase in cellularity. Depending on the state of fixation and other procedural factors, the capillaries may appear mildly dilated to severely engorged. Alveolar histiocytes contain hemosiderin pigment, consistent with hemorrhage. H&E stain.

VI. Pulmonary Artery Aneurysms, Arteriovenous Malformations, and Arterial Dissection

Pulmonary artery aneurysms (PAAs) are rare and may affect any part of the arterial tree from trunk to periphery, although more than 80% are identified in the pulmonary trunk (21). The classification of PAAs is not well established in the literature; however, Bartter and colleagues (81) suggest dividing these lesions into those with and without arteriovenous communication. Most PAAs are acquired lesions secondary to inflammation (infection and Behçet disease), trauma (penetrating/blunt injury and iatrogenic catheter-related perforation), or pulmonary hypertension (81–83). Rasmussen's aneurysm arises in association with tuberculous cavities (81) and is characteristically peripheral in location as are most mycotic PAAs. Pulmonary arterial dissection also appears to arise in the same clinical setting as PAA, although there is not complete documentation that every case occurs in an aneurysmally dilated artery. Most dissections occur in the pulmonary trunk, and features of cystic medial degeneration and pulmonary artery ectasia are usually present (84).

Pulmonary arteriovenous malformations (PAVM) may appear as single, dilated vessel or a labyrinthine, telangiectatic vascular conglomerate (16). Because of exposure to sustained abnormal pressures and turbulence, the walls of these vessels are often difficult to differentiate as either arterial or venous in origin; some may be thrombosed. Most PAVM are single and in the range of 3 to 8 mm in diameter; up to 42% may be bilateral (17). Eighty-two percent of patients with PAVM have hereditary hemorrhagic telangiectasia (HHT, Osler-Weber-Rendu syndrome) (16). PAVM may be associated with significant right-to-left shunting resulting in exercise intolerance and cerebral abscess. One percent of patients have pulmonary hypertension.

References

1. Harris P, Heath D. The Human Pulmonary Circulation: Its Form and Function in Health and Disease. 3rd ed. New York: Churchill Livingstone 1986.
2. Brenner O. Pathology of the pulmonary circulation. Arch Intern Med 1935; 56:211–237.
3. Andrews R, Colloby P, Hubner PJB. Pulmonary artery dissection in a patient with idiopathic dilation of the pulmonary artery. Br Heart J 1993; 69:268–269.
4. Edwards J. Congenital pulmonary vascular disorders. In: Moser K, ed. Pulmonary Vascular Diseases. New York: Marcel Dekker, 1979.
5. Sondergaard T. Coarctation of the pulmonary artery. Dan Med Bull 1954; 1:46–48.
6. Collett RW, Edwards JE. Persistent truncus arteriosus: a classification according to anatomic types. Surg Clin North Am 1949; 29:1245–1270.
7. Neufeld HN, Lester RG, Adams P Jr., et al. Aorticopulmonary septal defect. Am J Cardiol 1962; 9:12–25.
8. Sotomora RF, Edwards JE. Anatomic identification of so-called absent pulmonary artery. Circulation 1978; 57:624–633.
9. D'cruz I, Agustsson M, Bicoff J, et al. Stenotic lesions of the pulmonary arteries: clinical and hemodynamic findings in 84 cases. Am J Cardiol 1964; 13:441–450.
10. Alagille D, Estrada A, Hadchouel M, et al. Syndromic paucity of interlobular bile ducts, Alagille syndrome or arteriohepatic dysplasia. J Pediatr 1987; 110:195–200.
11. Wagenwoort CA. Misalignment of lung vessels: a syndrome causing persistent neonatal pulmonary hypertension. Hum Pathol 1986; 17:727–730.

12. Langston C. Misalignment of pulmonary vessels and alveolar capillary dysplasia. Pediatr Pathol 1991; 11:163–170.
13. Kiely B, Filler J, Stone S, et al. Syndrome of anomalous venous drainage of the right lung to the inferior vena cava: a review of 69 reported cases and three new cases in children. Am J Cardiol 1967; 20:102–116.
14. Sun C-C, Doyle T, Ringel R. Pulmonary vein stenosis. Hum Pathol 1995; 26:880–886.
15. Burke CM, Safai C, Nelson DP, et al. Pulmonary arteriovenous malformations: a critical update. Am Rev Respir Dis 1986; 134:334–339.
16. Lee DW, White RI, Egglin TK, et al. Embolotherapy of large pulmonary arteriovenous malformations: long term results. Ann Thorac Surg 1997; 64:930–940.
17. Kay JM. Vascular disease. In: Thurlbeck WM, Churg AM, eds. Pathology of the Lung. New York: Thieme, 1995:931–1066.
18. Wagenwoort CA, Wagenwoort N. Age changes in muscular pulmonary arteries. Arch Pathol 1965; 79:524–528.
19. Galie N, Torbicki A, Barst R, et al. Guidelines on diagnosis and treatment of pulmonary arterial hypertension. The Task Force on Diagnosis and Treatment of Pulmonary Arterial Hypertension of the European Society of Cardiology. Eur Heart J 2004; 25:2243–2278.
20. Simmoneau G, Nazzareno G, Rubin LJ, et al. Clinical classification of pulmonary hypertension. J Am Coll Cardiol 2004; 43:5S–12S.
21. Heath D. Pulmonary vascular disease. In: Hasleton PS, ed. Spencer's Pathology of the Lung. New York: McGraw-Hill, 1996:649–693.
22. Jamison BM, Michel RP. Different distribution of plexiform lesions in primary and secondary pulmonary hypertension. Hum Pathol 1995; 26:987–993.
23. Smith P, Heath D. Electron microscopy of the plexiform lesion. Thorax 1979; 34:177–186.
24. Heath D, Wood EH, Dushane JW, et al. The relation of age and blood pressure to atheroma in the pulmonary arteries and thoracic aorta in congenital heart disease. Lab Invest 1960; 9: 259–272.
25. Yousem SA, Burke CM, Billingham ME. Pathologic pulmonary alterations in long-term human heart-lung transplantation. Hum Pathol 1985; 16:911–923.
26. Yousem SA, Paradis IL, Dauber JH, et al. Pulmonary arteriosclerosis in long-term human heart-lung transplant recipients. Transplantation 1989; 47:564–569.
27. Wagenwoort CA, Wagenwoort N. Pathology of Pulmonary Hypertension. New York: Wiley, 1977.
28. Yamaki S, Wagenwoort CA. Plexogenic pulmonary arteriopathy: significance of medial thickness with respect to advanced pulmonary vascular lesions. Am J Pathol 1981; 105:70–75.
29. Wagenwoort CA, Mooi WJ. Biopsy Pathology of the Pulmonary Vasculature. London: Chapman and Hall, 1989.
30. Rabinovitch M, Haworth SG, Castaneda AR, et al. Lung biopsy in congenital heart disease: a morphometric approach to pulmonary vascular disease. Circulation 1978; 58:1107–1122.
31. Heath D, Edwards JE. The pathology of hypertensive pulmonary vascular disease: a description of six grades of structural changes in the pulmonary arteries with special reference to congenital cardiac septal defects. Circulation 1958; 18:533–547.
32. Berk J, O'Regan A, Skinner M. Pulmonary and tracheobronchial amyloidosis. Semin Respir Crit Care Med 2002; 23:155–165.
33. Shiue S-T, McNall DP. Pulmonary hypertension from prominent vascular involvement in diffuse amyloidosis. Arch Intern Med 1988; 148:687–689.
34. Pai U, McMahon J, Tomashefski JF. Mineralizing pulmonary elastosis in chronic cardiac failure: endogenous pneumoconiosis revisited. Am J Clin Pathol 1994; 101:22–28.
35. Smith P, Heath D, Rodgers B, et al. Pulmonary vasculature in Fabry's disease. Histopathology 1991; 19:567–569.
36. Brown L, Miller A, Bhuptani A, et al. Pulmonary involvement in Fabry disease. Am J Respir Crit Care Med 1997; 155:1004–1010.

37. Stocker J. Pathologic features of long-standing "healed" bronchopulmonary dysplasia: a study of 28 3- to 40-month-old infants. Hum Pathol 1986; 17:943–961.
38. Murphy J, Rabinovitch M, Goldstein J, et al. The structural basis of persistent pulmonary hypertension of the newborn infant. J Pediatr 1981; 98:962–967.
39. Aiello V, Higuchi MDL, Gutierrez P, et al. Adventitial layer enlargement correlates with the percentage of medial thickness in peripheral pulmonary arteries from patients with congenital heart defects. Cardiovasc Pathol 1997; 6:213–217.
40. Chazova I, Loyd JE, Zhdaov V, et al. Pulmonary artery adventitial changes and venous involvement in primary pulmonary hypertension. Am J Pathol 1995; 146:389–397.
41. Olsen E. Perivascular fibrosis in lungs in mitral valve disease: a possible mechanism of production. Br J Dis Chest 1966; 60:129–136.
42. Stenmark K, Davie NJ, Frid MG, et al. Role of the adventitia in pulmonary vascular remodeling. Physiology 2005; 21:134–145.
43. Takemura T, Matsui Y, Saiki S, et al. Pulmonary vascular involvement in sarcoidosis: a report of 40 autopsy cases. Hum Pathol 1992; 23:1216–1223.
44. Arciniegas E, Coates E. Massive pulmonary arterial thrombus following pneumonectomy. J Thorac Cardiovasc Surg 1971; 61:487–489.
45. Tsao M-S, Schraufnagel D, Wang NS. Pathogenesis of pulmonary infarction. Am J Med 1982; 72:599–606.
46. Dalen J, Haffajee C, Alpert J, et al. Pulmonary embolism, pulmonary hemorrhage and pulmonary infarction. N Engl J Med 1977; 296:1431–1435.
47. Hoeper MM, Mayer E, Simmoneau G, et al. Chronic thromboembolic pulmonary hypertension. Circulation 2006; 113:2011–2020.
48. Hampton AO, Castleman B. Correlation of postmortem chest teleroentgenograms with autopsy findings with special reference to pulmonary embolism and infarction. AJR Am J Roentgenol 1940; 43:305–325.
49. Fedullo P, Auger W, Kerr K, et al. Chronic thromboembolic pulmonary hypertension. Semin Respir Crit Care Med 2003, 24:273–285.
50. Moser K, Auger WR, Fedullo PF, et al. Chronic thromboembolic pulmonary hypertension: clinical picture and surgical treatment. Eur Respir J 1992; 5:334–342.
51. Kim N. Assessment of operability in chronic thromboembolic pulmonary hypertension. Proc Am Thorac Soc 2006; 3:584–588.
52. Moser K, Bloor CM. Pulmonary vascular lesions occurring in patients with chronic major vessel thromboembolic pulmonary hypertension. Chest 1993; 103:685–692.
53. Pietra GG, Capron F, Stewart S, et al. Pathologic assessment of vasculopathies in pulmonary hypertension. J Am Coll Cardiol 2004; 43:25S–32S.
54. Mandel J, Mark EJ, Hales CA. Pulmonary veno-occlusive disease. Am J Respir Crit Care Med 2000; 162:1964–1973.
55. Dorfmuller P, Humbert M, Perros F, et al. Fibrous remodeling of the pulmonary venous system in pulmonary hypertension associated with connective tissue diseases. Hum Pathol 2007; 38: 893–902.
56. Petitpretz P, Brenot F, Azarian R, et al. Pulmonary hypertension in patients with human immunodeficiency virus infection: comparison with primary pulmonary hypertension. Circulation 1994; 89:2722–2727.
57. Chazova I, Robbins IM, Loyd JE, et al. Venous and arterial changes in pulmonary venoocclusive disease, mitral stenosis and fibrosing mediastinitis. Eur Respir J 2000; 15:116–122.
58. Lantuéjoul S, Sheppard MN, Corrin B, et al. Pulmonary veno-occlusive disease and pulmonary capillary hemangiomatosis: a clinicopathologic study of 35 cases. Am J Surg Pathol 2006; 30:850–857.
59. Glassroth J, Adams G, Schnoll S. The impact of substance abuse on the respiratory system. Chest 1987; 91:596–602.

60. Tomashefski JF, Felo J. The pulmonary pathology of illicit drug and substance abuse. Current Diagn Pathol 2004; 10:413–426.
61. Kringsholm B, Christoffersen P. The nature and the occurrence of birefringent material in different organs in fatal drug addiction. Forensic Sci Int 1987; 34:53–62.
62. Lamb D, Roberts G. Starch and talc emboli in drug addicts' lungs. J Clin Pathol 1972; 25: 876–881.
63. Schmidt R, Glenny R, Godwin J, et al. Panlobular emphysema in young intravenous Ritalin abusers. Am Rev Respir Dis 1991; 143:649–656.
64. Tomashefski JF, Hirsch CS. The pulmonary vascular lesions of drug abuse. Hum Pathol 1980; 11:133–145.
65. Overland ES, Nolan A, Hopwell PC. Alteration of pulmonary function in intravenous drug misusers. Am J Med 1980; 68:231–237.
66. Dimmick J, Bove K, McAdams A, et al. Fibre embolization: a hazard of cardiac surgery and catheterization. N Engl J Med 1975; 292:685–687.
67. Tang T, Chambers C, Gallen W, et al. Pulmonary fibre embolism and granuloma. JAMA 1978; 239:948–950.
68. Orenstein J, Sato N, Aaron B, et al. Microemboli observed in death following cardiopulmonary bypass surgery: silicone antifoam agents and polyvinyl chloride tubing as sources of emboli. Hum Pathol 1982; 13:1082–1090.
69. Roberts K, Hamele-Bena D, Saqi A, et al. Pulmonary tumour embolism: a review of the literature. Am J Med 2003; 115:228–232.
70. Soares FA, Pinto AP, Landell GA, et al. Pulmonary tumor embolism to arterial vessels and carcinomatous lymphangitis: a comparative clinicopathological study. Arch Pathol Lab Med 1993; 117:827–831.
71. Franquet T, Gimenez A, Prats R, et al. Thrombotic microangiopathy of pulmonary tumours: a vascular cause of tree-in-bud pattern on CT. AJR Am J Roentgenol 2002; 179:897–899.
72. Von Herbay A, Illes A, Waldherr R, et al. Pulmonary tumor thrombotic microangiopathy with pulmonary hypertension. Cancer 1990; 66:587–592.
73. Shields D, Edwards W. Pulmonary hypertension attributable to neoplastic emboli: an autopsy study of 20 cases and a review of the literature. Cardiovasc Pathol 1992; 1:279–287.
74. Marcus B, Collins K, Harley R. Ancillary studies in amniotic fluid embolism: a case report and review of the literature. Am J Forensic Med Pathol 2005; 26:92–95.
75. Dudney TM, Elliott CG. Pulmonary embolism from amniotic fluid, fat, and air. Prog Cardiovasc Dis 1994; 36:447–474.
76. Abromowsky CR, Pickett JP, Goodfellow BC, et al. Comparative demonstration of pulmonary fat emboli by "en bloc" osmium tetroxide and oil red O methods. Hum Pathol 1981; 12:753–755.
77. Frazier A, Galvin J, Franks T, et al. Pulmonary vasculature: hypertension and infarction. Radiographics 2000; 20:491–524.
78. Tron V, Magee F, Wright JL, et al. Pulmonary capillary hemangiomatosis. Hum Pathol 1986; 17: 1144–1150.
79. Ishii H, Iwabuchi K, Kameya T, et al. Pulmonary capillary hemangiomatosis. Histopathology 1996; 29:275–278.
80. Havlik DM, Massie LW, Williams WL, et al. Pulmonary capillary hemangiomatosis-like foci: an autopsy study of 8 cases. Am J Clin Pathol 2000; 113:655–662.
81. Bartter T, Irwin R, Nash G. Aneurysms of the pulmonary arteries. Chest 1988; 94:1065–1075.
82. Castaner E, Gallardo X, Rimola J, et al. Congenital and acquired pulmonary artery anomalies in the adult: radiologic overview. Radiographics 2006; 26:349–371.
83. Coard R, Martin M. Ruptured saccular pulmonary artery aneurysm associated with persistent ductus arteriosus. Arch Pathol Lab Med 1992; 116:159–161.
84. Walley V, Virmani R, Silver M. Pulmonary arterial dissections and ruptures: to be considered in patients with pulmonary arterial hypertension presenting with cardiogenic shock or sudden death. Pathology 1990; 22:1–4.

19
Vasculitis

ABIDA K. HAQUE
Weill College of Cornell University, New York, New York; The Methodist Hospital, Houston; and San Jacinto Methodist Hospital, Baytown, Texas, U.S.A.

I. Introduction

Vasculitis is defined as destructive inflammation of blood vessels. It may involve pulmonary arteries, veins, or capillaries, and therefore, the terms vasculitis, arteritis, and angiitis have been used interchangeably. Pulmonary vasculitides are often a component of a heterogeneous group of systemic diseases (1,2). Pulmonary vasculitis almost always presents as pulmonary hemorrhage, with the patients manifesting hemoptysis, anemia, and consolidation or densities on chest radiographs. In addition to the histologic findings, clinical presentation, other systemic manifestations, radiographic features, and serologic tests are important in arriving at a diagnosis.

The diseases associated with pulmonary vasculitis may be categorically divided into those associated with immune complex–mediated diseases, antineutrophil cytoplasmic antibodies (ANCA)-associated vasculitis, Goodpasture's syndrome (GPS), cell-mediated vasculitis, idiopathic vasculitis, and infection-associated vasculitis (Table 1). Of these entities, most common are those that preferentially involve small vessels and include Wegener's granulomatosis (WG), microscopic polyangiitis (MPA), Churg-Strauss syndrome (CSS), cryoglobulinemic vasculitis, Henoch-Schonlein purpura, drug-induced vasculitis, and GPS (3). Large vessel vasculitis or cell-mediated vasculitis only occasionally affects the lung, and medium-sized vessel vasculitis such as polyarteritis nodosa and Kawasaki disease rarely affect the lungs. The patients may have manifestations of the underlying multisystem disease and present with pulmonary-renal syndrome, acute glomerulonephritis, palpable purpura, and mononeuritis multiplex. The Chapel Hill Consensus Conference on the Nomenclature of Systemic Vasculitis Criteria and Nomenclature to Categorize the Different Vasculitides have proved useful in defining these entities with different clinical manifestations (4).

The pulmonary-renal syndromes manifest as diffuse alveolar hemorrhage with pulmonary capillaritis, and glomerulonephritis, and include ANCA-associated vasculitides, GPS with antiglomerular basement membrane (anti-GBM)-associated antibody, and systemic lupus erythematosus (SLE). Serologic tests are essential in confirming these diagnoses.

Table 1 Classification of Pulmonary Vasculitis

I. Immunologically mediated vasculitis
A. Immune complex–mediated vasculitis
Lupus vasculitis
Rheumatoid vasculitis
Henoch-Schonlein purpura
Cryoglobulinemic vasculitis
Serum sickness vasculitis
Infection-induced vasculitis
Drug-induced vasculitis
B. ANCA-mediated vasculitis
Wegener's granulomatosis
Microscopic polyangiitis
Churg-Strauss syndrome
Antithyroid drug-induced vasculitis
C. Goodpasture's syndrome
D. Cell-mediated vasculitis
Giant cell arteritis
Takayasu's arteritis
Kawasaki disease
II. Idiopathic vasculitis syndromes
Polyarteritis nodosa
Necrotizing sarcoid granulomatosis
Behcet's syndrome
III. Infection-associated vasculitis
Bacterial vasculitis
Rickettsial vasculitis
Fungal vasculitis
Viral vasculitis
Mycobacterial vasculitis
Spirochetal vasculitis

II. Etiology and Pathogenesis

Almost all pulmonary vasculitis syndromes have an underlying antigen-antibody reaction as the basis of the vascular inflammation (5). The antibodies are most commonly of immunoglobulin G (IgG) or IgM class. In Henoch-Schonlein purpura, IgA antibody is implicated. The influx and activation of inflammatory cells as a result of the immune reaction is manifested in vasculitis. In many instances, there is formation of autoantibodies against known or unknown antigens, and in other cases there is formation of antibodies against drugs. Direct infection of the vessel by a number of pathogens can also cause vasculitis. In case of GPS, formation of specific antiglomerular basement membrane (anti-GBM) that bind to the alveolar basement membranes result in alveolar capillaritis. In Behcet's disease and Takayasu's arteritis, large vessel vasculitis develops with autoreactive T cells against heat-shock protein (HSP) 60. In other instances, patients develop autoantibodies against cytoplasmic components of neutrophils, specifically, against a 29-kDa neutral serine protease known as proteinase-3 (PR3) of the azurophil granules and myeloperoxidase (MPO), resulting in ANCA-associated vasculitis (5).

ANCA are important serologic markers, with established clinical utility in not only the diagnosis, but in monitoring the disease activity and response to treatment of systemic vasculitis. ANCA is comprised of several autoantibodies and detected by indirect immunofluorescence assays using the patient's serum and ethanol-fixed human neutrophils. Two common fluorescent staining patterns are seen: cytoplasmic (C-ANCA) with specificity directed against PR3 and perinuclear (P-ANCA) with specificity directed mainly against MPO, and rarely against other granular components such as lysozyme, elastase, cathepsins, and lactoferrin (LF). The C-ANCA pattern is highly specific for WG, while P-ANCA pattern is seen in MPA and CSS, as well as in a few other vasculitis with or without glomerulonephritis. ANCA are predominantly IgG isotype, but may be also IgM and IgA (5).

A. Immunogenesis of ANCA

The mechanism of induction of ANCA is not known, however, there are many hypotheses. One hypothesis is the activation by environmental factors, such as infectious agents, since patients often report flu-like symptoms. There are reports of possible association with arbovirus and *Staphylococcus aureus* infections and bacterial endocarditis (6–9). The molecular mimicry between the ANCA antigens and the antigens present on infectious agents could be the trigger for ANCA induction. However, the structural similarity between the ANCA antigens and microbial proteins is limited. Another proposed mechanism for induction of ANCA implicates complementary PR3 (cPR3) as the initial trigger for autoimmune response to PR3. The immune response to cPR3 induces anti-cPR3 antibodies (idiotypic antibodies) that initiate a second immune response, reacting with PR3 (10).

Both PR3-ANCA and MPO-ANCA contribute to development of vascular inflammation. ANCA IgG has been shown to activate neutrophils and monocytes with resultant oxidative burst and release of enzymes, including the ANCA antigens themselves, from the intracellular stores (11). ANCA-mediated monocyte and neutrophil activation has also been shown to induce the expression and secretion of proinflammatory cytokines such as interleukins (IL)-1, IL-6, IL-8, and tumor necrosis factor (TNF), as well as chemokines (monocyte chemoattractant protein-1) (12). The cytokine-primed neutrophils may then generate reactive oxygen radicals and degranulate with resultant inflammation producing vasculitis (13). There is intensive research in progress to understand the mechanisms underlying ANCA-mediated neutrophil and monocyte activation. So far, most studies have shown that neutrophils require priming with proinflammatory stimuli, especially TNF, for activation. Neutrophil priming with TNF induces translocation of the ANCA antigens, PR3 and MPO, to the cell surface, thus making them accessible for interaction with ANCA (14,15). This laboratory observation fits the clinical experience that in patients suffering from systemic vasculitis, exacerbations are often preceded by episodes of infections, which may be associated with release of proinflammatory mediators.

B. T Cells and ANCA

The role of T cells in ANCA-associated diseases is also under investigation. Several markers associated with T-cell activation are also increased in ANCA-associated vasculitis, including soluble IL-2 receptor, soluble CD4 and CD8 (5,16). Also, activated CD4- and CD8-positive T cells are increased in patients with WG. In active ANCA-associated vasculitis syndromes, the cellular infiltrates consist primarily of macrophages and T and B lymphocytes, suggesting that T cells may be actively involved in ANCA-associated vasculitis. Majority of these cells are T4 positive, with a predominant T cell helper-1 (Th1) profile with significant interferon-gamma (IFN-γ) production (17,18). Recently, it was also demonstrated that a substantial number of these CD4-positive cells are CD28 negative, a major source of IFN-γ and TNF-α (19). This particular subset of T cells is also present in the granulomatous lesions of WG and may be active in the formation of granulomas in this disease.

C. Anti-GBM Antibody and ANCA

Anti-GBM disease or GPS is associated with ANCA. In approximately 25% of patients with anti-GBM antibodies, a positive ANCA titer, mostly anti-MPO (P-ANCA), is seen (20). The primary target of anti-GBM antibody is a component of type IV collagen, and the pathogenic epitope is in noncollagenous 1 (NC1) domain of the α-3 chain of type IV collagen. Interestingly, the pathogenic antigen in the lungs is only exposed to the anti-GBM antibody when there is an underlying injury to the endothelial cells, such as smoking or lung infection, since the alveolar endothelial cells lack fenestrations. There is a strong human leukocyte antigen (HLA) association, with greater than 80% of the patients with anti-GBM disease carrying HLA-DR15 and DR4 alleles, while the DR7 locus seems to have a protective character (21). This suggests a possible role for T cells in the pathogenesis of autoimmune response in anti-GBM disease.

III. Treatment

The treatment of ANCA-associated vasculitis depends on the severity of the disease, patient's age, and renal function. With effective induction treatment, almost 80% patients achieve remission. Patients with WG, MPA, and CSS with one or more poor prognostic factors often respond to a combination of corticosteroids and cyclophosphamide to induce remission. Once remission is induced, less toxic immunosuppressants such as azathioprine and methotrexate are used for maintenance therapy (22). Plasma exchange is indicated as an adjuvant therapy if there is evidence of severe renal function impairment. Biologic therapies may be tried in patients who are refractory to conventional therapy. Anti-TNF-α, anti-CD20, anti-IL5, and anti-IgE monoclonal antibodies may be useful; however, their optimal regimens have not yet been defined.

The clinical presentation, and radiologic and histologic features of the common vasculitis-associated pulmonary diseases are discussed in the following paragraphs. A summary of key diagnostic features and main pathologic features of the common vasculitides are presented in Tables 2 and 3.

IV. Wegener's Granulomatosis

A. Clinical Presentation

WG is a multisystem disease, characterized by granulomatous vasculitis involving the upper and lower respiratory tract and kidneys.

It predominantly affects males, with mean age at 40 years. Patients present with chronic sinusitis and/or rhinitis refractory to usual therapy, with or without hemoptysis,

Table 2 Key Diagnostic Features of Pulmonary Vasculitides

Wegener's granulomatosis:
Granulomatous vasculitis involving pulmonary arteries, veins, venules, and capillaries
Polymorphous inflammatory infiltrate consisting of lymphocytes, plasma cells, neutrophils, macrophages, and multinucleated giant cells
Geographic necrosis with vascular necrosis and "microabscesses"
In some cases only alveolar capillaritis may be seen
An organizing pneumonia—BOOP-like pattern may be seen at the periphery of the necrosis
C-ANCA positive

Collagen vascular disease–associated vasculitis:
SLE; alveolar capillaritis and interstitial fibrosis, pulmonary arteriopathy, no granulomas or geographic necrosis
Rheumatoid arthritis; vasculitis, necrotizing granulomas, and pulmonary vasculopathy
PSS; interstitial fibrosis, pulmonary vasculopathy
MCTD; UIP like fibrosis and pulmonary vasculopathy
P-ANCA positive and C-ANCA negative

Goodpasture's syndrome:
Necrotizing alveolar capillaritis with hemorrhage
No granulomatous vasculitis or geographic necrosis
Alveolar and capillary basement membranes show linear IgG and C3 deposits on immunofluorescence
Anti-GBM antibody positive

Microscopic polyangiitis:
Small- to medium-sized pulmonary artery vasculitis without chronic inflammation
Necrotizing vasculitis, may be severe with extensive pulmonary hemorrhage
No immune deposits on immunofluorescence
P-ANCA positive

Churg-Strauss syndrome:
Small vessel vasculitis with or without vessel wall necrosis
Predominantly eosinophil infiltrate, mixed with other inflammatory cells
Eosinophilic abscesses
Peripheral eosinophilia, asthma, and allergic rhinitis
P-ANCA positive

Drug-induced vasculitis:
Small vessel vasculitis with or without vessel wall necrosis
No granulomatous inflammation
P-ANCA positive
History of receiving antithyroid drugs (propylthiouracil or methimazole)

Behcet's disease:
Large vessel vasculitis
Lymphocytic and necrotizing vasculitis with pulmonary infarcts
Vascular thrombosis and recanalization
Pulmonary artery aneurysms

Abbreviations: BOOP, bronchiolitis obliterans with organizing pneumonia; C-ANCA, cytoplasmic-antineutrophil cytoplasmic antibodies; P-ANCA, perinuclear cytoplasmic-antineutrophil cytoplasmic antibodies; SLE, systemic lupus erythematosus; MCTD, mixed connective tissue disease; UIP, usual interstitial pneumonia; Ig, immunoglobulin; GBM, glomerular basement membrane.

Table 3 Pathologic Features of Pulmonary Vasculitides

Diagnosis	Capillaritis	Venulitis	Arteritis	Geo. nec.	Giant cells	Eos.	Alv. Fibr.	Aneuryms	Recan Th.
WG	+	+	+	+	+	+/−	−	−	−
MPA	+	+	+/−	−	−	+	−	−	−
CSS	+	+	+	−	+/−	++	−	−	−
CVD	+	+/−	−	−	−	−	+/−	−	−
DIV	+	+	−	−	−	−	+/−	−	−
GPS	+	−	−	−	−	−	+	−	−
BD	+	+	+	−	−	−	−	+	+

Abbreviations: WG, Wegener's granulomatosis; MPA, microscopic polyangiitis; CSS, Churg-Strauss syndrome; CVD, collagen vascular–associated vasculitis; DIV, drug-induced vasculitis; GPS, Goodpasture's syndrome; BD, Behcet's disease; Geo. Nec., geographic necrosis; Eos., eosinophils; Alv. Fibr., alveolar fibrin deposits; Recan Th., recanalized thrombi.

nasal bleeding, and microscopic hematuria. Almost 95% of patients have pulmonary disease. Mild anemia without peripheral eosinophilia and elevated erythrocyte sedimentation rate may be seen. Serology is positive for C-ANCA antibody in more than 90% patients with active WG. Computed tomograms usually demonstrate multiple bilateral pulmonary nodules with occasional cavitation. Lesions are often pleural based. A definitive diagnosis can be established by lung or nasal biopsy.

B. Pathologic Features

Grossly, multiple pulmonary nodules with central cavitation and geographic necrosis are commonly seen. Solid nodular zones of consolidation with focal punctuate necrosis are also seen. Rarely, a bronchocentric distribution and a solitary nodule may be seen (23).

Histologically, the hallmark of WG is granulomatous vasculitis involving pulmonary arteries, veins, venules, and capillaries. The inflammatory infiltrate centered on the blood vessels is polymorphous, consisting of lymphocytes, plasma cells, neutrophils, macrophages, multinucleated giant cells, and occasional eosinophils. The vasculitis is associated with vascular necrosis and "microabscesses," which coalesce to form the areas of geographic necrosis (Figs. 1–3).

The histologic features may be divided into major and minor manifestations. The major manifestations include vasculitis, parenchymal necrosis, and granulomatous inflammation. The parenchymal necrosis may be seen as either neutrophilic microabscesses or geographic necrosis with irregular and serpiginous borders. Granulomatous inflammation with clusters of multinucleated giant cells, palisading histiocytes, or palisading micrgranulomas is centered on or around the blood vessels. Tightly packed sarcoid-like granulomas are rare, and if present, should initiate search for other diagnoses such as necrotizing sarcoidosis or infection. Vasculitis is often focal and eccentric, and may be confined to the endothelium. Capillaritis is histologically similar to MPA. The minor histologic features of WG are nonspecific and include a large variety of histologic changes, including alveolar hemorrhage, interstitial fibrosis, organizing pneumonia, chronic bronchitis and bronchiolitis

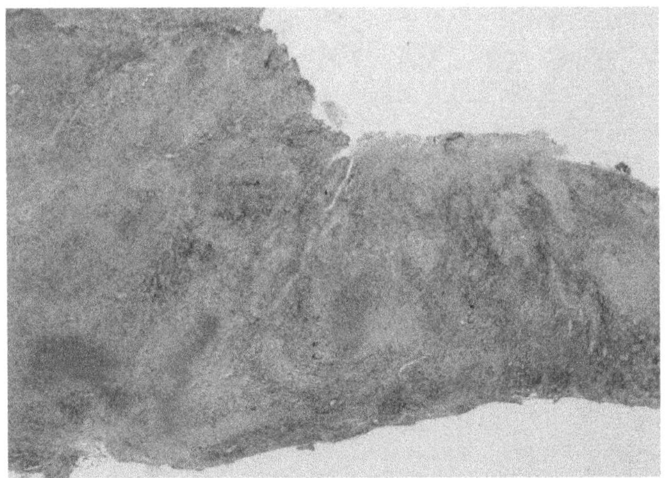

Figure 1 Wegener's granulomatosis shows microabscesses surrounded by inflammatory infiltrate.

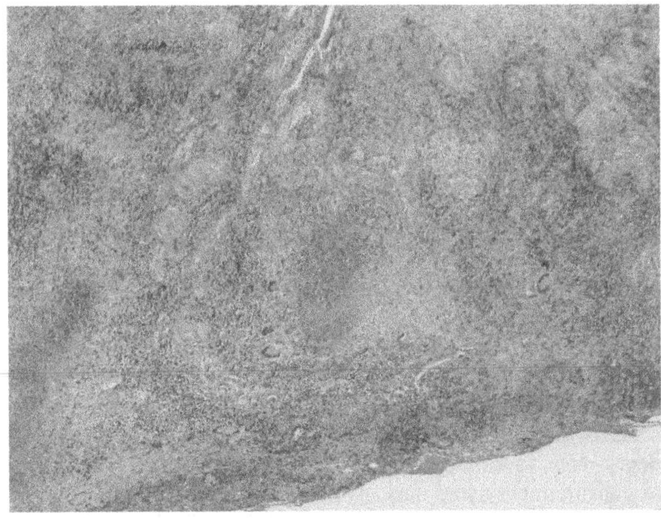

Figure 2 Wegener's granulomatosis with geographic necrosis, surrounded by inflammatory cells including multinucleated giant cells. The vessel wall is completely destroyed by the inflammation.

and follicular bronchitis, and bronchial stenosis (24). Atypical presentation, particularly alveolar capillary infiltration by neutrophils or "capillaritis" with necrosis and diffuse pulmonary hemorrhage with neutrophil spillover, may be the only lesion present in some cases (3). In these cases, clinical, radiologic, and serologic correlation is essential for a definitive diagnosis.

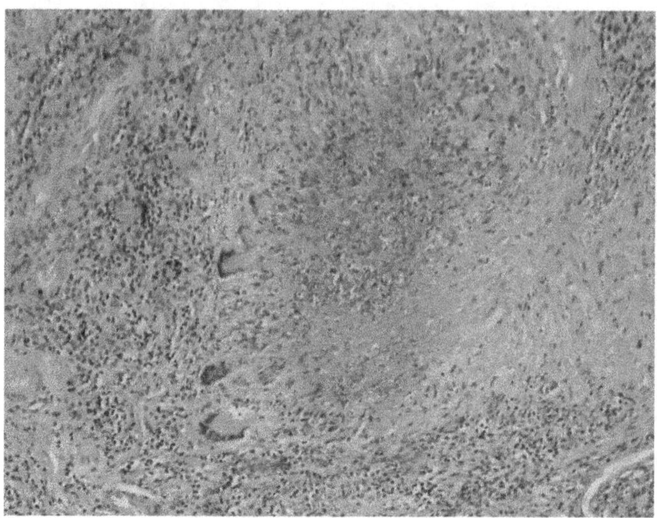

Figure 3 Higher magnification shows the inflammation, necrosis, and multinucleated giant cells characteristic of Wegener's granulomatosis.

Differential diagnosis includes lymphomatoid granulomatosis, necrotizing sarcoid granulomatosis, bronchocentric granulomatosis, rheumatoid nodule, CSS, and infection-induced vasculitis.

V. Microscopic Polyangiitis (Microscopic Polyarteritis)

A. Clinical Presentation

MPA is defined as necrotizing vasculitis that involves small vessels and has few or no immune deposits. It is a multisystem disease of middle-aged to older age group, with the vasculitis involving the skin, lungs, and kidney. Other synonyms include systemic necrotizing vasculitis, leukocytoclastic vasculitis, and hypersensitivity vasculitis. Clinical, epidemiologic, and pathologic differences warrant the separation of MPA from polyarteritis nodosa on the basis of absence of small vessel vasculitis in the latter (25). MPA is the most common cause for pulmonary-renal vasculitic syndrome (25). There is often a long prodromal phase with severe constitutional symptoms. Almost all patients develop rapidly progressive pauci-immune necrotizing and crescentic glomerulonephritis. Severe and extensive pulmonary involvement may result in fatal pulmonary hemorrhage. It is associated with P-ANCA antibody in approximately 75% to 80% of patients. Bilateral pulmonary opacities and consolidations may be seen on computed tomograms.

B. Pathologic Features

The vasculitis involves arterioles, venules, capillaries, and small arteries, although occasionally it can also involve medium-sized arteries. Typical histologic features include

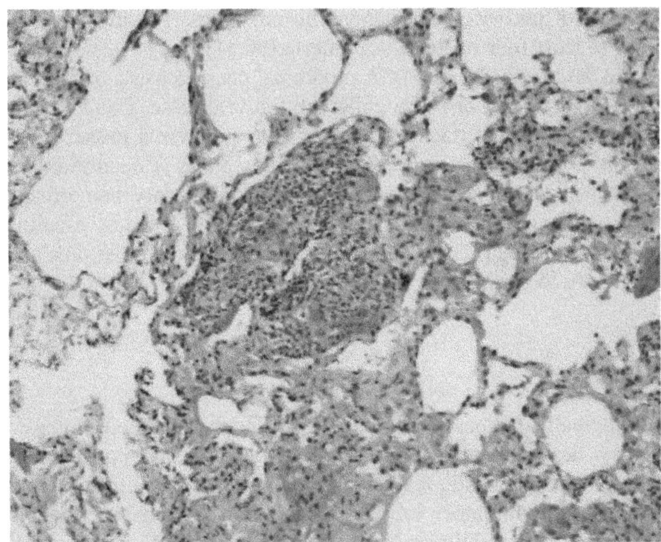

Figure 4 Microscopic polyangiitis has a dense neutrophil infiltrate of the alveolar capillaries spilling into the adjacent alveolar wall.

alveolar capillaritis with hemorrhage (3,26). There is patchy infiltration of capillary and alveolar walls by neutrophils associated with focal thickening and necrosis (Fig. 4). In severe cases, there may be a dense alveolar neutrophilic infiltrate resembling an infectious pneumonia; however, the presence of capillaritis, associated alveolar necrosis, and hemosiderin-filled macrophages should help in the diagnosis of MPA. Intra-alveolar hemorrhage, fibrinous exudates, and hyaline membranes resembling diffuse alveolar damage may be present (27). Venulitis, arteriolitis, and small vessel arteritis may be seen. The absence or paucity of Ig localization in vessel walls distinguishes MPA from immune complex–mediated small vessel vasculitis such as Henoch-Schonlein purpura and cryoglobulinemic vasculitis (25).

Differential diagnosis includes WG, drug-induced vasculitis, lupus-associated vasculitis, GPS, CSS, Henoch-Schonlein purpura, and cryoglobulinemic vasculitis.

VI. Allergic Angiitis and Granulomatosis (CSS)

A. Clinical Presentation

Allergic angiitis and granulomatosis (AAG), also known as Churg-Strauss syndrome (CSS), is a distinct multisystem disease of unknown etiology, characterized by asthma, peripheral blood eosinophilia, and systemic vasculitis involving upper airways, lungs, kidneys, heart, skin, and nerves (28,29). It is strongly associated with P-ANCA positivity. Most patients are middle aged. The diagnostic criteria include asthma, peripheral eosinophilia of at least 10%, mono- or polyneuropathy, radiologic evidence of migrating pulmonary infiltrates, allergic rhinitis, and histologic evidence of perivascular eosinophilic infiltrates. The diagnosis of CSS requires the presence of at least four of these six criteria (30,31).

Three clinical phases are described (29,32–34). A prodromal phase consists of asthma, peripheral eosinophilia, allergic rhinitis, and/or eosinophilic infiltrative disease. There may be eosinophilic pneumonia and gastrointestinal tract eosinophilia. The prodromal phase is followed by the vasculitis and the postvasculitis phase. The vasculitis phase is manifested by mononeuritis multiplex and cutaneous leukocytoclastic vasculitis. Pulmonary hemorrhage and glomerulonephritis are less common than in other forms of vasculitis. The postvasculitis phase is characterized by hypertension and peripheral neuropathy, associated with asthma and allergic rhinitis. Death is often due to cardiac complications.

B. Pathologic Features

The prodromal phase is histologically characterized by tissue eosinophilia and eosinophilic abscesses (28,33). There may be an associated asthmatic bronchitis and eosinophilic pneumonia. Vasculitic phase has the diagnostic features of small vessel vasculitis affecting arteries, veins, or capillaries. The inflammatory infiltrate consists of lymphocytes, plasma cells, epithelioid cells, giant cells, neutrophils, and abundant eosinophils (Figs. 5 and 6). The vasculitis may be necrotizing or nonnecrotizing. Chronic eosinophilic pneumonia with or without eosinophilic abscesses is present. There may be extravascular granulomas consisting of a central eosinophilic abscess surrounded by palisading histiocytes and giant cells. Postvasculitic phase has healed vasculitis with thrombosed vessels and decreased or absent tissue eosinophilia. Patients who had steroid therapy also show a decreased or absent eosinophilic infiltrate.

Differential diagnosis includes MPA, chronic eosinophilic pneumonia, WG, collagen vascular diseases, and drug-induced vasculitis.

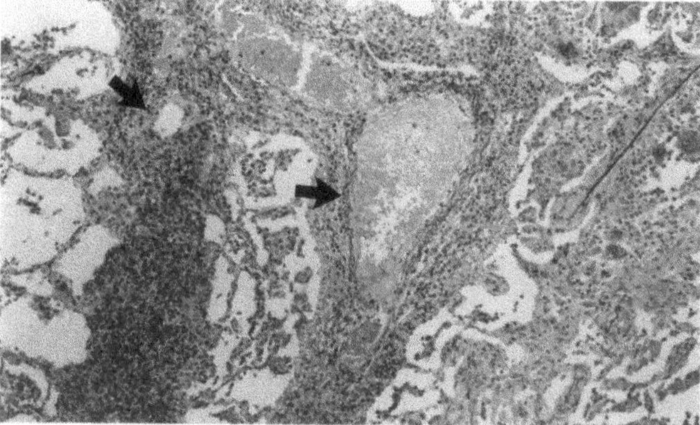

Figure 5 Churg-Strauss granulomatosis, low-power micrograph. H&E stain shows thickening of the arterial wall by an eosinophilic vasculitis (*arrows*). Eosinophilic and giant cell infiltrates are present in the interstitium and in airspaces.

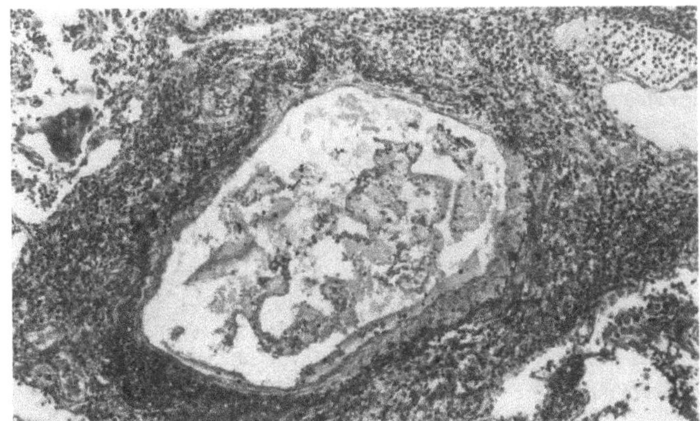

Figure 6 Churg-Strauss granulomatosis. H&E stain demonstrates eosinophilic vasculitis involving a medium-sized artery.

VII. Collagen Vascular Disease–Associated Vasculitis

This heterogeneous group is comprised of many diseases, with autoimmunity as the common underlying etiology. The majority of pulmonary complications in patients with collagen vascular diseases are related to the lung parenchyma. Occasionally, however, vasculitis may be seen. The common collagen vascular diseases include SLE, rheumatoid arthritis (RA), mixed connective tissue disease (MCTD), progressive systemic sclerosis (PSS), and Sjogren's disease. While any of these diseases may develop pulmonary lesions, vasculitis and alveolar hemorrhage are not a common complication, except in SLE (35,36). SLE-associated pulmonary vasculitis may be associated with approximately 50% fatality. Approximately 29% of patients with SLE are P-ANCA positive (with specificity directed against LF and lysozyme). In a study of 131 serum samples from 79 patients with SLE, RA, PSS, polymyositis/dermatomyositis (PM/DM), and idiopathic crescentic glomerulonephritis, and 36 healthy controls, both MPO and LF-ANCA were found in RA, SLE, and PSS, but not in PM/DM (37). Recent data suggest that presence of ANCA in SLE may be associated with serositis, venous thrombosis, and arthritis (38). Hemoptysis, anemia, fever, and dyspnea may be superimposed on the other systemic manifestations of the underlying collagen vascular disease.

Bilateral pulmonary infiltrates corresponding to the alveolar hemorrhages may be seen on chest radiograph or computed tomograms. Interstitial pulmonary fibrosis or rheumatoid nodules may be seen, depending on the underlying collagen vascular disease.

A. Pathologic Features

Histologic features of the collagen vascular disease–associated pulmonary disease include alveolar capillaritis, septal necrosis, alveolar hemorrhage, and hemosiderin-filled macrophages (Figs. 7 and 8). Occasionally, hemorrhage without capillaritis may be seen. The pneumonitis in SLE predominantly involves the alveolar septa, however, occasionally it may be secondary to vasculitis (Fig. 9) (35). In some patients, necrotizing arteritis with infiltration of the arterial wall by mononuclear cells may be present. In a small percentage

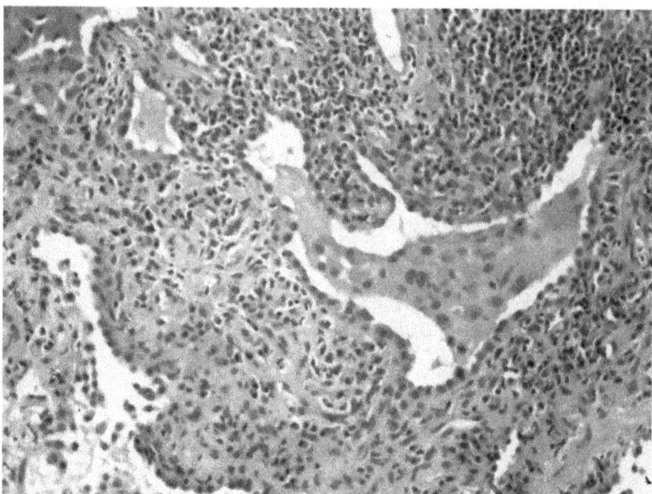

Figure 7 Systemic lupus erythematosus shows infiltration of the alveolar septa by chronic inflammatory cells including lymphocytes, plasma cells, and histiocytes, with expansion of the alveolar septa. There is alveolar pneumocyte hyperplasia and clusters of alveolar macrophages.

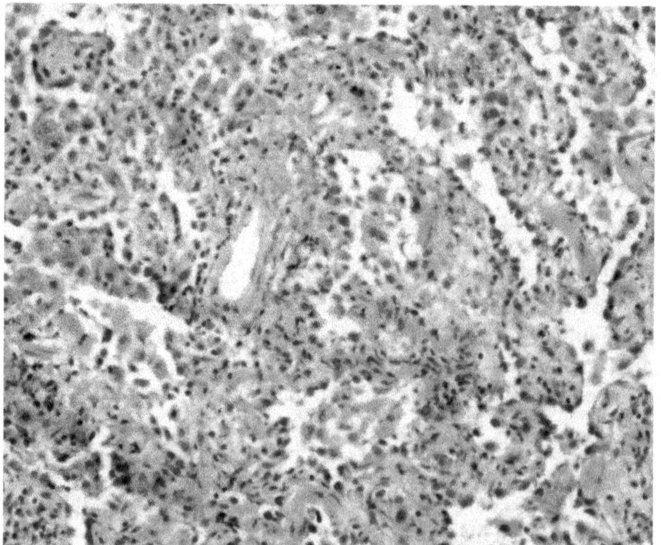

Figure 8 Systemic lupus erythematosus has septal thickening, alveolar pneumocyte hyperplasia, and many hemosiderin-laden alveolar macrophages, indicating old hemorrhage.

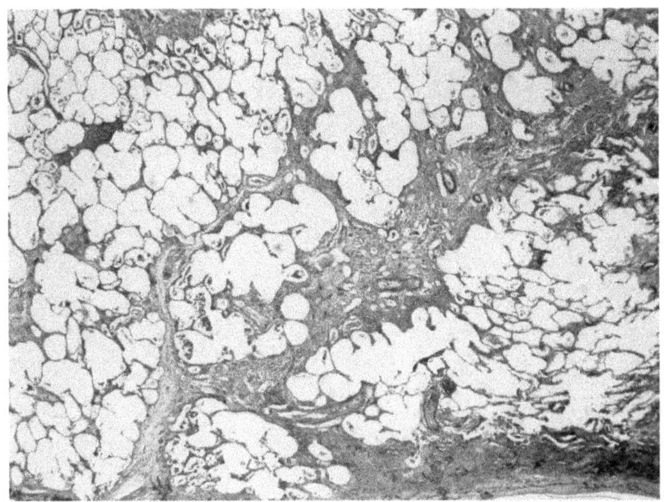

Figure 9 Movat pentachrome–stained section of systemic lupus erythematosus shows alveolar septal thickening with minimal inflammation.

of patients with SLE (14%), pulmonary hypertension secondary to pulmonary arteriopathy with plexiform lesions may be seen (39,40). These patients also reportedly have a higher prevalence of Raynaud's phenomenon and antiphospholipid antibodies (41).

The patients with rheumatoid arthritis may also develop pulmonary hypertension secondary to similar lesions as those seen in SLE (Fig. 10) (42). Less commonly, vasculitis and necrotizing granulomas may be seen in association with rheumatoid arthritis (35).

PSS may be associated with vasculopathy, with or without interstitial pulmonary fibrosis (43). The lungs may have changes of pulmonary hypertension with intimal fibrosis and medial hypertrophy of arteries and less commonly the veins. In one series of patients with PSS, pulmonary hypertension was present with only grade 2 or 3 vasculopathy (43). Pulmonary vasculitis, plexiform lesions, and onionskin pattern of vascular sclerosis are uncommon in the lungs in PSS.

MCTD is clinically characterized by a combination of signs and symptoms of SLE, PSS, and PM/DM. Patients may develop usual interstitial pneumonia (UIP) like interstitial fibrosis and severe pulmonary hypertension with plexiform vascular lesions (44).

Differential diagnosis includes MPA, WG, GPS, and UIP.

VIII. Drug-Induced Vasculitis

Recently, the development of an autoimmune disease with pulmonary vasculitis is described following treatment with antithyroid drugs (ATD), namely propylthiouracil and methimazole (45,46). The clinical and serologic profiles of idiopathic MPA and

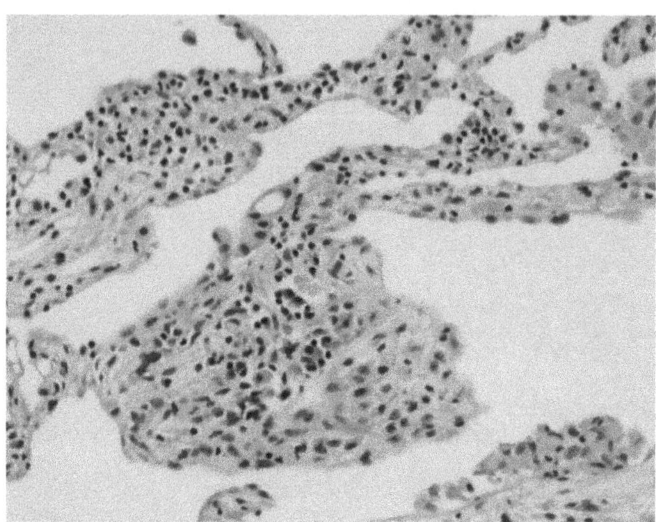

Figure 10 Rheumatoid arthritis demonstrates widened and thickened alveolar septa with moderate chronic inflammatory infiltrate including lymphocytes, plasma cells, and histiocytes. There is also an increase in alveolar macrophages.

ATD-induced vasculitis are very similar. Patients with ATD-induced autoimmune disease can have renal and skin lesions, in addition to pulmonary lesions.

A. Clinical Presentation

In a small series of 16 patients who became P-ANCA positive during treatment with ATD, 12 patients developed lupus-like disease and 4 developed pulmonary vasculitis (46). Clinically, ANCA-positive ATD-treated patients can be divided into two groups. First, those who develop drug-induced WG or microscopic polyarteritis resembling idiopathic systemic vasculitis, and second, consisting of those who develop SLE-like disease. The ATD-induced disease appears to have a milder course compared to idiopathic systematic vasculitis. The radiologic manifestations of ATD-induced vasculitis are not well defined.

B. Pathologic Features

Histologically, the lungs may show MPA-like vasculitis with neutrophil infiltration of alveolar capillaries associated with septal necrosis and alveolar hemorrhage (Fig. 11). Alternately, there may be granulomatous vasculitis resembling WG. Histologic findings should be correlated with the clinical history of drug intake, radiologic features, and clinical manifestations of the underlying disease (46).

Differential diagnosis includes MPA, WG, Henoch-Schonlein purpura, cryoglobulinemic vasculitis, CSS, lupus-associated vasculitis, and GPS.

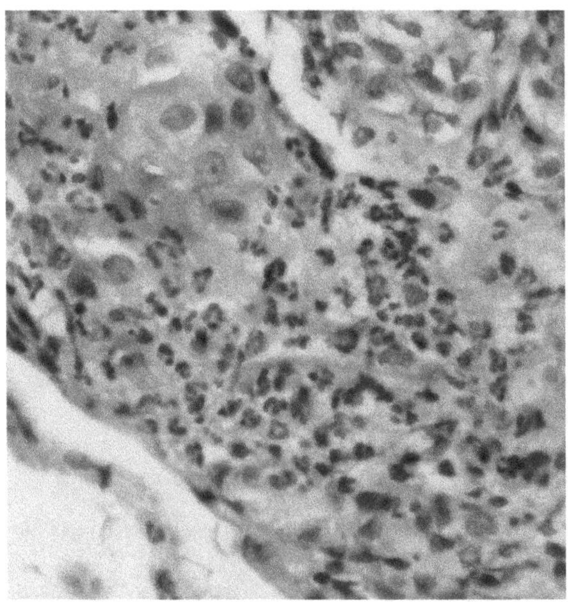

Figure 11 Drug-induced microscopic polyangiitis has histologic features indistinguishable from idiopathic microscopic polyangiitis, with infiltration of the alveolar capillaries by neutrophils and congestion and widening of the alveolar septa.

IX. Goodpasture's Syndrome (Anti-GBM Antibody Disease)

A. Clinical Presentation

GPS or anti-GBM antibody disease is a primary immune complex–mediated vasculitis characterized by pulmonary and renal disease. Pulmonary involvement alone is rare and often occurs prior to the renal disease. Approximately 50% of patients with anti-GBM renal disease have pulmonary involvement (5). It is a relatively rare disease, with an incidence of approximately one case per 2 million/yr in European Caucasians (47). ANCA-associated disease is approximately 10 times more common. GPS has a peak incidence in young adult men and a second peak in the sixth and seventh decade, which is equally seen in men and women. Environmental factors such as exposure to hydrocarbons and smoking may play a role in etiology (48). Pulmonary hemorrhage is almost exclusively seen in current smokers. Hemoptysis, mild anemia, shortness of breath, and microscopic or gross hematuria may be the presenting complaints. Serologic tests can detect the anti-GBM antibody. Approximately 25% of patients with GPS also have positive P-ANCA. Immunofluorescence of the renal or lung biopsy can also establish the diagnosis. Chest radiographs may show patchy, alveolar infiltrates in early stages; whiteout of the lung fields with massive pulmonary hemorrhage may be seen later.

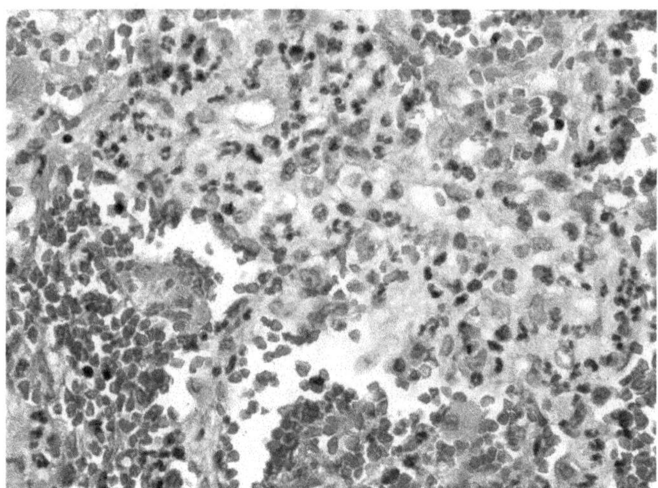

Figure 12 Goodpasture's syndrome has a dense neutrophil infiltrate of the alveolar septa surrounding the capillaries and associated with alveolar hemorrhage.

B. Pathologic Features

The characteristic histologic feature of GPS is necrotizing vasculitis with infiltration of the alveolar septa by neutrophils associated with alveolar necrosis, edema, and hemorrhage (Fig. 12). The alveoli are filled with red blood cells, fibrin, few neutrophils, and hemosiderin-filled macrophages. Rarely, hyaline membranes may be present. No large vessel vasculitis or granulomatous inflammation is seen. Immunofluorescence shows linear IgG and C3 deposits. Focal alveolar septal fibrosis may be seen in later healing stage. Differential diagnosis includes MPA, CSS, lupus-associated vasculitis, WG, and infection-associated vasculitis.

C. Henoch-Schonlein Purpura

Although often considered in the differential diagnosis of pulmonary vasculitides, pulmonary involvement in Henoch-Schonlein purpura is uncommon. The histologic features include a capillaritis similar to the MPA (49). IgA deposits in the alveolar septal capillaries were reported in one case (50).

X. Large Vessel Vasculitides

Behcet's disease and Takayasu's arteritis are chronic autoimmune diseases with vasculitis affecting primarily large blood vessels. The underlying pathogenetic mechanism of vasculitis involves autoreactive T cells against HSP 60. Pulmonary and coronary vessels are predominantly involved in Behcet's disease, and aorta is more frequently involved in Takayasu's arteritis. Pulmonary aneurysms are a major complication of Behcet's disease and may be fatal with massive hemoptysis. Pulmonary involvement is rare in Takayasu's arteritis.

A. Behcet's Disease

Behcet's disease is relatively more common than Takayasu's arteritis. Vascular inflammation in Behcet's disease involves the pulmonary arteries, veins, capillaries, and superior vana cava and may spread to the pleura and mediastinum. Pulmonary involvement is seen in 5% to 10% of patients. The classic presentation is the triad of oral and genital ulcerations and uveitis. Genetic factors and immune complexes are postulated to play a role in pathogenesis (51). The most common pulmonary symptom is hemoptysis. Patients develop multifocal necrotizing vasculitis with diffuse pulmonary hemorrhages, infarction, and organizing pneumonia. Pulmonary hypertension and infarcts can cause fever, malaise, and weight loss (52). Pulmonary consolidation and alveolar infiltrates may be seen. Imaging techniques such as MRI and tomodensitometry can demonstrate the pulmonary vascular lesions.

Histologically, there is transmural necrotizing vasculitis of medium and small pulmonary vessels, with destruction of the wall, replacement by granulation tissue, fibrosis, and resultant aneurysms formations of pulmonary vessels (Figs. 13 and 14). There is venous and arterial thrombosis with recanalization of lumen and associated pulmonary hemorrhages and infarcts. Later, arteriobronchial fistulas secondary to pulmonary arterial aneurysms may develop, with rupture of aneurysm and fatal massive hemoptysis.

B. Takayasu's Arteritis

Takayasu's arteritis primarily affects the thoracic and abdominal aorta and its main branches. In one study, however, abnormal pulmonary arteries were demonstrated in 70% of cases with Takayasu's arteritis (53). The abnormalities included arterial stenosis or

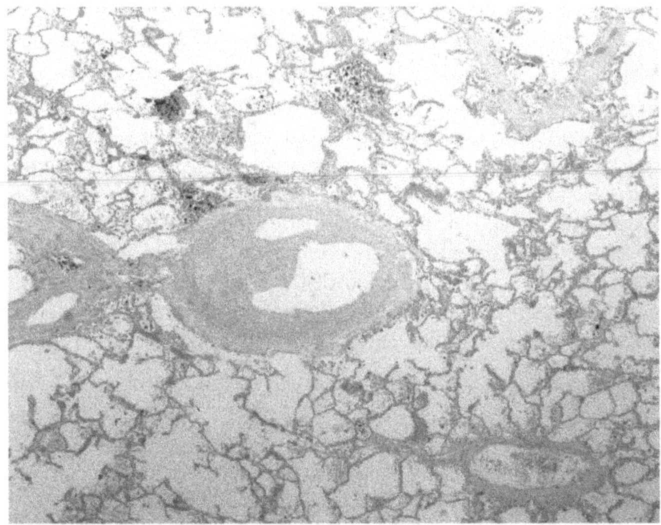

Figure 13 Behcet's disease has a thickened pulmonary artery with a recanalized lumen. The surrounding lung shows recent and old hemorrhage.

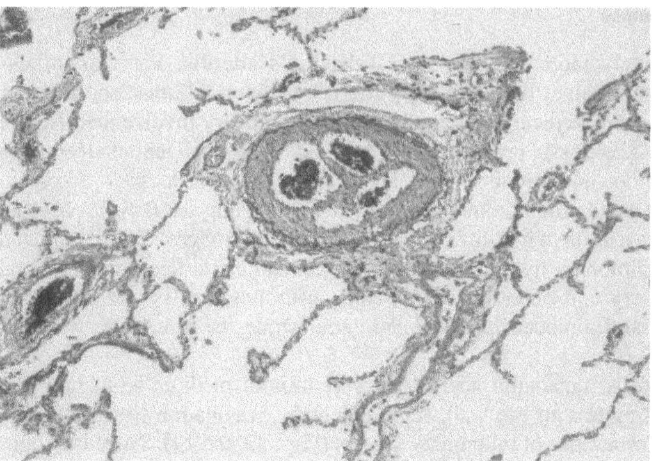

Figure 14 Movat pentachrome–stained section shows Behcet's disease with a thickened and fibrosed pulmonary artery with recanalized lumen, and a small pulmonary vein with mildly thickened wall.

occlusion of the segmental branches and, less commonly, of the subsegmental branches. The elastic pulmonary arteries in another autopsy study showed intimal fibrosis, thinning and disruption of media, and band-like fibrosis of adventitia (54). Some of the larger elastic pulmonary arteries were occluded by loose fibrous tissue while others demonstrated a stenosis recanalization lesion. In this study, some of the muscular branches of pulmonary artery also showed concentric intimal fibrosis.

C. Necrotizing Sarcoid Granulomatosis

Vasculitis, associated with sarcoid-like granulomas, and nodules showing central necrosis are the characteristic features of pulmonary necrotizing sarcoid granulomatosis (NSG). The sarcoid-like granulomas may be adjacent to the necrotizing nodules or may demonstrate the lymphatic distribution often seen in pulmonary sarcoidosis. The granulomatous vasculitis typically involves both arteries and veins, sparing the capillaries (55). There may be total effacement of the vessel wall by the sarcoid-like granulomas. Alternately, a giant cell vasculitis resembling temporal arteritis with destruction of the elastic lamina or a mononuclear infiltrate of intima and media may be seen. There are sarcoid-like granulomas in the adjacent airway walls, which help distinguish this entity from WG (56).

References

1. Franks TJ, Koss MN. Pulmonary capillaritis. Curr Opin Pulm Med 2000; 6:430–435.
2. Schwartz MI, Brown KK. Small vessel vasculitis of the lung. Thorax 2000; 55:502–510.
3. Travis WD. Pathology of pulmonary vasculitis. Semin Respir Crit Care Med 2004; 25:475–482.
4. Jennette JC, Falk RJ, Andrassy K, et al. Nomenclature of systemic vasculitides: the proposal of an international consensus conference. Arthritis Rheum 1994; 37:187–192.

5. Heeringa P, Schreiber A, Falk RJ, et al. Pathogenesis of pulmonary vasculitis. Semin Respir Crit Care Med 2004; 25:465–474.
6. Davies DJ, Moran JE, Niall JF, et al. Segmental necrotizing glomerulonephritis with anti-neutrophil antibody: possible arbovirus etiology? Br Med J (Clin Res Ed) 1982; 285:606.
7. Wucherpfennig KW. Mechanisms for the induction of autoimmunity by infectious agents. J Clin Invest 2001; 108:1097–1104.
8. Choi HK, Lamprecht P, Niles JL, et al. Subacute bacterial endocarditis with positive cytoplasmic antineutrophil cytoplasmic antibodies and anti-proteinase 3 antibodies. Arthritis Rheum 2000; 43:226–231.
9. Stegeman CA, Tervaert JW, Sluiter WJ, et al. Association of chronic nasal carriage of Staphylococcus aureus and higher relapse rate in Wegener granulomatosis. Ann Intern Med 1994; 120:12–17.
10. Pendergraft WF, Preston GA, Shah RR, et al. Autoimmunity is triggered by cPR-3(105-201), a protein complementary to human autoantigen proteinase-3. Nat Med 2004; 10:72–79.
11. Jennette JC, Falk RJ. Pathogenesis of the vascular and glomerular damage in ANCA-positive vasculitis. Nephrol Dial Transplant 1998; 13(suppl 1):16–20.
12. Hattar K, Bickenbach A, Csernok E, et al. Wegener's granulomatosis: antiproteinase 3 antibodies induce monocyte cytokine and prostanoid release-role of autocrine cell activation. J Leukoc Biol 2002; 71:996–1004.
13. Schultz DR, Diego JM. Antineutrophil cytoplasmic antibodies (ANCA) and systemic vasculitis: update of assays, immunopathogenesis, controversies, and report of a novel de novo ANCA-associated vasculitis after kidney transplantation. Semin Arthritis Rheum 2000; 29:267–285.
14. Falk RJ, Terrell RS, Charles LA, et al. Anti-neutrophil cytoplasmic antibodies induce neutrophils to degranulate and produce oxygen radicals in vitro. Proc Natl Acad Sci U S A 1990; 87: 4115–4119.
15. Csernok E, Ernst M, Schmitt W, et al. Activated neutrophils express proteinase 3 on their plasma membrane in vitro and in vivo. Clin Exp Immunol 1994; 95:244–250.
16. Popa ER, Stegeman CA, Bos NA, et al. Differential B- and T- cell activation in Wegener's granulomatosis. J Allergy Clin Immunol 1999; 103:885–894.
17. Csernok E, Trabandt A, Muller A, et al. Cytokine profiles in Wegener's granulomatosis: predominance of type 1 (Th1) in the granulomatous inflammation. Arthritis Rheum 1999; 42:742–750.
18. Muller A, Trabandt A, Gloeckner-Hofmann K, et al. Localized Wegener's granulomatosis: predominance of CD26 and IFN-gamma expression. J Pathol 2000; 192:113–120.
19. Komocsi A, Lamprecht P, Csernok E, et al. Peripheral blood and granuloma CD4(+)CD28(−) T cells are a major source of interferon-gamma and tumor necrosis factor-alpha in Wegener's granulomatosis. Am J Pathol 2002; 160:1717–1724.
20. Kalluri R, Meyers K, Mogyorosis A, et al. Goodpasture syndrome involving overlap with Wegener's granulomatosis and anti-glomerular basement membrane disease. J Am Soc Nephrol 1997; 8:1795–1800.
21. Fisher M, Pusey CD, Vaughan RW, et al. Susceptibility to antiglomerular basement membrane disease is strongly associated with HLA-DRB1 genes. Kidney Int 1997; 51:222–229.
22. Langford CA. Small vessel vasculitis: therapeutic management. Curr Rheumatol Rep 2007; 9:328–335.
23. Travis WD, Hoffman GS, Leavitt RY, et al. Surgical pathology of the lung in Wegener's granulomatosis: review of 87 open-lung biopsies from 67 patients. Am J Surg Pathol 1991; 15:315–333.
24. Uner AH, Rozum-Slota B, Katzenstein AL. Bronchiolitis obliterans-organizizng pneumonia (BOOP)-like variant of Wegener's granulomatosis: a clinicopathologic study of 16 cases. Am J Surg Pathol 1996; 20:794–801.
25. Jennette JC, Thomas DB, Falk RJ. Microscopic polyangiitis (microscopic polyarteritis). Semin Diagn Pathol 2001; 18:3–13.

26. Jennette JC, Falk RJ. Small vessel vasculitis. N Engl J Med 1997; 337:1512–1523.
27. Akikusa B, Kondo Y, Irabu N, et al. Six cases of microscopic polyarteritis exhibiting acute interstitial pneumonia. Pathol Int 1995; 45:580–588.
28. Churg J, Strauss L. Allergic granulomatosis, allergic angiitis and periarteritis nodosa. Am J Pathol 1951; 27:277–294.
29. Chumbley LC, Harrison EG Jr., DeRemee RA. Allergic granulomatosis and angiitis (Churg-Strauss syndrome): report and analysis of 30 cases. Mayo Clin Proc 1977; 52:477–484.
30. Masi AT, Hunder GG, Lie JT, et al. The American College of Rheumatology 1990 criteria for the classification of Churg-Strauss syndrome (allergic granulomatosis and angiitis). Arthritis Rheum 1990; 33:1094–1100.
31. Churg A. Recent advances in the diagnosis of Churg-Strauss syndrome. Mod Pathol 2001; 14:1284–1293.
32. Noth I, Strek ME, Leff AR. Churg-Strauss syndrome. Lancet 2003; 361:587–594.
33. Lanham JG, Churg J. Churg-Strauss syndrome. In: Churg A, Churg J, eds. Systemic vasculitides. New York: Igaku-Shoin, 1991:101–120.
34. Specks U, DeRemee RA. Granulomatous vasculitis. Wegener's granulomatosis and Churg-Strauss syndrome. Rheum Dis Clin North Am 1990; 16:377–397.
35. Hunninghake GW, Fauci AS. Pulmonary involvement in collagen vascular diseases. Am Rev Respir Dis 1979; 119:471–503.
36. Gross M, Esterly JR, Earle RH. Pulmonary alterations in systemic lupus erythematosus. Am Rev Respir Dis 1972; 105:572–577.
37. Chikazawa H, Nishiya K, Matsumori A, et al. Immunoglobulin isotypes of anti-myeloperoxidase and anti-lactoferrin antibodies in patients with collagen diseases. J Clin Immunol 2000; 20: 279–286.
38. Galeazzi M, Morozzi G, Sebastiani GD, et al. Anti-neutrophil cytoplasmic antibodies in 566 European patients with systemic lupus erythematosus: prevalence, clinical associations and correlation with other autoantibodies. European Concerted Action on the immunogenetics of SLE. Clin Exp Rheumatol 1998; 16:541–546.
39. Simonson JS, Schiller NB, Petri M, et al. Pulmonar hypertension in systemic lupus erythematosus. J Rheumatol 1989; 16:918–925.
40. Goldman J, Edwards WD. Plexogenic pulmonary hypertension in systemic lupus erythematosus: report of two cases and review of the literature. Cardiovasc Pathol 1994; 3:65–69.
41. Asherson RA, Higenbottam TW, Xuan ATD, et al. Pulmonary hypertension in a lupus clinic: experience with twenty four patients. J Rheumatol 1990; 17:1292–1298.
42. Shimosato Y, Miller RR. Biopsy Interpretation of the Lung. New York: Raven Press, 1995: 114–161.
43. Yousem SA. The pulmonary pathologic manifestations of the CREST syndrome. Hum Pathol 1990; 21:467–474.
44. Weiner-Kronish JP, Solinger AM, Warnock ML, et al. Severe pulmonary involvement in mixed connective tissue disease. Am Rev Respir Dis 1981; 124:449–503.
45. Choi HK, Merkel PA, Tervaert JW, et al. Alternating antineutrophil cytoplasmic antibody specificity: drug-induced vasculitis in a patient with Wegener's granulomatosis. Arthritis Rheum 1999; 42:384–388.
46. Bonaci-Nikolic B, Nikolic MM, Andrejevic S, et al. Antineutrophil cytoplasmic antibody (ANCA)-associated autoimmune diseases induced by antithyroid drugs: comparison with idiopathic ANCA vasculitides. Arthritis Res Ther 2005; 7:R1072–R1081.
47. Kluth DC, Rees AJ. Anti-glomerular basement membrane disease. J Am Soc Nephrol 1999; 10:2446–2453.
48. Bombassei GJ, Kaplan AA. The association between hydrocarbon exposure and anti-glomerular basement membrane antibody-mediated disease (Goodpasture's syndrome). Am J Ind Med 1992; 21:141–153.

49. Roth DA, Wilz DR, Theil GB. Schonlein-Henoch syndrome in adults. Q J Med 1985; 55: 145–152.
50. Kathuria S, Cheifec G. Fatal pulmonary Henoch-Schonlein syndrome. Chest 1982; 82:654–656.
51. Slavin RE, de Groot WJ. Pathology of the lung in Behcet's disease. Am J Surg Pathol 1981; 5:779–788.
52. Hirohata S, Kikuchi H. Behcet's disease. Arthritis Res Ther 2003; 5:139–146.
53. Yamada I, Shibuya H, Matsubara O, et al. Pulmonary artery disease in Takayasu's arteritis: angiographic findings. AJR Am J Roentgenol 1992; 159:263–269.
54. Matsubara O, Yoshimura N, Tamura A, et al. Pathologic features of the pulmonary artery in Takayasu's arteritis. Heart Vessels 1992; 7(suppl):18–25.
55. Liebow AA. The J Burns Amberson lecture: pulmonary angiitis and granulomatosis. Am Rev Respir Dis 1973; 108:1–18.
56. Koss MN, Hochholzer L, Feigin DS, et al. Necrotizing sarcoid-like granulomatosis: clinical, pathologic, and immunopathologic findings. Hum Pathol 1980; 11(suppl):510–519.

20
Clinical Diagnosis of Pulmonary Vascular Disease

LEWIS J. RUBIN
University of California, San Diego School of Medicine, La Jolla, California, U.S.A.

I. Introduction

Pulmonary hypertension is not a disease per se but rather a hemodynamic abnormality common to many conditions that are treated quite differently. Accordingly, it is crucial for the clinician to establish the etiology of pulmonary vascular disease before embarking on a course of therapy. While this can usually be accomplished on the basis of clinical grounds, examination of pathological material may be necessary. This chapter reviews the diagnostic approach to patients with pulmonary vascular disease.

Most patients with pulmonary vascular disease will present with dyspnea, usually exertional, reflecting the inability to increase right ventricular output in response to the demands of activity, because of the increased resistance in the pulmonary vascular bed. The nonspecific nature of this typical complaint often results in a delay in establishing the diagnosis. In the National Institutes of Health Registry on primary pulmonary hypertension (PPH, now referred to as idiopathic pulmonary arterial hypertension, IPAH), the mean time from the onset of symptoms to the establishment of the diagnosis was greater than two years (1). More severe symptoms, which are indicative of a greater degree of hemodynamic compromise, include syncope (often with exertion or immediately postexertion) and lower extremity edema. The diagnosis of pulmonary vascular disease in a patient with established underlying lung disease poses an even greater challenge, as these patients already have dyspnea because of impaired lung function. Worsening dyspnea in the face of unchanged parameters of lung function should suggest the possibility of concomitant pulmonary vascular compromise.

The findings of pulmonary hypertension on physical examination are usually subtle and nonspecific; they include a prominent right ventricular impulse, an accentuated pulmonic component of the second heart sound, and a murmur of tricuspid regurgitation. Patients with parenchymal lung disease, congenital heart disease, and the portal-pulmonary hypertension syndrome may have digital clubbing, which is a helpful clue to the etiology. Abnormal breath sounds may suggest the presence of parenchymal lung disease, and intrapulmonary bruits may be audible in areas of intraluminal thrombosis in patients with chronic thromboembolic disease. Patients with occult connective tissue disease may have cutaneous telangiectasia, acrocyanosis, or other skin and joint features of collagen vascular disease. Hepatomegaly, ascites, and edema are usually indicative of right heart failure—a late feature of pulmonary hypertension.

Table 1 Secondary Causes of Pulmonary Hypertension

Lung disease
Parenchymal lung diseases
Disorders of ventilation
Congenital anomalies
Altitude
Heart disease
Disorders of left heart filling
Congenital intracardiac shunts
Obstruction of the pulmonary vessels
Chronic thromboembolic disease
Mediastinal fibrosis
Congenital pulmonary artery stenoses
Foreign bodies
Tumor
Parasitic diseases
Connective tissue diseases and pulmonary vasculitis
Exogenous substances
Anorexigens
Cocaine
Methamphetamine
HIV infection
Portal hypertension

Once the presence of pulmonary hypertension is suspected on clinical grounds, the approach shifts to clarifying the etiology (Table 1). A careful history may reveal important clues to the etiology. A family history of pulmonary hypertension suggests the possibility of familial PAH (which accounts for approximately 10% of cases of this condition) or chronic thromboembolic disease related to a hereditary thrombophilic disorder (deficiencies of antithrombin III or proteins C or S). A history of excessive alcohol use or infectious hepatitis raises the possibility of the portal-pulmonary hypertension syndrome, and a history of intravenous drug use suggests either human immunodeficiency virus (HIV)-associated pulmonary hypertension or talc-induced granulomatous pulmonary vasculopathy. Prior use of anorexigens, particularly if recent and for periods exceeding three months, has been associated with a 20-fold increased incidence of PPH (2). The agents most frequently implicated are the serotonin reuptake inhibitors fenfluramine and dexfenfluramine, although amphetamine-like diet suppressants have also been implicated. In addition, both cocaine and methamphetamine use have been implicated as causes of exogenous pulmonary hypertension.

A variety of laboratory studies are helpful in both establishing the presence of pulmonary hypertension and clarifying its etiology. Indeed, no patient in the National Institutes of Health Registry was found by pathological examination to have a condition other than PPH when a comprehensive clinical diagnostic approach was followed (3). The widespread availability of echocardiography has resulted in this noninvasive test commonly providing the first suggestion of the presence of pulmonary hypertension in a patient with unexplained dyspnea. The typical findings of right ventricular pressure overload on echocardiogram include flattening or paradoxical motion of the interventricular septum, enlargement of the right heart chambers, and increased thickness of the right ventricular wall. Doppler interrogation may disclose evidence of tricuspid regurgitation, and the pulmonary artery systolic pressure may be estimated by the magnitude of the tricuspid regurgitant jet. Evidence of an intracardiac shunt may be disclosed using contrast echocardiography; this finding may provide meaningful information regarding etiology. Additionally, its presence urges caution with the administration of vasodilator agents, since worsening hypoxemia may result from any treatment, which could increase shunting. Although physicians frequently rely on the echocardiographic parameters to follow patients on therapy, it should be emphasized that the estimates of pulmonary artery pressure by Doppler study tend to underestimate the invasively measured hemodynamic parameters (4). Nevertheless, echocardiographic evidence of regression of right ventricular hypertrophy and reduction in right heart chamber size have been observed in patients who are responsive to treatment (5).

The sensitivity of echocardiography in identifying the presence of mild pulmonary hypertension is unknown. On occasion, patients with mild pulmonary hypertension may present with exertional dyspnea and oxygen desaturation and have a normal echocardiogram; in this setting, echocardiography or hemodynamic study during exercise may demonstrate abnormalities in hemodynamics or right heart function that indicate the presence of early, exercise-induced increases in pulmonary artery pressure.

An assessment of pulmonary function is appropriate in the evaluation of a patient with evidence of pulmonary vascular disease to exclude significant airway or parenchymal lung disease. In patients with chronic airflow obstruction, the presence and severity of pulmonary hypertension correlates with the degree of airflow obstruction. Most patients with a forced expiratory volume in one second (FEV_1) below 1 L will have pulmonary hypertension, although the degree of hemodynamic abnormality is usually modest compared with conditions that primarily affect the pulmonary circulation (IPAH, chronic thromboembolic disease, connective tissue disease) (6). Patients with interstitial lung disease develop secondary pulmonary hypertension once both a significant impairment in intrapulmonary gas exchange [diffusing capacity of lung for carbon monoxide (DLCO) less than 50% of predicted] and restriction in lung volume (forced vital capacity less than 50% predicted) are present. For all forms of parenchymal lung disease, significant hypoxemia correlates with the presence and severity of pulmonary hypertension, consistent with the known effects of hypoxia on pulmonary vasoreactivity and remodeling. Pulmonary function studies may be mildly abnormal in patients with PPH or chronic thromboembolic pulmonary hypertension (CTEPH). A mild restrictive ventilatory defect may be observed and the DLCO may be moderately to severely reduced. The latter abnormality is because of the reduction in cross-sectional vascular surface area and the diminution in pulmonary blood volume that are characteristic of these conditions.

A variety of laboratory studies are useful in clarifying the etiology of pulmonary vascular disease:

1. Connective tissue serological studies can suggest the presence of a collagen vascular disease. However, these tests must be interpreted cautiously, since patients with IPAH may have positive antinuclear antibody studies, albeit usually in a low titer.
2. Testing for antibodies to the HIV is recommended for all patients with unexplained pulmonary hypertension, since there appears to be an increased risk of pulmonary hypertension in HIV-positive individuals, even in the absence of the acquired immune deficiency syndrome (AIDS) (7).

3. Liver function studies may disclose abnormalities suggesting the presence of hepatic cirrhosis, with resulting portal-pulmonary hypertension.
4. In patients with suspected chronic thromboembolic disease, assays of antithrombin III, proteins C and S, factor V Leiden, and anticardiolipin antibodies may disclose a thrombophilic trait.
5. In patients suspected of having a vasculitis, determination of the erythrocyte sedimentation rate as well as antinuclear and antinuclear cytoplasmic antibodies may provide supportive data. In most patients with pulmonary vasculitis, however, angiography and lung biopsy will be necessary to confirm the diagnosis.

Perhaps the single most important and often most difficult distinction is between chronic thromboembolic disease and IPAH. Patients with both conditions can present at any age, and both disorders present with signs and symptoms of severe pulmonary hypertension and right heart failure. However, treatments for the two conditions are quite different. CTEPH may be amenable to pulmonary thromboendarterectomy, a procedure that has been shown to result in dramatic hemodynamic improvement when performed in carefully selected patients in highly specialized centers (8). While most patients with IPAH have a normal-appearing perfusion pattern on ventilation perfusion (V/Q) lung scanning and patients with CTEPH have multiple perfusion defects (Fig. 1), the scan may not be definitive. Furthermore, V/Q scanning underestimates the extent of organized thrombus in patients with CTEPH. Accordingly, patients with equivocal or abnormal V/Q scans should undergo conventional pulmonary arteriography, both to establish the diagnosis and to assess the extent and location of chronic thrombus if present. The abnormalities of CTEPH on arteriogram are quite different from those seen with acute pulmonary embolism (Fig. 2), and experience in their appearance is crucial for optimal interpretation. Recently, helical computed tomographic scanning has been used to disclose the presence of organized thrombus, particularly in the larger (main and lobar) pulmonary arteries.

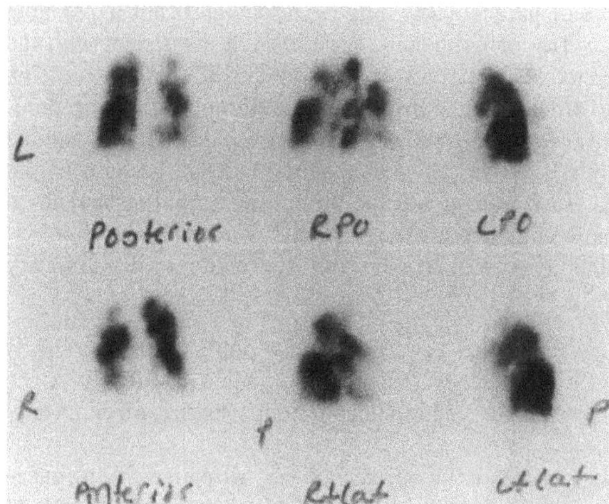

Figure 1 Perfusion lung scan from a patient with chronic thromboembolic pulmonary hypertension, showing multiple segmental perfusion defects.

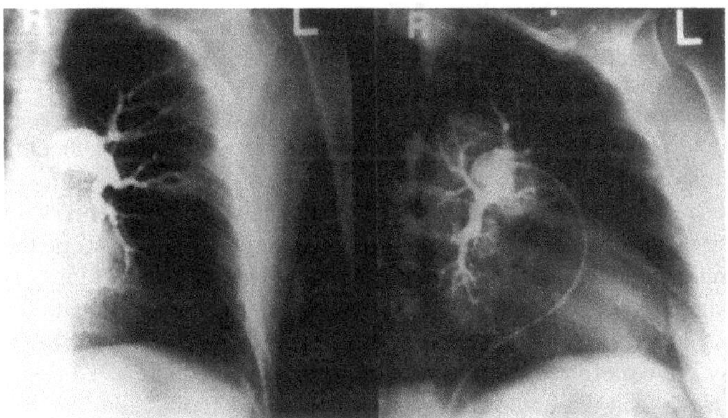

Figure 2 Pulmonary arteriogram from a patient with chronic thromboembolic pulmonary hypertension showing large areas of diminished or absent perfusion, narrowing of lobar vessels because of organized thrombus, and dilatation of the main pulmonary artery.

Complete cardiac catheterization is ultimately necessary to confirm the presence and severity of pulmonary vascular disease; to evaluate for the presence of congenital intracardiac shunts, valvular disease, or disorders of left ventricular filling; and to assess the responses to acute vasoactive agents to develop a strategy for management. Testing of pulmonary vasoreactivity is usually performed using potent short-acting vasodilator agents such as intravenous prostacyclin or adenosine and inhaled nitric oxide. The response to these agents, which has been correlated with the degree of muscularization of pulmonary arteries on biopsy specimens (9), is fairly predictive of the likelihood of a sustained beneficial response to oral vasodilator therapy. Patients who experience a fall in pulmonary artery pressure and vascular resistance with the acute administration of these agents can be treated with oral agents, typically calcium channel blockers, while nonresponders will require more aggressive and complex therapies, such as oral endothelin receptor antagonists or phosphodiesterase inhibitors, or continuous intravenous or subcutaneous prostacyclin analogues or lung/heart-lung transplantation (10).

While most etiologies of pulmonary vascular disease can be determined without the need for histological evaluation, several forms of pulmonary hypertension are difficult to diagnose on clinical grounds alone. Pulmonary veno-occlusive disease (PVOD), an unusual form of pulmonary hypertension, may be suggested by the finding of Kerley's B lines on the chest radiograph in the absence of left ventricular failure and a patchy perfusion pattern on V/Q scan. Measurement of pulmonary capillary wedge pressure is usually normal in PVOD, although measurements at multiple sites may disclose isolated elevations in regions of the circulation that are more severely involved. The acute administration of prostacyclin may result in acute pulmonary edema in PVOD, owing to an increased pulmonary blood flow in the face of downstream vascular obstruction (11). Pulmonary capillary hemangiomatosis, the least common and the most lethal form of pulmonary hypertension, may be suggested by the radiographic appearance of a diffuse, prominent vascular pattern coupled with severe hypoxemia because of widespread intrapulmonary shunting. Ultimately, however, this diagnosis is established only at autopsy or the pathologic examination of explanted lungs at the time of lung transplantation. The pulmonary vasculitides may be suspected on the basis of laboratory and imaging studies, but pathological confirmation of the type of vasculitis is often required to devise a therapeutic plan. Some forms of pulmonary vasculitis, such as sarcoidal angiitis and Churg-Strauss vasculitis, are responsive to high-dose corticosteroids; others, such as systemic lupus erythematosis and Wegener's granulomatosis, appear to respond better to more aggressive immunosuppressive therapy with azathioprine or cyclophosphamide.

Lung biopsy carries an increased risk of serious complications in patients with pulmonary vascular disease and should be performed in a center with expertise in the management of these complex, hemodynamically fragile patients. Transbronchial biopsy is not recommended, since the size of the tissue specimen obtained is usually inadequate for the pathologist to establish a diagnosis, and there is a risk of uncontrollable hemorrhage. Thoracoscopic lung biopsy is the preferred approach, since it provides adequate-sized tissue specimens and is less invasive than the traditional approach of thoracotomy. Additionally, in the event intraoperative complications arise, such as hemorrhage, the procedure can be quickly converted to a full thoracotomy.

In summary, establishing the presence and etiology of pulmonary vascular disease can usually be accomplished on clinical grounds following a rigorous algorithm of diagnostic testing (Fig. 3). When a diagnosis remains obscure despite this approach or when

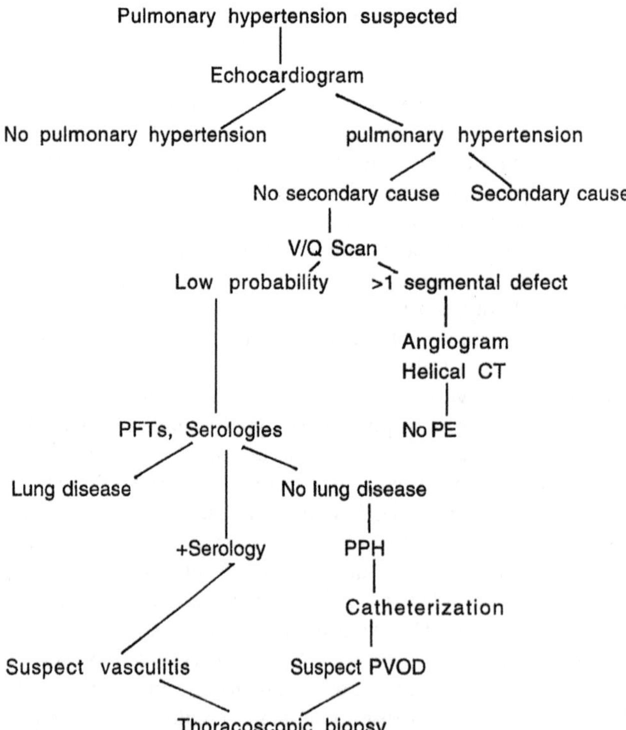

Figure 3 Algorithm for the diagnosis of pulmonary hypertension. *Abbreviations*: V/Q, ventilation perfusion lung scan; PFTs, pulmonary function tests; PVOD, pulmonary veno-occlusive disease.

vasculitis is suspected, thoracoscopic biopsy may be necessary to clarify the etiology. Communication between the clinician and pathologist is crucial in this setting to put the clinical and pathological data into a comprehensive perspective.

References

1. Rich S, Dantzker DR, Ayres SM, et al. Primary pulmonary hypertension. A national prospective study. Ann Intern Med 1987; 107:216–223.
2. Abenhaim L, Moride Y, Brenot F, et al. Appetite-suppressant drugs and the risk of primary pulmonary hypertension. N Engl J Med 1996; 335:609–616.
3. Pietra GG, Edwards WD, Kay JM, et al. Histopathology of primary pulmonary hypertension: a qualitative and quantitative study of pulmonary blood vessels from 58 patients in the National Heart, Lung, and Blood Institute primary pulmonary hypertension registry. Circulation 1989; 80:1198–1206.
4. Hinderliter AL, Willis PW, Barst RJ, et al. Echocardiographic effects of prostacyclin in primary pulmonary hypertension. Circulation 1997; 5:1479–1486.
5. Galiè N, Hinderliter AL, Torbicki A, et al. Effects of the oral endothelin-receptor antagonist bosentan on echocardiographic and doppler measures in patients with pulmonary arterial hypertension. J Am Coll Cardiol 2003; 41:1380–1386.
6. Macnee W. Pathophysiology of cor pulmonale in chronic obstructive pulmonary disease. Am J Respir Crit Care Med 1994; 150:833–852.
7. Opravil M, Pechere M, Speich R, et al. HIV-associated primary pulmonary hypertension. Am J Respir Crit Care Med 1997; 155:990–995.
8. Hoeper M, Meyer E, Simonneau G, et al. Chronic thromboembolic pulmonary hypertension. Circulation 2006; 113:2011–2020.
9. Palevsky HI, Schloo BL, Pietra GG, et al. Primary pulmonary hypertension: vascular structure, morphometry, and responsiveness to vasodilator agents. Circulation 1989; 80:1207–1221.
10. Rubin LJ, Badesch DB. Evaluation and management of the patient with pulmonary arterial hypertension. Ann Intern Med 2005; 143:282–292.
11. Badesch DB, Abman SH, Simonneau G, et al. Medical therapy for pulmonary arterial hypertension: updated ACCP evidence-based clinical practice guidelines. Chest 2007; 131(6):1917–1928.

21
Diagnostic Approach to the Patient with Necrosis on Lung Biopsy

STEVEN H. KIRTLAND and SOUMYA PARIMI
Virginia Mason Medical Center, Seattle, Washington, U.S.A.

I. Introduction

Necrosis is the morphologic change indicative of cell death, characterized by the breakdown of cell membranes. The histological appearance of necrosis depends on differences in the amounts of proteolysis, protein coagulation, and calcification. There are three recognized variants of necrosis found in the lung. Coagulation necrosis, the most common, is characterized by amorphic cell content from denaturization of cellular proteins after death with preservation of a pale, swollen, eosinophilic cell outline. Pulmonary embolus with infarction and some lung cancers produce this type of necrosis. Liquefaction necrosis is characterized by neutrophils in the central area of an amorphic region. This necrosis is because of the release of hydrolytic enzymes. Granulation tissue and fibroblasts start at the periphery of the lesion and move centrally as the lesion heals. Bacterial infection with abscess formation is the principal cause of this type of necrosis. Finally, caseating necrosis is a combination of coagulation and liquefaction. It results in yellow-white, sharply circumscribed, amorphous granular debris surrounded by epithelioid macrophages and multinucleated giant cells, with an outer rim of fibroblasts, plasma cells, lymphocytes, and histiocytes. Fungal and mycobacterial infections are usually responsible for this form of necrosis.

The pulmonary illnesses commonly associated with necrosis are listed in Table 1. Causes include infection, malignancy, or noninfectious inflammation, generally related to autoimmune vasculitic processes. This list is not all-inclusive, as rare diseases or diseases rarely associated with necrosis are not included.

The finding of necrosis on a lung biopsy can be perplexing to the clinician. Caseating necrosis and liquefaction necrosis are often recognized by the histologic reaction surrounding the necrotic focus and not by distinct features of the necrosis per se. A biopsy with *only* necrosis has little or no diagnostic specificity and raises a number of questions for the clinician: (*i*) Does the demonstration of necrosis narrow the diagnostic possibilities? (*ii*) Should the lung biopsy be repeated at the periphery of the lesion? (*iii*) Is there an accessible extrathoracic biopsy site that might provide a histological diagnosis?

The clinical approach to the patient with necrosis on lung biopsy does not lend itself to simple algorithms. The clinician must sift through numerous clinical details in developing the most direct and efficient route of diagnosis. Particular attention is paid to the patient's demographics, symptoms, physical examination, and chest roentgenographic and computed tomographic findings. A detailed search for evidence of multisystem disease

Table 1 Pulmonary Diseases That May Produce Necrosis on Lung Biopsy

- Malignancy
  - Primary bronchogenic cancer (6)
  - Metastatic cancer (6)
  - Atypical carcinoid tumor (7)
  - Lymphoma (8)
  - Lymphomatoid granulomatosis (5)
- Infection
  - Tuberculosis (9)
  - Atypical Mycobacteria (10)
  - Bacterial
    - *Staphylococcus including MRSA* (11,12)
    - *Streptococcus pneumoniae* (13)
    - *Pseudomonas* (14)
    - *Klebsiella* (15)
    - *Nocardia* (16)
    - *Legionella* (17)
  - Anaerobic bacteria (18)
    - *Pneumocystis jirovecii* (19)
  - Fungal
    - *Aspergillus* (20)
    - *Histoplasma* (21)
    - *Coccidioides immitis* (21)
    - *Blastomycoses* (21)
    - *Cryptococcus* (19)
  - Viral
    - Adenovirus (22)
    - Herpes simplex pneumonitis (23)
    - Varicella-zoster virus pneumonia (24)
- Noninfectious inflammation
  - Wegener's granulomatosis (5,25)
  - Churg-Strauss syndrome (allergic granulomatosis and angiitis) (5)
  - Polyarteritis nodosa (26)
  - Hypersensitivity vasculitis (26)
  - Necrotizing sarcoid granulomatosis (27,28)
  - Eosinophilic pneumonia (3)
  - Necrotizing rheumatoid lung nodules (29)
  - Silicosis (30)
  - Pulmonary emboli/infarction (31)

should be undertaken. We recommend the following initial database be obtained in all patients evaluated for the diagnostic possibilities listed in Table 1.

1. Characterization of the presenting illness, including duration of symptoms, rate of disease progression, presence or absence of fever, hemoptysis, extrathoracic symptoms and any history of immunosuppression.
2. A careful search for exposures that can produce pneumoconiosis.
3. Survey for extrathoracic abnormalities on the physical examination.
4. Careful review of the chest imaging studies.

5. Laboratory tests to include a complete blood count with differential, creatinine, aspartate amino transferase (AST) alkaline phoshatase, urinalysis, and in some patients, rheumatoid factor and antineutrophil cytoplasmic antibody (ANCA). In selected patients, sputum analysis for gram stain and acid-fast bacilli stain and culture may be helpful.

   A careful review of these data allows the clinician to narrow the differential diagnosis and proceed in a directed fashion to sort through the remaining possibilities.

II. Patient Demographics

The patient's age, sex, smoking history, occupational history, and history of exposure to infection, particularly tuberculosis or endemic fungal infection, are very important. For example, a patient who is a nonsmoker, age 30, and lives in the San Joaquin Valley who has a solitary pulmonary nodule and necrosis will most likely have *Coccidioides immitis* infection. In contrast, a 60-year-old patient with a 100-pack-per-year history of smoking who lives in the Pacific Northwest and has a solitary pulmonary nodule and necrosis will have a much greater likelihood of malignancy. The occupational history, detailing the patient's specific duties, should begin with the first job and continue chronologically through the entire career up to the present. When possible, a list of agents to which patients may have been exposed should be compiled. Particular attention should be given to any history of immunosuppression including HIV risk factors, chronic steroid or other immunosuppressive medication use, or known malignancy.

III. Symptoms and Signs

Pulmonary symptoms have little diagnostic specificity. The local symptoms produced in response to pulmonary disease (cough, dyspnea, chest pain, and hemoptysis) are common to most of the illnesses listed in Table 1. Similarly, constitutional symptoms such as weight loss and malaise have no specificity. However, the presence or absence of fever can be helpful. Infection, lymphoma, and noninfectious inflammation are commonly associated with fever. Most patients with lung cancer are free of fever except when secondary infection complicates an obstructing endobronchial lesion.

The presence of symptoms or signs of extrathoracic disease must not be missed, as it is often the only differentiating information. Skin rash, arthritis, lymphadenopathy, hepatosplenomegaly, ocular inflammation, and central or peripheral nervous system involvement, when present, help to narrow the differential diagnosis. Sarcoidosis, Wegener's granulomatosis (WG), Churg-Strauss syndrome (CSS), rheumatoid arthritis, and lymphoma are typically multisystem illnesses. Lung cancer and tuberculosis may sometimes present as multisystem disease but most often have just thoracic manifestations. The presence of upper respiratory symptoms, renal disease, arthritis, skin rash, and/or ocular inflammation is all-compatible with WG. Arthritis, erythema nodosum an iridiocyclitis are frequently presenting features in patients with sarcoidosis. Symptoms of central and peripheral nervous system involvement may be seen with CSS, WG, metastatic lung cancer, lymphomatoid granulomatosis, military tuberculosis, fungal infection, and, uncommonly, sarcoidosis. Mononeuritis multiplex is a typical manifestation of CSS.

IV. Physical Examination

The thoracic physical examination has little diagnostic specificity. Extrathoracic physical examination findings are directive but not diagnostic. Hepatosplenomegaly and lymphadenopathy are most common manifestations of sarcoidosis but may be seen with lymphoma, metastatic lung cancer, military tuberculosis, as well as a variety of infections. Skin rash, while not specific, may direct the clinician toward a noninfectious inflammatory cause such as sarcoidosis, WG, or CSS.

V. Roentgenographic Appearance of the Chest

The chest roentgenograph is a primary dictate of the differential diagnosis and diagnostic sequence. Table 2 lists the roentgenographic findings that are helpful diagnostically. Patients with a solitary pulmonary nodule <3 cm in diameter may be either fungal, mycobacterial, or malignant. The patient's exposure to endemic fungal infections and/or tuberculosis markedly affects the prevalence of granulomatous disease. Bilateral diffuse parenchymal disease is most common in sarcoidosis, silicosis, viral infection, and WG, but other diseases can produce this picture, as detailed in Table 2. Unilateral hilar lymphadenopathy is frequently associated with lung cancer, but lymphoma and tuberculosis should also be considered. Bilateral hilar adenopathy (BHA) raises a strong suspicion of sarcoidosis, although multiple diseases including lymphoma, metastatic cancer, tuberculosis, and silicosis may produce BHA. Disease localized to an anatomical segment or lobe fits best with a primary bacterial pneumonia. However, endobronchial tumor with postobstructive infection or noninfectious bronchocentric inflammation with stenosis in disease such as WG may also result in segmental or lobar airspace disease.

Table 2 Common Roentgenographic Patterns (30–33)

- Nodular Pattern
  - Single or multiple nodules
    - Lung cancer
    - Silicosis
    - Sarcoidosis
    - Wegener's granulomatosis
    - Lymphoma
    - Fungal infection
    - Rheumatoid nodules
    - Multiple pulmonary emboli, both septic and bland
  - Perilymphatic nodules
    - Sarcoidosis
    - Lymphangitic carcinomatosis
    - Silicosis
  - Diffuse/perivascular nodules
    - Tuberculosis
    - Fungal infections
    - Hematogenous metastases
  - Cavity
    - Necrotizing pneumonia
    - Tuberculosis

Table 2 Common Roentgenographic Patterns (30–33) (*Continued*)

-
  - Rheumatoid nodules
  - Wegener's granulomatosis
  - Pulmonary emboli/infarcts
  - Lung cancer
  - Metastatic cancer
  - Fungal infections
- Parenchymal Opacities
  - Lobar/segmental infiltrates
    - Chronic eosinophilic pneumonia (usually in lung periphery)
    - Pulmonary embolus/infarction
    - Bacterial pneumonia
    - Fungal pneumonia
    - Postobstructive pneumonia/atelectasis
    - Lymphoma
    - Hemorrhage
  - Upper-lobe predominant iinfiltrates
    - Tuberculosis
    - Silicosis
    - Sarcoidosis
  - Diffuse parenchymal infiltrates
    - Sarcoidosis
    - Wegener's granulomatosis
    - Periarteritis nodosa
    - Hypersensitivity vasculitis
    - Lymphoma
    - Fungal infection
    - Tuberculosis
    - Bacterial infection
    - Viral infection
    - Multiple pulmonary emboli
    - Silicosis
  - Ground-glass opacities
    - Pneumocystis jirovecii pneumonia
    - Viral pneumonias
    - Acute Eosinophilic pneumonia
- Hilar/Mediastinal Adenopathy
  - Sarcoidosis
  - Lymphoma
  - Lung cancer
  - Tuberculosis
  - Silicosis
- Pleural Effusion
  - Lung cancer
  - Rheumatoid lung disease
  - Tuberculosis
  - Bacterial pneumonia
  - Pulmonary emboli/infarction
  - Sarcoidosis (rare)

VI. Computed Tomography

Imaging of the thorax has been greatly improved by the computed tomography (CT) scan. High-resolution CT (HRCT) cuts are required to best examine the lung parenchyma for evaluation of interstitial disease. Conventional CT of the chest is best at detecting pulmonary nodules, adenopathy, and endobronchial and pleural disease. HRCT uses variable protocols that utilize thin cuts (usually 1 mm collimation) at wide intervals through the parenchyma to best assess diffuse parenchymal disease. However, the study may be limited to an involved area to evaluate focal lung processes. Prone scanning may be utilized to differentiate posterobasal lung disease from dependent atelectasis and edema.

Typical HRCT scan patterns have been described for many diseases including idiopathic pulmonary fibrosis, sarcoidosis, lymphangetic tumor, hypersensitivity pneumonia, pulmonary alveolar proteinosis, chronic eosinophilic pneumonia and bronchiectasis. The diagnostic specificity of these patterns and the clinical utility of HRCT in the workup of diffuse pulmonary disease vary widely. Silicosis is characterized by reticulonodular lesions with small perilymphatic nodules with or without eggshell calcification (30). Pneumocystis pneumonia (PCP) typically has ground-glass opacities on HRCT: a normal HRCT has a nearly 100% negative predictive value for ruling out PCP (32). Mycobacterial and fungal diseases may be associated with multiple cavitary or noncavitary nodules typically >10 mm in size while smaller noncavitary nodules are often seen in viral pneumonias. Larger cavitary nodules as well as scattered alveolar opacities can be seen in patients with WG. The "halo sign" and "reversed halo sign" on HRCT have been associated with specific diseases. The "halo sign" is a rim of ground-glass opacity completely encircling a central nodule or mass and is seen with invasive fungal infections, WG, and malignancies. The reversed halo sign is relatively specific but insensitive for cryptogenic organizing pneumonia (COP) (32,33).

VII. Laboratory Evaluation

In certain patients where infection is suspected, evaluation could include fungal serologies and urine antigen identification in addition to sputum analysis. These, in general, are fairly specific but insensitive. Note that many of the atypical mycobacteria and nocardia may take up to four weeks to grow in culture. Peripheral eosinophilia (>10%) may be found in CSS or chronic eosinophilic pneumonia. An abnormal urine sediment and/or elevated serum creatinine should direct attention to WG, other vasculitides, and, much less frequently, CSS. ANCA to diagnose WG should be ordered only in patients with compatible syndromes and not used as a screening test for all patients. Abnormal liver function tests indicate a hepatopathy and are nonspecific. Hyponatremia, often indicative of the syndrome of inappropriate antidiuretic hormone, can be seen with any of the diseases listed in Table 1.

VIII. Fiberoptic Bronchoscopy

Fiberoptic bronchoscopy (FOB) is safe, well tolerated, and a cornerstone diagnostic procedure in the evaluation of most of the lung diseases listed in Table 1. Major complications are rare (0.5%), and include pneumothorax [0.16% overall, 4% in transbronchial biopsies (tbbx)], pulmonary hemorrhage (0.12% overall, 2.8% in tbbx), and respiratory failure

(0.12% overall) (34). Minor complications include laryngospasm, epistaxis, and bronchospasm. Visual findings are usually meager, but an endobronchial salted or cobblestoning pattern with multiple 1 to 3 mm white nodules is virtually diagnostic of endobronchial sarcoidosis. WG may cause inflammation and stricture of the major airways.

In most patients undergoing FOB for the diseases listed in Table 1, tbbx should be obtained. Approximately 85% of patients with sarcoidosis, 80% of patients with lung cancer >3 cm in diameter, and most patients with pulmonary tuberculosis, or fungal infection can be recognized by this technique. In some cases, the pathology, while not specific, can be combined with the clinical picture to provide a confident diagnosis.

Quantitative culture of either a protected specimen brush, unprotected cytology brush or bronchoalveolar lavage fluid (BALF) is both sensitive and specific for recognizing bacterial lower respiratory tract infection and should be performed at FOB in any patient suspected of having a bacterial infection (1). The brush is passed under direct supervision into a segmental or smaller airway in the area of radiographic abnormality. The brush is advanced 2 to 3 cm beyond the tip of the FOB, rotated to collect secretions, and then withdrawn into the sheathing catheter. Processing of the brush begins by aseptically dropping the brush into 1 mL of trypticase soy broth. The solution is vortexed for 30 seconds and loops containing 0.01 mL of solution are plated onto various media for culture. Following incubation of one to three days, the plates are assessed for bacterial or fungal growth. Each distinct colony is counted separately, multiplied by 100, and recorded as colony-forming units per brush. Greater than 1000 colony-forming units per protected specimen brush and >4000 units per unprotected brush confirms bacterial infection. Similar to urine culture, this quantitative technique differentiates infection from colonization.

Bronchoalveolar lavage (BAL) samples the soluble constituents and cells in the airspaces distal to the reach of the FOB (2). As many as 1×10^6 alveoli may be sampled during a typical procedure. The specimen identifies the resident cell population in the lung parenchyma and samples a large surface area for infection and malignancy. In patients with diffuse lung disease, the right middle lobe or lingula is preferred because the horizontal position of the bronchi in the supine position facilitates return. The bronchoscope is gently wedged into a subsegmental or smaller bronchus. Normal saline at room temperature is instilled in 20 to 50 mL aliquots and gently aspirated without any dwell time. The first aliquot is discarded to eliminate contamination from material in proximal airways. The subsequent aliquots are then collected and pooled. The total volume of lavage varies from 100 to 500 mL. The most common volume is 100 to 150 mL. Larger lavages are associated with a higher incidence of post-procedure fever but no significant difference in cell differential counts. When a tbbx is performed, it should be done after the BAL and in a different subsegment to lessen the chance of bleeding.

The pooled specimen can be submitted to the laboratory unaltered if the analysis is performed within four hours. If a greater delay is necessary, the specimen should be centrifuged and the pellet resuspended in a buffered cell culture medium. The specimen can then be shipped on ice to a central processing laboratory. In the laboratory, a small portion is set aside for appropriate bacterial, AFB, and fungal cultures. Quantitative analysis is followed similar to the PSB but a threshold of 1×10^5 CFU is required to confirm a bacterial infection. A total cell count is performed with a hemocytometer on the remaining specimen. The total number of cells varies with lavage volume, but an average 60 mL sample from a nonsmoker contains 15 million cells (2). Two to five times as many cells may be recovered from a smoker. A cell differential is performed using a Wright-Giemsa stain. A normal differential count of 200 cells in nonsmokers is 85% macrophages, ≤2% polymorphonuclear neutrophil (PMNs) leukocytes <1% eosinophils, 7% to 12% lymphocytes, ≤5% ciliated epithelial cells, and <5% red blood cells (2). If the total number of lymphocytes is increased, the cells are incubated with fluroescein conjugated monoclonal antibodies against CD4 and CD8 antigens and analyzed by flow cytometry. The normal CD4/CD8 ration is 1.5 (2).

Special stains for fungi, acid-fast bacilli, and Legionella can be performed on BALF. Viral inclusions, vacuolated or hemosiderin-laden macrophages, asbestos bodies and intracellular organisms are noted. Diagnostically, BAL is most useful when it defines the presence of material or cell populations that are not normally present in the lung (3). Isolation of *Pneumocystis jirovecii*, *Legionella pneumophila*, or *Mycobacterium tuberculosis* from BAL fluid is diagnostic of infection. However, the same is not necessarily true of respiratory bacteria, *Herpes simplex*, Aspergillus, and atypical mycobacteria. Histiocytosis X can be confirmed when the percentage of cells expressing the CD1a antigen is >5% (3). Pulmonary alveolar proteinosis is associated with abundant amorphous material that is periodic acid-Schiff (PAS) positive, has a negative mucin-stain reaction, and no microorganisms. Asbestos exposure can be documented when there are several asbestos bodies per milliliter of lavage fluid. This correlates pathologically with more than 1000 asbestos bodies per gram of lung tissue (3). Cytologic examination of cells obtained by BAL can also be useful in the diagnosis of primary bronchogenic carcinoma and metastatic disease, in particular, lymphangitic carcinomatosis.

Alterations in BAL cell populations can provide clues to diagnosis but are rarely definitive in themselves. When there are increased T lymphocytes, an analysis of helper and suppressor subsets should be performed. A CD4/CD8 ratio >2 is seen in sarcoidosis, tuberculosis, and fungal infections. A BAL fluid CD4/CD8 ratio >2 with <3% neutrophils and <1% eosinophils in a patient with a clinical illness compatible with sarcoidosis has the same specificity in recognizing sarcoid as multiple noncaseating granuloma on transbronchial biopsy (4). Elevated PMN counts are seen with numerous illnesses. Chronic eosinophilic pneumonia is usually associated with BAL eosinophil counts >30%, while CSS produces counts >50% (3,5). Hemosiderin-laden macrophages are nonspecific markers of chronic hemorrhage.

IX. Extrathoracic Biopsy

A number of extrathoracic sites may provide diagnostic histologic specimens. Although insensitive, a positive biopsy of the upper airway can establish the diagnosis of WG. A kidney biopsy could be diagnostic in WG, as well as in CSS and polyarteritis nodosum in the presence of renal disease. Lymphomatoid granulomatosis produces characteristic changes in the biopsy of involved skin and peripheral lymph nodes (3). When CSS involves the peripheral nervous system, the histology is characteristic (3). Liver biopsy is positive in 75% of patients with sarcoidosis; biopsy of palpable lymph nodes and infiltrative skin lesions are also frequently diagnostic.

X. Surgical Lung Biopsy

In situations where transbronchial biopsy is non-diagnostic and other testing inconclusive, surgical lung biopsy may be necessary, especially in those patients with a solitary pulmonary nodule or mass. The options include limited thoracotomy and video-assisted thoracoscopic surgery (VATS). VATS requires two to three incisions <1 cm each for percutaneous insertion of a thoracoscope. It is performed under general anesthesia with single lung ventilation. A partially collapsed lung on the side of the biopsy is required to safely insert the thoracoscope. Thus, the procedure is contraindicated in patients with severe hypoxemia requiring mechanical ventilation with PEEP who will be unable to maintain adequate oxygenation with single lung ventilation (38). It is also contraindicated in the presence of pleural adhesions and lack of a pleural space to introduce the scope. Although the rate of diagnostic accuracy is comparably high in both, VATS may be associated with a shorter length of stay and a lower morbidity and mortality rate when compared to limited thoracotomy (35–37). Nonetheless, a familiarity with the fine points of clinical presentations, use of appropriate serologies, FOB with BAL, and a careful search for extrathoracic biopsy sites will serve to decrease the need for surgical lung biopsy.

XI. Illustrative Cases

The following cases illustrate our diagnostic approach to the patient with necrosis on lung biopsy. The presentation format parallels the diagnostic sequence beginning with the history and physical examination, imaging studies, laboratory results, and finally FOB. As you read the cases, use Tables 1, 2, and 3 as references. Table 1 lists illnesses that commonly demonstrate necrosis on lung biopsy, Table 2 helps to narrow the differential by chest imaging patterns, and Table 3 provides the diagnostic criteria for some of the diseases considered. The diagnostic criteria for malignancy and infection are not part of Table 3. Patients with malignancy require a histological diagnosis at either a thoracic or extrathoracic site.

Patient 1

The patient is a 49-year-old female with a 2 cm spiculated solitary pulmonary nodule in the posterior segment of the right upper lobe discovered during evaluation for an upper respiratory infection. The nodule was new since an X ray only two years previously. The patient smoked 2.5 packs per day for 25 years and had quit smoking four days prior to the examination.

Table 3 Diagnostic Criteria for Noninfectious, Inflammatory Pulmonary Diseases Commonly Associated with Necrosis

	Diagnostic criteria	Reference
1. Wegener's granulomatosis	Vasculitis—either tissue or angiographically demonstrated and any two of the following four findings: 1. Painful or painless nasal ulcers or purulent or bloody nasal discharge 2. Abnormal findings on chest radiograph (nodules, fixed infiltrates, or cavities) 3. Abnormal urine sediment (Red cell casts or >5 red blood cells per high-power field) 4. Histological changes showing granulomatous inflammation within the wall of an artery or in the perivascular or extravascular area	38

(Continued)

Table 3 Diagnostic Criteria for Noninfectious, Inflammatory Pulmonary Diseases Commonly Associated with Necrosis (*Continued*)

	Diagnostic criteria	Reference
2. Allergic granulomatosis and angiitis (Churg-Strauss syndrome)	In a patient with documented vasculitis, the presence of four or more of the following: 1. Asthma 2. >10% eosinophilia on peripheral white blood cell count differential 3. Mononeuropathy (including multiplex) or polyneuropathy 4. Migratory pulmonary infiltrates on roentgenography 5. Paranasal sinus abnormality 6. Biopsy containing a blood vessel with extravascular eosinophils	39
3. Necrotizing sarcoid granulomatosis	1. Compatible clinical and radiographic manifestations 2. Demonstration of noncaseating granuloma on biopsy 3. Exclusion of all other diseases that can mimic sarcoidosis	27
4. Chronic eosinophilic pneumonia	1. Peripheral pulmonary infiltrates 2. An increase in peripheral blood eosinophils 3. Bronchoalveolar lavage fluid eosinophilia 4. Transbronchial biopsy showing an eosinophilic parenchymal infiltrate	3
5. Necrotizing rheumatoid lung nodules	1. Presence of rheumatoid arthritis 2. Exclusion of pulmonary infection and malignancy	28
6. Silicosis	1. History of exposure to silica (ore processing, quarrying, and stoneworking, tunneling, abrasive polishing, ceramic and pottery production, firebrick, and use of ground silica flour) 2. Plain chest X rays or CT showing upper lung nodular infiltrates and hilar/mediastinal lymphadenopathy; 5% to 15% have eggshell calcification outlining the peripheral margin of mediastinal lymph nodes	
7. Pulmonary emboli/ infarction	1. In a patient with demonstrated DVT and typical clinical presentation, a clinical diagnosis can be made 2. If none of the above, pulmonary angiography typically is required 3. A high-probability ventilation/perfusion scan along with a high clinical suspicion	30

The patient's only symptom was cough, which had resolved with a course of antibiotics. There was no fever, hemoptysis, or weight loss. Physical examination was normal.

A CT scan of the thorax revealed a 2.2 × 2.3 cm nodule in right upper lobe (Fig. 1A). There were neither hilar nor mediastinal lymph node enlargement. No pleural disease was

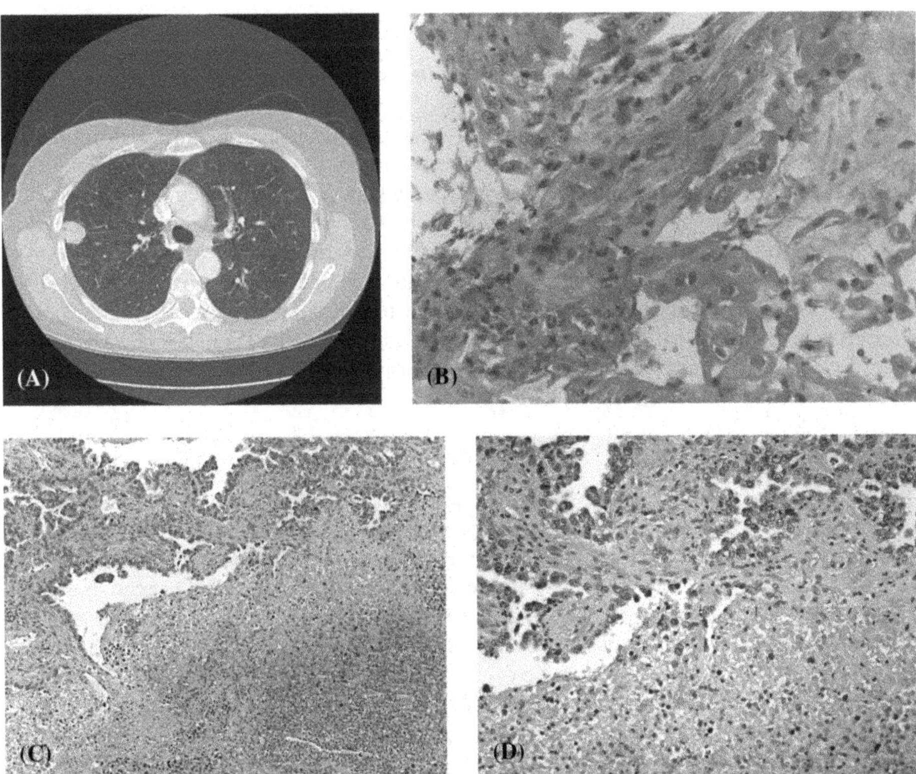

Figure 1 Patient 1: (**A**) CT scan demonstrates a right upper lobe nodule in the posterior segment of the right upper lobe. No hilar or mediastinal adenopathy is present. (**B**) The tranbronchial biopsy illustrated extensive necrosis with no specific pathologic diagnosis. (**C**) Thoracoscopic resection proved this to be a moderately well-differentiated adenocarcinoma. Necrosis can be seen adjacent to the tumor. (**D**) Higher-power magnification demonstrating adenocarcinoma.

present. The upper abdomen was normal. Positron emission tomography demonstrated increased uptake in the right upper lobe nodule with a standard uptake value of 13.8 without hilar, or mediastinal uptake, and no evidence of uptake outside the chest.

Laboratory results: WBC 8.4 with a normal differential, hematocrit 40%. The urinalysis and creatinine were normal.

Fiberoptic bronchoscopy was visually normal. A BAL in the posterior segment of the right upper lobe returned 16.8 million nucleated cells with a differential showing 76% macrophages, 4% lymphocytes, 16% polys, 3% bronchoepithelial cells, and 1% eosinophils. A transbronchial biopsy from the same area showed multiple fragments of bronchial wall with chronic inflammation and adjacent necrotic cells (Fig. 1B). There was no evidence of malignancy and special stains for microorganisms were negative.

Discussion

The patient had a solitary pulmonary nodule that showed only necrosis on tranbronchial biopsy. The chest roentgenographic pattern focused the differential on lung cancer, limited WG, lymphoma, invasive aspergillus, fungal infection, rheumatoid nodule, and pulmonary emboli (Table 1). The patient had no history of exposure to endemic fungal infection. The BAL cell population revealed inflammation, but the pattern was nonspecific and compatible with most of the diagnoses being considered. There was no evidence of rheumatoid arthritis. The patient was immunocompetent and invasive Aspergillus is rare in such patients.

Since malignancy remained a major concern, the patient went on to video-assisted wedge resection. Frozen section analysis demonstrated a moderately differentiated adenocarcinoma and the patient went onto a completion lobectomy (Fig. 1C, D). The patient has done well without evidence of recurrent disease.

Patient 2

A 49-year-old previously healthy Native American male computer software developer had a four-week history of a productive cough and malaise but without fever, sweats, or hemoptysis. He was in good physical shape. He had traveled extensively across the United States and Alaska and has vacationed in Mexico. He was previously PPD negative. He had worked as a day laborer in the past but denies any history of sandblasting. He has only a five pack year history of smoking; he had quit smoking at age 26.

Initial chest X ray revealed vague densities in the right upper and lower lobes (Fig. 2A). A CT scan revealed a right upper lobe density with associated bronchiectasis and scattered areas of consolidation in the left lower lobe, right middle lobe, and right lower lobe. He was treated with a seven-day course of clarithromycin and his symptoms resolved. Repeat chest CT two months later at the time of consultation revealed complete clearing of the scattered areas of consolidation but with persistence of the right upper lobe linear opacities and bronchiectasis (Fig. 2B).

The physical examination was normal with clear lung fields. The patient was not clubbed. There was no lymphadenopathy, hepatosplenomegaly, synovitis, skin rash, or ocular inflammation.

White blood cell count was 6200 with a normal differential, hematocrit 45%, creatinine 1.1, and liver function tests normal. PPD testing demonstrated 20 mm of induration. Three sputums for AFB were smear negative. HIV testing was negative.

Fiberoptic bronchoscopy was performed. The study was visually normal. Bronchoalveolar lavage from the right upper lobe demonstrated 1.9 million nucleated cells with a differential of 40% macrophages, 41% lymphocytes, 7% polys, and 12% bronchoepithelial cells. Biopsy from the right upper lobe revealed ischemic necrosis with small granuloma formation (Fig. 2C). Special stains for AFB and fungus failed to reveal any organisms.

Discussion

The patient's history of tuberculin positivity, and possible exposure to tuberculosis, Native American origin, and upper lobe radiographic changes all favored tuberculosis. Lung cancer would be unlikely in a near nonsmoker. He was started on four drug antituberculosis therapy. The bronchoalveolar lavage obtained at bronchoscopy eventually grew out

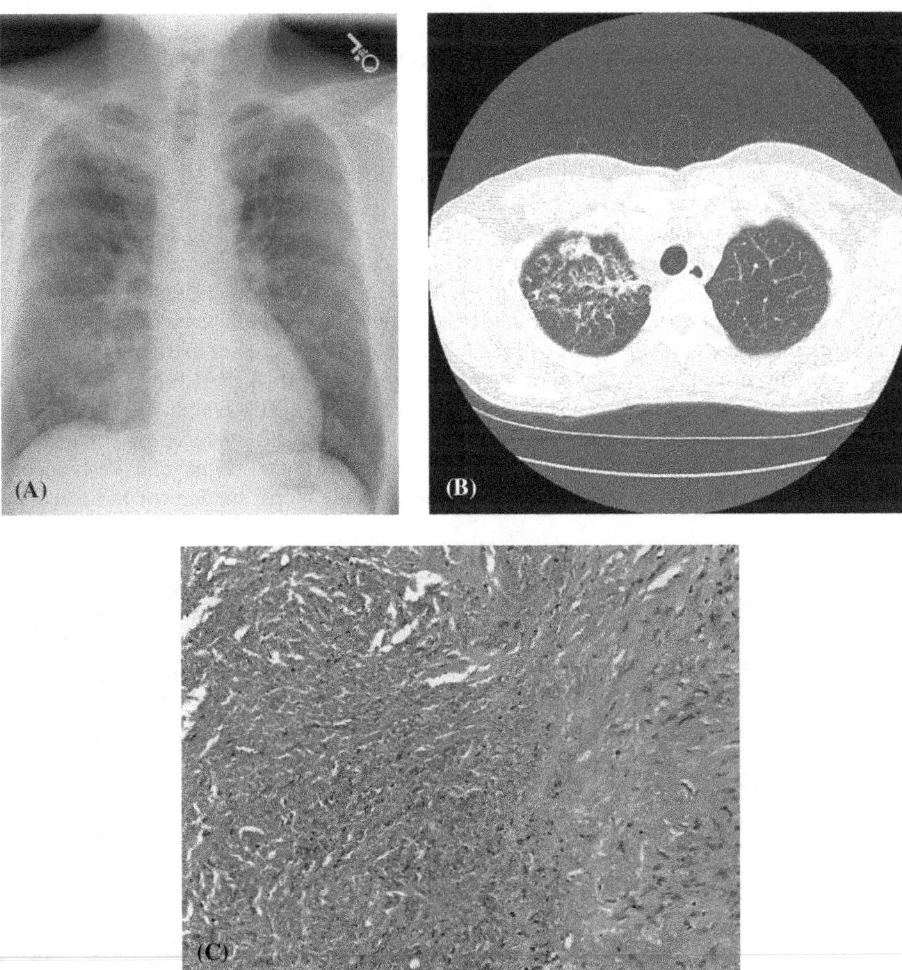

Figure 2 Patient 2: (**A**) Plain chest roentgenogram shows a fibronodular opacity in the apex of the right upper lobe. (**B**) The CT scan reveals a rounded opacity in the right apex superimposed on existing bronchiectatic changes and irregular parenchymal strand-like densities. (**C**) Transbronchial biopsy shows necrotizing granulomatous inflammation. The special stains were negative for microorganisms but the culture grew out *Mycobacterium tuberculosis.*

Mycobacterium tuberculosis at four weeks. The patient has shown significant radiographic improvement with antituberculous treatment.

Patient 3

77-year-old woman referred for a nonproductive cough of several months duration. She denied hemoptysis, shortness of breath, weight loss, or malaise. Her past medical history includes hypertension, hyperlipidemia, hypothyroidism, and osteoarthritis. She had no prior history of malignancy. She had a 20 pack year history of smoking but had quit 40 years ago. No occupational or tuberculosis exposures. Medications included ranitidine, atorvastatin, atenolol, and aspirin.

Physical examination revealed a normal lung exam, and only trace edema of the lower extremities.

Laboratory exam: WBC 10.4 with normal differential, HCT 36%. Urinalysis was normal. Creatinine was 1.2

Chest X ray demonstrated a 9 cm opacity in the right mid-lung field (Fig. 3A). A chest X ray from one year ago was normal. CT scan showed a large mass in the lateral segment of the right middle lobe (Fig. 3B). There was no mediastinal adenopathy or extrathoracic findings. Positron emission tomography showed intense increased uptake in the right lung mass (SUV 7.6) but without evidence of mediastinal or extrathoracic uptake.

Airway inspection at fiberoptic bronchoscopy was normal. BALF had 10.8 million nucleated cells with a differential showing 51% macrophages, 31% lymphocytes, 9% polys, 8% bronchoepithelial cells, and 1% eosinophils. There was no evidence of hemorrhage. Stains and cultures for bacteria, fungi, and mycobacteria were all negative. Transbronchial biopsy showed nonspecific inflammatory changes. Needle biopsy demonstrated focal areas

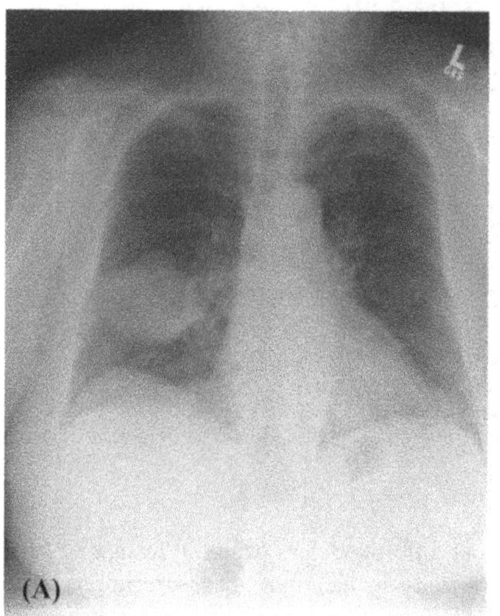

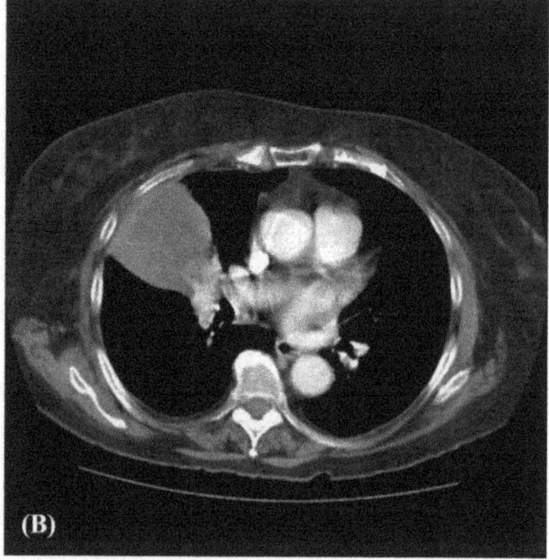

Figure 3 Patient 3: (**A**) Plain chest roentgenogram shows a large rounded radiodensity in the right middle lobe measuring over 9 cm. (**B**) CT scan confirms the presence of the large mass involving the right middle lobe and inferior aspect of the right upper lobe. It extends to the pleural surface laterally, and medially extends into contact with the vascular structures in the right hilum. It has fairly diffuse low density centrally consistent with necrosis. (**C**) Needle biopsy demonstrates focal areas of necrosis (*on left*) and acute inflammation. (**D**) Higher-power magnification of necrosis on needle biopsy. (**E**) (**1** and **2**) Surgical-resection specimen demonstrates extensive necrosis (at ×10 and ×20 magnification). (**F**) Surgical resection specimen with evidence of acute and chronic vasculitis.

(Continued)

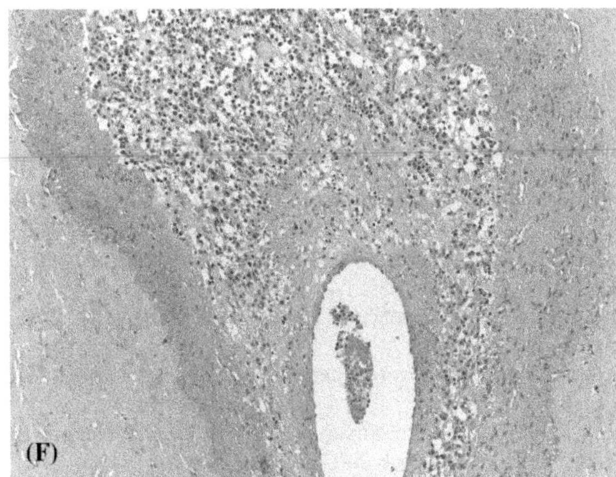

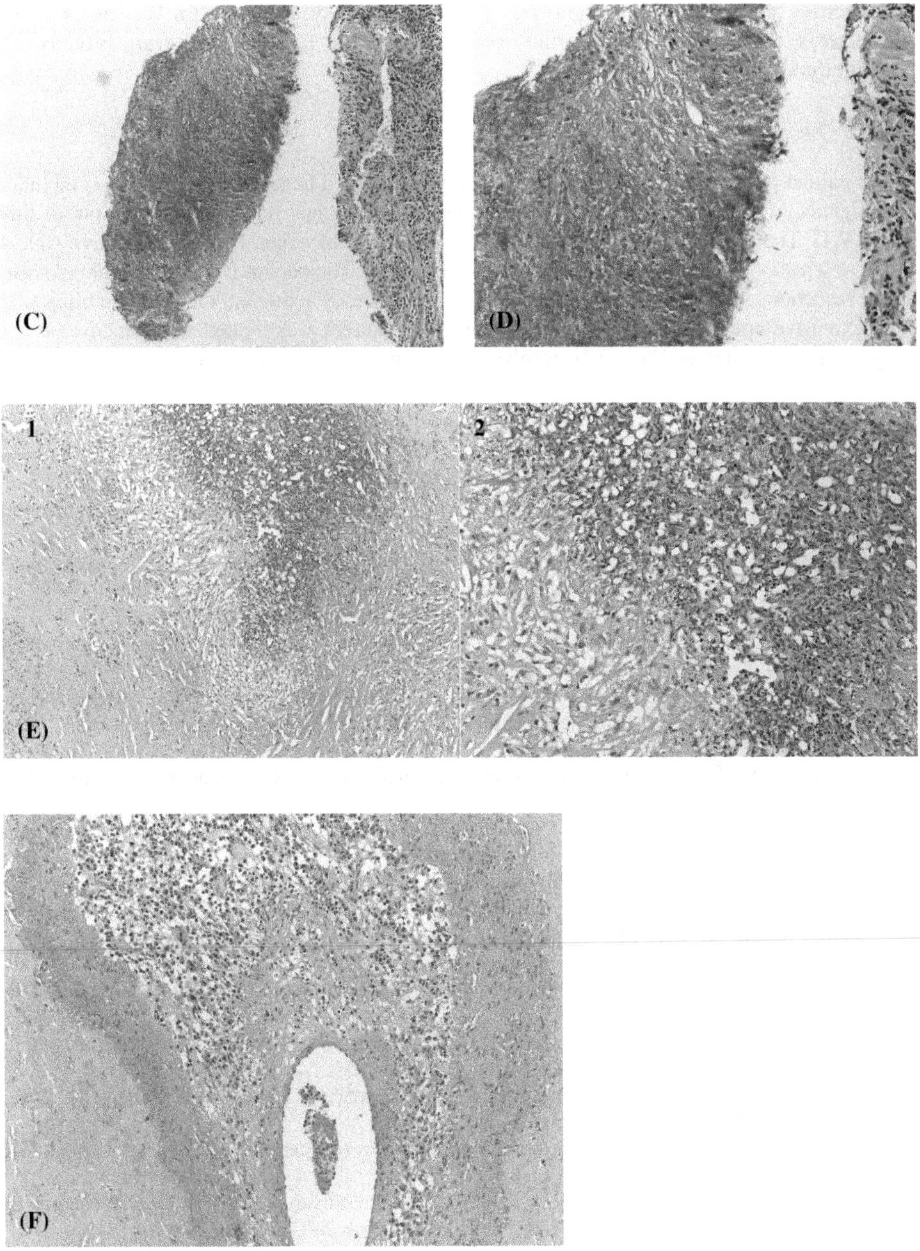

Figure 3 *(Continued)*

of necrosis and acute inflammation (Fig. 3C, D). Because of a concern for Wegener's granulomatosis, an ANCA was performed but was negative for both antiserum protease III antibody and antimyeloperoxidase.

Discussion

The patient presented with a rapidly enlarging lung mass. The differential diagnosis included malignancy (either primary or metastatic), sarcoidosis, fungal or bacterial infection, or limited WG. The FOB and BAL failed to identify an infectious agent. Despite a negative ANCA and absence of renal disease, WG was still a possibility. The patient went on to a thoracotomy and resection of the mass. Pathology revealed evidence of acute and chronic vasculitis with an extensive amount of necrosis (Fig. 3E, F). The patient was treated with prednisone and cyclophosphamide and the cough resolved. She remains in clinical remission.

References

1. Winterbauer RH, Hutchinson JF, Reinhardt GN, et al. The use of quantitative cultures in antibody coating of bacteria to diagnose bacterial pneumonia by fiberoptic bronchoscopy. Am Rev Respir Dis 1983; 128:98–103.
2. Winterbauer RH, Wu R, Springmeyer SC. Fractional analysis of the 120 mm bronchoalveolar lavage: determination of the best specimen for diagnosis of sarcoidosis. Chest 1993; 104:344–351.
3. DePaso WJ, Winterbauer RH. Interstitial lung disease. Dis Mon 1991; 37:63–133.
4. Winterbauer RH, Lammert J, Selland M, et al. Bronchoalveolar lavage cell populations in the diagnosis of sarcoidosis. Chest 1993; 104:352–361.
5. Winterbauer RH. Wegener's granulomatosis and other pulmonary vasculitides. In: Bone RC, ed. Pulmonary and Critical Care Medicine (electronic version). St. Louis: Mosby–Year Book, 1998: M6-1-7.
6. Pugatch RD. Radiologic evaluation in chest malignancies: a review of imaging modalities. Chest 1995; 107(6 suppl):294S–297S.
7. Hage R, Brutel de la Rivière A, Seldenrijk CA, et al. Update in pulmonary carcinoid tumors: a review article. Ann Surg Oncol 2003; 10(6):697–704.
8. Berkman N, Breuer R. Pulmonary involvement in lymphoma. Respir Med 1993; 87:85–92.
9. Schluger NW, Ron WN. Current approaches to the diagnosis of active pulmonary tuberculosis. Am J Respir Crit Care Med 1994; 149:264–267.
10. Griffith DE, Aksamit T, Brown-Elliott BA, et al. An official ATS/IDSA statement: Diagnosis, treatment and prevention of nontuberculosis mycobacterial disease. Am J Respir Crit Care Med 2007; 175:367
11. Woodhead MA, Radvan J, Macfarlane JT. Adult community-acquired staphylococcal pneumonia in the antibiotic era: a review of 61 cases. Q J Med 1987; 64:783–790.
12. Bradley SF. Staphylococcus aureus pneumonia: emergence of MRSA in the community. Semin Respir Crit Care Med 2005; 26(6):643–649.
13. Taylors SN, Sanders CV. Unusual manifestations of invasive pneumococcal infection. Am J Med 1999; 107(1A):12S–27S.
14. Crnich CJ, Gordon B, Andes D. Hot tub-associated necrotizing pneumonia due to Pseudomonas aeruginosa. Clin Infect Dis 2003; 36(3):e55–e57 ; [Epub 2003 Jan 20].
15. Wang JL, Chen KY, Fang CT, et al. Changing bacteriology of adult community-acquired lung abscess in Taiwan: *Klebsiella pneumoniae* versus anaerobes. Clin Infect Dis 2005; 40(7): 915–922.
16. Marrie TJ. Pneumonia caused by Nocardia species. Semin Respir Infect 1994; 9:207–213.

17. Winn WC Jr., Myerowitz RL. The pathology of the Legionella pneumonias: A review of 74 cases and the literature. Hum Pathol 1981; 12:401–422.
18. Bartlett JG. The role of anaerobic bacteria in lung abscess. Clin Infect Dis 2005; 40(7):923–925.
19. Aviram G, Fishman JE, Sagar M. Cavitary lung disease in AIDS: etiologies and correlation with immune status. AIDS Patient Care STDS. 2001; 15(7):353–361.
20. Herbert PA, Bayer AS. Fungal pneumonia: Part 4. Invasive pulmonary aspergillosis. Chest 1981; 80:220–225.
21. Sarosi GA. Community acquired fungal diseases. Clin Chest Med 1991; 12:337–347.
22. Hogg JC, Hegele RG. Adenovirus and Epstein-Barr virus in lung disease. Semin Respir Infect 1995; 10:244–253.
23. Ramsey PG, Fife KH, Hackman RC, et al. Herpes simplex virus pneumonia: clinical, virologic, and pathologic features in 20 patients. Ann Intern Med 1982; 97:813–820.
24. Feldman S. Varicella-zoster virus pneumonitis. Chest 1994; 106(1 suppl):22S–27S.
25. Winterbauer RH, Corley DE. Recent advances in interstitial lung disease. In: Bone RC, Petty TL, eds. Yearbook of Pulmonary Medicine. Chicago: Mosby-Year Book, 1996:321–327.
26. Leavitt RY, Fauci AS. Pulmonary vasculitis. Am Rev Respir Dis 1986; 134:149–166.
27. Chittock DR, Mariamma GJ, Paterson NAM, et al. Necrotizing sarcoid granulomatosis with pleural involvement: clinical and radiographic features. Chest 1994; 106:672–676.
28. Hsu RM, Connors AF Jr., Tomashefski JF. Histologic, microbiologic and clinical correlates of the diagnosis of sarcoidosis by transbronchial biopsy. Arch Pathol Lab Med 1996; 120:364–368.
29. Corley DE, Winterbauer RH. Collagen vascular diseases as mimics of pneumonia. Semin Respir Infect 1995; 10:65–77.
30. Chong S, Lee KS, Chung MJ, et al. Pneumoconiosis: comparison of imaging and pathologic findings. Radiographics 2006; 26(1):59–77.
31. Stein PD. Acute pulmonary embolism. Dis Mon 1994; 40:467–523.
32. Raoof S, Naidich DP. Imaging of unusual diffuse lung diseases. Curr Opin Pulm Med 2004; 10(5): 383–389.
33. Zompatori M, Bnà C, Poletti V, et al. Diagnostic imaging of diffuse infiltrative disease of the lung. Respiration 2004; 71(1):4–19.
34. CA Pue, ER Pacht. Complications of fiberoptic bronchoscopy at a university hospital. Chest 1995; 107:430–432.
35. Miller JD, Urschel JD, Cox G, et al. A randomized, controlled trial comparing thoracoscopy and limited thoracotomy for lung biopsy in interstitial lung disease. Ann Thorac Surg 2000; 70(5): 1647–1650.
36. Bensard DD, McIntyre RC Jr., Waring BJ, et al. Comparison of video thoracoscopic lung biopsy to open lung biopsy in the diagnosis of interstitial lung disease. Chest 1993; 103(3):765–770.
37. Carrillo G, Estrada A, Pedroza J, et al. Preoperative risk factors associated with mortality in lung biopsy patients with interstitial lung disease. J Invest Surg 2005; 18:39–45
38. Lettieri CJ, Veerappan GR, Helman DL, et al. Outcomes and safety of surgical lung biopsy for interstitial lung disease. Chest 2005; 127:1600–1605.
39. Leavitt RY, Fauci AS, Bloch DA. The American College of Rheumatology 1990 criteria for the classification of Wegener's granulomatosis. Arthritis Rheum 1990; 33:1101–1107.

22
Transplant-Related Pathology

FAQIAN LI, CHI K. LAI, JEFFREY TRUELL, and MICHAEL C. FISHBEIN
David Geffen School of Medicine, University of California, Los Angeles, California, U.S.A.

W. DEAN WALLACE
Cedars-Sinai Medical Center, Los Angeles, California, U.S.A.

I. Introduction

Pathology of the lung is common in transplant recipients and may be related to the patient's underlying disease, donor-transmitted disease, acute and chronic allograft rejection, and complications of immunosuppression and other therapeutic interventions (1). These processes may have similar clinical and radiological findings that may require transbronchial or wedge biopsies for the correct diagnosis. Since the differential diagnosis may be broad and the histopathological findings may overlap, transplant-related lung pathology can be quite challenging for the anatomic pathologist.

II. Pathology of Lung Transplantation

A. Introduction

According to the 2007 International Society for Heart and Lung Transplantation (ISHLT) Registry, a total of 23,716 adult lung and 3262 combined heart-lung transplantation procedures have been performed worldwide (2). Through innovative surgical techniques, better organ preservation, enhanced immunosuppressive therapy, and comprehensive prophylactic regimens for infection, the survival and quality of life after transplantation have continued to improve (3). The overall survival of lung transplant recipients at one- and five-year post-transplant has increased from 74% to 81% and 47% to 52% between the periods of 1995 to 1999 and 2000 to 2005, respectively (2). However, the long-term effectiveness of lung transplantation is limited by infection, acute and chronic rejection, and the potential development of malignancies (2–4).

Certain post-transplant pulmonary complications have a tendency to occur at particular times after transplantation. Therefore, they can be classified by postoperative time intervals to facilitate the selection of diagnostic tests and to narrow the differential diagnosis (4,5). From a practical standpoint, three postoperative time intervals are considered: perioperative (<7 days), early (7 days to 3 months), and late (>3 months).

Perioperative Complications (<7 days)

Surgical complications may occur in the first 24 hours after the operation. The unavoidable period of ischemia between organ harvest and implantation predisposes the lung allograft to ischemia/reperfusion injury.

Early Complications (7 days to 3 months)

Acute rejection is the main concern during this period. Bacterial infections are the most common cause of pulmonary infections during the first postoperative month.

Late Complications (>3 months)

Opportunistic infections are the main concerns due to ongoing and occasionally enhanced immunosuppression to prevent and treat acute rejection. Bronchiolitis obliterans (BO) and post-transplant lymphoproliferative disorders (PTLDs) may develop and lead to significant morbidity and mortality. In addition, certain diseases may potentially recur in the lung allografts.

B. Perioperative Complications

Reimplantation Response

The reimplantation response is a mild, self-limited, but inevitable transplant-related injury that in most cases is of little clinical consequence. It typically occurs in the early post-operative period and has been attributed to surgical trauma; graft ischemia; and disruption of lymphatics, blood vessels, and nerves (6). Clinically, it presents with hypoxemia, decreased lung compliance, and perihilar infiltrates on chest radiographs (7). Histological findings include alveolar and interstitial edema with scattered neutrophils (8). The diagnosis of reimplantation response is made by exclusion of other causes such as rejection, infection, and cardiogenic pulmonary edema.

Ischemia/Reperfusion Injury

Ischemia/reperfusion injury is a fairly common finding in early post-transplant transbronchial lung biopsies and results from the obligatory ischemic time that accompanies procurement and implantation of the donor lungs. The ischemic interval begins with removal of the lungs from the donor and ends with the reestablishment of circulation. During this period of ischemia and reperfusion following re-anastomosis of the pulmonary vessels in the lung transplant recipient, a variety of cellular events occur that culminate in lung tissue damage. These include upregulation of cell surface molecules, release of pro-inflammatory mediators, leukocyte activation, and generation of free radicals (9). When the ischemia/reperfusion injury results in severe and persistent allograft dysfunction with increased oxygen requirements and prolonged mechanical ventilatory support, the term "primary graft failure" is used. The latter has been estimated to occur in 11% to 60% of lung transplant recipients and is associated with a high mortality rate, lengthy hospitalization, and longer intensive care unit (ICU) stays (10).

Clinical manifestations typically occur within 72 hours of transplantation and include poor oxygenation, markedly decreased lung compliance, and diffuse pulmonary infiltrates

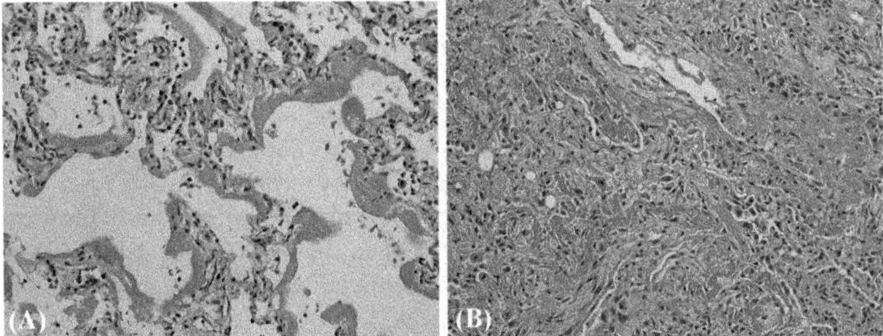

Figure 1 Ischemia/reperfusion injury. (**A**) Exudate phase of DAD with characteristic hyaline membranes lining the alveolar spaces (H&E, 200×). (**B**) Proliferative phase of DAD exhibiting fibroblastic proliferation and incorporation of the hyaline membranes into the alveolar walls. Note also the presence of prominent type 2 pneumocyte hyperplasia (H&E, 200×). *Abbreviations*: DAD, diffuse alveolar damage; H&E, hematoxylin-eosin.

on chest radiographs (9,10). Histologically, ischemia/reperfusion injury is characterized by varying stages of diffuse alveolar damage (DAD). The early exudative phase consists of interstitial edema, hyaline membranes lining alveolar spaces, occasional fibrin thrombi, and scattered neutrophils in the alveolar septa (Fig. 1A). Later, the proliferative phase is characterized by type 2 pneumocyte hyperplasia and intra-alveolar fibroblastic proliferation (Fig. 1B). In most cases, DAD may resolve without any clinical sequela, but occasionally, DAD may progress to parenchymal fibrosis.

Like the reimplantation response, the diagnosis of ischemia/reperfusion injury is made by exclusion of other causes of graft dysfunction including hyperacute rejection (HAR), acute cellular rejection (ACR), infection, cardiogenic pulmonary edema, and pulmonary venous and arterial anastomotic complications (10). HAR can be excluded by the absence of alveolar septal immunoglobulin (Ig) and complement deposition on immunofluorescent studies as well as a negative cross-match and ABO compatibility. ACR is usually not seen in the immediate post-transplant period and may be assessed using the transbronchial lung biopsy. Infections, predominantly bacterial, may occur in the early postoperative period and may give rise to histopathological changes of DAD. Special histochemical stains and tissue cultures are necessary to exclude an infectious etiology. Hemodynamic monitoring and transesophageal echocardiography may be used to evaluate cardiac function as well as anastomotic complications.

C. Acute Rejection

HAR

HAR is an extremely rare and potentially fatal cause of graft dysfunction in the immediate post-transplant period with only a few reported cases in the literature (11–14). Graft dysfunction typically occurs within minutes to hours after implantation of the donor lungs into the recipient and is characterized by rapid onset pulmonary edema with copious production of frothy, pink fluid from the allograft bronchial orifice, severe hypoxemia, and extensive pulmonary infiltrates on chest radiographs.

HAR results from deposition of preformed antibodies, usually against HLA or ABO antigens, in the allograft vasculature and subsequent complement activation via the classical pathway. Eventually, there is destruction of capillary endothelial cells resulting in pulmonary edema, hemorrhage, thrombosis, and necrosis of the allograft.

Histopathological findings include marked pulmonary congestion and edema, alveolar hemorrhage, interstitial neutrophilia, extensive fibrin thrombi, small vessel vasculitis, and changes of DAD. The diagnosis can be confirmed using immunofluorescent studies to demonstrate deposition of Ig and complement in the alveolar septa as well as presence of serum anti-donor antibodies. The main differential diagnostic consideration is ischemia/reperfusion injury as was previously discussed.

ACR

ACR is a cell-mediated form of alloimmune injury typically involving the vasculature and airways of the lung allograft. It may occur at any time during the post-transplant period; however, it is most frequently seen in the first year after transplantation, particularly within the first three months. According to the 2007 ISHLT Registry, approximately 45% to 55% of adult lung transplant recipients (stratified by maintenance immunosuppression) between 2000 and 2006 were treated for rejection in the first year post-transplant (2). Moreover, acute rejection accounted for 4.7% of deaths in the first 30 days, 2.0% from 31 days to 1 year, 1.9% from 1 to 3 years, 0.8% from 3 to 5 years, 0.7% from 5 to 10 years, and 0% at greater than 10 years. Clinically, lung transplant recipients may be asymptomatic or present with dyspnea, cough, low-grade fever, greater than 10% decrease in force expiratory volume in one second (FEV_1), hypoxemia, and pulmonary infiltrates on chest radiographs. A transbronchial biopsy is usually necessary to confirm the clinical suspicion of ACR and to exclude an infectious etiology.

The ISHLT working formulation for the classification of lung rejection was first established in 1990 in order to standardize the pathological diagnosis of rejection in lung transplant biopsies (15). This was further revised in 1995 (16) and in 2006 (17). According to the latest revision of the working formulation, at least five pieces of well-expanded alveolar lung tissue are required for a reliable assessment of acute rejection. A grade of "AX" is given when there are fewer than five pieces. However, a specific diagnosis from the available tissue should be reported whenever possible. The transbronchial lung biopsy specimens should be gently agitated in 10% neutral buffered formalin in order to inflate the alveolar spaces. Histological examination is performed on hematoxylin-eosin (H&E) stained slides of serial sections from at least three levels. A trichrome stain for connective tissue is useful in the evaluation of submucosal fibrosis of BO and vascular changes of transplant vasculopathy. Since infections can often mimic acute rejection, special histochemical stains for microorganisms, including silver stains for fungi and *Pneumocystis*, and immunohistochemical stain for cytomegalovirus (CMV) should be performed to exclude an infectious etiology. At our institution, the frequency of findings of infection is quite low, so we have abandoned routine staining for microorganisms, and only order them when there is suspicion of infection.

Acute rejection is diagnosed primarily on the presence of perivascular and interstitial mononuclear cell infiltrates, the intensity and distribution of which determine the histological grade (17). When more than one focus of rejection is present, the biopsy is graded

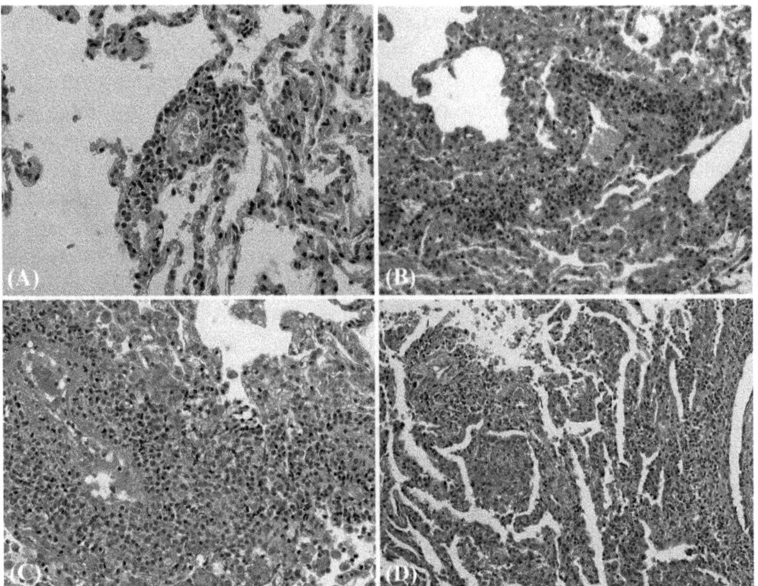

Figure 2 Acute cellular rejection. (**A**) Grade A1 acute rejection demonstrates circumferential, perivascular mononuclear cell infiltrate without eosinophils, endothelialitis, and epithelial damage (H&E, × 400). (**B**) Grade A2 acute rejection exhibits prominent perivascular mononuclear cell infiltrate with endothelialitis (H&E, 200×). (**C**) Grade A3 acute rejection shows infiltration of adjacent alveolar septae in addition to a prominent perivascular mononuclear cell infiltrate (H&E, 200×). (**D**) Grade A4 acute rejection demonstrates perivascular and interstitial polymorphous inflammatory infiltrates with prominent epithelial damage and intra-alveolar fibrinous exudate and macrophages (H&E, 200×). *Abbreviation*: H&E, hematoxylin-eosin.

according to the worst area. Moreover, inflammatory cell infiltrates around submucosal vessels of airways are not considered to represent acute rejection.

No acute rejection (grade A0) is characterized by normal alveolated parenchyma without features of acute rejection.

Minimal acute rejection (grade A1) exhibits occasional, scattered foci of mononuclear infiltrates in the alveolated lung parenchyma that typically form a circumferential cuff around blood vessels, particularly venules (Fig. 2A). The infiltrate is two to three cells in thickness and comprised of small round, plasmacytoid and activated lymphocytes. Eosinophils, endothelialitis, and pneumocyte damage are not present. Asymptomatic grade A1 acute rejection is usually not treated by some clinicians, in contrast to the other histological grades.

Mild acute rejection (grade A2) is characterized by thicker, denser, and more frequent perivascular mononuclear cell infiltrates surrounding venules and arterioles (Fig. 2B). These infiltrates are easily recognized at low (scanning) magnification and consist of both small and activated lymphocytes, macrophages, and eosinophils. Subendothelial mononuclear cell infiltration with associated reactive endothelial cell changes (or endothelialitis) is often present. Coexistent lymphocytic bronchiolitis (LB) is more commonly associated with grade

A2 than with grade A1 acute rejection. Moreover, unlike the higher grades of rejection, extension into the adjacent alveolar septae and pneumocyte damage are not observed.

Moderate acute rejection (grade A3) shares similar histological features with grade A2 rejection including the presence of dense perivascular mononuclear cell infiltrates with eosinophils and endothelialitis (Fig. 2C). However, there are some notable differences, particularly the contiguous extension of the inflammatory cell infiltrate into the adjacent alveolar septae and airspaces, which may contain intra-alveolar macrophages and exhibit type 2 pneumocyte hyperplasia. Occasional neutrophils are also commonly present.

Severe acute rejection (grade A4) consists of diffuse perivascular, interstitial, and airspace infiltration by mononuclear cells with endothelialitis and prominent alveolar pneumocyte damage (Fig. 2D). The latter typically manifests as DAD with intra-alveolar necrotic debris, macrophages, hyaline membranes, hemorrhage, and neutrophils. Parenchymal necrosis, infarction, or necrotizing vasculitis may also be seen.

The main differential diagnostic considerations of acute rejection are infections and PTLDs. Distinguishing infection from acute rejection can be a difficult task and is further complicated by the fact that the two may coexist. In the latter scenario, the dominant histological pattern should be conveyed to the clinician so as to guide patient management. Features that favor infection include greater alveolar septal inflammation than perivascular infiltrates; presence of necrosis with microabscesses (CMV); frothy, eosinophilic exudates within alveolar spaces (*Pneumocystis* infection); nuclear or cytoplasmic inclusions and/or multinucleation (viral infections); granulomatous inflammation (mycobacterial, fungal, or *Pneumocystis* infection); and abundant eosinophils (fungal infection). PTLD can be distinguished from acute rejection by the presence of an intense monomorphous or polymorphous inflammatory infiltrate that may exhibit large, atypical cells. Moreover, there may be destruction and replacement of the lung parenchyma. Immunophenotyping, in situ hybridization for Epstein-Barr virus (EBV) genome, and molecular studies for Ig gene rearrangements may be helpful in difficult cases.

LB

LB is recognized as a form of alloreactive immune injury that affects the airways and is considered to be a risk factor for the development of BO (18,19). Although LB is not used in the assessment of acute rejection, this finding should still be included in the pathology report (17).

The 1990 working formulation recommended that airway inflammation be reported as being either present or absent. Subsequently, the 1995 classification recommended that airway inflammation be categorized into four grades: B0 (no airway inflammation), B1 (mild airway inflammation), B2 (moderate airway inflammation), and B4 (severe airway inflammation) (16). However, not all members of the lung rejection study group accepted this grading system for a variety of reasons including poor inter- and intraobserver reproducibility, frequent coexistence of LB with airway infection, and frequent problems with adequate sampling of airways and with technical issues such as tangential sectioning. The latest revision of the working formulation simplified the grading of airway inflammation from the 1995 classification to low grade (grade B1R) and high grade (grade B2R) with the "R" indicating the "revised grade" (17).

No airway inflammation (grade B0) indicates that bronchiolar inflammation is not present in the biopsy.

Low-grade airway inflammation (grade B1R) includes previous grades B1 and B2 and exhibits patchy or circumferential bronchiolar submucosal mononuclear infiltrates with scattered eosinophils. No epithelial damage is evident.

High-grade airway inflammation (grade B2R) includes previous grades B3 and B4 and exhibits bronchiolar submucosal mononuclear infiltrates comprised of larger and activated lymphocytes and more eosinophils. In addition, there is evidence of epithelial damage, which consists of necrosis and metaplasia and considerable intra-epithelial mononuclear cell infiltration. The most severe forms of airway inflammation are characterized by mucosal ulceration with associated necrotic debris and fibrinopurulent exudate. However, a disproportionate number of neutrophils within the submucosa and epithelium should raise the possibility of an infectious process rather than rejection.

Ungradeable bronchiolar inflammation (grade BX) is assigned to biopsies in which airway inflammation cannot be evaluated due to sampling and technical issues such as tangential sectioning, infection, or other artifact.

The differential diagnosis of LB includes infections, aspiration, and bronchus-associated lymphoid tissue (BALT). Infections need to be excluded by use of histochemical and immunohistochemical stains for microorganisms. The presence of foreign material with an associated foreign-body giant cell reaction supports the diagnosis of aspiration. BALT is usually well circumscribed, contains tingible body macrophages, and is generally found in larger airways underneath the epithelium. No epithelial injury or eosinophils are present.

Antibody-Mediated Rejection

Antibody-mediated rejection (AMR) is a well-documented yet incompletely characterized clinicopathological entity in solid organ transplants (20). The clinical, histopathological, and immunological criteria are best defined in heart and kidney transplants. In these two organs, capillary deposition of C4d, the final split product derived from C4 during activation of the classical complement pathway, is a sensitive and specific marker to diagnose AMR(21).

The diagnosis and recognition of AMR in the lung, however, is still poorly defined and controversial. C4d deposition, when present in lung allografts, is usually weak and patchy in nature, and lacks sensitivity and specificity (3,22) The presence of C4d in the microvasculature of lung allografts does not correlate with the appearance of panel-reactive antibodies or the development of acute or chronic rejection (22,23). However, a recent study showed that the detection of serum anti-HLA antibodies correlated with complement deposition in alveolar tissue following transplantation (24). In addition, C4d deposition has been associated with pulmonary functional deterioration and septal capillary necrosis and fibrin deposition (23,25). Moreover, plasmapheresis appears to improve pulmonary function and reduce complement and Ig deposition in these patients, suggesting a role for humoral immune responses in lung transplantation (23). “Capillaritis,” defined as an increase in alveolar septal capillary neutrophils with necrosis of alveolar septae, has also been reported as a marker of AMR, but the specificity and significance of this finding has been questioned (23).

There is no reason why AMR should not occur in lung transplant recipients. Unfortunately, there is currently no consensus on the histopathological and immunological features to diagnose AMR in lung allografts. To better define AMR in lung transplants, more studies that correlate the clinical, immunological, and pathological findings with therapeutic interventions and clinical outcomes are needed.

D. Chronic Rejection

BO

Advances in surgical techniques, immunosuppressive therapy, and management of acute complications have made lung transplantation a realistic option for patients with end-stage lung disease. However, long-term survival lags behind results of other solid organ transplantation such as heart, kidney, or liver transplantation. The average five-year survival for lung transplantation is approximately 50% (2), while the five-year survival for other solid organ transplants is greater than 70%. There is no doubt that the major obstacle to long-term survival after lung transplantation is BO, clinically termed bronchiolitis obliterans syndrome (BOS). BO is the leading cause of late mortality after lung transplantation. First reported in heart-lung recipients at Stanford in 1984 (26), BO represents a progressive fibroinflammatory process resulting in obstruction of small airways in the transplanted lung. BO has been reported as early as three months after transplantation. Fortunately, for some patients, the onset of BO may be many years after transplantation. While BO is uncommon during the first year after transplantation, the reported prevalence at five years ranges from 50% to 80%. Once BOS is diagnosed, three-year mortality exceeds 50%. While the course is somewhat variable, most patients progressively deteriorate and die during follow-up. Moreover, an earlier onset of BOS is associated with a worse outcome.

Clinical Manifestations

Patients with BO experience shortness of breath and decreased exercise tolerance. Pulmonary function tests demonstrate a decrease in FEV_1. Indeed, the FEV_1 is the most reliable and consistent measure of overall graft function. The severity of the clinical manifestations of BO is graded in large part by the severity of the FEV_1 abnormality (27). Patients with BOS may have characteristic high resolution computed tomographic abnormalities, increased risk of infection, and increased neutrophils and mediators of inflammation in bronchoalveolar lavage (BAL) fluid as well (28).

Risk Factors

A great deal of effort has been made to identify risk factors for the development of BO. There is general agreement that acute allograft rejection is the most potent risk factor (29). The more episodes of rejection, the greater the severity of rejection, and the late occurrence of rejection are associated with BO. The relationship between acute rejection and BO is not intuitive since the former is primarily a perivascular process, not a peribronchiolar process. More recently, it has been confirmed that LB is also a risk factor for BO. Other risk factors have been suggested, but there are conflicting data. These potential risk factors include CMV infection, HLA mismatch, airway ischemia (30), infections other than CMV, gastroesophageal reflux disorder (GERD) among others (29).

Pathogenesis

Studies in humans and experimental animals have shed light on the cells and mediators of BO (31). Both alloimmune-dependent and independent processes appear to be involved. However, the actual pathogenesis of BO is still unknown. Certainly T cells play a pivotal role, but other inflammatory cells are also involved, particularly alveolar macrophages and neutrophils. Inflammatory cytokines and growth factors have been identified that would seem to play an important role in the eventual fibrosis that occurs. The cellular proliferation that eventually obstructs the airways involves the interaction of the bronchial epithelial cells, inflammatory cells, and mesenchymal cells, namely smooth muscle cells, fibroblasts, and endothelial cells.

Pathology

The initial morphological abnormality appears to be an infiltrate of chronic inflammatory cells, primarily lymphocytes and macrophages that injure the bronchiolar wall and epithelium (Fig. 3A). This initial inflammatory process is followed by a fibroproliferative phase (Fig. 3B, C). The early proliferative phase is characterized by abundant granulation tissue that is eventually replaced by dense fibrotic tissue that totally obliterates the small airway, hence the other term for BO, "vanishing airway disease" (Fig. 3D–F).

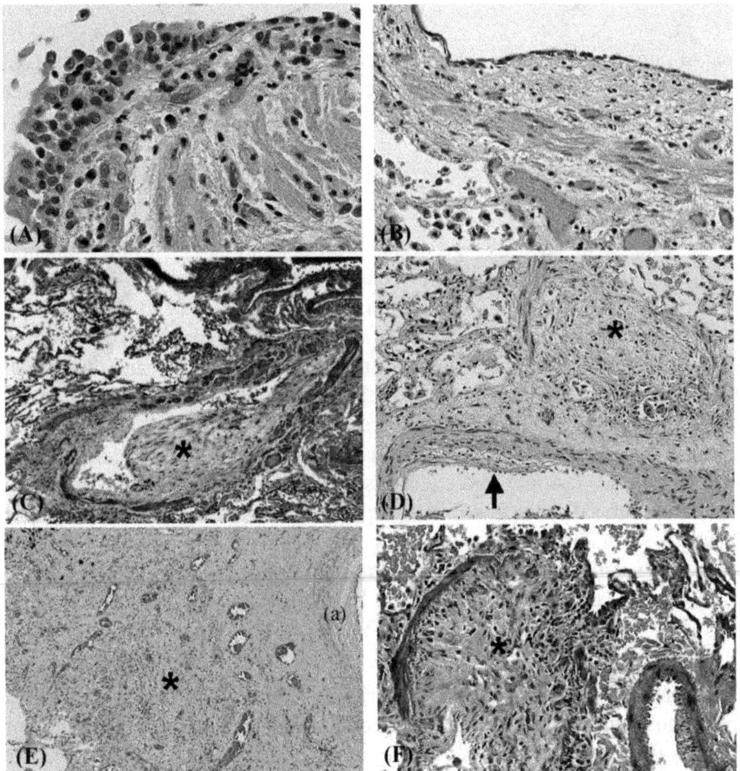

Figure 3 Bronchiolitis obliterans. (**A**) Early lesion consisting of chronic inflammation and neovascular proliferation beneath the bronchiolar epithelium (H&E, 200×). (**B**) Slightly more mature lesion with a fibrotic layer with few inflammatory cells beneath an atrophic epithelial layer (H&E, 100×). (**C**) Obstructive lesion with fibrous tissue [plug (*) protruding into airway (trichrome, 100×)]. (**D**) Airway is completely obliterated by fibrous tissue (*). Note slight neointimal infiltrate of foam cells in adjacent artery (*arrow*) (H&E, 100×). (**E**) Airway has vanished and is replaced by scar tissue adjacent to an artery (a) with intimal hyperplasia (H&E, 100×). (**F**) Trichrome stain showing residual smooth muscle of bronchiole indicating site of vanished airway (*) (trichrome, 100×). *Abbreviation*: H&E, hematoxylin-eosin.

Because of the sampling error of small transbronchial biopsies, and because the small airways actually disappear, the transbronchial biopsy has a very poor sensitivity for the diagnosis of BO, even in patients who clearly demonstrate clinical manifestations of small airway obstruction. It is this difficulty in confirming the diagnosis pathologically that has led to the clinical term and concept of BOS.

In transbronchial biopsies, an increase in collagen deposition with and without chronic inflammatory cell infiltrate between the bronchiolar smooth muscle and the epithelial layer may be appreciated. Collagen plugs filling the airways may be seen, but not often. In lung wedge biopsies, usually obtained for other reasons, these airway changes can be more readily appreciated. An actual decrease in the number of airways is apparent. Numerous small nonspecific scars adjacent to pulmonary arteries mark the sites from which the airways have vanished.

Therapy

There is a great deal of ongoing clinical research to identify therapeutic strategies to prevent or slow the progression of BO. To date, no therapeutic intervention has been shown to alter the course and outcome of BO.

Chronic Vascular Rejection

The Achilles heel to long-term success of cardiac transplantation is chronic vascular rejection. In the lung allograft, chronic vascular rejection shares many similarities with cardiac allograft vasculopathy and BO: (*i*) it is an fibro-inflammatory process; (*ii*) it obstructs the lumen of the structure; (*iii*) it has a number of allogenic dependent and independent causes and risk factors; (*iv*) it is present in most patients five years after organ transplantation; (*v*) its pathogenesis is not completely understood; and (*vi*) there is no therapy to completely prevent its occurrence or progression. Chronic rejection also affects the blood vessels in the lung, yet the vasculopathy has not received as much attention as BO, mainly because BO appears sooner and exerts its detrimental effects on the graft and patient long before the vascular disease is clinically apparent. In the lung, chronic vascular rejection and BO share similar risk factors, pathogenesis, pathology, lack of effective therapy, and difficulty in seeing the lesion on transbronchial biopsy. Just like BO, these vascular abnormalities are clearly apparent in wedge biopsies from lung allografts.

Pathology

Chronic vascular rejection affects large and small arteries as well as veins in the lung. Early lesions (Fig. 4A) and those with an accelerated progression may demonstrate a prominent chronic inflammatory infiltrate that can affect one or more layers of the vascular wall. As the lesions evolve, there is progressive fibromuscular intimal hyperplasia that compromises the vascular lumen (Fig. 4B, C). Older lesions tend to have more collagen deposition and fewer smooth muscle and inflammatory cells (Fig. 4D–F). In a study of University of California, Los Angeles (UCLA) cases, we have noted marked involvement of small veins in interlobular septae, a finding not previously emphasized (unpublished observations).

As stated previously, the consensus of opinion has been that the vascular changes of chronic rejection occur long after the allografts are compromised by other processes, most notably BO. However, clinical pulmonary hypertension does occur in lung transplant

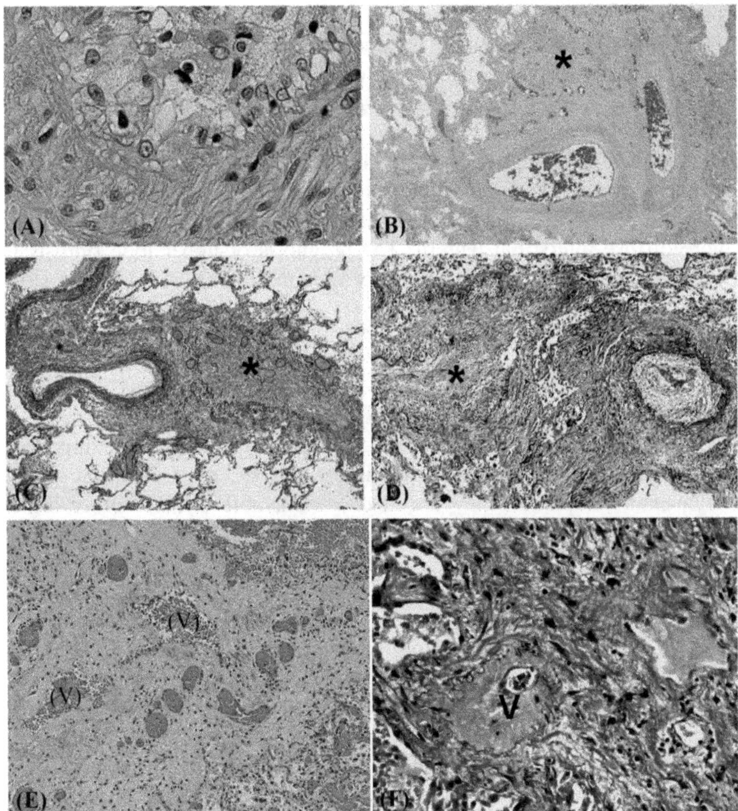

Figure 4 Chronic vascular rejection. (**A**) Early lesion with numerous foam cells in neointima of artery (H&E, 400×). (**B**) Arteries with mild fibrous thickening of intima, note adjacent obliterated airway (*) (H&E, 40×). (**C**) Trichrome stain showing eccentric, mild neointimal thickening of artery with adjacent obliterated airway (*) (40×). (**D**) Trichrome stain showing near total occlusion of an artery adjacent to an obliterated airway (*) (40×). (**E**) Veins (V) in interlobular septum with thickened wall. Due to fibrosis of interlobular septum, it is difficult to appreciate thickening of the vein that is more apparent with trichrome stain, shown in (**F**) (**E**, H&E, 100×; **F**, trichrome, 100×). *Abbreviation*: H&E, hematoxylin-eosin.

recipients. No doubt, the changes observed in the vasculature in chronic rejection contribute to the clinical sequelae of pulmonary hypertension in these patients.

E. Upper Lobe Fibrosis

Another recently described form of chronic allograft dysfunction in lung transplant recipients is upper lobe fibrosis (32). Although BO and upper lobe fibrosis may coexist, the latter appears uniquely different from the former in terms of its physiology, natural history, and imaging findings. The reported incidence of upper lobe fibrosis is approximately 1.9%.

The etiology and pathogenesis of this entity require further clarification from multicenter studies. Similar to BO, upper lobe fibrosis may represent a final common manifestation of lung injury initiated by a variety of factors such as infection, alloimmunity, and aspiration. Clinically, patients are initially asymptomatic, but eventually develop exertional dyspnea frequently accompanied by dry cough and weight loss. Radiologically, the upper lobes first show nonspecific interstitial thickening that may evolve into honeycomb change, traction bronchiectasis, and focal or diffuse fibrosis (4,32). Transbronchial biopsies are often nondiagnostic. Lung wedge biopsies exhibit either focal dense fibrosis with alveolar obliteration or a more diffuse interstitial pattern. The prognosis of upper lobe fibrosis is poor with lack of effective treatment. Augmentation of immunosuppression does not slow the disease progression.

F. Post-transplant Infections

Infections remain the leading cause of mortality after lung transplantation in spite of decreasing rates of infections due to prophylactic antimicrobial therapy and improved immunosuppressive regimens (5). The lungs represent not only the most common site of infection in lung transplant recipients; they are also a vulnerable site for other organ transplant patients. The latter are at risk for almost the entire spectrum of respiratory tract pathogens. The rates of pulmonary infections are lower in bone marrow and renal transplant recipients than those with solid organ transplants.

During the first postoperative month, as lung transplant patients recover from surgery in the ICU and begin their immunosuppressive regimen, they are exposed to a variety of nosocomial pathogens. The vast majority of these are bacterial with gram-negative and staphylococcal species being the most common. From one to six months, patients often live in their normal environment and the risk of bacterial infection decreases. During this period, however, patients attain their maximal level of immunosuppression and have residual effects of induction therapy. Consequently, the opportunistic pathogens such as CMV and *Aspergillus* emerge as the causative agents of pulmonary infections. Beyond six months, the level of immunosuppression is often reduced and patients are less susceptible to opportunistic pathogens except during periods of enhanced immunosuppression to treat acute and chronic rejection. Community-acquired pathogens become more common including *Haemophilus influenzae*, *Streptococcus pneumoniae*, and *Legionella* species (1).

G. Post-transplant Malignancies

Recipients of solid organ and bone marrow/stem cell transplantation (SCT) have a higher incidence of malignancies compared with the nontransplant population, primarily as a result of chronic immunosuppression. In heart and/or lung transplant recipients, there is a 7.1-fold increase in the incidence of malignancies (33). Overall, lymphoid neoplasms are the most common type of malignancy in transplant patients. However, skin cancers are the most frequent in lung transplant recipients by the fifth year after transplantation (2).

PTLD

PTLD is an abnormal lymphoid proliferation occurring in solid organ and bone marrow/SCT recipients (34). Most cases are associated with EBV infection, which results in polyclonal activation and proliferation of B lymphocytes. Under normal circumstances, the latter are controlled by EBV-specific cytotoxic T lymphocytes. However, antirejection therapy suppresses T-cell surveillance, and thus, permits the persistence of EBV-infected B cells and the eventual development of PTLD (35). The reported incidence of PTLDs after solid organ and bone marrow/SCT ranges from less than 1% to 20%. This significant variation may reflect differences in diagnostic criteria, patient population, immunosuppressive regimens, and type of organ transplanted. Data from multicenter studies have shown that the overall incidence of PTLDs is less than 2% (36,37). The incidence of PTLDs in lung and heart-lung recipients is 2.5% to 3.3% (38,39).

Clinical Manifestations

PTLDs typically occur in the first year following transplantation (37,40). In early polyclonal B-cell proliferation, patients may exhibit infectious mononucleosis-like symptoms. Tonsillar and lymphoid tissues around Waldeyer's ring are often involved, especially in children. Monomorphic PTLDs often presents with mass lesions, lymphadenopathy, allograft dysfunction, fever, and other constitutional symptoms. The distribution and extent of mass lesions and lymphadenopathy depend on the allograft type. With the exception of lung allografts, PTLDs usually develop in the vicinity of the transplanted organs, but often spares the allograft (37). The thorax, abdomen, and head and neck region may all be involved (38,41). Lung allograft recipients have the highest involvement of thoracic organs with solitary or multiple lung nodules and mediastinal lymphadenopathy (38,39). PTLDs in lung transplant patients often occur earlier after transplantation and have a shorter survival (38). This may partly be due to the relatively higher level of required immunosuppression and limited options in decreasing therapy in these patients. Polymorphic PTLDs can show features that overlap with early lesions and monomorphic PTLDs (34). Despite the low incidence of PTLDS, careful and close clinical surveillance of lung transplant recipients is warranted due to the poor outcome of patients once these complications develop (38).

Risk Factors

EBV infection is a well-established risk factor for PTLDs. The risk for PTLDs in seronegative patients is increased 76-fold when compared with seropositive patients (42). In particular, children exhibit a higher incidence and earlier occurrence of PTLDs, as they are often negative for EBV prior to transplantation (36). The incidence of PTLDs is also influenced by the type of organ transplanted and type of immunosuppressive regimen. Lung, together with intestinal and heart, transplant recipients have the highest incidence of PTLDs (36) while renal transplant patients have the lowest occurrence. Immunosuppressive regimens with FK506, OKT3, or ATG increase the risk of PTLDs (37,42).

Pathogenesis

EBV infection plays a central role in the pathogenesis of PTLDs; however, the exact molecular mechanism of EBV oncogenesis remains elusive. Most of the supporting data are derived from epidemiological studies (34). EBV is present in almost all PTLDs that develop in the early post-transplant period with EBV titers being increased in patients prior to the development of PTLDs. More importantly, EBV viral DNA is often clonally integrated in tumor cells of monoclonal PTLDs, which suggests viral presence at the time of malignant transformation. Treatment with EBV-specific T cells can result in tumor reduction (43). EBV proteins, LMP1 and 2A, have been shown to possess transforming activity by mimicking B-cell receptors to activate prosurvival signals (44). Nevertheless, some PTLDs

(20%) are negative for EBV markers. In these cases, it is hypothesized that EBV is involved in early events, but gradually disappears during the evolution of PTLDs. Certainly, other factors such as antigen stimulation and suppressed T-cell function in transplant patients may also have direct roles in the development of PTLDs (35). Genetic alterations in myc, bcl-6, N-ras, and p53 have been found in PTLDs with the most common being the bcl-6 mutation. In solid organ transplants, PTLDs are derived from recipient lymphoid tissues; however, they are donor derived in bone marrow/SCT recipients (34,35).

Pathology

PTLDs are a heterogeneous group of lymphoid and plasmacytic lesions ranging from early polyclonal reactive proliferations to late frank monoclonal lymphomas. The latest WHO classification of hematopoietic and lymphoid tumors divides PTLDs into four major categories: early lesions, polymorphic PTLD, monomorphic PTLD, Hodgkin's lymphoma (HL) and HL-like PTLD (40). It is not entirely clear whether HL-like PTLD is truly a form of HL or a subtype of B-cell PTLD (45). Monomorphic PTLDs can be derived from either B or T cells and are classified according to their respective classifications for B- and T-cell neoplasms in nontransplant patients. Non-HL B-cell monomorphic PTLD is the most common type and often presents as a diffuse large B-cell lymphoma (Fig. 5). HL only accounts for 1.8% to 3.4% of all PTLDs (35). Clinical, histological, immunophenotypic, and molecular features of PTLDs are summarized in Table 1. The predominant histological type in allograft lungs is

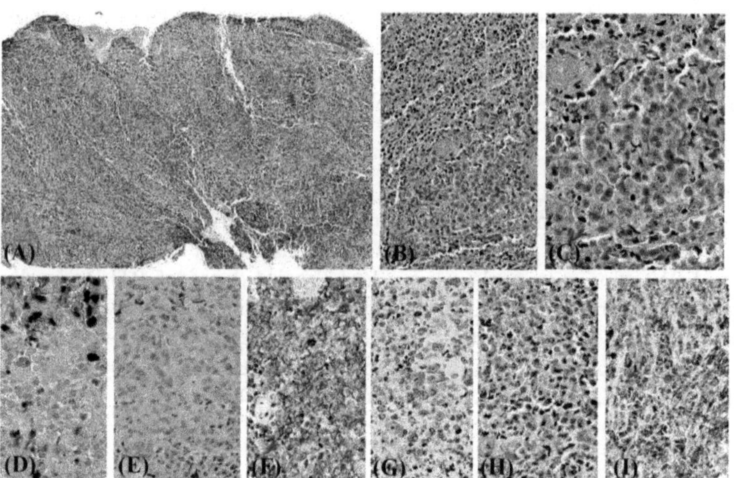

Figure 5 Monomorphic PTLD (diffuse large B cell lymphoma) two and a half months after bilateral lung transplantation. (**A**) Endobronchial biopsy shows bronchial wall diffusely infiltrated by lymphocytes (H&E, 40×). (**B**) Sheets of large lymphocytes with areas of necrosis (H&E, 200×). (**C**) Large lymphocytes have vesicular nuclei and prominent nucleoli with abundant cytoplasm (H&E, 400×). (**D**) In situ hybridization demonstrates EBV-encoded RNA. Large lymphocytes are negative for CD3 (**E**) and lambda light chain (**H**) and positive for CD20 (**F**), BCL2 (**G**), and kappa chain (**I**) (**D** to **I**, 200×). *Abbreviations*: H&E, hematoxylin-eosin; PTLD, post-transplant lymphoproliferative disorder; EBV, Epstein-Barr virus.

Table 1 Clinical, Microscopic, Immunophenotypic and Molecular Features of PTLDs

PTLD type	Clinical	Microscopic	Immunophenotypic	Molecular
Early lesion: IM-like and PCH	Occur in younger and EBV-negative patients; virtually all positive for EBV; often regress after the reduction of immunosuppression	Preservation of tissue architecture. IM-like: paracortical expansion with numerous immunoblasts. PCH: sheets and clusters of plasma cells	Mixture of B, T, and plasma cells; immunoblasts, $CD30^+$; Ig, polytypic (no chain restriction)	EBV and IgH, polyclonal or oligoclonal; no mutati on in bcl-6, N-ras, p53.
Polymorphic	Majority positive for EBV; half regress after the reduction of immunosuppression; others progress to monomorphic lymphoma	Destructive lesion with immunoblasts, plasma cells, and small- to intermediate-sized lymphocytes	Ig, polytypic or monotypic (chain restriction) B lymphocytes positive for pan-B cell markers; immunoblasts, $CD30^+$	EBV and IgH, clonal; 40% show bcl-6 mutation.
Monomorphic: B, T, or NK cells	B and NK cells usually positive, and T cells often negative for EBV; often fail reduction of immunosuppression	Destructive lesion and morphologically malignant; often pleomorphic rather than monotonous cells	Ig, monotypic B cells: usually $CD20^+$, $PAX5^+$, $CD79a^+$, and variable for CD10, bcl-6, MUM-1/IRF-4, and CD138. T cells: pan-T cell and immaturity markers. NK cells: $CD56^+$, $CD3^-$, cytotoxic markers positive	EBV, clonal. B cell: clonal for IgH, 90% show bcl-6 mutation, may have mutation in N-ras, myc, and p53. T and NK cells: clonal for TCR
HL and HL-like	Often positive for EBV, occur late in transplantation, and variable response to the reduction of immunosuppression	RS cells in classic HL background.	Mixture of B and T cells HL: RS cells, $CD30^+$, $CD15^+$, $CD20^{+/-}$, $CD45^-$ HL-like: RS cells, $CD30^{+/-}$, $CD15^-$, $CD20^+$, $CD45^+$	IgH, varies and may be clonal; EBV, clonal

Abbreviations: EBV, Epstein-Barr virus; HL, Hodgkin's lymphoma; Ig, immunoglobulin; IgH, immunoglobulin heavy chain; IM, infectious mononucleosis; NK, natural killer; PCH, plasma cell hyperplasia; PTLD, post-transplantation lymphoproliferative disorders; RS, Reed-Sternberg; TCR, T cell receptor.

monomorphic B-cell PTLD, similar to other solid organ recipients (38). Other rare histological subtypes include B cell not further classified and anaplastic T-cell lymphomas (39).

Polymorphic PTLD contains small to large lymphocytes, plasma cells, and immunoblasts. Monomorphic PTLD is histologically malignant and characterized by diffuse sheets of pleomorphic large lymphoid cells. In the more common diffuse, large B-cell type of PTLD, the malignant cells are usually positive for pan-B cell markers, CD20, CD79a, and PAX5. They are also variably positive for CD10, bcl-6, MUM-1/IRF-4 or CD138, depending on their histogenetic maturation.

Therapy

The one-year mortality in renal and heart transplant patients with lymphoma is approximately 40% and 50%, respectively (37). The outcome for lung transplant recipients is significantly worse with mortality rates higher than 60% and a median survival of 4.6 months (39). Patients developing PTLDs within the first six months after transplantation have a significantly better survival than those developing PTLDs more than six months after lung transplant (46). Treatment for PTLDs requires a multidisciplinary approach that includes surgery, radiation, rituximab, and cytotoxic chemotherapy (39,43). The first therapeutic option may be reduction of immunosuppression; however, monomorphic PTLDs rarely respond to reduced immunosuppression alone (39). Pulmonary retransplantation has been performed in two patients for PTLD with no evidence of recurrence at 23 and 36 months postoperatively (46).

Other Types of Malignancies

Cutaneous malignancies including squamous cell and basal cell carcinomas are the second most common type of malignancies in transplant patients after PTLDS (2,33). The head and neck region is the most common site (2,33). In lung transplant recipients surviving for five years after transplantation, skin cancers are the most frequent malignancies (2). Lung cancer is the third most common tumor type in heart and/or lung transplant patients. Non–small cell carcinoma is the predominant histological type. The incidence of lung cancer is especially higher in the native lung of single-lung transplant recipients (47). The prognosis of patients with post-transplant malignancies is often worse than their nontransplant counterparts. Most patients present with advanced disease and a rapidly progressive clinical course despite close clinical surveillance.

H. Recurrent Disease in Lung Allografts

Certain native lung diseases leading to lung transplantation can recur in the transplanted lungs. Lymphangioleiomyomatosis and sarcoidosis typically recur in allografts without significant functional consequence (48–50). In contrast, recurrence of Langerhans' cell histiocytosis often leads to clinical symptoms. Survival in patients with recurrent disease is similar to patients transplanted for nonrecurrent lung diseases (50). Sarcoidosis is the most frequent recurrent disease in lung allografts with development of granulomata in up to 80% of patients (48) and recurrence observed as early as three months after transplantation. Garve et al. reported four of seven patients with recurrent bronchioloalveolar carcinoma in the donor lungs after complete removal of native lung tissue during transplantation (51). Bronchiectasis, emphysema, cystic fibrosis, and diffuse interstitial lung diseases have also been reported to recur in the lung allograft.

I. Aspiration

GERD is common after lung transplantation in both adults and children (52). There are a number of possible causes of GERD after lung transplantation that include effects of medication on lower esophageal sphincter function, vagus nerve injury after surgery, and changes in intra-abdominal and intrathoracic pressure. The true incidence is unknown because most patients are asymptomatic. In these patients, GERD has been documented by 24-hour pH testing and by finding increased bile acids and pepsin in BAL fluid. These studies are abnormal in up to 76% of patients 12 months after lung transplantation (53). GERD after lung transplantation is important because it is associated with an increased risk of both acute rejection and BO. In the denervated lung, the normal cough and mucociliary reflexes may be lacking, predisposing to aspiration. The aspirated gastric content is not only directly toxic to the bronchial tissue, but also alters surfactant proteins and phospholipids that stimulate an immune response that is thought to contribute to the increased risk of acute and chronic rejection in lung transplant patients with GERD (54). Early fundoplication prevents the deleterious effects of GERD on the lung allograft (53). Unfortunately, transbronchial biopsy is not a sensitive technique for making this diagnosis. The biopsy may be normal, or only exhibit a nonspecific pneumonia pattern. Rarely, foreign food material may be observed.

III. Lung Pathology After Other Solid Organ and Hematopoietic SCT

A. Introduction

Although the lungs may not be the transplanted organs, they are affected by a variety of disorders primarily due to immunosuppressive therapy or other therapeutic interventions. These disorders include direct pulmonary complications of the specific therapies, infections, and increased risk of malignancies. In patients with SCT, the pathology is further complicated by the possibility of graft versus host disease (GVHD).

SCT has been used for the treatment of solid and hematopoietic malignancy and less often for benign hematopoietic and congenital immunodeficiency disorders. Lung pathology is a common cause of morbidity and mortality in this population. In particular, the lung and other organs may be affected by a group of noninfectious disorders collectively referred to as "graft versus host-associated disease." Unlike GVHD in other organs that have well-defined pathological lesions, there is no specific lesion in pulmonary GVHD (55).

The differential diagnosis of pulmonary disorders in SCT recipients is different in the acute setting (less than 90 days after transplantation) than in the chronic setting (greater than 90 days after transplantation). The most common diagnoses include acute pneumonia (bacterial, fungal, viral, and parasitic), diffuse alveolar hemorrhage (DAH), DAD, pulmonary fibrosis related to irradiation and drug toxicity, BO, organizing pneumonia, and recurrent leukemia and lymphoma.

B. Pulmonary Drug Toxicity and Radiation Changes

Prior to SCT, patients commonly undergo myeloablative therapy consisting of total body irradiation and/or cytotoxic chemotherapy. These are known to induce short- and long-term morbidity and rarely mortality (56–58). The spectrum of possible histological changes and clinical findings is broad. Table 2 summarizes the more common cytotoxic drugs used in

Table 2 Common Myeloablative Drugs with Associated Pulmonary Pathology

Drugs	Histologic pattern(s)
Busulfan	Diffuse alveolar damage, chronic interstitial pneumonia, pulmonary alveolar proteinosis, ossification
Cyclophosphamide	Diffuse alveolar damage, chronic interstitial pneumonia, usual interstitial pneumonia, bronchiolitis obliterans organizing pneumonia, hemorrhage
Carmustine	Diffuse alveolar damage, chronic interstitial pneumonia, pulmonary veno-occlusive disease
Lomustine	Diffuse alveolar damage, bronchiolitis obliterans
Bleomycin	Diffuse alveolar damage, pleural fibrosis, eosinophilic pneumonia, bronchiolitis obliterans organizing pneumonia, pulmonary veno-occlusive disease
Methotrexate	Chronic interstitial pneumonia (with granulomas), hypersensitivity pneumonitis, bronchiolitis obliterans organizing pneumonia (with granulomas), diffuse alveolar damage

SCT with their associated histological patterns of injury (59). Any drug may cause more than one histological pattern of injury and many drugs may result in the same pattern, making specific etiological diagnoses difficult, if not, impossible.

Acute radiation toxicity presents with cough, fever, and occasionally, hemoptysis. It typically presents in the first few weeks of therapy. The most common histological pattern is acute and organizing DAD. Chronic radiation toxicity typically presents with interstitial fibrosis and thickened arteries with intimal fibrosis. The hallmark of radiation fibrosis is the sharp demarcation between the irradiated fibrotic area and the uninvolved lung parenchyma.

C. Infections After Hematopoietic SCT

Infection is most common in the early period after SCT, but it may occur any time after transplantation. The pathogenic microorganisms and histopathology overlap with those seen in other immunocompromised populations. Retrospective studies of microbial cultures from BAL and autopsy lung specimens commonly show infection with *Staphylococcus* species, *Pseudomonas aeruginosa*, *Enterococcus* species, *Enterobacter* species, *Mucormycosis*, *Aspergillus, Candida* species, CMV, respiratory syncytial virus, adenovirus, *Toxoplasma gondii*, and *Pneumocystis jiroveci* (60,61). In autopsied patients, infection is often associated with concurrent DAH and/or DAD. Autopsy studies have shown that only 24% to 48% of decedents will have an organism identified by culture or histology. Thus, the offending organism cannot be identified in the majority of cases. Moreover, only 50% of microorganisms identified postmortem have been identified antemortem (60,61).

D. Noninfectious Diseases After Hematopoietic SCT

DAD

DAD is the most common noninfectious disease diagnosed after hematopoietic SCT. DAD is found in approximately 40% to 50% of patients at the time of autopsy (60,61). As in the nonhematopoietic SCT setting, DAD may be idiopathic or associated with numerous etiologies. In the SCT setting, DAD is commonly associated with infection, DAH, and idiopathic pulmonary syndrome (IPS) (62).

IPS

IPS is defined clinically as evidence of widespread alveolar injury without evidence of an infectious agent by tissue culture, special histochemical stains, or cytological evaluation. Histologically, there are changes of DAD, interstitial pneumonitis, and acute or organizing pneumonia. IPS occurs in the autologous or allogeneic SCT setting, typically within weeks of transplantation, with an incidence of approximately 5% to 10% (60,62,63). Furthermore, there is no effective treatment, and prognosis is poor with a mortality rate of greater than 75% in most studies (62,63).

DAH

The "DAH" syndrome was defined in 1989 as diffuse pulmonary infiltrates, fever, hypoxemia, thrombocytopenia, and renal insufficiency in the setting of increasingly bloody BAL fluid and negative microbial cultures (64). DAH was originally described in patients who had undergone autologous SCT, but further described in patients who had undergone allogeneic SCT as well as in nontransplant patients (65). Multiple studies have found an incidence of approximately 5% to 35% in hematopoietic SCT recipients (61,64,65). Focal or widespread alveolar hemorrhage associated with or without an identifiable infectious organism is commonly seen after autologous and allogeneic hematopoietic SCT. DAH is seen at time of autopsy in 15% to 40% of hematopoietic SCT recipients (60,61). BAL specimens show blood and hemosiderin-laden macrophages while histological sections of lung show these cells within alveoli, without capillaritis, vasculitis, or other distinct histopathological findings. The prognosis is poor, with reported mortality rates of 50% to 100% (55,64). The pathogenesis of DAH is uncertain, but believed to be related to total body irradiation, pretransplant chemotherapy, severe acute GVHD, and infection.

BO

BO is the most common, late-onset, noninfectious pulmonary complication after allogeneic hematopoietic SCT and is strongly associated with concurrent chronic GHVD (62,63). It is almost always seen after three months of transplantation. Histologically, there is fibrous obliteration of the small airways, which may not be present on small biopsy specimens. Allogeneic hematopoietic SCT patients with new onset airflow obstruction in the absence of asthma, smoking history, and viral or bacterial pneumonia are clinically diagnosed as having "BOS." BO is seen in 2% to 26% of patients in various retrospective studies (62,63). The etiology is unclear, but an increased risk of BO is associated with the presence of chronic GVHD, history of acute GVHD, busulfan-based conditioning regimen, peripheral blood SCT, long duration to transplantation, female donor to male recipient, and prior episode of interstitial pneumonitis. Generally, the course of BO is one of progressive decline in pulmonary function. Controlling the underlying GVHD stabilizes the pulmonary function, providing further evidence that this is a true manifestation of pulmonary GVHD.

Bronchiolitis Obliterans Organizing Pneumonia

There are numerous case reports of bronchiolitis obliterans organizing pneumonia (BOOP) in the setting of allogeneic and syngeneic SCT (66,67). BOOP in the transplant patient has the same histological features and clinical course of idiopathic BOOP occurring in the non-SCT setting. Most patients with BOOP have a history of acute or chronic GVHD (68).

In the nontransplant population, the term for idiopathic "BOOP" has been replaced by "COP" for cryptogenic organizing pneumonia.

Pulmonary Veno-occlusive Disease

Pulmonary veno-occlusive disease (PVOD) after hematopoietic SCT is an infrequent but well-recognized finding (69,70). Clinically, the patients present with an insidious onset of shortness of breath and fatigue. Histologically, one sees intimal proliferation and fibrous obliteration of the pulmonary veins. PVOD is also seen after radiation and chemotherapy. Therefore, it is possible that PVOD develops in the post hematopoietic SCT setting as a result of preconditioning chemotherapy and/or irradiation.

PTLD

The incidence of PTLDs is lower in hematopoietic SCT than in solid organ transplants (35). The risk of HL, however, is relatively increased after hematopoietic SCT. In contrast to solid organ transplants, PTLDs in hematopoietic SCT recipients are donor rather than recipient derived.

Recurrent Disease

Primary diseases of the recipient such as leukemia and lymphoma can recur in the lung.

References

1. Kotloff RM, Ahya VN, Crawford SW. Pulmonary complications of solid organ and hematopoietic stem cell transplantation. Am J Respir Crit Care Med 2004; 170:22–48.
2. Trulock EP, Christie JD, Edwards LB, et al. Registry of the International Society for Heart and Lung Transplantation: twenty-fourth official adult lung and heart-lung transplantation report—2007. J Heart Lung Transplant 2007; 26:782–795.
3. Marboe CC. Pathology of lung transplantation. Semin Diagn Pathol 2007; 24:188–198.
4. Krishnam MS, Suh RD, Tomasian A, et al. Postoperative complications of lung transplantation: radiologic findings along a time continuum. Radiographics 2007; 27:957–974.
5. Stewart S. Pulmonary infections in transplantation pathology. Arch Pathol Lab Med 2007; 131:1219–1231.
6. Prop J, Ehrie MG, Crapo JD, et al. Reimplantation response in isografted rat lungs. Analysis of causal factors. J Thorac Cardiovasc Surg 1984; 87:702–711.
7. Khan SU, Salloum J, O'Donovan PB, et al. Acute pulmonary edema after lung transplantation: the pulmonary reimplantation response. Chest 1999; 116:187–194.
8. Tazelaar HD, Yousem SA. The pathology of combined heart-lung transplantation: an autopsy study. Hum Pathol 1988; 19:1403–1416.
9. de Perrot M, Liu M, Waddell TK, et al. Ischemia-reperfusion-induced lung injury. Am J Respir Crit Care Med 2003; 167:490–511.
10. Carter YM, Davis RD. Primary graft dysfunction in lung transplantation. Semin Respir Crit Care Med 2006; 27:501–507.
11. Zander DS, Baz MA, Visner GA, et al. Analysis of early deaths after isolated lung transplantation. Chest 2001; 120:225–232.
12. Choi JK, Kearns J, Palevsky HI, et al. Hyperacute rejection of a pulmonary allograft. Immediate clinical and pathologic findings. Am J Respir Crit Care Med 1999; 160:1015–1018.

13. Frost AE, Jammal CT, Cagle PT. Hyperacute rejection following lung transplantation. Chest 1996; 110:559–562.
14. Bittner HB, Dunitz J, Hertz M, et al. Hyperacute rejection in single lung transplantation—case report of successful management by means of plasmapheresis and antithymocyte globulin treatment. Transplantation 2001; 71:649–651.
15. Yousem SA, Berry GJ, Brunt EM, et al. A working formulation for the standardization of nomenclature in the diagnosis of heart and lung rejection: Lung Rejection Study Group. The International Society for Heart Transplantation. J Heart Transplant 1990; 9:593–601.
16. Yousem SA, Berry GJ, Cagle PT, et al. Revision of the 1990 working formulation for the classification of pulmonary allograft rejection: Lung Rejection Study Group. J Heart Lung Transplant 1996; 15:1–15.
17. Stewart S, Fishbein MC, Snell GI, et al. Revision of the 1995 working formulation for the standardisation of nomenclature in the diagnosis of lung rejection. J Heart Lung Transplant 2007; 26:1229–1242.
18. Hirt SW, You XM, Moller F, et al. Development of obliterative bronchiolitis after allogeneic rat lung transplantation: implication of acute rejection and the time point of treatment. J Heart Lung Transplant 1999; 18:542–548.
19. Yousem SA. Lymphocytic bronchitis/bronchiolitis in lung allograft recipients. Am J Surg Pathol 1993; 17:491–496.
20. Michaels PJ, Fishbein MC, Colvin RB. Humoral rejection of human organ transplants. Springer Semin Immunopathol 2003; 25:119–140.
21. Michaels PJ, Espejo ML, Kobashigawa J, et al. Humoral rejection in cardiac transplantation: risk factors, hemodynamic consequences and relationship to transplant coronary artery disease. J Heart Lung Transplant 2003; 22:58–69.
22. Wallace WD, Reed EF, Ross D, et al. C4d staining of pulmonary allograft biopsies: an immunoperoxidase study. J Heart Lung Transplant 2005; 24:1565–1570.
23. Magro CM, Deng A, Pope-Harman A, et al. Humorally mediated posttransplantation septal capillary injury syndrome as a common form of pulmonary allograft rejection: a hypothesis. Transplantation 2002; 74:1273–1280.
24. Ionescu DN, Girnita AL, Zeevi A, et al. C4d deposition in lung allografts is associated with circulating anti-HLA alloantibody. Transpl Immunol 2005; 15:63–68.
25. Astor TL, Weill D, Cool C, et al. Pulmonary capillaritis in lung transplant recipients: treatment and effect on allograft function. J Heart Lung Transplant 2005; 24:2091–2097.
26. Burke CM, Theodore J, Dawkins KD, et al. Post-transplant obliterative bronchiolitis and other late lung sequelae in human heart-lung transplantation. Chest 1984; 86:824–829.
27. Estenne M, Maurer JR, Boehler A, et al. Bronchiolitis obliterans syndrome 2001: an update of the diagnostic criteria. J Heart Lung Transplant 2002; 21:297–310.
28. Belperio JA, Lake K, Tazelaar H, et al. Bronchiolitis obliterans syndrome complicating lung or heart-lung transplantation. Semin Respir Crit Care Med 2003; 24:499–530.
29. Sharples LD, McNeil K, Stewart S, et al. Risk factors for bronchiolitis obliterans: a systematic review of recent publications. J Heart Lung Transplant 2002; 21:271–281.
30. Luckraz H, Goddard M, McNeil K, et al. Microvascular changes in small airways predispose to obliterative bronchiolitis after lung transplantation. J Heart Lung Transplant 2004; 23:527–531.
31. Neuringer IP, Chalermskulrat W, Aris R. Obliterative bronchiolitis or chronic lung allograft rejection: a basic science review. J Heart Lung Transplant 2005; 24:3–19.
32. Pakhale SS, Hadjiliadis D, Howell DN, et al. Upper lobe fibrosis: a novel manifestation of chronic allograft dysfunction in lung transplantation. J Heart Lung Transplant 2005; 24:1260–1268.
33. Roithmaier S, Haydon AM, Loi S, et al. Incidence of malignancies in heart and/or lung transplant recipients: a single-institution experience. J Heart Lung Transplant 2007; 26:845–849.
34. Tsao L, Hsi ED. The clinicopathologic spectrum of posttransplantation lymphoproliferative disorders. Arch Pathol Lab Med 2007; 131:1209–1218.

35. Said JW. Immunodeficiency-related Hodgkin lymphoma and its mimics. Adv Anat Pathol 2007; 14:189–194.
36. Dharnidharka VR, Tejani AH, Ho PL, et al. Post-transplant lymphoproliferative disorder in the United States: young Caucasian males are at highest risk. Am J Transplant 2002; 2:993–998.
37. Opelz G, Dohler B. Lymphomas after solid organ transplantation: a collaborative transplant study report. Am J Transplant 2004; 4:222–230.
38. Ramalingam P, Rybicki L, Smith MD, et al. Posttransplant lymphoproliferative disorders in lung transplant patients: the Cleveland Clinic experience. Mod Pathol 2002; 15:647–656.
39. Reams BD, McAdams HP, Howell DN, et al. Posttransplant lymphoproliferative disorder: incidence, presentation, and response to treatment in lung transplant recipients. Chest 2003; 124:1242–1249.
40. Harris NL, Swerdlow SH, Frizzera G, et al. Post-transplant lymphoproliferative disorders. In. Jaffe ES, Harris NL, Stein H, et al., eds. Pathology and Genetic of Tumours of Haematopoietic and Lymphoid Tissue. Lyon, France: IARC Press, 2001:264–269.
41. Wilde GE, Moore DJ, Bellah RD. Posttransplantation lymphoproliferative disorder in pediatric recipients of solid organ transplants: timing and location of disease. AJR Am J Roentgenol 2005; 185:1335–1341.
42. Walker RC, Paya CV, Marshall WF, et al. Pretransplantation seronegative Epstein-Barr virus status is the primary risk factor for posttransplantation lymphoproliferative disorder in adult heart, lung, and other solid organ transplantations. J Heart Lung Transplant 1995; 14:214–221.
43. Frey NV, Tsai DE. The management of posttransplant lymphoproliferative disorder. Med Oncol 2007; 24:125–136.
44. Bechtel D, Kurth J, Unkel C, et al. Transformation of BCR-deficient germinal-center B cells by EBV supports a major role of the virus in the pathogenesis of Hodgkin and posttransplantation lymphomas. Blood 2005; 106:4345–4350.
45. Pitman SD, Huang Q, Zuppan CW, et al. Hodgkin lymphoma-like posttransplant lymphoproliferative disorder (HL-like PTLD) simulates monomorphic B-cell PTLD both clinically and pathologically. Am J Surg Pathol 2006; 30:470–476.
46. Raj R, Frost AE. Lung retransplantation after posttransplantation lymphoproliferative disorder (PTLD): a single-center experience and review of literature of PTLD in lung transplant recipients. J Heart Lung Transplant 2005; 24:671–679(review).
47. Dickson RP, Davis RD, Rea JB, et al. High frequency of bronchogenic carcinoma after single-lung transplantation. J Heart Lung Transplant 2006; 25:1297–1301.
48. Johnson BA, Duncan SR, Ohori NP, et al. Recurrence of sarcoidosis in pulmonary allograft recipients. Am Rev Respir Dis 1993; 148:1373–1377.
49. Nine JS, Yousem SA, Paradis IL, et al. Lymphangioleiomyomatosis: recurrence after lung transplantation. J Heart Lung Transplant 1994; 13:714–719.
50. Boehler A. Lung transplantation for cystic lung diseases: lymphangioleiomyomatosis, histiocytosis x, and sarcoidosis. Semin Respir Crit Care Med 2001; 22:509–516.
51. Garver RI Jr., Zorn GL, Wu X, et al. Recurrence of bronchioloalveolar carcinoma in transplanted lungs. N Engl J Med 1999; 340:1071–1074.
52. Benden C, Aurora P, Curry J, et al. High prevalence of gastroesophageal reflux in children after lung transplantation. Pediatr Pulmonol 2005; 40:68–71.
53. Cantu E III, Appel JZ III, Hartwig MG, et al. J. Maxwell Chamberlain Memorial Paper. Early fundoplication prevents chronic allograft dysfunction in patients with gastroesophageal reflux disease. Ann Thorac Surg 2004; 78:1142–1151; discussion 1142–1151.
54. D'Ovidio F, Mura M, Ridsdale R, et al. The effect of reflux and bile acid aspiration on the lung allograft and its surfactant and innate immunity molecules SP-A and SP-D. Am J Transplant 2006; 6:1930–1938.

55. Watkins TR, Chien JW, Crawford SW. Graft versus host-associated pulmonary disease and other idiopathic pulmonary complications after hematopoietic stem cell transplant. Semin Respir Crit Care Med 2005; 26:482–489.
56. Jantunen E, Itala M, Lehtinen T, et al. Early treatment-related mortality in adult autologous stem cell transplant recipients: a nation-wide survey of 1482 transplanted patients. Eur J Haematol 2006; 76:245–250.
57. Wadehra N, Farag S, Bolwell B, et al. Long-term outcome of Hodgkin disease patients following high-dose busulfan, etoposide, cyclophosphamide, and autologous stem cell transplantation. Biol Blood Marrow Transplant 2006; 12:1343–1349.
58. Neve V, Foot AB, Michon J, et al. Longitudinal clinical and functional pulmonary follow-up after megatherapy, fractionated total body irradiation, and autologous bone marrow transplantation for metastatic neuroblastoma. Med Pediatr Oncol 1999; 32:170–176.
59. Myers JL. Pathology of drug-induced lung disease. In: Katzenstein AI, ed. Katzenstein and Askins Surgical Pathology of Non-neoplastic Lung Disease. Philadelphia: WB Saunders, 1997: 81–111.
60. Sharma S, Nadrous HF, Peters SG, et al. Pulmonary complications in adult blood and marrow transplant recipients: autopsy findings. Chest 2005; 128:1385–1392.
61. Roychowdhury M, Pambuccian SE, Aslan DL, et al. Pulmonary complications after bone marrow transplantation: an autopsy study from a large transplantation center. Arch Pathol Lab Med 2005; 129:366–371.
62. Afessa B, Litzow MR, Tefferi A. Bronchiolitis obliterans and other late onset non-infectious pulmonary complications in hematopoietic stem cell transplantation. Bone Marrow Transplant 2001; 28:425–434.
63. Kantrow SP, Hackman RC, Boeckh M, et al. Idiopathic pneumonia syndrome: changing spectrum of lung injury after marrow transplantation. Transplantation 1997; 63:1079–1086.
64. Witte RJ, Gurney JW, Robbins RA, et al. Diffuse pulmonary alveolar hemorrhage after bone marrow transplantation: radiographic findings in 39 patients. AJR Am J Roentgenol 1991; 157:461–464.
65. Agusti C, Ramirez J, Picado C, et al. Diffuse alveolar hemorrhage in allogeneic bone marrow transplantation. A postmortem study. Am J Respir Crit Care Med 1995; 151:1006–1010.
66. Baron FA, Hermanne JP, Dowlati A, et al. Bronchiolitis obliterans organizing pneumonia and ulcerative colitis after allogeneic bone marrow transplantation. Bone Marrow Transplant 1998; 21:951–954.
67. Hayes-Jordan A, Benaim E, Richardson S, et al. Open lung biopsy in pediatric bone marrow transplant patients. J Pediatr Surg 2002; 37:446–452.
68. Freudenberger TD, Madtes DK, Curtis JR, et al. Association between acute and chronic graft-versus-host disease and bronchiolitis obliterans organizing pneumonia in recipients of hematopoietic stem cell transplants. Blood 2003; 102:3822–3828.
69. Hackman RC, Madtes DK, Petersen FB, et al. Pulmonary venoocclusive disease following bone marrow transplantation. Transplantation 1989; 47:989–992.
70. Williams LM, Fussell S, Veith RW, et al. Pulmonary veno-occlusive disease in an adult following bone marrow transplantation. Case report and review of the literature. Chest 1996; 109:1388–1391.

23
Clinical Complications of Lung Transplantation

RAJEEV SAGGAR and DAVID J. ROSS
David Geffen School of Medicine, Ronald Reagan UCLA Medical Center,
University of California, Los Angeles, California, U.S.A.

I. Gastrosophageal Reflux Disease

Gastrointestinal (GI) complaints are common before and after lung transplantation (1–5). In patients with end-stage lung disease (ESLD) awaiting lung transplantation, the prevalence of gastrosophageal reflux disease (GERD) ranges between 32% and 68% (2–5).

In lung transplant recipients (LTRs), GERD has been shown to worsen after surgery in LTRs and is associated with increased incidence of acute rejection, earlier onset of chronic rejection, and higher mortality (4,6,7). GERD has been implicated as an important cause of respiratory disease either by aspiration of refluxed gastric contents or by neurally mediated reflux bronchoconstriction secondary to irritation of the esophageal mucosa. These mechanisms may contribute to deterioration in spirometric indices, worsening lung disease, dysphagia, strictures, and emesis-induced malnutrition.

Several factors may explain the occurrence of GERD in LTRs. GI side effects, including gastritis and ulceration, have been reported with commonly used posttransplant immunosuppressive medications, such as prednisone or calcineurin inhibitors (8,9). Also, vagal nerve damage during lung transplantation may cause or exacerbate GERD, chronic aspiration, or delayed gastric empyting (6,8). The causes of GERD and delayed gastric emptying in ESLD are complex. In addition to problems with lower esophageal mechanics, systemic diseases such as scleroderma and cystic fibrosis can further diminish esophageal motility (10).

Several researchers have suggested a relationship between GERD and the development of lung allograft injury and bronchiolitis obliterans syndrome (BOS) in LTRs (6,11–13). Allommune-mediated injury directed against endothelial and epithelial structures has been thought to be the underlying cause of bronchiolitis obliterans; however, a growing body of literature suggests a strong link between BOS and nonalloimmune mechanisms of airway injury and inflammation, leading to airway fibrosis, such as viral infections, ischemic injury, and BOS (14,15). Two forms of obliterative bronchiolitis (OB) have been identified in heart-lung transplant recipients: an acellular concentric fibrosing process limited to the terminal bronchioles, and a focal and cellular process, extending into the distal alveolar spaces, associated with aspirated material and foreign body-type giant cells (16). The latter of the two is pathologically supportive of a possible role of GERD in the development of OB. Young and colleagues showed that the presence of acid reflux prior to transplantation was strongly associated with posttransplant reflux (17). In addition, seven patients (21%) had normal esophageal pH probe studies pretransplant but acquired GERD after transplantation. Interestingly, the majority of patients with posttransplant GERD were asymptomatic. Acid contact time by 24-hour pH probe was increased by a mean of 3.7% after transplantation ($p = 0.035$); the greatest increase occurred during supine position compared with upright acid contact time (17).

Investigators at Duke Hospital retrospectively analyzed 42 patients (56.8%) pretransplant and 119 (74.9%) posttransplant patients with abnormal pH probe studies. Of the patients with concomitant pH probe studies pre- and posttransplantation, 48.6% had abnormal pH studies pretransplant, whereas 74.3% demonstrated abnormal pH studies posttransplant, ($p = 0.005$; odds ratio = 2.24).

Elevated levels of bronchoalveolar lavage (BAL) pepsin, a biomarker of gastric aspiration, have been recently shown to be present in lung allograft recipients and the highest levels were seen in patients with greater than and equal to grade A2 acute rejection (18). This study, however, did not show an association between higher pepsin levels and BOS. Nevertheless, pepsin was not detected in healthy volunteers or control subjects with chronic cough and GERD. There is also increasing evidence using BAL bile salts, a biomarker of duodenal-gastroesophageal reflux and aspirate, to correlate with the development of BOS in lung allografts (14). The authors concluded that nonalloimmune injury may contribute to lung injury and occult aspiration may be an ongoing source of continuous injury (14,18).

Several uncontrolled studies in LTRs with GERD and decline in lung function have reported a delayed onset, improvement, or even reversal of BOS following surgical fundoplication (5,7,10,19,20). Davis et al. performed 43 fundoplication procedures in LTRs with abnormal pH probe studies, of which 26 patients (60%) also met criteria for BOS (20). Sixteen patients improved their BOS grades, with 13 (81.2%) no longer meeting spirometric criteria for BOS. Six-month follow-up disclosed an increase in forced expiration volume in one second (FEV_1) of 24.1% in those patients who underwent antireflux surgery (20). Furthermore, survival after six months, as determined by Kaplan-Meier, was significantly higher in patients with a normal vis-à-vis abnormal pH study ($p = 0.047$) and in the "fundoplication group" compared with "routine transplant population" ($p = 0.013$) (20). Intraoperative and postoperative complication rates of fundoplication procedures were 0% to 3% (10,20). These studies have several important limitations, including their retrospective analysis, small sample size, selection bias, and inability to control for all covariates.

Other severe GI complications of chronic immunosuppression described after lung transplantation have included cholecystitis, diverticulitis, colitis (infectious or ischemic), pancreatitis, intestinal obstruction, perforation, and malignancy (21). A high index of suspicion is therefore warranted to establish a timely diagnosis and appropriate intervention.

II. Posttransplant Lymphoproliferative Disorder and Other Malignancies

There is a reported increased incidence of certain malignancies, particularly skin cancers, non-Hodgkin's lymphoma, and posttransplant lymphoproliferative disorder (PTLD), after lung transplantation. Although the data are limited for LTRs, the prevalence of common cancers such as lung, breast, and colon appear to be higher (2- to 4-fold) in solid organ recipients than in the general population (21,22). Nonmelanotic skin cancers are the most commonly reported de novo malignancies in solid organ transplant (SOT) recipients, with their incidence varying in proportion to the degree of sun exposure (23,24). The most common-encountered skin cancers are squamous cell (SCC) and basal cell (BCC) carcinomas. The increasing recognition of malignancy risk likely is attributed to two variables, improved graft function and increased patient survival, and the mean age of recipients has risen by 10 years over the past 15 years. The incidence of malignancy has been estimated at 20% after 10 years and 30% after 20 years of chronic immunosuppression (25–28). In 2004 and 2005, the International Society for Heart and Lung Transplant (ISHLT) reported the overall incidence of malignancy after lung transplantation as 3.8% and 13% for survivors at one and five years, respectively (29,30). Lymphoid malignancies have the highest incidence during the first year, and skin cancers are more common in patients more than five years posttransplant (30).

PTLD is considered to represent a spectrum ranging from Epstein-Barr virus (EBV)-associated mononucleosis to polyclonal lymphoid hyperplasia to monoclonal lymphoma. The incidence of PTLD after lung transplant has ranged between 2.5% and 20% (31–35). Most cases of PTLD present during the initial year posttransplant and appear to be associated with EBV infection. Most represent B-cell origin (36); however, T-cell proliferation comprises up to 14% of PTLD (37,38) and natural killer (NK) cells comprise 1% (39). One major risk factor for development of PTLD has been "primary" EBV infection in a seronegative allograft recipient (40). In fact, in fewer than 10% of cases, the lymphoid cells are donor in origin, suggesting that these passenger cells can survive and undergo malignant transformation in some patients (41–43). Nevertheless, some patients with PTLD show no evidence of concurrent EBV viremia or viral expression (34,44). Native lung chronic obstructive pulmonary disease (COPD) and recipient age greater than 55 years appear to be additional risk factors for development of PTLD (34).

In the majority of cases of PTLD associated with EBV, virus can be identified using molecular techniques such as quantitative polymerase chain reaction (PCR) immunochemical analysis of EBV latent membrane protein (LMP-1) or nuclear antigen [Epstein Barr Virus Nuclear Antigen-2 (EBNA-2)] (45,46). Detection of EBV in peripheral blood in suspected cases of PTLD can be used only as a surrogate marker or adjunct to the histopathologic evaluation with immunohistochemistry.

Recent evidence has indicated that newer immunosuppressive agents are associated with an improved side-effect profile, protecting against graft rejection while potentially inhibiting tumor growth (47,48). Maintenance with tacrolimus rather than cyclosporine has been linked with reduced incidence of cancers (49). More recently, combination therapy with tacrolimus and sirolimus has been reported to reduce frequency of skin cancers compared with tacrolimus/mycophenolate and mycophenolate/cyclosporine in heart transplant recipients (50). Further studies and novel approaches are required to further refine the immunosuppressive protocols to retard allograft rejection with less propensity for development of malignancy.

The clinical manifestations of PTLD are diverse (51). Early cases of PTLD often present with only constitutional symptoms or infectious mononucleosis-like illness; later, the disease may be nodal or extranodal, thoracic or widely disseminated, often mimicking an acute abdomen or associated with recurrent spiking fevers (51). In LTRs, PTLD involves the thorax in up to 89% of cases (52,53); the next most common site is within the abdomen, ranging from 20% to 34% (54–56). In LTRs, PTLD typically presents within the initial year, with a predilection for the allograft (33). Later-onset PTLD (>1 year posttransplant) is less likely to involve the graft and carries a worse prognosis (57).

In the appropriate clinical setting, radiographic findings can be strongly suggestive of the diagnosis of PTLD. Computed tomographic (CT) imaging is used to determine the extent of intrathoracic PTLD. Typical features include pulmonary nodules, infiltrates, and intrathoracic lymphadenopathy (56,58). Positron emission tomography (PET) has been utilized as an adjunct to CT imaging, in particular to evaluate potential extrathoracic sites, and can be used to assess response to therapy (59). Clinical approaches to therapy for PTLD entail a reduction in immunosuppression (60); however, this approach may be associated with an increased risk of allograft rejection (61). Antiviral agents (e.g., acyclovir, valgancyclovir, ganciclovir) are routinely used; however, their efficacy has not been established. Other treatment modalities include rituxan, multiagent chemotherapy, surgery, radiation therapy, and gamma interferon. Other experimental treatment regimens have included alemtuzumab, hydroxyurea, and everolimus.

III. Primary Graft Dysfunction

Primary graft dysfunction (PGD) likely represents lung ischemic-reperfusion injury (LIRI) usually occurring within the first 72 hours posttransplant (62–65). PGD is arguably the most common early complication of lung transplantation, occurring in as high as 11% to 25% of patients and contributes to significant morbidity and mortality (62,66). In fact, Christie and colleagues described PGD as contributing up to 43% of early mortality within 30 days of lung transplantation (62). In addition, survivors of PGD had worse survival extending beyond the first year of transplantation (62).

PGD is characterized by transient hypoxemia associated with diffuse roentgenographic alveolar infiltrates, decreased pulmonary compliance, and increased pulmonary vascular resistance. Severe cases may present with life-threatening acute alveolar damage requiring aggressive intervention, including extracorporeal membrane oxygenation (ECMO) support (67,68).

There are many cellular and molecular events underlying the development of PGD, and both donor and recipient factors play a role (69). In severe cases, histologic examination of the lungs reveals diffuse alveolar damage. However, diagnostic criteria for PGD have been previously inconsistent because of a lack of standardized criteria (63,70,71). As a result, the ISHLT Working Group on primary graft dysfunction has reported standardized consensus criteria to define PGD on the basis of recipient arterial oxygenation tension/fraction of inspired oxygen (PaO_2/FiO_2) ratios and chest radiographic findings (Table 1) (69,72). The result of the ISHLT efforts have provided improved reporting of incidence and clinical outcomes (69).

The presence of nonspecific diffuse alveolar damage, reactive type II pneumocyte hyperplasia, parenchymal edema, and even endothelitis can be present on histologic evaluation of the affected lung. Nevertheless, one must exclude other diagnoses with potentially similar clinical presentations. Hemodynamic monitoring with a pulmonary artery catheter can be used to confirm the presence of noncardiogenic edema, pulmonary capillary wedge pressure (PCWP) less than 18 mm Hg, and often documenting elevated pulmonary vascular resistance up to threefold normal values (73). A transesophageal echocardiogram (TEE) may be useful in assessment of cardiac function and visualizing the

Table 1 Recommendations for Grading of Primary Graft Dysfunction

PGD severity		
Grade	PaO_2/FiO_2	Radiographic infiltrates consistent with pulmonary edema
0	>300	Absent
1	>300	Present
2	200–300	Present
3	<200	Present

Abbreviations: PGD, primary graft dysfunction; PaO_2/FiO_2, arterial oxygenation tension/fraction of inspired oxygen.
Source: From Ref. 85.

pulmonary arteries and veins for potential vascular anastomosis complications. Finally, flexible bronchoscopy provides a rapid ability to assess the bronchial anastomosis to evaluate for strictures, torsion, or dehiscence as well as BAL for detection of infection.

Translational research continues to be important in determining the molecular and cellular paradigm causing PGD. The depth of data is beyond the scope of this article; however, a few key concepts will be addressed. Early tissue injury is largely dependent on donor organ alveolar macrophages activation of endothelial and epithelial cells (74). Through autocrine and paracrine transcriptional activation, cytokine and chemokine production facilitates leukocyte activation and further tissue injury (74–76). A second (later) phase of ischemic reperfusion injury requires recipient neutrophil and lymphocyte activation and recruitment into the allograft (74). Certain patterns of chemokine elaboration have also been demonstrated in LIRI (77). In BAL from human lung recipients, increased levels of tumor necrosis factor (TNF)-α, interleukin (IL)-10, IL-12, and IL-18 have been detected during ischemia, while IL-8 had increased predominantly after reperfusion (78). In contrast, IL-10 and IL-4 have been shown to protect against tissue injury in animal models (78). Finally, nitric oxide (NO) may play a critical role in vascular homeostasis by inhibiting neutrophil adhesion and platelet aggregation and maintaining endothelial integrity. Although prophylactic-inhaled NO does not prevent LIRI, it may blunt the downstream sequelae if LIRI exists (79).

The specific characteristics that result in PGD is complex and may involve a series of donor-related insults (Table 2), procurement or transplant as well as issues pertaining to the recipient (Table 3) after reperfusion (80). The impact of donor factors, however, is dependent on the intrinsic characteristics of the donor lung as well those acquired during and subsequent to death. Female gender, African-American race and age have been shown to independently affect the frequency of PGD (81). Christie et al. found that donor ages less than 21 years and greater than 45 years were more frequently associated with PGD; however, other groups have successfully used older donors (82–84). According to ISHLT Registry data, donor age greater than 45 years and ischemic time greater than seven to eight hours were associated with higher 30-day mortality after lung transplant (83). Donor smoking may also impact long-term outcomes, but it does not appear to increase incidence of PGD (85).

Acquired lung donor factors that may contribute to PGD include brain death, prolonged mechanical ventilation, aspiration, trauma, pneumonia, multiple blood transfusions, or hemodynamic instability (81,86). Techniques that have been instituted to improve donor management and lung preservation include retrograde flush, pretreatment with

Table 2 Donor-Related Risk Factors

Inherent donor factors:
Female gender
African-American
Age >45 yr + ischemia time >7–8 hr
Age <21 yr
Acquired donor factors:
Brain death, pneumonia, trauma
Increased IL-6, IL-8 levels
Decreased IL-10 levels
Lung
Preservation
Low-potassium preservate (Perfadex®)
Ischemia time + other risk factors
Retrograde flush + PGE_1

Table 3 Recipient-Associated Risk Factors

Definitive association:
Diagnosis of PPH
Modified reperfusion technique
Strong associated risk factors
Hepatic dysfunction (bilirubin >2 mg/dL)
Complicated pleural space
Weak associated risk factors
Renal disease
Secondary pulmonary hypertension
Elevated anti-HLA antibodies
Left heart disease

Abbreviation: PPH, primary pulmonary hypertension.

prostaglandin E_1 (87,88), temperature and volume of preservation solution, as well as inflation, temperature, and oxygenation of the lung during storage (81).

Currently, the most clearly established *recipient* risk factor for PGD is the diagnosis of primary pulmonary hypertension (PPH) (63,66,80,82). Christie and investigators found that the underlying diagnosis of PPH and not the severity of pulmonary hypertension was strongly associated with developing allograft failure after transplantation in a multivariate analysis of 255 lung transplant procedures (adjusted relative risk = 9.24; $p = 0.009$) (82). Meticulous surgical technique, attention to hemodynamic parameters, and use of a modified reperfusion protocol (80,89) may decrease the incidence of LIRI. The UCLA group studied 100 lung transplant procedures using a modified reperfusion technique with leukocyte-depleted and nutrient-enriched reperfusate associated with low reperfusion pressure after implantation (89). This technique was associated with a 2% incidence of PGD and a 30-day survival of 97% (89). Using this protocol, Schnickel et al. were able to show that the incidence of PDG, early mortality, and one-year survival was similar, whether using higher-risk "non-standard" criteria for lungs compared with "standard" donors (89).

Although lacking conclusive evidence, other associated risk factors that may contribute to the development of PGD include hepatic dysfunction (bilirubin >2mg/dL) (90), increased risk of postoperative bleeding from pleural adhesions, and/or prior lung surgery (91,92). Other additional factors that possibly contribute to the development of PGD include secondary pulmonary hypertension (82,93,94), elevated anti-HLA antibodies, left heart disease, and renal impairment (80).

IV. Infections in Lung Transplantation

Mycobacterial infections (MBIs) [due to both *Mycobacterium tuberculosis* and non-tuberculosis mycobacteria (NTM)] are rare but potentially lethal complications of hematopoietic stem cell or solid organ transplantation (95–101). Posttransplant MBIs may reflect acquisition of new infections (because of the intensity of immunosuppression) (99), reactivation of latent disease (particularly *M. tuberculosis*) within the recipients (100,101), or receipt of infected organs (99,102–104). Environmental sources are the reservoir for most human infections due to NTM (23,105,106), whereas human-to-human transmissions or reactivation of latent infections are the critical factors for development of infections due to *M. tuberculosis* (100). The incidence of MBIs depends on the intensity of immunosuppression, the prevalence of mycobacteria (both typical and NTM) in the region of country, type of transplanted organ, and risk factors and exposures to mycobacteria.

The incidence of tuberculosis (TB) in transplant recipients is 20- to 70-fold higher than in the general population (98,100). The incidence of TB following lung transplantation ranges from less than 1% to 6.5% (99,100,102). In areas that are endemic to TB, such as Asia, the development of TB posttransplant is a genuine concern, especially transmission via the donor lungs (99,107,108). To reduce the risk of TB among LTRs, the following steps are critical: (*i*) the explanted lungs must be examined for granulomata or evidence of TB; (*ii*) BAL fluid from the donor and recipient bronchi should be sent for mycobacterial cultures; and (*iii*) isoniazid (INH) prophylaxis should be routinely given to candidates for lung transplantation with any of the following criteria: positive tuberculin skin test, anergy but increased risk for TB, or evidence for old granulomatous disease on chest radiographs.

NTM infections are uncommon but potentially lethal complications of SOT (95–97,101,109–112). A comprehensive review of the English language literature from 1996 to 2003 detected 276 cases of NTM infections, 66% in SOT recipients (95). More than half of NTM infections involved the skin, soft tissue or joints; lung involvement occurred in 25% (95,97). The most common species of NTM in SOT recipients are *Micobacterium avium* complex (MAC), *Micobacterium fortuitum-chelonei-abscessus* group, *Micobacterium kansassi*, and *Micobacterium haemophilum* (95,101,113,114). Clinical manifestations of NTM are protean and include localized or disseminated cutaneous infections, pulmonary involvement, wound infections, and intestinal involvement (95). CT scans may be invaluable in detecting localized disease, which may be amenable to biopsy and microbiologic sampling (95). Treatment of NTM needs to be individualized depending on the specimen, site of infections, and degree of immunosuppression (95). In general, treatment of NTM disease requires the use of combinations of antimicrobial agents for prolonged periods (6–24 months) (95).

V. Bacterial Infections and Pneumocystis Infections

Bacterial infections are the most common pathogens after lung transplant and may relate to preexisting colonization of the donor or recipient, surgical complications, community-acquired or nosocomial exposure (115–118). In two different single-center studies, bacterial pneumonia constituted over 40% of all posttransplant-related deaths, the majority often due to gram-negative organisms (117–119). Three-fourths of all bacterial pneumonias occur within the first six months of transplantation (117,120).

Careful assessment of the donor and recipient is essential to assure adequate prophylactic or presumptive therapy. Both the donor and recipient undergo a standard panel of serological testing, which serves to define the risk more precisely and to guide pre- and posttransplant interventions. Often lung donors are intubated for presumed aspiration risk and subsequently initiated on antibiotics. It has been reported that over 40% of donors are colonized with *Staphylococcus aureus*, including methicillin-resistant *S. aureus* strains (MRSA), and almost 50% are colonized with gram-negative bacilli (121). As a result, many large centers routinely perform sampling of the donor lung intraoperatively as well as posttransplant using fiber-optic bronchoscopy (FOB). Avolonitis et al. showed a close relationship between increased bacterial colonization of donor lung and rates of subsequent pulmonary infections (121). Although most centers recommend initiating broad-spectrum antibiotics in the postoperative period, the benefits of pretransplant antibiotic therapy are still unknown.

Pulmonary infections in lung recipients are often difficult to diagnose, the clinical presentation may mimic rejection or even posttransplant edema. Bronchoscopy with BAL and transbronchial biopsy is often warranted to differentiate between an infectious process and rejection. Chan and investigators evaluated BAL, protected specimen brushings, and transbronchial biopsies that were performed in 83 lung recipients (120). The diagnostic yield in isolating bacteria increased from 17.5% (BAL alone) to over 90% with the addition of a protected specimen brushing (120). Even with this aggressive approach, a pathogen is often not isolated in the setting of clinical infection.

Cystic fibrosis (CF) patients are often chronic carriers with multidrug-resistant bacteria; the most common organism is *Pseudomonas aeruginosa*. The Duke group reported that 86% lung recipients with CF were infected with *P. aeruginosa* pretransplant, 24% with MRSA, and 19% with *Stenotrophomonas*. However, pretransplant colonization, including multidrug-resistant *P. aeruginosa*, is not a contraindication to transplant (122–126). Despite posttransplant antibiotic prophylaxis, *Pseudomonas* may develop either early or later, often with identical strains isolated pretransplantation. The University of North Carolina compared the types of infections among lung recipients with CF and without CF (124). The group with CF tended to have a higher rate of bacterial sinusitis, however, overall both groups experienced similar rates of pneumonia or bronchitis after transplantation (124). This has led some institutions to examine the role of sinus surgery, a presumed reservoir for these pathogens, in CF-transplant recipients (127,128). Although the studies contain small numbers and are nonrandomized, at least one study suggested a reduced frequency of tracheobronchitis (128). Current treatment modalities include antipseudomonal agent, inhaled tobramycin, inhaled colistin, and systemic aminoglycosides. The risk of nephrotoxicity is a major concern, especially in concert with calcineurin inhibitors.

Colonization of *Burkholderia cepacia*, a gram-negative rod, often found in soil and water, appears to be a major risk factor of posstransplant morbidity and mortality in CF patients (129). Various studies have documented poor outcomes in lung recipients with

CF who are infected with *B. cepacia* pretransplant (130,131). Chaparro et al. reported a three-year survival outcome in 53 CF lung recipients, in 45% of patients with *B. cepacia* compared with 86% of those without *B. cepacia* infection, ($p < 0.01$) (130). Acquired *B. cepacia* in lung recipients is also associated with higher mortality, and the most common isolate is genomovar III (131–133). Given the increased risk of mortality in many centers, *B. cepacia*, especially genomovar III strain, is considered a relative contraindication to lung transplantation (132,133).

Prophylaxis with trimthoprim-sulfamethoxazole (TMP-SMX) has dramatically reduced the incidence of *Pneumocystis jiroveci*- (formally *carinii*) associated respiratory illnesses. All organ transplant recipients are at increased risk of developing *Pneumocystis* pneumonia, usually within the first six months of transplantation (134). Lung recipients appear to be more susceptible to *P. jiroveci*, and the need for lifelong prophylaxis may be indicated, especially in those patients with augmented immunosuppression (134–136). For those patients intolerant or allergic to sulfa drugs, aerosolized pentamidine (137) dapsone (138) or atovaquone are alternative agents (139).

Nocardia spp, a gram-positive bacterium, is now less often seen after lung transplantation, especially after the universal use of TMP-SMX. Nocardiosis usually infects the lungs but can involve the brain, skin, soft tissue, and bones. Two separate reviews identified nocardiosis in 1.85% to 2.1% of lung recipients, respectively (140,141). Typical lung involvement is characterized by consolidation, nodules, and, less often, cavitations.

Bacterial infections may also be acquired as a consequence of early posttransplant mechanical complications. Pleural complications, including empyema, are rarely reported. The Pittsburg group identified 14 (3.9%) empyema cases of 392 lung recipients, with 79% of the cases secondary to bacterial pathogens. Typical bacterial infections include *Staphylococcus*, *Enterobacter* sp, *Klebsiella* sp, *Enterococcus* sp, and *Escherichia coli* (142). Similar pathogens are seen in other wound sites, including thoracotomy, sternotomy, or other clamshell incision, but may occasionally be caused by fungal, atypical *Mycobacterium*, and *Mycoplasma hominis* (143,144).

Many bacterial infections can occur in either nosocomial or community settings, seen both immediately pretransplant and in later stages of the posttransplant period. Immunosuppression and increasing resistant organisms appear to enhance the risk and development of increasing complications, including isolates of MRSA and extended spectrum β-lactamase producing gram-negative enteric rods, multidrug-resistant *Pseudomonas*, *Acinetobacter*, and *Stenotrophomonas*. *Legionella pneumophilia* can also occur in the nosocomial setting. It is increasingly diagnosed by urinary antigen testing (*L. pneumophila* serotype 1), although isolation from sputum or BAL fluid is still the gold standard. The majority of cases will present as pneumonia, although extrapulmonary manifestations are common in immunosuppressed individuals. Risk factors include hospital water systems, air conditioners, as well as pleural effusions, lung abscesses, and cavitations.

VI. Fungal Infections: Aspergillosis, Coccidiomycosis, Cryptococcus, Endemic Mycosis

Fungal infections can occur in lung recipients and typically occur in conjunction to pretransplant colonization, to community and nosocomial exposures, and to airway and anastomotic complications.

Aspergillus infections are characterized by several distinct clinical syndromes. Airway colonization after lung transplantation is common and usually detected on survellaince bronchoscopy or routine screening (145). Posttransplant colonization is considered a risk factor to developing subsequent invasive disease, and treatment is warranted (146). *Aspergillus* tracheobronchitis is almost exclusively seen in lung recipients and typically occurs within the first three months of transplantation (147). Invasive pulmonary aspergillosis and bronchial anastomotic infections are the most feared complications and carry a high mortality (148). Disseminated disease occurs in 10% of lung recipients and may involve almost any organ (149). Successful treatment of aspergillosis varies from center to center but usually requires early- and high-dose systemic antifungal agents and modification in immunosuppression (150).

Coccidiomycosis is a geographically limited fungal infection, occurring in the southwestern United States and Mexico. The incidence of coccidiomycosis is reported ranging from 0.3% to 10% in renal, liver, and heart-lung transplant recipients from endemic areas (151). Pretransplant colonization with cocciodioides in SOT recipients appears to be a risk factor for reactivation posttransplant. Donor transmission of coccidiomycosis has also resulted in fulminant multiorgan failure and rapid dissemination (152,153). Pulmonary manifestations include multiple nodules, cavitations, pleural thickening, and effusions. Extrapulmonary sites may include the meninges, cutaneous sites, joints, lymph nodes, or other areas. A comprehensive pretransplant screen is warranted to determine the extent of disease and dissemination. Effective antifungal therapy is warranted prior to listing if active disease is suspected, and even "cured" recipients should be considered for prolonged suppressive therapy after transplantation (154).

Cryptococcus infection is associated with bird droppings and predominantly affects immunocompromised hosts (155). The incidence of *Cryptococcus* in SOT ranges from 0% to as high as 6%, although lung recipients tend to have a lower incidence compared with other solid organ recipients (156–159). The central nervous system (CNS) is the most common site of infection in SOT recipients. Other common sites affected include the lung (10%), skin, bone, soft tissue (13%), and other sites. The diagnosis can be made by culture, direct microscopic examination (India ink), and detection of polysaccharide antigen in fluid or tissue. The mortality rate due to *Cryptococcus* is high, with rates from 40% to 50% with crytpococcal meningitis (160). A high index of suspicion warrants rapid administration of antifungal therapy with a reduction in immunosuppression.

Significant mold infections in LTRs include *Fusarium*, the dermatiaceous mold, and zygomycetes. In particular, zygomycetes (*Mucor*, *Rhizopus*, Rhizomucor) are very aggressive with potential for invasion and dissemination and are associated with high mortality. Typically, these molds are resistant to azole antibiotics, with the exception of posaconazole. Standard treatment consists of high dose amphotericin in conjuction with surgical debriedment.

Finally, other fungi that cause significant morbidity and mortality include histoplasmosis, blastomycosis, and scedosporium.

VII. Chronic Rejection

The intermediate results of lung transplantation are suboptimal with less than 50% survival at five years. (161). The major limitation is the occurrence of OB, which is thought to represent chronic allograft rejection. Bronchiolitis obliterans was first described in 1984 after heart-lung transplant recipients showed a progressive decline in FEV_1 (162). Lung biopsies from these patients showed intraluminal polyps comprised of fibomyxoid granulation tissue and plaques of dense submucosal scar that tended to obliterate the lumens of the terminal bronchioles (162).

Because of the marginal response to medical therapy, OB has emerged as the leading cause of late mortality and the major obstacle to long-term success after lung transplantation (163). In this chapter, we give an overview of the incidence, risk factors, and diagnosis of OB.

A. Incidence and Prevalence of OB/BOS

Bronchiolitis obliterans (histology) and its clinical correlate BOS affect up to 50% to 60% of patients who survive five years after transplantation (164,165).

B. Pathogenesis

OB is an intraluminal scarring process that occludes the small airways of the lung allograft (166). In 2001, the ISHLT consensus definition agreed that the presence of a lymphocytic submucosal infiltrate or intraluminal granulation tissue is insufficient for a diagnosis of OB (167). Furthermore, the obliterative lesions are temporally heterogeneous with some airways considered "active" if associated with fibrosis and mononuclear infiltrates or "inactive" if demonstrated by fibrosis only (167). Histopathologic features suggest that inflammation and injury to epithelial and subepithelial structures of the small airways lead to augmented fibroproliferation and ineffective tissue repair (166,168). The salient feature of the fibrous scarring can be eccentric or concentric in distribution, reducing the bronchiolar lumen and, in severe cases, causing complete obliteration (167). The initial pathologic insult seen involves lymphocytic infiltration of the submucosa of the epithelium and airways, known as lymphocytic bronchiolitis (LB) (169). In fact, Ross et al. have described the association with refractory airflow obstruction in association with isolated LB, suggesting its role as the progenitor lesion (170). OB likely represents the "final common pathway" (163) lesion from various insults and suggests alloimmune-dependent and independent mechanisms acting alone or in concert (171).

C. Risk Factors for Chronic Rejection

Alloimmune-Dependent Risk Factors

The single most important risk factor for OB is acute rejection characterized by perivascular infiltration of lymphocytes into the graft. Previous studies suggested that recurrent acute rejection of histologic grade II or more or at least one episode of grade III or IV acute rejection or late onset of acute rejection were significant risk factors for the development of OB in over 90% of recipients (172–174). However, more recent literature suggests that minimal (A1) rejection (175–177) and even LB, in the absence of acute vascular injury, are independent markers of OB (170). Although treatment largely leads to histologic resolution, there is scant evidence that augmented treatment of acute rejection prevents BOS.

The role of alloreactivity toward mismatches at specific loci of the major histocompatibility complex (MHC) is controversial. The largest series from the United Network for Organ Sharing (UNOS)/ISHLT Registry, which included 3459 lung transplants, found no association between HLA and the development of BOS (178). However, several small single-center studies have shown association between BOS and other anti-HLA class I and class II antibodies (179,180). The cause and effect relationship between anti-HLA antibodies and BOS needs to be better elucidated in future studies.

D. Alloimmune-Independent Risk Factors

Nonalloimmunologic inflammatory conditions have been reported as risk factors for BOS. GI complaints are common before and after lung transplantation (1–5). As described earlier in this chapter, GERD has been associated with increased incidence of acute rejection, earlier onset of chronic rejection, and higher mortality (4,6,7), while a therapeutic role for gastric fundoplication has been proposed.

Cytomegalovirus (CMV) infection, pneumonitis, and CMV serologic mismatching have been associated with BOS in several earlier studies (172,174). However, since the introduction of ganciclovir prophylaxis and CMV hyperimmune globulin treatment, the association of CMV pneumonitis and BOS has diminished (181). Intriguingly, an emerging body of literature has been published reporting the association between non-CMV viral infections (respiratory syncytial virus, *Human herpesvirus-6*, *Chlamydia pneumonia*, adenovirus, parainfluenza), bacterial, and fungal infections and BOS (172,174,182–185). As the risk environment changes because of the use of prophylactic antimicrobial agents (186), changes in immunosuppressive approaches, and/or improving management strategies, the degree of association to BOS will need to be further elucidated.

The potential role of other risk factors for BOS, such as older donor age, longer graft ischemic time, and donor antigen-specific reactivity, remains controversial (174,187,188).

E. Diagnosis/Staging

The diagnosis of OB is based on histology; however, because of the patchy nature of this disease transbronchial biopsy (TBB) often has a poor yield. In fact, the sensitivity of TBB for OB was 28% and specificity was 75% (189). As such, in 1993, a consensus definition of BOS was proposed by the ISHLT on the basis ofchanges in pulmonary function criteria, specifically FEV_1 (164). On the basis of these criteria, BOS was divided into four stages, BOS stage 0 indicating stable posttransplant FEV1; progressive deterioration in FEV_1 is defined by the progressive stages of BOS from 1 to 3 (Table 4). Also, if no biopsy was concomitantly performed or no OB was identified on biopsy, a notation of "a" is

Table 4 BOS Stages Based on Percentage of the Best Postoperative FEV_1

BOS stage	FEV_1 (%)
0	80 or more
1	66–79
2	51–65
3	<50

Abbreviations: BOS, bronchiolitis obliterans; FEV_1, forced expiratory volume in one second.
Source: From Ref. 162.

Table 5 Revised BOS Classification of the Best Postoperative FEV_1

BOS stage	FEV_1 (%)
0	FEV_1 >90 and FEF $_{25–75}$ >75
potential BOS	FEV_1 81–90 and/or FEF $_{25–75}$ <76
1	FEV_1 66–80
2	FEV_1 51–65
3	FEV_1<50

Abbreviations: BOS, bronchiolitis obliterans; FEV_1, forced expiratory volume in one second; $FEF_{25–75}$, forced midexpiration flow rate.
Source: From Ref. 165.

designated; "b" indicates OB has been identified (164). Although BOS is a clinical descriptor of OB, clearly not all patients with airflow obstruction develop OB. In fact, other confounding factors such as infections, acute rejection, anastomotic complications, native lung hyperinflation, aging, pleural manifestations, and pain often mimic BOS and needs to be addressed (164,167). In a recent revision of these BOS criteria, FEF_{25-75} (midexpiratory flow rates) has also been included in the staging parameters (167), as evidence suggested this measure was more sensitive, primarily in bilateral transplant recipients, than FEV_1 for early detection of obstructive airflow in BOS (190–192). In addition, the original guidelines defined BOS 1 as a >20% decrease in FEV_1 from baseline, possibly lacking sensitivity to address small and potentially important early changes in spirometric indices. Therefore, in the revised criteria (Table 5), a *potential* BOS stage (BOS 0-p) was added to increase the sensitivity of physiologic change for the diagnosis of BOS (167). Since the revised criteria were formulated, one study provided contrary evidence supporting the superiority of FEV_1 to that of the $FEF_{25–75}$ in predicting BOS 1, in single LTRs with underlying restrictive physiology (193). Similarly, Hachem et al. reported the superior positive predictive value and negative predictive value of FEV_1 criterion of stage BOS 0-p to predict development of BOS 1 over $FEF_{25–75}$ criterion of BOS 0-p (194).

F. High Resolution CT Scan

Findings associated with chronic rejection and OB/BOS on chest radiographs include hyperinflation, decreased peripheral vascular markings, segmental atelectasis, increased linear opacities, and bronchiectasis (195,196). Conventional and thin slice CT has been used to characterize the early and late manifestations of OB/BOS. Air trapping is detected on expiratory CT as mosaic attenuation of the lung (defined as heterogeneous areas of lung attenuation), bronchiectasis, and bronchial wall thickening have all been suggested to be predictive of OB (197–200). A cutoff of 32% of air trapping was the threshold in distinguishing between patients with and without BOS with a sensitivity of 83% and a specificity of 89% (201). Other surrogate markers such as spirometrically gated CT (198) and hyperpolarized ^{3}He magnetic imaging have limited clinical role in evaluating BOS (202).

G. Exhaled Nitric Oxide

There is increasing interest in exhaled nitric oxide (eNO) as a noninvasive marker of airway inflammation after lung transplantation. Previous studies have shown that lung recipients with BOS exhibit an increased fractional excretion of NO (FE_{NO}) compared with normal nonsmoking healthy controls and stable lung transplant patients (203–205). Interestingly, eNO levels tend to be higher in patients with early BOS (grade 1) compared with more severe stages of BOS (2 and 3) (203,205). More recently, Van Muylem and colleagues assessed the performance of eNO, eCO, and single-breath washout-derived S_{He} for the early detection of BOS stages 0-p and 1. The results indicated that S_{He} had a higher sensitivity than either eNO or eCO, alone or in combination, for detection of chronic rejection. However, combining all three biomarkers increased the sensitivity to 86% and 94%, respectively, for BOS 0-p and BOS 1 (206). Future studies are needed to evaluate early therapeutic intervention during episodes of persistent elevations in these surrogate markers such that it may halt or even prevent the progression of BOS.

References

1. Tobin RW, et al. Increased prevalence of gastroesophageal reflux in patients with idiopathic pulmonary fibrosis. Am J Respir Crit Care Med 1998; 158(6):1804–1808.
2. Sweet MP, et al. Prevalence of delayed gastric emptying and gastroesophageal reflux in patients with end-stage lung disease. Ann Thorac Surg 2006; 82(4):1570; author reply 1570–1571.
3. Raghu G, et al. High prevalence of abnormal acid gastro-oesophageal reflux in idiopathic pulmonary fibrosis. Eur Respir J 2006; 27(1):136–142.
4. D'Ovidio F, et al. Prevalence of gastroesophageal reflux in end-stage lung disease candidates for lung transplant. Ann Thorac Surg 2005; 80(4):1254–1260.
5. Cantu E III, et al. J. Maxwell Chamberlain Memorial Paper. Early fundoplication prevents chronic allograft dysfunction in patients with gastroesophageal reflux disease. Ann Thorac Surg 2004; 78(4):1142–1151 (discussion 1142–51).
6. Berkowitz N, et al. Gastroparesis after lung transplantation. Potential role in postoperative respiratory complications. Chest 1995; 108(6):1602–1607.
7. Hartwig MG, Appel JZ, Davis RD. Antireflux surgery in the setting of lung transplantation: strategies for treating gastroesophageal reflux disease in a high-risk population. Thorac Surg Clin 2005; 15(3):417–427.
8. Arcasoy SM, Wilt J. Medical complications after lung transplantation. Semin Respir Crit Care Med 2006; 27(5):508–520.
9. Verleden GM, Besse T, Maes B. Successful conversion from cyclosporine to tacrolimus for gastric motor dysfunction in a lung transplant recipient. Transplantation 2002; 73(12):1974–1976.
10. Gasper WJ, et al. Antireflux surgery for patients with end-stage lung disease before and after lung transplantation. Surg Endosc 2008; 22(2):495–500.
11. Reid KR, et al. Importance of chronic aspiration in recipients of heart-lung transplants. Lancet 1990; 336(8709):206–208.
12. Au J, et al. Upper gastrointestinal dysmotility in heart-lung transplant recipients. Ann Thorac Surg 1993; 55(1):94–97.
13. Rinaldi M, et al. Gastro-esophageal reflux as cause of obliterative bronchiolitis: a case report. Transplant Proc 1995; 27(3):2006–2007.
14. D'Ovidio F, et al. Bile acid aspiration and the development of bronchiolitis obliterans after lung transplantation. J Thorac Cardiovasc Surg 2005; 129(5):1144–1152.
15. Hadjiliadis D, et al. Gastroesophageal reflux disease in lung transplant recipients. Clin Transplant 2003; 17(4):363–368.
16. Abernathy EC, et al. The two forms of bronchiolitis obliterans in heart-lung transplant recipients. Hum Pathol 1991; 22(11):1102–1110.
17. Young LR, et al. Lung transplantation exacerbates gastroesophageal reflux disease. Chest 2003; 124(5):1689–1693.
18. Stovold R, et al. Pepsin, a biomarker of gastric aspiration in lung allografts: a putative association with rejection. Am J Respir Crit Care Med 2007; 175(12):1298–1303.

19. O'Halloran EK, et al. Laparoscopic Nissen fundoplication for treating reflux in lung transplant recipients. J Gastrointest Surg 2004; 8(1):132–137.
20. Davis RD Jr., et al. Improved lung allograft function after fundoplication in patients with gastroesophageal reflux disease undergoing lung transplantation. J Thorac Cardiovasc Surg 2003; 125(3): 533–542.
21. Adami J, et al. Cancer risk following organ transplantation: a nationwide cohort study in Sweden. Br J Cancer 2003; 89(7):1221–1227.
22. Buell JF,Gross TG, Woodle ES. Malignancy after transplantation. Transplantation 2005; 80(suppl 2):S254–S264.
23. Dreno B, et al. Skin cancers in transplant patients. Adv Nephrol Necker Hosp 1997; 27:377–389.
24. Gupta AK,Cardella CJ, Haberman HF. Cutaneous malignant neoplasms in patients with renal transplants. Arch Dermatol 1986; 122(11):1288–1293.
25. Buell JF, et al. Donor transmitted malignancies. Ann Transplant 2004; 9(1):53–56.
26. Buell JF, et al. De novo breast cancer in renal transplant recipients. Transplant Proc 2002; 34(5): 1778–1779.
27. Buell JF, et al. Incidental diagnosis of gastric cancer in transplant recipients improves patient survival. Surgery 2002; 132(4):754–758 (discussion 758–60).
28. Trofe J, et al. Posttransplant malignancy. Prog Transplant 2004; 14(3):193–200.
29. Trulock EP, et al. The Registry of the International Society for Heart and Lung Transplantation: twenty-first official adult lung and heart-lung transplant report–2004. J Heart Lung Transplant 2004; 23(7):804–815.
30. Trulock EP, et al. Registry of the International Society for Heart and Lung Transplantation: twenty-second official adult lung and heart-lung transplant report–2005. J Heart Lung Transplant 2005; 24(8):956–967.
31. Levine SM, et al. A low incidence of posttransplant lymphoproliferative disorder in 109 lung transplant recipients. Chest 1999; 116(5):1273–1277.
32. Bakker NA, et al. Early onset post-transplant lymphoproliferative disease is associated with allograft localization. Clin Transplant 2005; 19(3):327–334.
33. Ramalingam P, et al. Posttransplant lymphoproliferative disorders in lung transplant patients: the Cleveland Clinic experience. Mod Pathol 2002; 15(6):647–656.
34. Reams BD, et al. Posttransplant lymphoproliferative disorder: incidence, presentation, and response to treatment in lung transplant recipients. Chest 2003; 124(4):1242–1249.
35. Gao SZ, et al. Post-transplantation lymphoproliferative disease in heart and heart-lung transplant recipients: 30-year experience at Stanford University. J Heart Lung Transplant 2003; 22(5): 505–514.
36. Shroff R, Rees L. The post-transplant lymphoproliferative disorder-a literature review. Pediatr Nephrol 2004; 19(4):369–377.
37. Lundell R, Elenitoba-Johnson KS, Lim MS. T-cell posttransplant lymphoproliferative disorder occurring in a pediatric solid-organ transplant patient. Am J Surg Pathol 2004; 28(7): 967–973.
38. Sebire NJ, Malone M, Ramsay AD. Posttransplant lymphoproliferative disorder presenting as CD30+, ALK+, anaplastic large cell lymphoma in a child. Pediatr Dev Pathol 2004; 7(3):290–293.
39. Bustillo M, et al. High grade lymphoma in a post-renal transplant patient. Description of a case and literature review. Nephron 2000; 84(2):189–191.
40. Ho M, et al. Epstein-Barr virus infections and DNA hybridization studies in posttransplantation lymphoma and lymphoproliferative lesions: the role of primary infection. J Infect Dis 1985; 152(5): 876–886.
41. Caillard S, et al. Posttransplant lymphoproliferative disorders after renal transplantation in the United States in era of modern immunosuppression. Transplantation 2005; 80(9):1233–1243.
42. Randhawa PS, Yousem SA. Epstein-Barr virus-associated lymphoproliferative disease in a heart-lung allograft. Demonstration of host origin by restriction fragment-length polymorphism analysis. Transplantation 1990; 49(1):126–130.

43. Larson RS, et al. Microsatellite analysis of posttransplant lymphoproliferative disorders: determination of donor/recipient origin and identification of putative lymphomagenic mechanism. Cancer Res 1996; 56(19):4378–4381.
44. Collins MH, et al. Post-transplant lymphoproliferative disease in children. Pediatr Transplant 2001; 5(4):250–257.
45. Gulley ML, et al. Tumor origin and CD20 expression in posttransplant lymphoproliferative disorder occurring in solid organ transplant recipients: implications for immune-based therapy. Transplantation 2003; 76(6):959–964.
46. Pallesen G, et al. Expression of Epstein-Barr virus replicative proteins in AIDS-related non-Hodgkin's lymphoma cells. J Pathol 1991; 165(4):289–299.
47. Koehl GE, et al. Rapamycin protects allografts from rejection while simultaneously attacking tumors in immunosuppressed mice. Transplantation 2004; 77(9):1319–1326.
48. Guba M, et al. Rapamycin inhibits primary and metastatic tumor growth by antiangiogenesis: involvement of vascular endothelial growth factor. Nat Med 2002; 8(2):128–135.
49. Bustami RT, et al. Immunosuppression and the risk of post-transplant malignancy among cadaveric first kidney transplant recipients. Am J Transplant 2004; 4(1):87–93.
50. Kobashigawa JA, et al. Tacrolimus with mycophenolate mofetil (MMF) or sirolimus vs. cyclosporine with MMF in cardiac transplant patients: 1-year report. Am J Transplant 2006; 6(6): 1377–1386.
51. Preiksaitis JK. New developments in the diagnosis and management of posttransplantation lymphoproliferative disorders in solid organ transplant recipients. Clin Infect Dis 2004; 39(7):1016–1023.
52. Armitage JM, et al. Posttransplant lymphoproliferative disease in thoracic organ transplant patients: ten years of cyclosporine-based immunosuppression. J Heart Lung Transplant 1991; 10(6):877–886 (discussion 886–7).
53. Siegel MJ, et al. CT of posttransplantation lymphoproliferative disorder in pediatric recipients of lung allograft. AJR Am J Roentgenol 2003; 181(4):1125–1131.
54. Hachem RR, et al. Abdominal-pelvic lymphoproliferative disease after lung transplantation: presentation and outcome. Transplantation 2004; 77(3):431–437.
55. Lim GY, et al. Posttransplantation lymphoproliferative disorder: manifestations in pediatric thoracic organ recipients. Radiology 2002; 222(3):699–708.
56. Pickhardt PJ, Siegel MJ. Posttransplantation lymphoproliferative disorder of the abdomen: CT evaluation in 51 patients. Radiology 1999; 213(1):73–78.
57. Paranjothi S, et al. Lymphoproliferative disease after lung transplantation: comparison of presentation and outcome of early and late cases. J Heart Lung Transplant 2001; 20(10): 1054–1063.
58. Scarsbrook AF, et al. Post-transplantation lymphoproliferative disorder: the spectrum of imaging appearances. Clin Radiol 2005; 60(1):47–55.
59. Marom EM, et al. Positron emission tomography with fluoro-2-deoxy-D-glucose (FDG-PET) in the staging of post transplant lymphoproliferative disorder in lung transplant recipients. J Thorac Imaging 2004; 19(2):74–78.
60. Hurwitz M, et al. Complete immunosuppressive withdrawal as a uniform approach to post-transplant lymphoproliferative disease in pediatric liver transplantation. Pediatr Transplant 2004; 8(3):267–272.
61. Aull MJ, et al. Experience with 274 cardiac transplant recipients with posttransplant lymphoproliferative disorder: a report from the Israel Penn International Transplant Tumor Registry. Transplantation 2004; 78(11):1676–1682.
62. Christie JD, et al. The effect of primary graft dysfunction on survival after lung transplantation. Am J Respir Crit Care Med 2005; 171(11):1312–1316.
63. Thabut G, et al. Primary graft failure following lung transplantation: predictive factors of mortality. Chest 2002; 121(6):1876–1882.

64. Meyers BF, et al. Primary graft dysfunction and other selected complications of lung transplantation: A single-center experience of 983 patients. J Thorac Cardiovasc Surg 2005; 129(6): 1421–1429.
65. Oto T, et al. Definitions of primary graft dysfunction after lung transplantation: differences between bilateral and single lung transplantation. J Thorac Cardiovasc Surg 2006; 132(1):140–147.
66. King RC, et al. Reperfusion injury significantly impacts clinical outcome after pulmonary transplantation. Ann Thorac Surg 2000; 69(6):1681–1685.
67. Dahlberg PS, et al. Medium-term results of extracorporeal membrane oxygenation for severe acute lung injury after lung transplantation. J Heart Lung Transplant 2004; 23(8):979–984.
68. Oto T, et al. Extracorporeal membrane oxygenation after lung transplantation: evolving technique improves outcomes. Ann Thorac Surg 2004; 78(4):1230–1235.
69. Christie JD, et al. Report of the ISHLT Working Group on Primary Lung Graft Dysfunction part II: definition. A consensus statement of the International Society for Heart and Lung Transplantation. J Heart Lung Transplant 2005; 24(10):1454–1459.
70. Christie JD, et al. Primary graft failure following lung transplantation. Chest 1998; 114(1):51–60.
71. Khan AS, et al. Hantavirus pulmonary syndrome in Florida: association with the newly identified Black Creek Canal virus. Am J Med 1996; 100(1):46–48.
72. Christie JD, et al. Report of the ISHLT Working Group on Primary Lung Graft Dysfunction part I: introduction and methods. J Heart Lung Transplant 2005; 24(10):1451–1453.
73. Fehrenbach H, et al. Pulmonary ischemia/reperfusion injury: a quantitative study of structure and function in isolated heart-lungs of the rat. Anat Rec 1999; 255(1):84–89.
74. Fiser SM, et al. Lung transplant reperfusion injury involves pulmonary macrophages and circulating leukocytes in a biphasic response. J Thorac Cardiovasc Surg 2001; 121(6):1069–1075.
75. Clark SC, et al. Controlled reperfusion and pentoxifylline modulate reperfusion injury after single lung transplantation. J Thorac Cardiovasc Surg 1998; 115(6):1335–1341.
76. Keshavjee S, et al. A randomized, placebo-controlled trial of complement inhibition in ischemia-reperfusion injury after lung transplantation in human beings. J Thorac Cardiovasc Surg 2005; 129(2):423–428.
77. Farivar AS, et al. Alpha chemokines regulate direct lung ischemia-reperfusion injury. J Heart Lung Transplant 2004; 23(5):585–591.
78. de Perrot M, et al. Impact of human interleukin-10 on vector-induced inflammation and early graft function in rat lung transplantation. Am J Respir Cell Mol Biol 2003; 28(5):616–625.
79. Ardehali A, et al. A prospective trial of inhaled nitric oxide in clinical lung transplantation. Transplantation 2001; 72(1):112–115.
80. Barr ML, et al. Report of the ISHLT Working Group on Primary Lung Graft Dysfunction part IV: recipient-related risk factors and markers. J Heart Lung Transplant 2005; 24(10):1468–1482.
81. de Perrot M, et al. Report of the ISHLT Working Group on Primary Lung Graft Dysfunction part III: donor-related risk factors and markers. J Heart Lung Transplant 2005; 24(10):1460–1467.
82. Christie JD, et al. Clinical risk factors for primary graft failure following lung transplantation. Chest 2003; 124(4):1232–1241.
83. Novick RJ, et al. Influence of graft ischemic time and donor age on survival after lung transplantation. J Heart Lung Transplant 1999; 18(5):425–431.
84. Pierre AF, et al. Marginal donor lungs: a reassessment. J Thorac Cardiovasc Surg 2002; 123(3): 421–427 (discussion, 427–8).
85. Oto T, et al. A donor history of smoking affects early but not late outcome in lung transplantation. Transplantation 2004; 78(4):599–606.
86. de Perrot M, et al. Strategies to increase limited donor resources. Eur Respir J 2004; 23(3):477–482.
87. Struber M, et al. Surfactant function in lung transplantation after 24 hours of ischemia: advantage of retrograde flush perfusion for preservation. J Thorac Cardiovasc Surg 2002; 123(1):98–103.
88. Chen CZ, et al. Retrograde flush and cold storage for twenty-two to twenty-five hours lung preservation with and without prostaglandin E1. J Heart Lung Transplant 1997; 16(6):658–666.

89. Schnickel GT, et al. Modified reperfusion in clinical lung transplantation: the results of 100 consecutive cases. J Thorac Cardiovasc Surg 2006; 131(1):218–223.
90. Kramer MR, et al. Clinical significance of hyperbilirubinemia in patients with pulmonary hypertension undergoing heart-lung transplantation. J Heart Lung Transplant 1991; 10(2):317–321.
91. Arcasoy SM, et al. Characteristics and outcomes of patients with sarcoidosis listed for lung transplantation. Chest 2001; 120(3):873–880.
92. Hadjiliadis D, et al. Outcome of lung transplantation in patients with mycetomas. Chest 2002; 121(1):128–134.
93. Bando K, et al. Impact of pulmonary hypertension on outcome after single-lung transplantation. Ann Thorac Surg 1994; 58(5):1336–1342.
94. Conte JV, et al. Lung transplantation for primary and secondary pulmonary hypertension. Ann Thorac Surg 2001; 72(5):1673–1679 (discussion 1679–80).
95. Doucette K, Fishman JA. Nontuberculous mycobacterial infection in hematopoietic stem cell and solid organ transplant recipients. Clin Infect Dis 2004; 38(10):1428–1439.
96. Patel R, Paya CV. Infections in solid-organ transplant recipients. Clin Microbiol Rev 1997; 10(1): 86–124.
97. Patel R, et al. Infections due to nontuberculous mycobacteria in kidney, heart, and liver transplant recipients. Clin Infect Dis 1994; 19(2):263–273.
98. Munoz P, Rodriguez C, Bouza E. Mycobacterium tuberculosis infection in recipients of solid organ transplants. Clin Infect Dis 2005; 40(4):581–587.
99. Winthrop KL, et al. Transmission of mycobacterium tuberculosis via lung transplantation. Am J Transplant 2004; 4(9):1529–1533.
100. Singh N, Paterson DL. Mycobacterium tuberculosis infection in solid-organ transplant recipients: impact and implications for management. Clin Infect Dis 1998; 27(5):1266–1277.
101. John GT, Shankar V. Mycobacterial infections in organ transplant recipients. Semin Respir Infect 2002; 17(4):274–283.
102. Ridgeway AL, et al. Transmission of Mycobacterium tuberculosis to recipients of single lung transplants from the same donor. Am J Respir Crit Care Med 1996; 153(3):1166–1168.
103. Lattes R, et al. Tuberculosis in renal transplant recipients. Transpl Infect Dis 1999; 1(2):98–104.
104. Kiuchi T, et al. Experience of tacrolimus-based immunosuppression in living-related liver transplantation complicated with graft tuberculosis: interaction with rifampicin and side effects. Transplant Proc 1996; 28(6):3171–3172.
105. Wolinsky E. Mycobacterial diseases other than tuberculosis. Clin Infect Dis 1992; 15(1):1–10.
106. Wolinsky E. Nontuberculous mycobacteria and associated diseases. Am Rev Respir Dis 1979; 119(1):107–159.
107. Dye C, et al. Consensus statement. Global burden of tuberculosis: estimated incidence, prevalence, and mortality by country. WHO Global Surveillance and Monitoring Project. Jama 1999; 282(7):677–686.
108. Lee J, et al. Multidrug-resistant tuberculosis in a lung transplant recipient. J Heart Lung Transplant 2003; 22(10):1168–1173.
109. Chocarra A, et al. Disseminated infection due to Mycobacterium malmoense in a patient infected with human immunodeficiency virus. Clin Infect Dis 1994; 19(1):203–204.
110. Hellinger WC, et al. Localized soft-tissue infections with Mycobacterium avium/Mycobacterium intracellulare complex in immunocompetent patients: granulomatous tenosynovitis of the hand or wrist. Clin Infect Dis 1995; 21(1):65–69.
111. Cooper JF, et al. Mycobacterium chelonae: a cause of nodular skin lesions with a proclivity for renal transplant recipients. Am J Med 1989; 86(2):173–177.
112. Kiehn TE, White M. Mycobacterium haemophilum: an emerging pathogen. Eur J Clin Microbiol Infect Dis 1994; 13(11):925–931.
113. Fairhurst RM, et al. Mycobacterium haemophilum infections in heart transplant recipients: case report and review of the literature. Am J Transplant 2002; 2(5):476–479.

114. Stelzmueller I, et al. Mycobacterium chelonae skin infection in kidney-pancreas recipient. Emerg Infect Dis 2005; 11(2):352–354.
115. Kramer MR, et al. Infectious complications in heart-lung transplantation. Analysis of 200 episodes. Arch Intern Med 1993; 153(17):2010–2016.
116. Brooks RG, et al. Infectious complications in heart-lung transplant recipients. Am J Med 1985; 79(4):412–422.
117. Maurer JR, et al. Infectious complications following isolated lung transplantation. Chest 1992; 101(4):1056–1059.
118. Dauber JH, Paradis IL, Dummer JS. Infectious complications in pulmonary allograft recipients. Clin Chest Med 1990; 11(2):291–308.
119. Zander DS, et al. Analysis of early deaths after isolated lung transplantation. Chest 2001; 120(1): 225–232.
120. Chan CC, et al. Diagnostic yield and therapeutic impact of flexible bronchoscopy in lung transplant recipients. J Heart Lung Transplant 1996; 15(2):196–205.
121. Avlonitis VS, et al. Bacterial colonization of the donor lower airways is a predictor of poor outcome in lung transplantation. Eur J Cardiothorac Surg 2003; 24(4):601–607.
122. Dobbin C, et al. The impact of pan-resistant bacterial pathogens on survival after lung transplantation in cystic fibrosis: results from a single large referral centre. J Hosp Infect 2004; 56(4): 277–282.
123. Aris RM, et al. The effects of panresistant bacteria in cystic fibrosis patients on lung transplant outcome. Am J Respir Crit Care Med 1997; 155(5):1699–1704.
124. Flume PA, et al. Infectious complications of lung transplantation. Impact of cystic fibrosis. Am J Respir Crit Care Med 1994; 149(6):1601–1607.
125. Egan TM, et al. Improved results of lung transplantation for patients with cystic fibrosis. J Thorac Cardiovasc Surg 1995; 109(2):224–234 (discussion 234–5).
126. Frist WH, et al. Cystic fibrosis treated with heart-lung transplantation: North American results. Transplant Proc 1991; 23(1 Pt 2):1205–1206.
127. Lewiston N, et al. Cystic fibrosis patients who have undergone heart-lung transplantation benefit from maxillary sinus antrostomy and repeated sinus lavage. Transplant Proc 1991; 23(1 pt 2): 1207–1208.
128. Holzmann D, et al. Effects of sinus surgery in patients with cystic fibrosis after lung transplantation: a 10-year experience. Transplantation 2004; 77(1):134–136.
129. Snell GI, et al. Pseudomonas cepacia in lung transplant recipients with cystic fibrosis. Chest 1993; 103(2):466–471.
130. Chaparro C, et al. Infection with Burkholderia cepacia in cystic fibrosis: outcome following lung transplantation. Am J Respir Crit Care Med 2001; 163(1):43–48.
131. Aris RM, et al. Lung transplantation for cystic fibrosis patients with Burkholderia cepacia complex. Survival linked to genomovar type. Am J Respir Crit Care Med 2001; 164(11):2102–2106.
132. De Soyza A, et al. Burkholderia cepacia complex genomovars and pulmonary transplantation outcomes in patients with cystic fibrosis. Lancet 2001; 358(9295):1780–1781.
133. LiPuma, JJ. Burkholderia cepacia complex: a contraindication to lung transplantation in cystic fibrosis? Transpl Infect Dis 2001; 3(3):149–160.
134. Dummer JS. Pneumocystis carinii infections in transplant recipients. Semin Respir Infect 1990; 5(1):50–57.
135. Kramer MR, et al. Trimethoprim-sulfamethoxazole prophylaxis for Pneumocystis carinii infections in heart-lung and lung transplantation—how effective and for how long? Transplantation 1992; 53(3):586–589.
136. Gordon SM, et al. Should prophylaxis for Pneumocystis carinii pneumonia in solid organ transplant recipients ever be discontinued? Clin Infect Dis 1999; 28(2):240–246.
137. Nathan SD, et al. Utility of inhaled pentamidine prophylaxis in lung transplant recipients. Chest 1994; 105(2):417–420.

138. Souza JP, et al. High rates of Pneumocystis carinii pneumonia in allogeneic blood and marrow transplant recipients receiving dapsone prophylaxis. Clin Infect Dis 1999; 29(6):1467–1471.
139. Meyers B, Borrego F, Papanicolaou G. Pneumocystis carinii pneumonia prophylaxis with atovaquone in trimethoprim-sulfamethoxazole-intolerant orthotopic liver transplant patients: a preliminary study. Liver Transpl 2001; 7(8):750–751.
140. Husain S, et al. Nocardia infection in lung transplant recipients. J Heart Lung Transplant 2002; 21(3):354–359.
141. Roberts SA, et al. Nocardia infection in heart-lung transplant recipients at Alfred Hospital, Melbourne, Australia, 1989–1998. Clin Infect Dis 2000; 31(4):968–972.
142. Nunley DR, et al. Empyema complicating successful lung transplantation. Chest 1999; 115(5): 1312–1315.
143. Steffenson DO, et al. Sternotomy infections with Mycoplasma hominis. Ann Intern Med 1987; 106(2):204–208.
144. Lee J, et al. Delayed sternotomy wound infection due to Paecilomyces variotii in a lung transplant recipient. J Heart Lung Transplant 2002; 21(10):1131–1134.
145. Cahill BC, et al. Aspergillus airway colonization and invasive disease after lung transplantation. Chest 1997; 112(5):1160–1164.
146. Minari A, et al. The incidence of invasive aspergillosis among solid organ transplant recipients and implications for prophylaxis in lung transplants. Transpl Infect Dis 2002; 4(4):195–200.
147. Singh N, Husain S. Aspergillus infections after lung transplantation: clinical differences in type of transplant and implications for management. J Heart Lung Transplant 2003; 22(3):258–266.
148. Hadjiliadis D, et al. Anastomotic infections in lung transplant recipients. Ann Transplant 2000; 5(3):13–19.
149. Cunha BA. Central nervous system infections in the compromised host: a diagnostic approach. Infect Dis Clin North Am 2001; 15(2):567–590.
150. Gordon SM, Avery RK. Aspergillosis in lung transplantation: incidence, risk factors, and prophylactic strategies. Transpl Infect Dis 2001; 3(3):161–167.
151. Kubak BM. Coccidioidomycosis after solid organ transplant. In: Ross JLa.D. ed. Lung and Heart-Lung Transplantation. New York, NY: Taylor & Francis Group, 2006:527–556.
152. Miller MB, Hendren R, Gilligan PH. Posttransplantation disseminated coccidioidomycosis acquired from donor lungs. J Clin Microbiol 2004; 42(5):2347–2349.
153. Wright PW, et al. Donor-related coccidioidomycosis in organ transplant recipients. Clin Infect Dis 2003; 37(9):1265–1269.
154. Galgiani JN, et al. Practice guideline for the treatment of coccidioidomycosis. Infectious Diseases Society of America. Clin Infect Dis 2000; 30(4):658–661.
155. Hoang LM, et al. Cryptococcus neoformans infections at Vancouver Hospital and Health Sciences Centre (1997–2002): epidemiology, microbiology and histopathology. J Med Microbiol 2004; 53(pt 9):935–940.
156. Singh N, et al. Clinical spectrum of invasive cryptococcosis in liver transplant recipients receiving tacrolimus. Clin Transplant 1997; 11(1):66–70.
157. Jabbour N, et al. Cryptococcal meningitis after liver transplantation. Transplantation 1996; 61(1): 146–149.
158. Wu G, et al. Cryptococcal meningitis: an analysis among 5,521 consecutive organ transplant recipients. Transpl Infect Dis 2002; 4(4):183–188.
159. Singh N, Husain S. Infections of the central nervous system in transplant recipients. Transpl Infect Dis 2000; 2(3):101–111.
160. Husain SSF. Invasive fungal infections complicating lung and solid organ transplantation. In: JLa.D. Ross, ed. Aspergillosis, Cryptococcosis, and Molds, in Lung and Heart-Lung Transplantation. New York, NY: Taylor & Francis Group, 2006:556–586.
161. Hosenpud JD, et al. The Registry of the International Society for Heart and Lung Transplantation: eighteenth Official Report-2001. J Heart Lung Transplant 2001; 20(8):805–815.

162. Burke CM, et al. Post-transplant obliterative bronchiolitis and other late lung sequelae in human heart-lung transplantation. Chest 1984; 86(6):824–829.
163. Estenne M, Hertz MI. Bronchiolitis obliterans after human lung transplantation. Am J Respir Crit Care Med 2002; 166(4):440–444.
164. Cooper JD, et al. A working formulation for the standardization of nomenclature and for clinical staging of chronic dysfunction in lung allografts. International Society for Heart and Lung Transplantation. J Heart Lung Transplant 1993; 12(5):713–716.
165. Boehler A, et al. Bronchiolitis obliterans after lung transplantation: a review. Chest 1998; 114(5): 1411–1426.
166. Yousem SA, et al. Revision of the 1990 working formulation for the classification of pulmonary allograft rejection: Lung Rejection Study Group. J Heart Lung Transplant 1996; 15(1 pt 1):1–15.
167. Estenne M, et al. Bronchiolitis obliterans syndrome 2001: an update of the diagnostic criteria. J Heart Lung Transplant 2002; 21(3):297–310.
168. Verleden GM. Chronic allograft rejection (obliterative bronchiolitis). Semin Respir Crit Care Med 2001; 22(5):551–558.
169. Yousem SA. Lymphocytic bronchitis/bronchiolitis in lung allograft recipients. Am J Surg Pathol 1993; 17(5):491–496.
170. Ross DJ, et al. "Refractoriness" of airflow obstruction associated with isolated lymphocytic bronchiolitis/bronchitis in pulmonary allografts. J Heart Lung Transplant 1997; 16(8):832–838.
171. Knoop C, Estenne M. Acute and chronic rejection after lung transplantation. Semin Respir Crit Care Med 2006; 27(5):521–533.
172. Kroshus TJ, et al. Risk factors for the development of bronchiolitis obliterans syndrome after lung transplantation. J Thorac Cardiovasc Surg 1997; 114(2):195–202.
173. Bando K, et al. Obliterative bronchiolitis after lung and heart-lung transplantation. An analysis of risk factors and management. J Thorac Cardiovasc Surg 1995; 110(1):4–13; (discussion 13–4).
174. Heng D, et al. Bronchiolitis obliterans syndrome: incidence, natural history, prognosis, and risk factors. J Heart Lung Transplant 1998; 17(12):1255–1263.
175. Hachem RR, et al. The significance of a single episode of minimal acute rejection after lung transplantation. Transplantation 2005; 80(10):1406–1413.
176. Khalifah AP, et al. Minimal acute rejection after lung transplantation: a risk for bronchiolitis obliterans syndrome. Am J Transplant 2005; 5(8):2022–2030.
177. Hopkins PM, et al. Association of minimal rejection in lung transplant recipients with obliterative bronchiolitis. Am J Respir Crit Care Med 2004; 170(9):1022–1026.
178. Quantz MA, et al. Does human leukocyte antigen matching influence the outcome of lung transplantation? An analysis of 3,549 lung transplantations. J Heart Lung Transplant 2000; 19(5): 473–479.
179. Palmer SM, et al. Development of an antibody specific to major histocompatibility antigens detectable by flow cytometry after lung transplant is associated with bronchiolitis obliterans syndrome. Transplantation 2002; 74(6):799–804.
180. Jaramillo A, et al. Development of ELISA-detected anti-HLA antibodies precedes the development of bronchiolitis obliterans syndrome and correlates with progressive decline in pulmonary function after lung transplantation. Transplantation 1999; 67(8):1155–1161.
181. Ruttmann E, et al. Combined CMV prophylaxis improves outcome and reduces the risk for bronchiolitis obliterans syndrome (BOS) after lung transplantation. Transplantation 2006; 81(10): 1415–1420.
182. Billings JL, et al. Respiratory viruses and chronic rejection in lung transplant recipients. J Heart Lung Transplant 2002; 21(5):559–566.
183. Khalifah AP, et al. Respiratory viral infections are a distinct risk for bronchiolitis obliterans syndrome and death. Am J Respir Crit Care Med 2004; 170(2):181–187.
184. Neurohr C, et al. Human herpesvirus 6 in bronchalveolar lavage fluid after lung transplantation: a risk factor for bronchiolitis obliterans syndrome? Am J Transplant 2005; 5(12):2982–2991.

185. Glanville AR, et al. Chlamydia pneumoniae infection after lung transplantation. J Heart Lung Transplant 2005; 24(2):131–136.
186. Gerhardt SG, et al. Maintenance azithromycin therapy for bronchiolitis obliterans syndrome: results of a pilot study. Am J Respir Crit Care Med 2003; 168(1):121–125.
187. McSherry C, et al. Sequential measurement of peripheral blood allogeneic microchimerism levels and association with pulmonary function. Transplantation 1996; 62(12):1811–1818.
188. Husain AN, et al. Analysis of risk factors for the development of bronchiolitis obliterans syndrome. Am J Respir Crit Care Med 1999; 159(3):829–833.
189. Pomerance A, et al. Transbronchial biopsy in heart and lung transplantation: clinicopathologic correlations. J Heart Lung Transplant 1995; 14(4):761–773.
190. Patterson GM, et al. Physiologic definitions of obliterative bronchiolitis in heart-lung and double lung transplantation: a comparison of the forced expiratory flow between 25% and 75% of the forced vital capacity and forced expiratory volume in one second. J Heart Lung Transplant 1996; 15(2):175–181.
191. Reynaud M, et al. Objective diagnosis of alcohol abuse: compared values of carbohydrate-deficient transferrin (CDT), gamma-glutamyl transferase (GGT), and mean corpuscular volume (MCV). Alcohol Clin Exp Res 2000; 24(9):1414–1419.
192. Ouwens JP, et al. Bronchiolar airflow impairment after lung transplantation: an early and common manifestation. J Heart Lung Transplant 2002; 21(10):1056–1061.
193. Lama VN, et al. Prognostic value of bronchiolitis obliterans syndrome stage 0-p in single-lung transplant recipients. Am J Respir Crit Care Med 2005; 172(3):379–383.
194. Hachem RR, et al. The predictive value of bronchiolitis obliterans syndrome stage 0-p. Am J Respir Crit Care Med 2004; 169(4):468–472.
195. Morrish WF, et al. Bronchiolitis obliterans after lung transplantation: findings at chest radiography and high-resolution CT. The Toronto Lung Transplant Group. Radiology 1991; 179(2): 487–490.
196. Kramer MR, et al. The diagnosis of obliterative bronchiolitis after heart-lung and lung transplantation: low yield of transbronchial lung biopsy. J Heart Lung Transplant 1993; 12(4):675–681.
197. Leung AN, et al. Bronchiolitis obliterans after lung transplantation: detection using expiratory HRCT. Chest 1998; 113(2):365–370.
198. Knollmann FD, et al. Bronchiolitis obliterans syndrome in lung transplant recipients: use of spirometrically gated CT. Radiology 2002; 225(3):655–662.
199. Siegel MJ, et al. Post-lung transplantation bronchiolitis obliterans syndrome: usefulness of expiratory thin-section CT for diagnosis. Radiology 2001; 220(2):455–462.
200. Konen E, et al. Bronchiolitis obliterans syndrome in lung transplant recipients: can thin-section CT findings predict disease before its clinical appearance? Radiology 2004; 231(2):467–473.
201. Bankier AA, et al. Bronchiolitis obliterans syndrome in heart-lung transplant recipients: diagnosis with expiratory CT. Radiology 2001; 218(2):533–539.
202. Gast KK, et al. (3)He-MRI in follow-up of lung transplant recipients. Eur Radiol 2004; 14(1): 78–85.
203. Fisher AJ, et al. Cross sectional study of exhaled nitric oxide levels following lung transplantation. Thorax 1998; 53(6):454–458.
204. Verleden GM, et al. Exhaled nitric oxide after lung transplantation: impact of the native lung. Eur Respir J 2003; 21(3):429–432.
205. Gabbay E, et al. Post-lung transplant bronchiolitis obliterans syndrome (BOS) is characterized by increased exhaled nitric oxide levels and epithelial inducible nitric oxide synthase. Am J Respir Crit Care Med 2000; 162(6):2182–2187.
206. Van Muylem A, Knoop C, Estenne M. Early detection of chronic pulmonary allograft dysfunction by exhaled biomarkers. Am J Respir Crit Care Med 2007; 175(7):731–736.

24
Intracellular and Extracellular Structures

ROSE C. ANTON and PHILIP T. CAGLE
Weill Medical College of Cornell University, New York, New York,
and The Methodist Hospital, Houston, Texas, U.S.A.

I. Endogenous Structures

Endogenous structures present in pulmonary biopsy, resection, or cytological specimens include both those unique to the lung and those that may also be recognized in other organ sites. Many are nonspecific findings with unknown clinical significance. While none are pathognomonical of a specific diagnosis, their presence can be suggestive of certain disease conditions. Additionally, the identification of endogenous structures may have therapeutic and medicolegal consequences (1).

Asteroid bodies are needle shaped, eosinophilic inclusions within giant cells (Fig. 1). They range in size from 5 to 30 μm and are composed of cell organelles in a stellate configuration. Since asteroid bodies may be present as a component of granulomatous inflammation, they are at best suggestive but not diagnostic of sarcoidosis. However, one should bear in mind that the list of etiologies of granulomatous inflammation in the lung is extensive and that granulomas may also be produced by infectious organisms or inhalation of foreign material.

Intra-alveolar basophilic *blue bodies* are a nonspecific finding, consisting of rare to multiple laminated, calcified concretions ranging from 15 to 40 μm in size (Fig. 2). Blue bodies are formed exclusively within macrophages and/or giant cells. Special stains that may identify blue bodies include periodic acid–Schiff (PAS) and alcian blue; the outer laminations stain with iron. On unstained sections, blue bodies are birefringent.

PAS-positive eosinophilic, intranuclear inclusions may occasionally be seen in bronchioloalveolar carcinoma. Immunohistochemical staining shows immunoreactivity of these inclusions with surfactant apoprotein.

Calcifications are a nonspecific finding and have a basophilic, finely granular to sheet-like appearance on H&E stain. Additional special stains that help to identify these structures are the von Kossa and alizarin red stains. Deposition of dystrophic calcifications occurs as part of a healing response to any one of numerous causes of inflammatory reactions in the lung. These calcifications do little more than to identify sites of previous injury to the lung and hilar lymph nodes and usually have no clinical significance. On the other hand, metastatic calcifications are frequently markers for any disease that alters serum levels of calcium and phosphate including bone, renal, or parathyroid disease. These calcifications are located in the alveolar septa and vascular walls and may be either an isolated finding or more diffuse in nature.

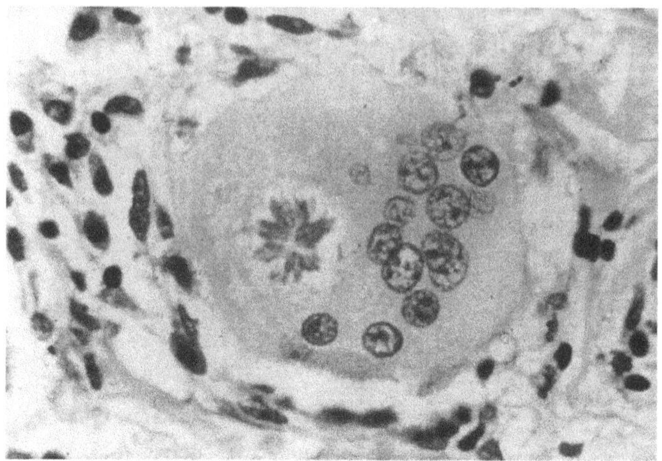

Figure 1 Asteroid body showing cell organelles in a stellate configuration within multi-nucleated giant cell.

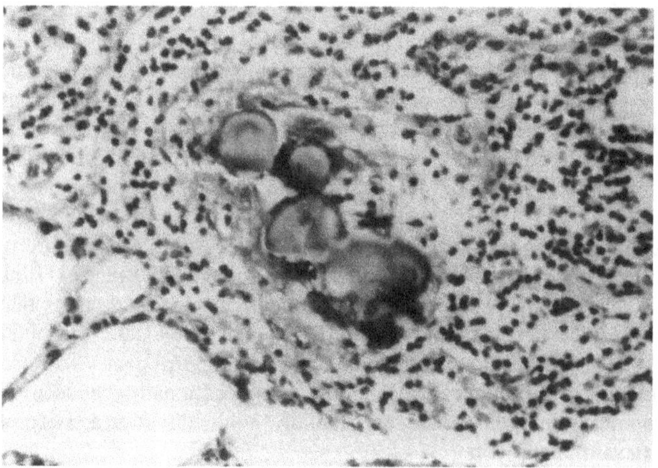

Figure 2 Multiple laminated, calcified blue bodies within giant cells.

Calcium oxalate crystals may also be seen within giant cells associated with granulomatous inflammation and may be present adjacent to blue bodies. These crystals are evident within the giant cells as glassy, irregular sheets with sharp edges; they range in size from 1 to 20 μm. Although optically clear, they are birefringent and easily identifiable under polarized light (Fig. 3). *Aspergillus niger* is unique to the *Aspergillus* sp. in that it may produce calcium oxalate crystals. A careful examination should be performed to prevent these crystals from being confused with foreign bodies.

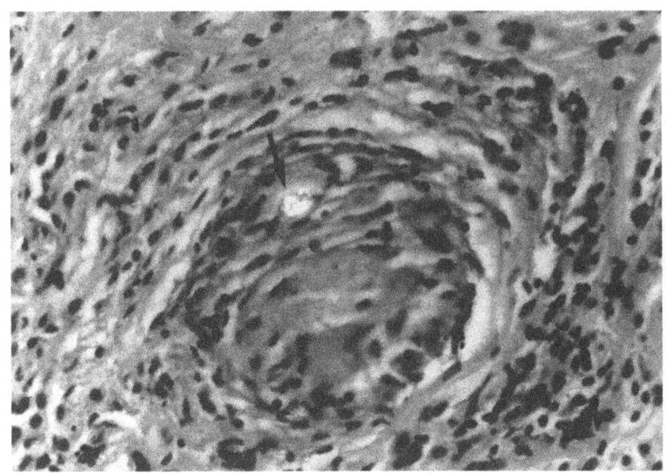

Figure 3 Calcium oxalate crystal (*arrow*) evident within granulomatous inflammation under polarized light.

Calcospherites and *psammoma bodies* are calcified basophilic concretions with a laminated appearance and may be seen in papillary malignancies (psammoma bodies) or in benign conditions such as tuberculosis or pulmonary alveolar microlithiasis (multiple calcospherites ranging from 0.1–0.3 mm present in 25–80% of alveoli) The central portion of the calcospherite may be PAS-positive, with the surrounding layers staining with the von Kossa stain. Occasionally, the calcospherites are birefringent and may be demonstrated under a polarizing microscope by a "Maltese cross" pattern.

Charcot-Leyden crystals are needle-shaped crystals present within macrophages (Fig. 4). The formation of these crystals occurs following ingestion of eosinophilic debris

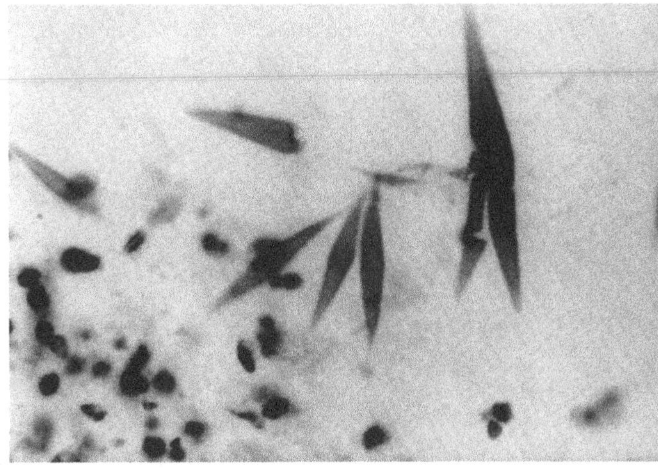

Figure 4 Multiple needle-shaped Charcot-Leyden crystals in bronchial wash.

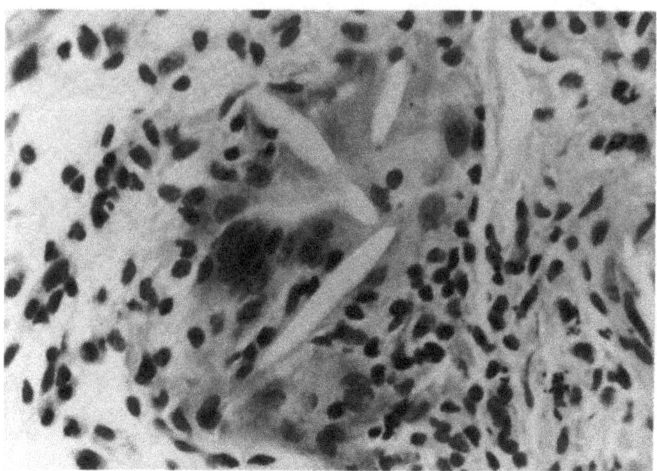

Figure 5 Multinucleated giant cell containing cholesterol clefts.

by macrophages and accumulation of the material within these macrophages. Charcot-Leyden crystals are associated with hypersensitivity and may be seen in cases of asthma, eosinophilic pneumonia, paragonimiasis, or any other disease with a high turnover of eosinophils.

Inclusions of *cholesterol clefts* can be present within giant cells in hypersensitivity pneumonitis and can be mistaken for foreign bodies (Fig. 5).

Corpora amylacea are pale pink, laminated, round to oval concretions present within alveoli and alveolar walls (Fig. 6). They can range in size from 30 to 200 μm and may have

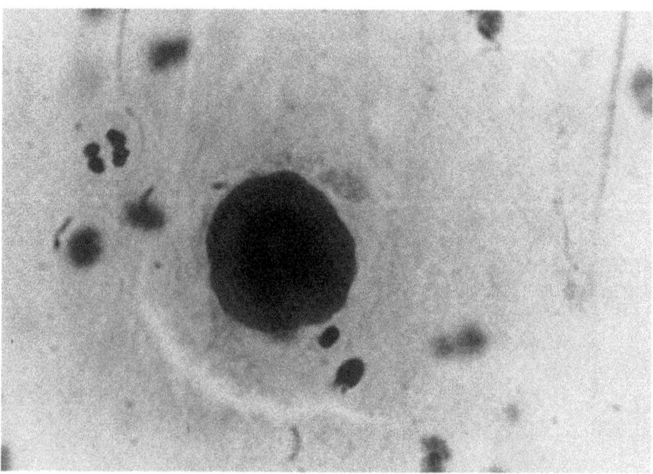

Figure 6 Corpora amylacea containing multiple laminations.

an associated histiocytic reaction. A birefringent central core may occasionally be demonstrated under polarized light; however, unlike calcospherites, they are not usually calcified. Corpora amylacea are also PAS-positive and have no known clinical significance. They are associated with congestive heart failure or other disorders that result in pulmonary edema.

Hemosiderin is a golden brown, granular pigment that may accumulate within macrophages (siderophages) or be deposited in the interstitial tissues. This pigment is formed following phagocytosis of red cell debris by macrophages, which then convert the hemoglobin into hemosiderin. Accumulation of hemosiderin can be seen following any hemorrhagic condition or in specific disorders including lymphangioleiomyomatosis. The golden colors of lipofuscin and of melanin may be confused with hemosiderin; only the latter will stain with Prussian blue.

Lipid-laden macrophages, or foam cells, are macrophages that have ingested lipid from exogenous sources (e.g., nose drops) or endogenous sources originating from injured or degenerating cells, which results in a bubbly cytoplasm. These cells will stain with oil-red-O and are present in a variety of conditions including lipoid pneumonia, infections, and malignancy.

Dystrophic ossification may be seen in association with dystrophic calcification and therefore may also be seen in areas of previous tissue injury (Fig. 7). Heterotopic or metaplastic bone may also have associated marrow elements.

Reactive type II pneumocytes may contain intracytoplasmic, eosinophilic hyaline inclusions as a response to various forms of injury, including viral infection, organizing pneumonia (OP), infarct, diffuse alveolar damage, and asbestosis. They may also be present adjacent to bronchioloalveolar carcinoma.

Schaumann bodies are concentrically laminated concretions composed of calcium, iron, and mucopolysaccharide and are present within giant cells as a component of granulomatous disease (Fig. 8). These calcospherites are basophilic on H&E stain, range in size from 25 to 200 μm, have irregular shapes, and may be associated with calcium oxalate

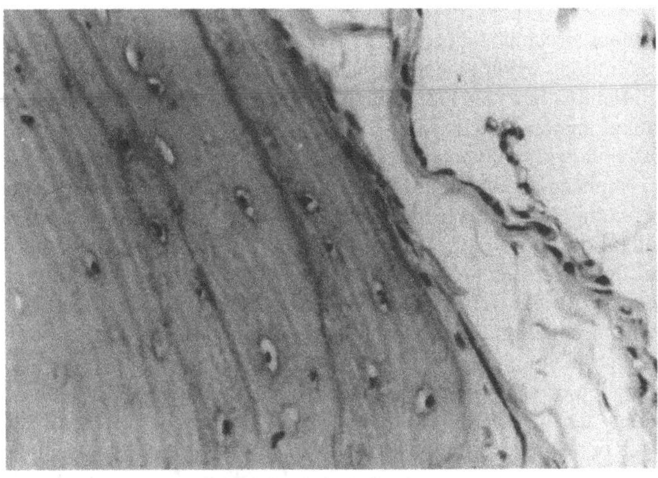

Figure 7 Focus of dystrophic ossification.

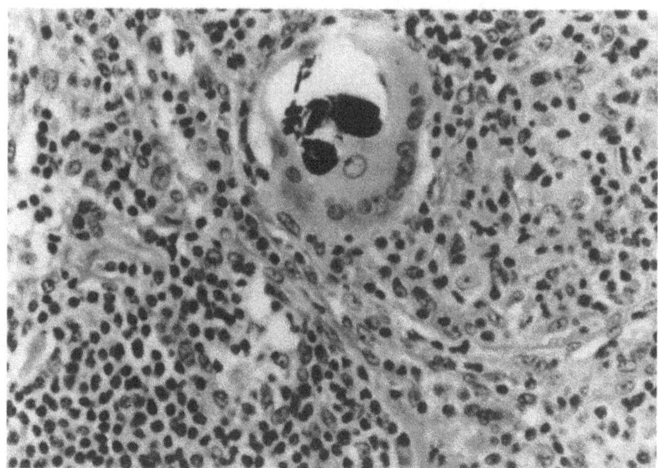

Figure 8 Schaumann body present within giant cell as a component of granulomatous inflammation.

crystals. Schaumann bodies may be present adjacent to blue bodies. Interstitial Schaumann bodies may be the only marker to identify sites of resolved granulomatous inflammation. Schaumann bodies may also be demonstrated by von Kossa, alizarin red, and iron stains. They are occasionally birefringent, usually when in association with calcium oxalate crystals, and can be confused with foreign material. Similar to asteroid bodies, Schaumann bodies are suggestive of but not pathognomonical for sarcoidosis.

II. Exogenous Structures

The identification of exogenous structures in pulmonary tissue indicates exposure to foreign materials by inhalation, aspiration, or intravenous administration. Their presence can produce a nonspecific host inflammatory response, which ranges from simple ingestion by macrophages to severe granulomatous reaction.

Anthracotic pigment, both within alveolar macrophages and freestanding within scar tissue, accumulates in a lymphangitic distribution following exposure to carbon or coal dust. It is a nonspecific finding that can be identified following inhalation of tobacco smoke, pollution, and mineral dusts.

The presence of oral flora and squamous epithelial cells suggests *aspiration.* Foreign materials, including vegetable particles (refractile cell walls), meat fibers (cross striations), and pills may also be evidence of aspiration. Foreign-body giant cells and OP or bronchiolitis obliterans organizing pneumonia (BOOP) are associated findings.

Intravenous administration of narcotics can produce embolization of foreign material to the pulmonary capillaries accompanied by a foreign-body reaction to the insoluble material, interstitial fibrosis, or vascular thrombosis. The foreign-body reaction can range from individual giant cells to severe granulomatous reaction. Injection of a narcotic that is primarily intended for oral consumption produces the latter response owing to large amounts of insoluble filler material such as talc, cornstarch, or microcrystalline cellulose. Since the material is frequently birefringent, the presence of the foreign crystals may be illustrated either within or adjacent to giant cells, regardless of the inflammatory reaction, by the use of polarized light. *Talc*, or magnesium silicate, has a large, irregular, plate-like structure. It is pale yellow on H&E stain. *Starch*, also present in surgical gloves, is a crystal that can be recognized by its round shape and characteristic "Maltese cross" pattern under polarized light. It is slightly eosinophilic on H&E stain and is PAS positive. *Microcrystalline cellulose* is demonstrated on special stains (Congo red, methenamine silver, and digested PAS) as attenuated crystals.

Silica dust is present initially either free or within macrophages. Eventually, silicosis is represented microscopically as nodules with an acellular, hyaline core surrounded by fibrous tissue and macrophages. Silica crystals are evident as small, birefringent particles at the periphery of these nodules under polarized light.

A. Ferruginous Bodies

All ferruginous bodies consist of a core mineral surrounded by layers of glycoprotein and hemosiderin and appear golden-yellow on hematoxylin and eosin (H&E) stain. These layers are furnished over the core mineral by macrophages. The specific ferruginous body is named after the type of mineral within the core. Ferruginous bodies may be identified either on H&E or Prussian blue stains. *Siderosis* represents deposition of iron on fragmented elastin fibers and can sometimes be confused with ferruginous bodies.

Asbestos bodies have a straight, thin, colorless core and characteristic dumbbell configuration (Fig. 9). These bodies are formed following inhalation of asbestos fibers, which are phagocytized by free alveolar macrophages and coated with ferritin and proteins. Occasionally, branching or curving of the core may be seen. Usually, their size ranges from 20 to 50 μm in length by 2 to 5 μm in diameter. Asbestos bodies are not pathognomonical of

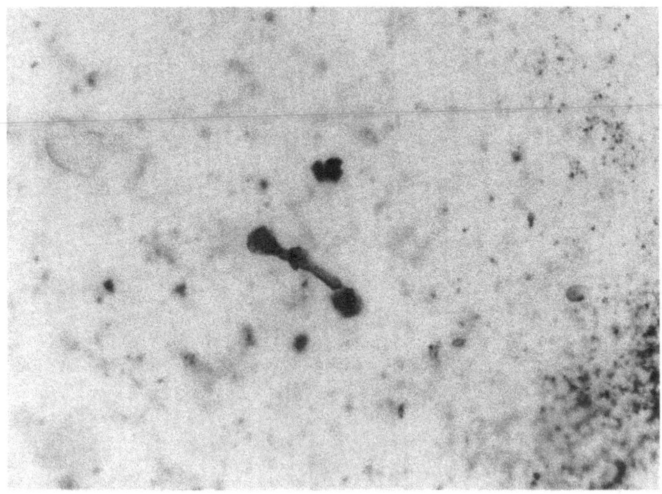

Figure 9 Asbestos body with characteristic dumbbell shape.

asbestosis; they are simply markers of exposure, while asbestosis is a diffuse, mature interstitial fibrosis due to asbestos exposure. Asbestos bodies are used to confirm the diagnosis of asbestosis when the characteristic pattern of diffuse, mature interstitial fibrosis is present.

Additionally, there are many nonasbestos mineral fibers that may form ferruginous bodies. *Coal/carbon* particles have an irregular, black, plate-like shape (Fig. 10). *Coal fly ash* (mullite) consists of lacy, black spheres (Fig. 11). These particles may also be identified without the glycoprotein coat, either free or within macrophages. *Iron* particles are small, round, and solid black. *Rutile* (titanium dioxide) are black fibers (Fig. 12). *Sheet silicates*

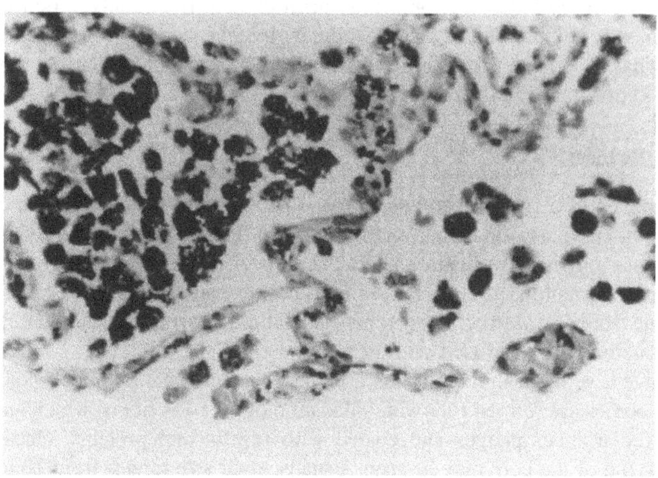

Figure 10 Coal particles within free alveolar macrophages.

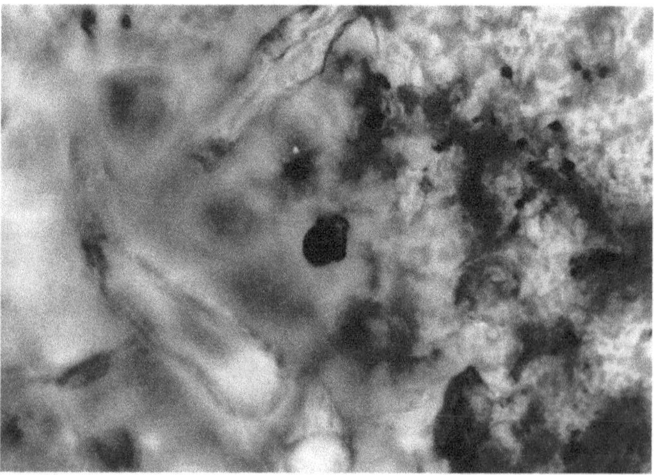

Figure 11 Black sphere characteristic of coal fly ash.

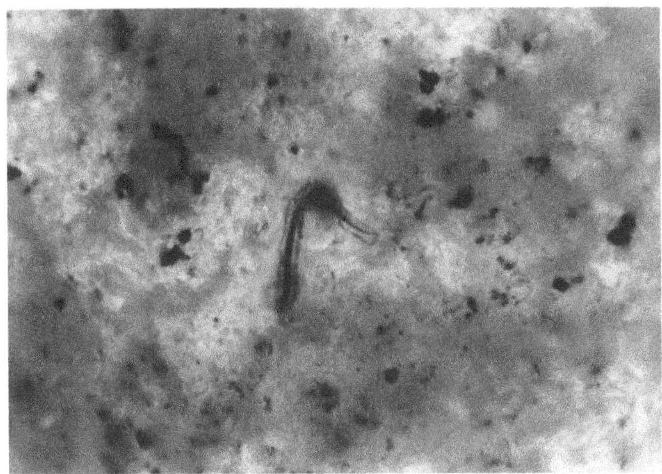

Figure 12 Black fiber characteristic of titanium dioxide.

(mica, talc, etc.) are irregular, broad, yellow plates or fibers. The yellow staining of the core is paler than that of the coat. *Silicon carbide* takes the form of black fibers. These fibers may result in diffuse interstitial fibrosis (2).

III. Organisms

Pulmonary tissue obtained for histological or cytological examination may include any one of a number of infectious organisms. Viruses and fungi are commonly present in specimens obtained from immunocompromised or immunosuppressed hosts and are readily recognizable on routine or special stains. Fungi may produce a host granulomatous response and should be considered in the differential of necrotizing granulomas.

A. Viruses

Adenovirus may cause two types of inclusions within the bronchial epithelial cells. The larger and more numerous inclusion is called a smudge cell because of the basophilic appearance of the entire cell (Fig. 13). The second inclusion is a smaller eosinophilic intranuclear inclusion surrounded by a clear halo; it can be confused with herpesvirus.

Cytomegalovirus (CMV) infection produces enlargement (up to 40 μm) of involved epithelial cells, endothelial cells, and/or macrophages. Both nuclear and cytoplasmic inclusions should be demonstrated. The chromatin becomes marginated and a large, central intranuclear inclusion of variable staining is separated from the nuclear rim by a white halo (Fig. 14). Following evolution of the nuclear inclusion, intracytoplasmic granules develop.

Herpesvirus also generates slight enlargement of epithelial cells, although not nearly as striking as that of CMV. Fusion produces multinucleate cells with nuclear molding (Figs. 15 and 27B). Initially, as the virions multiply, the nucleus enlarges and develops a "ground glass"

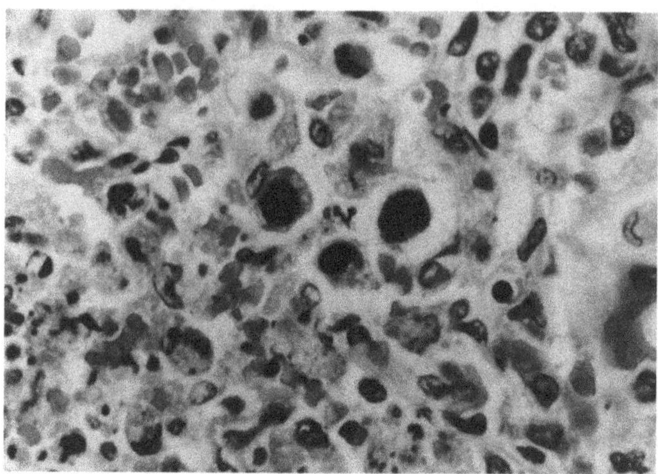

Figure 13 Epithelial cells infected with adenovirus showing large, basophilic inclusion (smudge cell). *Source*: Courtesy of Dr. Claire Langston, Baylor College of Medicine, Houston, Texas, U.S.A.

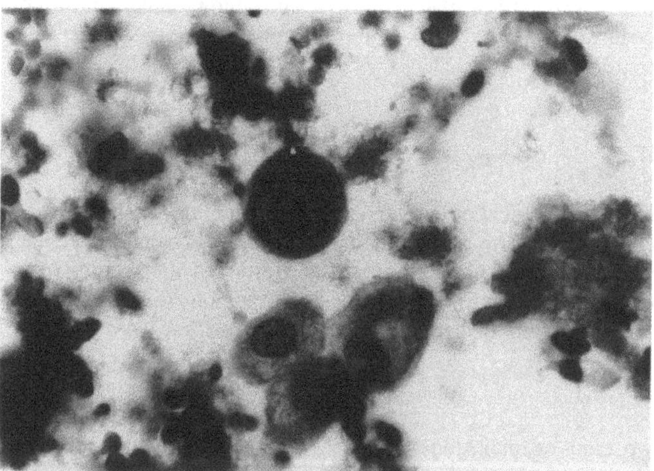

Figure 14 Cytomegalovirus in bronchial wash with large central, intranuclear inclusion.

appearance with margination of the chromatin at the nuclear membrane. Eventually, the center of the nucleus develops a central eosinophilic inclusion surrounded by a white halo (Cowdry type A). This inclusion can be mistaken for one of the types of adenovirus inclusions.

Measles virus can generate both intranuclear and intracytoplasmic inclusions in the epithelial cells. Initially, intracytoplasmic inclusions form around the nucleus, enlarge, and assume an eosinophilic hue. These inclusions are not easily identifiable and may not be seen. Intranuclear inclusions originating as eosinophilic particles evolve into a single eosinophilic inclusion surrounded by a modest halo. Measles also produces multinucleate cells (Fig. 16).

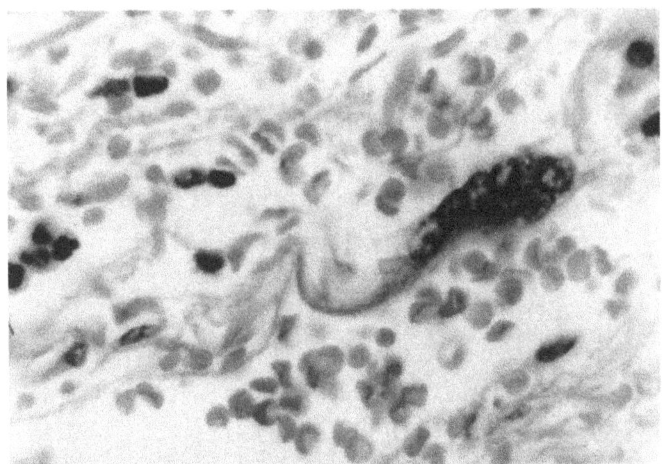

Figure 15 Multinucleated cell of herpesvirus exhibiting nuclear molding and a "ground-glass" appearance of the nuclei with margination of the chromatin at the nuclear membrane.

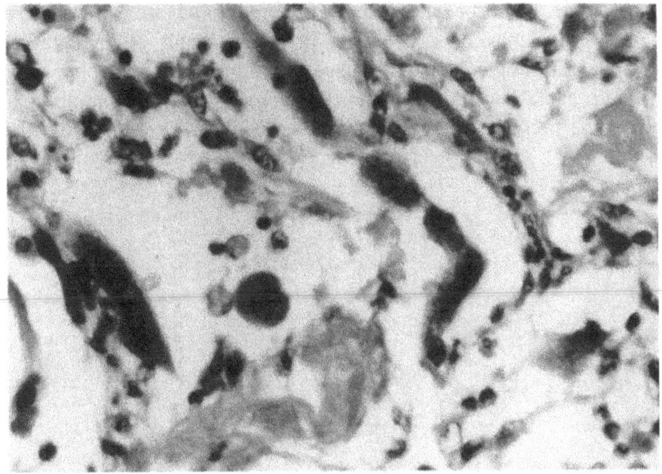

Figure 16 Multinucleated cells of measles virus. *Source*: Courtesy of Dr. Claire Langston, Baylor College of Medicine, Houston, Texas, U.S.A.

Intracytoplasmic inclusions of *respiratory syncytial virus* (RSV) may occasionally be demonstrated within epithelial cells as eosinophilic, round inclusions (Fig. 17). These inclusions may also be evident on Giemsa stain. The giant cells produced by RSV are formed from multinucleate, syncytial aggregates of respiratory cells.

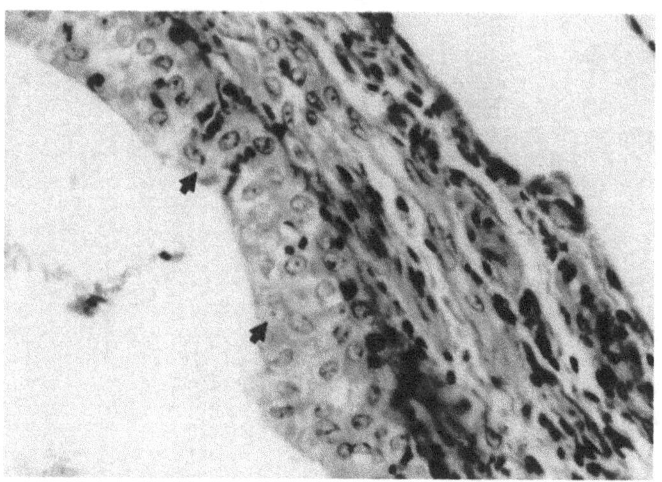

Figure 17 Eosinophilic round, intracytoplasmic inclusions of respiratory syncytial virus (*arrows*). *Source*: Courtesy of Dr. Claire Langston, Baylor College of Medicine, Houston, Texas, U.S.A.

B. Fungi

Several members of the *Aspergillus* sp., especially *Aspergillus fumigatus*, are known to be pathogenical in humans. *Aspergillus* may be a colonizer in the bronchus or an invasive organism. The fungus may appear as single, isolated hyphae or a large body of hyphae. The hyphae are 3 to 10 μm in width and show septation and dichotomous branching at approximately 45° angles (Fig. 18). The presence of septa help differentiate *Aspergillus* from the

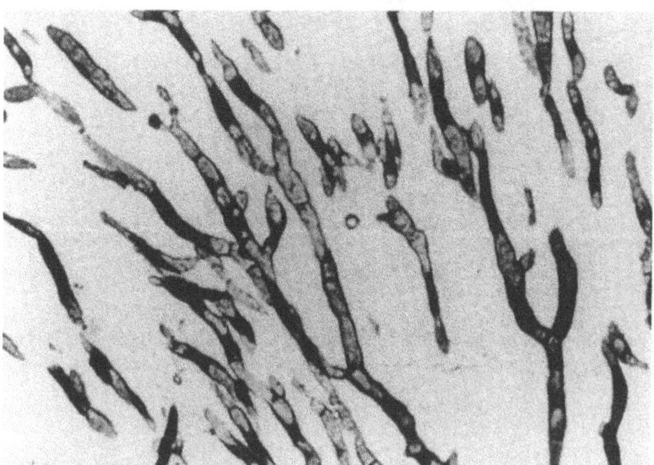

Figure 18 Hyphae exhibiting septation and dichotomous branching at approximately 45° angles consistent with *Aspergillus*.

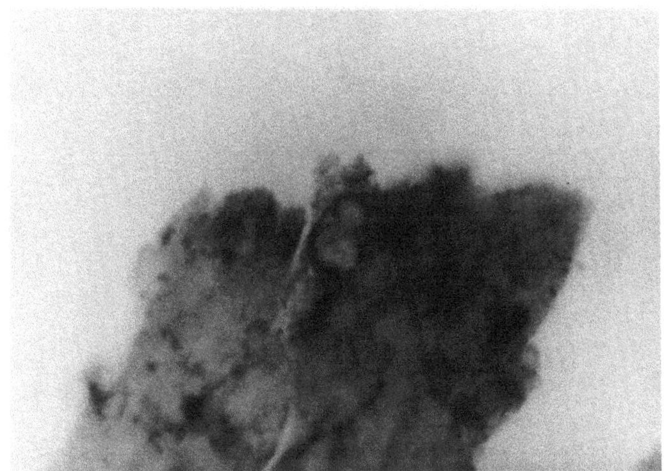

Figure 19 *Blastomyces* showing broad-based budding.

Zygomycetes or *Candida*. The hyphae are often arranged in a parallel manner. The conidiophore or fruiting body must be seen to make a definitive diagnosis of aspergillosis. Unfortunately, they are rarely evident on histological sections and only a presumptive identification of *Aspergillus* sp. can be given. The exact species of *Aspergillus* cannot be determined on histological sections unless birefringent calcium oxalate crystals, which are produced only by *Aspergillus niger*, are identified under polarized light. The fungus may be better appreciated on special stains, including Grocott's methanamine silver (GMS) and PAS.

Yeast of *Blastomyces* may be present within histiocytes or scattered within granulomatous inflammation. They are uniform, round yeasts averaging 8 to 15 μm but can measure up to 25 μm in diameter with broad-based budding averaging 4 to 5 μm in diameter (Fig. 19). The basophilic protoplasm is encompassed by a thick, refractile (double-contoured) cell wall. Special stains (GMS and PAS) may also aid in identifying the fungus.

Candida sp. can be identified in either nonbranching pseudohyphae or budding yeast (blastoconidia). Pseudohyphae consist of elongated blastoconidia linked together in a chain-like fashion. These pseudohyphae do not display true septations. Blastoconidia are round to oval with a diameter of up to 5 μm and bud off from the pseudohyphae. Special stains (GMS, PAS, and Gram) highlight the *Candida*.

Coccidioides may be identified by spherules, ranging from 20 to 60 μm in diameter, which have thick, refractile walls. These spherules may be empty or filled with round endospores, each measuring 1 to 5 μm (Fig. 20). Hyphal forms may also be seen. The fungus is best appreciated on GMS, PAS, and H&E stains. Calcifications may be confused with the spherules of *Coccidioides*; however they will not stain with GMS.

Cryptococcus is a round to oval yeast averaging 5 to 10 μm in diameter. Yeast can be identified on histological sections where they appear as pale blue structures surrounded by a thick mucoid capsule (Fig. 21). On routine H&E-stained sections, the capsule is visualized as a clear halo, which is actually an artifact of processing, producing shrinkage of the capsule. GMS and PAS highlight the yeast; mucin stains, preferably mucicarmine, are used to identify the capsule (bright red on mucicarmine stain). The capsule, when present, allows

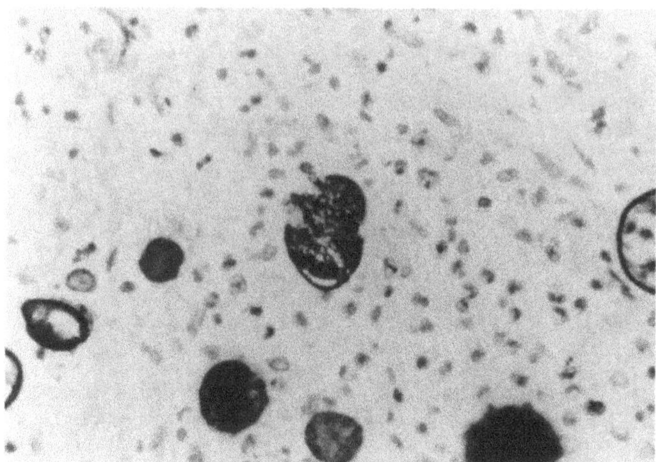

Figure 20 Endospores within a ruptured spherule of *Coccidioides*.

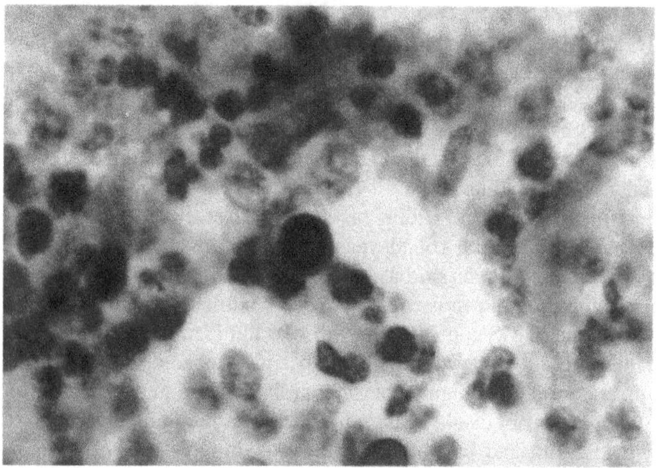

Figure 21 Thick, mucoid capsule of *Cryptococcus* highlighted by PAS stain.

the *Cryptococcus* to be distinguished from other small yeast. Budding is unequal and, unlike *Blastomyces, Cryptococcus* has a narrow base.

Histoplasma is a small, ovoid budding yeast ranging from 2 to 5 μm in diameter (Fig. 22). The yeast has a basophilic core surrounded by a clear halo and reside within macrophages. The fungus is best appreciated with GMS stain.

Nocardia are branching, filamentous, gram-positive organisms and produce necrotic, nongranulomatous inflammation (Fig. 23). These organisms are not visible on routine H&E-stained sections but are weakly acid-fast and therefore evident on modified acid-fast stains as well as Gram and GMS stains. *Nocardia* can be mistaken for mycobacteria; special stains help differentiate the two organisms.

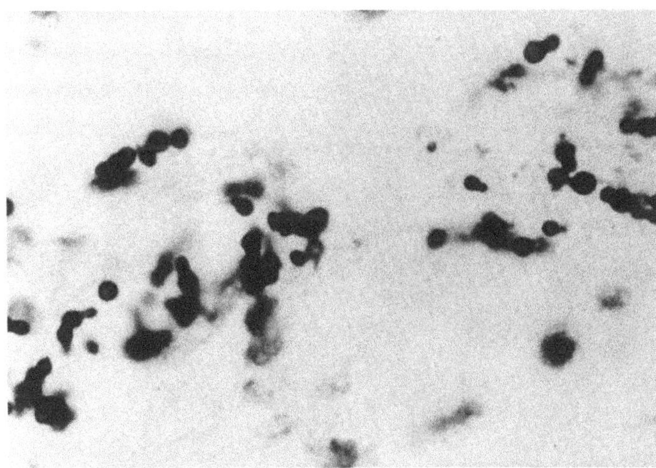

Figure 22 Small ovoid, budding yeast of *Histoplasma*.

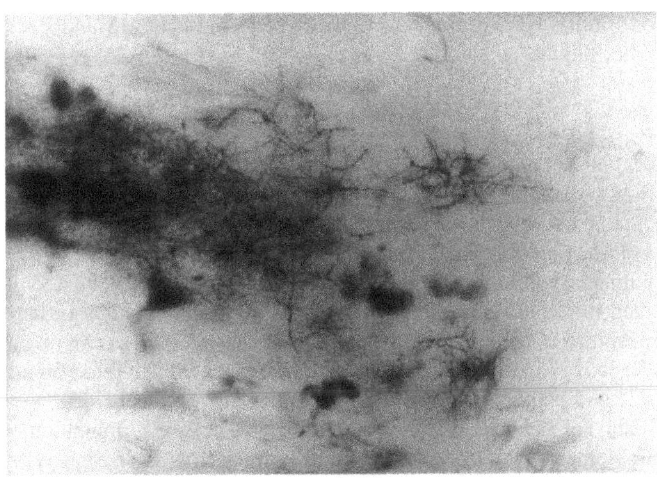

Figure 23 Long, branching, filamentous organisms of *Nocardia*.

Pneumocystis jiroveci reside within intra-alveolar, pink-staining foamy material that resembles edema fluid. The cysts and trophozoites are unable to be seen on routine H&E-stained sections. Initially thought to be a parasite, the organism is now believed to be a fungus. The cyst (4–8 μm) is best appreciated on GMS stain, showing the typical "cup-shaped" appearance, often with a central black dot (Fig. 24). Up to eight trophozoites measuring 0.5 to 1.0 μm in diameter may be present in each cyst. These trophozoites can be seen on Romanovsky stain as tiny purple dots, but they cannot be seen on GMS. Additional stains, including toluidine blue and Giemsa, may be employed to demonstrate the organism.

Zygomycosis consists of irregular, nonseptate, basophilic hyphae ranging from 6 to 50 μm in width. Yeast forms are not present. The hyphae often have wide-angle branching

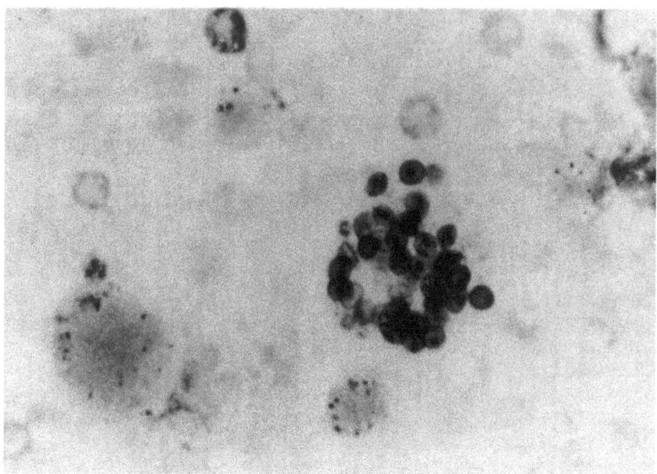

Figure 24 *Pneumocystis jiroveci* with typical "cup-shaped" appearance and central black dot.

(90°) and appear empty on routine H&E-stained sections. Special stains (GMS and PAS) are helpful in identifying the fungus.

C. Parasites

Larval migration of *Ascaris lumbricoides* through the lungs can produce an inflammatory reaction. The eggs are yellow-brown, have a thick shell, and measure up to 1 mm in length. Refractile granules are contained within the eggs.

Embolization of *Dirofilaria immitis* larvae into a branch of the pulmonary artery can produce a small, nodular pulmonary infarct, usually at the periphery of the lung. The nodule consists of a necrotic center surrounded by either nonspecific or granulomatous inflammation at the periphery. Examination of the vasculature within the necrotic areas can reveal more than one organism. When seen in cross section, *Dirofilaria* ranges from 100 to 300 μm and contains somatic muscle and pathognomonical internal cuticular ridges (Fig. 25).

Parasitic cysts or hydatids of *Echinococcus granulosus* develop following migration of larvae to the lungs. A central lumen of the cyst contains fluid surrounded at the periphery by two layers: an inner, nucleated layer of germinal epithelium and an outer laminated, non-nucleated layer, which serves as a protective coat. After several months, the germinative layer of the hydatid cysts produces cellular buds ("brood capsules"), which enlarge and become daughter cysts (ranging from barely visible to 2 to 3 cm in diameter). Scolices develop and are characteristically invaginated into their own bodies. Eventually, the brood capsules separate from the germinal layer and float in the central hydatid fluid, where they are referred to as "hydatid sand." The cysts can measure several centimeters in diameter and are encompassed by a host reaction of mononuclear and eosinophilic cells, giant cells, and fibroblasts.

Entamoeba histolytica trophozoites are spherical and range in size from 10 to 60 μm. The nucleus contains a small, single, and usually central karyosome and a chromatin pattern that is usually uniformly distributed and granular. The cytoplasm is finely granular and may contain ingested red blood cells. The trophozoites are usually located on histological sections

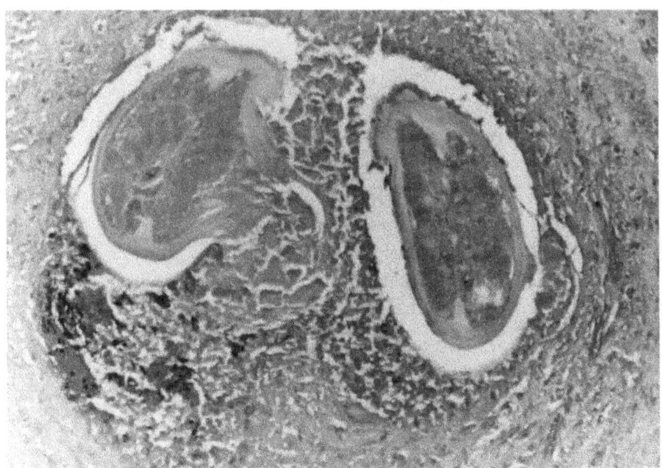

Figure 25 Cross section of necrotic *Dirofilaria immitis*.

at the junction of necrotic and viable lung. The organism may be more easily identified using the trichrome stain. Red blood cells can be highlighted by the iron-hematoxylin stain.

Adult worms of the genus *Paragonimus* migrate to the lungs, where they become encapsulated into cystic spaces by a host inflammatory reaction, initially consisting of numerous eosinophils and histiocytes. Usually one or two adult worms (7.5–12 mm × 4–6 mm) and mucinous fluid are contained within each cyst. These cysts are often multiple and can measure up to several centimeters in size. The parasites then extrude numerous ovoid, thick-shelled eggs (80–120 μm × 45–70 μm) from the cysts. The eggs have a prominent, thick, flat operculum at one end and a thick, round shell at the opposite end. Eggs may be seen in sputum samples. The eggs and the wall of the cysts induce a host granulomatous reaction.

Several species of *schistosomes* are known to produce pulmonary damage. The eggs measure up to 150 μm in length (Fig. 26). A spine may or may not be present. Schistosome eggs may embolize to the pulmonary vasculature and become impacted within it. A granulomatous inflammatory reaction develops, and granulomas may be seen disrupting the arterial elastic lamina. The eggs are extruded into the adjacent tissue and surrounded by an inflammatory reaction. Adult worms may also be identified. Progressive pulmonary hypertension may follow the obliterative arteriolitis.

Filariform larvae of *Strongyloides stercoralis* migrate through pulmonary capillaries and into alveoli, with associated hemorrhage but often with minimal inflammatory reaction. The larvae are approximately 500 μm long and display a notched tail (Fig. 27A and B). Adult worms measure approximately 2.5 mm × 35 μm and can develop within the lung.

Toxoplasma gondii is an obligate intracellular parasite; these organisms can be recognized as free trophozoites or as tissue cysts. Division of trophozoites occurs within host cells, which rupture releasing the organisms. Free trophozoites are crescent shaped, with one tapered and a blunt end. They measure 4 to 8 μm long and 2 to 3 μm wide and have a large, darkly stained nucleus. Intracellular cysts range from 5 to 1000 μm in diameter and are filled with numerous organisms. The organisms are evident on routine H&E-stained sections as well as Giemsa and PAS stains. The nucleus stains red and the

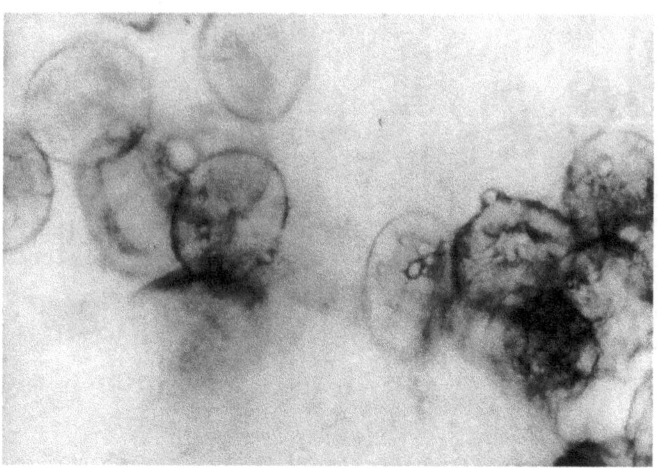

Figure 26 Large, pale, translucent, nonoperculate schistosome eggs. *Source*: Courtesy of Ms. Patricia Cernoch, The Methodist Hospital, Houston, Texas, U.S.A.

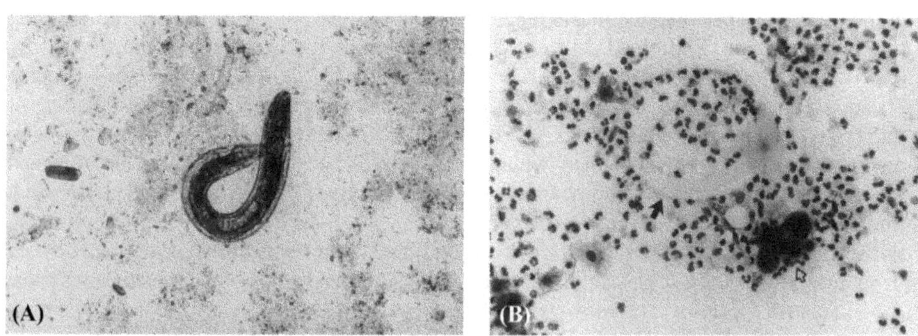

Figure 27 (**A**) Larva of *Strongyloides stercoralis*. (**B**) Sputum sample containing *Strongyloides stercoralis* (*closed arrow*). Note adjacent multinucleated cells of herpesvirus (*open arrow*). *Source*: (**A**) Courtesy of Ms. Patricia Cernoch, The Methodist Hospital, Houston, Texas, U.S.A.

cytoplasm blue on Romanovsky stain. Free tachyzoites may be difficult to find and should be differentiated from *Histoplasma* and *Pneumocystis* (3).

References

1. Laga AC, Allen TC, Bedrossian C, et al. Noncellular structures. In: Cagle PT, ed. Color Atlas and Text of Pulmonary Pathology, 2nd ed. Philadelphia: Lippincott, Williams and Wilkins, 2008:25–28.
2. Churg A. Nonneoplastic disease caused by asbestos. In: Churg A, Green FHY, eds. Pathology of Occupational Lung Disease, 2nd ed. Baltimore: Williams and Wilkins, 1998:277–338.
3. Specific infectious agents. In: Cagle PT, ed. Color Atlas and Text of Pulmonary Pathology, 2nd ed. Philadelphia: Lippincott, Williams and Wilkins, 2008:405–470.

25
The Molecular Diagnosis of Pulmonary Infections

GARY W. PROCOP
Cleveland Clinic Foundation and the Cleveland Clinic Lerner College of Medicine, Cleveland, Ohio, U.S.A.

I. Introduction

The innate defenses of the immune system are particularly important in anatomic areas of the body that make contact with the environment. The skin, the gastrointestinal tract, and the respiratory tract are such areas. It is in these regions that interactions with commensal, opportunistic, and obligate pathogenic microorganisms occur. Although the respiratory tract has numerous innate host defenses, such as the mucociliary escalator and a readily mobilized innate cellular immunity, it is arguably the most vulnerable of these organ systems to infection. The proximal most aspect of the lungs, after all, consists of only a few lipid bilayers (i.e., the cell membranes of the type I pneumocyte and capillary endothelial cell) that separate the outside world from the bloodstream.

Numerous different types of infections occur in the lungs. There are several types of bacterial pneumonias. Lobar pneumonia is typified by *Streptococcus pneumoniae*. Of increasing importance are ventilator-associated pneumonia, which may be caused by a variety of different types of bacteria, such *Klebsiella pneumoniae* and other members of the Enterobacteriaceae, *Pseudomonas aeruginosa*, and often a mixture of anaerobic bacteria. In addition, there are the so-called "atypical pneumonias," caused by organisms that are difficult to cultivate in the laboratory (e.g., *Mycoplasma pneumoniae*), that require a cell-line for propagation (e.g., *Chlamydophila pneumoniae*), or that require special media for cultivation (e.g., *Legionella pneumophila*). There are significant challenges for the use of molecular techniques for the detection of disease caused by some of these pathogens, such as *S. pneumoniae*, since the organism is often part of the human normal microbiota of the upper respiratory tract. Conversely, in some instances nucleic acid amplification detection methods are likely superior to traditional methods of detection of the causes of atypical pneumonia, as discussed further below.

The mycobacteria are another type of bacteria that may infect the lungs. These infections range from tuberculosis (i.e., pulmonary disease caused by *Mycobacterium tuberculosis*) to diseases caused by nontuberculous mycobacteria species, which often produce disease in patients with underlying diseases such as bronchiectiasis. Related bacteria, such as *Nocardia* species, are also important causes of pulmonary infections in patients with underlying disease, particularly patients with compromised immune systems secondary to transplantation. *Nocardia* infections are particularly important to recognize, since dissemination from the lungs to the brain is common in this patient population.

Nucleic acid amplification methods are particularly useful for the rapid detection of certain pathogens, such as *M. tuberculosis*, whereas DNA sequencing is now considered the gold standard by many for the classification of *Mycobacterium* and *Nocardia* species.

All humans experience viral infections of the lungs. Many of these infections are contacted annually or every few years in the human population, such as influenza, parainfluenza, and respiratory syncytial virus. Some viruses, such as cytomegalovirus (CMV), may be contracted anytime during life but remain latent following infection and may reactivate at a later time. CMV reactivation results in the most severe disease, which includes CMV pneumonitis, in immunocompromised patients, particularly patients with advanced HIV (i.e., AIDS) and immunosuppression secondary to transplantation. The use of molecular methods for the detection, identification, and characterization of viral infections is becoming commonplace. It is likely that these methods will replace standard viral culture for the routine detection of these pathogens in the near future.

Fungi also cause a variety of pulmonary infections. These range from infections caused by endemic fungi, such as *Histoplasma capsulatum* and *Coccidioides immitis*, which may occur in the human host regardless of their immune status, to opportunistic infections that occur in the immunocompromised host. A myriad of fungi may cause infection in the immunocompromised host, but common pathogens include *Aspergillus* species, members of the zygomycetes, and *Fusarium* species among many others. There are a number of challenges regarding the timely and accurate diagnosis of such infections, some of which will likely be addressed using new molecular methods.

There are a number of parasitic infections that involve the lung to varying degrees. Many of these only transiently involve the lung as the infecting parasite completes its life cycle (e.g., *Ascaris lumbricoides*), whereas some involve the lung as part of a systemic disease (e.g., *Plasmodium* species). Less commonly, some parasites, such as *Paragonimus* species, migrate to the lung, wherein maturation and reproduction are accomplished. *Echinococcus* species cause another parasitic infection that manifests with infections that involve either the lungs or the liver. Molecular methods have not been employed very commonly for the detection and characterization of parasitic diseases that involve the lungs, in part because these infections are readily diagnosed and characterized by traditional morphologic and serologic methods.

II. Diagnosing Pulmonary Infections Using Traditional Methods

The detection of pulmonary infections is often accomplished through the recognition of clinical signs and symptoms of disease, as well as radiographic changes. The identification of the causative agent of infection, however, is often quite difficult. Every method available if fraught with diagnostic hazards of difficulties, and many of the pitfalls that confound traditional testing also complicate molecular diagnostic testing for similar reasons. Therefore, it is useful to briefly review the traditional methods used for the detection of pulmonary infection and to examine corollaries with regard to molecular testing.

The culture of respiratory secretions, the mainstay for the diagnosis of typical bacterial pneumonia, is actually a poor test. In some instances, the causative agent of the pneumonia may be present in low quantities and overgrown by normal flora. In other instances members of the normal microbiota that are *potential* pathogens, such as *S. pneumonia* or *Haemophilus influenzae*, may be misconstrued as the etiologic agent of a pneumonia that is, in fact, caused by another microorganism. The challenge to molecular diagnostics in the first instance is to be able to detect potentially low quantities of nucleic acid from the pathogenic microorganism in a background of vast quantities of human and bacterial DNA (i.e., DNA derived from normal cellular elements and normal microbiota in the clinical specimen). In the second instance, one would need to be able to distinguish pathogenic bacteria from commensal bacteria, which is challenging, since many bacteria that normally colonize the oropharynx may also cause pneumonia (e.g., *S. pneumoniae*).

The common respiratory viruses are not part of the normal human flora and if detected, whether by traditional viral culture, direct immunofluorescence, or advanced molecular methods, are deemed true pathogens. Although traditional viral culture has been the gold standard diagnostic method for years, many virologists would contend that molecular methods are superior. Direct immunofluorescent antigen detection (DFA) and enzyme immunoassays are other non–nucleic acid based methods for the detection of the common respiratory viruses. The DFA, although quite sensitive and highly specific, is labor intensive and requires a fluorescent microscope and a skilled microscopist. The immunoassay cards, which resemble the rapid "Strep" tests often performed in a physician's office, have become popular within the last five years given the rapid availability of the result and the ease of use. There have, however, been significant issues raised regarding the diagnostic reliability of some of these products (1–3). Issues of particular concern are limited sensitivity and insufficient positive predictive value when these are used in instances of low prevalence (i.e., outside of normal respiratory virus season). The users of such products are, therefore, advised to thoroughly research this topic, before committing to the diagnostic "path of least resistance." Fortunately, the rapid detection of many of the common respiratory viruses, such as Influenza A, Influenza B, and respiratory syncytial virus, is being addressed using molecular methods that produces clearly superior results.

Infections caused by mycobacteria and certain fungi, such as *H. capsulatum*, may not be identified in a timely manner since these agents grow slowly. Molecular methods may prove useful adjuncts for the more timely detection and characterization of such pathogens. Whether such methods will ever replace culture remains to be determined through well-controlled comparative studies. Although some fungi that cause infections in humans grow relatively rapidly, particularly many of the opportunistic fungi that infect the immunocompromised hosts, it may be difficult to determine whether these represent true pathogens, transient colonizers, or specimen contaminants. This challenge remains to be addressed for both traditional and molecular approaches to diagnosis.

The parasites that cause infections that involve the lungs are less commonly encountered in North America and other developed countries. These are usually detected and identified using morphologic methods, which will likely remain the standard for quite awhile, but niche applications for molecular diagnostics may occur.

Many of the same difficulties that are impediments to achieving an identification of the etiologic agent of pulmonary infections using traditional methods transcend into the molecular realm. There are, however, notable exceptions wherein molecular diagnostics represent true advances in the diagnosis of pulmonary infections. The following sections, although limited, examine the advances and challenges of the use of molecular diagnostics for the detection and characterization of pulmonary infections. Regardless of the method used, the goal of rapid diagnostics remains to identify the cause of disease in the most timely manner so that appropriate, directed therapy may be employed (4).

III. Fresh Vs. Formalin-Fixed, Paraffin-Embedded Tissues

The paraffin boundary has been crossed, but there are distinct limitations regarding the recovery of DNA and particularly RNA from formalin-fixed, paraffin-embedded (FFPE) tissues. We now have the ability to microdissect areas of interest in FFPE tissues to examine even single cells. Although this is possible using advance methods, such as laser capture microdissection, even a simplified approach may prove effective. We have employed a method wherein the area that contains the highest quantity of microorganism is identified by the pathologist, the block is cleaned with an alcohol pad and allowed to dry, and the area is punched out of the block using a sterile, disposable punch biopsy tool of the dermatologist (Fig. 1). Thereafter, the tissue is deparaffinized, digestion is accomplished using protease K, and the DNA is extracted using standard methods. The molecular diagnostic assays of choice may then be used to target the microorganism of interest. A limitation of any approach that uses FFPE tissues is that these tissues have not been handled in an aseptic manner. Common reagents and containers are used (i.e., most tissue processors retain the cassettes, which in turn retain the patient tissues, in common containers that are then flooded with common reagents). Therefore, it would be expected that contaminating environmental bacteria, including rapidly growing mycobacteria, as well as the spores from environmental fungi are likely present in the tissue block. This places significant limitations on the ability to use broad-range bacterial and fungal PCR primers, since a myriad of targets will be present and amplified. Currently, species-specific primers are preferred in such instances, although sophisticated methods of post-amplification analysis may address some of these limitations.

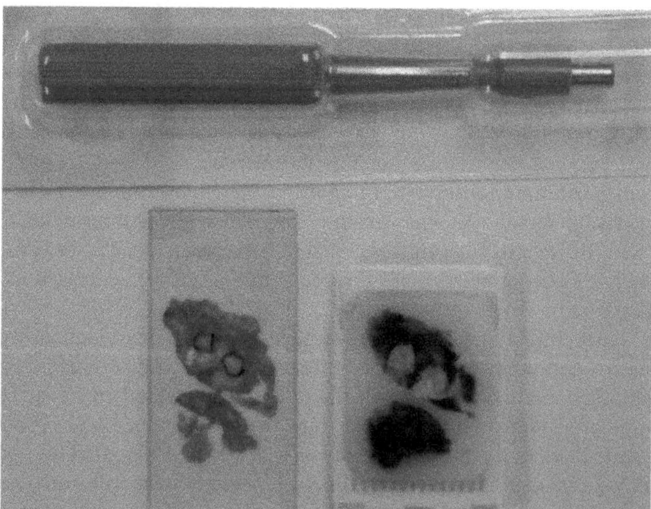

Figure 1 A simplified approach to microdissection is demonstrated. The foci that contain the highest quantity of microorganisms are identified through microscopic examination (i.e., the circled area). After cleaning the block with an alcohol pad, the area of interest is removed using a punch biopsy. This approach minimizes the amount of human DNA and any potential contaminants that might be in the paraffin used for embedding.

Another approach that has been found particularly useful is to correlate the histopathologic finding in surgical pathology specimens with the residual tissue submitted for culture to the microbiology laboratory. It is common practice for most microbiology laboratories to refrigerate and retain excess clinical material that is submitted for culture for 7 to 10 days. These specimens are usually obtained from the same anatomic site as the tissue submitted for histologic studies. Gross anatomy skills may be used to guide the pathologist to the area most likely to contain the microorganisms of interest. A portion of tissue may then be taken from this area and submitted for digestion, DNA extraction, and PCR. The advantage of this approach is that the tissue has not been fixed using common reagents and embedded in paraffin, whereas the disadvantage is that one does not have microscopic evidence that the area submitted for molecular studies does not contain the highest quantity of microorganisms. An additional advantage of this approach is that it fosters interactions between the microbiologist and the pulmonary pathologist, which often translates into the best medical practice.

IV. Bacterial Infections

A. Typical Bacterial Pneumonia

Many of the issues that confound culture as a method of determining the cause of bacterial pneumonia are also problematic when molecular methods are used. In current and traditional practice, semiquantitative and quantitative cultures are used to help determine the likelihood that a bacterial species present in a respiratory culture may be the cause of a pulmonary infection. Although this approach is not perfect, it is the best method available to help differentiate potential pathogens from respiratory flora. Newer technologies that employ homogeneous PCR with or without post-amplification analysis may be able to provide results comparable to respiratory cultures, but these are not yet available and are likely cost prohibitive compared with culture.

Many of the bacteria that may cause pneumonia, such as *S. pneumoniae, H. influenzae,* and *Moraxella catarrhalis*, are also normal flora in the oropharynx. Qualitative PCR results for the detection of these bacteria may detect normal oropharyngeal inhabitants and thereby produce misleading results, which may in turn lead to inappropriate antimicrobial therapy. For example, suppose a patient with legionellosis had a PCR qualitative for *S. pneumoniae* PCR that was truly positive, but as a result of oropharyngeal contamination of the respiratory specimen. The patient, in this example, could erroneously be treated with a β-lactam antibiotic, which is not effective against the intracellular legionellae.

Therefore, highly sensitive qualitative nucleic acid amplification assays may be positive in the absence of disease (i.e., colonization was detected). For these reasons, quantitative molecular approaches are being examined as methods to differentiate colonization from infection (5–7). Although examined in the setting of meningitis, Carrol et al. have shown a positive correlation between *S. pneumoniae* DNA loads and mortality in children (8). Many are hopeful of the success of such approaches, given the success of quantitative PCR, in contrast to qualitative PCR for the detection of disease versus reactivation of several of the medically important herpesviruses.

There are added difficulties in hospitalized patients, particularly those that are intubated, since nosocomial pathogens, such as *Staphylococcus aureus, P. aeruginosa*, and members of the Enterobacteriaceae rapidly colonize endotracheal tube and upper respiratory tract of these patients. Finally, aspiration pneumonias are typically caused by a variety of bacteria from the respiratory and gastrointestinal tract, including anaerobes.

The etiologic agents of ventilator-associated pneumonia and aspiration pneumonia are more complicated to determine from both a traditional and molecular perspective because any of the wide variety of bacteria that may colonize the upper respiratory tract may be the cause of lower respiratory tract disease. Furthermore, some of these may be difficult to impossible to culture using standard methods but have been detected using molecular methods (9). Recent studies have shown that the types of bacteria responsible for pneumonia in such settings are grossly underestimated, and that uncultivable bacteria may play a significant role (9). There is some evidence, however, that early-onset ventilator-associated pneumonia, in many instances, may be caused by the same bacteria that cause community-acquired pneumonia for which quantitative PCR assays have been developed (10). Such studies suggest that molecular methods may play a role in the future in the more rapid and accurate determination of the causes of aspiration and ventilator-associated pneumonia, but this remains to be determined.

B. Atypical Bacterial Pneumonia

The determination of the cause of what has been termed an atypical pneumonia has always been challenging. The microorganisms that cause these infections are fastidious and difficult to cultivate, and are difficult to visualize in histopathologic sections and/or pulmonary secretions. A number of molecular diagnostic assays have been developed for the detection of the most common causes of atypical bacterial pneumonia. The causes of atypical bacterial pneumonia are *Legionella* species, most commonly *L. pneumophila, Mycoplasma pneumoniae*, and *C. pneumoniae*, among others (11).

The importance of *L. pneumophila* came to light with the outbreak of legionellosis at the Legionnaire's convention in Philadelphia in 1976. Although *L. pneumophila* is the most common cause of legionellosis, other *Legionella* species many also cause the disease (12–15). It is important to differentiate legionellosis from other causes of atypical bacterial pneumonia, since the disease is often more severe with legionellosis, and there may be an environmental source associated with an outbreak that can be addressed. Traditionally, the detection of *Legionella* has been made through culture and/or the demonstration of bacilli in pulmonary secretions or pulmonary biopsy that stain poorly with Gram's stain but well with a modified silver stain, such as a Warthin-Starry stain (16,17). The antigen-based detection of *L. pneumophila* in respiratory secretions through direct microscopy (i.e., direct immunofluorescence antigen detection) or the enzyme-immunoassay-based detection of antigen shed in the urine (i.e., *L. pneumophila* urinary antigen) are also currently used methods for the establishment of legionellosis. These antigen-based assays are limited to the detection of *L. pneumophila,* but fail to disclose other *Legionella* species. A variety of nucleic acid amplification assays have been designed for the detection of *L. pneumophila* (18–22). These include a few rapid-cycle (i.e., real-time) PCR assays. Others have devised assays that detect the *Legionella* genus to detect all patients with legionellosis, rather than just those infected by *L. pneumophila.* In addition to laboratory designed assays, there is an Food and Drug Administration (FDA)-approved product for the detection of *L. pneumophila* that utilizes strand-displacement amplification (i.e., BD ProbeTec™ ET *L. pneumophila* DNA Amplified Assay, BD Diagnostic systems, Sparks, Maryland, U.S.).

It is difficult to detect the presence of *C. pneumoniae* and *Mycoplasma pneumoniae* using traditional culture and anatomic pathology methods. Molecular detection methods are superior to traditional microbiologic methods for the detection of these agents, given the difficulty needed to cultivate these microorganisms. In addition, noninvasive specimens, like a throat swab, may be used successfully for the detection of *Mycoplasma pneumoniae*, as demonstrated by Liu et al. (23). Although Morozumi et al. showed PCR to be only slightly superior to recovery by culture, it is faster and less complex than culture (24). In this study, Morozumi et al. confirmed the utility of serology for the confirmation of infection by demonstrating a rise in antibody titer in almost all infected individuals tested (24). However, Kim et al. suggest that these methods may be superior to serology in the very young and the immunocompromised (25). Regardless, serologic assays remain the mainstay for the diagnosis of infections caused by these pathogens. The optimal detection of infection by these pathogens is likely achieved through the use of both serology and a molecular diagnostic test in the appropriate clinical setting (i.e., some will be detected by serology and not PCR, and vice versa) (26).

Although many molecular assays are designed to detect these pathogens, none have been approved by the FDA. In addition, they are rarely ordered by clinicians, in the experience of this author, who tend to begin empiric therapy, culture for typical bacterial pathogens, assess the patient for *Legionella*, and assess the patient using serologic methods for *Chlamydophila pneumophila* and *Mycoplasma pneumoniae*, if clinically indicated. This may be because most infections caused by these microorganisms are usually self-limited, although significant morbidity and some mortality have been observed in certain hosts, such as the elderly (27).

A number of excellent studies that examine the use of a variety of molecular methods for the detection of bacterial pathogens of pneumonia are available for those who would like to read further on this subject (28–31). Methods that are more advanced than single pathogen detection are likely to be used to more fully characterize patients with pneumonia in the future. These methods may incorporate either multiple amplification reactions (e.g., a multiplex PCR) or incorporate broad-range PCR. The character of the amplified products following either multiplex or broad-range PCR will then be differentiated using a variety of post-amplification detection methods, which may include reverse hybridization methods, solid or liquid microarrays, and possibly DNA sequencing. For example, Wang et al. examined a promising assay that combined multiplex PCR and reverse hybridization to detect a variety of commonly occurring bacterial pathogens that cause lung disease (32). The pathogens in this assay included easily cultivated bacteria, such as *S. pneumoniae* and *M. catarrhalis*, as well as fastidious bacteria or slow-growing microorganisms, such as *L. pneumophila, Bordetella pertussis,* and *M. tuberculosis*, which demonstrate the wide range of organisms that may be detected using such assays (32). Such methods will be important for the accurate characterization of the full spectrum of the etiologic agents of pneumonia, as both community and hospital-associated pneumonias may be caused by more than one microorganism (33). In addition, molecular methods of detection may prove superior to culture in instances wherein the patient has received antimicrobial therapy (34). The near-term future will likely hold the continued assessment of a variety of molecular methods for the more rapid detection of the causes of bacterial pneumonia, and in some instances they will be incorporated into routine testing. The assessment of these assays will by necessity be compared with traditional methods, which have their own strengths and limitations. Most importantly, it will be necessary to demonstrate that the use of these assays, which are usually more expensive than traditional methods, will contribute significantly to the health improvement of patients with pneumonia and an improvement of the healthcare system overall.

C. Mycobacteria

The mycobacteria, particularly *M. tuberculosis*, are excellent candidates for detection by molecular methods and numerous assays have been devised (e.g., a search of PubMed for mycobacteria and PCR yielded 4012 manuscripts). Most mycobacteria are slow-growing, some cause severe disease, and for the most part are morphologically indistinguishable. When these microorganisms grow in culture, they are usually either identified using a species-specific probe or using biophysical characterization. The use of species-specific probes was one of the first advances in the routine implementation of molecular testing in mycobacteriology (35,36). Although these truly represented an advance in diagnostic testing, the limitation of such testing is that they simply identify or exclude the presence of the single microorganism for which they are designed to detect. False-negative reactions may occur using this technology if too few organisms are present or poor probe design, whereas false-positives have rarely been reported due to cross-hybridization of *Mycobacterium* species with a high degree of DNA sequence homology (37,38). The limitations of these assays have been addressed, and they remain commonly used for the rapid identification of the most commonly occurring clinically important mycobacteria.

The majority of the molecular assays in this category have been designed for the detection and identification of *M. tuberculosis*. As noted above, one of the most successful product is the AccuProbe *M. tuberculosis* complex (Gen-Probe, Inc., San Diego, California, U.S.), a genetic probe that hybridizes to the rRNA of cultivated mycobacteria of a particular species. A signal is then generated that utilizes a proprietary chemistry, which denotes probe/target hybridization. These probes are useful only for the identification of mycobacteria in culture, since a relatively large quantity of organisms is necessary to perform this test. In situ hybridization is another signal-amplification methodology that has been used for the identification of *M. tuberculosis* and other *Mycobacterium* species (39,40). One of the potential advantages of this technology is that a single assay could be used for assessing respiratory specimens that contain acid-fast bacilli, anatomic pathology and cytology specimens, as well as positive cultures. This method, although demonstrated to be feasible, is not commonly used.

The detection of non-tuberculous mycobacteria has not proven as pressing a clinical issue as the detection of *M. tuberculosis*, since these microorganisms are not transmissible in the same manner as *M. tuberculosis* and often the disease is not as progressive or severe. Many of the non-tuberculous mycobacteria, however, cause pulmonary infections, some of which may be severe. Petrini has recently reviewed the nature of infections caused by non-tuberculous mycobacteria (41). The identification of the non-tuberculous mycobacteria that is responsible for a particular infection may be achieved traditionally through an evaluation of its biophysical profile or through the use of a number of molecular tools. Genetic probes are commercially available for the identification of *M. avium, M. intracellulare, M. kansasii,* and *M. gordonae*. Individual nucleic acid assays have also been designed to detect some of the more commonly occurring non-tuberculous mycobacteria, but these are less commonly used in clinical practice compared with those designed to detect *M. tuberculosis*. More recently, multiplex assays and broad-range PCR assays have been created that detect and differentiate the most clinically important mycobacteria (see below).

A large number of nucleic acid amplification assays for the detection of *M. tuberculosis* have also been devised. The majority of these are suggested for the direct detection of *M. tuberculosis* from respiratory specimens, such as sputa or bronchoalveolar lavage (BAL). Two commercially available products are FDA approved, whereas third is not FDA approved, but commonly used in Europe and elsewhere outside the United States. These use three different types of nucleic acid amplification chemistry, namely, PCR, transcription-mediated amplification, and strand-displacement amplification. These products have not been cleared for use on pulmonary biopsies, but some of the laboratory-designed assays have been used in this manner. Commentaries regarding the most appropriate use of these assay are available for further review (42–44).

The types of laboratory-designed and analyte-specific reagents (ASRs) consist of monoplex species-specific, multiplex, and broad-range (i.e., "pan-mycobacteria") assays. The monoplex assays have proven useful for determining the identity of acid-fast bacilli present in a clinical specimen, and limited utility on "smear-negative" specimens. These are used in a manner similar to the FDA-approved assays, but many do not include internal controls, which is a significant limitation. The multiplex assays usually contain one reaction to detect *M. tuberculosis* in addition to other commonly encountered mycobacteria, such as *M. avium* and *M. intracellulare* (45–47). In addition, these often contain an internal amplification control. Broad-range PCR linked with one of several methods of post-amplification analysis is another method to detect more than one species of *Mycobacterium* and to effectively differentiate these into clinically important categories (e.g., *M. tuberculosis* complex). Broad-range PCR and post-amplification melt-curve analysis has been designed to detect and differentiate *M. tuberculosis* complex from non-tuberculous mycobacteria, which is the most important clinical differentiation (48) (Fig. 2).

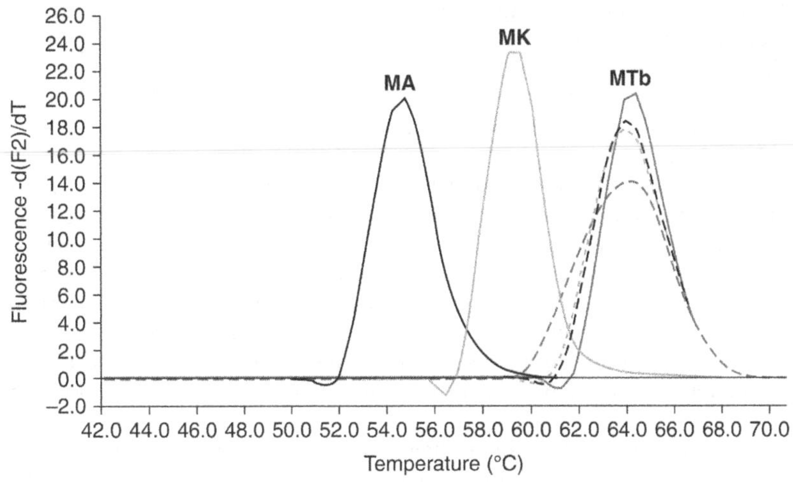

Figure 2 Numerous isolates of *M. tuberculosis* (MTb), one of which is the control stain, are differentiated from the control strains of *M. kansasii* (MK) and *M. avium* (MA) by post-amplification melt-curve analysis.

The same type of approach may be linked with methods that achieve more specific species-level differentiation such as reverse hybridization, microarray analysis, and traditional or pyrosequencing (49–54). These molecular tools may also be used to assay for molecular determinants of antimicrobial resistance in addition to achieving accurate identification (51,55,56).

Molecular tools are commonly used in the routing mycobacteriology laboratory for the detection and identification of medically important mycobacteria. The expanded use of these techniques will likely include the routine identification of mycobacteria that are detected in fixed and processed tissues and cytology specimens. In addition, assays of higher complexity, such as microarrays, will likely become more commonly used, as the costs of these assays declines.

V. Viral Infections

The virologists are usually in the forefront of molecular diagnostics. Viruses, in many instances, are difficult to cultivate and several cell culture lines must be inoculated with a clinical specimen to optimize virus recovery. Even with such extensive measures, there are viruses that often remain undetected in such culture systems, such as the newly recognized human metapneumovirus. Therefore, clinical virologists have derived assays for the detection of virtually all clinically important viruses. How these assays will be used on a daily basis in the clinical laboratories remains to be determined. In some instances, laboratories have substantially if not entirely replaced traditional virologic methods with novel molecular tests. In addition to adding the possibility of detecting more viruses than with traditional methods, these assays are more sensitive than traditional methods, and are by design highly specific.

One of the initial challenges that needed to be addressed was that a monoplex assay was needed for each virus. It is not possible to design a single broad-range (i.e., pan-viral) PCR assay that detects all clinically important viruses, as these organisms are too evolutionary or taxonomically distinct. Broad-range assays have, however, been designed to detect and differentiate certain groups of viruses (e.g., the Herpesviridae). The use of numerous monoplex assays is too labor intensive and cost prohibitive to be used in the routine laboratory for all viruses. Fortunately, newer technologies and advanced assays have addressed this issue.

Multiplex assays have been designed that detect and differentiate some of the most common respiratory viruses, Influenza A, Influenza B, and respiratory syncytial virus (57). Other assays have added the most commonly occurring parainfluenza viruses, adenovirus, and some of the causes of atypical bacterial pneumonia among other viruses (58,59). A variety of assays have also been derived that detect all or the most clinically important subtypes of adenovirus, which can cause severe disease in immunocompromised hosts (60–62). In addition to the viruses mentioned above, there is emerging evidence that other viruses, such as rhinovirus, may be important causes of community-acquired pneumonia in children (63).

Rapid-cycle PCR and reverse transcription (RT) PCR methods have been instrumental in the detection of emerging viral pathogens, as well as the characterization of the prevalence of newly recognized pathogens. Although traditional methods, such as electron microscopy are often the initial methods used to help recognize the class of virus causing a disease (e.g., the SARS epidemic), it is molecular methods including rapid genomic sequencing and rapid-cycle RT-PCR were then used to fully characterize this pathogen and rapidly detect infected patients (64,65). Similarly, it is rapid-cycle RT-PCR that has been used to evaluate the prevalence and investigate the range and severity of disease caused by the human metapneumovirus (66,67). The use of molecular methods is particularly important for the investigation of viral infections that are caused by agents that fail to grow or do not grow well in commonly used cell culture systems.

Multiplex assays have currently been developed that amplify and detect so many viral pathogens that they exceed the detection capabilities of the real-time PCR instruments available (i.e., there are a limited number of channels available for fluorescent detection on these instrument). Therefore, researchers and manufacturers have turned to microarrays as means by which to detect these products of amplification. A variety of solid-phase microarrays have been derived, but possibly the most user-friendly are the bioelectric arrays. These have been designed to detect the products of amplification of the most commonly occurring respiratory viruse denoted above (68). Importantly, this type of technology readily detects co-infections, which may be important in disease severity. One of the most exciting areas of multiple analyte detection is the liquid-base microsphere technology. These methods of post-amplification analysis may follow complex multiplex reactions needed for the detection of a variety of potential viral agents. For example, Mahony et al. reported a highly effective approach that interrogates specimens for 20 respiratory viruses simultanteously (69). The FDA has recently cleared an assay similar to the one reported in this study for use clinical laboratories.

The detection of viruses is largely becoming a molecular endeavor in many institutions. Several of these methods are FDA approved and other groups are seeking such approval. The modification of such assays for use on fixed tissue and cytologic specimens is possible. The evolution of viral diagnostics will continue to move away from culture-based methods in many instances and involve the investigation and implementation of more rapid molecular methods to detect the causative agents of viral infections.

VI. Fungal Infections

The lungs are an important portal of entry for fungi, since many fungal spores are small enough to remain suspended in the air and avoid innate respiratory defenses, such as nasal hairs and the mucociliary escalator. The rare fungal spore from most molds that reaches the alveolus will be addressed by pulmonary macrophages and will not cause disease. If, however, a large bolus is inhaled then an allergic-type reaction will follow (i.e., the so-called “bronchopulmonary aspergillosis”). This process also occurs after one encounters any large bolus of either spores or cellular fragments or the aerobic actinomycetes, and is not limited to spore from *Aspergillus*.

When the spores of certain pathogens reach the terminal alveolus, then disease invariably ensues. These pathogens include the endemic fungi, *H. capsulatum, C. immitis,* and *Blastomyces dermatitidis*, in the United States. The infections caused by these pathogens, particularly disease caused by *H. capsulatum* and *C. immitis*, are often self-limited. Pulmonary disease caused by *B. dermatitidis* is more likely to become progressive, but resolution may occur in some patients. The confirmation of identity of these isolate once they grow in culture is usually achieved through the use of species-specific hybridization probes (i.e., AccuProbe assays), as describe for the mycobacteria above.

The ability to accurately identify the dimorphic fungal pathogens in histologic section has been explored using in situ hybridization. The number of possible fungi that appear as yeast and yeast-like forms in tissue is substantial. The histopathologist differentiates these fungi by examining the type of inflammatory response present, the size of the fungal forms and other morphologic features (e.g., the broad-based bud of *B. dermatitidis*), and other features (e.g., the capsule of *Cryptococcus neoformans* or the spherule of *C. immitis*). Hayden et al. have demonstrated the utility of in situ hybridization to differentiate these fungi, which is particularly useful when considering morphologically similar species (70). Accurate morphologic identification may be useful, since some of these species, such as *H. capsulatum*, are slow-growing fungi.

There have been a number of nucleic acid amplification assays that have been described for the detection of the dimorphic molds. Real-time PCR assays specific for *H. capsulatum* have been described, but these are rarely used in practice (71,72). Although the presence of *H. capsulatum* may be detected in the peripheral blood of the patient with disseminated histoplasmosis, the utility of this assay for the detection of this disease and its comparative performance with *Histoplasma* antigen testing remains to be determined. The detection of *H. capsulatum* using a rapid PCR method is particularly attractive, given the slow growth of this fungus. Similarly, PCR and real-time PCR assays have been developed to detect *B. dermatitidis* and *C. immitis* (73,74). Researchers have applied the *C. immitis/C. posadasii* PCR assay to the identification of fungal forms in histologic sections, since the identification of coccidioidomycosis may be particularly challenging if intact spherules are not seen (75,76).

There is a large population of people with compromised immune systems that are living longer because of advances in modern medicine. The immunocompromised host is at risk for a variety of opportunistic infections, among which are fungal infections. The type of deficit in the immune system is associated with the risk for certain types of infections. For example, patients with end-stage HIV infection (i.e., AIDS) are at risk for infections by *Candida* species and may develop disseminated histoplasmosis, but less commonly develop an invasive infection by a hyaline septate mold or a zygomycete. The profoundly neutropenic hosts, however, is at significant risk for all types of fungal infections. The immune status of the host, therefore, is likely the most important determinant of the risk for fungal infections (77).

Aspergillus fumigatus and *Candida albicans* are the most important fungal pathogens of the immunocompromised host (77). However, a number of other molds, such as *Fusarium* sp., *Pseudallescheria boydii, Acremonium* sp., and members of the zygomycetes, among others, are also important causes of fungal infections in this population. Similarly, non-*albicans Candida* species are becoming increasingly important pathogens in this group, and other yeast or yeast-like fungi, such as *Trichosporon, Blastoschizomyces,* and *Rhodotorula* species may also cause clinically significant infections.

It is not practical to approach fungal molecular diagnostics using monoplex assays, given the great variety of different fungi that may cause human disease. Two methods that hold the greatest promise for the detection and characterization of fungal infections utilize either a multiplex or a broad-range (i.e., "pan-fungal") amplification reaction in conjunction with some type of advanced post-amplification analysis. The methods of post-amplification analysis may include reverse hybridization, DNA sequencing, or solid or liquid microarray analysis, as described above for the mycobacteria. The advantage of such an approach is that the broad-range PCR will detect any infecting fungus, whereas the post-amplification analysis affords the opportunity to identify the presence of a wide variety of pathogens. One of the limitations of broad-range PCR for fungi is the possibility contamination, since fungi are ubiquitous in the environment. This is concerning, since if inappropriately addressed, this could result in false-positive reactions.

There are many challenges regarding the rapid diagnosis of fungal infections. Antigen detection assays, such as galactomannan and *Histoplasma* urinary antigen, have proven quite useful for the detection of *Aspergillus* and *Histoplasma* infections, respectively in certain populations. How multiplex and broad-range nucleic acid amplification assays will compete with these assays remains to be determined? Regardless, molecular methods will continue to be evaluated and some be routinely implemented in the mycology laboratory of the future.

VII. Parasitic Infections

There are a wide variety of helminthic parasites that involve the lungs at some stage in their life cycle. However, many of these involve the lungs only transiently. The pathologic results of these transient migrations are minimal and do not often result in a biopsy. *Strongyloides stercoralis* is one of the geohelminths that transmigrates the lungs as part of its normal life cycle, but for other reasons deserves special mention. The larvae, rather than the eggs of *S. stercoralis*, are passed in the feces, unlike other geohelminths. In addition, the filariform larvae of *S. stercoralis* have the ability to penetrate the perianal skin and gastrointestinal mucosa resulting in an autoinfection of the host. The degree of autoinfection, which may persist for decades, is minimized in the immunocompetent host. Hyperinfections, however, may occur in the immunocompromised or elderly patient, which have a high associated mortality. Currently, diagnosis for exposure relies on serology, whereas diagnosis of active infection relies upon microscopic morphologic detection of larvae in the stool, transmigrating larvae in the lung or respiratory secretions (i.e., BAL or sputum), or the demonstration of the adult in an upper gastrointestinal biopsy. PCR-based assays that detect the presence of *S. stercoralis* have been developed (78), but these are not commonly used in routine practice.

Parasites that infect in the lung and primarily occupying this location are less common. These include *Paragonimus* and the *Echinococcus* species. There have been a number of molecular tests designed to detect and or characterize these parasites, but these also have not been adopted most clinical practices. This may be because of the infrequency of these infections, especially in North America, as well as the high degree of diagnostic accuracy that may be achieved using the combination of morphologic and serologic studies.

Molecular assays targeting *Paragonimus* could potentially come into use in select reference centers as a diagnostic test, since egg detection in the stool and sputum by morphologic methods is insensitive (79). Intapan et al. designed a PCR assay that detected five eggs of *Paragonimus heterotremus* in 0.6 g of feces, which suggests that such an assay may be useful as a diagnostic test (80). Conversely, serology is an excellent means of documenting infection in patents suspected of having paragonimiasis; it is superior to morphologic methods and may prove superior to molecular methods too (79). To date, molecular methods have been used most extensively to more accurately define the taxonomic relationships of the various *Paragonimus* species than as diagnostic tests, although exceptions exist (81–85).

Similarly, molecular tools have been developed for the detection and differentiation of *Echinococcus* species (86). These, however, are not routinely used in most centers, which commonly rely predominantly on radiologic findings, morphology, and serology to achieve a definitive diagnosis (87). The use of molecular testing for the diagnosis of echinococcosis is more challenging than for *Paragonimus*, since the human host is essentially acting as an intermediate host and parasitic elements are not shed in the stool or sputum. Therefore, invasive methods, such as biopsy or fine-needle aspiration, are needed to obtain the clinical specimen for morphologic or molecular studies. The diagnosis is often clinically suspected and morphologically confirmed, which leaves little need for molecular diagnostics.

VIII. Summary and Conclusion

The lungs are a common portal of entry for a variety of microorganisms. Bacteria, mycobacteria, viruses, fungi, and parasites all cause pulmonary infections. The bacterial pathogens are sundry and range from the routine pathogens, like *S. pneumoniae*, to less commonly encountered bacteria that are more fastidious such as *L. pneumophila*. Molecular methods designed to detect bacteria such as *L. pneumophila* are relatively simple to design and implement, since these organisms are virtually always considered pathogens in a clinical specimen and are not part of the human microbiota. Conversely, the qualitative assays for bacteria such as *S. pneumoniae* and *H. influenzae* are not particularly useful, since these are normally present in the oropharynx and are likely to be normally present in respiratory specimens. The use of quantitative assays for such potential pathogens holds promise as a means of differentiating colonization from disease.

Molecular diagnostic testing is becoming commonplace in the virology and mycobacteriology laboratories. Molecular diagnostic assays may soon replace viral culture in many laboratories. Although such methods are unlikely to replace mycobacterial culture, they will become more commonly utilized to achieve rapid identification. Qualitative assays are useful of detecting viruses such as influenza and respiratory syncytial virus, and mycobacteria such as *M. tuberculosis*. Multiplex assays with post-amplification methods of amplicon segregation hold promise as assays that can detect a number of different viruses simultaneously. Similarly, broad-range PCR followed by DNA sequencing or another method of post-amplification characterization has changed the way mycobacteria are identified. Each of these advances has implications with respect to patient care, laboratory utilization, turn-around time, and cost.

There is an increased interest in the molecular detection of fungal infections. Although there may be certain instances wherein qualitative species-specific assays for particular fungi, such as the dimorphic fungal pathogens, may be useful, it is likely that quantitative broad-range assays or multiplex assays that target the most commonly occurring fungal pathogens will more likely prove useful. These assays, like in situ hybridization, may prove useful for the differentiation of morphologically similar fungi.

Molecular assays are progressively being introduced into molecular microbiology and molecular pathology laboratories. Many of these assays target agents responsible for pulmonary infections. The future will likely hold the implementation of many assays that have already been designed, particularly for obligate pathogens, such as *L. pneumophila*, *M. tuberculosis*, Influenza A and B, and others. In addition, we will also likely see the implementation of novel approaches to diagnosing pneumonia caused by microorganisms that may be normal microbiota or potential environmental contaminants or transient flora.

References

1. Fader RC. Comparison of the Binax NOW Flu A enzyme immunochromatographic assay and R-Mix shell vial culture for the 2003–2004 influenza season. J Clin Microbiol 2005; 43(12): 6133–6135.
2. Reina J, Padilla E, Alonso F, et al. Evaluation of a new dot blot enzyme immunoassay (directigen flu A+B) for simultaneous and differential detection of influenza A and B virus antigens from respiratory samples. J Clin Microbiol 2002; 40(9):3515–3517.
3. Goodrich JS, Miller MB. Comparison of Cepheid's analyte-specific reagents with BD directigen for detection of respiratory syncytial virus. J Clin Microbiol 2007; 45(2):604–606.
4. Stralin K. Usefulness of aetiological tests for guiding antibiotic therapy in community-acquired pneumonia. Int J Antimicrob Agents 2008; 31(1):3–11.
5. Johansson N, Kalin M, Giske CG, et al. Quantitative detection of Streptococcus pneumoniae from sputum samples with real-time quantitative polymerase chain reaction for etiologic diagnosis of community-acquired pneumonia. Diagn Microbiol Infect Dis 2008; 60(3):255–261 [Epub November 26, 2007].
6. Abdeldaim GM, Stralin K, Olcen P, et al. Toward a quantitative DNA-based definition of pneumococcal pneumonia: a comparison of Streptococcus pneumoniae target genes, with special reference to the Spn9802 fragment. Diagn Microbiol Infect Dis 2008; 60(2):143–150 [Epub 2007 October 3, 2007].
7. Kais M, Spindler C, Kalin M, et al. Quantitative detection of Streptococcus pneumoniae, Haemophilus influenzae, and Moraxella catarrhalis in lower respiratory tract samples by real-time PCR. Diagn Microbiol Infect Dis 2006; 55(3):169–178.
8. Carrol ED, Guiver M, Nkhoma S, et al. High pneumococcal DNA loads are associated with mortality in Malawian children with invasive pneumococcal disease. Pediatr Infect Dis J 2007; 26(5):416–422.
9. Bahrani-Mougeot FK, Paster BJ, Coleman S, et al. Molecular analysis of oral and respiratory bacterial species associated with ventilator-associated pneumonia. J Clin Microbiol 2007; 45(5): 1588–1593.
10. Apfalter P, Stoiser B, Barousch W, et al. Community-acquired bacteria frequently detected by means of quantitative polymerase chain reaction in nosocomial early-onset ventilator-associated pneumonia. Crit Care Med 2005; 33(7):1492–1498.
11. Cunha BA. The atypical pneumonias: clinical diagnosis and importance. Clin Microbiol Infect 2006; 12(suppl 3):12–24.
12. Muder RR, Yu VL. Infection due to Legionella species other than L. pneumophila. Clin Infect Dis 2002; 35(8):990–998.
13. Taylor TH, Albrecht MA. Legionella bozemanii cavitary pneumonia poorly responsive to erythromycin: case report and review. Clin Infect Dis 1995; 20(2):329–334.
14. Harrington RD, Woolfrey AE, Bowden R, et al. Legionellosis in a bone marrow transplant center. Bone Marrow Transplant 1996; 18(2):361–368.
15. Lode H, Kemmerich B, Schafer H, et al. Significance of non-pneumophila Legionella species in adult community-acquired and nosocomial pneumonias. Klin Wochenschr 1987; 65(10): 463–468.
16. Greer PW, Chandler FW, Hicklin MD. Rapid demonstration of Legionella pneumophila in unembedded tissue. An adaptation of the Gimenez stain. Am J Clin Pathol 1980; 73(6):788–790.
17. Pounder DJ. Warthin-Starry for Legionella. Am J Clin Pathol 1983; 80(2):276.
18. Wilson DA, Yen-Lieberman B, Reischl U, et al. Detection of Legionella pneumophila by real-time PCR for the mip gene. J Clin Microbiol 2003; 41(7):3327–3330.

19. Koide M, Higa F, Tateyama M, et al. Detection of Legionella species in clinical samples: comparison of polymerase chain reaction and urinary antigen detection kits. Infection 2006; 34(5):264–268.
20. McDonough EA, Barrozo CP, Russell KL, et al. A multiplex PCR for detection of Mycoplasma pneumoniae, Chlamydophila pneumoniae, Legionella pneumophila, and Bordetella pertussis in clinical specimens. Mol Cell Probes 2005; 19(5):314–322.
21. Pinar A, Bozdemir N, Kocagoz T, et al. Rapid detection of bacterial atypical pneumonia agents by multiplex PCR. Cent Eur J Public Health 2004; 12(1):3–5.
22. Diederen BM, Kluytmans JA, Vandenbroucke-Grauls CM, et al. The utility of real-time PCR for the diagnosis of Legionnaires' disease in routine clinical practice. J Clin Microbiol 2008; 46 (2):671–677.
23. Liu FC, Chen PY, Huang FL, et al. Rapid diagnosis of Mycoplasma pneumoniae infection in children by polymerase chain reaction. J Microbiol Immunol Infect 2007; 40(6):507–512.
24. Morozumi M, Ito A, Murayama SY, et al. Assessment of real-time PCR for diagnosis of Mycoplasma pneumoniae pneumonia in pediatric patients. Can J Microbiol 2006; 52(2): 125–129.
25. Kim NH, Lee JA, Eun BW, et al. Comparison of polymerase chain reaction and the indirect particle agglutination antibody test for the diagnosis of Mycoplasma pneumoniae pneumonia in children during two outbreaks. Pediatr Infect Dis J 2007; 26(10):897–903.
26. Oktem IM, Ellidokuz H, Sevinc C, et al. PCR and serology were effective for identifying Chlamydophila pneumoniae in a lower respiratory infection outbreak among military recruits. Jpn J Infect Dis 2007; 60(2–3): 97–101.
27. Troy CJ, Peeling RW, Ellis AG, et al. Chlamydia pneumoniae as a new source of infectious outbreaks in nursing homes. JAMA 1997; 277(15):1214–1218.
28. Bayram A, Kocoglu E, Balci I, et al. Real-time polymerase chain reaction assay for detection of Streptococcus pneumoniae in sputum samples from patients with community-acquired pneumonia. J Microbiol Immunol Infect 2006; 39(6):452–457.
29. Hohenthal U, Vainionpaa R, Meurman O, et al. Aetiological diagnosis of community acquired pneumonia: utility of rapid microbiological methods with respect to disease severity. Scand J Infect Dis 2007:1–8.
30. Sohn JW, Park SC, Choi YH, et al. Atypical pathogens as etiologic agents in hospitalized patients with community-acquired pneumonia in Korea: a prospective multi-center study. J Korean Med Sci 2006; 21(4): 602–607.
31. Saito A, Kohno S, Matsushima T, et al. Prospective multicenter study of the causative organisms of community-acquired pneumonia in adults in Japan. J Infect Chemother 2006; 12(2):63–69.
32. Wang Y, Kong F, Gilbert GL, et al. Use of a multiplex PCR-based reverse line blot (mPCR/RLB) hybridisation assay for the rapid identification of bacterial pathogens. Clin Microbiol Infect 2008; 14:155–160.
33. Jennings LC, Anderson TP, Beynon KA, et al. Incidence and characteristics of viral community-acquired pneumonia in adults. Thorax 2008; 63(1):42–48.
34. Stralin K, Korsgaard J, Olcen P. Evaluation of a multiplex PCR for bacterial pathogens applied to bronchoalveolar lavage. Eur Respir J 2006; 28(3):568–575.
35. Lebrun L, Espinasse F, Poveda JD, et al. Evaluation of nonradioactive DNA probes for identification of mycobacteria. J Clin Microbiol 1992; 30(9):2476–2478.
36. Evans KD, Nakasone AS, Sutherland PA, et al. Identification of Mycobacterium tuberculosis and Mycobacterium avium-M. intracellulare directly from primary BACTEC cultures by using acridinium-ester-labeled DNA probes. J Clin Microbiol 1992; 30(9):2427–2431.
37. Somoskovi A, Hotaling JE, Fitzgerald M, et al. False-positive results for Mycobacterium celatum with the AccuProbe Mycobacterium tuberculosis complex assay. J Clin Microbiol 2000; 38(7): 2743–2745.

38. Tortoli E, Simonetti MT, Lavinia F. Evaluation of reformulated chemiluminescent DNA probe (AccuProbe) for culture identification of Mycobacterium kansasii. J Clin Microbiol 1996; 34(11): 2838–2840.
39. Lefmann M, Schweickert B, Buchholz P, et al. Evaluation of peptide nucleic acid-fluorescence in situ hybridization for identification of clinically relevant mycobacteria in clinical specimens and tissue sections. J Clin Microbiol 2006; 44(10):3760–3767.
40. Scanga CA, Bafica A, Sher A. Viral gene expression in HIV transgenic mice is activated by Mycobacterium tuberculosis and suppressed after antimycobacterial chemotherapy. J Infect Dis 2007; 195(2):246–254.
41. Petrini B. Non-tuberculous mycobacterial infections. Scand J Infect Dis 2006; 38(4):246–255.
42. Minh VD, Hanh LQ, Vu M. Clinical use of nucleic-acid-amplification tests. Chest 2000; 118(3): 574–575.
43. Nucleic acid amplification tests for tuberculosis. MMWR Morb Mortal Wkly Rep 1996; 45(43): 950–952.
44. Rapid diagnostic tests for tuberculosis: what is the appropriate use? American Thoracic Society Workshop. Am J Respir Crit Care Med 1997; 155(5):1804–1814.
45. Mokaddas E, Ahmad S. Development and evaluation of a multiplex PCR for rapid detection and differentiation of Mycobacterium tuberculosis complex members from non-tuberculous mycobacteria. Jpn J Infect Dis 2007; 60(2–3):140–144.
46. Gomez MP, Herrera-Leon L, Jimenez MS, et al. Comparison of GenoType MTBC with RFLP-PCR and multiplex PCR to identify Mycobacterium tuberculosis complex species. Eur J Clin Microbiol Infect Dis 2007; 26(1):63–66.
47. Soo PC, Horng YT, Hsueh PR, et al. Direct and simultaneous identification of Mycobacterium tuberculosis complex (MTBC) and Mycobacterium tuberculosis (MTB) by rapid multiplex nested PCR-ICT assay. J Microbiol Methods 2006; 66(3):440–448.
48. Shrestha NK, Tuohy MJ, Hall GS, et al. Detection and differentiation of Mycobacterium tuberculosis and nontuberculous mycobacterial isolates by real-time PCR. J Clin Microbiol 2003; 41(11):5121–5126.
49. Tuohy MJ, Hall GS, Sholtis M, et al. Pyrosequencing as a tool for the identification of common isolates of Mycobacterium sp. Diagn Microbiol Infect Dis 2005; 51(4):245–250.
50. Miller N, Infante S, Cleary T. Evaluation of the LiPA MYCOBACTERIA assay for identification of mycobacterial species from BACTEC 12B bottles. J Clin Microbiol 2000; 38(5):1915–1919.
51. Tortoli E, Mariottini A, Mazzarelli G. Evaluation of INNO-LiPA MYCOBACTERIA v2: improved reverse hybridization multiple DNA probe assay for mycobacterial identification. J Clin Microbiol 2003; 41(9):4418–4420.
52. Fukushima M, Kakinuma K, Hayashi H, et al., Detection and identification of Mycobacterium species isolates by DNA microarray. J Clin Microbiol 2003; 41(6):2605–2615.
53. Chemlal K, Portaels F. Molecular diagnosis of nontuberculous mycobacteria. Curr Opin Infect Dis 2003; 16(2):77–83.
54. Roberts GD, Bottger EC, Stockman L. Methods for the rapid identification of mycobacterial species. Clin Lab Med 1996; 16(3):603–615.
55. Ahmad S, Araj GF, Akbar PK, et al. Characterization of rpoB mutations in rifampin-resistant Mycobacterium tuberculosis isolates from the Middle East. Diagn Microbiol Infect Dis 2000; 38(4):227–232.
56. Yang Z, Durmaz R, Yang D, et al. Simultaneous detection of isoniazid, rifampin, and ethambutol resistance of Mycobacterium tuberculosis by a single multiplex allele-specific polymerase chain reaction (PCR) assay. Diagn Microbiol Infect Dis 2005; 53(3):201–208.
57. Legoff J, Kara R, Moulin F, et al. Evaluation of the one-step multiplex real-time reverse transcription-PCR ProFlu-1 assay for detection of influenza A and influenza B viruses and respiratory syncytial viruses in children. J Clin Microbiol 2008; 46:789–791.

58. Brittain-Long R, Nord S, Olofsson S, et al. Multiplex real-time PCR for detection of respiratory tract infections. J Clin Virol 2008; 41(1):53–56.
59. Yoo SJ, Kuak EY, Shin BM. Detection of 12 respiratory viruses with two-set multiplex reverse transcriptase-PCR assay using a dual priming oligonucleotide system. Korean J Lab Med 2007; 27(6):420–427.
60. Pehler-Harrington K, Khanna M, Waters CR, et al. Rapid detection and identification of human adenovirus species by adenoplex, a multiplex PCR-enzyme hybridization assay. J Clin Microbiol 2004; 42(9):4072–4076.
61. Xu W, McDonough MC, Erdman DD. Species-specific identification of human adenoviruses by a multiplex PCR assay. J Clin Microbiol 2000; 38(11):4114–4120.
62. Xu W, Erdman DD. Type-specific identification of human adenovirus 3, 7, and 21 by a multiplex PCR assay. J Med Virol 2001; 64(4):537–542.
63. Camps M, Pumarola T, Moreno A, et al. Virological diagnosis in community-acquired pneumonia in immunocompromised patients. Eur Respir J 2008; 31(3):618–624 [Epub October 24, 2007].
64. Peiris JS, Yuen KY, Osterhaus AD, et al. The severe acute respiratory syndrome. N Engl J Med 2003; 349(25):2431–2441.
65. Kiechle FL, Zhang X, Holland-Staley CA. The -omics era and its impact. Arch Pathol Lab Med 2004; 128(12):1337–1345.
66. Percivalle E, Sarasini A, Visai L, et al. Rapid detection of human metapneumovirus strains in nasopharyngeal aspirates and shell vial cultures by monoclonal antibodies. J Clin Microbiol 2005; 43(7):3443–3446.
67. Maertzdorf J, Wang CK, Brown JB, et al. Real-time reverse transcriptase PCR assay for detection of human metapneumoviruses from all known genetic lineages. J Clin Microbiol 2004; 42(3):981–986.
68. Li H, McCormac MA, Estes RW, et al. Simultaneous detection and high-throughput identification of a panel of RNA viruses causing respiratory tract infections. J Clin Microbiol 2007; 45 (7):2105–2109.
69. Mahony J, Chong S, Merante F, et al. Development of a respiratory virus panel test for detection of twenty human respiratory viruses by use of multiplex PCR and a fluid microbead-based assay. J Clin Microbiol 2007; 45(9):2965–2970.
70. Hayden RT, Qian X, Roberts GD, et al. In situ hybridization for the identification of yeastlike organisms in tissue section. Diagn Mol Pathol 2001; 10(1):15–23.
71. Martagon-Villamil J, Shrestha N, Sholtis M, et al. Identification of Histoplasma capsulatum from culture extracts by real-time PCR. J Clin Microbiol 2003; 41(3):1295–1298.
72. Guedes HL, Guimaraes AJ, Muniz Mde M, et al. PCR assay for identification of histoplasma capsulatum based on the nucleotide sequence of the M antigen. J Clin Microbiol 2003; 41(2): 535–539.
73. Bialek R, Gonzalez GM, Begerow D, et al. Coccidioidomycosis and blastomycosis: advances in molecular diagnosis. FEMS Immunol Med Microbiol 2005; 45(3):355–360.
74. Bialek R, Cirera AC, Herrmann T, et al. Nested PCR assays for detection of Blastomyces dermatitidis DNA in paraffin-embedded canine tissue. J Clin Microbiol 2003; 41(1):205–208.
75. Binnicker MJ, Buckwalter SP, Eisberner JJ, et al. Detection of Coccidioides species in clinical specimens by real-time PCR. J Clin Microbiol 2007; 45(1):173–178.
76. Bialek R, Kern J, Herrmann T, et al. PCR assays for identification of Coccidioides posadasii based on the nucleotide sequence of the antigen 2/proline-rich antigen. J Clin Microbiol 2004; 42(2):778–783.
77. Procop GW, Roberts GD. Emerging fungal diseases: the importance of the host. Clin Lab Med 2004; 24(3):691–719, vi–vii.
78. Melville LA, Sykes AM, McCarthy JS. The beta-tubulin genes of two Strongyloides species. Exp Parasitol 2006; 112(3):144–151.

79. Blair D, Xu ZB, Agatsuma T. Paragonimiasis and the genus Paragonimus. Adv Parasitol 1999; 42: 113–222.
80. Intapan PM, Wongkham C, Imtawil KJ, et al. Detection of Paragonimus heterotremus eggs in experimentally infected cats by a polymerase chain reaction-based method. J Parasitol 2005; 91(1):195–198.
81. Blair D, Davis GM, Wu B. Evolutionary relationships between trematodes and snails emphasizing schistosomes and paragonimids. Parasitology 2001; 123(suppl):S229–S243.
82. Le TH, Van De N, Blair D, et al. Paragonimus heterotremus Chen and Hsia (1964), in Vietnam: a molecular identification and relationships of isolates from different hosts and geographical origins. Acta Trop 2006; 98(1):25–33.
83. Chang ZS, Wu B, Blair D, et al. Gene sequencing for identification of Paragonimus eggs from a human case. Zhongguo Ji Sheng Chong Xue Yu Ji Sheng Chong Bing Za Zhi 2000; 18(4):213–215.
84. Schuster H, Agada FO, Anderson AR, et al. Otitis media and a neck lump—current diagnostic challenges for Paragonimus-like trematode infections. J Infect 2007; 54(2):e103–e106.
85. Devi KR, Narain K, Bhattacharya S, et al. Pleuropulmonary paragonimiasis due to Paragonimus heterotremus: molecular diagnosis, prevalence of infection and clinicoradiological features in an endemic area of northeastern India. Trans R Soc Trop Med Hyg 2007; 101(8):786–792.
86. Siles-Lucas MM, Gottstein BB. Molecular tools for the diagnosis of cystic and alveolar echinococcosis. Trop Med Int Health 2001; 6(6):463–475.
87. Garcia HH, Moro PL, Schantz PM. Zoonotic helminth infections of humans: echinococcosis, cysticercosis and fascioliasis. Curr Opin Infect Dis 2007; 20(5):489–494.

26
Nonmalignant Versus Malignant Proliferations on Lung Biopsy

ARMANDO E. FRAIRE
Department of Pathology, University of Massachusetts Medical School, Worcester, Massachusetts, U.S.A.

I. Introduction

The establishment of a tissue diagnosis holds a very special place in clinical chest medicine (1). This is particularly true in atypical (borderline) epithelial or mesenchymal proliferations of the lung. The purpose of this chapter is twofold. First, it discusses the histopathology of cell proliferations that may be seen by the diagnostic surgical pathologist on lung tissue biopsy on course of his or her daily practice, and second, it provides the surgical pathologist with histopathologic hints that may be useful in differentiating nonmalignant from malignant tissue proliferations. This differentiation between malignant and nonmalignant cell proliferations may range from the exquisitely simple, i.e., differentiating a squamous papilloma from an invasive squamous cell carcinoma, to the extremely difficult, i.e., differentiating an atypical alveolar cell hyperplasia from a low-grade bronchioloalveolar cell carcinoma.

The chapter is limited to three major categories of cell proliferations: (*i*) squamous cell proliferations, (*ii*) alveolar cell proliferations, and (*iii*) spindle cell proliferations. In each of these categories emphasis is laid on the task of differentiating such cell proliferations from their malignant prototypical counterparts, namely, squamous cell carcinoma and spindle cell carcinomas and sarcomas. Benign epithelial neoplasms, spindle cell neoplasms, biphasic neoplasms, and other uncommon endobronchial neoplasms are further discussed elsewhere in this volume. Also, the important differentiation between atypical adenomatous hyperplasia (AAH) and adenocarcinoma is described in chapter 30 of this volume.

II. Squamous Cell Proliferations

A. Squamous Cell Metaplasia

Squamous metaplasia in interstitial pulmonary fibrosis occurs as isolate mounds or aggregates of cytologically bland squamous epithelial cells, lining remodeled air spaces in case of organizing stage of diffuse alveolar damage, well-established interstitial pulmonary fibrosis, older pulmonary infarctions, and bronchiectasis. These squamous proliferations present no major diagnostic challenge to the pathologist unless they occur in a florid, extensive fashion and are associated with cytologic atypia. In these instances, careful attention to the histopathology of the underlying lesion should facilitate differentiation from

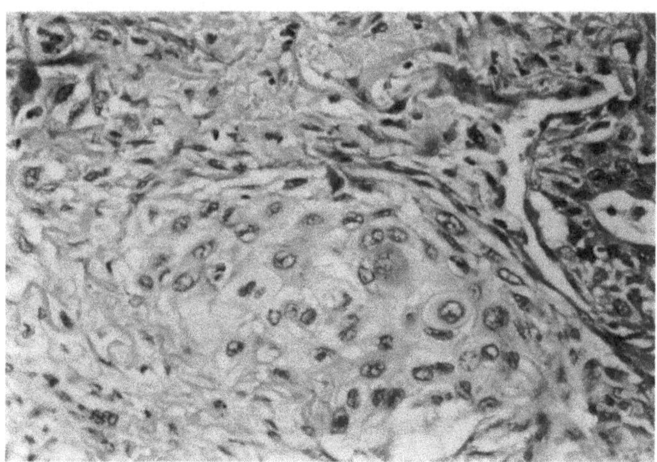

Figure 1 Squamous metaplasia arising in the setting of interstitial pulmonary fibrosis. Note aggregate of bland looking squamous epithelial cells (Hematoxylin and eosin, 200×).

a well-differentiated squamous cell carcinoma. Necrosis and keratin pearl formations generally do not occur and invasion of the surrounding parenchyma is not seen (Fig. 1). A potential diagnostic pitfall is the regenerative atypical squamous metaplasia that appears secondary to repetitive injury (i.e., biopsy sites) (2). This lesion is similar to the necrotizing sialometaplasia that occurs in salivary gland tissue of the palate and must be differentiated from ordinary squamous metaplasia. It is associated with necrosis and focal atypia and occurs in a background of epithelial ulceration. A distinctive histopathologic feature seen in this condition is occlusion of mucous bronchial glands by plugs of squamous epithelium.

B. Squamous Cell Papilloma and Papillomatosis

The family of squamous cell papillary lesions encompasses benign endobronchial, sometimes intrapulmonary, lesions that occur as single or multiple lesions. Distinction between squamous cell papilloma and squamous cell carcinoma is usually made with no difficulty. However, cases of florid squamous cell papillomatosis may pose a problem. Solitary squamous cell papillomas are wart-like lesions that protrude in the bronchial lumen. Microscopically, squamous cell papillomas are made up of fine papillae containing bland nonkeratinizing or minimally keratinizing squamous epithelial cells and do not differ from those encountered in the skin and mucous membranes (Fig. 2). The squamous epithelial cells, often multilayered, line fibrovascular stalks containing minimal amount of chronic inflammatory cells (3,4). Although, generally bland and nonatypical, squamous papillomas may contain focal areas of condylomatous atypia (Figs. 3–5) (4). Squamous papillomas are noninvasive lesions.

Papillomatosis of the larynx and tracheobronchial tree is a much more aggressive lesion. Virtual bronchoscopy is a new diagnostic tool for viewing helical/spiral computed tomographic images of the tracheobronchial tree and has proven useful in the localization, sampling, and eventual diagnosis of this important lesion (5). This lesion differs from

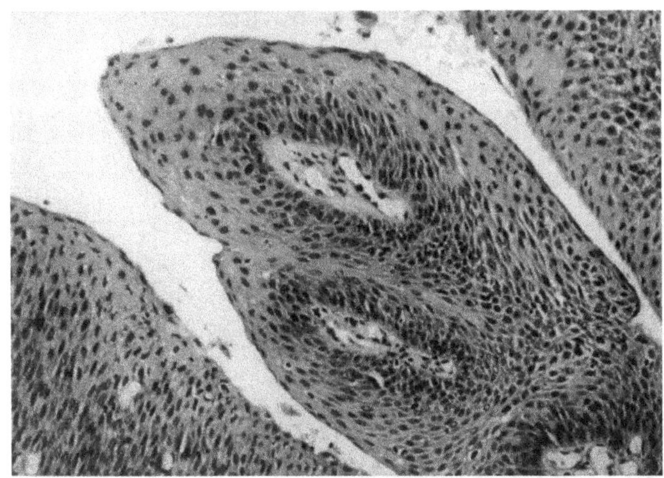

Figure 2 Squamous papilloma. Note fibrovascular cores lined by proliferating squamous epithelia (Hematoxylin and eosin, 100×). *Source*: Courtesy of Dr. P. Cagle.

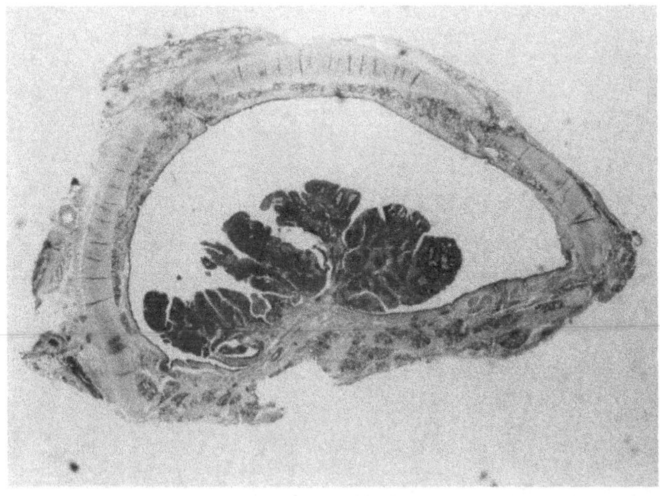

Figure 3 Cross section of surgically resected right upper lobe bronchus showing (condylomatous) papilloma partially obstructing lumen (Hematoxylin and eosin, 50×). *Source*: From Ref. 4.

solitary squamous cell papilloma in regard to its multiplicity and in regard to the greater degree of cytologic atypia and the development of carcinoma in up to 3% of patients. Histologically, however, most cases of squamous cell papillomatosis retain the mature nonkeratinizing or minimally keratinizing squamous epithelium, which is also seen in solitary squamous cell papillomas. Although locally aggressive, these lesions do not

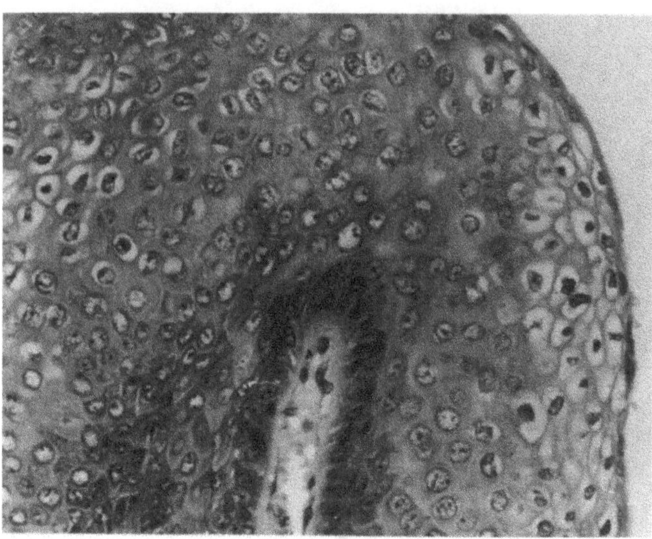

Figure 4 Condylomatous papilloma. Note papillary frond with marked koilocytic atypia (Hematoxylin and eosin, 400×). *Source*: From Ref. 4.

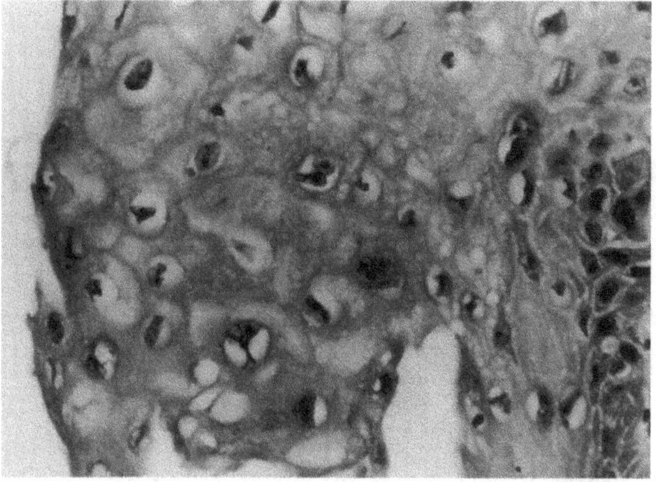

Figure 5 Condylomatous papilloma. Note stratified squamous epithelium showing greater detail of koilocytic cells with marked nuclear atypia (Hematoxylin and eosin, 500×). *Source*: From Ref. 4.

metastasize. As shown in Table 1, there is some overlap between the histologic features of squamous papillomas, papillomatosis, and squamous cell carcinoma. Features favoring benignancy include a single or solitary lesion and a papillary architecture that does not differ significantly from that seen in cutaneous papillomas. A lesion confined to the

Table 1 Squamous Cell Papilloma Vs. Squamous Papillomatosis Vs. Well-differentiated Squamous Cell Carcinoma

Papilloma	Papillomatosis	Squamous carcinoma
Exophytic	Exo and endophytic	Exo and endophytic
Fine papillae	Fine papillae	Broad papillae
Nonkeratinizing or minimally keratinizing	Nonkeratinizing or minimally keratinizing	Keratinizing and nonkeratinizing
No atypia	Atypia if present is slight and constant throughout	Atypia is increased at base
Noninvasive	Noninvasive	Invasive

Source: From Ref. 11.

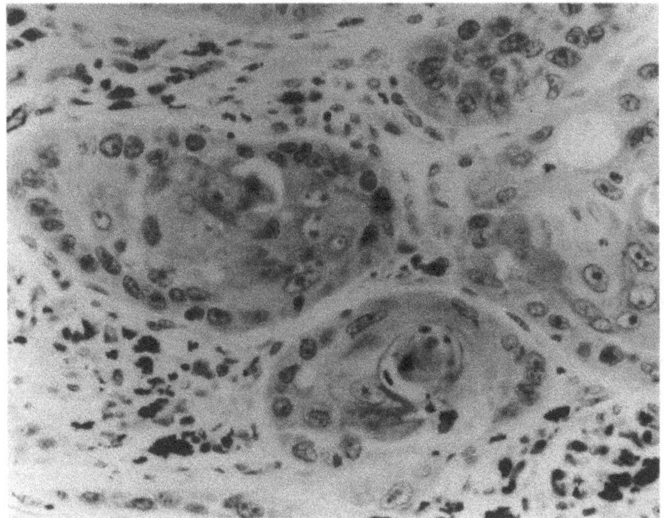

Figure 6 Squamous cell carcinoma. Note nesting pattern and formation of keratin pearls (Hematoxylin and eosin, 400×). *Source*: Courtesy of Dr. Barbara Banner.

epithelium and koilocytic changes suggesting human papilloma virus (HPV) infection further support benignancy. In problematic cases, in situ hybridization and polymerase chain reaction for HPV DNA may be of help (6). On the other hand, extension of a papillary lesion over a broad surface, multiplicity of lesions, and presence of necrosis or significant cellular atypia will favor malignancy. Intercellular bridging, squamous pearl formation, individual cell keratinization, and growth in a pavement-like fashion are the major histopathologic features of squamous cell carcinoma (Fig. 6). Intercellular bridges exhibit regular spacing that resembles railroad tracks (Fig. 7). This useful histologic feature helps to distinguish squamous cell carcinoma from nonspecific intercellular extensions found in carcinomas of various types (7). In well-differentiated carcinomas these features are readily apparent, but in poorly differentiated tumors they maybe difficult to ascertain. There are

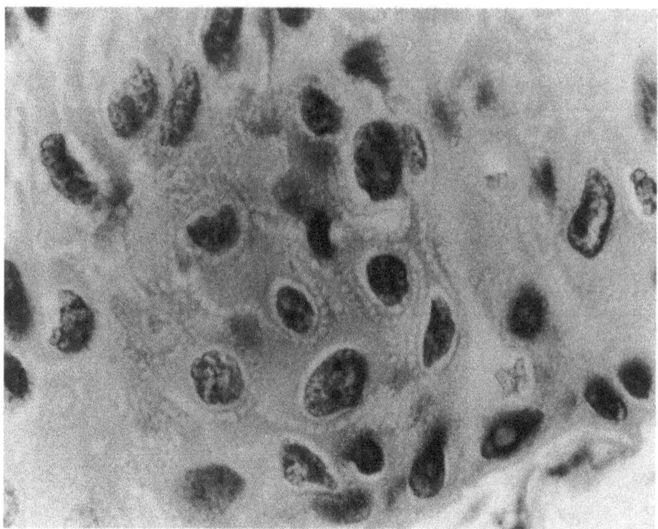

Figure 7 Squamous cell carcinoma. Intercellular bridging shows regular spacing resembling railroad tracks (Hematoxylin and eosin, 600×).

several unusual histologic subtypes of squamous cell carcinoma, including small cell, basaloid variant, and the exophytic endobronchial types, that differ from conventional squamous cell carcinoma and are likely to present diagnostic difficulties. In these instances, attention to architecture and cellular features will facilitate the diagnosis. Invasion of subepithelial lamina and spread to adjoining structures or regional lymph nodes are further unequivocal features favoring a malignant cell proliferation (Table 1).

C. Transitional Cell Papillomas

These rare benign growths are characterized histologically by fibrovascular cores lined by transitional epithelium similar to that seen in papillary growths of the urothelium and nasopharynx. Invasion was not observed in any of three cases cited in the literature (8). Transitional cell papillomas are said to be inherently more prone to undergo malignant change, but this assertion is based on individual case reports only. In cases of transitional cell papillomas occurring in association with local spread and/or cytologic atypia of any degree, the main task of the pathologists will be to differentiate such lesions from metastasizing transitional cell carcinomas to the lung. In these instances, a previous diagnosis of urothelial carcinoma and/or focal necrosis may help to make the distinction. Necrosis is distinctly uncommon in transitional cell papillomas.

D. Mixed Cell Papillomas

These benign neoplasms differ from squamous and transitional papillomas in that they contain epithelial elements of diverse nature, including columnar, cuboidal, ciliated, and

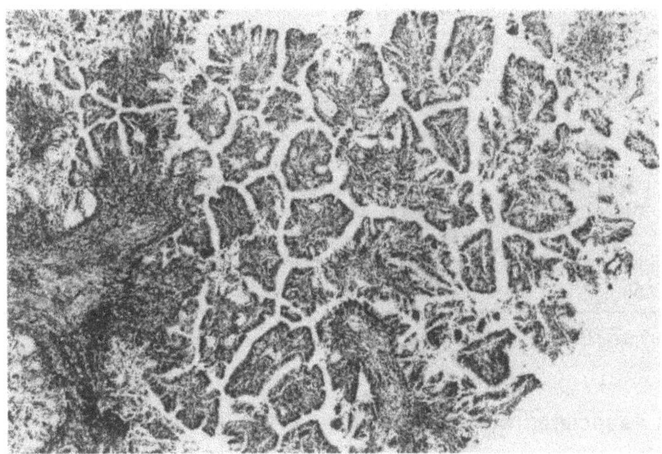

Figure 8 Papillary variant of low-grade mucoepidermoid carcinoma. Note papillary growth almost completely obstructing the bronchial lumen (Hematoxylin and eosin, 30×). *Source*: From Ref. 10.

squamous epithelia. The underlying (subepithelial) tissue consists of a fibrous stroma with foci of hyalinization and granulation tissue (8). Papillomas lined entirely by columnar epithelium do occur. In a series of eight such cases, some were lined by columnar ciliated epithelium, and others showed combinations of cuboidal and columnar epithelia, with or without stratification (9). In a reported case of columnar papilloma, the cells were aligned as a single layer, with most cells having basal nuclei and clear cytoplasm. Mitotic activity and mucicarminophilia were not detected (9). Mixed cell papillomas further need to be differentiated from the papillary variant of low-grade mucoepidermoid carcinoma, a tumor with clear papillary architecture and prominent mucus-secreting cellular components (10,11) (Fig. 8).

III. Alveolar Cell Proliferations

Atypical alveolar cell hyperplasias unassociated with fibrotic, inflammatory, or neoplastic lung conditions are rare, but do occur. In a study of 100 consecutive patients who came to autopsy without any known clinical or radiographic pulmonary disease, two had atypical alveolar cell hyperplasia. In that study, the criteria used to define hyperplasia included absence of any significant fibrosis or inflammation, a single row of cells, and atypical alveolar cells at least double the size of neighboring nonatypical cells. The hyperplastic foci were minute, were not visible at gross inspection, and showed greater than 10% positivity of the atypical cells when studied with C-erb-2 and p53 protein immunostains, suggesting a neoplastic potential (12). Most other atypical alveolar cell hyperplasias occur in association with diffuse alveolar damage (13) or coexistence with adenocarcinoma of lung (14–16), but a few have been reported following chemotherapy in adolescent cancer patients (17) and rarely in association with tuberous sclerosis (18,19).

Table 2 RA of the Peripheral Alveolar Epithelium Vs. BAC

RA	BAC
Associated with parenchymal damage or fibrosis larger than area of epithelial atypia	Interstitial desmoplasia is minimal and limited to septae lined by neoplastic cells
Mixed cell types	Uniformity of cell type
Mixed degrees of cytologic atypia	Uniformity of cytologic atypia
Rare, small intranuclear inclusions	Frequent, large intranuclear inclusions
Cilia may be present	Cilia not present
Blends into adjacent epithelium	More abrupt demarcation from adjacent epithelium
Attached to septa in single row	Projecting tufts or buds

Abbreviations: RA, reactive atypias; BAC, bronchoalveolar carcinoma. *Source*: From Ref. 20.

A. Hyperplasias Associated with Diffuse Alveolar Damage

The acute lung injury syndrome is characterized in part by severe atypical hyperplasia of type II pneumocytes. These hyperplastic cells line distal air spaces, where they protrude into the lumen in a hobnail fashion. Diffuse alveolar damage is a histologic term used to describe acute lung injury syndrome and encompasses two phases, exudative and organizing (13,20). Although these two phases overlap, some reactive cells such as type II pneumocytes are more likely to be present in the organizing stage. Most often these alveolar cell proliferations are associated with injuries related to viral infection and chemotherapy. Differentiating reactive proliferations of the peripheral epithelium from bronchioloalveolar carcinoma on a lung biopsy can be challenging and particularly worrisome at frozen section. Reactive type II pneumocytes and metaplastic epithelium with or without cytologic atypia often line airspace interstitium in lung injuries associated with interstitial inflammation and fibrosis. The reactive type II pneumocytes are cuboidal to columnar, with enlarged, sometimes hobnailed, nuclei (20). Histologic features most helpful in distinguishing reactive atypias such as seen in diffuse alveolar damage and bronchioloalveolar carcinoma are listed in Table 2. Nonatypical cuboidal metaplasia of the alveolar epithelium may occur in association with diffuse interstitial fibrosis or localized areas of fibrosis of varying etiology. These metaplastic processes can be recognized because of the orderly uniform appearance of the alveolar epithelial cells. These metaplastic cells lack significant atypia, and their presence amid fibrotic scars facilitates their recognition.

B. Atypical Hyperplasias Associated with Adenocarcinoma

Atypical alveolar cell hyperplasias most often occur in association with a coexisting adenocarcinoma, usually bronchioloalveolar carcinoma, but may present de novo. These proliferations are now recognized by the World Health Organization as precancerous lesions and are currently known as AAH (21–23). As noted earlier, AAH and related lesions are discussed at greater length in chapter 30 of this volume.

C. Alveolar Adenomas

Adenomas of peripheral lung are much less frequently encountered than reactive atypias and thus play a lesser role in the differential diagnosis of bronchioloalveolar carcinoma.

These rare lesions characteristically present as incidental solitary peripheral coin lesions, which are usually excised to rule out cancer (20). Adenomas differ fundamentally from atypical hyperplasias in that they are discrete, well-defined lesions. The most important consideration is to be aware that these rare entities exist (20). If difficulty in categorizing a peripheral lung mass is encountered, alveolar adenoma should be included in the differential. Most alveolar adenomas are well-circumscribed nodular lesions. They may be mucinous, papillary, or bronchioloalveolar in type. Alveolar adenomas are generally detected clinically as asymptomatic coin lesions with an average diameter of 1.8 cm. They are well defined and display a characteristic central cystic area with multiple smaller cysts that are lined by type II pneumocytes (24,25). Alveolar adenomas differ from sclerosing hemangioma in that the latter shows an interstitial proliferation of distinct round cells within the stroma. Hamartomas, which may also contain spaces lined by type II pneumocytes, are easily recognized by the presence of adipose or chondroid tissue components. Lymphangiomas, on the other hand, may represent a difficult diagnostic problem. In these benign tumors, prominent endothelial cells may be mistaken as attenuated pneumocytes. In these instances, CD31, CD34, and factor VIII immunostains may help to resolve the issue. Mucinous cystadenomas consist of well-circumscribed unilocular or multilocular thin-walled macrocysts filled with abundant mucin and lined by nonciliated, columnar goblet cells with abundant apical mucin (26). Rare mucinous cystadenocarcinomas may also occur and are characterized by cytologic and architectural atypia. Peripheral papillary adenomas are well-circumscribed lesions made up of uniform nonciliated cuboidal to columnar cells lining multiple branching papillary fronds with delicate fibrovascular cores. Papillary adenoma of type II pneumocytes occurs as a well-circumscribed papillary tumor made up of cuboidal and sometimes Clara and ciliated cells (27) (Fig. 9). Immunocytochemically, this tumor reacts positively with antibodies to surfactant apoproteins A and B and carcinoembryonic antigen (26). Bronchioloalveolar carcinomas may have predominant papillary

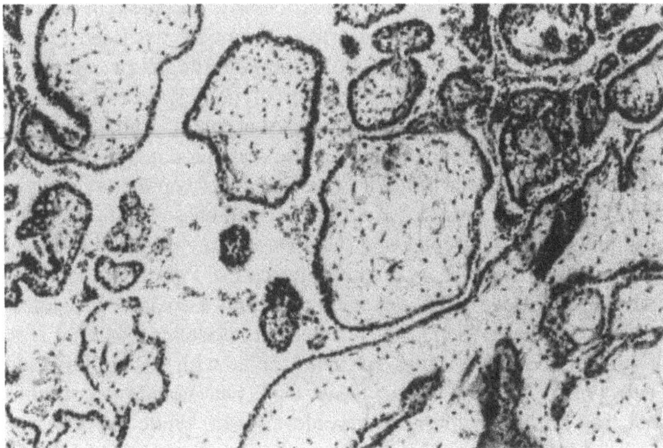

Figure 9 Papillary adenoma of type II pneumocytes. Note papillary growth with edematous fibrous cores and cuboidal, uniform looking cell lining the fibrous cores (Hematoxylin and eosin, 33×). *Source*: From Ref. 23.

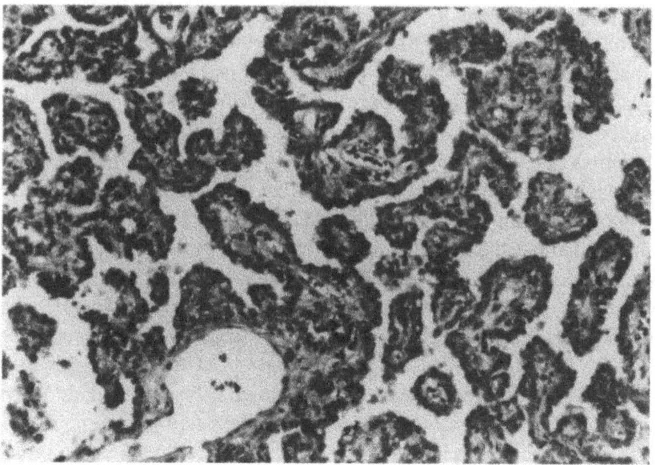

Figure 10 Bronchoalveolar carcinoma with predominant papillary pattern. Note uniformity of tumor cells lining fibrovascular cores (Hematoxylin and eosin, 100×).

architecture with a bland, cytologic appearance (Fig. 10). In these instances, invasion of the surrounding stroma will facilitate separation from papillary adenoma. However, in the case reported by Mori et al., the adenoma was associated with transbronchial dissemination and vascular invasion suggesting a malignant potential for this tumor (27). Bronchioloalveolar adenomas show atypical hyperchromatic nuclei, occasional small intranuclear inclusions, and sometimes striking cytologic atypia (28). Metaplastic epithelium taking the form of bronchiolar, squamous, or goblet cell types of epithelium may also simulate malignant epithelial cell proliferations. Metaplastic epithelium is particularly common in scarred interstitium around airways, where it has been referred to as Lambert sis based on the hypothesis that the epithelium has spread to the alveolar septa through the canals of Lambert. These nonspecific changes are part of the limited stereotypic response of the lung to a wide variety of injuries. Metaplastic epithelium and reactive atypia of epithelium may be found in focal scars, in diffuse interstitial fibrosis and diffuse alveolar damage of known cause, as well as in acute interstitial pneumonia of unknown cause. These epithelial changes are important for two reasons: (*I*) benign reactive atypias and metaphases should not be misdiagnosed as carcinomas, and (*ii*) these atypias and metaphases are suspected of being precursors to carcinomas which may arise in scars in some cases. Pulmonary nodules resembling bronchi alveolar carcinoma were reported by Travis and associates in adolescent cancer patients following chemotherapy (17). The lesions were nodular, 1.0 cm or less, and were histologically characterized by atypical epithelial cells with a papillary and growth pattern and were surrounded by normal lung tissue (17). One nodule was immunoreactive to antibodies reacting with the carcinoembryonic antigen, while another was aneuploid, suggesting that these lesions were early cancers, despite the unusual clinical context (17). A peculiar multifocal micronodular proliferation of type II pneumocytes was reported in patients with tuberous sclerosis (18). In this case, the nodules were small, 1.6 mm or less, and were composed of thickened fibrotic alveolar septae lined by pleomorphic type II pneumocytes (18). The type II pneumocyte were immunoreactive for cytokeratin, surfactant, and Ber-Ep4, but negative for an antibody recognizing Clara cell antigens, suggesting an epithelial origin from type II pneumocytes (18). While rare, this type of alveolar cell proliferation must be kept in the differential diagnosis of this lesion with atypical alveolar cell hyperplasia, which may be a precursor of adenocarcinoma. Similar pneumocyte proliferations without nuclear atypia were reported earlier in patients with tuberous sclerosis (19). Other lesions that may be confused with multifocal micronodular pneumocyte proliferations include papillary adenoma of type II pneumocyte, alveolar adenoma, and chemodectoma-like bodies. Papillary adenoma of type II pneumocytes and alveolar adenoma tend to be larger, solitary lesions. Minute meningothelial-like nodules (so-called chemodectomas) may be multiple and tend to be perivenular in location and to have a "zellballen"-like arrangement. Further, they stain with epithelial membrane antigen, but not with keratin (18).

IV. Spindle Cell Proliferations

A. Mesenchymal Cystic Hamartoma

This rare benign form of spindle fibrous cell proliferation is likely to have a peripheral subpleural location and occurs primarily in children. Its closeness to the pleura may result in the development of spontaneous pneumothorax, and in this instance, the histopathology may be complicated or obscured by changes secondary to the pneumothorax. The stroma of the cystic lesion is made up of poorly differentiated mesenchymal cells, while the cystic component is lined by epithelial, cuboidal to low columnar cells with and without cilia. Importantly, the cystic cavity may be in continuity with the lumen of small airways (29,30). Mesenchymal cystic hamartoma must be differentiated from fibrochondromatous hamartomas with predominance of fibrous tissue component, benign metastasizing leiomyomas, fibrohistiocytic tumors, and metastasizing sarcomas, particularly low-grade endometrial stromal sarcomas and lymphangioleiomyomatosis (LAM) (29,30). Histopathologic features helpful in separating mesenchymal cystic hamartomas from the aforementioned entities include fibrous hamartomas, which on multiple sectioning may show minimal fat or cartilage and are unlikely to show cystic change. Benign metastasing leiomyomas occur exclusively in women and are made up of smooth muscle fibers with blunt-ended nuclei and show immunoreactivity to pan-actin and smooth muscle actin. Fibrohistiocytic tumors may have foamy histiocytic cells, which are not seen in mesenchymal cystic hamartoma. Markers of histiocytic differentiation such as CD 68, lyzozyme, α-1-antitrypsin, and α-1-antichymotrypsin may be of help, if positive, in differentiating fibrohistiocytic tumors from mesenchymal cystic hamartomas. Metastasizing sarcomas to the lung and particularly low-grade endometrial sarcomas must also be differentiated from cystic mesenchymal hamartoma. In this instance, the clinical history and immunostaining with CD10 (which is positive in endometrial stromal sarcomas) may be of help. Metastatic sarcomas from the uterus may be estrogen and/or progesterone positive. As was the case with benign metastasizing leiomyomas, LAM occurs almost exclusively in women. In LAM, the spindle cell proliferation occurs primarily around lymphatics and small airways and subpleurally. Nuclei are generally bland and mitosis is not seen. Immunoreactivity to S-100 protein, melanoma-specific antigen (HMB-45), and estrogen and progesterone receptors are of value in identifying this lesion (31,32).

B. Inflammatory Pseudotumor

Also known as plasma cell granuloma and fibrous histiocytoma, inflammatory pseudotumor of the lung is a benign lung tumor that is histologically characterized by a mixture of spindle cell mesenchymal cells and variable numbers of inflammatory mononuclear cells. This mixture of cell types has led to the formulation of clinically useful histopathologic classifications. For example, Matsubara et al. studied 32 cases and grouped them as follows: organizing pneumonia pattern (44%), fibrous histiocytoma pattern (44%), and lymphoplasmacytic pattern (12%). These classifications are believed to be useful, as they allow for comparisons to be made among cases from diverse institutions (33).

Recent data derived from immunohistochemical and ultrastructural studies have suggested a hybrid myofibroblastic origin of this tumor. The term inflammatory myofibroblastic tumor has been recently proposed and appears to be gaining acceptance (20). The tumoral stroma is made up primarily of bland-appearing spindle cells with variable numbers of inflammatory cells, including plasma cells, lymphocytes, and eosinophils. Glandular-like elements resembling bronchiolar epithelium may be seen but generally represent entrapped epithelium. Necrosis and mitotic activity are generally not seen, and if prominent, they would argue against the diagnosis. The spindle cells are negative for the S-100 protein CD34 and cytokeratin but react strongly with antibodies directed toward vimentin and actin (34–36). Expression of ALK1 and p80 occurs in about 40% of the cases (36). On the other hand, p53 immunoreactivity is rare but clinically significant in positive cases because of the possibility of recurrence or malignant transformation (36).

Inflammatory pseudotumors must be differentiated from bronchiolitis obliterans organizing pneumonia (BOOP). BOOP differs from inflammatory pseudotumors in that the spindle cell proliferation of BOOP involves airspaces, and the underlying pulmonary framework is preserved rather than destroyed. Organization of a prior necrotizing pneumonia may be difficult to differentiate from inflammatory pseudotumor. However, at the periphery, active inflammatory exudate can be seen and changes of BOOP can also be seen. Inflammatory fibrosarcoma is an aggressive tumor capable of metastasizing in about 10% of the cases. Histologically, increased cellularity, mitotic activity, and multifocal necrosis are features that help to distinguish between these two conditions. Malignant fibrous histiocytoma (MFH), currently regarded as an undifferentiated sarcoma, should also be considered in the differential diagnosis of inflammatory pseudotumor. In this pleomorphic malignant tumor, the main distinguishing features are the cellular pleomorphism, large cells with bizarre nuclei, and foamy cytoplasm. Immunoreactivity with the so-called histiocytic markers represent added differentiating features, with most MFHs being positive for CD-68, α-1-antitrypsin, and α-1-anti-chymotrypsin. Inflammatory pseudotumor also needs to be differentiated from malignant intrapulmonary solitary fibrous tumor (SFT). A rare neoplasm, SFT may occur either in the lung or the overlying pleura. SFTs enter the differential diagnosis of inflammatory pseudotumor primarily on the basis of its occasional intrapulmonary location. Nearly 10% of SFTs have distinct histologic malignant features. Most SFTs do not stain with cytokeratin. Most SFTs do stain positively with vimentin, while only few stain with desmin, actin, CD34, and α-1-anti-chymotrypsin. Rarely, inflammatory pseudotumors may occur in association with invasive fungal organisms. Figure 11 shows an inflammatory pseudotumor removed from a 14-year old girl at the University of Massachusetts Medical Center. In this patient, the inflammatory pseudotumor was centrally cavitated and contained numerous aspergilli. Table 3 shows major histopathologic features that help to separate inflammatory pseudotumor from pulmonary sarcoma and sarcomatoid carcinoma.

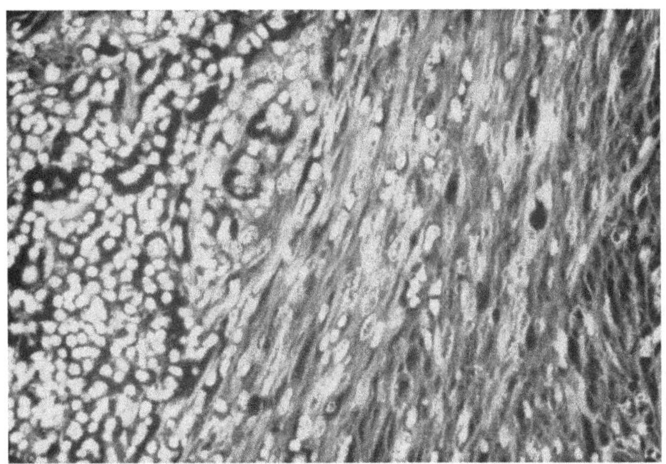

Figure 11 Inflammatory pseudotumor. Note inflammatory lymphoplasmacytic component on the left and myofibroblastic component on the right (Hematoxylin and eosin, 100×).

Table 3 Spindle Cell Lesions of the Lung

Histologic features	Inflammatory pseudotumor	Pulmonary sarcoma	Sarcomatoid carcinoma
Atypia in spindle cells	No	Yes	Yes
Necrosis	No	Yes	Yes
Mitosis	Variable	Yes	Yes
Inflammatory infiltrate	Yes	No	No
Keratin + (spindle cells)	No	Variable	Yes
Vimentin + (spindle cells)	Yes	Yes	Yes
P53 + (spindle cells)	No	Yes	Yes

Source: From Ref. 20.

C. Kaposi's Sarcoma

Pulmonary involvement by Kaposi's sarcoma is commonly seen in the setting of the AIDS epidemic and is said to be less common in slow-growing, classic non-HIV-associated cases. Currently, most cases occur primarily in HIV-positive homosexual and bisexual men infected with herpes virus 8, which is also called KS-associated herpes virus (37,38). Kaposi's sarcoma typically spreads in a lymphangitic pattern along bronchovascular septae and in the pleura. Subtle involvement may be missed, particularly in the presence of intercurrent infection or hemorrhage. Discrete nodular lesions are uncommon and enter a differential diagnosis with other primary pulmonary sarcomas, the most common of which are fibrosarcoma, leiomyosarcoma, and malignant fibrous histiocytoma. Kaposi's sarcoma is recognized, as at other sites, by slit-like channels containing erythrocytes and hyaline globules. The endothelial nature may be confirmed in equivocal cases by immunoreactivity for CD 31. With the exception of AIDS-related Kaposi's sarcoma, primary pulmonary sarcomas are very rare; therefore, metastatic sarcoma, sarcomatoid carcinoma, either primary or metastatic (e.g., renal cell carcinoma), and inflammatory pseudotumor must be excluded on the basis of clinical, pathologic, and immunohistochemical features (37,38).

Kaposi's sarcoma and other spindle cell proliferations in the lung need to be differentiated from inflammatory pseudotumor. Inflammatory pseudotumors are recognized by the presence of cytologically bland spindle cells with plump nuclei, histiocytes, fibrosis, and a prominent lymphoplasmacytic inflammatory infiltrate; however, occasional cases may show a predominance of the spindle cells with higher mitotic activity and mild-to-moderate atypia. Thus they may be confused with Kaposi's sarcoma, MFH, or monophasic sarcomatoid carcinomas. In these cases, absence of immunoreactivity with keratin is helpful in excluding the latter. Immunoreactivity to the p53 protein product is absent in inflammatory pseudotumors but present in two-third of pulmonary sarcomas, suggesting a utility for p53 immunostaining in this differential diagnosis. Further, the differential diagnosis of spindle cell proliferations of the lung must also include pleomorphic carcinoma. This rare neoplasm may have both giant and spindle cell components (39,40). While the giant cell component can be easily recognized, the spindle cell component might represent a diagnostic problem. In this instance, immunostaining for the p53 protein product may be of help, as it is likely to be positive in the spindle cell component of pleomorphic carcinomas (40). This positivity, however, does not help to discriminate pleomorphic carcinoma from spindle-shaped areas of squamous cell carcinoma, which are also immunohistochemically positive for the p53 protein product (40).

References

1. Underwood JCE. Introduction to biopsy interpretation and surgical pathology. New York: Springer Verlag, 1990.
2. Chandraratnam EA, Henderson DW, Meredith DJ, et al. Regenerative atypical squamous metaplasia in fibre optic bronchial biopsy sites—A lesion liable to misinterpretation as carcinoma on rebiopsy. Report of 5 cases. Pathology 1987; 19:419–424.
3. Dail DH. Uncommon tumors. In: Dail DH, Hammar SP, eds. Pulmonary Pathology. New York: Springer Verlag, 1994:847–972.
4. Trillo A, Guha A. Solitary condylomatous papilloma of the bronchus. Arch Pathol Lab Med 1988; 112:731–733.
5. Chang CH, Wang HC, Wu MT, et al. Virtual bronchoscopy for diagnosis of recurrent respiratory papillomatosis. Formos Med Assoc 200;105:508–511.
6. Popper HH, El-Shabrawi Y, Wockel W, et al. Prognostic importance of human papilloma viral typing in squamous cell papilloma of the bronchus. Hum Pathol 1994; 25:1191–1197.
7. Hasleton PS. Spencer's pathology of the lung. New York, St. Louis: McGraw-Hill, 1996:1024.
8. Saldaña MJ, Mones JM. Papillary tumors of surface epithelium. In: Saldana MJ, ed. Pathology of Pulmonary Disease. Philadelphia: JB Lippincott Co., 1994:609–615.
9. Basheda S, Gephart GN, Stoller JK. Columnar papillomas of the bronchus. Case report and literature review. Amer Rev Respir Dis 1991; 144:1400–1402.
10. Guillou L, Deluze P, Zysset F, et al. Papillary variant of low grade mucoepidermoid carcinoma—An unusual bronchial neoplasm. Am J Clin Pathol 1994; 101:269–274.
11. Mark EJ. Lung biopsy interpretation. Baltimore, London: Williams and Wilkins, 1984:192–194.
12. Sterner DJ, Mori M, Roggli VL, et al. Prevalence of pulmonary atypical alveolar cell hyperplasia in an autopsy population. A study of 100 cases. Mod Pathol 1997; 10:469–473.
13. Stanley MW, Henry-Stanley MJ, Gajl-Peczalska KJ, et al. Hyperplasia of type II pneumocytes in acute lung injury. Cytologic findings of sequential bronchoalveolar lavage. Am J Clin Pathol 1992; 97:669–677.

14. Nakanishi K. Alveolar epithelial hyperplasia and adenocarcinoma of the lung. Arch Pathol Lab Med 1990; 114:363–368.
15. Rao S, Fraire AE. Alveolar cell hyperplasia in association with adenocarcinoma of lung. Mod Pathol 1995; 8:165.
16. Mori M, Chiba R, Takahashi T. Atypical adenomatous hyperplasia of the lung and its differentiation from adenocarcinoma. Characterization of atypical cells by morphometry and multivariates cluster analysis. Cancer 1993; 72:2331.
17. Travis WD, Linnoila RI, Horowitz M, et al. Pulmonary nodules resembling bronchioloalveolar carcinoma in adolescent cancer patients. Mod Pathol 1988; 1:372–377.
18. Guinee D, Singh R, Azumi N, et al. Multifocal micronodular pneumocyte hyperplasia: a distinctive pulmonary manifestation of tuberous sclerosis. Mod Pathol 1995; 8:902–906.
19. Popper HH, Juettner-Smolle FM, Pongratz MG. Micronodular hyperplasia of type II pneumocytes — A new lung lesion associated with tuberous sclerosis. Histopathology 1991; 18: 347–354.
20. Cagle PT, Brown RW, Greenberg SD. Handout, Pulmonary Pathology Course, "Diagnostic Dilemmas in Pulmonary Neoplasia" American Society of Clinical Pathology, Chicago, IL, 1995.
21. Kerr KM, Carey FA, King G, et al. Atypical alveolar hyperplasia: relationship with pulmonary adenocarcinoma, p53 and c-erB-2 expression. J Pathol 1994; 174:249.
22. Cagle PT, Fraire AE, Greenberg SD, et al. Potential utility of p53 immunopositivity in differentiation of adenocarcinomas from reactive epithelial atypias of the lung. Hum Pathol 1996; 27:1198–1203.
23. Mori M, Tezuka F, Chiba R, et al. Atypical adenomatous hyperplasia and adenocarcinoma of the human lung. Their heterology in form and analogy in immunohistochemical characteristics. Cancer 1996; 77:665.
24. Yousem SA, Hochholzer L. Alveolar adenoma. Hum Pathol 1986; 17:1066–1071.
25. Cakan A, Samancilar O, Nart D, et al. Alveolar adenoma: an unusual lung tumor. Interact Cardiovasc Thorac Surg 2003; 2:345–347.
26. Kragel PJ, Devaney KO, Meth BM, et al. Mucinous cystadenoma of the lung. Arch Pathol Lab Med 1990; 114:1053–1056.
27. Mori M, Chiba R, Tezuka F, et al. Papillary adenoma of type II pneumocytes may have malignant potential. Virchows Arch 1996; 428:195–200.
28. Miller RR, Nelems B, Evans KG, et al. Glandular neoplasia of the lung. A proposed analogy to colonic tumors. Cancer 1988; 61:1009.
29. Mark EJ. Mesenchymal cystic hamartoma of the lung. N Engl J Med 1986; 315:1255–1259.
30. Glezos J, Toppin D, Cooney T. Mesenchymal cystic hamartoma. Can Respir J 2003; 10:280–281.
31. Bonetti F, Chioder L, Pea M. Transbronchial biopsy in lymphangioleimyomatosis of the lung. HMB for Diagnosis. Am J Surg Pathol 1993; 17:1092–1102.
32. Berger U, Khaghans A, Pomerance A, et al. Pulmonary lymphangioleiomyomatosis and steroid receptors. An immunocytochemical study. Am J Clin Pathol 1990; 93:609–614.
33. Matsubara O, Tan-Liu NS, Kenney RM, et al. Inflammatory pseudotumors of the lung. Progression from organizing pneumonia to fibrous histiocytoma or to plasma cell granuloma in 32 cases. Hum Pathol 1988; 19:807.
34. Pettinato G, Manival JC, DeRosa N, et al. Inflammatory myofibroblastic tumor (plasma cell granuloma). Clinicopathologic study of 20 cases with immunohistochemical and ultrastructural observations. Am J Clin Pathol 1990; 94:538.
35. Calamari S, Brown RW, Cagle PT. p53 immunostaining in the differentiation of inflammatory pseudotumor of the lung from sarcoma. Lab Invest 1994;70:149A (abstract).
36. Yousem SA, Tazelaar HD, Manabe T, et al. Inflammatory myofibroblastic tumour. In: Travis WD, Brambilla T, Müller-Hermelink HK, et al. eds. World Health Organization Classification of Tumours. Pathology and Genetics. Tumours of the Lung, Pleura, Thymus and Heart. Lyon: IARC Press 2004:105–106.

37. Aboulafia DM. The epidemiologic, pathologic and clinical features of AIDS-Associated Pulmonary Kaposis Sarcoma. Chest 2000; 117:1128–1145.
38. Purdy LJ, Colby TV, Yousem SA, et al. Pulmonary Kaposi's sarcoma. Am J Surg Pathol 1986; 10:301.
39. Fishback NF, Travis WD, Moran CS, et al. Pleomorphic (spindle/giant Cell) carcinoma of the lung. Cancer 1994; 73:2936–2945.
40. Przygodski RM, Koss MN, Moran CA, et al. Pleomorphic (giant and spindle cell) carcinoma is genetically distinct from adenocarcinoma and squamous cell carcinoma by K-*ras* and p53 analysis. Am J Clin Pathol 1996; 106:487–492.

27
Preneoplastic and Preinvasive Lesions

KEITH M. KERR
Department of Pathology, Aberdeen University Medical School and
Aberdeen Royal Infirmary, Aberdeen, U.K.

I. Introduction

This chapter focuses on the three putative precursors of invasive malignancy recognized in the WHO classification of lung tumors (1), the diagnostic features of the respective lesions, and their differential diagnosis. The lesions in question are squamous dysplasia and carcinoma in situ (SD/CIS), atypical adenomatous hyperplasia (AAH), and diffuse idiopathic pulmonary neuroendocrine cell hyperplasia (DIPNECH). For each of these lesions there are a number of differential diagnoses that may have to be considered, some neoplastic, possibly even malignant lesions, others are benign reactive conditions. The diagnosis of a pulmonary preinvasive condition carries with it some complexity. The patient is given a diagnosis, which is neither truly benign nor malignant. A diagnosis of a preinvasive precursor lesion implies risk of developing life-threatening invasive disease, yet for the above three lesions, the degree of risk is uncertain and clear treatment strategies have yet to emerge. It is thus important that the pathologist is aware of the implications, both for patient and pulmonologist, when making such a diagnosis. There are a number of other pulmonary diseases or lesions, for example, asbestosis and other diffuse fibroinflammatory parenchymal disease and congenital cystic adenomatoid malformation, which increase the risk of lung cancer in those with this condition. These diseases have been reviewed elsewhere and are beyond the scope of this chapter (2).

As with any problem of differential diagnosis, it is of utmost importance when dealing with a case of possible preinvasive lung disease that the pathologist is aware of the relevant clinical history, radiological findings, and the context in which the lesion in question has occurred. Clinicopathological correlation is key to reaching the correct diagnosis. The preinvasive lesions under discussion here are most frequently encountered as incidental findings in lung tissue removed for the diagnosis or treatment of other, usually malignant, conditions. These findings may alter the significance of any diagnosis of preinvasive disease. However, preinvasive lesions may constitute the primary diagnosis in some situations. SD/CIS may be encountered as the only pathological abnormality in bronchial biopsy samples, especially if the bronchoscopist is using autofluorescence bronchoscopy (AFB). AAH lesions, at least those larger examples, will be among the range of small parenchymal lesions identified and removed as part of a lung cancer screening program using high-resolution spiral CT scanning (3). Thus the pathologist's exposure to pulmonary preinvasive lesions depends, to some extent, on local clinical practice.

II. Bronchial SD/CIS

SD/CIS is a lesion arising, for all practical purposes, in the epithelium lining the major bronchi and, to a lesser extent, small bronchi and bronchioles. This group of lesions comprises a spectrum of change within an epithelium showing squamous differentiation, ranging from mild dysplasia to CIS (4). It is believed to be a precursor lesion for bronchogenic carcinomas, principally squamous cell carcinoma but possibly others, including some small cell carcinomas.

These lesions are generally invisible on gross examination of the bronchial mucosa either by the bronchoscopist or pathologist. Some CIS lesions, however, may cause mucosal roughening, pallor, and loss of the rugal mucosal folds and pits, rendering up to 40% of CIS lesions visible to the experienced observer, especially on the spurs of bronchial carinae (5). Thus, most of these lesions are incidental findings in bronchoscopic biopsy material or accompanying features in the airways in lung specimens resected for squamous carcinoma in particular, but may appear in any bronchial samples, especially from tobacco smokers. SD/CIS will be found more frequently in centers, which utilize AFB, either as a routine diagnostic procedure or as part of a lung cancer screening program. AFB is a very sensitive but relatively much less specific modality for detecting mucosal abnormality, and while this may generate many bronchial biopsies with a range of SD/CIS lesions, it will also generate many more nondysplastic, inflamed, or even normal mucosal samples which had abnormal AFB appearances (6). SD/CIS lesions are generally small but may exist as multiple patches in the bronchial epithelium. There is evidence from AFB studies that patches of SD are usually around 1 to 3 mm in diameter, while CIS lesions tend to be larger, measuring 4 to 12 mm (7).

In the WHO classification of lung tumors, SD and CIS are, by definition, lesions which occur within a full thickness squamous epithelium (4). The lesions are graded as mild, moderate, or severe dysplasia, and CIS according to the degree of atypia (cytological abnormality) and the extent of change from the basal layer of the epithelium toward the epithelial luminal surface (architectural abnormality). The main distinguishing features of these four categories are as follows:

Mild dysplasia is characterized by minimal abnormality. Abnormal squamous cells show slight increase in size and pleomorphism, nuclear angulation is minimal, chromatin is finely granular, and mitoses are virtually absent. Such abnormal, vertically orientated nuclei are confined to the lower third of a minimally thickened epithelium which otherwise retains a prickle cell zone and matures completely to a layer of flattened cells on the surface (Fig. 1).

Moderate dysplasia shows more nuclear changes with grooves and angulations, but chromatin remains finely granular and nucleoli remain inconspicuous. Cells are larger and more variable, mitoses are seen in the lower third of the epithelium, and the abnormal cell zone with vertically orientated nuclei extends to the middle third of the epithelium. Prickle cells and maturation are seen in the superficial zone (Fig. 2).

In severe dysplasia cellular and nuclear changes are marked. Cells are often enlarged and pleomorphism is the norm. Nuclei show marked irregularity but chromatin is coarse and uneven, and nucleoli may be conspicuous. Although there may be some maturation and flattening of cells, a prickle cell layer is rare, and the zone of abnormal cells occupies at least the lower two-thirds of the epithelium, which may be markedly thickened. Mitoses may be found throughout this zone (Fig. 3).

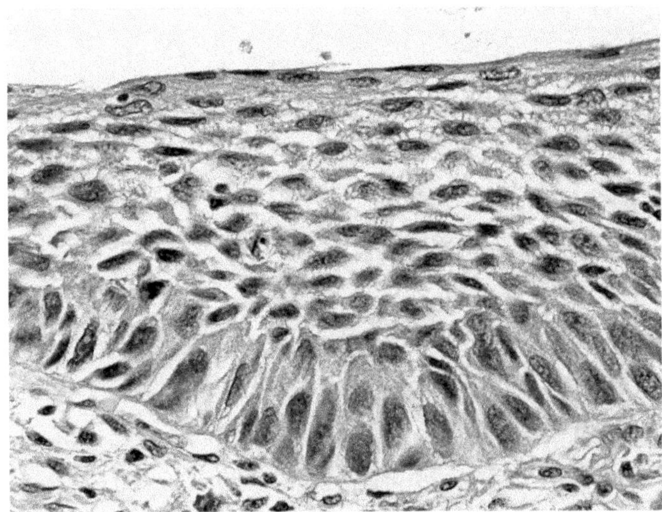

Figure 1 Mild dysplasia showing vertically oriented atypical nuclei in a basal location but most of the epithelium above this demonstrates maturation (400×).

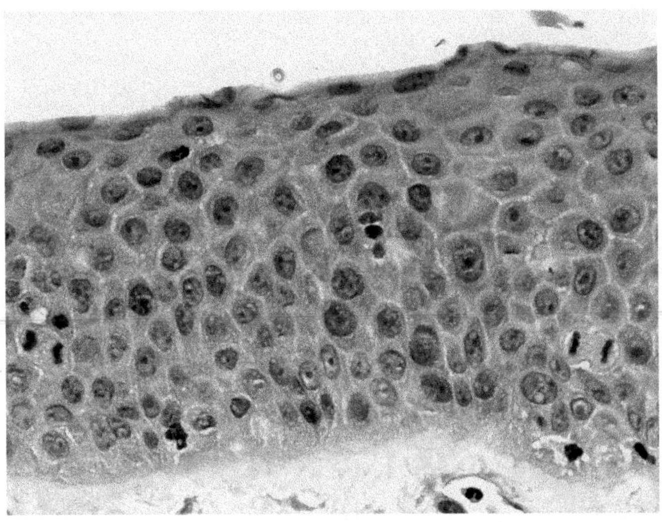

Figure 2 Despite the relatively prominent nucleoli, this is best classified as moderate dysplasia. Mitoses are evident in the basal third of the epithelium (400×).

CIS is characterized by the most marked cytological and architectural abnormality so that the epithelium may be described as chaotic, with no evidence of maturation, and identical extreme cellular abnormality including mitoses at all levels. While many examples of CIS show thick multilayered epithelium, other examples are only a few cells thick (Fig. 4).

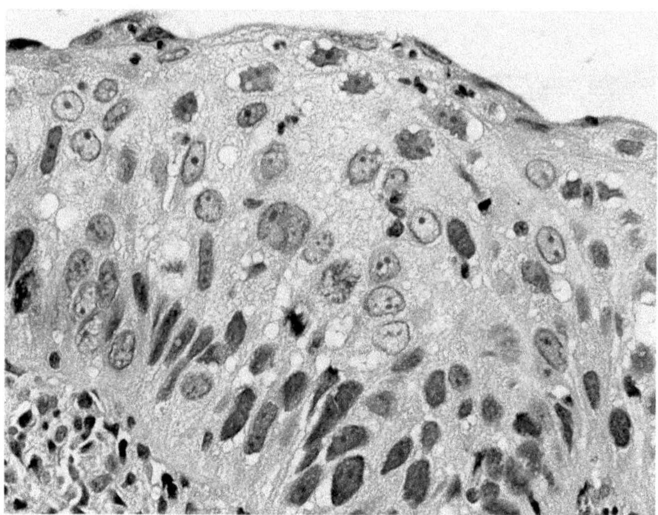

Figure 3 This is severe dysplasia. In contrast to mild or moderate dysplasia, nuclear changes here are marked. There is some evidence of maturation. Mitoses are present in the middle third of the epithelium (400×).

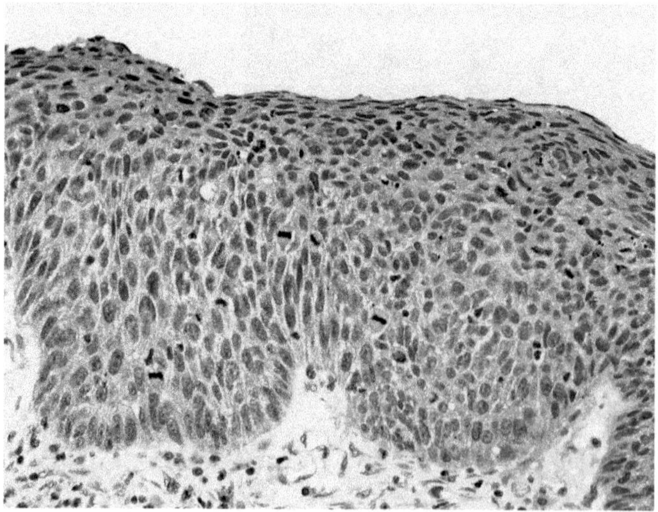

Figure 4 Carcinoma in situ may show considerable thickening of the epithelium, as in this case. Pleomorphism is marked at all levels, even superficially where there is flattening of cells which retain abnormal nuclei. The epithelium has a haphazard character (200×).

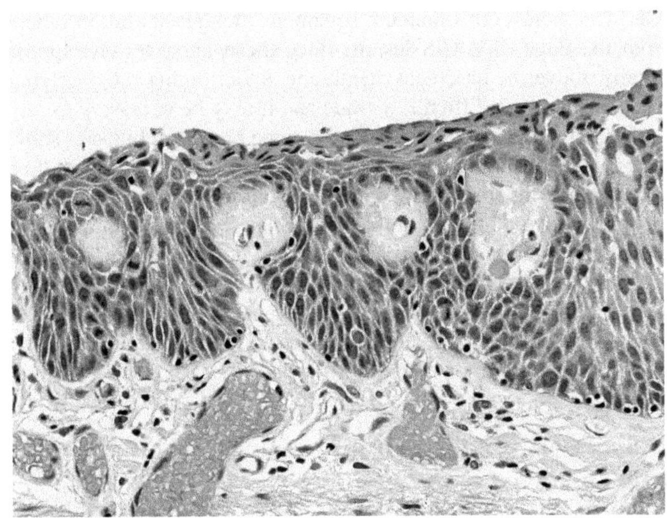

Figure 5 There is cytological atypia, mitoses are evident but note the architecture of the epithelium and the associated vascularity beneath and in the fibrous cores invaginating into the epithelium. This is known as angiogenic squamous dysplasia (400×).

Epithelial basement membrane tends to thicken as SD develops but at the CIS stage the basement membrane may vary remarkably in thickness.

An unusual and particular variant of SD called angiogenic squamous dysplasia (ASD) has been described, which shows protrusions of subepithelial tissue, rich in capillaries embedded in a variably atypical squamous epithelium, so that the apices of the vascular projections are covered by only a thin layer of epithelium, giving the whole mucosa a rather papillomatous appearance (8) (Fig. 5). These vascular pegs often show excess basement membrane material. It has been suggested that the angiogenic character of this lesion may be a herald of invasion but the true clinical significance of ASD is unknown. The author has also seen examples of such vascular budding into nonsquamous respiratory epithelium.

There are a number of factors that may cause problems in the diagnosis of SD/CIS. The discussion above described the 'full house' of features and it must be remembered that these are artificial categories derived in an attempt to describe, grade, and bring consistency of diagnosis to what is, in fact, a continuum of biological change in patches of bronchial mucosa. All the features described may not be present in every case. Lesions of different grade will merge, even in the same high-power field, and grade of disease will vary, sometimes markedly, between areas in the same airway. Diagnosis then involves a description of the range of abnormality, emphasizing the most advanced grade of change. Despite the definition of SD/CIS requiring a full-thickness squamous epithelium, atypical features undoubtedly occur where the 'metaplastic' transformation of normal respiratory epithelium to squamous epithelium is incomplete. In such circumstances, atypical cells, variably identifiable as squamous, may be covered by differentiated columnar ciliated or mucous cells. In some cases, this situation probably represents dysplasia arising within basal cell hyperplasia (BCH) (see below) or immature squamous metaplasia, but in others could reflect sampling from the edge of a CIS lesion, since these latter lesions appear occasionally to spread laterally above the basement membrane, undermining the overlying respiratory epithelium. These changes are difficult to grade and it may be necessary to rely on the cytological features rather than architecture. Similarly, some bronchial biopsies show a lining of a few layers of atypical cells and a rather ragged surface, probably the result of loss of the superficial cells to instrument trauma or mucosal brushing/washing before biopsy. It is important to acknowledge that in some cases the material is inadequate, with insufficient features for diagnosis. Again a descriptive report may be appropriate, perhaps, describing dysplasia but indicating that the material is insufficient for confident grading. In some difficult cases, it may be appropriate to classify dysplasia as low or high grade without being more specific. There is some molecular evidence to support the inclusion of moderate and severe dysplasia in a high-grade category (9).

III. Differential Diagnosis of SD/CIS from Nondysplastic Lesions

Reference has already been made to the idea that SD is preceded in the proposed sequential progression of this disease by a stage of full-thickness nondysplastic squamous metaplasia. In this lesion, there is a prominent prickle cell layer, cells have abundant eosinophilic cytoplasm, the basal cell layer is a monolayer with small basal nuclei, and there may be keratinization on the surface. Despite the traditional view of the place of squamous metaplasia in bronchial carcinogenesis, in the author's experience these lesions are relatively infrequent, at least in the context of bronchial biopsy samples taken for investigation of possible bronchial malignancy. This may be a reflection of relatively recent changes in tobacco manufacturing, smoke content, and smoking habits in current smokers (10,11). Squamous metaplasia is often seen overlying long-standing endobronchial lesions (carcinoid tumors, hamartoma, benign tumors) and may be markedly thickened or remarkably thin. It may also be seen in chronically inflamed airways (bronchiectasis, draining chronic sepsis) or lung cavities (tuberculosis etc). There is much less evidence to support any suggestion that squamous metaplasia arising in these circumstances is preinvasive. When squamous metaplasia occurs on a background of chronic inflammation or sepsis, cytological atypia may occur but this is usually mild, and the nondysplastic nature of the lesion is suggested by accompanying inflammation of the epithelium itself and an understanding of the clinical context.

BCH is a more frequent finding. It is present when the basal cell layer is three or more layers thick. This may be a precursor for full-blown squamous metaplasia as described earlier, since it is not unusual to see a transitional lesion rather like BCH, but with a central prickle (squamous) cell zone, still surmounted by a layer of differentiated columnar cells. In the author's opinion, such lesions may become atypical and deserve diagnosis as dysplasia, without ever passing through a phase of true squamous metaplasia. Similar transitional lesions have been described by others but more studies are required before diagnostic criteria can be established (12). It may be extremely difficult to distinguish BCH from mild dysplasia, especially if one accepts that full thickness squamous change is not an obligatory phase in this process. This is often a matter of fine judgment based on slight differences in cytological characteristics. Tangential cutting of a normal respiratory epithelium can mimic

BCH, but such overdiagnosis can be avoided by observing similar cross cutting of superficial differentiated cells and subepithelial structures and a curious thickening and spreading of the epithelial basement membrane. Respiratory epithelial basal cells stain with cytokeratins 5/6 and 34 betaE12.

To conclude this section it is worth remembering that cytological atypia may also occur in at least two other circumstances. Atypical nonsquamous respiratory epithelial cells or bronchial glandular cells may occur in the respiratory mucosa damaged by radiotherapy, cytotoxic chemotherapy, or in severe viral infection. Atypical squamous metaplastic epithelium may occur in the alveolar lining in cases of usual interstitial pneumonia (UIP) or diffuse alveolar damage (DAD) and care should be taken not to overdiagnose squamous cell carcinoma in these circumstances.

IV. Differential Diagnosis of SD/CIS from Invasive Carcinoma

There are no cytological features to distinguish in situ from invasive squamous carcinoma as diagnosis of the latter relies on the identification of invasion itself. Confident diagnosis of invasion requires the presence of some subepithelial connective tissue stroma or other tissue such as cartilage that can be seen to be infiltrated by tumor. The presence of a fibroblastic stromal reaction may be a useful clue to invasion, as may vasoproliferation. Not infrequently, bronchial biopsy samples show disaggregated fragments of cytologically malignant squamous epithelium devoid of fibroblastic stroma. Distinction between a strip of CIS and invasive carcinoma may be very difficult in these circumstances. CIS tends to give relatively even, straight or curved strips of epithelium with a straight or undulating surface and base, whereas fragments of invasive tumor are often more irregular and convoluted. CIS does not show necrosis. Small tumor islands strongly suggest invasive disease. Invasive disease and CIS may both be present in the same biopsy sample, further complicating the diagnostic process. In some cases there will remain doubt as to the presence of invasion and the pathologist must convey the fact that the diagnosis is that of 'at least CIS' but if invasion is absent in the biopsy, even if the bronchoscopist is confident that a tumor was seen, the pathologist should resist the temptation, or even pressure, to diagnose more advanced disease than is present in the biopsy examined.

CIS extending downward along bronchial gland ducts and replacing bronchial gland acini may be confused with mucosal invasive disease. This overdiagnosis of invasive disease may be avoided by appreciating the preservation of the lobular architecture of the bronchial glands replaced by CIS, their proximity to bronchial cartilage, and sometimes observing residual glandular epithelial cells within the atypical cellular nodules. Although, strictly speaking, not invasion in the usual sense, this pattern of disease extension is often associated with true invasion elsewhere in the affected bronchus.

Noninvasive exophytic squamous papillary lesions with or without atypia may rarely be encountered in the bronchus. True benign squamous papillomas are rare lesions and comprise delicate fronds of vascular connective tissue covered by extremely regular nondysplastic squamous epithelium. Some of these lesions are associated with human papilloma virus (HPV) infection and koilocytes may be seen. Papillary lesions showing high-grade cytological atypia may be seen and, while some accept the existence of papillary CIS (13), in the current WHO classification, such papillary lesions are considered, by definition, to be invasive carcinomas (14).

V. SD/CIS: Implications of Diagnosis

As mentioned in the introduction, the importance of the diagnosis of SD/CIS is the implied risk of developing invasive life-threatening malignancy. Those reactive mimics of SD/CIS apparently carry no such risk. The major problem in assessing the degree of risk faced by the patient is that good data on likelihood of progression of SD/CIS to invasive disease are scarce and much of the literature is controversial. While AFB studies have allowed, at least to some extent, the necessary longitudinal studies to be carried out, there is no clear-cut conclusion. It seems probable that if SD is to progress, many years must elapse before invasive disease appears. Limited studies have, however, shown intervals of between six months and six years between first diagnosis of SD and development of invasive carcinoma (15). There is no inevitability about progression of SD/CIS, and several recent studies suggest that many cases of even high-grade disease may regress completely or wax and wane between low- and high-grade disease (16,17). Studies of outcome in resected lung cancer where CIS is identified at the bronchial resection margin describe conflicting findings though more favor no adverse prognosis if CIS is identified (18–20). Although there is some literature on molecular markers which may be associated with progressive disease, none of these are good enough to be used in a prognostic fashion in individual patients (21–25).

In some cases, the recognition of SD in particular may be difficult and frequently grading of SD/CIS is a challenge. While there are studies which show that SD/CIS can be consistently graded (26), others recognize that this is not always the case (27).

VI. Atypical Adenomatous Hyperplasia

AAH is a localized proliferation of bronchioloalveolar cells lining several alveoli usually in a centriacinar location and is thought to be a possible precursor lesion for the development of many, perhaps most, peripheral parenchymal-type adenocarcinomas of the lung (28).

The vast majority of AAH lesions are encountered clinically in lung specimens, which are resected for the treatment of primary carcinoma. Of course they may be encountered in any sample of alveolated lung, even, at least in theory, in a transbronchial biopsy, although, in this circumstance, a definitive diagnosis will be almost impossible. Sometimes, if the lung specimen is well inflated and fixed prior to sectioning, and carefully examined, AAH lesions may be visible on the cut surface of lung parenchyma as small pale yellowish tan to grey colored rather indistinct foci within which individual alveolar spaces may give some lesions a stippled or pitted appearance. Occasionally some lesions are fibrotic enough to be palpable on the lung cut surface but most are impalpable. Prospective sampling of all such areas seen when lung wedge biopsies, lobectomies and so on are sectioned will improve the yield of AAH lesions. However, many of the foci so identified on gross examination prove to be nonspecific fibrotic or inflammatory lesions. Most AAH lesions encountered in diagnostic practice are incidental histological findings. Lesions range in size from tiny foci involving only a few adjacent alveoli to uncommon examples up to 15 mm or more in diameter. In the author's own series, around 64% of lesion measured less than 3 mm, 17% measured between 3 and 5 mm, 9% between 5 and 10 mm, and 10% measuring between 10 and 19 mm in diameter (9). Similar data have been reported from Japanese patient cohorts (29). It is now clear that despite earlier descriptions, AAH lesions over 5 mm in diameter can and do occur.

As mentioned above, AAH lesions are most often found, and are probably most prevalent in lungs bearing a primary lung cancer, especially an adenocarcinoma. Of the five most complete prospective studies reporting prevalence of AAH lesions, three Japanese studies reported an average prevalence of around 20% for AAH in primary lung cancer resections (29–31), while in two other studies from Canada (32) and Scotland (33), the mean prevalence was just over 11%. In adenocarcinoma-bearing lungs the figures were 34% and 19% for the two groups, respectively, while for squamous cell carcinoma resections, it was 17% and 3%, respectively. A few autopsy studies have attempted to determine a 'background' prevalence of AAH in noncancer-bearing lungs and have suggested figures of between 2% (U.S.A.) and 4% (Japan) (34,35). AAH lesions are more frequent in females, in the upper lobes, and in subpleural alveolated lung. In most studies, identified AAH lesions are singular in half of the cases, most of the remainder yielding two to five lesions, but exceptional cases with over 100 lesions are also encountered (33,36). Often these latter cases also show multiple pure nonmucinous bronchioloalveolar carcinomas (BAC, see below) and sometimes multiple synchronous primary adenocarcinomas. AAH numbers will almost always be underestimated because of gross undersampling of the lung.

Histologically, AAH shows slightly thickened alveolar walls lined by plump rounded, cuboidal, or low columnar cells distributed in an interrupted layer with notable gaps between cells (Figs. 6 and 7). Cells may vary quite considerably in size or shape but nuclear atypia is generally mild, mitotic figures are almost never seen, and nuclear inclusions are frequent. Nuclei are generally oval with a smooth outline and an even chromatin pattern.

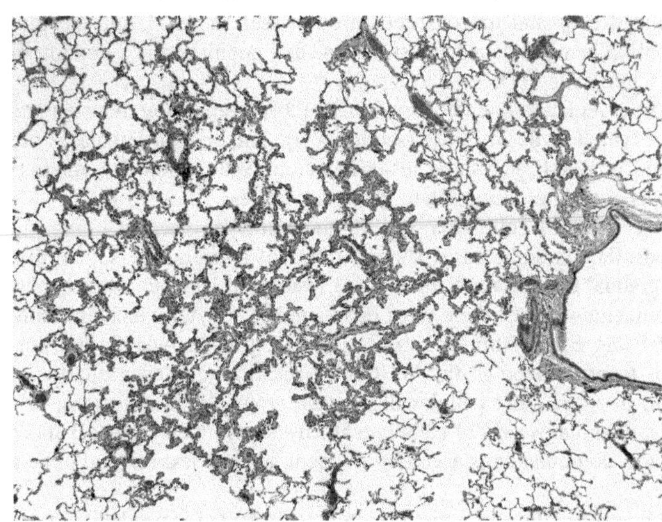

Figure 6 At low power AAH lesions can often be identified arising in the centriacinar region close to a terminal or respiratory bronchiole. These lesions almost certainly represent abnormal epithelial cellular proliferation within the so-called terminal respiratory unit (20×). *Abbreviation*: AAH, atypical adenomatous hyperplasia.

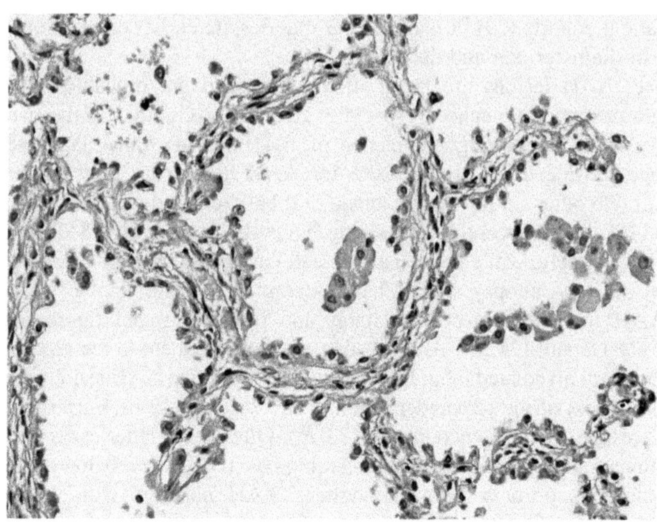

Figure 7 AAH lesions may show mild alveolar wall thickening. Note the interrupted cell layer lining the alveoli. Individual cells are rather bland (200×). *Abbreviation*: AAH, atypical adenomatous hyperplasia.

Some nuclei are hyperchromatic. Occasional cells with double nuclei, often found in the apex of the cell, are not uncommon and some cells may have apical snouts; these are probably Clara cells. Ciliated cells and mucous cells are not seen in AAH, and electron microscopic and immunohistochemical data suggest that the cell population is a mixture of type 2 pneumocytes and Clara cells (37).

The thickening of the alveolar walls may vary considerably from lesion to lesion and some lesions may show a lymphocytic infiltrate (section VII). The alveolar airspaces are frequently focally enlarged in AAH, and some lesions have a cystic or emphysematous character. Alveolar macrophages often accumulate in the air spaces.

AAH lesions show a range of cellularity and atypia. Variation may be limited to lesions in the same patient, though some cases show a range of appearances. Given that there is believed to be a gradual transition, in some AAH lesions, at least, to a lesion best regarded as localized nonmucinous BAC, there must be examples of AAH which are more cellular, yet fall short of being BAC. Although the concept of grading AAH is not universally accepted and not recommended in the WHO classification, around a quarter of AAH lesions probably fall into this more cellular high-grade group. In these lesions, cellularity is increased so that continuous runs of cells line at least some alveoli, there is more obvious cell-cell contact, low columnar cells are more frequent, and the lesions tend to be a little larger. (Fig. 8)

AAH lesions may be very subtle, and optimally prepared material is needed for their identification. Emphysema and background pulmonary fibrosis can make them impossible to identify and the author generally tends not to diagnose AAH in these circumstance. Similarly, the range of fibroinflammatory changes seen in the pulmonary parenchyma distal to a tumor obstructing an airway may mask the presence of AAH.

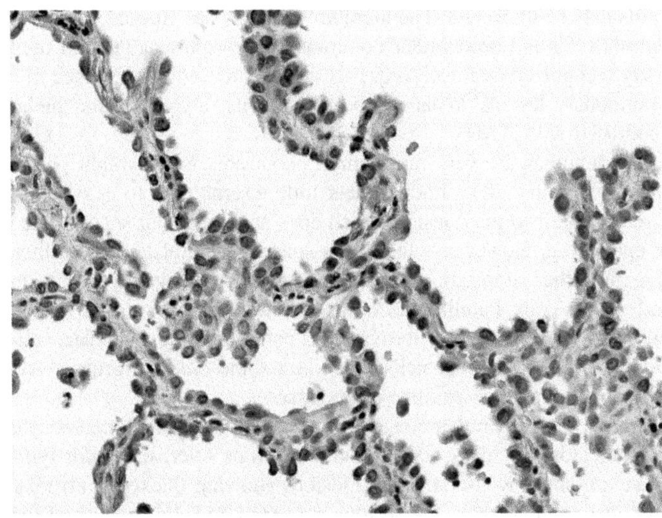

Figure 8 A higher power view of the lesion shown in Figure 6. This is a more cellular AAH. Cell shape and size is still variable, occasional gaps between cells are still visible but cell and nuclear size is greater than in the lesion in Figure 7. This lesion falls short of features sufficient to merit a diagnosis of BAC (200×). *Abbreviations*: AAH, atypical adenomatous hyperplasia; BAC, bronchioloalveolar carcinomas.

VII. Differential Diagnosis of AAH from Reactive or Other Proliferations and Benign Tumors

Reactive hyperplasia of type 2 pneumocytes is a common change in many circumstances where there has been alveolar injury. There is potential for this change to be confused with AAH and the WHO definition of AAH qualifies the definitive description of the alveolar cell proliferation in AAH with the statement 'generally in the absence of underlying interstitial inflammation and fibrosis' (28). As alluded to above, AAH lesions may have slightly thickened fibrotic alveolar walls and even some lymphocytic infiltration. This is always limited to the lesion itself and does not extend beyond the edge of the lesion defined by the epithelial cell component. AAH lesions are distinctive, localized lesions. In reactive lesions, the fibroinflammatory process is the dominant pathological feature, which is usually not localized, and epithelial cell proliferation is a patchy localized phenomenon within a larger ill-defined zone of inflammation and fibrosis. In addition, reactive epithelial proliferations often lack the interrupted heterogeneous cell lining, instead comprising a more homogeneous population of small regular cuboidal cells in a continuous single layer.

In the parenchyma close to lung cancers, small focal lesions comprising several alveoli and perhaps a terminal bronchiole may show airspaces filled with a mixture of macrophages and acute inflammatory cells, while the epithelial lining of the airspaces appears cellular and hyperplastic. This is not AAH. Another common lesion to be distinguished from AAH is peribronchiolar metaplasia. In this lesion, a terminal bronchiole usually shows fibrosis and the surrounding alveoli are lined by a bronchiolar-type epithelium including obvious ciliated columnar cells. Alveolar walls may be thickened. The literature contains descriptions of lesions termed columnar cell dysplasia (12) and bronchiolar columnar cell dysplasia (38), but until these lesions are more widely recognized and accepted, it is difficult to know their place in a discussion of preinvasive pulmonary lesions. Whatever be their nature, atypia in bronchiolar epithelium should not be confused with AAH.

Alveolar and papillary adenomas are very rare benign neoplasms which might potentially enter a differential diagnosis with AAH, although bear little resemblance to it. Alveolar adenoma is a discrete, well-circumscribed mass lesion which does have 'alveolar spaces' lined by a simple low columnar epithelium. However, while these spaces recapitulate alveoli, they are not native lung airspaces but rather neoplastic structures, also associated with a prominent stroma of myxoid tissue and spindle cells. Papillary adenomas are well-defined, circumscribed neoplasms comprising well-defined papillae with fibrovascular cores lined by a regular, continuous population of cuboidal or low columnar cells, including some ciliated forms. AAH lesions may have small cellular tufts but true papillae are not seen.

A much rarer lesion, morphologically rather closer to AAH, is micronodular pneumocyte hyperplasia (39,40). Seen either alone or in association with tuberous sclerosis and/or lymphangioleiomyomatosis, these are small well-demarcated lesions showing thickened alveolar walls lined by plump nonatypical pneumocytes. The lesions appear more solid because of the alveolar wall thickening, collapse of the architecture, and macrophage infiltration. AAH lesions do not have this collapsed or solid character and show more atypia.

VIII. Differential Diagnosis of AAH from BAC and Other Malignancies

AAH has already been described as a precursor lesion in lung adenocarcinogenesis as it is thought, in some cases, to transform into localized nonmucinous bronchioloalveolar carcinoma (LNMBAC). The latter is now considered to be essentially adenocarcinoma in situ, and alveolar collapse and neofibroplasia in LNMBAC herald the onset of invasive adenocarcinoma (41,42). LNMBAC is thus very similar to AAH in its architecture but differs in the degree of cytological atypia and cellularity seen in both lesions. The distinction between the two can be difficult, especially when AAH is at the cellular (high-grade) end of the spectrum, and at this level, the distinction is arbitrary. Criteria have been proposed as an aid to separating AAH from LNMBAC (Table 1) (3,41), but the discrimination may, in some cases, be subjective. Lesions do occur where some areas appear AAH-like while other areas are more like BAC; and even invasion may be found. Final diagnosis will be determined by the most advanced stage seen in the lesion. Interstitial fibrosis, lymphoplasmacytic inflammation, and elastosis are more frequent and not unusual in LNMBAC. LNMBAC lesions with a normal, expanded alveolar architecture are sometimes referred to as Noguchi type A lesions (42). When the alveolar architecture is collapsed and compressed and there is increased elastosis, a Noguchi type B lesion may be diagnosed. Types A and B are still considered pure BAC lesions lacking any evidence of invasion, and as such have a 100% five-year survival when resected. An elastic stain is helpful in showing the retention of the alveolar wall elastic pattern, even in the collapsed areas. AAH may sometimes show increased fibrosis in alveolar walls and the alveolar spaces, as a result, may be reduced in size. It is probable that some cases may become rather sclerotic and their epithelial cells lost, although it is very difficult to prove that these lesions were previously conventional

Table 1 Criteria to Distinguish AAH from LNMBAC

LNMBAC shows three or more of the following five features while AAH rarely shows more than one:
High cell density with prominent nuclear overlapping
Marked cell stratification
Prominent nucleoli and coarse chromatin
Increased tumor cell height, exceeding that of normal terminal bronchiolar columnar cells
True papillae or cells growing in 'picket fence' pattern
Additional points worth noting are:
BAC cell population is usually more homogeneous than that of AAH
Often a sharp transition at the edge of BAC to normal lung
Most BAC lesions measure over 10 mm in diameter
Large BAC lesions often show alveolar collapse

Abbreviations: AAH, atypical adenomatous hyperplasia; LNMBAC, localized nonmucinous bronchioloalveolar carcinoma; BAC, bronchioloalveolar carcinomas.

AAH lesions. The author has occasionally encountered lesions apparently in transition, with part of the lesion straightforward AAH and part showing sclerotic, fibrotic alveolar walls and loss of epithelium. The epithelial cell cytology and organization remains the key to differentiating AAH from LNMBAC.

LNMBAC is actually a relatively rare lesion in thoracic surgical histopathology practice, but is more often seen in Japan than in western, Caucasian cohorts. Greater experience of LNMBAC has been afforded through these early asymptomatic lesions being discovered in spiral CT-based lung cancer screening programs where the localized ground-glass opacity on CT is associated, although not exclusively, with the BAC pattern of disease (43–45). LNMBAC is just as likely to be encountered as an incidental, additional lesion (or lesions) in a lung specimen resected for an invasive adenocarcinoma, more often than not accompanied by AAH lesions, as it is to be the primary lesion for which surgery was performed.

AAH lesions do not contain mucinous cells. Localized mucinous BAC is, certainly in the author's experience, an exceptionally rare lesion. Small foci of mucigenic cells are described within alveoli adjacent to congenital cystic adenomatoid malformation type 1, and are believed to be the possible source of mucinous BAC seen in some patients with this developmental abnormality (46). These mucinous lesions should not be confused with AAH.

Metastatic adenocarcinomas may rarely adopt a BAC-like lepidic growth pattern in the lung (47). Once again, the presence of mucin-containing cells and the pleomorphism usually seen in metastatic carcinoma makes confusion with AAH extremely unlikely.

IX. AAH: Implications of Diagnosis

There are no data on the risk and rate of progression of AAH to LNMBAC and invasive adenocarcinoma. The author's extensive follow up of over 150 patients with AAH over many years has, in a detailed case-control study, failed to show any adverse effect on postoperative survival, although there are hints that patients with larger numbers of AAH may have decreased survival (48). Longitudinal studies of AAH are almost impossible to perform since they are almost impossible to detect radiologically and diagnosis requires excision. Refinements in CT scanning technology may allow some such study in the future as there are studies purporting to discriminate AAH from BAC on high resolution CT scanning but, given the difficulty that may arise for the pathologist in achieving this distinction, a healthy skepticism needs to prevail over these studies (49). More studies with long follow up are needed in patients with well-characterized AAH burdens in their resected lung, to understand better the risk that AAH may have, albeit in the context of patients in whom a diagnosis of usually adenocarcinoma has already been made, and in whom it is assumed that AAH lesions remain in the unresected lung.

X. Diffuse Idiopathic Pulmonary Neuroendocrine Cell Hyperplasia

DIPNECH is an extremely rare lesion, which is characterized by a widespread, diffuse bilateral hyperplasia of pulmonary neuroendocrine cells (PNEC), giving a range of findings in an affected lung (50). The hyperplasia manifests itself as increased numbers of single PNEC in the basal layers of the airway respiratory epithelium, short runs of contiguous PNEC, clusters and nodules of cells, sometimes referred to as neuroendocrine bodies, and carcinoid tumorlets. The latter are discrete, small airway-based nodules comprising nests, clusters, and cords of PNEC, often with a rather plump spindle cell morphology and small hyperchromatic nuclei, which appear to have extended beyond the limits of the associated bronchiole (Figs. 9 and 10). These lesions also show dense collagenous tissue between foci of PNEC. The small

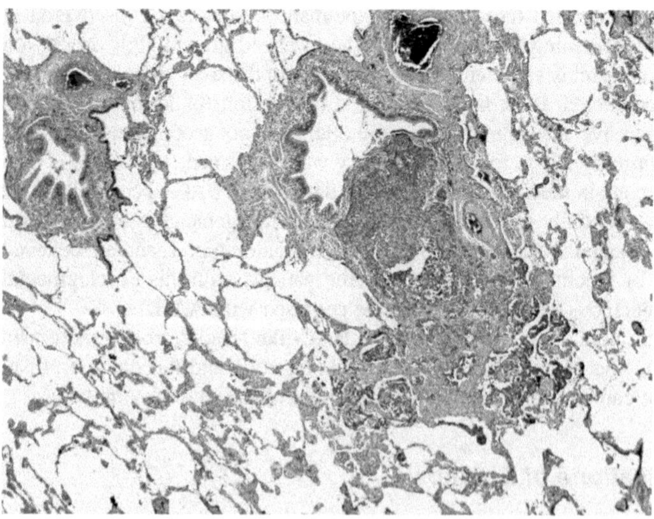

Figure 9 This patient with DIPNECH had dozens of carcinoid tumorlets in a wedge lung biopsy. In this example, the tumorlet impinges on the bronchiolar lumen, whilst the extra-bronchiolar component shows fibrosis surrounding nests of PNEC (20×). *Abbreviations*: DIPNECH, diffuse idiopathic pulmonary neuroendocrine cell hyperplasia; PNEC, pulmonary neuroendocrine cells.

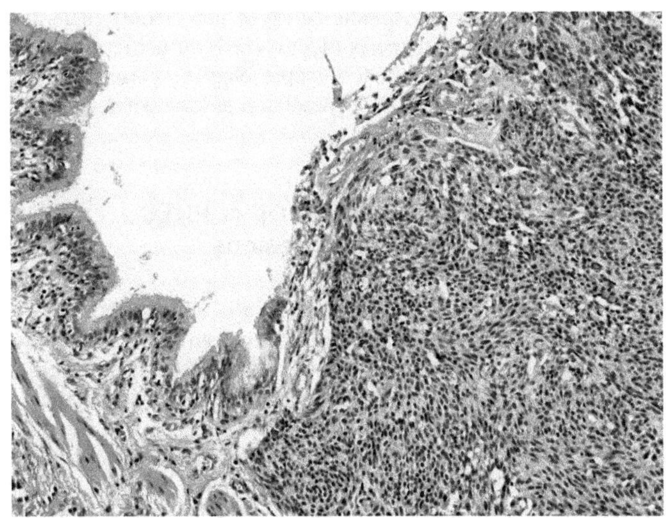

Figure 10 Higher power view of the lesion in Figure 9 showing the typical spindle cell morphology in the tumorlets of DIPNECH (100×). *Abbreviation*: DIPNECH, diffuse idiopathic pulmonary neuroendocrine cell hyperplasia.

airways may be narrowed by larger neuroendocrine bodies or even obliterated by tumorlets. Tumorlets and PNEC nodules are quite characteristic on H&E stained sections but anti-chromogranin immunohistochemistry is excellent in highlighting more extensive PNEC hyperplasia in the background in small airways. Many cases of DIPNECH also show one or more carcinoid tumors, hence the inclusion of DIPNECH in the list of preinvasive pulmonary lesions. A carcinoid tumorlet is defined as a nodule of PNEC extending beyond the limits of its parent bronchiole but measuring no more than 5 mm in diameter (51). Lesions over 5 mm are defined as carcinoid tumors, and in cases of DIPNECH, several such lesions may be found depending on the nature and size of the lung tissue available for examination. While this proposal rather blurs the distinction between hyperplasia and neoplasia, we probably require to be pragmatic around this issue and accept that whatever the true biological nature of these lesions, this is a workable criterion. Smaller tumors are structurally similar to tumorlets, but larger lesions tend to have less fibrosis and are conventional spindle cell typical carcinoid tumors.

When DIPNECH was first described it was seen in the context of patients who presented with small-airways obstruction and asthma-like symptoms, because of the widespread narrowing of small airways as described above (52). Radiology shows anything from very little beyond localized (subsegmental) air trapping to diffuse nodules and/or tumors. It is a moot point as to whether one should diagnose DIPNECH in the absence of such symptoms, but a recent report suggests that 50% of cases are asymptomatic (53). There are also no clearly established criteria for how much PNEC hyperplasia, tumorlets, or tumors must be present for a diagnosis of DIPNECH; most individual pathologists' experience of DIPNECH is limited. In the absence of a typical presentation of DIPNECH as described above, in a case where the pathological examination shows widespread PNEC hyperplasia, tumorlets, and perhaps one or more spindle cell type peripheral typical carcinoid tumors, the author suggests the likely diagnosis of DIPNECH in his report to the physician or surgeon. Final diagnosis will require clinicopathological correlation and exclusion of, as far as possible, other causes of PNEC hyperplasia, at least when carcinoid tumors are absent (see below).

XI. Differential Diagnosis of DIPNECH from Other PNEC Hyperplasias and Nonneuroendocrine Lesions

The WHO definition of DIPNECH acknowledges that lesions are, as described above, 'sometimes accompanied by intra- and extra-luminal fibrosis of involved airways, but other pathology (inflammatory or fibrous lesions) that might induce reactive PNC hyperplasias is absent' (50). It is well recognized that fibroinflammatory diseases of the lung may induce PNEC hyperplasia including tumorlets and these changes are well recognized, for example, in bronchiectasis (54). A diagnosis of DIPNECH would thus be difficult to substantiate if there was a plausible alternative cause for PNEC hyperplasia. However, we have no idea whether previous but resolved inflammation could account for PNEC hyperplasia, and extremely common conditions like chronic obstructive pulmonary disease (COPD) have been suggested as possible causes, adding to our difficulty when faced with such lesions in a lung biopsy. Equally, none of the reported series of carcinoid tumorlets associated with inflammatory disease describe carcinoid tumors in the cases, so when the latter are present, in the appropriate background, DIPNECH may be the more likely diagnosis. It is also recognized that in lung resected for peripheral spindle cell carcinoid tumor, additional carcinoid tumorlets are often found in the absence of fibroinflammatory disease (55), and it was thus suggested that these may be subclinical cases or formes frustes of DIPNECH. Similarly, multiple foci of PNEC and tumorlets may appear in resected lung lacking either fibroinflammatory disease or a carcinoid tumor. Is this a subclinical DIPNECH? We still have much to learn about this area of pulmonary pathology.

Carcinoid tumorlets or neuroendocrine bodies are unlikely to be confused with any other lesion in the lung. Although the cells in tumorlets in particular may be hyperchromatic, distinction from small foci of small-cell lung carcinoma or lymphoid aggregates should be straightforward, taking into account clinical history and context, nuclear morphology if preserved, mitotic and apoptotic activity (absent in tumorlets), and relevant immunochemistry such as chromogranin and CD45. Minute meningothelial nodules present as small clusters of plump spindle cells in alveolated lung, which could be confused with tumorlets. However, these lesions lack fibrosis, the cells tend to be distributed interstitially, are not associated with bronchioles and instead occur in proximity to pulmonary veins, show more pale open nuclei than carcinoid tumorlets, and lack chromogranin.

XII. Conclusion

This chapter has reviewed the surgical pathological features of three putative precursors of invasive malignant disease in the lung; SD/CIS of bronchial mucosa, AAH of the terminal respiratory unit, and DIPNECH, again a lesion of small airways. Each lesion has a number of differential diagnoses which have been described, and an indication has been given of how to distinguish between preinvasive disease and its potential mimics. When any such preinvasive condition is diagnosed, it is important to appreciate the significance of this both for the patient and for the pulmonologist, who will have to follow-up the patient. The diagnosis of preinvasive disease implies a risk of developing invasive, life-threatening malignancy, yet the degree of risk is extremely difficult to quantify.

References

1. Travis WD, Brambilla E, Muller-Hermelink HK, et al., eds. World Health Organization Classification of Tumours. Pathology and Genetics of Tumours of the Lung, Pleura, Thymus and Heart. Lyon: IARC Press, 2004.
2. Kerr KM, Fraire AE. Preinvasive diseases of the lung. In: Tomashefski J, Farver C, Cagle P, Fraire A, eds. Dail and Hammer's Pulmonary Pathology, Vol 2, 3rd ed. New York: Springer, 2008: pp.158–215.
3. Kerr KM, Noguchi M. Pathology of screen-detected lesions. In: Hirsch FR, Bunn PA Jr., Kato H, et al., eds. IASLC Textbook on Prevention and Early Detection of Lung Cancer. London, UK: Martin Dunitz Publisher, 2005:245–267.
4. Franklin WA, Wistuba II, Geisinger K, et al. Squamous dysplasia and carcinoma in situ. In: Travis WD, Brambilla E, Muller-Hermelink HK, et al., eds. World Health Organization Classification of Tumours. Pathology and Genetics of Tumours of the Lung, Pleura, Thymus and Heart. Lyon: IARC Press, 2004:68–72.
5. Lam S, MacAulay C, LeRiche JC, et al. Detection and localization of early lung cancer by fluorescence bronchoscopy. Cancer 2000; 89:2468–2473.
6. Lam S, Kennedy T, Unger M, et al. Localization of bronchial intraepithelial lesions by fluorescence bronchoscopy. Chest 1998; 113:696–702.
7. Lam S, LeRiche JC, Zheng Y, et al. Sex-related differences in bronchial epithelial changes associated with tobacco smoking. J Natl Cancer Inst 1999;91:691–696.
8. Keith RL, Miller YE, Gemmill RM, et al. Angiogenic squamous dysplasia in bronchi of individuals at high risk for lung cancer. Clin Cancer Res 2000; 6:1616–1625.
9. Kerr KM. Morphology and genetics of preinvasive pulmonary disease. Curr Diag Pathol 2004; 10:259–268.
10. Thun MJ, Lally CA, Flannery JT, et al. Cigarette smoking and changes in the histopathology of lung cancer. J Natl Cancer Inst 1997; 89:1580–1586.
11. Strauss GM, Jemal A, McKenna MB, et al. The epidemic of smoking-related adenocarcinoma of the lung: the role of the tobacco industry and filtered and low-tar cigarettes. J Thorac Oncol 2007; 2(suppl 4):S305.
12. Wang GF, Lai MD, Yang RR, et al. Histological types and significance of bronchial epithelial dysplasia. Mod Pathol 2006; 19:429–437.
13. Spencer H, Dail DH, Arneaud J. Non-invasive bronchial epithelial papillary tumors. Cancer 1980; 45:1486–1497.
14. Hammar SP, Brambilla C, Pugatch R, et al. Squamous cell carcinoma. In: Travis WD, Brambilla E, Muller-Hermelink HK, et al., eds. World Health Organisation Classification of Tumours. Pathology and Genetics of Tumours of the Lung, Pleura, Thymus and Heart. Lyon: IARC Press, 2004:26–30.
15. Banerjee AK, Rabbitts PH, George J. Lung cancer 3: fluorescence bronchoscopy: clinical dilemmas and research opportunities. Thorax 2003; 58:266–271.
16. Venmans BJ, van Boxem TJ, Smit EF, et al. Outcome of bronchial carcinoma in situ. Chest 2000; 117:1572–1576.
17. Bota S, Auliac J-B, Paris C, et al. Follow-up of bronchial precancerous lesions and carcinoma in situ using fluorescence endoscopy. Am J Crit Care 2001; 164:1688–1693.

18. Tan KK, Kennedy MM, Kerr KM, et al. Patient survival and bronchial resection line status in primary lung carcinoma. Thorax 1995; 50:437P.
19. Pasic A, GrÏnberg K, Mooi W, et al. The natural history of carcinoma in situ involving bronchial resection margins. Lung Cancer 2005; 49(suppl 2):S57.
20. Aubert A, Moro-Sibilot D, Diab S, et al. Prognostic significance of carcinoma in situ in the vicinity of non small cell resected lung cancer in stage I to IIIA. Lung Cancer 2005; 49(suppl 2):S57.
21. Jeanmart M, Lantuejoul S, Fievet F, et al. Value of immunohistochemical markers in preinvasive bronchial lesions in risk assessment of lung cancer. Clin Cancer Res 2003; 9:2195–2203.
22. Ponticiello A, Barra E, Giani U, et al. P53 immunohistochemistry can identify bronchial dysplastic lesions proceeding to lung cancer: a prospective study. Eur Respir J 2000; 15:547–552.
23. Sozzi G, Oggionni M, Alasio L, et al. Molecular changes track recurrence and progression of bronchial precancerous lesions. Lung Cancer 2002; 37:267–270.
24. Brambilla E, Gazzeri S, Lantuejoul S, et al. p53 mutant immunophenotype and deregulation of p53 transcription pathway (bcl2, bax and waf1) in precursor bronchial lesions of lung cancer. Clin Cancer Res 1998; 4:1609–1618.
25. Brambilla E, Gazzeri S, Moro D, et al. Alterations of Rb pathway (Rb-p16INK4-cyclin D1) in preinvasive bronchial lesions. Clin Cancer Res 1999; 5:243–250.
26. Nicholson AG, Perry LJ, Cury PM, et al. Reproducibility of the WHO/IASLC grading system for pre-invasive squamous lesions of the bronchus: a study of inter-observer and intra-observer variation. Histopathology 2001; 38:202–208.
27. Venmans BJ, van Boxem TJ, Smit EF, et al. Outcome of bronchial carcinoma in situ. Chest 2000; 117:1572–1576.
28. Kerr KM, Fraire AE, Pugatch B, et al. Atypical adenomatous hyperplasia. In: Travis WD, Brambilla E, Muller-Hermelink HK, et al., eds. World Health Organisation Classification of Tumours. Pathology and Genetics of Tumours of the Lung, Pleura, Thymus and Heart. Lyon: IARC Press, 2004:73–75.
29. Weng SY, Tsuchiya E, Kasuga T, et al. Incidence of atypical bronchioloalveolar cell hyperplasia of the lung: relation to histological subtypes of lung cancer. Virchows Arch A Pathol Anat Histopathol 1992; 420:463–471.
30. Koga T, Hashimoto S, Sugio K, et al. Lung adenocarcinoma with bronchioloalveolar carcinoma component is frequently associated with foci of high-grade atypical adenomatous hyperplasia. Am J Clin Pathol 2002; 117:464–470.
31. Nakahara R, Yokose T, Nagai K, et al. Atypical adenomatous hyperplasia of the lung : a clinicopathological study of 118 cases including cases with multiple atypical adenomatous hyperplasia. Thorax 2001; 56:302–305.
32. Miller RR. Bronchioloalveolar cell adenomas. Am J Surg Pathol 1990; 14:904–912.
33. Chapman AD, Kerr KM. The association between atypical adenomatous hyperplasia and primary lung cancer. Br J Cancer 2000; 83:632–636.
34. Sterner DJ, Masuko M, Roggli VL, et al. Prevalence of pulmonary atypical alveolar cell hyperplasia in an autopsy population: a study of 100 cases. Mod Pathol 1997; 10:469–473.
35. Yokose T, Doi M, Tanno K, et al. Atypical adenomatous hyperplasia of the lung in autopsy cases. Lung Cancer 2001; 33:155–161.
36. Anami Y, Matsuno Y, Yamada T, et al. A case of double primary adenocarcinoma of the lung with multiple atypical adenomatous hyperplasia. Pathol Int 1998; 48:634–640.
37. Kitamura H, Kameda Y, Ito T, et al. Cytodifferentiation of atypical adenomatous hyperplasia and bronchioloalveolar lung carcinoma: immunohistochemical and ultrastructural studies. Virchows Arch 1997; 431:415–424.
38. Ullman R, Bongiovanni M, Halbwedl I, et al. Bronchiolar columnar cell dysplasia – genetic analysis of a novel preneoplastic lesion of peripheral lung. Virchows Arch 2003; 442:429–436.
39. Muir TE, Leslie KO, Popper H, et al. Micronodular pneumocyte hyperplasia. Am J Surg Pathol 1998; 22:465–472.

40. Lantuejoul S, Ferretti G, Negoescu A, et al. Multifocal alveolar hyperplasia associated with lymphangioleiomyomatosis in tuberous sclerosis. Histopathol 1997; 30:570–575.
41. Colby TV, Noguchi M, Henschke C, et al. Adenocarcinoma. In: Travis WD, Brambilla E, Muller-Hermelink HK, et al., eds. World Health Organisation Classification of Tumours. Pathology and Genetics of Tumours of the Lung, Pleura, Thymus and Heart. Lyon: IARC Press, 2004:35–44.
42. Noguchi M, Morokawa A, Kawasaki M, et al. Small adenocarcinoma of the lung. Histologic characteristics and prognosis. Cancer 1995; 75:2844–2852.
43. Travis WD, Garg K, Franklin WA, et al. Evolving concepts in the pathology and CT imaging of lung adenocarcinoma and bronchioloalveolar carcinoma. J Clin Oncol 2005; 23:3279–3287.
44. Travis WD, Garg K, Franklin WA, et al. Bronchioloalveolar carcinoma and lung adenocarcinoma: the clinical importance and research relevance of the 2004 WHO Pathologic criteria. J Thorac Oncol 2006; 1(9):S13–S19.
45. Flieder DB, Vasquez M, Carter D, et al. Pathologic findings of lung tumors diagnosed on baseline CT screening. Am J Surg Pathol 2006; 30:606–613.
46. Sheffield EA, Addis BJ, Corrin B, et al. Epithelial hyperplasia and malignant change in congenital lung cysts. J Clin Pathol 1987; 40:612–614.
47. Dail DH, Cagle PT, Marchevsky AM, et al. Metastases to the lung. In: Travis WD, Brambilla E, Muller-Hermelink HK, et al., eds. World Health Organisation Classification of Tumours. Pathology and Genetics of Tumours of the Lung, Pleura, Thymus and Heart. Lyon: IARC Press, 2004:122–124.
48. Kerr KM, Devereux G, Chapman AD, et al. Is survival after surgical resection of lung cancer influenced by the presence of atypical adenomatous hyperplasia (AAH)? J Thorac Oncol 2007; 2 (suppl 4):S401.
49. Nomori H, Ohtsuka T, Naruke T, et al. Differentiating between atypical adenomatous hyperplasia and bronchioloalveolar carcinoma using the computed tomography number histogram. Ann Thorac Surg 2003; 76:867–871.
50. Gosney JR, Travis WD. Diffuse Idiopathic Pulmonary Neuroendocrine Cell Hyperplasia. In: Travis WD, Brambilla E, Muller-Hermelink HK, et al., eds. World Health Organisation Classification of Tumours. Pathology and Genetics of Tumours of the Lung, Pleura, Thymus and Heart. Lyon: IARC Press, 2004:76–77.
51. Colby TV, Koss MN, Travis WD. Carcinoid and other neuroendocrine tumours. In: Tumours of the Lower Respiratory Tract. Washington: AFIP, 1994:290–294.
52. Aguayo SM, Miller YE, Waldron JA, et al. Idiopathic diffuse hyperplasia of pulmonary neuroendocrine cells and airway disease. N Engl J Med 1992; 327:1285–1288.
53. Davies SJ, Gosney JR, Hansell DM, et al. Diffuse idiopathic pulmonary neuroendocrine cell hyperplasia: an under-recognised spectrum of disease. Thorax 2007; 62:248–252.
54. Churg A, Warnock ML. Pulmonary tumourlet. A form of peripheral carcinoid. Cancer 1976; 37:1469–1477.
55. Miller RR, Muller NL. Neuroendocrine cell hyperplasia and obliterative bronchiolitis in patients with peripheral carcinoid tumours. Am J Surg Pathol 1995; 19:653–658.

28
Clinical Diagnosis of Pulmonary Neoplasms

SHANDA BLACKMON
The Methodist Hospital, Houston, Texas, U.S.A.

I. Incidence and Mortality

Lung cancer is the leading cause of cancer death in both men and women in the United States. In 1987, it surpassed breast cancer to become the leading cause of cancer deaths in women (1). Lung cancer causes more deaths than the next three most common cancers combined (colon, breast, and prostate). An estimated 160,390 deaths from lung cancer will occur in the United States during 2007 (2). Between 1979 and 2003 lung cancer deaths increased by 60%. The age-adjusted death rate for lung cancer in men was 74% greater than the rate seen in women. The age-adjusted death rate in the African-American population was 12% greater than the rate in the Caucasian population (3). An estimated 351,344 Americans are living with lung cancer (4).

II. Clinical Evaluation

Patients who present with lung cancer have an approximate average age of 60 years and frequently have other medical comorbidities. Many patients are symptomatic for several months prior to seeking medical treatment. Specific problems that affect thoracic surgical patients are performance status, age, cardiac status, poor pulmonary reserve, comorbidities, malnutrition, weight loss, and neoadjuvant chemotherapy or radiation therapy.

A. History and Physical Examination

The history and physical examination is the single most important part of the assessment of a patient with lung cancer. No imaging modality, laboratory assessment, or new technology can replace the physical exam. The patient must be examined completely, and every organ system must be reviewed to eliminate the involvement of other systems. Cancers from other primary sites often metastasize to the lungs. This is because the body's entire blood volume must pass through the lungs and cancer cells from other primary sites are often trapped in the pulmonary capillaries. Bronchial artery tumor embolization is noted much less frequently (5).

B. Symptoms

The symptoms of lung cancer range from severe to none. Those more commonly associated with lung cancer are: coughing, shortness of breath or dyspnea, fatigue, pain located in the chest, shoulder, upper back, or arm, repeated pneumonia or bronchitis, blood in sputum (hemoptysis), loss of appetite, weight loss, general pain, hoarseness, wheezing, and swelling in the face or neck.

When reviewing symptoms, cough is primarily the main complaint by the time a patient presents with symptoms. Any form of cancer involving the lungs may be associated with cough. However, cough is more likely to indicate involvement of the airways than the lung parenchyma because of the location of cough receptors (6). Adenocarcinoma of the lung usually occurs in the periphery of the lung, and it may not cause cough as an early symptom (7,8). Cancer cell types that are centrally located in the airways (i.e., squamous cell carcinoma and small cell undifferentiated lung cancer) are more likely to cause cough at the time of presentation (8). Carcinoid tumors, mucoepidermoid carcinoma, and adenoid cystic carcinoma usually arise in the more central conducting airways (9), and cough is often a presenting symptom for these less common airway neoplasms. Bronchoalveolar cell carcinoma, a type of primary lung cancer that is parenchymal in location, accounts for 2% to 4% of all primary lung cancers (8). This cell type may be confused with pneumonia because of its airspace opacification pattern that is apparent on a chest radiograph. While cough, which is productive of large amounts of thin sputum, is the paradigm often used to characterize the clinical presentation of patients with bronchoalveolar cell carcinoma, most patients with this type of lung cancer have a nonproductive cough (10).

Smoking tobacco causes 90% of primary lung cancers (11). Thus, heavy cigarette smokers who have a new onset of cough, a change in the characteristics of a preexisting cough, and the presence of hemoptysis (usually a small volume, often only streaks) should promote consideration of cancer as the cause of cough (12). Among other important points in a person's medical history that lead to a higher index of suspicion for primary lung cancer are passive cigarette smoke exposure; exposure to asbestos, radon, and selected other carcinogens; COPD; and a family history of lung cancer. A personal history of cancer in another body site raises the possibility of metastatic cancer involving the lung.

Cough is present in greater than 65% of patients at the time lung cancer is diagnosed, and productive cough is present in greater than 25% of patients (13). While cough as a presenting symptom of lung cancer is common, many studies (14–19) have shown that lung cancer is the cause of chronic cough in less than or equal to 2% of all patients who present with a chronic cough. Normal chest radiograph findings markedly reduce, but do not eliminate, the likelihood that cough is due to a neoplasm (20). Conversely, those abnormalities on the chest radiograph that are typical for a neoplasm should make the clinician place cancer at the top of the list as a cause for cough.

Dyspnea often accompanies the cough caused by a cancer in the airway, regardless of whether the tumor is a primary lung cancer or a metastasis to the bronchus from another site. Intraluminal tumor involvement, particularly if it is in the trachea or a main stem bronchus, will stimulate cough receptors and also obstruct airflow to produce the sensation of dyspnea. Extraluminal compression of a large airway is more likely to cause dyspnea without associated cough, but cough is not infrequent in this setting. Obstruction of the airway may lead to postobstructive pneumonia, which may accentuate the cough. Specific, tumor-related complications, such as massive hemoptysis and tracheoesophageal fistula, may also accentuate cough and be amenable to problem-directed treatment approaches. Additionally, comorbid diseases such as obstructive chronic bronchitis, not just the tumor itself, may be independent or contributing causes to cough. Treatment that is directed at the comorbid process may ameliorate the complaint of cough (21). In a patient with cough who has risk factors for lung cancer or has a known or suspected cancer in another site that may metastasize to the lungs, a chest radiograph should be obtained. In patients with a suspicion of airway involvement by a malignancy (e.g., smokers with hemoptysis), even when the chest radiograph findings are normal, bronchoscopy is indicated.

A chest radiograph should be obtained when a patient with cough has risk factors for lung cancer or a known or suspected cancer in another site that may metastasize to the lungs. A computed tomography (CT) scan of the chest is often needed to further characterize abnormalities that are seen on the plain chest radiograph. Occasionally, a central airway cancer will not be visible on a plain chest radiograph, yet will be quite evident on assessment of the airways via CT imaging or at the time of bronchoscopy (20). Precise data are not available for the increased yield from CT imaging over plain chest radiographs for central airway tumors that are endoscopically visible, but are not visible on the plain chest radiograph.

Cytologic examination of sputum may provide a definitive diagnosis of lung cancer. However, bronchoscopy is usually indicated when there is suspicion of an airway malignancy. Shure (20) found completely obstructing lung cancers in the central airways (segmental or larger) in 36 of 81 endobronchial lesions (44%) with no radiographic signs of obstruction. The chest radiograph findings were normal in 13 patients (16%). All 13 patients had risk factors for and symptoms suggestive of bronchogenic carcinoma (20). Thus, for a smoker who has both cough and hemoptysis that persist after antimicrobial treatment for bronchitis, bronchoscopy is indicated even when the chest radiograph finding is normal.

Wheezing, seen with partial occlusion of a proximal bronchus, occurs when the airway is narrowed to less than 50% of its normal diameter. In proximal main stem bronchial involvement, an inspiratory stridor may be present instead of a wheeze. Pneumonic symptoms occur as a result of bronchitis, atelectasis, or postobstructive pneumonia. These may then cause the patient to complain of fever. Progression of these can lead to a lung abscess from the necrotic tumor cavity, which occurs more frequently with squamous or large cell anaplastic cancer.

When the tumor or enlarged lymph nodes directly invade contiguous structures, pain or neurologic deficits (Horner's syndrome, diaphragmatic dysfunction, recurrent laryngeal nerve loss causing hoarseness), venous insufficiency (superior vena cava syndrome), pericardial effusions, or esophageal dysmotility or obstruction may result. For a complete list of clinical manifestations of extrathoracic paraneoplastic syndromes, please refer to Table 1.

When assessing a person's prognosis, performance status as well as mental attitude is taken into consideration. There are three basic performance status scales; Performance Status Score, Karnofsky Score, and Zubrod Score. These scoring systems serve to follow someone clinically through the course of therapy and serve as prognostic indicators as well.

Other factors that should be taken into consideration when evaluating lung cancer patients clinically include other comorbidities, malnutrition, the degree of weight loss, any neoadjuvant therapy they may have received before evaluation or from other tumors, previous surgery, family history, and history of exposures (tobacco or carcinogens).

A thorough pulmonary assessment should also be performed which should always include spirometry if the patient is considered a surgical candidate (Fig. 1). Patients who are not surgical candidates, but may have stereotactic radiation, should also have quantitative analysis of their lung function to ensure that they will tolerate a necessary volume loss of the lung for treatment.

Table 1 Clinical Findings in Extrathoracic Paraneoplastic Syndromes

General
- Fatigue
- Malaise

Endocrine
- Cushing's syndrome
- Inappropriate antidiuretic hormone secretion (hyponatremia)
- Carcinoid syndrome
- Hypoglycemia
- Ectopic PTH-induced hypercalcemia
- Gynecomastia
- Hypercalcitonemia
- Elevated growth hormone
- Elevated prolactin, FSH, or LH
- Hyperthyroidism

Skeletal
- Clubbing
- Hypertrophic pulmonary osteoarthropathy

Neuromuscular (more common with small cell carcinoma)
- Polymyositis
- Eaton-Lambert syndrome (myasthenia-like syndrome)
- Peripheral neuropathy
- Subacute cerebellar degeneration
- Encephalopathy
- Optic neuritis

Vascular
- Vascular thrombophlebitis

Hematologic
- Anemia
- Leukemoid reactions
- Thrombocytosis
- Thrombocytopenia
- Eosinophilia
- Pure red cell aplasia
- Leukoerythroblastosis
- Disseminated intravascular coagulation

Cutaneous
- Hyperkeratosis
- Dermatomyositis
- Acanthosis nigricans
- Hyperpigmentation
- Erythema gyratum repens
- Hypertrichosis languinosa acquisita

Other
- Nephrotic syndrome
- Hypouricemia
- Secretion of VIP with diarrhea

1. Performance Status Score

   0 Fully active, able to carry on all predisease performance without restriction

   1 Restricted in physically strenuous activity but ambulatory and able to carry out work of a light or sedentary nature, e.g., light house work, office work

Table 1 Clinical Findings in Extrathoracic Paraneoplastic Syndromes (*Continued*)

2 Ambulatory and capable of all self-care but unable to carry out any work activities. Up and about more than 50% of waking hours
3 Capable of only limited self-care, confined to bed or chair more than 50% of waking hours
4 Completely disabled. Cannot carry on any self-care. Totally confined to bed or chair
5 Dead

2. Karnofsky Performance status score

100 Normal, no evidence of disease
90 Able to perform normal activity with only minor symptoms
80 Normal activity with effort, some symptoms
70 Able to care for self but unable to do normal activities
60 Requires occasional assistance, cares for most needs
50 Requires considerable assistance
40 Disabled, requires special assistance
30 Severely disabled
20 Very sick, requires active supportive treatment
10 Moribund

3. ECOG/Zubrod Score Performance Status (the Zubrod score is similar to the "performance status")

0 Asymptomatic
1 Symptomatic, fully ambulatory
2 Symptomatic, in bed < 50% of the day
3 Symptomatic,in bed > 50% of the day but not bedridden
4 Bedridden
5 Dead

Source: From Ref. 55.
Abbreviations: FSH, folicle stimulating hormone; LH, luteinising hormone; ECOG, Eastern Cooperative Oncology Group.

Average Risk:	*High Risk:*	*Prohibitive Risk:*
ppoFEV1% >40	ppoFEV1% 20–40	ppoFEV1% <20
ppoDLCO% >40	ppoDLCO% 20–40	ppoDLCO% <20
pO2 >60	pO2 45–60	pO2 <45
pCO2 <45	pCO2 45–60	pCO2 >60
VO2max >15	VO2max 10–15	VO2max <10

Figure 1 Pulmonary evaluation for lung resection.

C. Smoking

Smoking is the most important cause of lung cancer in the United States. It is estimated that 90% lung cancer cases are caused by smoking. Lung cancer incidence rates are declining in men and appear to be plateauing in women after increasing for many decades. The lag in the temporal trend of lung cancer incidence rates in women compared with men reflects historical differences in cigarette smoking between men and women; cigarette smoking in women peaked about 20 years later than in men.

Table 2 Causes of Lung Cancers

Classification:	Agent:
Group 1	Arsenic
	Asbestos
	Beryllium
	Bis (chloromethyl) Ether
	Cadmium
	Chromium
	Nickel
	Polycyclic aromatic hydrocarbons
	Radon
	Vinyl Chloride
Group 2A	Acrylonitrile
	Formaldehyde
	Diesel Exhaust
Group 2B	Acetaldehyde
	Silica
	Welding fumes

Source: From Refs. 52–54.

D. Other Environmental Causes

Other causes include radon, asbestos, and air pollution (22). For a more extensive listing of causative agents, please see Table 2.

E. Genetic Factors

Inherited factors may determine why some patients smoke and develop lung cancer but others do not. Family clusters of lung cancer have been documented (23). It has yet to be determined whether or not a specific gene is responsible for the development of lung cancer. The cytochrome P-450 oxidase system, which is responsible for the body's fight against carcinogens, may be responsible for a higher level of activated carcinogens. Molecular pathology includes detection of mutations in oncogenes, loss or mutations in tumor suppression genes, and determination of overexpression of oncogenes. It also includes the assessment of cytogenetic abnormalities and clonality, determining the susceptibility to cancer by means of linkage analysis, molecular profiling, and development of screening tests. Microsatellite alterations, such as loss of heterozygosity in a short arm of chromosomes 3, 9, and 5, have been reported. K-RAS mutations have been found in as high as 30% of lung cancers (24,25). Mutation of the p53 gene is one of the most common genetic abnormalities found in all types of human tumors (26,27), although they are more common in small cell (90%) (28) than non-small cell (50%) (29) lung tumors. The progression from squamous metaplasia to atypia to carcinoma in situ to invasive cancer is well documented for patients with squamous cell cancer of the lung (30). Please refer to Table 3 for a list of growth factors on oncogenes and tumor suppressor genes commonly associated with thoracic oncology.

Table 3 Molecular Biology of Thoracic Oncology

Growth factors	GRP (small cell lung cancer) PDGF (adenocarcinoma)
Oncogenes	IGF TGF-alpha EGFR Erb-2 Cyclin D K-ras MYC bcl-2
Tumor suppressor genes	3p Rb p53 p16

Abbreviations: PDGF, Platelet-derived growth factor; TGF, transforming growth factor; IGF, insulin-like growth factor; EGFR, epidermal growth factor receptor.

F. Gender and Race

Overall, men have higher rates of lung cancer than women. In 2003, 78.5 per 100,000 men compared to 51.3 per 100,000 women were diagnosed with lung cancer in the United States (31). However, lung cancer incidence rates have been significantly decreasing among men. The rate has been stable since 1998 in women after a long period of increasing (32). In 2003, the lung cancer incidence rate in black men was 50% higher than that of white men. Rates were similar among black and white women (33). Lung cancer surpassed breast cancer as the leading cause of cancer death in women in 1987 (Fig. 2). Lung cancer is expected to account for 26% of all female cancer deaths in 2007. Death rates for all cancer sites combined decreased by 1.6% per year from 1993 to 2003 in males and by 0.8% per year in females. Mortality rates have continued to decrease across all four major cancer sites in men and in women, except for female lung cancer, in which rates continued to increase by 0.3% per year from 1995 to 2003.

G. Location

In 2002, in United States, Kentucky had the highest age-adjusted lung cancer incidence rates in both males (133.8 per 100,000) and females (73.0 per 100,000). Utah had the lowest age-adjusted cancer incidence rates in both males and females (38.1 per 100,000 and 20.9 per 100,000, respectively). These state-specific rates were parallel to smoking prevalence rates (34).

H. Diet

It was not until a Norwegian study detected the presence of an unusually high dietary intake of vitamin A that dietary factors were considered a part of the development of lung cancer (35).

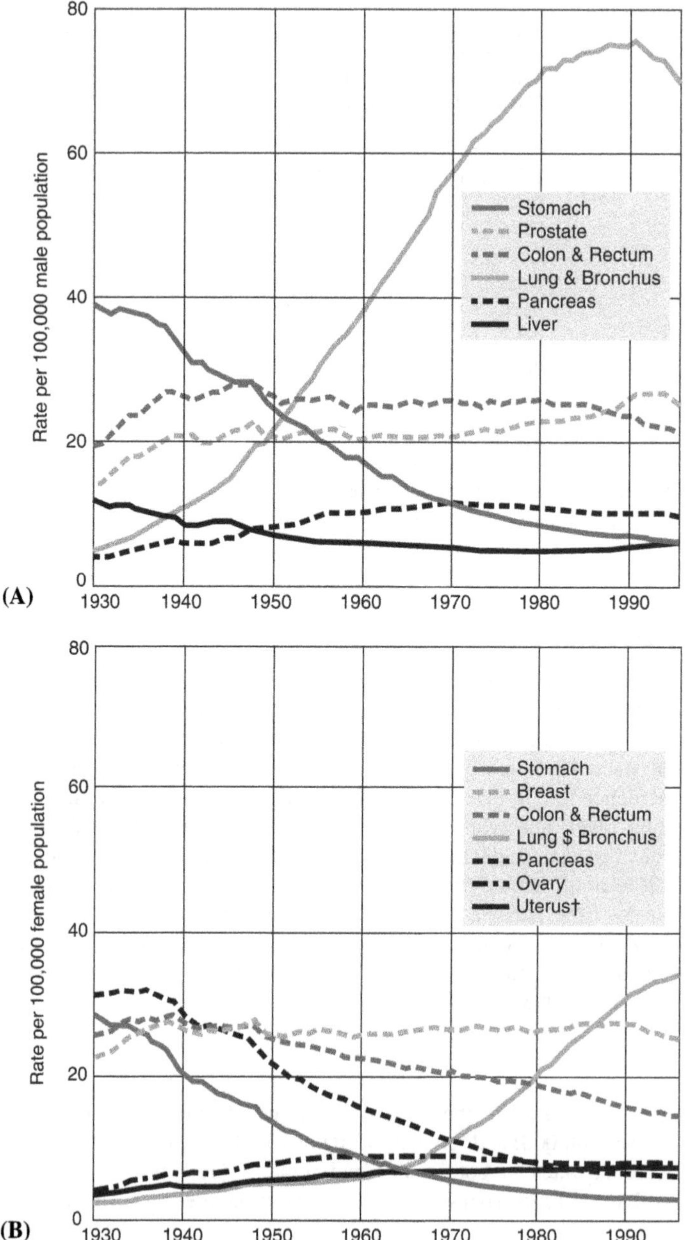

Figure 2 (**A**) Male deaths from cancer according to type. (**B**) Female deaths from cancer according to type.

Since then, we have discovered that dietary intake of certain fruits and vegetables are associated with a reduced risk of lung cancer, regardless of the smoking status (36).

I. Laboratory Investigations

All patients should have a complete metabolic profile, liver function testing, coagulation profiling, and a complete blood cell count as a baseline upon initial evaluation. The role of immunohistochemistry to detect occult metastasis in lung cancer is controversial, but many institutions have found this helpful. Success has been reported with the specific monoclonal antibodies Ber-EP4 (37) and CK18 (38) and using the RT-PCR technique (39). The normal clearance of these cells through the blood stream versus true metastasis makes clinical significance of this technology unclear.

J. Radiographic Evaluation

Please refer to the section on radiologic assessment from chapter 29 for a complete review of radiographic assessment of patients with pulmonary disease including the solitary pulmonary nodule. Regarding lung cancer screening, the current evidence does not support screening for lung cancer with chest radiography or sputum cytologic examination. Frequent chest radiography might be harmful. Further, methodologically rigorous trials are required before any new screening methods are introduced into clinical practice.

K. Histologic Classification

There are two major types of lung cancer. Non-small cell lung cancer (NSCLC) is much more common. It usually spreads to different parts of the body more slowly than small cell lung cancer (SCLC). Squamous cell carcinoma, adenocarcinoma, and large cell carcinoma are three types of NSCLC. SCLC, also called "oat cell cancer," accounts for less than 20% of all lung cancer (40). Please see Table 4 for a list of World Health Organization/International Association for the Study of Lung Cancer (WHO/IASLC) histologic classification of lung tumors.

III. Classification by Disease and Stage

Evaluation of patients with suspected lung cancer includes both a diagnosis of the primary tumor and an evaluation of the extent of spread to regional or distant lymph nodes or to other structures. The current system for staging lung cancer is based on the TNM classification (Table 5, and Fig. 3) (41,42). The staging of lung cancer patients not only provides important prognostic information with regard to survival (Fig. 4), but also guides the decision-making process with regard to choosing optimal treatment modality.

Mediastinal lymph node involvement is found in 26% of newly diagnosed lung cancer patients, and extrathoracic metastases are found in 49% (Fig. 5) (43). In patients with NSCLC, those with mediastinal lymph node involvement are classified as having stage III disease and those with extrathoracic metastases as having stage IV disease. Induction therapy followed by surgery is the primary treatment modality for stage IIIA NSCLC (44–46). For patients with SCLC, both types of patients would be classified as having extensive disease. The remainder of newly diagnosed lung cancer patients who

Table 4 1999 WHO/IASLC Histologic Classification of Lung and Pleural Tumors

1. Epithelial tumors
    - 1.1 Benign
        - 1.1.1 Papillomas
        - 1.1.2 Adenomas
    - 1.2 Preinvasive tumors
    - 1.3 Invasive malignant
        - 1.3.1 Squamous cell carcinoma
        - 1.3.2 Small cell carcinoma
        - 1.3.3 Adenocarcinoma
        - 1.3.4 Large cell carcinoma
        - 1.3.5 Adenosquamous carcinoma
        - 1.3.6 Carcinoma with pleomorphic, sarcomatoid, or sarcomatous elements
        - 1.3.7 Carcinoid tumor
        - 1.3.8 Carcinomas of salivary gland type
        - 1.3.9 Unclassified carcinoma
2. Soft tissue tumors
    - 2.1 Localized fibrous tumor
    - 2.2 Epithelioid hemangioendothelioma
    - 2.3 Pleuropulmonary blastoma
    - 2.4 Chondroma
    - 2.5 Calcifying fibrous pseudotumor of the pleura
    - 2.6 Congenital peribronchial myofibroblastic tumor
    - 2.7 Diffuse pulmonary lymphangiomatosis
    - 2.8 Desmoplastic small round cell tumor
    - 2.9 Other
3. Mesothelial tumors
    - 3.1 Benign
        - 3.1.1 Adenomatoid tumor
    - 3.2 Malignant
        - 3.2.1 Epithelioid mesothelioma
        - 3.2.2 Sarcomatoid mesothelioma
        - 3.2.3 Biphasic mesothelioma
        - 3.2.4 Other
4. Miscellaneous tumors
5. Lymphoproliferative diseases
6. Secondary tumors
7. Unclassified tumors
8. Tumor-like lesions
    - 8.1 Tumorlet
    - 8.2 Multiple meningothelioid nodules
    - 8.3 Langerhans cell histiocytosis
    - 8.4 Inflammatory pseudotumor
    - 8.5 Organizing pneumonia
    - 8.6 Amyloid tumor
    - 8.7 Hyalinizing granuloma
    - 8.8 Lymphangioleiomyomatosis
    - 8.9 Multifocal micronodular pneumocyte hyperplasia
    - 8.10 Endometriosis
    - 8.11 Bronchial inflammatory polyps
    - 8.12 Others

Abbreviation: WHO/IASLC, World Health Organization/International Association for the Study of Lung Cancer.

present without mediastinal lymph node or extrathoracic metastases are said to have stage I or II NSCLC or limited-stage SCLC.

The evaluation of a patient who presents with newly suspected lung cancer includes a clinical evaluation to assess for the presence or absence of extrathoracic metastatic disease and imaging procedures. As the most common sites of lung cancer metastases are the brain, bones, liver, and adrenal glands, the neurologic clinical evaluation ordinarily includes an assessment for headache, focal neurologic deficits, seizures, or changes in personality that may suggest brain metastases, in addition to a complete neurologic exam for patients with stage II disease or greater. If a complete neurologic examination is not performed, then brain imaging should be performed to assess for metastases. Bone pain or pathologic fractures may suggest bone metastases, and abdominal or flank pain or serum enzyme levels may suggest liver metastases. Adrenal metastases are usually asymptomatic.

Table 5 Current ACCP/AJCC Staging System for Non-Small Cell Lung Cancer and Small Cell Lung Cancer

Primary tumor (T)	
Tis	Carcinoma in situ
TX	Tumor, which cannot be assessed or is not apparent radiologically or bronchoscopically (malignant cells in bronchopulmonary secretions)
T1	≤3 cm and surrounded by lung or visceral pleura or endobronchial tumor distal to the lobar bronchus
T2	>3 cm, extension to the visceral pleura, atelectasis, or obstructive pneumopathy involving less than 1 lung; lobar endobronchial tumor; or tumor of a main bronchus more than 2 cm from the carina
T3	Tumor at the apex, total atelectasis of 1 lung; endobronchial tumor of main bronchus within 2 cm of the carina but not invading it; or tumor of any size with direct extension to the adjacent structures such as the chest wall mediastinal pleura, diaphragm, pericardium parietal layer, or mediastinal fat of the phrenic nerve
T4	Invasion of the mediastinal organs, including the esophagus trachea, carina, great vessels and/or heart; obstruction of the superior vena cava; involvement of a vertebral body; recurrent nerve involvement; malignant pleural or pericardial effusion; or satellite pulmonary nodules within the same lobe as the primary tumor
Lymph nodes (N)	
Nx	Regional lymph nodes cannot be assessed
N0	No lymph nodes involved
N1	Ipsilateral bronchopulmonary or hilar nodes involved
N2	Ipsilateral mediastinal nodes or ligament involved
	Upper paratracheal and lower paratracheal nodes
	Pretracheal and retrotracheal nodes
	Aortic and aortic window nodes
	Para-aortic nodes
	Paraesophageal nodes
	Pulmonary ligament
	Subcarinal nodes
N3	Contralateral mediastinal or hilar nodes involved or any scalene or supraclavicular nodes involved
Distant metastasis (M)	
Mx	Metastasis cannot be assessed
M0	Absence of distant metastasis

(*Continued*)

Table 5 Current ACCP/AJCC Staging System for Non-Small Cell Lung Cancer and Small Cell Lung Cancer (*Continued*)

Primary tumor (T)	
M1	Presence of distant metastasis [separate metastatic tumor nodule(s) in the ipsilateral nonprimary tumor lobe(s) of the lung also are grouped as M1]
Stage grouping—TNM	
Subsets	
Stage 0 (TisN0M0)	
Stage IA (T1N0M0)	
Stage IB (T2N0M0)	
Stage IIA (T1N1M0)	
Stage IIB (T2N1M0, T3N0M0)	
Stage IIIA (T3N1M0), (T(1–3)N2M0)	
Stage IIIB (T4, Any N, M0) (Any T, N3M0)	
Stage IV (Any T, Any N, M1)	

Note:
1. UICC staging revision recommendations include reclassifying T2 tumors greater than 7 cm as T3, subclassifying T1and T2 tumors as T1a, T1b, T2a, and T2b, respectively, reclassifying T4 tumors by adding satellite nodules in the primary lobe of the lung as T3, reclassifying pleural dissemination as M1, and reclassifying M1 nodules in the ipsilateral lung in a different lobe than the primary as T4.
2. The staging system used more commonly for small cell lung cancer is a simplified two-stage system originally suggested by the Veterans Administration Lung Cancer Study Group;

Limited disease: (confined to one hemithorax and ipsilateral regional lymph nodes) Ipsilateral pleural effusions, laryngeal nerve involvement, and superior vena cava syndrome are considered limited.
Extensive Disease: Bilateral pulmonary involvement or pericardial involvement or any disease that cannot be treated with local radiation.
Abbreviations: ACCP, American College of Chest Physicians; AJCC, American Joint Committee on Cancer.

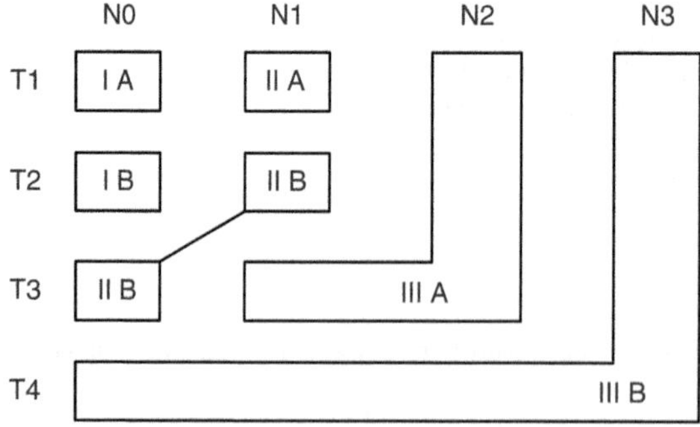

Figure 3 NSCLC Staging System.

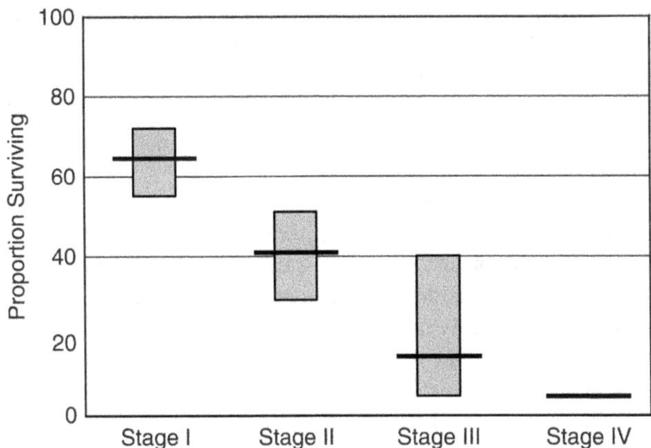

Figure 4 NSCLC: Survival by Stage.

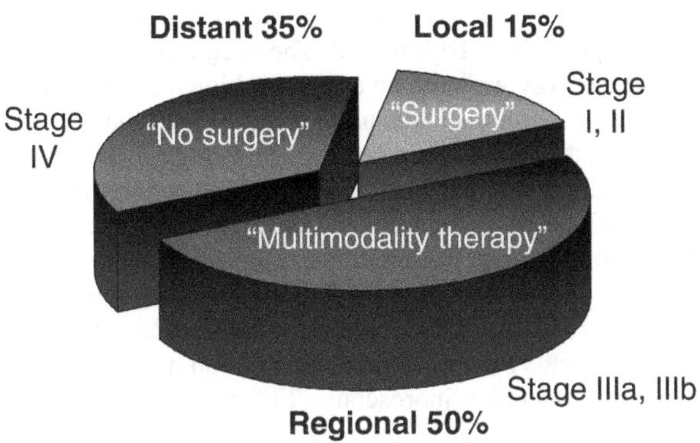

Figure 5 NSCLC Presentation.

Diagnosing a primary tumor can be performed through direct open surgical biopsy, video-assisted thoracic surgery (VATS), percutaneous biopsy, or one of the procedures more commonly used for nodal staging. Noninvasive techniques to evaluate mediastinal nodes rely on either lymph node size (CT, endoscopic ultrasound) or metabolism (positron emission tomography) to detect cancerous involvement. However, while noninvasive tests can identify nodes suspicious for cancer, they do not provide definitive tissue diagnosis and often are not sufficient for initiation of nonsurgical treatment. Thus, invasive tests are almost always required to further evaluate nonresectability. Decision about the status of a node should never be taken on the basis of imaging alone.

Invasive techniques utilize needle biopsy or surgical open biopsy to obtain tissue samples to confirm the diagnosis of metastatic disease. Needle biopsy techniques include transbronchial needle aspiration (TBNA), transthoracic needle aspiration (TTNA), endoscopic ultrasound-guided needle aspiration (EUS-NA), and endobronchial ultrasound (EBUS). Surgical open biopsy can be performed by standard cervical mediastinoscopy, extended cervical mediastinoscopy, or anterior mediastinotomy.

Bronchoscopy may suggest the optimal treatment which may relieve the cough and often relieve the dyspnea. The bronchoscopy findings may provide insights into the post-obstructive pneumonia and treatment of the obstruction may ameliorate the pneumonia.

In patients who are at low risk for lung cancer, for example nonsmokers, and with normal plain chest x-rays, bronchoscopy is usually negative for cancer. In two studies, chest x-rays had positive predictive values for airway malignancies of 36% and 38% and a negative predictive value of 100% whereas bronchoscopy had positive predictive values of 50% and 89% and a negative predictive value of 100%. Therefore, while bronchoscopy may be indicated for complete evaluation of a cough in a nonsmoker with normal chest x-ray, bronchoscopy should almost always be performed in a smoker with a new cough or change in a cough persisting for months, even if the chest x-ray is negative (47).

Bronchoscopy is used to execute a TBNA by passing a needle catheter through the bronchoscope's working channel. The needle catheter comes in varying gauges, with larger gauges used for acquiring a tissue core biopsy, and is directed to the part of the trachea or carina that overlies the mediastinal lymph node to be biopsied. The needle is inserted into the mediastinal lymph node through the airway wall and an aspiration biopsy is performed. This may require several passes in order to acquire an adequate specimen. Adequacy check is performed to confirm that diagnostic material has been obtained allowing for immediate feedback to the bronchoscopist regarding whether additional aspirations are needed. Possible complications with TBNA include those related to bronchoscopy, for example laryngospasm, and those related to performing biopsies, for example endobronchial bleeding. Limitations of TBNA include that it is performed "blind" and that only a few nodal stations can be readily sampled. Real-time CT-fluoroscopy, EBUS and other new imaging techniques which are undergoing study may provide better lymph node sampling.

Using guidance by CT or, less frequently, fluoroscopy, TTNA involves percutaneously inserting a biopsy needle into a mediastinal lymph node and performing an aspiration biopsy. Tissue cores may be acquired using larger gauge needles. Adequacy check may be performed to confirm that diagnostic material has been acquired and additional aspirations may be performed if needed. Complications of this procedure include intrathoracic bleeding and pneunothorax and limitations include that only a few nodal stations can be readily sampled.

Esophagoscopy with guidance by ultrasound is used to execute a EUS-NA by passing a needle catheter through the endoscope's working channel. The needle catheter comes in varying gauges, with larger gauges used for acquiring a tissue core biopsy, and is directed through the esophageal wall that overlies the mediastinal lymph node to be biopsied. The needle is inserted into the mediastinal lymph node through the esopahgeal wall and an aspiration biopsy is performed. This may require several passes in order to acquire an adequate specimen. Adequacy check is performed to confirm that diagnostic material has been obtained allowing for immediate feedback to the endoscopist regarding whether additional aspirations are needed. Evaluation of the mediastinal lymph nodes by ultrasound may help identify lymph nodes that have a higher probability of being positive for malignancy. However, like TBNA and TTNA, limitations of EUS-NA include that only a few nodal stations can be readily sampled. This type of nodal sampling is best when combined with EBUS and complete preoperative nodal staging is being performed.

EBUS uses radial scanning ultrasonic bronchofibrescope to enhance diagnosis of invasion or compression and carcinoma in situ through increased ultrasonic penetration, while a linear scanning ultrasonic bronchovideoscope is used for real-time EBUS with TBNA. By extending the view of the endoscopist beneath the inner surface of the airways, a more accurate sampling of lymphatic tissue can increase sensitivity of staging while avoiding an incision at the same time. General anesthesia is not required, but it is recommended for this procedure.

Virtual bronchoscopy uses three-dimensional images reconstructed from routine helical CT scans. The technology is much like a global positioning system and provides a map of the lungs through which the practitioner can steer a navigation catheter to reach smaller branches of the tracheobronchial tree and more peripheral lesions. This system can also be used to plan resections and minimally invasive approaches.

During standard cervical mediastinoscopy, a small surgical incision is made above the suprasternal notch of the manubrium and a mediastinoscope is inserted into the mediastinum after dissection down to the pretracheal fascia. Bilateral paratracheal and subcarinal blunt dissection allows direct visualization of the mediastinal lymph nodes and direct sampling of all four paratracheal lymph node stations (levels 2R, 2L, 4R and 4L) and the anterior subcarinal lymph node station (level 7). Potential complications of standard cervical mediastinoscopy include the risks of general anesthesia, bleeding and left laryngeal nerve injury. A benefit of this procedure is the ability to completely remove a node of interest for testing.

Biopsy of the aortopulmonary window lymph node station (level 5) and the preaortic lymph node station (level 6) can be achieved under direct visualization by extended cervical mediastinoscopy. Extended cervical mediastinoscopy is performed through the same surgical incision as a standard cervical mediastinoscopy by passing over the aortic arch between the brachiocephalic artery and the left carotid artery to the aortopulmonary window. Potential complications of extended cervical mediastinoscopy include bleeding and embolic stroke. Level 5 and 6 lymph nodes can also be sampled under direct visualization by anterior mediastinoscopy in which an additional parasternal incision is made, typically at the level of the second or third intercostal space. Potential complications of anterior mediastinoscopy include damage to the internal mammary artery and pleura. These procedures require general anesthesia as well.

Once the primary tumor type is known, the patient is staged according to the staging system appropriate for the tumor type, and once a preoperative evaluation have been completed, the treatment can begin. The overall five-year survival rate for patients with lung cancer is much less (15.5%) than the overall five-year survival rate for patients with colon cancer (64.8%), breast cancer (89%) or prostate cancer (99.9%). Only 24% of patients with lung cancer are diagnosed with early state disease and the five-year survival for lung cancer patients with localized disease at diagnosis is only 49.3%. The five-year survival rate for lung cancer patients with metastatic disease at diagnosis is only just over 2%. Of patients diagnosed with lung cancer, about 60% die within one year of diagnosis and 70 to 89% die within 2 years of diagnosis.

The presence of lymph node metastases is important as a predictor of survival in operable cases of NSCLC and for selecting the type and timing of adjuvant therapy. False positives may cause potentially curable patients to be misclassified as untreatable and false negatives may lead to unwarranted surgery. Mediastinoscopy is the gold standard for assessing lymph node status with a sensitivity of 89% and a specificity of nearly 100% (48), but is limited due to the fact that it is an invasive procedure that requires general anesthesia and does not permit easy evaluation of all lymph nodes. CT scan by itself has a sensitivity of only 63% and a specificity of only 57% and about 10% of patients with negative lymph nodes on CT scan are found to have N1 or N2 metastases with mediastinoscopy. On the other hand, the combination of CT scan and positron emission tomography (PET) scan has a sensitivity of 84% and a specificity for 94% for N2 metastases (49). Micrometastases can be missed on routine histopathologic examination of a lymph node and influence survival of stage I NSCLC (50,51)

IV. Summary

Once the patient has had a thorough history and physical evaluation, has been staged, has met all providers who will be administrating all planned parts of their possible multimodal therapy, and has a histologic diagnosis (if feasible), the practitioner can begin therapy. Selection of patients for surgery, chemotherapy, or radiation therapy, and the type of approach for each modality is practitioner dependent. The addition of clinical trials to investigate the utility of new modalities must also be considered when educating patients about their options.

References

1. American Cancer Society. Cancer Facts and Figures, 2006.
2. Jemal A, Tiwari RC, Murray T, et al. Cancer statistics. CA Cancer J Clin 2004; 54:8–29.
3. National Vital Statistics Report. Deaths: Final Data for 2003. Vol. 54(2), February 28, 2005.
4. Ries LAG, Eisner MP, Kosary CL, et al., eds. SEER Cancer Statistics Review, 1975–2003, National Cancer Institute. Bethesda, MD, 2006.
5. Braman SS, Whitcomb ME. Endobronchial metastasis. Arch Intern Med 1975; 135:543–547.
6. Sant'Ambrogio G. Afferent pathways for the cough reflex. Bull Eur Physiopathol Respir 1987; 23(suppl):19S–23S.
7. Mackay B, Lukeman JM, Ordonez NG. Adenocarcinoma. Mackay B, Lukeman JM, Ordonez NG, eds. Tumors of the Lung. Philadelphia, PA: WB Saunders, 1991:100–164.
8. Vaporciyan AA, Kies M, Stevens C, et al. Cancer of the lung. Kufa DW, Pollock RE, Weichselbaum RR, et al. eds. Cancer Medicine. BC Decker. Hamilton, ON, Canada, 2003: 1385–1445.
9. Schrump DS, Altorki NK, Henschke CL, et al. Non-small cell lung cancer. DeVita VT Jr, Hellman S, Rosenberg SA, eds. Cancer: Principles & Practice of Oncology 7th ed. Philadelphia, PA: Lippincott Williams & Wilkins, 2005:753–810.
10. Lee KS, Kim Y, Han J, et al. Bronchioloalveolar carcinoma: clinical, histopathologic, and radiologic findings. Radiographics 1997; 17:1345–1357.
11. Alberg AJ, Samet JM. Epidemiology of lung cancer. Chest 2003; 123(suppl):21S–49S.
12. Beckles MA, Spiro SG, Colice GL, et al. Initial evaluation of the patient with lung cancer: symptoms, laboratory tests, and paraneoplastic syndromes. Chest 2003; 123(suppl):97S–104S.
13. Vaaler AK, Forrester JM, Lesar M, et al. Obstructive atelectasis in patients with small cell lung cancer: incidence and response to treatment. Chest 1997; 111:115–120.
14. Irwin RS, Corrao WM, Pratter MR. Chronic persistent cough in the adult: the spectrum and frequency of causes and successful outcome of specific therapy. Am Rev Respir Dis 1981; 123:413–417.

15. Irwin RS, Curley FJ, French CL. Chronic cough: the spectrum and frequency of causes, key components of the diagnostic evaluation and outcome of specific therapy. Am Rev Respir Dis 1990; 141:640–647.
16. Smyrnios NA, Irwin RS, Curley FJ. Chronic cough with a history of excessive sputum production: the spectrum and frequency of causes and key components of the diagnostic evaluation, and outcome of specific therapy. Chest 1995; 108:991–997.
17. Pratter MR, Bartter T, Akers S, et al. An algorithmic approach to chronic cough. Ann Intern Med 1993; 119:977–983.
18. Poe RH, Israel RH, Utell MJ, et al. Chronic cough: bronchoscopy or pulmonary function testing? Am Rev Respir Dis 1982; 126:160–162.
19. Poe RH, Harder RV, Israel RH, et al. Chronic persistent cough: experience in diagnosis and outcome using an anatomic diagnostic protocol. Chest 1989; 95:723–738.
20. Shure D. Radiographically occult endobronchial obstruction in bronchogenic carcinoma. Am J Med 1991; 91:19–22.
21. Kvale PA. Chronic cough due to lung tumors: ACCP evidence-based clinical practice guidelines. Chest 2006; 129(1 suppl):147S–153S.
22. Alberg AJ, Samet J. Epidemiology of Lung Cancer. Chest 2003; 123(1 suppl):21S–49S (review).
23. Farber SM. Clinical appraisal of pulmonary cytology. JAMA 1961; 175:345–348.
24. Rodenhuis S, Slebos RJ, Boot AJ, et al. Incidence and possible clinical significance of K-ras oncogene activation in adenocarcinoma of the human lung. Cancer Res 1988; 48:5738–5741.
25. Suzuki Y, Orita M, Shiraishi M, et al. Detection of ras gene mutations in human lung cancers by single-strand conformation polymorphism analysis of polymerase chain reaction products. Oncogene 1990; 5:1037–1043.
26. Hollstein M, Sidransky D, Vogelstein B. p53 mutations in human cancers. Science 1991; 253: 49–53.
27. Harris CC, Hollstein M. Clinical implications of the p53 tumor suppressor gene. N Engl J Med 1993; 329:1318–1327.
28. Carbone D, Kratske R. RB1 and p53 genes. In: Pass HI, Mitchell J, Johnson D, et al., ed. Lung Cancer: Principles and Practice. Philadelphia, PA: Lippincott-Raven, 1996:107–121.
29. Lee JS, Yoon A, Kalapurakal SK, et al. Expression of p53 oncoprotein in non-small-cell lung cancer: a favorable prognostic factor. J Clin Oncol 1995; 13:1893–1903.
30. Saccomanno G, Archer VE, Auerbach O, et al. Development of carcinoma of the lung as reflected in exfoliated cells. Cancer 1974; 33:256–270.
31. Ries LAG, Eisner MP, Kosary CL, et al. eds. SEER Cancer Statistics Review, 1975–2003, National Cancer Institute. Bethesda, MD, 2006.
32. American Cancer Society. Cancer Facts and Figures, 2006.
33. Ries LAG, Eisner MP, Kosary CL, et al. eds. SEER Cancer Statistics Review, 1975–2003, National Cancer Institute. Bethesda, MD.
34. U.S. Cancer Statistics Working Group. United States Cancer Statistics: 2001 Incidence and Mortality. Department of Health and Human Services, Centers for Disease Control and Prevention and National Cancer Institute. Atlanta (GA), 2004.
35. Bjelke E. Dietary vitamin A and human lung cancer. Int J Cancer 1975; 15:561–565.
36. Ziegler RG, Mayne ST, Swanson CA. Nutrition and lung cancer. Cancer Causes Control 1996; 7: 157–177 (review).
37. Passlick B, Izbicki RJ, Kubuschok B, et al. Immunohistochemical assessment of individual tumor cells in lymph nodes of patients with non-small cell lung cancer. J Clin Oncol 1994; 12: 1827–1832.
38. Pantel K, Izbicki J, Passlick B, et al. Frequency and prognostic significance of isolated tumor cells in the bone marrow of patients with NSCLC without overt metastases. Lancet 1996; 347: 649–653.
39. Salerno CT, Frizelle S, Neihans GA, et al. Detection of occult micrometastases in non-small cell lung carcinoma by reverse transcriptase polymerase chain reaction. Chest 1998; 113:1526–1532.
40. American Cancer Society. All About Lung Cancer, 2005.

41. Mountain CF. Revisions in the International System for Staging Lung Cancer. Chest 1997; 111:1710–1717.
42. Fleming ID, Cooper JS, Henson DE, et al. AJCC Cancer Staging Handbook. 5th ed. Philadelphia, PA: Lippincott Williams & Wilkins, 1998.
43. Jemal A, Thomas A, Murray T, et al. Cancer Statistics, 2002. CA Cancer J Clin 2002; 52:23–47.
44. Rosell R, Gomez-Codina J, Camps C, et al. A randomized trial comparing preoperative chemotherapy plus surgery with surgery alone in patients with non-small-cell lung cancer. N Engl J Med 1994; 330:153–158.
45. Roth JA, Atkinson EN, Fossella F, et al. Long-term follow-up of patients enrolled in a randomized trial comparing perioperative chemotherapy and surgery with surgery alone in resectable stage IIIA non-small-cell lung cancer. Lung Cancer 1998; 21:1–6.
46. Roth JA, Fossella F, Komaki R, et al. A randomized trial comparing perioperative chemotherapy and surgery with surgery alone in resectable stage IIIA non-small-cell lung cancer. J Natl Cancer Inst 1994; 86:673–680.
47. Ries LAG, Eisner MP, Kosary CL, et al. eds. SEER Cancer Statistics Review, 1975–2003, National Cancer Institute. Bethesda, MD.
48. Investigation for mediastinal disease in patients with apparently operable lung cancer. Canadian Lung Oncology Group. Ann Thorac Surg 1995; 60:1382–1389.
49. Valk PE, Pounds TR, Hopkins DM, et al. Staging non-small cell lung cancer by whole-body positron emission tomographic imaging. Ann Thorac Surg 1995; 60:1573–1581; (discussion 81–82).
50. Osaki T, Oyama T, Gu CD, et al. Prognostic impact of micrometastatic tumor cells in the lymph nodes and bone marrow of patients with completely resected stage I non-small-cell lung cancer. J Clin Oncol 2002; 20:2930–2936.
51. Hashimoto T, Kobayashi Y, Ishikawa Y, et al. Prognostic value of genetically diagnosed lymph node micrometastasis in non-small cell lung carcinoma cases. Cancer Res 2000; 60:6472–6478.
52. Overall evaluations of carcinogenicity: an updating of IARC monographs 1–42 supplement 7. Lyon, France: International Agency for Research on Cancer (IARC), 1989.
53. Diesel and gasoline engine exhaust and some nitroarenes, monograph 46. Lyon, France: IARC, International Agency for Research on Cancer (IARC), 1989.
54. Beryllium, cadmuid, mercury and exposures in the glass manufacturing industry, monograph 58. Lyon, France: International Agency for Research on Cancer (IARC), 1989.
55. Oken MM, Creech RH, Tormey DC, et al. Toxicity and response criteria of the Eastern Cooperative Oncology Group. Am J Clin Oncol 1982; 5:649–655.

29
Radiologic Diagnosis of Pulmonary Neoplasms

JOE M. CHAN and MARC V. GOSSELIN
Oregon Health and Science University, Portland, Oregon, U.S.A.

I. Introduction

The greatest cause of cancer-related deaths in the United States is lung cancer. According to statistics from the American Cancer Society for 2006, 31% of all cancer-related deaths for men and 26% for women were due to lung cancer, which totaled an estimated 161,419 lives lost (1). One of the reasons for the high mortality associated with lung cancer is its late presentation. Once the diagnosis of lung cancer is made, the average patient can expect an estimated five-year survival of just 10% to 15% (2). For many patients, the diagnosis of lung cancer begins with radiographic imaging and the finding of a pulmonary nodule, either with chest radiographs or chest computed tomography (CT) (Fig. 1). According to the Nomenclature Committee of the Fleischner Society that organizes and defines terms to be used for thoracic radiology, a nodule is defined as a round opacity, at least moderately well marginated and no greater than 3 cm in maximum diameter. Over 150,000 patients a year present with pulmonary nodules found on chest radiographs, with 90% of them being completely incidental findings unrelated to their initial diagnostic workup (3). While it is the job of the pathologist to come up with a tissue diagnosis of lung cancer, it is the job of the radiologist to detect pulmonary nodules and identify characteristics that make them either benign or malignant. Correct identification by the radiologist of benignity can save the patient from further unnecessary evaluation and associated morbidity. Early detection of malignancy can potentially decrease patient mortality associated with lung cancer.

The purpose of this chapter is to characterize pulmonary neoplasms from a radiologist's perspective. It will begin with radiographic findings of pulmonary nodules, such as size, the presence of calcification, and attenuation, that make it more likely to be benign or malignant. Next will be a brief description of the more common pulmonary neoplasms and their collective radiographic characteristics. The chapter will conclude with a discussion on the role of radiology in lung cancer screening as well as in the management of detected pulmonary nodules.

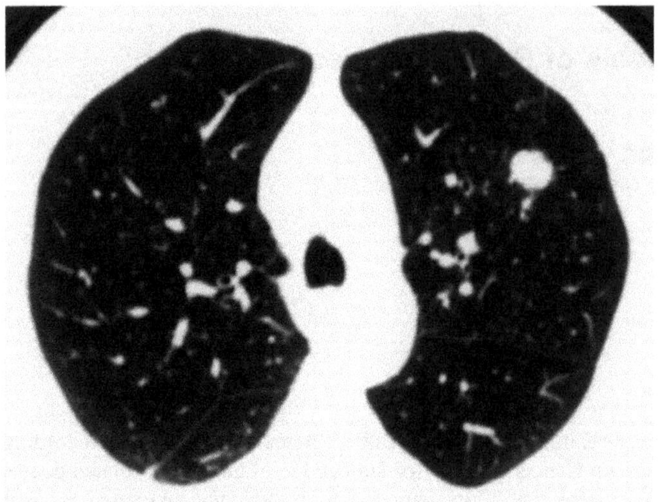

Figure 1 Nodule found on chest CT. *Abbreviation*: CT, computed tomography.

II. The Pulmonary Nodule: Benign or Malignant?

A. Clinical History

Once a pulmonary nodule is detected on chest radiograph or CT, the determination of whether or not it is more likely to be malignant or benign begins not with the radiologic findings but with the pertinent clinical history. Advanced age increases the risk of a pulmonary nodule being malignant. Recent trends in lung cancer mortality in the United States from the National Cancer Institute point out the ever-increasing incidence of lung cancer in patients older than 40 years (4). Increased smoking duration and amount, described as the number of pack-years, has long been an established risk factor for lung cancer. Every year on average, cigarette smoking accounts for nearly 23% of all carcinomas for women and 38% for men. Looking at lung cancer specifically, cigarette smoking contributes to approximately 85% of lung cancers in men and 47% in women (5). Other established clinical data that increase the risk of lung cancer include a history of pulmonary fibrosis, history of radiation exposure, as well as certain environmental exposures such as asbestos. While lung cancer in the past has traditionally been more common in men, recent data suggest that the incidence of lung cancer in women has nearly caught up with that of men (1). Intuitively, it also makes sense for patients with a history of known primary lung cancer or extrapulmonary neoplasm that a newly detected pulmonary nodule has an increased chance of also being malignant. Interestingly, patients with certain extrapulmonary malignancies can lend clues as to whether a new pulmonary nodule detected on chest CT or radiograph is likely to be a primary lung cancer or a metastasis. For example, patients with a history of head and neck squamous cell carcinoma have a nearly eightfold increase in their pulmonary nodule being a primary lung cancer as opposed to patients with melanoma or sarcoma who have a twofold higher likelihood of their pulmonary nodule being a metastasis (6).

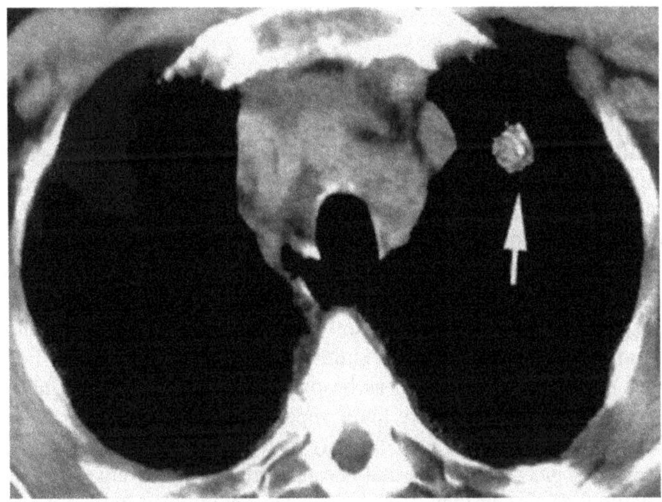

Figure 2 Hamartoma showing popcorn calcification pattern on CT. *Abbreviation*: CT, computed tomography.

B. Calcification and Fat

No single radiologic finding of pulmonary nodules can make the diagnosis of malignancy. It is the combination of multiple radiologic findings with clinical history that makes the radiologist confident in calling a nodule benign or malignant. One of the more helpful radiologic findings is the presence and pattern of distribution of calcification within pulmonary nodules. Nodules that are less than 1 cm in size are usually difficult to detect on chest radiographs unless they are diffusely calcified. Diffuse calcification along with other patterns including laminated, popcorn, and central nidus calcification are highly indicative of benignity for smoothly bordered nodules less than 3 cm (7). For the latter patterns of calcification, chest CT has been shown to be the most sensitive (Fig. 2). Frequently, hamartomas and certain infections such as histoplasmosis exhibit such benign patterns of nodule calcification.

Malignant pulmonary nodules usually show distinctive patterns of eccentric or stippled calcification, particularly in larger-sized nodules above 3 cm that are usually not smoothly bordered. Eccentric calcification usually results from a malignant pulmonary nodule that has extended to include a calcified benign nodule resulting in a more peripheral calcified appearance (7). Stippled calcification has been described to occur commonly in adenocarcinoma of the lung (8,9). Although both malignant and benign pulmonary nodules can exhibit the presence or absence of intrinsic calcification, characteristic benign calcification patterns, as described, can be very specific and help the radiologist make the more likely diagnosis of benignity.

The presence of fat in pulmonary nodules is detected through chest CT and the measurement of focal fat attenuation. With the exception of patients with a history of renal cell carcinoma or liposarcoma, fat indicates benignity and is most commonly found in hamartomas, lipomas, or focal areas of lipoid aspiration nodules (10).

C. Nodule Size and Location

Comparing all of a patient's prior imaging once a pulmonary nodule is detected is the radiologist's equivalent of a thorough chart review. This is especially important in assessing nodule size and rate of growth. For over 50 years now, it has been traditional thinking that any single pulmonary nodule that remains unchanged in over two years of follow-up, radiographic imaging from its initial detection makes benignity highly likely with no need for further diagnostic evaluation (3). In the past, measurement of nodule size could be problematic on standard chest radiography if peripheral lung reaction was erroneously included in the lung nodule measurement. With improved imaging technology and high-resolution chest CT, more accurate nodule size measurements can be made. In addition, improved understanding of certain pulmonary neoplasms and their growth behavior has challenged the label of benignity for nodules that exhibit no growth in two years. For example, well-differentiated adenocarcinomas such as bronchioloalveolar carcinoma tend to exhibit very slow rates of growth that can make them appear benign.

Although nodule size can be nonspecific for benignity or malignancy, particularly in the setting of metastatic disease, it has been shown that nodules smaller than 1 cm are most likely benign on average, while those larger than 2 cm in its largest axial diameter are more likely to be malignant (11). The Mayo Clinic CT Screening Trial reported that less than 1% of nodules less than 5 mm were malignant. Malignancy was present in 0.9% for nodules that were 4 to 7 mm while 18% was found in those that measured 8 to 20 mm. Malignancy was found in 50% of nodules larger than 2 cm (12).

Location alone provides the radiologist little help in distinguishing a malignant from a benign solitary pulmonary nodule despite epidemiologic evidence that showed primary pulmonary malignancies have a predilection for the upper lobes (13). However, in regions of the lung where there are indications of fibrosis, particularly in the peripheral lower lobes, the presence of a pulmonary nodule is more likely to be malignant, given the significantly increased risk of lung cancer development associated with pulmonary fibrosis.

D. Nodule Attenuation, Shape, and Margin

The composition and shape of a pulmonary nodule, whether it is ground glass and round, strictly solid and ovoid, or a mixture of the two with a polygonal or complex shape can be assessed using chest radiographs. This task has proven to be even easier using chest CT, where even the margins of a pulmonary nodule can be confidently seen to distinguish between those that are irregular and spiculated with those that are smoothly marginated. Nodule attenuation, shape, and margination factor significantly helps in deciding whether it is malignant or benign.

Ground-glass attenuation on chest CT means that a pulmonary nodule has nonsolid components where lung parenchyma and vessels can still be appreciated through the nodule (Fig. 3). Solid pulmonary nodules, however, completely obliterate the lung parenchyma. Results from the Early Lung Cancer Action Project using thin-section chest CT for lung cancer screening found that the majority of purely ground glass–appearing nodules or those with a mixture of both solid and ground-glass (Fig. 4) components were confirmed to be more likely malignant than those that were purely solid (14). While ground-glass attenuation intuitively represents inflammation or bronchioloalveolar hyperplasia, it is frequently the primary finding on chest CT of a nodule representing bronchioloalveolar carcinoma or

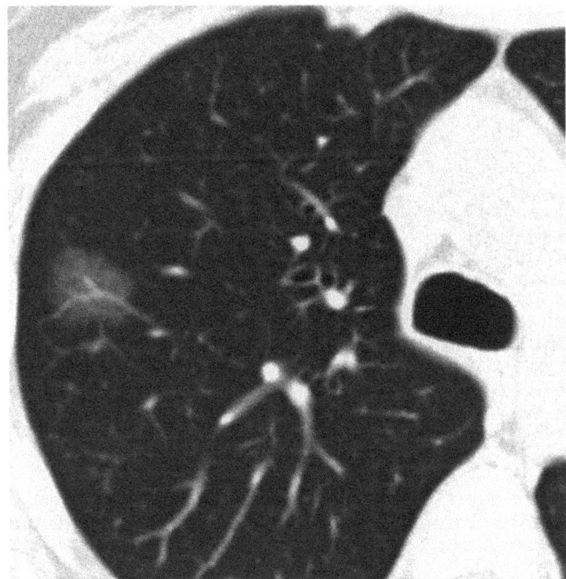

Figure 3 Ground-glass nodule representing bronchioloalveolar carcinoma.

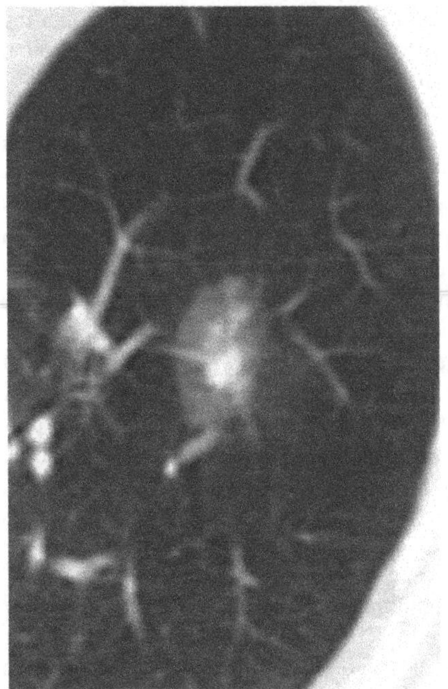

Figure 4 Part solid and ground-glass nodule as seen in a patient with adenocarcinoma.

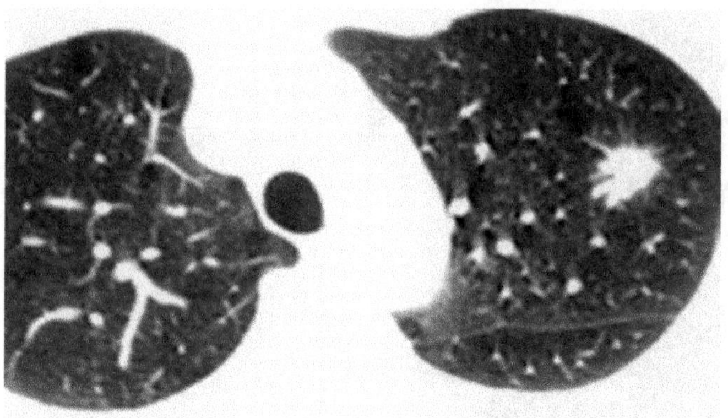

Figure 5 Spiculated nodule seen in adenocarcinoma.

adenocarcinoma with bronchioloalveolar features. The finding of a solid central nodule surrounded by ground-glass attenuation can represent hemorrhage around an invasive tumor or can represent severely compressed alveoli centrally, which is inadequately oxygenated with surrounding partially aerated alveoli that have thickened walls, resulting in a cloudy appearance (14). A recent study from Japan of 222 suspicious nodules that were followed up with diagnostic chest CT confirmed the increased frequency of malignancy in pulmonary nodules that display a mixture of both solid central attenuation and surrounding ground-glass components with a positive predictive value of 85%. In addition, it was found that among purely solid nodules, 77 out of 77 with smooth margins were benign (15).

Spiculated and irregularly marginated nodules are associated with malignancy (Fig. 5). Spiculation is most likely the result of malignant cell extension into the adjacent interlobular septa and blood vessels. It has been stated that spiculation and margin irregularity have a 90% positive predictive value for nodule malignancy (16). Irregular margination should not be confused with the "comet tail" sign found in rounded atelectasis on CT scan or the "rabbit ears" sign of a feeding artery and draining vein into a pulmonary arteriovenous malformation. The comet tail emanating from an apparent pulmonary nodule simply represents the compression of lung parenchyma and vasculature from atelectasis.

Not all smoothly marginated nodules are benign, however. Many can represent metastases that exhibit slow growth with less aggressive invasion. Another subset of smooth margination that can also represent malignancy is a lobulated shape to the pulmonary nodule. Lobulation is the result of heterogeneous rates of growth within the nodule itself, characteristic of malignant cells in primary lung cancer and less often in metastases.

E. Nodule Attenuation with Intravenous Contrast

Increased angiogenesis to support proliferating malignant cells is one of the reasons why many radiologists believe that CT with intravenous (IV) contrast is helpful in further characterizing pulmonary nodules. Swenson et al. concluded from their study that nodules with less than 15 Hounsfield units were more likely to be benign, whereas nodules with greater than 20 Hounsfield units were highly indicative of malignancy (17).

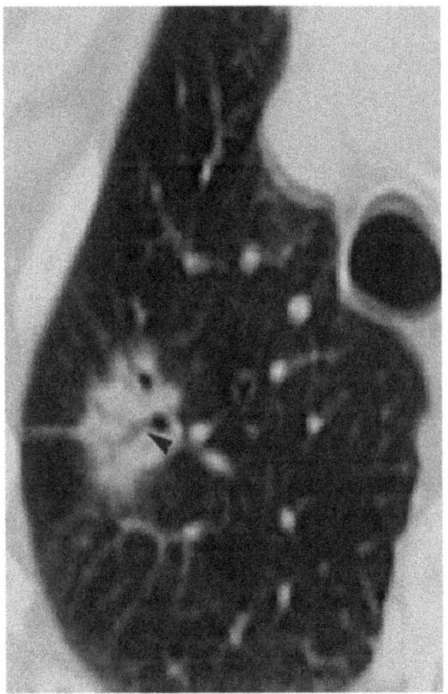

Figure 6 Pulmonary nodule exhibiting air bronchograms (*arrowhead*).

F. Air Bronchograms and Cavitation

The bronchial airways are usually invisible on chest radiographs and CT scans. Their appearance is called air bronchograms or air bronchiolograms (Fig. 6). For lung airways to appear on radiographic imaging, there must be air space consolidation present in the form of a pneumonia or nodule to provide enough surrounding contrast for the airways to stand out. Interestingly, a study conducted by Kuriyama et al. concluded that the presence of air bronchograms in a lung nodule helped to differentiate malignancy from benignity. They took 20 peripheral lung nodules that were confirmed to be lung cancer along with 20 benign lung nodules and scanned them all with thin-section chest CT. An air bronchogram or air bronchiologram was seen in 65% of malignant nodules, while only 5% were seen in benign nodules (18). These later would be termed "bubble-like lucencies" and are seen in up to 55% of bronchioloalveolar cell carcinomas (Fig. 7) (19).

The presence of cavitation within a pulmonary nodule is not as helpful for the radiologist. It can be seen equally in both tumors and in infection. In malignant tumors such as squamous cell carcinoma of the lungs, it represents central necrosis from breakdown of fragile and poorly constructed neovascularization (Fig. 8). Some have argued that cavity wall thickness can be helpful in distinguishing benign from malignant nodules. One follow-up study found that the majority of pulmonary nodules with cavity walls less than 5 mm were benign, while greater than 1.6 cm in wall thickness were usually associated with malignancy (20).

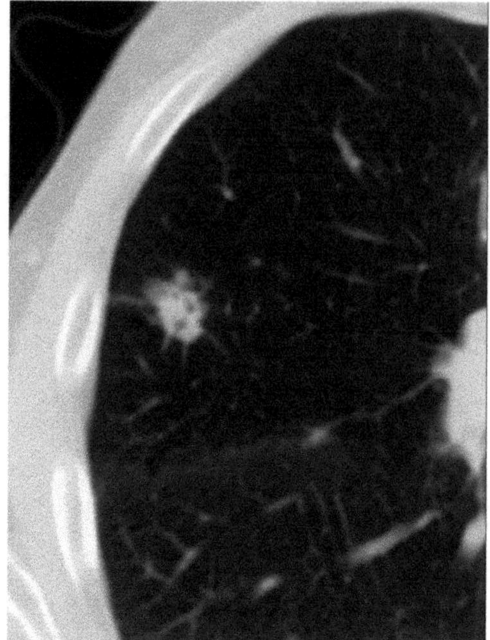

Figure 7 Adenocarcinoma with "bubble-like lucencies."

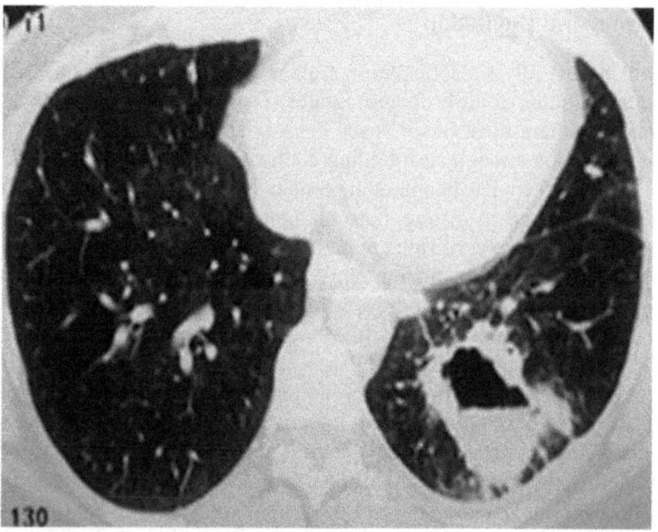

Figure 8 Cavitary nodule with air fluid level in squamous cell carcinoma.

III. Radiographic Findings of Common Pulmonary Neoplasms

A. Adenocarcinoma

The incidence of adenocarcinoma has risen dramatically since the 1980s to become currently the most common of all lung cancers, making up nearly half of all cases (21). Since adenocarcinoma more commonly occurs peripherally in the distal airways, many initially attributed its increased incidence to advances in chest CT, the use of flexible bronchoscopy, and improved histologic stains for mucin. Epidemiologic data from the American Cancer Society, however, revealed two more likely reasons for the rise in adenocarcinoma stemming from changes in cigarette design. The first is the change from unfiltered cigarettes to medium-yield filtertip cigarettes in the 1950s, allowing smoke to be inhaled more deeply and carcinogens to reach the bronchioloalveolar junction where adenocarcinomas are frequently found. The second design change to cigarettes, which also occurred in the 1950s, was the use of blended reconstituted tobacco with higher concentrations of nitrosamines derived from tobacco stems in place of purely tobacco leaves alone. Nitrosamines in the rodent model were shown to induce adenocarcinoma (22,23). In Connecticut, from 1959 through 1991, there was found to be a 17-fold increased incidence of adenocarcinoma in women and a 10-fold increase in men, both strongly associated with cigarette smoking (22). One other finding that remains unresolved is the increased incidence of adenocarcinoma among nonsmokers as well.

Radiographic features of adenocarcinoma, in addition to their typically peripheral and subpleural location on chest radiograph and CT scan, include the appearance of primarily a solitary nodule that can be lobulated or spiculated in margination. Nodule attenuation of adenocarcinoma can present radiographically as purely ground glass, purely solid, or as a mixture of both. Noguchi et al. classified adenocarcinoma of the lung into six histologic types (A-F) on the basis of lepidic (A-B) or invasive (C-F) tumor growth and its relation to patient prognosis. Type A (localized bronchioloalveolar carcinoma) and type B (localized bronchioloalveolar carcinoma with foci of structural collapse of alveoli) showed a 100% five-year survival while types C-F, which showed invasive areas with active fibroblastic proliferation, poorly differentiated tubular or papillary morphology, showed a less favorable prognosis. (24). Yang et al. successfully correlated four primary CT patterns of adenocarcinoma with the histologic Noguchi classification. They found that ground glass and heterogeneous low-attenuation nodules found on CT matched histologically to types A and B, while nodules with a central zone of high attenuation surrounded by ground glass and homogenous, soft tissue density nodules matched to types C and D, respectively (25).

B. Bronchioloalveolar Carcinoma

Most commonly, bronchioloalveolar carcinoma presents as a solitary nodule that is peripheral and subpleural in location. Known for its slow growth and good prognosis when it presents as a solitary nodule, it often appears ground glass in attenuation on CT scan because of its lepidic growth pattern. Fibrosis is frequently associated with bronchioloalveolar carcinoma development, and nearly 55% of cases are found with air bronchiolograms or bubble-like lucencies (19).

Bronchioloalveolar carcinoma can also present as two other forms on radiographic imaging. It can appear as an area of consolidation with multiple other nodules in different parts of the lung. This appearance is associated with poorer prognosis and occurs in 20% of cases (26). It can also appear as multiple ill-defined nodules on chest CT, which is the rarest of all the presentation forms.

C. Squamous Cell Carcinoma

Squamous cell carcinoma was the most common cell subtype of lung neoplasms in the 1950s. It is strongly associated with cigarette smoking where respiratory bronchi lined with respiratory mucosa undergo squamous metaplasia and eventually turn into invasive carcinoma. Its radiographic findings reflect its endobronchial growth. The majority of squamous cell carcinomas are found centrally near the proximal airways and are seen as a perihilar or hilar mass. Frequently, their endobronchial growth results in airway occlusion causing atelectasis and obstructive pneumonia more distally that can be seen on both chest radiograph and CT.

Squamous cell carcinoma grows rapidly by direct extension and often can be seen with central necrosis and cavitation on radiographic imaging. As the tumor expands, its increasing nutrient and oxygen demands place greater stress on more rapid angiogenesis. Frequently, the new vasculature that is constructed to meet the needs of the tumor is more fragile and its structure is easily compromised. Once this occurs, necrosis results and central cavitation is observed. Its rapid regional growth causes local extension to surrounding lymph nodes that can easily be seen on contrast-enhanced chest CT. Less frequently, squamous cell carcinoma presents peripherally and displays the same radiographic characteristics such as central necrosis and cavitation with thick walls. Classically, it is known to present in the superior sulcus and cause Pancoast syndrome. Tumor invasion into the chest wall and extension into the neck can best be seen also on contrast-enhanced CT.

D. Large Cell Neuroendocrine Carcinoma

Large cell neuroendocrine carcinomas grow by bronchial extension and occur peripherally. They are often very aggressive in growth and exhibit early metastases. Strongly associated with cigarette smoking, large cell neuroendocrine carcinomas typically present as large peripheral masses that can be seen on chest radiographs and CT scans. They are almost never found as pulmonary nodules. Masses that are 5 to 7 cm in diameter are not uncommon for large cell neuroendocrine carcinomas. Similar to squamous cell carcinomas, its rapid growth is associated with areas of necrosis and cavitation.

E. Small Cell Carcinoma

Associated with the highest mortality, small cell carcinoma almost always presents with extensive metastatic disease. Radiographically, it appears as a large central mass with diffuse adenopathy. Often, the presentation of a large central mass is accompanied by postobstructive findings on imaging from bronchial compression. Patients can present with symptoms of shortness of breath, facial swelling, and hoarseness that correspond with the radiographic findings of superior vena cava compression. The primary tumor is rarely visualized on chest radiograph alone. It is also difficult to distinguish tumor from surrounding adenopathy without the use of IV contrast on chest CT.

IV. Radiographic Findings of Other Primary Pulmonary Neoplasms

A. Lymphoma

Chest CT, often with IV contrast enhancement, is the primary radiographic modality for evaluation of both Hodgkin's and non-Hodgkin's lymphoma. The reason is primarily for staging and mediastinal lymph node involvement. Primary pulmonary Hodgkin's and non-Hodgkin's lymphomas are extremely rare. Should Hodgkin's be found within the lung parenchyma, it characteristically presents as ill-defined nodules and masses that fan out from the hilum in an orderly bronchovascular distribution, best appreciated on chest CT.

Non-Hodgkin's lymphoma presents differently on radiographic imaging of the thorax in that it is more random in distribution. It can present as a chest wall mass from mediastinal extension or involve the pleura with associated pleural effusions. Should non-Hodgkin's lymphoma involve the lung parenchyma, it can be seen on chest radiograph or CT as peripheral or central consolidative lesions, much like a severe multifocal pneumonia.

B. Carcinoid

Carcinoid tumors are one of the few more common primary pulmonary neoplasms that are not associated with cigarette smoking. They are known for their less aggressive nature and are associated with a good prognosis. Stemming from neuroendocrine cells, they are similar to squamous cell carcinoma in that they exhibit endobronchial growth and are typically found centrally as a hilar or perihilar mass on chest CT or radiography. Postobstructive pneumonitis and atelectasis are both associated with their endobronchial growth. Recurrent inflammation of the airways from obstruction can eventually lead to bronchiectasis or dilated bronchi from fibrosis found on chest CT.

Carcinoid tumors are occasionally found peripherally within the lungs. When they are found as solitary pulmonary nodules, their growth is slow and almost appear as unchanged on follow-up radiographic imaging. Nearly 30% of carcinoid tumors have internal calcification that can be best seen on thin-section chest CT (26).

C. Metastatic Disease to The Lungs

One of the primary roles of the lungs, besides their job in gas exchange, is to serve as the body's filter. Venous clots are saved from entering the systemic circulation because they are caught and eventually broken down in the lungs. Unfortunately, the lungs are also a common site for metastases. Metastases are deposited in the lungs through hematogenous, lymphangitic, or endobronchial spread. Unlike the solitary pulmonary nodule, metastatic disease to the lungs typically presents as multiple nodules. Most commonly, they occur from primary malignancies of the pancreas, breast, kidney, and skin. Endobronchial metastases are rare and typically are from primary tumors of the kidney and thyroid. Their radiographic findings are again a reflection of their pathophysiology resulting in post-obstruction from airway occlusion. In hematogenous spread, metastases in the lungs appear as round or ovoid nodules of varying size with sharp margins in a peripheral, bilateral distribution. More often, the metastases are more numerous in regions of greater blood flow, particularly in the lower lobes of the lungs. A miliary pattern of innumerable subcentimeter nodules can also occur in hematogenous spread and is known to occur in melanoma, renal cell carcinoma, and thyroid cancer.

Lymphangitic metastases are seen as a combination of interlobular septal thickening and small nodules on chest radiograph. On chest CT, these metastases are seen with associated septal thickening and nodules that track along the bronchovascular anatomy of the lungs to include the interlobular septa peripherally, giving them a beaded string appearance. Both lymphangitic and hematogenous metastases are often associated with mediastinal lymphadenopathy.

V. Staging of Pulmonary Neoplasms

Beyond identifying the radiographic characteristics of pulmonary neoplasms, the radiologist must also be able to accurately stage non-small cell lung cancers. The reason for staging is primarily for the opportunity for tumor resection, which conveys a much higher rate of survival for patients. On average, patients diagnosed with lung cancer in stage IA disease have a five-year survival following surgical resection of 61% to 75% (3,27). Staging of lung cancer is the primary determinant of available treatment courses and patient prognosis.

On the basis of the TNM staging system from the American Joint Committee on Cancer, between stage IIIA and stage IIIB is usually where thoracic surgeons decide is the cutoff for resection of lung cancers (28). Stage IIIB is assigned when tumor spread affects the contralateral mediastinal lymph nodes, whereas stage IIIA has metastases only to the ipsilateral mediastinal lymph nodes. Chest CT with IV contrast enhancement has been the preferred radiologic modality for assessing mediastinal involvement. CT scans are also useful in detecting distant metastases of lung cancers in common locations, such as the adrenal glands and liver.

VI. Lung Cancer Screening

It has been found that only 15% of lung cancers are diagnosed as stage I (11). The rest are usually in their advanced stages where metastases have already occurred and treatment options are limited. Given the significant difference in mortality early detection can have on lung cancer, the search is on to find the most effective screening modality. For a screening test to be successful, it must have high sensitivity as well as specificity. The potential harm from side effects of the screening test and/or its financial burden on societal resources must not outweigh the benefits it has on treatment of the disease and in decreasing mortality. Radiology has traditionally used the chest radiograph as a screening tool for the detection of lung cancer. However, the use of chest radiographs alone has proven to be too insensitive. A recent study from the Netherlands argued that the generally accepted miss rate for radiologic detection of lung cancer was unacceptable, and it tried to find reasons for why so many were missed on chest radiographs. Putting their own radiologists to the test from a major hospital, a total of 396 chest radiographs from patients with a known diagnosis of non-small cell lung cancer were analyzed. A 19% miss rate was found with many of the misses attributable to superimposition of structures along with small lesion size (29).

With chest CT scans, the issues that chest radiographs face are no longer significant. Current spatial and temporal resolution of CT scanners allow for the detection of structures less than 1 mm in size with negligible artifact. The axial images obtained on CT scans reduce, to a large degree, the problem of adjacent structure superimposition. Chest CT has greatly improved the sensitivity of lung cancer detection. The Lung Cancer Screening Study took over 3000 patients and randomized them to either chest radiograph or chest CT for lung cancer screening. Examinations were done at baseline and then again at follow-up after one year. Of the 60 lung cancers diagnosed, 40 were made with CT scans with nearly half being stage I cancers and amenable to surgical resection (30).

Despite the increased sensitivity of CT scans over chest radiographs, there is the concern of high radiation exposure to patients. Chest CT scans can be readjusted to have a lower dose of radiation. The trade-off is often decreased resolution. Another concern for CT scans is its high cost and availability. Many rural medical centers cannot afford the purchase and maintenance of CT scanners. Their high cost has caused many to argue for more effective financial resource allocation, such as investing in smoking prevention programs that will clearly have an effect on mortality associated with lung cancer. The other issue is CT scan specificity. CT scans can increase the frequency of false positives, when a benign nodule that would normally be missed on chest radiograph is labeled as potentially malignant. Currently, no evidence exists for the use of chest CT in screening and the reduction of lung cancer mortality.

The use of positron emission tomography (PET) as a screening tool for lung cancer has also not been ideal. Many lung nodules that are benign are inflammatory in nature and result in a false positive on PET. Studies have also shown that the sensitivity of PET drops dramatically as lung nodule size decreases, making its usefulness questionable at best for detecting lung cancers in their early stages (31).

VII. Management of Detected Pulmonary Nodules

Pulmonary nodules that are over 1 cm in diameter and exhibit radiographic findings suspicious for malignancy in patients with significant smoking histories are relatively easy to manage. Most likely, these high-risk nodules are biopsied or surgically resected. However, for nodules that are less than 1 cm with minimal radiographic findings suspicious for malignancy in low-risk patients, the follow-up and management becomes more unclear. The follow-up required for subcentimeter nodules relies solely on radiographic imaging to assess for any change in size and density that would make the diagnosis of malignancy more likely. Published guidelines from the American College of Chest Physicians detail the need for chest CT follow-up of pulmonary nodules at 3-, 6-, 12-, and 24-month intervals without any specifics on nodule size (3). No supporting evidence or specific reason is given for these proposed time intervals other than the goal of trying to detect lung malignancy as early as possible. The radiographic imaging frequency of pulmonary nodules that underlies many current recommendations most likely started from the Mayo Lung Project, which sought to show whether the combination of obtaining sputum cytology and chest radiographs every four months was an effective screening policy for lung cancer. Despite not showing an improvement in mortality, it did show at the time that chest radiographs were effective in detecting early-stage lung cancers (32). However, the same imaging standard using chest radiographs over two decades ago should not be applied today, given the

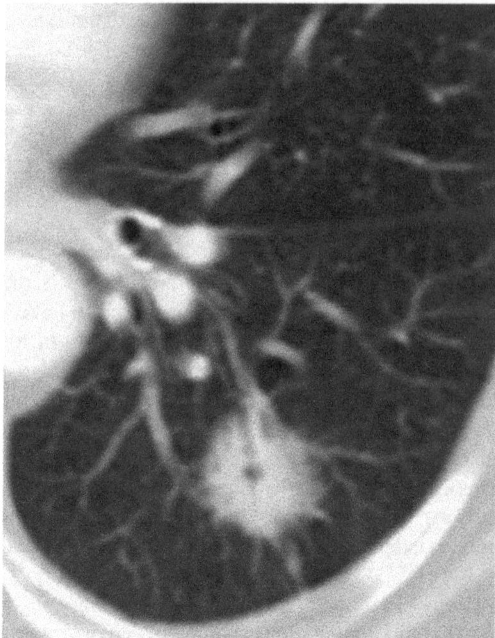

Figure 9 Pulmonary nodule at baseline.

existence of CT. Chest CT is clearly more sensitive in detecting lung nodules and is far superior in evaluating nodule characteristics in comparison with chest radiographs. Subjecting patients to CT scanning at increased frequencies without supportive evidence means unnecessary radiation exposure, which on a population basis can hurt more people than it is helping.

Our current understanding of lung cancer pathophysiology and the natural behavior of the tumor subtypes have increased significantly over the last few decades. With the use of advanced CT scanners, pulmonary nodules and masses are better characterized to the point where their tissue type, malignant potential, and growth can be predicted. The concept of tumor doubling time has been introduced with the growth of a nodule indicated not just by increases in diameter but also by density and volume (Figs. 9 and 10). Characteristic lung nodule attenuation on CT scan can mean differences in growth rate. This was observed in studies by Hasegawa et al., in which the growth rates of malignant lung nodules were measured and compared using CT scans. They found that ground-glass nodules had a mean volume doubling time of 813 days, whereas ground-glass nodules with a solid component had a mean volume doubling time of 457 days. Not surprisingly, solid nodules had the shortest mean volume doubling time of 149 days (33). More aggressive tumors have faster doubling times, which mean poorer prognosis. More indolent tumors with slow doubling times challenged the traditional two-year follow-up rule of pulmonary nodules. With advances in CT software technology on the horizon, volume changes can potentially be detected on follow-up in a growing nodule that otherwise would have measured equally in diameter using electronic calipers.

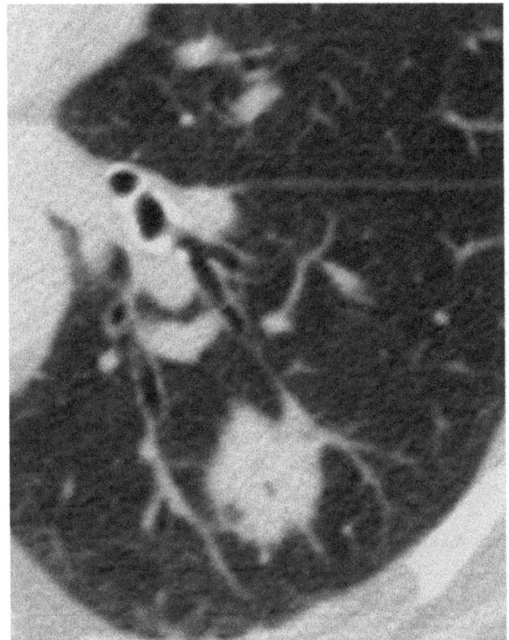

Figure 10 Pulmonary nodule at 12-month follow-up with unchanged size but increased density later found to be adenocarcinoma.

The combination of improved technology, better understanding of lung cancer behavior, and associated patient risk factors demands revised guidelines for the radiographic management of small pulmonary nodules. The Fleischner Society has made some recommendations that take these factors into account. For patients of low risk without any history of smoking or other known risk factors, no follow-up is needed for detected pulmonary nodules less than 4 mm. Nodules 4 to 6 mm in size need follow-up CT scanning in 12 months; if unchanged, no further follow-up is required. Follow-up CT at 6 to 12 months and then at 18 to 24 months is required if no change is observed for nodules measuring 6 to 8 mm. For nodules greater than 8 mm, follow-up CT with IV contrast is recommended at 3, 9, and 24 months. PET and biopsy should also be considered. For the high-risk patient with a significant history of smoking, the recommendations for CT scanning become more frequent for each nodule size interval. However, for nodules greater than 8 mm, the same recommendation applies to both low- and high-risk patients. Exceptions are made for patients with a history of known malignancy who are at greater risk and may need even more frequent CT follow-up. Patients younger than 35 years with no other risk factors who are at less than 1% chance of having a malignant nodule should have follow-up with a single CT scan at 12 months to look for nodule change. Also, given the improved understanding of some bronchioloalveolar and adenocarcinoma subtypes that tend to exhibit extremely slow growth, recommendations have been made for longer follow-up CT imaging (34).

References

1. American Cancer Society. Cancer facts and figures. Available at: www.cancer.org. Accessed July 2007.
2. Yankelvitz DF, Hensche CI. Lung cancers: small solitary pulmonary nodules. Radiol Clin North Am 2000; 38:1–9.
3. Tan BB, Flaherty KR, Kazerooni EA, et al. The solitary pulmonary nodule. Chest 2003; 123: 89S–96S.
4. Jemal A, Chu KC, Tarone RE. Recent trends in lung cancer mortality in the United States. J Natl Cancer Inst 2001; 93(4):277–283.
5. Shopland DR. Tobacco use and its contribution to early cancer mortality with a special emphasis on cigarette smoking. Environ Health Perspect 1995; 103(suppl 8):131–142.
6. Quint LE, Park CH, Iannettoni MD. Solitary pulmonary nodules in patients with extrapulmonary neoplasms. Radiology 2000; 217:257–261.
7. Zerhouni EA, Stitik FP, Siegelmann SS, et al. CT of the pulmonary nodule: a cooperative study. Radiology 1986; 160(2):319–327.
8. Mahoney MC, Shipley RT, Corcoran HL, et al. CT demonstration of calcification in carcinoma of the lung. Am J Roentgenol 1990; 154:255–258.
9. Webb WR. Radiologic evaluation of the solitary pulmonary nodule. Am J Roentgenol 1990; 154: 701–708.
10. Winer-Muram HT. The solitary pulmonary nodule. Radiology 2006; 239(1):34–49.
11. Henschke CI, McCauley DI, Yankelevitz DF, et al. Early lung cancer action project: overall design and findings from baseline screening. Lancet 1999; 354:99–105.
12. Midthun DE, Swenson SJ, Jett JR, et al. Screening for lung cancer with low-dose spiral computed tomography. Lung Cancer 2000; 29 (suppl 1):S241.
13. Byers TE, Vena JE, Rzepka TF. Predilection of lung cancer for the upper lobes: an epidemiologic inquiry. J Natl Cancer Inst 1984; 72:1271–1275.
14. Henschke CI, Yankelevitz DF, Mirtcheva R, et al. CT screening for lung cancer: frequency and significance of part solid and nonsolid nodules. Am J Roentgenol 2002; 178:1053–1057.
15. Li F, Sone S, Abe H, et al. Malignant versus benign nodules at CT screening for lung cancer: comparison of thin-section CT findings. Radiology 2004; 233:793–798.
16. Siegelmann SS, Khouri NF, Leo FP, et al. Solitary pulmonary nodules: CT assessment. Radiology 1986; 160(2):307–312.
17. Swenson SI, Brown LR, Colby TV, et al. Lung nodule enhancement at CT: prospective findings. Radiology 1996; 201:447–455.
18. Kuriyama K, Tateishi R, Doi O, et al. Prevalence of air bronchograms in small peripheral carcinomas of the lung on thin-section CT: comparison with benign tumors. Am J Roentenol 1991; 156:921–924.
19. Zwirewich CV, Vedal S, Miller RR, et al. Solitary pulmonary nodule: high resolution CT and radiographic-pathologic correlation. Radiology 1991; 179:469–476.
20. Woodring JH, Fried AM. Significance of wall thickness in solitary cavities of the lung: a follow up study. AJR Am J Roentgenol 1983; 140:473–474.
21. Travis WD, Travis LB, Devesa SS. Lung cancer. Cancer 1995; 75:191–202.
22. Thun MJ, Lally CA, Flannery JT, et al. Cigarette smoking and changes in the histopathology of lung cancer. J Natl Cancer Inst 1997; 89(21):1580–1586.
23. Hoffman D, Brunnemann KD, Prokopczyk B, et al. Tobacco-specific N-nitrosamines and Areca-derived N-nitrosamines: chemistry, biochemistry, carcinogenicity, and relevance to humans. J Toxicol Environ Health 1994; 41:1–52.
24. Noguchi M, Morikawa A, Kawasaki M, et al. Small adenocarcinoma of the lung: histologic characteristics and prognosis. Cancer 1995; 75:2844–2852.

25. Yang Z, Sone S, Honda T, et al. High-resolution CT analysis of small peripheral lung adenocarcinomas revealed on screening helical CT. Am J Roentgenol 2001; 176:1399–1407.
26. McLoud T. Pulmonary neoplasms. Thoracic Radiology: The Requisites, 1st ed. Boston, MA: Mosby, 1998:310–311.
27. Mountain CF. Revisions in the international system for staging lung cancer. Chest 1997; 111: 1710–1717.
28. Kazerooni EA, Gross BH. Lung cancer. Cardiopulmonary imaging, 1st ed. Philadelphia, PA: Lippencott Williams and Wilkins, 2004:143–164.
29. Quekel LG, Kessels AG, Goei R, et al. Miss rate of lung cancer on the chest radiograph in clinical practice. Chest 1999; 115:720–724.
30. Gohagan JK, Marcus PM, Fagerstrom RM, et al. Final results of the lung screening study, a randomized feasibility study of spiral CT versus chest X-ray screening for lung cancer. Lung Cancer 2005; 47:9–15.
31. Lowe VJ, Fletcher JW, Gobar L, et al. Prospective investigation of positron emission tomography in lung nodules. J Clin Oncol 1998; 16:1075–1084.
32. Fontana RS, Sanderson DR, Woolner LB, et al. Lung cancer screening: the Mayo program. J Occup Med 1986; 28(8):746–750.
33. Hasegawa M, Sone S, Takashima S, et al. Growth rate of small lung cancers detected on mass CT screening. Br J Radiol 2000; 73:1252–1259.
34. MacMahon H, Austin JHM, Gamsu G, et al. Guidelines for management of small pulmonary nodules detected on CT scans: a statement from the Fleischner society. Radiology 2005; 237: 395–400.

30
Nonmalignant Versus Malignant Proliferations on Pleural Biopsy

FRANÇOISE GALATEAU-SALLÉ
MESONAT Registry/ERI 3 INSERM CHU Caen University of Medicine, Caen, France

PHILIP T. CAGLE
Weill Medical College of Cornell University, New York, New York, and The Methodist Hospital, Houston, Texas, U.S.A.

I. Introduction

Three categories of pathology are commonly encountered on pleural biopsy: (*i*) benign reactive, inflammatory processes; (*ii*) metastatic malignancies; and (*iii*) primary malignancies that consist mostly of malignant mesotheliomas. These three categories often overlap in their gross presentation, with nodules, thickening, or encasement of the pleura and/or presence of pleural effusion; tissue examination is required to establish the diagnosis. Therefore, an adequate pleural biopsy is the "gold standard" for differentiating among these possibilities. However, because these lesions may overlap in their histopathological appearance, they present a challenge to the pathologist as well. The proliferating mesothelial cells and/or fibroblasts of pleuritis may strongly resemble malignancy, with florid cellularity, cytological atypia, and mitoses; they may even mimic invasion when benign mesothelial cells are entrapped within the pleuritis. In contrast, the malignant cells of a mesothelioma may be relatively bland. Therefore, determining whether or not a lesion is malignant may be more of a problem than determining a type of malignancy on some pleural biopsies (1–22).

The focus of this chapter is on the differential diagnosis of nonmalignant proliferations versus malignancies on pleural biopsy, but a word on the diagnosis of different types of malignancy in the pleura is warranted as part of the introduction. Metastatic malignancies are much more common in the pleura than primary mesothelioma, even in asbestos-exposed individuals. The wide variety of histopathological appearances of mesotheliomas means that carcinomas, sarcomas, melanomas, germ cell tumors, and other cancers may enter into the differential diagnosis of mesothelioma and vice versa. Mesotheliomas may be epithelioid, sarcomatoid, or biphasic (when both patterns are present in at least 10% of cells). Epithelioid and sarcomatoid mesotheliomas may be further subdivided into histopathological subsets. These major subsets are listed in Table 1 (15–28); the other types of cancer that may mimic them and vice versa are listed in Table 2 (15–39). Histochemical studies, immunohistochemical studies, and electron microscopy may be necessary to differentiate between the different types of malignancy (16–20). Each case reported in the French National Mesothelioma Surveillance Program undergoes a

Table 1 Histopathological Subsets of Mesothelioma

Epithelioid
Tubulopapillary
Sheet-like
Adenomatoid
Deciduoid
Sarcomatoid
Sarcomatoid (resembling fibrosarcoma or malignant fibrous histiocytoma)
Desmoplastic
Desmoplastic (mimicking organizing pleuritis) (23)
Biphasic
Mixed epithelioid (>10% of tumor) and sarcomatoid (>10% of tumor) and/or Desmoplastic
Rare variants
Sarcomatoid with heterologous elements (chondroid, osteoid, rhabdoid) (24)
Lymphohistiocytoid (mixed with heavy lymphoplasmacytic infiltrate) (25,26)
Clear cell (27)
Small cell (28)
Pleomorphic/giant cell

Table 2 Cancers Mimicking Mesothelioma on Pleural Biopsy

Mesothelioma	Malignant Mimickers
Epithelioid	Carcinomas (adenocarcinomas including solid, acinar, papillary, tubular; squamous cell; transitional cell), epithelioid sarcomas, melanomas, germ cell tumors, thymic carcinoma
Sarcomatoid	Sarcomas, sarcomatoid carcinomas (lung, renal cell, ENT, etc.), melanoma, thymic carcinoma
Biphasic	Biphasic carcinomas, carcinosarcomas, pulmonary blastomas, biphasic sarcomas, melanomas, thymic carcinoma

Abbreviation: ENT, ear nose throat.

standardized diagnostic confirmation procedure made by the Mesopath group that ruled out 13% of the initial diagnoses. Despite an extended immunohistochemical studies half of the 13% cases remains unclassified (40). Further details about the differential diagnosis of mesothelioma versus other malignancies are given in chapters (31–33,36,37,39).

II. Benign Vs. Malignant Epithelioid Lesions: Mesothelial Hyperplasia and Atypical Mesothelial Hyperplasia

Mesothelial cells may proliferate along the pleural surface in any type of pleural reaction or injury, often in association with pleural effusion, including infections, collagen-vascular diseases, drug reactions, pneumothorax, and subsequent to chest surgery or trauma, among many other conditions. On biopsy, fibrin, fibrin organizing into granulation tissue, and granulation tissue are present in many cases of pleuritis, and inflammation is also often present. However, the presence of fibrin, granulation tissue, or inflammation on pleural biopsy does not rule out a malignancy.

The mesothelial cells are generally cuboidal with round nuclei, prominent nucleoli, and abundant eosinophilic cytoplasm; depending on the severity of the reaction, these cells may exhibit cytological atypia, mitoses, and pseudoinvasion by entrapment in the fibrin and granulation tissue. Entrapped reactive mesothelial cells may also line gaps in pleural tissue planes or infoldings of pleural tissue. It is then that these cells may enter into the differential diagnosis of an epithelioid malignancy. Identification of true invasion into the adjacent lung or subpleural soft tissues is the most reliable finding to confirm a diagnosis of a well-differentiated malignancy, particularly mesothelioma.

In cases that are cytologically or architecturally worrisome, the diagnosis of atypical mesothelial hyperplasia is recommended. Atypical mesothelial hyperplasia ranges from highly reactive proliferations to proliferations that may represent malignancy but do not present conclusive finding of invasion. When an early, incipient, or adjacent malignancy cannot be ruled out, the diagnosis of atypical mesothelial hyperplasia should be followed by the phrase "of undetermined malignant potential" and close follow-up and/or additional tissue samples suggested. Although the concept of an "in situ" phase of mesothelioma is a useful theory, a diagnosis of pure in situ mesothelioma is not recommended at present, since the diagnosis cannot be made unless an adjacent invasive component is identified (10,41).

The mesothelial proliferation typically occurs along the surface or is entrapped within the thickened pleura (Fig. 1) and paralleled the pleural surface while full thickness involvement of the pleura is observed in malignant mesothelioma (Fig. 2). Papillary tufts of reactive mesothelial cells may be present along the pleural surface and have bland collagen cores (Fig. 3), but they lack the desmoplastic cores seen with papillary malignancies. Entrapped benign cells typically line large spaces representing clefts within the connective tissues and do not produce a desmoplastic reaction in the surrounding stroma. The major difficulty is encountered with a new concept of lesion of mesothelial origin, entilted "well-differentiated papillary mesothelioma" (WDPM), particularly on small biopsy samples. WDPM is a superficial mesothelial proliferation associated with an indolent clinical course

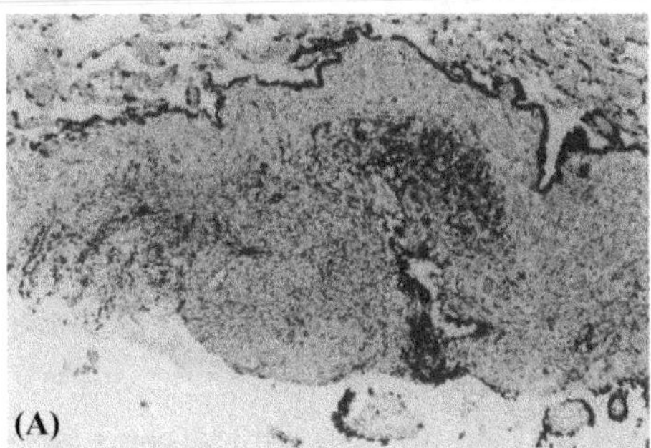

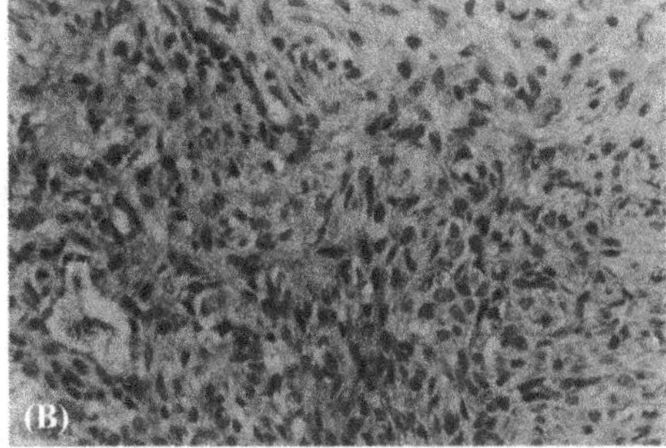

Figure 1 Orientation of florid reactive mesothelial proliferation toward pleural surface. (**A**) Low-power view of keratin immunostain showing orientation of cells within pleura. (**B**) High-power view showing proliferating mesothelial cells.

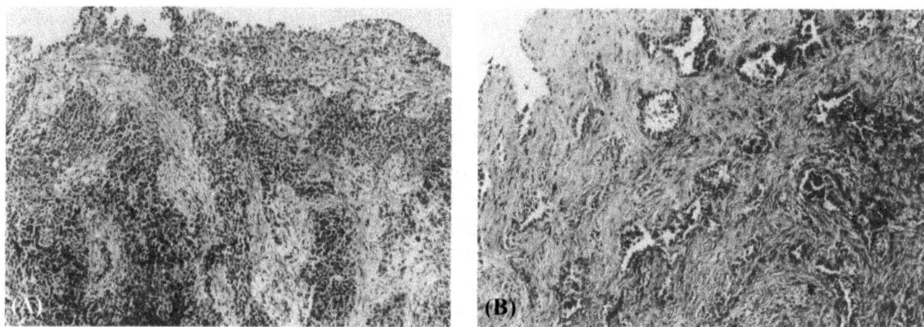

Figure 2 Full-thickness involvement of pleura by epithelioid mesothelioma. (**A**) Low-power view showing full thickness involvement. (**B**) High-power view showing epithelioid cells arranged in tubular structures with desmoplastic reaction.

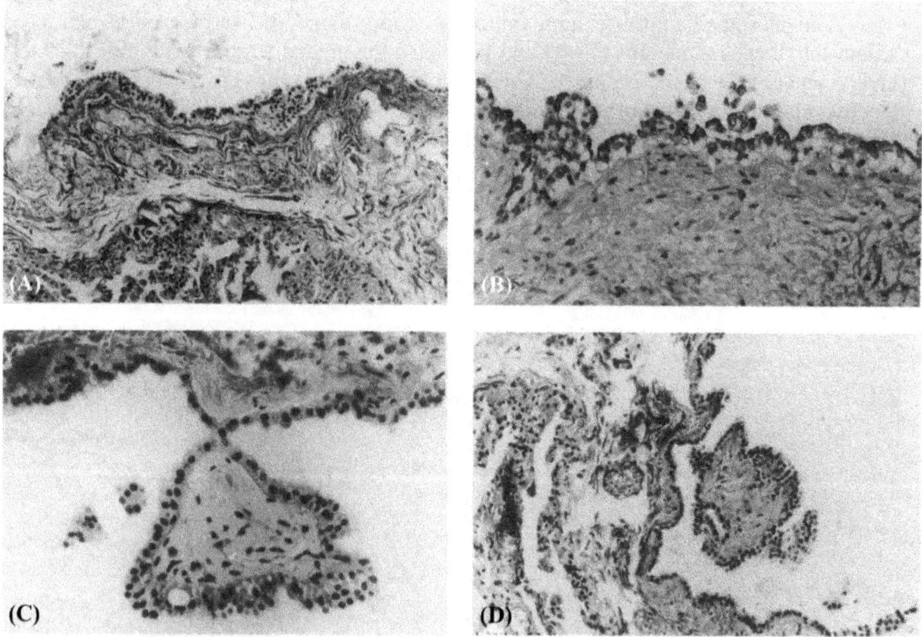

Figure 3 Reactive atypical mesothelial proliferation. (**A**) and (**B**) Low- and high-power views showing proliferation of cuboidal mesothelial cells with mild atypia along pleural surface. (**C**) High-power view showing papillary tufts of reactive mesothelial cells with bland collagenous cores. (**D**) High-power view showing papillary tufts of atypical mesothelial cells of undetermined malignant potential with desmoplastic cores.

and long survival. WDPMs present with a similar and radiographical presentation and a very similar histopathological appearance to atypical mesothelial hyperplasia except that the papillae show stout myxoid fibrovascular cores covered with a single layer of flattened mesothelial cells, with bland cytology (42).

The most reliable evidence that an equivocal epithelioid proliferation is malignant is invasion into the subpleural fat and muscle or lung tissue. Therefore, biopsies should be deep enough to include these tissues. Keratin immunostains may highlight the invasion of malignant cells into the fat or other tissues if needed (16–20).

Although certain immunohistochemical stains may be a useful adjunct study when strict criteria for immunopositivity are used, no immunohistochemical stain has been found to be reliable in differentiating mesothelial hyperplasias from malignancies. Immunopositivity for p53 in greater than 10% of atypical cells has been reported to support a diagnosis of malignancy as it has strong membranous staining for epithelial membrane antigen (EMA) (43–49). However, many mesotheliomas and other malignancies are negative for these markers and reactive processes may be positive. Variations in antibodies, laboratory techniques, and fixation and processing of tissue make standardization of these procedures difficult. Therefore, a diagnosis of malignancy should not be made only on the basis of a positive p53 or EMA stain. Very recently, it has been reported that GLUT 1, a member of the mammalian facilitative glucose transporter may be a sensitive immunohistochemical marker allowing separation of reactive mesothelial proliferation from a diffuse malignant mesothelioma (50). On histological preparations, Mesothelin a 40 kDa glycoprotein, and osteopontin a phophoprotein acting as a protein ligand of CD44, have been under investigation in both reactive and malignant mesothelioma, but ultimately, they were not helpful in determining reactive versus malignant mesothelial proliferations (51,52). However soluble mesothelin-related peptides (mesothelin) and osteopontin may be promising markers when measured either in the serum or in pleural effusion to predict malignancy, but additional extended studies are necessary to evaluate the usefulness of these biomarkers in the screening of early malignant mesothelioma (53,54).

Features of benign versus malignant epithelioid lesions of the pleura are listed in Table 3.

Table 3 Benign Vs. Malignant Epithelioid Lesions of the Pleura

Benign
Absence of deep invasion into lung or subpleural soft tissues
Cellularity oriented toward pleural surface
No desmoplastic reaction
Pseudoinvasion by entrapment within fibrin/granulation tissue or restricted along planes or infoldings of tissue
Mild to moderate cytological atypia
Normal mitoses
Malignant
Frank invasion into lung or subpleural soft tissues
Cellularity throughout pleura without orientation toward surface
Desmoplastic reaction
Frankly malignant cytological features
Abnormal mitoses
Bland necrosis

III. Benign Vs. Malignant Spindle Cell Lesions: Organizing and Fibrous Pleuritis

Benign reactive and inflammatory lesions of the pleura may be characterized by fibrinous pleuritis, in which there are fibrin deposits along a denuded pleural surface. This fibrin is organized by the ingrowth of granulation tissue composed of reactive fibroblasts and blood vessels. The reactive atypia of the fibroblasts or endothelial cells during this organization may mimic a sarcomatoid malignancy, including sarcomatoid mesothelioma (18–23,55).

Frankly malignant histological features such as striking pleomorphism, atypical mitoses, storiform pattern, and necrosis favor a diagnosis of malignancy. As with the epithelioid lesions, the orientation of the spindle cell proliferation may indicate the likely diagnosis. Organizing pleuritis is limited to or oriented along the pleural surface, whereas a sarcomatoid mesothelioma tends to involve the full thickness of the pleura. Deep invasion into the lung underlying the visceral pleura or soft tissues underlying the parietal pleura is diagnostic of malignancy. Since sarcomatoid mesotheliomas are generally keratin immunopositive, keratin immunostains may demonstrate this deep invasion (Fig. 4).

Keratin immunonegativity is consistent with malignant fibroblasts versus sarcomatoid mesothelioma, which is generally keratin immunopositive. Sarcomas and metastatic melanomas, which may be of the spindle cell type, are also typically keratin immunonegative. However, in addition to most sarcomatoid mesotheliomas, reactive mesothelial cells and reactive fibroblasts are keratin positive, as are most sarcomatoid carcinomas as well as some sarcomas. Therefore, the keratin stain should not be the sole basis for the diagnosis of a spindle cell proliferation in the pleura. A summary of the keratin immunostaining patterns of spindle cell lesions of the pleura is given in Table 4. Although strong immunopositivity for p53 is observed in many cases of sarcomatoid mesothelioma and other sarcomatoid malignancies, the same caveats regarding p53 apply to spindle cell lesions, as noted with the epithelioid lesions, and this marker cannot be relied on alone to make a diagnosis.

Features of benign versus malignant spindle cell lesions of the pleura are summarized in Table 5.

Desmoplastic mesotheliomas are difficult to differentiate from fibrous pleuritis, since both lesions have comparatively little cellularity in association with extensive collagen (23,55,56). This is the diagnostic area in which members of the United States Canadian Mesothelioma Reference Panel are most likely to be unable to form a consensus on a given case. It is particularly important in cases of desmoplastic mesothelioma to have adequate sampling of the pleura so as to look for cellular areas within the desmoplastic lesion and to examine for invasion of underlying tissues. A diagnosis of desmoplastic mesothelioma should be avoided on small biopsies. Features that favor malignancy in these lesions are areas of increased cellularity, frankly sarcomatoid features, foci of bland necrosis, and invasion of the underlying lung or soft tissues. It is recommended that at least two of these features be present in order to make a diagnosis of desmoplastic mesothelioma. Features diagnostic of desmoplastic mesothelioma as originally defined by Mangano et al. (23) are listed in Table 6. An additional criterion of distant metastases has been dropped for the evaluation of pleural biopsies.

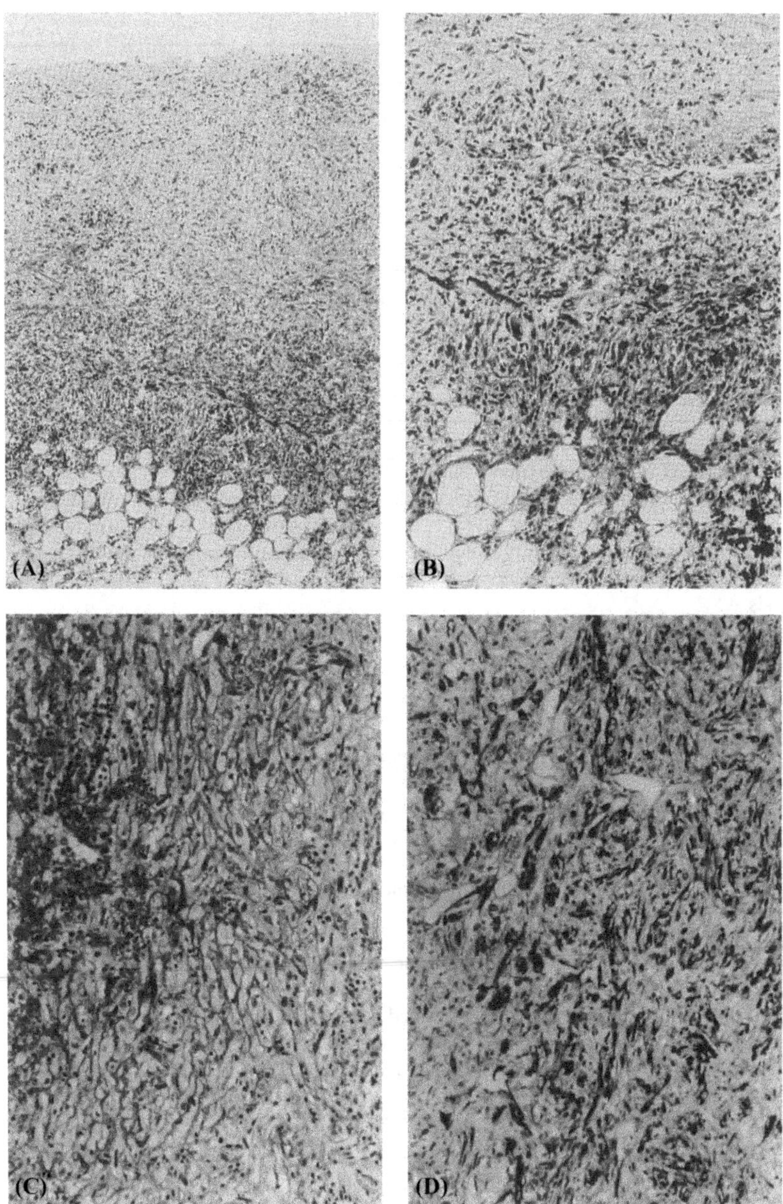

Figure 4 Sarcomatoid mesothelioma with frankly sarcomatous features of increased cellularity and pleomorphism. (**A**) and (**B**) Low- and high-power views showing full-thickness involvement of thickened pleura without orientation toward surface and with invasion of subpleural fat. (**C**) Higher-power view showing increased cellularity. (**D**) Higher-power view showing keratin immunopositivity of the pleomorphic spindle cells.

Table 4 Keratin Immunostaining Patterns in Spindle Cell Lesions of the Pleura

Cell Type	Keratin Immunostaining
Activated fibroblasts	Positive
Reactive mesothelial cells	Positive
Mesothelioma	Positive[a]
Sarcoma	Negative[a]
Sarcomatoid carcinoma	Positive[a]
Melanoma	Negative[a]

[a]Rare exceptions exist and require further close evaluation in those cases. Particularly, sarcomas may be immunopositive for keratin in some cases.

Table 5 Benign Vs. Malignant Spindle Cell Lesions of the Pleura

Features favoring malignancy:
- Invasion into underlying lung parenchyma or subpleural soft tissues
- Full-thickness involvement of pleura with atypical cells and lack of orientation toward pleural surface
- Frankly sarcomatous features including high cellularity, cytological pleomorphism, storiform pattern, and increased and/or atypical mitoses
- Bland necrosis

Features favoring benignity:
- No invasion into underlying tissues
- Orientation of cellularity toward pleural surface
- Mild to moderate cytological atypia
- Inflammatory and not bland necrosis
- Numerous capillaries almost completely traversing the thickened pleura perpendicular to pleural surface

Table 6 Features Diagnostic of Desmoplastic Malignant Mesothelioma

Storiform or patternless pattern in paucicellular fibrotic lesion with one or more of the following:
1. Invasion by the tumor into chest wall, skeletal muscle, and/or adipose tissue or invasion into the lung parenchyma
2. Areas of bland necrosis, defined as well-circumscribed areas, characterized by subtle areas in staining along with nuclear fragmentation and karyorrhexis
3. Frankly sarcomatoid areas with increased cellularity and nuclear atypia sufficient to suggest sarcomatoid lesion

Source: Ref. 42.

IV. Benign Neoplasms Vs. Mesothelioma

Primary benign neoplasms of the pleura are rare, but when present, they may enter into the differential diagnosis of malignancy, including mesothelioma. These are discussed in chapter 32.

References

1. Lillington GA, Gould MK. Identification of benign pulmonary nodules by needle biopsy. Chest 1998; 113:3–5.
2. Galateau-Salle F, Brambilla E, Cagle P, et al. Differential diagnosis: mesothelial proliferations.. In: Galateau-Salle F, eds. Pathology of Malignant Mesothelioma. London: Springer-Verlag, 2006:132–147.
3. Travis WD, Brambilla E, Muller–Hermelink HK, Harris CC, eds. World Health Organization Classification of Tumors. Tumors of the lung, pleura, thymus and heart. Lyon: IARC press, 2004:97–98.
4. Churg A, Colby T, Cagle P, et al. The separation of benign and malignant mesothelial proliferations. Am J Surg Pathol 2000; 24:1183–1200.
5. Silverman JF. Inflammatory and neoplastic processes of the lung: differential diagnosis and pitfalls in FNA biopsies. Diagn Cytopathol 1995; 13:448–462.
6. Loddenkemper R, Boutin C. Thoracoscopy: present and therapeutic indications. Eur Respir J 1993; 6:1544–1555.
7. Loddenkemper R. Thoracoscopy—state of the art. Eur Respir J 1998; 11:213–221.
8. Colt HG. Thoracoscopy: a prospective study of safety and outcome. Chest 1995; 108:324–329.
9. Boutin C, Viallat JR, Rey F. Thoracoscopy in the diagnosis, prognosis and treatment of mesothelioma. In: Antman A, ed. Asbestos Related Malignancy. Orlando, FL: Grune & Stratton, 1986:301–321.
10. Landreneau RJ, Mack MJ, Hazelrigg SR, et al. The role of thoracoscopy in the management of intrathoracic neoplastic processes. Semin Thorac Cardiovasc Surg 1993; 5:219–228.
11. Bensard DB, McIntyre RC, Waring BJ, et al. Comparison of video thoracic lung biopsy to open lung biopsy in the diagnosis of interstitial lung disease. Chest 1993; 103:765–770.
12. Hammar SP. The pathobioloy of benign and malignant pleural disease. Chest Surg Clin North Am 1994; 4:405–430.
13. Henderson DW, Shilkin KB, Whitaker D. Reactive mesothelial hyperplasia vs. mesothelioma including mesothelioma in situ. Am J Clin Pathol 1998; 110:397–404.
14. McCaughey WT, Al-Jabi M. Differentiation of serosal hyperplasia and neoplasia in biopsies. Pathol Annu 1986; 21(pt 1):271–294.
15. Colby TV. Malignancies in the lung and pleura mimicking benign processes. Semin Diagn Pathol 1995; 12:30–44.
16. Moran C, Suster S, Koss MN. The spectrum of histologic growth patterns in benign and malignant fibrous tumors of the pleura. Semin Diagn Pathol 1992; 9:169–180.
17. Carter D, Otis CN. Three types of spindle cell tumor of the pleura: fibroma, sarcoma, and sarcomatoid mesothelioma. Am J Surg Pathol 1988; 12:747–753.
18. Roggli VL, San Filippo F, Shelburne JD. Mesothelioma. In: Roggli VL, Greenberg SD, Pratt PC, eds. Pathology of Asbestos Associated Diseases. Boston: Little, Brown & Co., 1992:109–164.
19. Churg A. Neoplastic asbestos-induced disease. In: Churg A, Green FHY, eds. Pathology of Occupational Lung Disease. 2nd ed. Baltimore: Williams & Wilkins, 1998:339–392.
20. Hammar SP, Bolen JW. Pleural neoplasms. In: Dail DH, Hammar SP, eds. Pulmonary Pathology. New York: Springer-Verlag, 1994:1123–1278.
21. Hasleton PS. Pleural disease. In: Spencer's Pathology of the Lung, 5th ed. New York: McGraw-Hill, 1996:1111–1210.
22. Henderson DW, Commin CE, Harnmar SP, et al. Malignant mesothelioma of the pleura: current surgical pathology. In: Corrin B, ed. Pathology of Lung Tumors. New York: Churchill Livingstone, 1997:241–280.
23. Mangano WE, Cagle PT, Churg A, et al. The diagnosis of desmoplastic malignant mesothelioma and its distinction from fibrous pleurisy: a histological and immunohistochemical analysis of 31 cases including p53 immunostaining. Am J Clin Pathol 1998; 110:191–199.

24. Andrion A, Mazzucco G, Bernardi P. Sarcomatous tumor of the chest wall with ostechondroid differentiation: evidence of mesothelial origin. Am J Surg Pathol 1989; 13:707–712.
25. Henderson DW, Attwood HD, Constance TJ, et al. Lymphohistiocytoid mesothelioma: a rare lymphomatoid variant of predominantly sarcomatoid mesothelioma. Ultrastruct Pathol 1988; 12:367–384.
26. Galateau-Salle F, Attanoos R, Gibbs A, et al. Lymphohistiocytoid variant of malignant mesothelioma of the pleura: a series of 22 cases. Am J Surg Pathol 2007; 31:711–716.
27. Ordonnez NG, Myrhe M, Mackay B. Clear cell mesothelioma. Ultrastruct Pathol 1996; 20:331–336.
28. Mayall FG, Gibbs AR. The histology and immunohistochemistry of small cell mesothelioma. Histopathology 1992, 20:47–51.
29. England DM, Hochholzer L, McCarthy MJ. Localized benign and malignant fibrous tumors of the pleura. Am J Surg Pathol 1989; 13:64–658.
30. Moran CA, Suster S, Koss MN. Smooth muscle tumours presenting as pleural neoplasms. Histopathology 1995; 27:227–234.
31. Fletcher CDM. Haemangiopericytoma—a dying breed? Reappraisal of an entity and its variants: a hypothesis. Curr Diagn Pathol 1994; 1:19.
32. Zeren H, Moran CA, Suster S, et al. Primary pulmonary sarcoma with features of monophasic synovial sarcoma: a clinicopathological, immunohistochemical and ultrastructural study of 25 cases. Hum Pathol 1995; 26:474–480.
33. Gaertner E, Zeren H, Fleming MV, et al. Biphasic synovial sarcoma arising in the pleural cavity: clinicopathologic study of five cases. Am J Surg Pathol 1996; 20:36–45.
34. Lin BT, Colby TV, Gown AM, et al. Malignant vascular tumors of the serous membranes mimicking mesothelioma: a report of 14 cases. Am J Surg Pathol 1996; 20:1431–1439.
35. Cohn L, Hall AD. Extraosseous osteogenic sarcoma of the pleura. Ann Thorac Surg 1968; 5:545–549.
36. Wong WWW, Pluth JR, Grado GL, et al. Liposarcoma of the pleura. Mayo Clinic Proc 1994; 69:882–885.
37. Goetz SP, Robinson RA, Landas SK. Extraskeletal myxoid chondrosarcoma of the pleura: report of a case clinically simulating mesothelioma. Am J Clin Pathol 1992; 97:498–502.
38. Shih DF, Wang JS, Tseng HH, et al. Primary pleural thymoma. Arch Pathol Lab Med 1997; 121:79–82.
39. Moran CA, Travis DW, Rosado-de-Christenson M, et al. Thymomas presenting as pleural tumors: report of eight cases. Am J Surg Pathol 1992; 16:138–144.
40. Goldberg M, Imbernon E, Rolland P, et al. The French National Mesothelioma Surveillance Program. Occup Environ Med 2006;10:1–7.
41. Whitaker D, Henderson DW, Shilkin KB. The concept of mesothelioma in situ: implications for diagnosis and histogenesis. Semin Diagn Pathol 1992; 9:151–161.
42. Galateau-Salle F, Vignaud JM, Burke L, et al. Well-differentiated mesothelioma of the pleura: a series of 24 cases. Am J Surg Pathol 2004; 28:534–540.
43. Mayall FG, Goddard H, Gibbs AR. The frequency of p53 immunostaining in asbestos-associated mesotheliomas and non-asbestos-associated mesotheliomas. Histopathology 1993; 22:383–386.
44. Cagle PT, Brown RW, Lebovitz RM. p 53 immunostaining in the differentiation of reactive processes from malignancy in pleural biopsy specimens. Hum Pathol 1994; 25:443–448.
45. Kafiri G, Thomas DM, Krausz T, et al. p53 expression in malignant mesothelioma. Histopathology 1992; 21:331–334.
46. Mayall FG, Goddard H, Gibbs AR. p53 Immunostaining in the distinction between benign and malignant mesothelial proliferation using formalin-fixed paraffin sections. J Pathol 1992; 168:377–381.
47. Ramael M, Lemmens G, Eerdekens C, et al. Immunoreactivity for p53 protein in malignant mesothelioma and non-neoplastic mesothelium. J Pathol 1992; 168:371–375.

48. Mullick SS, Green LK, Ramzy I, et al. p53 gene product in pleural effusions. Acta Cytol 1996; 40:855–860.
49. Wolanski KD, Whitaker D, Shilkin KB, et al. The use of epithelial membrane antigen and silver stained nucleolar organizer regions testing in the differential diagnosis of mesothelioma from benign reactive mesothelioses. Cancer 1998; 82:583–589.
50. Kato Y, Tsuta K, Seki K, et al. Immunohistochmical detection of GLUT-1 can discriminate between reactive mesothelium and malignant mesothelioma. Mod Pathol 2007; 20:215–220.
51. Tigrani DY, Weydert JA. Immunohistochemical expression of osteopontin in epithelioid mesotheliomas and reactive mesothelial proliferations. Am J Clin Pathol 2007; 127:580–584.
52. Ordonnez NG. Value of mesothelin immunostaining in the diagnosis of mesothelioma. Mod Pathol 2003; 16:192–197.
53. Robinson BW, Creaney J, Lake R, et al. Mesothelin-family proteins and diagnosis of msothelioma. Lancet 2003; 15:1612–1616.
54. Bogdan-Dragos G, Scherpereel A, Devos P, et al. Utility of osteopontin and serum mesothelin in malignant pleural mesothelioma diagnosis and prognosis assessment. Clin Cancer Res 2007; 13:2928–2935.
55. Colby TV. The diagnosis of desmoplastic malignant mesothelioma. Am J Clin Pathol 1998; 110:135–136.
56. Wilson GE, Hasleton PS, Chatterjee AK. Desmoplastic malignant mesothelioma: a review of 17 cases. J Clin Pathol 1992; 45:295–298.

31
Clinical Diagnosis of Pleural Disease

RICHARD W. LIGHT
Vanderbilt University Medical Center, Nashville, Tennessee, U.S.A.

I. Introduction

Pleural effusions may develop as a complication of many diseases (Table 1). However, about a dozen diseases account for more than 90% of all pleural effusions (Table 2). The vigor with which one pursues a given diagnosis will depend upon the likelihood that a patient has that disease entity.

This chapter is organized such that the laboratory findings or the pathological findings serve as the starting point for each section. For example, one starting point is the finding of pleural fluid eosinophilia, while another starting point is the finding of non-specific pleuritis on a needle biopsy of the pleura.

II. Transudative Pleural Effusion

Pleural effusions are classically divided into transudates and exudates. By definition, a transudative effusion occurs when the systemic factors, hydrostatic or oncotic pressures, influencing the formation and reabsorption of pleural fluid are altered such that pleural fluid accumulates. In contrast, an exudative pleural effusion occurs when pleural fluid accumulates due to alterations in local factors. The first step in the clinical workup of a patient with a pleural effusion is to determine if the patient has a transudative or an exudative pleural effusion. If the patient has a transudative effusion, no additional diagnostic studies need be directed toward the pleura. Alternatively, if the patient has an exudative pleural effusion, additional efforts should be made to determine what disease process is affecting the pleura.

The separation of transudative from exudative pleural effusions is best made by simultaneous measurements of the protein and lactic acid dehydrogenase (LDH) levels in the pleural fluid and in the serum. If one or more of the following criteria are met, the patient probably has an exudative pleural effusion (1).

1. Pleural fluid protein/serum protein > 0.5
2. Pleural fluid LDH/serum LDH > 0.6
3. Absolute pleural fluid LDH > 2/3rds the upper limit of normal for serum

If none of these criteria are met, then the patient has a transudative pleural effusion.

Table 1 Differential Diagnoses of Pleural Effusion

Transudative pleural effusions
Congestive heart failure
Cirrhosis
Nephrotic syndrome
Superior vena caval obstruction
Fontan procedure
Urinothorax
Peritoneal dialysis
Glomerulonephritis
Myxedema
Exudative pleural effusions
Neoplastic disease
Metastatic disease
Mesothelioma
Infectious diseases
Bacterial infections
Tuberculosis
Fungal infections
Parasitic infections
Viral infections
Pulmonary embolization
Gastrointestinal disease
Pancreatic disease
Intra abdominal abscess
Esophageal perforation
After abdominal surgery
Diaphragmatic hernia
Endoscopic variceal sclerosis
After liver transplant
Collagen vascular disease
Rheumatoid pleuritis
Systemic lupus erythematosus
Drug-induced lupus
Immunoblastic lymphadenopathy
Sjogren's syndrome
Familial Mediterranean fever
Churg-Strauss syndrome
Wegener's granulomatosis
Drug-induced pleural disease
Nitrofurantoin
Dantrolene
Methysergide
Bromocriptine
Amiodarone
Procarbazine
Methotrexate
Miscellaneous diseases and conditions
Asbestos exposure

(*Continued*)

Table 1 Differential Diagnoses of Pleural Effusion (*Continued*)

Post cardiac injury syndrome
Meig' syndrome
Yellow nail syndrome
Sarcoidosis
Pericardial disease
After coronary artery bypass surgery
After lung transplant
Fetal pleural effusion
Uremia
Trapped lung
Radiation therapy
Postpartum pleural effusion
Amyloidosis
Electrical burns
Iatrogenic injury
Hemothorax
Chylothorax

Source: From Ref. 3.

Table 2 Approximate Annual Incidence of Various Types of Pleural Effusions in the United States

Congestive heart failure	500,000
Pneumonia (bacterial)	300,000
Malignant disease	200,000
Lung	60,000
Breast	50,000
Lymphoma	40,000
Other primaries	50,000
Pulmonary embolization	150,000
Viral disease	100,000
Cirrhosis with ascites	50,000
Gastrointestinal disease	25,000
Collagen vascular disease	6,000
Tuberculosis	2,500
Asbestos exposure	2,000
Mesothelioma	1,500

Source: From Ref. 3.

There above criteria (Light's criteria) identify almost all exudates correctly but falsely label about 25% of transudates as being exudates (2). If a patient appears to have a transudative effusion clinically, but the pleural fluid meets exudative criteria, the difference between the serum and pleural fluid protein levels should be assessed. If this difference is above 3.1 g/dL, the patient in all probability has a transudative effusion (2).

The primary etiologies for transudative pleural effusions are congestive heart failure, cirrhosis, nephrosis, hypoalbuminemia, and pulmonary embolization. If the patient has one of the first four of these diagnoses, no additional workup is to define the etiology of their pleural disease. If the patient does not have one of these diagnoses, a cardiac workup is indicated to determine if the patient has occult cardiac disease. An ultrasonic examination of the abdomen should also be obtained to ascertain whether the patient has ascites since the etiology of the fluid with ascites is the movement of free peritoneal fluid into the pleural space through defects in the diaphragm.

Transudates due to heart failure can be differentiated from other transudates etiologies by measuring the levels of aminoterminal probrain natriuretic peptide (NT-pro-BNP) in the pleural fluid or serum (3). When the ventricles are subjected to increased pressure or volume, brain natriuretic peptide (BNP) is released (4). The biologically active BNP and the NT-pro-BNP are released in equimolar amounts in the circulation (4). The pleural fluid levels of NT-pro-BNP are elevated in patients with heart failure. In one study of 117 patient including 44 with heart failure, 25 with malignancy, 20 with tuberculous pleurisy, and 10 with hepatic hydrothorax, the median pleural fluid level of NT-pro-BNP in patients with congestive heart failure was 6931 pg/mL compared with 551 pg/mL in patients with hepatic hydrothorax or 292 pg/mL in the 63 patients with exudative effusions (5). A cutoff level of 1500 pg/mL in the pleural fluid provided a sensitivity of 91% and a specificity of 93% in the diagnosis of heart failure (5). Two more recent studies (6,7) confirmed the results of the previous study and demonstrated that the levels of NT-pro-BNP were nearly identical in the serum and pleural fluid. It is important to emphasize that studies have not been performed evaluating the levels of BNP in the pleural fluid or serum in making the diagnosis of congestive heart failure. However, it should be noted that in general the level of NT-pro-BNP is approximately three times higher than that of BNP and the two values are not closely correlated (8).

There are several other entities that may have an associated transudative pleural effusion. Approximately 2% of patients undergoing continuous ambulatory peritoneal dialysis will develop large transudative pleural effusions due to the dialysate passing into the pleural space through defects in the diaphragm. Transudative pleural effusions also occur in patients with severe hypoproteinemia (AIDS or nephrotic syndrome), superior vena caval obstruction, and obstruction of a ureter (urinothorax).

III. Cloudy Pleural Fluid

Cloudiness or turbidity in pleural fluid can be due to either high lipid levels or high amounts of cells and debris suspended in the pleural fluid. To differentiate these two causes of turbidity, one needs only to centrifuge the pleural fluid and examine the supernatant. If the supernatant is clear, the cloudiness was due to cells and/or debris, while if the supernatant remains cloudy, the cloudiness was due to a high lipid level and the patient has either a chylothorax or a pseudochylothorax (3).

Chylothorax can usually be differentiated from pseudochylothorax on clinical grounds. A chylothorax is due to disruption of the thoracic duct. Chylothoraces are most commonly due to thoracic surgical procedures or malignant disease involving the thoracic duct. Lymphoma is the most common malignancy causing chylothorax. Patients with chylothorax usually have large pleural effusions and symptoms that are relatively acute. In contrast, a pseudochylothorax is a pleural effusion with a high lipid content (usually cholesterol), which is not related to disruption of the thoracic duct. The effusion has usually been present for at least five years. CT scan of the chest reveals markedly thickened pleural surfaces with pseudochylothorax and normal pleura with chylothorax. Measurement of the triglycerides in the pleural fluid is useful in making the differentiation. A pleural fluid triglyceride level above 110 mg/dL is highly suggestive of chylothorax. The finding of cholesterol crystals in the pleural fluid is diagnostic of pseudochylothorax.

IV. Bloody Pleural Fluid

There are occasions when the pleural fluid obtained appears to be blood. The fluid usually looks a lot bloodier than it really is. To quantitate the amount of blood present, a hematocrit on the pleural fluid should be obtained. If the hematocrit exceeds 50% that of the peripheral blood, the patient has a hemothorax. The most common causes of bloody pleural fluid are chest trauma, pleural malignancy, pulmonary embolus, or pneumonia. One can obtain an estimate of the hematocrit in the pleural fluid by taking the red cell count and dividing by 100,000. For example, a pleural fluid RBC of 1,000,000 yields a hematocrit of approximately 10%.

V. Eosinophilic Pleural Effusion

Pleural fluid eosinophilia exists when more than 10% of the cells in the pleural fluid are eosinophils. The two most common causes of pleural fluid eosinophilia are air and blood in the pleural space. Frequently the air is the result of a previous thoracentesis. If the patient has neither air nor blood in the pleural space, what is the likely etiology of an eosinophilic pleural effusion? In one review of 392 cases of eosinophilic pleural effusions not associated with pleural air and/or blood, the most common diagnosis was idiopathic (39.8%) followed by malignancy (17%), parapneumonic (12.5%), transudates (7.9%), pulmonary embolism (4.3%), and other (12.8%) (9). When a patient has pleural fluid eosinophilia, one should consider a drug reaction. The drugs most frequently associated with eosinophilic pleural effusions are dantrolene, bromocriptine, metronidazole, and methysergide. Two rare causes of eosinophilic pleural effusions are the Churg-Strauss syndrome (asthma with vasculitis) and paragonimiasis (oriental liver fluke). With these two diseases, the pleural fluid is characterized by a low pH and glucose. No other causes of eosinophilic pleural effusions have a low pH or glucose.

VI. Low Glucose Pleural Effusion

A pleural fluid glucose level should be obtained in all patients with exudative pleural effusions not only because a low pleural fluid glucose (<60 mg/dL) narrows the differential diagnosis but also because it provides prognostic information for patients with parapneumonic and malignant pleural effusions. The pleural fluid glucose may be reduced with complicated parapneumonic effusions, malignant pleural effusions, rheumatoid pleural effusions, tuberculous pleural effusions, paragonimiasis, the Churg-Strauss syndrome, hemothorax, and on occasion with lupus pleuritis. In patients with a parapneumonic effusion, the lower the glucose, the more likely the patient will need tube thoracostomy, thoracoscopy, or thoracotomy for resolution of the pleural effusion. Patients with malignant pleural effusions and a low pleural fluid glucose have a poor prognosis (mean life expectancy of 30 days) and are more likely to fail attempts at pleurodesis (10).

VII. Low-pH Pleural Effusion

In general, the same conditions that are associated with a low pleural fluid glucose are associated with a low pH (<7.20) and a high LDH (>3× normal serum) pleural effusion. If one wishes to use the pleural fluid pH diagnostically, it must be measured with the same care as the arterial pH. The fluid must be collected anaerobically and placed on ice for its transfer to the laboratory. The pH must be measured with a blood gas machine (11). Paper tapes are not sufficiently accurate. Systemic acidosis may influence the pleural fluid pH. Therefore, before any decision is made based only on a low pleural fluid pH, an arterial pH should be obtained to verify that the patient does not have systemic acidosis. With parapneumonic effusions, the pleural fluid pH falls before the pleural fluid glucose and is an early indication for the placement of chest tubes. With malignant pleural effusions, the prognosis is worse and pleurodesis is less likely to succeed if the pleural fluid pH is low.

VIII. High Amylase Pleural Effusion

If a patient with a pleural effusion is found to have a high pleural fluid amylase level, the list of possible etiologies for the pleural effusion is narrowed to four, namely, acute pancreatitis, chronic pancreatic disease, esophageal rupture, and malignant pleural effusion. Although most patients with acute pancreatitis present with abdominal symptoms, an occasional patient will present with predominantly chest symptoms. Pleuritic pain may arise from pleural irritation, and shortness of breath may arise from hypoxia. An elevated pleural fluid amylase in such patients is frequently the first clue that one is dealing with acute pancreatitis. Patients with a pancreatic pseudocyst may develop a sinus tract from their pseudocyst retroperitoneally through the diaphragm and into the mediastinum. Once the sinus tract reaches the mediastinum, it may rupture into either pleural space. The sinus tract allows the pseudocyst to drain into the pleural space and thus decompresses the pancreas. The patient may then present with chest pain and shortness of breath. Frequently these patients do not have abdominal pain. Most patients with this entity are chronically ill, and it appears as if they have cancer. Again the elevated pleural fluid amylase is the clue to the diagnosis.

Patients with esophageal rupture frequently develop a pleural effusion secondary to the intense mediastinitis that results from contamination of the mediastinum by saliva with its high bacterial count. Patients with esophageal rupture are extremely ill with severe chest pain and signs of sepsis. A clue to this diagnosis is again an elevated pleural fluid amylase. In this case the amylase is of salivary origin.

About 10% of patients with a malignant pleural effusion will have an elevated pleural fluid amylase. The primary carcinoma in patients with a malignant pleural effusion and a high amylase level is usually not the pancreas. With a malignant pleural effusion, the amylase level is usually only moderately elevated. If doubt exists whether the patient has a malignancy or chronic pancreatic disease, the differentiation can be made with amylase isoenzymes. The amylase in patients with malignant pleural effusions is mostly the salivary type (12).

IX. LDH Increasing with Serial Thoracentesis

The level of LDH in the pleural fluid is a reliable indicator of the degree of pleural inflammation; the higher the LDH, the more inflamed the pleural surfaces (3). Therefore, if the level of LDH increases with successive thoracenteses, the process in the pleural space is becoming more intense and one should be more aggressive in pursuing a diagnosis. If there are predominantly polymorphonuclear leukocytes in the pleural fluid, it is likely that the patient has an infection either in their chest or in their peritoneal cavity. A CT scan of both the chest and the abdomen should be obtained. Abdominal abscesses including subphrenic, intrahepatic, and intrasplenic are notoriously difficult to diagnosis. Their presence should be specifically sought for on the CT scan of the abdomen.

X. Pleural Fluids with Predominantly Mononuclear Cells

The presence of predominantly mononuclear cells in the pleural fluid suggests either malignancy or chronic infection, usually tuberculosis. A good screening test for tuberculosis is the level of adenosine deaminase (ADA) in the pleural fluid. If the ADA level is below 40 IU/L, it is quite unlikely that the patient has tuberculosis (13). If the ADA level is above 40 IU/L, the patient in all probability has tuberculous pleuritis. The pleural fluid level of interferon-γ is also useful in establishing the diagnosis of tuberculous pleuritis. Greco and associates (14) reviewed all English language studies from 1978 until November 2000. These studies included 4738 patients on whom ADA was measured and 1189 patients on whom interferon-γ was measured. These researchers reported that the maximum joint sensitivity and specificity for ADA was 93%, which was 96% for interferon-γ (14). Since there is not much difference in the performance of the two tests and since ADA is much less expensive, ADA appears to be the preferred test. Another test that has been advocated by some is the polymerase chain reaction (PCR) for tuberculous DNA. The sensitivity and the specificity for PCR in the diagnosis of pleural tuberculosis are inferior to those of the pleural fluid ADA and interferon-γ, and therefore this test is not recommended.

If there are predominantly mononuclear cells in the pleural fluid and if the pleural fluid ADA is below 40 IU/L, then the patient probably has malignancy. Pleural fluid cytology is an excellent means to establish the diagnosis of a malignant pleural effusion. However, the pleural fluid cytology will be negative in approximately 25% of patients with a malignant pleural effusion. If the pleural fluid cytology is negative and serial LDHs are increasing, the next diagnostic procedure should probably be thoracoscopy. Thoracoscopy can establish the diagnosis of malignancy in more than 90% of cases. Needle biopsy of the pleura is another alternative, but it is positive in less than 25% of patients with a malignant pleural effusion and negative cytology.

XI. Positive Pleural Fluid Cytology

If the pleural fluid cytology is positive for malignant cells, how diligent should one be in searching for the primary tumor? Metastatic lung carcinoma is the leading cause of malignant pleural effusion and accounts for approximately 30% of cases. Metastatic breast carcinoma is the second leading cause accounting for approximately 25%, while the lymphoma-leukemia group is the third accounting for approximately 20%. All other tumors account for the remaining 25%. In approximately 5%, the primary tumor is never discovered even at autopsy.

The prognosis of patients with malignant pleural effusions is poor. The median life expectancy after diagnosis is approximately 90 days. If the pleural fluid glucose or pH is reduced, then the median life expectancy is only about 30 days. The presence of a malignant pleural effusion indicates that the tumor has metastasized to the pleura and that the patient cannot be cured by surgery. The great majority of tumors that cause malignant pleural effusions do not respond well to chemotherapy. In view of the above, it is unreasonable to keep the patient in the hospital for an extended period in an attempt to discover the primary tumor.

If the pleural fluid cytology is positive and if the site of the primary tumor is unknown, what tests should be obtained? A chest CT with cuts of the upper abdomen is indicated since lung cancer is the most common cause of a malignant pleural effusion. If the CT scan is positive, it is reasonable to attempt to get a tissue diagnosis from the positive site. Women should have a mammogram and a careful pelvic examination. If the patient is anemic or has occult blood in the stool, the gastrointestinal tract should be studied. If the urinalysis is abnormal, the urinary tract should be studied. If all of these tests are negative and if the patient has no localizing symptoms, no addition workup is recommended.

XII. Mesothelioma or Metastatic Adenocarcinoma?

The possibility of a malignant mesothelioma should be considered whenever a patient's pleural fluid cytologic study or pleural biopsy suggests a metastatic adenocarcinoma, because the epithelial form of malignant mesothelioma is frequently misdiagnosed as adenocarcinoma on cytologic examination or pleural biopsy. There are several tests that are useful in making this differentiation. Electron microscopic examination with particular attention to the microvilli is useful diagnostically. The microvilli with metastatic adenocarcinoma are sparse, short, and stubby. In contrast, the microvilli with mesothelioma are abundant, long, and thin.

Immunohistochemical tests using monoclonal antibodies directed against various antigens are also useful in distinguishing metastatic adenocarcinoma from mesothelioma. The most useful monoclonal antibodies for identifying adenocarcinoma are carcinoembryonic antigen (CEA) and MOC-31 (or B72.3, Ber-EP4, or BG8) while the best markers for mesothelioma appear to be calretinin and cytokeratin 5/6 (15). When one attempts to differentiate adenocarcinoma from mesothelioma with immunohistochemistry, a panel of monoclonal antibodies including two that stain with mesothelioma and two that stain with adenocarcinoma should be used (15).

Two histochemical tests are useful for the differentiation of mesothelioma from adenocarcinoma. The Alcian blue stain detects the acid mucins characteristic of mesothelioma. It is positive in about 50% of patients with mesothelioma but is rarely positive in patients with metastatic adenocarcinoma. The periodic acid-Schiff stain after diastase digestion (PAS-D) detects neutral mucins, which are diagnostic of adenocarcinoma. It is positive in approximately 60% of patients with adenocarcinomas. In summary, if the specimen stains positively with the Alcian blue stain, the patient in all probability has mesothelioma, while if the specimen stains positively with the PAS-D stain, the patient has metastatic adenocarcinoma, but if the specimen is positive for neither, no conclusion can be made.

XIII. Granulomas on Pleural Biopsy

The great majority of patients who have granulomas on pleural biopsy have tuberculosis. Nearly 100% of patients with caseous necrosis or positive acid fast bacilli stains have pleural tuberculosis. On rare occasions other entities such as fungus diseases, sarcoidosis, or rheumatoid pleuritis can produce granulomatous pleuritis, and these possibilities should be kept in mind when granulomatous pleuritis is discovered.

XIV. Nonspecific Pleuritis on Needle Biopsy

There are several options available when the needle biopsy of the pleura reveals nonspecific pleuritis, and the cytology of the pleural fluid is nondiagnostic. Certainly one diagnosis that should be considered is pulmonary embolization. This entity is the fourth leading cause of pleural effusion in the United States, and the patient should be evaluated for this possibility with a CT angiogram. The CT angiogram will also demonstrate pleural parenchymal and mediastinal lesions, which will dictate the next procedure if no pulmonary embolus is present. Options available when the needle biopsy reveals nonspecific pleuritis, and the diagnosis of pulmonary embolism has been eliminated including observation, repeat needle biopsy of the pleura, bronchoscopy, thoracoscopy, and thoracotomy with open biopsy.

Observation is probably the best option if the patient is improving. A diagnosis is never obtained in 10% to 20% of patients with pleural effusions. If these patients have prolonged follow-up, only rarely does an etiology for the pleural effusion become apparent (16). It is likely that many of these effusions are due to viral illnesses. If one elects this option, it is important to rule out the diagnosis of tuberculosis. Although only a small percentage of pleural effusions in the United States is due to tuberculosis at the present time, it is important to exclude this diagnosis. The pleural effusion with tuberculous pleuritis will resolve spontaneously, but subsequently the majority of patients will develop pulmonary or extrapulmonary tuberculosis. One good way to exclude the diagnosis of tuberculous pleuritis is to measure the pleural fluid ADA level. If the pleural fluid ADA level is below 40 IU/L, the diagnosis of tuberculosis is virtually excluded. If ADA or interferon-γ assays are not available, then the tuberculin skin test is useful diagnostically. If the skin test is positive, the patient should be treated for pleural tuberculosis. If the skin test is negative, it should be repeated in six to eight weeks. If the skin test has converted on this repeat testing, the patient should be treated for tuberculous pleuritis. The reasoning behind this approach is that approximately 30% of patients with tuberculous pleuritis will have a negative skin test when they are first evaluated, but the skin test will become positive in virtually all of the patients within six weeks.

A second option is to repeat the needle biopsy of the pleura. This option can be utilized when the suspicion for tuberculosis is very high, but the initial pleural biopsy was not diagnostic. However, if the patient is young with a lymphocytic pleural effusion and either a positive tuberculin skin test or an elevated pleural fluid ADA level, the patient should be treated for tuberculosis regardless of the outcome of the second pleural biopsy, and therefore the performance of the second pleural biopsy is extraneous. A second pleural biopsy is rarely diagnostic if the patient has a disease other than pleural tuberculosis.

A third option is to perform bronchoscopy. Bronchoscopy is indicated if the patient has either a concurrent pulmonary infiltrate or hemoptysis, because if either of these is present bronchoscopy will yield a diagnosis in approximately 80% of the patients (17). Bronchoscopy is probably also indicated if the patient has a large (occupying more than three-fourths of the hemithorax) pleural effusion. Bronchoscopy will be diagnostic in approximately 50% of such patients. However, if the patient does not have a parenchymal infiltrate, hemoptysis, or a large pleural effusion, bronchoscopy is not indicated because it is rarely diagnostic (18).

A fourth option is to perform thoracoscopy. Thoracoscopy is an excellent means to establish the diagnosis of pleural malignancy or tuberculosis. Thoracoscopy establishes the diagnosis of pleural malignancy in approximately 90% of cases including mesothelioma. The diagnosis of tuberculous pleuritis can also be established in almost all patients with tuberculosis. However, only rarely are other diagnoses established. Thoracoscopy is recommended for the patient with an undiagnosed pleural effusion in whom the diagnosis of malignancy or tuberculosis is suspected, and in whom the pleural fluid cytology and a pleural fluid test for tuberculosis (ADA or interferon-γ) are negative or equivocal. In addition, thoracoscopy is recommended only if the effusion is not resolving. It should be noted that less than 10% of patients who present with a pleural effusion will meet these criteria and therefore need a thoracoscopy (19). When thoracoscopy is done for diagnostic purposes, it is important for the operator to be prepared to perform a procedure to create a pleurodesis at the time of the surgery. Our preferred method is pleural abrasion.

The fifth option is to perform a thoracotomy and do an open biopsy of the pleura. In recent years, open thoracotomy with direct biopsy of the pleura has been supplanted by video-assisted thoracoscopy in most institutions. If both thoracoscopy and thoracotomy are available, thoracoscopy is the preferred procedure because it is associated with less morbidity.

XV. Nonspecific Pleuritis with Thoracoscopy or Open Thoracotomy

A definite diagnosis is not always obtained with thoracoscopy or open biopsy of the pleura. In one older series from the Mayo Clinic, no diagnosis was established in 51 patients who underwent open pleural biopsy for an undiagnosed pleural effusion (20). In 31 of the patients (61%), there was no recurrence of the pleural effusion, and no cause for the effusion ever became apparent. However, 13 of the patients were eventually proven to have malignant disease (6 lymphomas, 4 mesotheliomas, and 3 other types of malignancy). In view of the above, it appears that patients with a nondiagnostic thoracoscopy or open thoracotomy are best managed with observation.

References

1. Light RW, MacGregor MI, Luchsinger PC, et al. Pleural effusions: the diagnostic separation of transudates and exudates. Ann Intern Med 1972; 77:507–513.
2. Romero-Candeira S, Fernandez C, Martin C, et al. Influence of diuretics on the concentration of proteins and other components of pleural transudates in patients with heart failure. Am J Med 2001; 110:681–686.
3. Light RW. Pleural Diseases. 5th ed. Philadelphia: Lippincott Williams and Wilkins, 2007.
4. Porcel JM. The use of probrain natriuretic peptide in pleural fluid for the diagnosis of pleural effusions resulting from heart failure. Curr Opin Pulm Med 2005; 11:329–333.
5. Porcel JM, Vives M, Cao G, et al. Measurement of pro-brain natriuretic peptide in pleural fluid for the diagnosis of pleural effusions due to heart failure. Am J Med 2004; 116:417–420.
6. Tomcsányi J, Nagy E, Somlói M, et al. NT-brain natriuretic peptide levels in pleural fluid distinguish between pleural transudates and exudates. Eur J Heart Fail 2004; 6:753–756.
7. Kolditz M, Halank M, Schiemanck S, et al. High diagnostic accuracy of NT-proBNP for cardiac origin of pleural effusions. Eur Respir J 2006; 24:144–150.
8. Sanz MP, Borque L, Rus A, et al. Comparison of BNP and NT-proBNP assays in the approach to the emergency diagnosis of acute dyspnea. J Clin Lab Anal 2006; 20:227–232.
9. Kalomenidis I, Light RW. Eosinophilic pleural effusions. Curr Opin Pulm Med 2003; 9:254–260.
10. Rodriguez-Panadero F, Lopez-Mejias J. Low glucose and pH levels in malignant pleural effusions. Am Rev Respir Dis 1989; 139:663–667.
11. Cheng DS, Rodriguez RM, Rogers J, et al. Comparison of pleural fluid pH values obtained using blood gas machine, pH meter, and pH indicator strip. Chest 1998; 114:1368–1372.
12. Kramer MR, Cepero RJ, Pitchenik AE. High amylase in neoplasm-related pleural effusion. Ann Intern Med 1989; 110:567–569.
13. Valdes L, Alvarez D, San Jose E, et al. Tuberculous pleurisy: a study of 254 patients. Arch Intern Med 1998; 158:2017–2021.
14. Greco S, Girardi E, Masciangelo R, et al. Adenosine deaminase and interferon gamma measurements for the diagnosis of tuberculous pleurisy: a meta-analysis. Int J Tuberc Lung Dis 2003; 7:777–786.
15. Ordonez NG. The immunohistochemical diagnosis of mesothelioma: a comparative study of epithelioid mesothelioma and lung adenocarcinoma. Am J Surg Pathol 2003; 27:1031–1051.
16. Ferrer JS, Munoz XG, Orriols RM, et al. Evolution of idiopathic pleural effusion. A prospective, long-term follow-up study. Chest 1996; 109:1508–1513.
17. Chang S-C, Perng RP. The role of fiberoptic bronchoscopy in evaluating the causes of pleural effusions. Arch Intern Med 1989; 149:855–857.
18. Poe RH, Levy PC, Israel RH, et al. Use of fiberoptic bronchoscopy in the diagnosis of bronchogenic carcinoma. A study in patients with idiopathic pleural effusions. Chest 1994; 105:1663–1667.
19. Kendall SW, Bryan AJ, Large SR, et al. Pleural effusions: is thoracoscopy a reliable investigation? A retrospective review. Respir Med 1992; 86:437–440.
20. Ryan CJ, Rodgers RF, Unni KK, et al. The outcome of patients with pleural effusion of indeterminate cause at thoracotomy. Mayo Clin Proc 1981; 56:145–149.

References

32
Radiologic Diagnosis of Pleural Disease

BRETT BURBRIDGE and MARC V. GOSSELIN
Oregon Health and Science University, Portland, Oregon, U.S.A.

I. Anatomical Considerations

The word pleura comes from the Greek word *pleura* meaning "the side of the body or the ribs." The parietal pleura lines the thoracic cavity and the visceral pleura lines the lungs, following each lobe intimately. This thin layer of tissue develops after the 24th week of gestation from splanchnic mesenchyme, which grows to join the body wall mesenchyme and in turn becomes contiguous with the parietal pleura, which is derived from somatic mesoderm. Visceral pleura lines the interior aspect of the thoracic cavity, upper aspect of the diaphragm, spine, and lateral mediastinal wall. Because of normal hydrostatic pressures in the parietal pleural vasculature, capillary leakage produces pleural fluid at the rate of 0.01 mL/kg of body weight per hour. The parietal pleural lymphatic system absorbs this fluid and returns it to the systemic circulation via the thoracic duct. Under normal physiologic conditions, approximately 10 mL of pleural fluid occupies the pleural space and provides lubrication for the two tissue layers to slide past one another during the continuous morphing of the lung due to respiration.

The hydrogen bonding between water molecules provides dynamic adhesion between the layers. Disruption of this force results in an increase in volume of the potential space, which is then filled with air or fluid of varying origins and consistencies.

II. Types of Imaging

A. Radiographs

Radiographs have been the primary modality of investigating the state of the pleura (1) and are frequently preferred to initially detect and subsequently track the progress of pleural disease. An important anatomical correlate to keep in mind is that the radiograph only "sees" the visceral pleura on the edge as it curves from deep to shallow or vice versa and during the remainder of their course around the lungs (visceral) or thorax for (parietal) they are invisible (2), overwhelmed by the scatter from the lungs, bones, and soft tissue. As such, many of the disorders of pleura or pleural fluid manifest as displacement of neighboring structures such as lung parenchyma or soft tissue or by approaching the same density of neighboring structures creating a silhouette sign (3). Furthermore, pleural fluid may appear to occupy the entire lung zone when in fact it is confined to the pleural space. By remaining distinctly physically separate from structures of similar density, the fluid will not blur the pulmonary vasculature, as in the case of pulmonary edema, but will instead simply "drop a veil" over the lung zone, while the pulmonary vessels, separate from that fluid collection, remain distinct.

B. Computed Tomography

Computed tomography (CT) scans play a central role in the detection and differential diagnosis of pleural disease. As technology has advanced, newer multidetector scanners have increased resolution and decreased scan times. CT scans detect healthy pleura as they fold around lobes (2) and reveal anatomical relationships as well as vascularity if contrast is used. The pleura is rarely visualized in the absence of disease but often thickens, either focally or diffusely, in the presence of disease.

C. Ultrasound

Although radiographs and CT remain the mainstay of pleural imaging modalities, ultrasound can add information to the clinical picture with relatively low cost and invasiveness. Obstacles inherent to thoracic ultrasound include the ribs and intercostal muscles scattering the beam between the lungs and the transducer as well as the air within the lung itself scattering the sound waves. Tumors of either bone or soft tissue of the thorax may be well represented on ultrasound. Imaging of deeper structures such as the pleura may also be possible. The pleuras are normally visualized as two small closely approximated hyperechoic lines and can be seen to slide past each other during respiration. Additionally, ultrasonographic needle guidance for both diagnostic and therapeutic aspirations of masses and fluid collections is both safe and accurate and eliminates radiation exposure to both provider and patient.

D. Magnetic Resonance Imaging

Currently, magnetic resonance (MR) has limited clinical utility in evaluating and treating pleural disease (2,4), mainly answering specific questions about anatomical extension of malignancy to the chest wall.

III. Pleural Effusion

A. Histopathology and Clinical Features

A pleural effusion is an excessive accumulation of fluid in the pleural space. This fluid accumulates as a result of five different processes, which may be present alone or in combination. Transudative effusions result from either decreased oncotic pressure or increased hydrostatic pressure in the vasculature. Accumulation of fluid due to leakage from a disturbed capillary membrane or decreased lymphatic clearance is termed an exudative effusion. An infection in the pleural space results in an empyema and may result from untreated or poorly treated pneumonia. Lastly, bleeding into the pleural space can cause a hemothorax.

Pleural effusion can be suspected clinically in the presence of dyspnea, cough, or pleuritic chest pain. On physical examination, one may appreciate dullness to percussion of the thorax or decreased lung sounds. Advanced effusions may create a compressive mass effect on the mediastinum, resulting in tracheal deviation, compression of the great vessels, decreased venous return, and increased peripheral venous congestion. Alternately, small pleural effusions frequently produce no signs and few symptoms.

Pleural effusions should also be considered as part of a spectrum of concomitant diseases that may be more clinically apparent or known a priori in the patient's medical history. Examples include congestive heart failure, cirrhosis, nephrotic syndrome, peritoneal dialysis, myxedema, neoplasms including mesothelioma and metastatic disease, and gastrointestinal or collagen vascular disease. Iatrogenic causes may follow vascular access, vascular surgery, or coronary artery bypass. Trauma including hemothorax and pulmonary contusion may cause pleural effusion, as can thoracic radiation exposure. Any loss of anatomical integrity of neighboring structures can introduce fluid into the pleural space causing effusion or form neighboring cavities through partitions such as from the abdomen through the diaphragm. The etiology, differential diagnosis, and pleural fluid analysis of pleural effusion are covered in detail in Chapter 31.

B. Imaging Findings

The predominant imaging modality useful in the assessment of pleural effusion involves a combination of the two-view chest radiograph and the CT scan. Ultrasound may be useful in quantifying the amount of fluid present (5).

Radiographs

Often the first to be obtained, frontal chest radiographs will show blunting of the costophrenic angles in the case of moderate-sized effusions or incomplete-to-nearly complete opacification of the entire lung zone in the case of massive effusions. The lateral chest radiograph in an upright patient will show blunting of the posterior costophrenic angles. In the case of massive effusions, the entire lung zone may be opacified, introducing the possibility that the pathology lies not in the pleural space but in the lung parenchyma itself. Careful inspection of the pulmonary vasculature can resolve this confusion. Although the vasculature is slightly more difficult to see, the vessel margins still remain radiographically sharp, placing it outside the lung parenchyma (Fig. 1A, B).

Patient positioning represents a crucial factor in evaluating radiographs for effusion. The spectrum ranges from upright posterior anterior (PA) films, prevalent in the outpatient setting, to supine portable anterior posterior (AP) films in the intensive care unit. Because the pleural space, barring any loculations, ranges from the lower posterior thorax to just beneath the clavicles, the fluid will shift to follow gravity depending on patient position. This dynamic introduces important considerations. First, an upright PA film in a patient with an effusion of less than 500 mL (1) may show none of the expected findings of lateral costophrenic angle blunting. However, the lateral projection does demonstrate the effusion much earlier, and as little as 150 cc of fluid will be visible in the posterior sulcus. Second, if the patient is supine, as in the case of the ICU patient, even a small effusion will layer along the posterior aspect of the thorax and opacify most or all of the lung zone. In order to overcome these confounders, changing patient placement into a lateral recumbent or

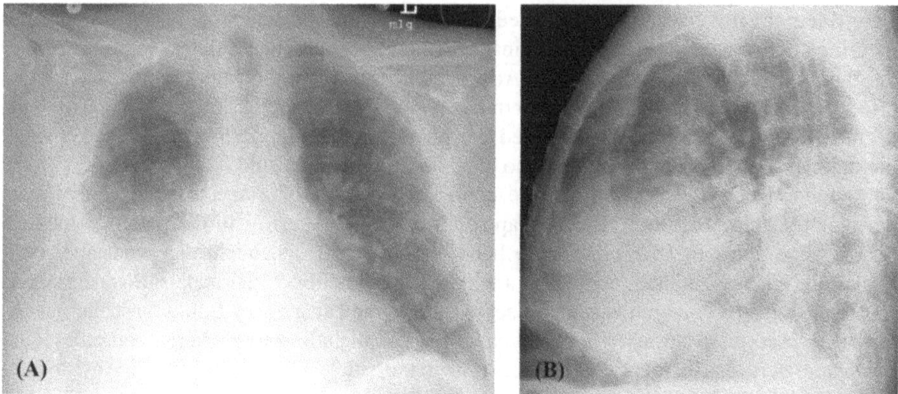

Figure 1 (**A**) PA chest and (**B**) lateral chest radiograph. Large, partially loculated, right-sided effusion with evidence of multiple pulmonary and pleural nodules bilaterally. Thoracocentesis demonstrated extensive lymphocytes. The patient was diagnosed on pleural biopsy with lymphoma.

semi-upright position if supine and repeating the film will allow true effusions to shift and reveal a more accurate extent. As little as 5 to 10 cc of free fluid may be appreciated on a lateral decubitus film (6). If such manipulations are not possible, then alternate imaging such as CT or ultrasound may be beneficial.

Fluid may also collect in the subpulmonic region in an upright or semi-upright patient and may only be visible as an increased apparent distance between the gastric bubble and the left hemidiaphragm. Additionally, fluid may hide within a fissure, mimicking a lung mass. Obtaining a radiograph in a different position such as lateral decubitus may allow the fluid to track out of the fissure, resolving the "mass."

Computed Tomography

Small effusions not appreciated on radiographs will first appear in the posterior recesses of the thorax. CT can better define the location and extent of the effusions. Though not particularly helpful in differentiating transudative versus exudative, CT can better define the location and extent of the effusion (1). In the case of loculated effusions, CT can better define the presence and extent of loculations as compared with radiographs. The use of Hounsfield unit measurements of fluid density as well as the presence or absence of pleural enhancement can be quite helpful in determining transudative and exudative effusions. The exudative effusions tend to be of a higher density and demonstrate enhancement secondary to the development of granulation tissue along the parietal and visceral pleura.

Ultrasound

Pleural effusions increase the distance between these two lines, which are then separated by a variably hypoechoic line representing the pleural fluid, which may be relatively dark as in a transudative effusion or somewhat echoic as in the case of an exudative effusion. Doppler modes can assist in differentiation of apparent masses from vascular structures. Sonography may also prove useful in quantifying an effusion and may be superior to a lateral decubitus radiograph in estimating the quantity of pleural fluid by measuring the thickness of the effusion lamella (5). Sonography is well suited for detecting loculations and septations in pleural fluid. Sonography is technically limited by interfering structures such as bone and air-filled lung.

IV. Empyema

A. Histopathology and Clinical Features

Empyema is defined as the presence of pus in the pleural cavity. Most commonly, pneumonia is the cause of this parapneumonic effusion (7), also termed pyothorax. The lobar infection grows to become contiguous with the visceral pleura, and breaches the pleural space. Introduction of bloodstream products into this space, combined with local activation of local mesothelial cells potentially releasing cytokines, creates a proinflammatory state that in turn coats both pleura with polymorphonuclear neutrophils and fibrin or granulation tissue. The resulting loculations and peels create a rind-like coating along the parietal and, more importantly, the visceral pleura. Such fibrosis prevents the lung from fully expanding and can provide valuable diagnostic information following thoracocentesis or chest tube insertion. The coated lung will not be able to adequately reinflate following introduction of air into the pleural space because of the fibrotic restrictions of the visceral pleura. Should a pneumothorax persist following access to the pleural space, a chronic exudative process is assuredly present such as an empyema among others, including malignancy or chronic hemothorax.

Empyema should be considered in any patient with a bacterial pneumonia (8) and may be associated with generalized sepsis (9). The differential diagnosis of empyema is discussed in detail in Chapter 31.

B. Imaging Findings

Radiographs and CT provide the majority of diagnostic information useful in the detection and management of empyema. Ultrasound can demonstrate fluid echogenicity and loculations aiding in the differentiation between simple pleural effusion and empyema.

Radiographs

Standard PA and lateral projections will demonstrate a cavitary opacity with an air fluid level, adjacent pleural thickening, and, most likely, a pleural effusion. The excess pleural fluid associated with empyema may be unilateral or bilateral. If bilateral, the affected side usually has a greater volume (7). Typical findings include a peripheral lens-shaped opacity that forms an obtuse angle with the chest wall, simulating a "ball under the carpet." This appearance puts the location outside of the lung parenchyma, which can be particularly useful in differentiating cavitary lucencies that could represent a lung abscess versus empyema. Additionally, careful comparison of two perpendicular views may reveal two different lengths of an air fluid level depending on the view. Such a difference places the finding squarely in the pleural space, as an abscess confined to the lung parenchyma would be roughly spherical and have the same appearance regardless of the angle of view.

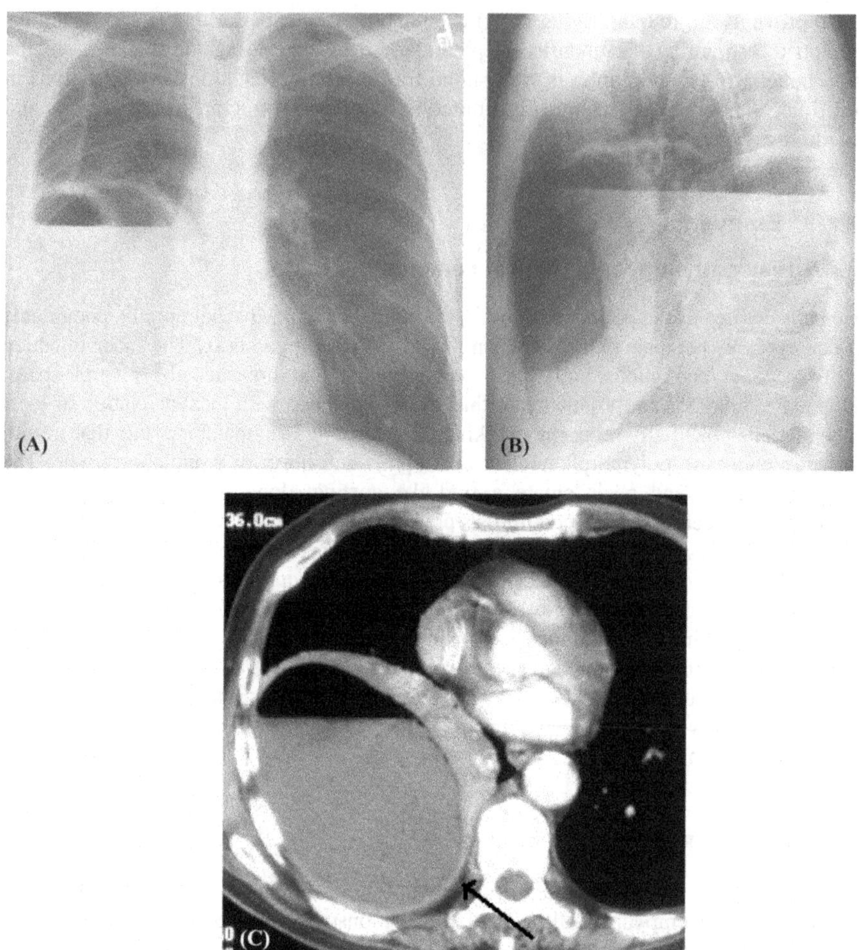

Figure 2 (**A, B**) PA and lateral chest radiograph. Large, predominately loculated, pleural effusion status post pleurocentisis. There is an air fluid level of unequal length on the two-view chest radiograph, confirming the pleural location. The pleural tap yielded klebsiella. (**C**) Axial computed tomography scan with contrast demonstrates the thick enhancing pleura (*arrow*) and the compression and atelectasis of the right lower lobe, characteristic of an empyema.

Computed Tomography

Cavitary opacities with adjacent pleural effusion and thickening predominate. Compression of neighboring lung is consistent with empyema. Should lung parenchyma be directly involved, abscess should be considered instead (Fig. 2A, B, C). Radiographs and ultrasound are generally sufficient for diagnosis and drainage (7), but CT may further aid in needle location or otherwise complicated cases. Should the pleural thickening include or cross the mediastinum, tumor should be strongly considered (see the section "Pleural malignancy").

C. Clinical Management

Thoracocentesis, both diagnostic and therapeutic, is indicated for the treatment of empyema. Once an empyema is confirmed with imaging, early aggressive drainage is paramount in addition to antimicrobial administration to minimize the extent of pulmonary fibrosis that can occur following a parapneumonic infection. Decortication should be considered early in cases of resistance (8), generally within the first five-to-seven days.

V. Pleural Malignancy

A. Histopathology and Clinical Features

Ninety-five percent of pleural tumors are metastatic, and the vast majority are adenocarcinomas. Others include lymphoma, and occasionally, invasive thymoma.

The most common primary pleural malignancy is mesothelioma. Although most pleural tumors are not primary cancers, malignant mesothelioma is a primary tumor of the pleural mesoderm and most often a result of asbestos exposure. Asbestos-related pleural disease is bilateral. The pleural plaques most often occur as a result of a distant history (>20 years) of asbestos exposure. As with many long-standing acquired structures in the body, the plaques typically become calcified over time. They generally involve the posterior and lateral aspects of the pleura (2,7), following the posterior ribs seven through ten. The apices and costophrenic angles are generally free of plaques.

Localized fibrous tumors of the pleura are not related to asbestos exposure. The vast majority of these tumors are benign, but a small number may be malignant. They are often amenable to surgical resection.

B. Imaging Findings

The predominant mode of radiographic analysis in pleural malignancy is the CT scan. The tumor may be incidentally discovered on radiographs.

Radiographs

Plaques typically appear as smooth straight-to-curvilinear opacities less than 1 cm in thickness that parallel the chest wall. They involve the posterior and lateral aspects of ribs seven through ten and the lateral aspects of ribs six through nine. Evidence of diaphragmatic calcification can be considered nearly pathognomonic for prior asbestos exposure (10). These plaques may be indistinguishable from extrapleural fat, a structure that can be differentiated with high-resolution computed tomography (HRCT).

Computed Tomography

CT is best at differentiating benign disease from malignant disease (9). Malignant mesothelioma generally shows unilateral pleural thickening with irregular contours of the lung border (Fig. 3). HRCT best assesses the extent of pleural plaque formation and differentiates extrapleural fat from adjacent composite shadows. Tumor appearance depends on its tissue origin and varying degrees of enhancement of nodularity. Pleural tumors cross the

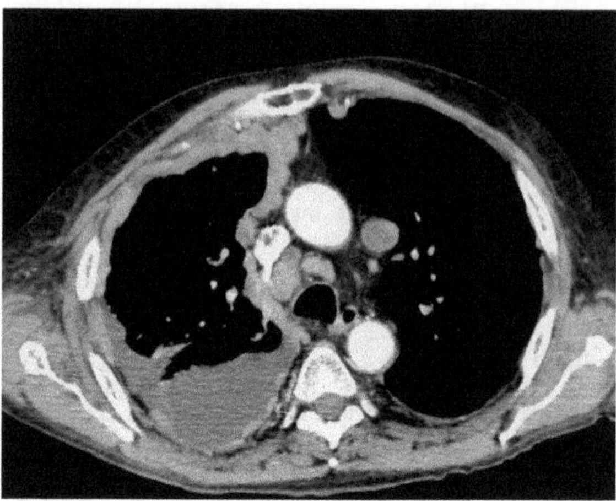

Figure 3 Axial CT scan through the mid chest. Mesothelioma. CT scan demonstrates a circumferential, enhancing, right-nodular mesothelioma. Note the mediastinal pleural involvement, highly characteristic of malignant pleural disease. *Abbreviation*: CT, computed tomography.

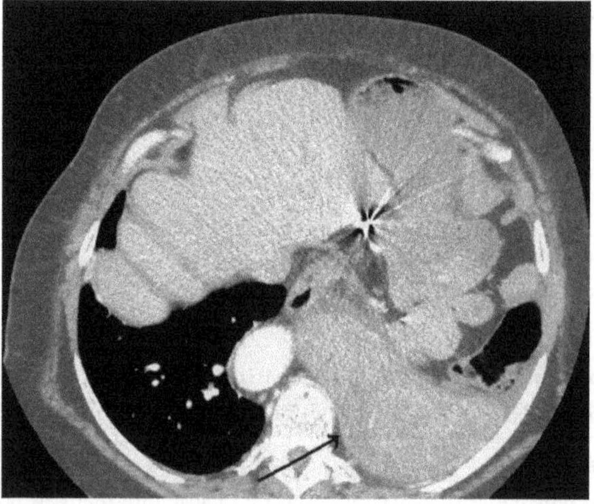

Figure 4 Axial CT scan through lower lobes. A 52-year-old female demonstrates a left posterior enhancing pleural mass measuring 10 cm × 14 cm. On surgical resection, a localized fibrous tumor of the pleura was diagnosed. *Abbreviation*: CT, computed tomography.

mediastinal pleura, whereas empyemas do not. Any lesion that involves or crosses the mediastinum should be considered cancer until proven otherwise. Figure 4, in contrast, demonstrates a left posterior enhancing pleural mass measuring 10 × 14 cm. Upon surgical resection, a localized fibrous tumor of the pleura was diagnosed.

Magnetic Resonance Imaging

The role of magnetic resonance imaging (MRI) in pleural disease has not been established, though there is evidence that it is useful in differentiating normal from pathologic pleura and may be superior to CT in detecting pleural thickening (11). Additionally, in certain circumstances, MR can provide more anatomical detail while assessing the extent of chest wall involvement in the case of malignancy, aiding in prognosis or surgical planning.

C. Clinical Management

Pleural biopsy is generally required for diagnosis of malignant mesothelioma or metastatic pleural tumor. Early disease is generally amenable to surgery alone or in combination with chemotherapy and radiation. Advanced (stages III, IV) disease is generally managed with palliative care.

VI. Pneumothorax

A. Histopathology and Clinical Features

Pneumothorax is defined as air in the pleural space. Air may be introduced from the thorax externally as in the case of penetrating thoracic trauma, iatrogenically during instrumentation of the thorax, in the presence of bronchopleural fistula, or may be spontaneous, either idiopathic or as a result of poor pleural adhesion from recurrent spontaneous pneumothoracies. Other causes include catamenial, pneumocystis, and acupuncture.

Pneumothorax may be clinically suspected in the setting of trauma or recent surgical instrumentation. Symptoms may include pleuritic chest pain, dyspnea, or in more subtle settings, isolated tachypnea. Signs may be absent in small pneumothorax, but with larger or progressive cases, there may be decreased tactile fremitus, hyperresonance, and decreased or absent breath sounds. Progression to a tension pneumothorax can be accompanied by distended jugular veins, hypotension, narrow pulse pressure, tracheal deviation, and a critically ill patient.

B. Imaging Findings

Pneumothorax is nearly exclusively discovered on frontal radiographs. Clinical suspicion should prompt investigation with this rapid diagnostic modality, often at the bedside with a portable machine. Those found on CT should merely confirm previously gained knowledge.

Radiographs

Typically, the chest radiograph reveals a separation of visceral pleura and its associated lung parenchyma from the surrounding structures. Small pneumothoracies may not be readily apparent, located only in the apex and partially obscured by the osseous structures. Careful inspection of the apices in an upright film and the costophrenic angles in the supine patient are critical to detecting smaller air collections. The appearance of a white line (Fig. 5A, B) representing the visceral pleura on edge is a common finding in pneumothorax. Skin folds (Fig. 6A, B) will show different densities on either side of the apparent line, which in fact appears more like a stripe. The pneumothorax will show similar or identical dark lucencies on either side of a thin white visceral pleural line. Skin folds are more

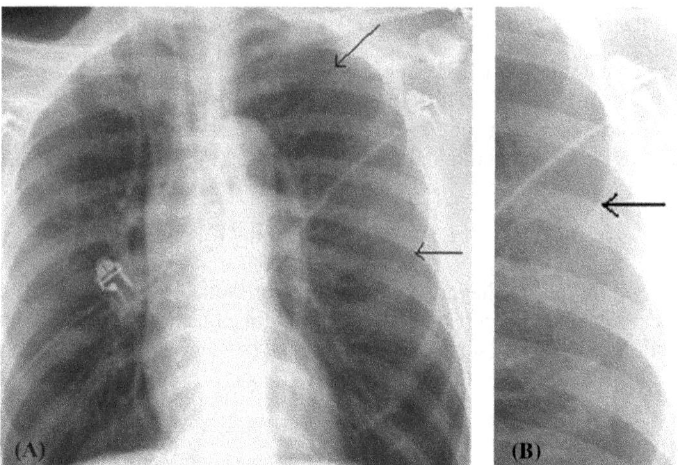

Figure 5 White line, deep sulcus, skin fold. (**A**) Frontal radiograph and (**B**) close up. A 30-year-old male s/p trauma. There is a left-sided moderate pneumothorax (*arrow*). Close up (**B**) demonstrates the thin white line of the visceral pleura.

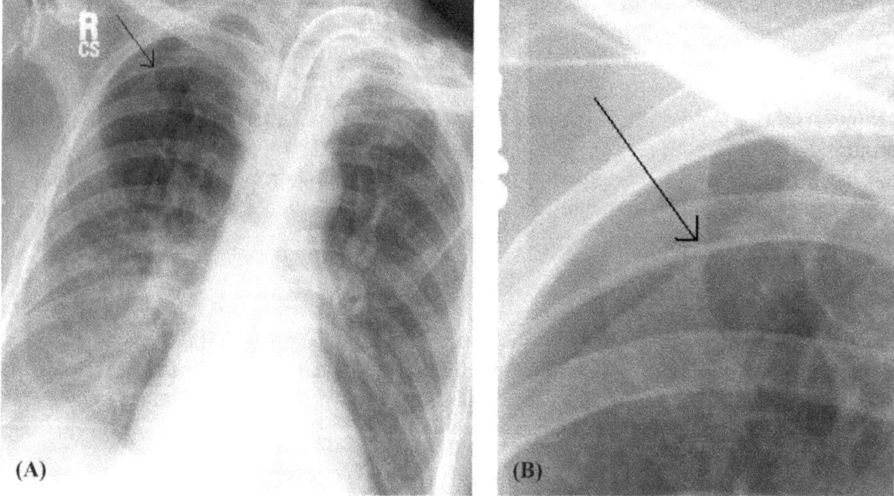

Figure 6 (**A**) AP chest radiograph and (**A**) close up. Skin fold. A 55-year-old male, ventilator dependent. Has an apparent line overlying the right upper hemithorax (*arrow*). Close inspection (**B**) demonstrates there is no white line but rather a white stripe with vasculature extending beyond it. This is characteristic of a skin fold.

common in thinner individuals as the reduced amount of tissue results in less attenuation of photons, allowing increased contrast. If the upright frontal radiograph does not demonstrate a pneumothorax in the setting of high clinical suspicion, a lateral decubitus view (2,7) may reveal smaller air collections.

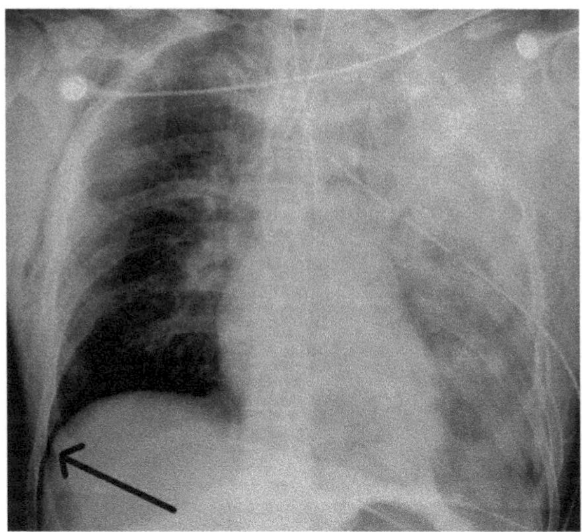

Figure 7 Frontal radiograph. Deep sulcus. A 35-year-old male had a severe motor vehicle accident w/multiple injuries and fractures. AP supine radiograph demonstrates presence of air extending into the right costophrenic sulcus (*arrow*), diagnostic of anterior inferior pneumothorax.

In the supine patient, air will migrate to the anterior chest as the lungs settle posteriorly because of gravity. Contrasted with an upright patient who will likely demonstrate a pneumothorax in the apices, the supine patient should have unusually deep costophrenic angle(s) on the frontal radiograph, termed the "deep sulcus sign" (Fig. 7).

Larger pneumothoracies and tension pneumothoracies are generally more apparent as absence of lung parenchyma within the lung zone rather than appreciation of the displaced visceral pleura. Tension pneumothorax may include tracheal or mediastinal deviation away from and depression of the hemidiaphragm on the affected side. Such radiographs are commonly termed "the forbidden radiographs" as the clinical presentation of extremis should obviate the need for imaging, which should be replaced with emergent decompression via needle or tube thoracostomy.

Computed Tomography

Subtle pneumothoracies may be incidentally revealed from CT imaging when compared with radiographs. Also, it could help define any ancillary findings that may be associated with or the cause of the pneumothorax. CT is particularly helpful in evaluating bronchopleural fistulas, which may result from cardiothoracic surgery, penetrating trauma, bronchial instrumentation, infection, or malignancy.

C. Clinical Management

Evacuation of the trapped pleural air via needle or chest tube thoracostomy is indicated for most pneumothoracies. Smaller events (15%) can be managed conservatively (12) as the air is reabsorbed. Smoking cessation and strict avoidance of dynamic pressure environments (diving, air travel) should be avoided. Recurrent cases may require the services of a thoracic surgeon to encourage reattachment of the pleura.

References

1. Muller NL, Fraser RS, Colman NC. Radiologic Diagnosis of Diseases of the Chest. Philadelphia: Saunders, 2001.
2. Qureshi N, Gleeson FV. Imaging of pleural disease. Clin Chest Med 2006; 27(2):193–213.
3. Goodman LR. Felson's Principles of Chest Roentgenology. 2nd ed. Milwaukee: Saunders, 1999.
4. Muller NL. Imaging of the pleura. Radiology 1993; 186(2):297–309.
5. Eibenberger KL, Dock WI, Ammann ME, et al. Quantification of pleural effusions: sonography versus radiography. Radiology 1994; 191(3):681–684.
6. Moskowitz H, Platt RT, Schachar R, et al. Roentgen visualization of minute pleural effusion. An experimental study to determine the minimum amount of pleural fluid visible on a radiograph. Radiology 1973; 109(1):33–35.
7. Hanna JW, Reed JC, Choplin RH. Pleural infections: a clinical-radiologic review. J Thorac Imaging 1991; 6(3):68–79.
8. Kasper DL, Braunwald E, Fauci AS, et al. Harrison's Principles of Internal Medicine. 16th ed. New York: McGraw Hill, 2005.
9. Kaiser LR, Singal S. Essentials of Thoracic Surgery. Philadelphia: Elsevier, Mosby, 2004.
10. Leung AN, Muller NL, Miller RR. CT in differential diagnosis of diffuse pleural disease. AJR Am J Roentgenol 154:487–492.
11. Weber MA, Bock M, Plathow C, et al. Asbestos-related pleural disease: value of dedicated magnetic resonance imaging techniques. Invest Radiol 2004; 39(9):554–564.
12. Tierney LM, McPhee SJ, Papadakis MA. Current Medical Diagnosis and Treatment. 44th ed. New York: McGraw Hill, 2005.

33
Malignant Epithelial Neoplasms

KIRK D. JONES
Department of Anatomic Pathology, University of California San Francisco,
San Francisco, California, U.S.A.

I. Introduction

The malignant epithelial neoplasms or carcinomas comprise a large group of tumors of the lung characterized by cells that are often polygonal to columnar with round-to-oval enlarged nuclei and moderate amounts of cytoplasm. Derived from the various glandular and surface epithelia, these tumors can be differentiated by architectural features such as gland formation and by cytologic features including keratinization. Recent advances in immunohistochemistry have led to the development of several stains that can aid in differentiation of these lesions and in particular can be useful in distinguishing metastatic tumors from primary pulmonary lesions and true epithelial tumors from so-called epithelioid tumors.

II. Malignant Epithelial Neoplasms of Lung Origin

A. Classification

Classification of neoplasms allows for the possibility of a more focused treatment of a specific disease. Although some may mourn the loss of the simple classification system of Hippocrates that involved only four humors, our current classification has evolved by observation of morphologic, histochemical, and genetic features of pulmonary neoplasms. The World Health Organization (WHO) Classification of Tumors of the Lung, published in 2004, divides pulmonary neoplasms into several categories based on histologic features (1). This classification is summarized in Table 1. The current classification has broadened the recognition of tumors with microscopically heterogeneous appearances by defining entities such as adenosquamous carcinoma and mixed-type adenocarcinomas. Even with this recognition, however, some tumors may be difficult to classify because of heterogeneity in their appearance (2). Use of immunohistochemistry and other supportive tests may help pin down the diagnosis in these cases.

Squamous Cell Carcinoma

Squamous cell carcinoma is recognized histologically by keratinization of tumor cells and/or presence of intercellular bridges (Fig. 1). These cancers frequently grow in rounded or angulated aggregates organized with more poorly differentiated anaplastic cells at the

Table 1 World Health Organization Histological Classification of Epithelial Malignant Neoplasms

Squamous cell carcinoma
Papillary
Clear cell
Small cell
Basaloid
Small cell carcinoma (see chap. 34)
Adenocarcinoma
Acinar
Papillary
Bronchioloalveolar
Nonmucinous
Mucinous
Solid with mucus formation
Mixed subtype
Large cell carcinoma
Large cell neuroendocrine carcinoma (see chap. 34)
Basaloid carcinoma
Lymphoepithelioma-like carcinoma
Clear cell carcinoma
Large cell with rhabdoid phenotype
Adenosquamous carcinoma
Sarcomatoid carcinoma (see chap. 36)
Carcinoid tumor (see chap. 34)
Salivary gland tumors (see chap. 38)

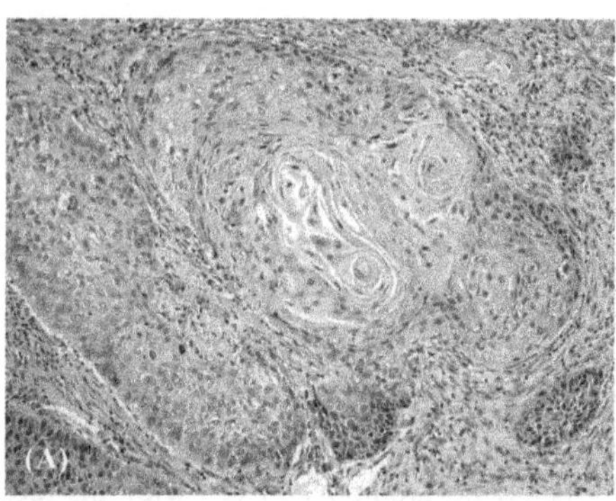

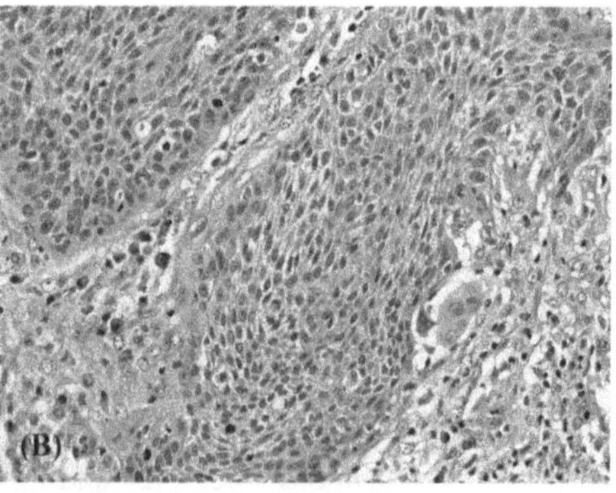

Figure 1 Characteristics of squamous cell carcinoma. (**A**) Squamous cell carcinoma showing characteristic keratin pearl formation in the central region of differentiation. (**B**) Squamous cell carcinoma showing intercellular bridges.

periphery and a central "keratin pearl" formed by layers of flattened keratinized epithelium with an anucleate keratin core. Single-cell keratinization is more difficult to recognize, and one may be deceived by solitary degenerating necrotic cells with eosinophilic cytoplasm. Proper identification requires recognition of a laminated or concentric ring of eosinophilia around a viable nucleus (3). Intercellular bridging is distinguished by relatively uniformly spaced linear connections spanning adjacent cells, resulting in a train-track appearance. This morphologic finding is the result of desmosomes connecting adjacent tumor cells. Uniform spacing of cells without direct connection is often noted in large cell carcinomas and should not be misinterpreted as bridging. It should be noted that the criteria for designation of squamous differentiation in these lesions is more strict than those used in some other organ systems. The presence of an "epithelioid" growth pattern in tumors showing distinct cell borders, eosinophilic cytoplasm, and a central nucleus is insufficient for classification as squamous cell carcinoma.

Histologic Variants of Squamous Cell Carcinoma

The current WHO classification identifies four special variants of squamous cell carcinoma. Papillary variant of squamous cell carcinoma is characterized by tumor growth in an exophytic or endophytic papillary pattern with fibrovascular cores and focal invasion. Clear cell variant of squamous carcinoma is characterized by a predominance of cells with cytoplasmic clearing and focal keratinization (4). Small cell variant of squamous carcinoma demonstrates cells with ovoid-to-round nuclei and markedly increased nuclear-to-cytoplasmic ratios that resemble small cell carcinoma but have focal keratinization and nuclear features more consistent with non–small cell tumors. Basaloid variant of squamous cell carcinoma shows prominent peripheral palisading of tumor cell nuclei within tumor cell nests. Identification of focal keratinization is necessary to differentiate between a basaloid variant of large cell carcinoma.

Immunohistochemical Profile of Squamous Cell Carcinoma

Squamous cell carcinoma typically stains with low–molecular weight keratins such as cytokeratin 5 but does not stain for the glandular keratins cytokeratin 7, 19, or 20 (5,6). These tumors tend to be negative for thyroid transcription factor-1 (7, 8). Nuclear staining for p63 is typical (9,10); these findings are summarized in Table 2.

Adenocarcinoma

Adenocarcinomas are tumors derived from secretory-type epithelium and thus show gland formation, mucin production, or composition by the secretory surface cells of the lung (type 2 pneumocytes or Clara cells).

Histologic Variants of Adenocarcinoma

The WHO Classification of Tumours distinguishes four major variants of adenocarcinoma: acinar, papillary, bronchioloalveolar, and solid with mucin production (Fig. 2). Acinar tumors are composed of angular neoplastic glands within a fibrotic or desmoplastic stroma. Papillary tumors show tumor cell growth within a papillary architecture with fibrovascular

Table 2 Immunohistochemical Profiles of Squamous Cell Carcinoma and Adenocarcinoma of the Lung

	CK 5/6	CK 7	MOC-31	P63	TTF-1
Squamous cell carcinoma	++	−/+	++	++	−
Adenocarcinoma	−	++	++	−/+	++

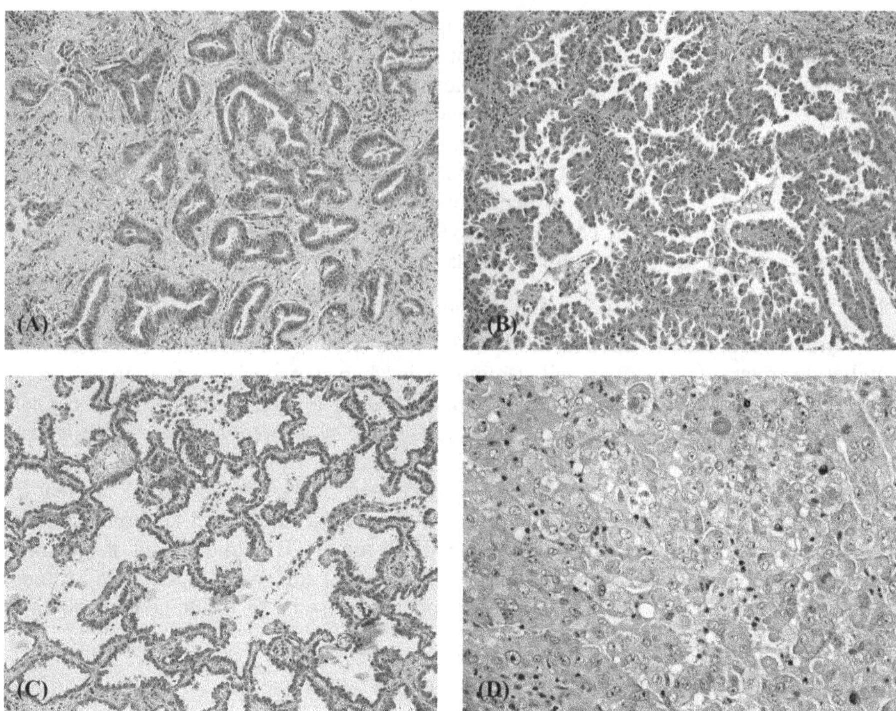

Figure 2 Major variants of adenocarcinoma. (**A**) Acinar carcinoma with angulated glands within fibrous stroma. (**B**) Papillary carcinoma with branching papillae with fibrovascular cores. (**C**) Bronchioloalveolar carcinoma with surface alveolar growth (lepidic growth). (**D**) Solid type with mucin production.

cores. Bronchioloalveolar carcinoma shows simple surface lining of alveolar surfaces without vascular, stromal, or pleural invasion (so-called lepidic growth, from the Greek *lepis*, meaning "scale" or "membrane," not from Lepidoptera, as is often stated). Bronchioloalveolar carcinoma is further divided into nonmucinous and mucinous subtypes. Solid-type adenocarcinoma with mucus production grows with a sheet-like pattern showing five or more tumor cells with intracytoplasmic mucin in each of two high-power fields on staining. In lung tumor pathology, the periodic acid Schiff stain with enzyme digestion (PAS-D) is preferred over mucicarmine staining, as up to 25% of mesotheliomas will show mucicarmine positivity (11). The current classification also recognizes the common occurrence of mixed forms of adenocarcinoma that show combinations of the above types of tumor. The mixed subtype is found in over three-quarters of adenocarcinomas, as many tumors with central invasion or solid growth will show a bronchioloalveolar growth pattern at the periphery. In these cases, the diagnosis of "adenocarcinoma, mixed type" is appropriate, with a listing of the various components in the diagnosis line.

Since the recognition of invasion in adenocarcinoma precludes rendering the diagnosis of bronchioloalveolar carcinoma, it is important to be able to separate focal septal fibrosis from desmoplasia. Clues for the presence of central scarring (and probable acinar-type adenocarcinoma) include fused glands, cribriform growth pattern, angulated glands, absence of alveolar macrophages within glands, solid growth pattern, single-cell infiltration, necrosis, or destruction of elastic tissue or epithelial basement membrane (12–15). Small adenocarcinomas that lack invasion have a better prognosis than tumors with invasion. In addition, tumors with microinvasion (central scarring less than 5 mm in diameter) appear to have an improved prognosis over those with larger regions of central invasion (16–19).

Immunohistochemical Profile of Adenocarcinoma

Adenocarcinomas of the lung stain with the glandular keratins cytokeratin 7 and 19, but do not express cytokeratin 20 (5,20). These tumors are generally negative for cytokeratins 5 and 6. Strong nuclear staining for thyroid transcription factor-1 is present in most cases of adenocarcinoma, as shown in Figure 3 (21); however, this staining is often absent in mucinous bronchioloalveolar carcinomas (22).

Adenosquamous Carcinoma

Adenosquamous carcinoma is defined as containing foci of both adenocarcinoma and squamous cell carcinoma, with both components representing at least 10% of the total tumor. The criteria for squamous and glandular differentiation are the same as for the aforementioned malignancies.

Large Cell Carcinoma

Although it might seem reasonable, large cell carcinoma is not the same entity as non–small cell carcinoma. It is important to acknowledge that while non–small cell carcinoma is a category of neoplasms, the WHO does not recognize it as a definitive diagnosis. In small biopsies, where one is unable to separate a tumor into a more specific category, the term

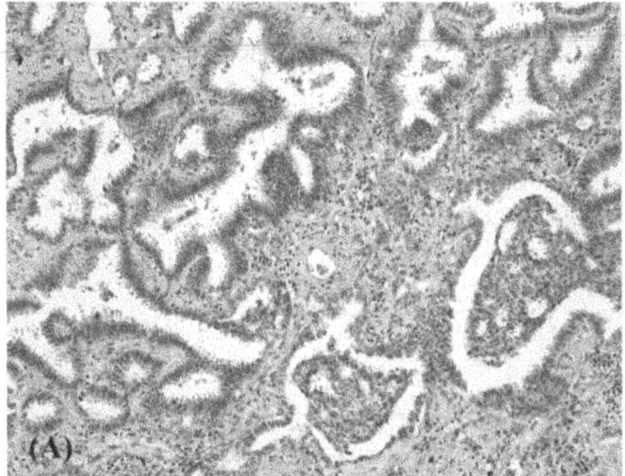

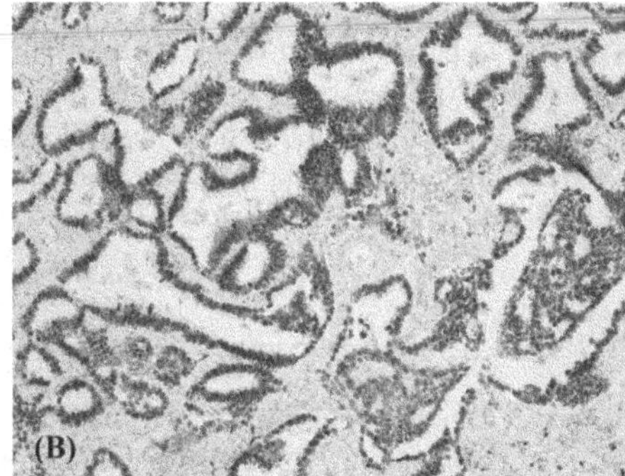

Figure 3 (**A**) Adenocarcinoma (central acinar portion of a mixed-type tumor). (**B**) Characteristic strong nuclear staining for thyroid transcription factor-1.

"non–small cell carcinoma" is appropriate; however, in resection specimens, one must make a decision. If a carcinoma lacks features of squamous or glandular differentiation and lacks the cytologic features of small cell carcinoma, it should be diagnosed as large cell carcinoma.

Histologic Variants of Large Cell Carcinoma

The current WHO classification identifies five variants of large cell carcinoma. When none of these characteristics are identified, a diagnosis of large cell undifferentiated carcinoma may be made. Clear cell carcinoma shows tumors with clear cytoplasm and are negative for mucin stains. Large cell neuroendocrine carcinoma shows characteristic morphology with tumor cells arranged in an organoid fashion and reveals neuroendocrine immunohistochemical markers (see chap. 34). Basaloid carcinoma of the lung shows tumor cell nests with peripheral palisading of cells with increased nuclear-to-cytoplasmic ratios, nuclear hyperchromasia, and inconspicuous nucleoli. Lymphoepithelial carcinoma shows sheets of large cell with prominent nucleoli within a dense lymphocytic background. Large cell carcinoma with rhabdoid phenotype shows at least 10% of cells containing large eosinophilic cytoplasmic inclusions composed of intermediate filaments (which may stain for vimentin or keratin).

Immunohistochemical Profile of Large Cell Carcinoma

The immunohistochemical staining of large cell carcinomas reflects the fact that most of these tumors probably represent the extreme spectrum of poorly differentiated squamous cell carcinomas, adenocarcinomas, and neuroendocrine carcinomas. In keeping with this, some subtypes (e.g., basaloid) will show an immunohistochemical profile similar to squamous cell carcinoma, while others will have profiles more consistent with adenocarcinomas (22,23).

III. Differentiation of Primary Lung Carcinoma from Metastasis

The unique position of the lungs within the circulatory system makes them susceptible to metastasis from nearly all varieties of tumors. The question facing the pathologist is often not "What type of lung carcinoma is this?" but rather "Is this a carcinoma of the lung?" or even "Is this a carcinoma?" Use of clinical history, gross and histologic appearances, and immunohistochemical studies can help in rendering a correct diagnosis.

A. Clues for Tumor Origin

Tumors can metastasize to or within the lung through numerous routes, including blood vascular permeation (both bronchial and pulmonary vascular systems), lymphatic vascular spread, and extension within bronchi, along alveolar walls or within the interstitium (24). The result is a variety of tumor growth patterns, all of which may overlap with the architectural patterns of primary lung carcinomas. The most common appearance of metastatic malignancy is the finding of multiple bilateral masses. Occasionally, these tumors will show a distinct color such as brown or black metastatic melanoma or yellow metastatic renal cell carcinoma, or a distinct consistency such as the cartilaginous matrix in metastatic chondrosarcoma or the hemorrhagic appearance of metastatic choriocarcinoma. Diagnostic confusion is most typically encountered when the metastasis presents as a solitary mass in the absence of a known malignancy. Metastatic malignancies comprise 3% to 9% of surgically resected solitary pulmonary nodules (25). The primary sites that most commonly produce a solitary nodule are melanoma, sarcoma, colon and breast adenocarcinoma, renal cell carcinoma, urothelial carcinoma, and nonseminomatous germ cell tumors of the testis (25). The most common sites of origin of metastases to the lungs are listed in Table 3.

Clinical history is essential in differentiating a solitary metastasis from a second primary malignancy. The patient presenting with a metastatic pulmonary lesion in the absence of a known malignancy is less common than the patient with a history of malignancy who later presents with a pulmonary lesion. Younger patients with a history of melanoma or sarcoma will most often have a metastasis in this setting. However, older patients with a history of carcinoma often end up showing a second primary (25). This likelihood increases if the patient has a significant smoking history or if the disease-free interval between diagnoses is greater than five years. Depending on the primary site, resection of a truly solitary metastasis may result in prolonged survival; therefore, the ability of the pathologist to reach a definitive diagnosis assumes much greater significance (26–28).

Metastatic tumors to the lung may show some characteristic, yet nonspecific, histologic features. These are summarized in Table 4 and illustrated in Figure 4.

Table 3 Common Sites of Origin of Metastases to the Lungs

Genitourinary
Kidney, ovary, prostate, uterus, bladder
Gastrointestinal
Colon, pancreas, stomach
Breast
Skin (melanoma)
Thyroid
Soft tissue (sarcomas)

Table 4 Nonspecific Histological Features Suggesting Metastasis

Multifocality
Pushing rounded border
Lack of central anthracotic or elastotic sclerosis
Prominent lymphocytic permeation
Nuclear pleomorphism
Dirty necrosis
Diffuse lymphatic involvement

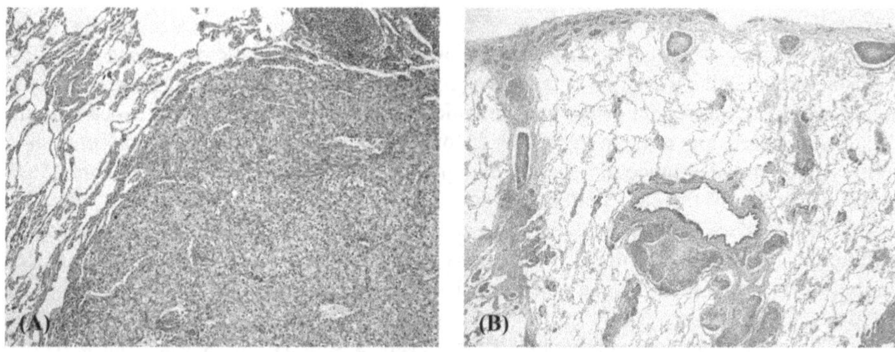

Figure 4 Histological features suggesting metastasis. (**A**) Metastatic renal cell carcinoma with rounded pushing margin demarcating tumor from normal lung. Lepidic spread is absent. (**B**) Extensive lymphatic permeation by metastatic gastric adenocarcinoma showing tumor in bronchovascular bundle, subpleural, and interlobular septal lymphatics.

B. Primary Squamous Cell Carcinoma Vs. Metastasis

The conundrum of whether a squamous cell carcinoma is primary or metastatic is most commonly encountered in patients with prior head and neck squamous cell carcinomas.

There are currently no immunohistochemical markers that can differentiate between pulmonary and head and neck squamous cell carcinomas. Various clinical and histologic standards have been developed incorporating criteria of tumor type and grade, multifocality of lesions, and location of lesions. However, even in series where clinical indicators suggest that metastasis is more likely, molecular analysis has supported a diagnosis of primary carcinoma of the lung in many cases (29). An exception to the rule that squamous cell carcinomas are negative for cytokeratin 7 is squamous carcinoma of the uterine cervix (5).

C. Primary Adenocarcinoma Vs. Metastasis

Tumors with Mucinous and Glandular Features

Adenocarcinoma of the colon is the most common metastasis with mucinous morphology, often presenting as an apparently solitary nodule (Fig. 5A). Histologic features that are helpful in identifying these lesions as metastases include the presence in glandular lumina of karyorrhectic debris ("dirty necrosis") and the segmental absence of epithelium, resulting in "incomplete glands." Metastatic colon adenocarcinoma also tends to show a nodular architecture and often lacks a peripheral bronchioloalveolar growth pattern (30). Immunohistochemistry for the nuclear protein CDX2 is useful in differentiating tumors of colonic origin from pulmonary adenocarcinomas (31). In addition, the reciprocal cytokeratin profiles of the lung (CK7+, CK20−) and colon (CK7−, CK20+) are also useful in recognition of metastases (5). An unusual variant of pulmonary adenocarcinoma with intestinal-type morphology has been described (32). This tumor shows architectural similarities to metastatic colon adenocarcinoma with a garland-like glandular growth pattern and central necrosis. However, the tumor shows a typical pulmonary adenocarcinoma immunohistochemical

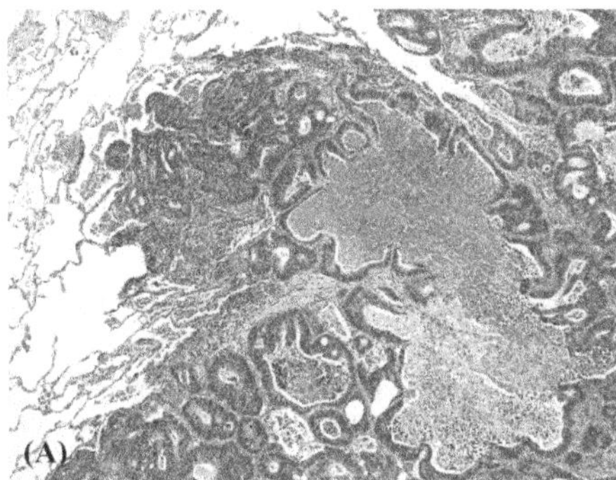

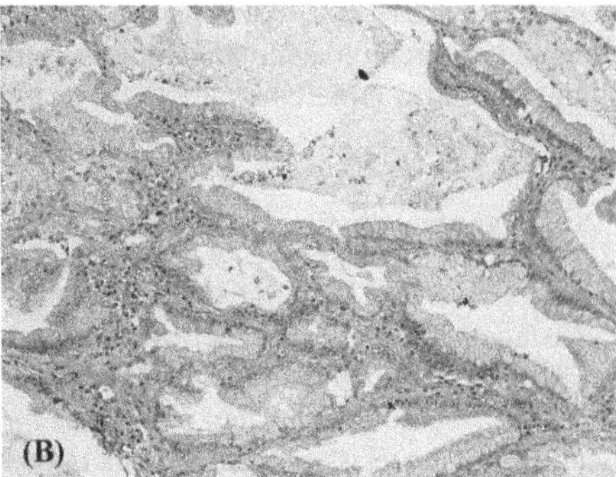

Figure 5 Patterns of metastases. (**A**) Metastatic colon adenocarcinoma. Characteristic incomplete glands and dirty necrosis. (**B**) Metastatic pancreatic carcinoma. Mucinous tumor cells show a bronchioloalveolar growth pattern along alveolar septa.

profile (TTF-1+, CDX2−, CK7+, CK20−). Primary lung carcinomas showing signet ring cell morphology that may be mistaken for gastric neoplasms and mucinous carcinomas with tumor cell aggregates within pools of mucin that mimic breast or colon carcinomas have been described (33,34). Some of these tumors show immunohistochemical overlap with colon carcinoma, and it is important to rule out metastasis through clinical testing.

Tumors with Papillary Features

Papillary-type adenocarcinoma of the lung should be distinguished from metastatic papillary carcinoma of the ovary and thyroid, its two most common nonpulmonary mimics. Morphologic clues such as intranuclear cytoplasmic inclusions and psammoma bodies are nonspecific and may be observed in both primary and metastatic lesions. Histochemical staining for PAS-D may show cytoplasmic mucin in lung and ovarian tumors; however, thyroid tumors will lack this expression. Immunohistochemical staining can aid in the differentiation of primary pulmonary papillary adenocarcinoma and metastatic lesions. Ovarian serous papillary carcinomas do not express TTF-1 or CEA, but will show staining with vimentin, WT-1, and CA125 (35). Primary lung tumors show the reciprocal immunohistochemical profile (TTF-1+, CEA+, vimentin−, WT-1−, CA125−). TTF-1 cannot be used to differentiate metastatic papillary thyroid carcinoma from lung cancer, but thyroid carcinoma can be recognized by the expression of thyroglobulin and S-100 (36).

Tumors with Bronchioloalveolar Features

Mucinous bronchioloalveolar carcinoma typically shows multifocality and is thought to metastasize aerogenously. These features make it difficult to differentiate it from metastatic tumors that show surface alveolar growth, such as adenocarcinomas of the pancreas (Fig. 5B), stomach, and colon. As mentioned previously, mucinous bronchioloalveolar carcinoma does not show a typical immunohistochemical profile: often coexpressing cytokeratin 7 and 20 while lacking expression of TTF-1 (21,22). This close morphologic mimicry of metastatic disease and atypical staining pattern necessitates that the differential diagnosis of mucinous bronchioloalveolar carcinoma must always include metastasis. In these cases, it is often prudent to undertake radiologic imaging or endoscopic studies to exclude metastases from stomach, pancreas, or colon.

Tumors with Clear Cell Features

Clear cell variant of large cell carcinoma of the lung must be differentiated from both metastatic renal cell carcinoma and benign clear cell tumor of the lung (4). Many clear cell carcinomas, on adequate histologic examination, do not meet criteria for clear cell variant of large cell carcinoma. They may show focal keratinization or mucin production and thus would be better classified as variants of squamous cell carcinoma or adenocarcinoma. The lung is the most frequent distant metastatic site for renal cell carcinoma; therefore, metastatic renal cell carcinoma, either secondary to a known primary or as a first presentation, is a much more frequently encountered clear cell tumor in the lung than either clear cell carcinoma or benign clear cell tumor.

Renal cell carcinoma has several immunohistochemical markers that may aid in diagnosis. The majority of clear cell carcinomas will show staining with RCC marker, PAX2, and CD10 (37,38). Vimentin is positive in renal cell carcinoma and tends to be negative in pulmonary carcinomas. In addition, renal cell carcinomas are typically negative for cytokeratin 7 and 20 (5).

Benign clear cell tumor or "sugar tumor" is a rare neoplasm with perivascular epithelioid cell differentiation. These well-circumscribed lesions are composed of nests of polygonal cells with abundant clear PAS-positive glycogen-rich cytoplasm. They show a thin-walled sinusoidal vascular network that differs from the usual thick-walled vessels of the clear cell carcinomas. Like other perivascular epithelioid cell tumors (or PEComas), these tumors express immunohistochemical markers for HMB-45, S-100, and actin, but are negative for keratin and epithelial membrane antigen (39,40).

Poorly Differentiated Carcinomas

Many of the most common lesions that metastasize to the lung, including ductal carcinoma of the breast, melanoma, renal cell carcinoma (non–clear cell types), urothelial carcinoma, and nonseminomatous germ cell tumors, particularly embryonal carcinoma, will produce pulmonary nodules with no histologic features to suggest site of origin. These lesions are typically composed of large cells in solid sheets with moderate pleomorphism, prominent necrosis, and pushing margins. Differentiation from primary carcinomas of the lung depends on careful review for features favoring metastasis, as described previously, and on a careful history. When these are unrevealing, it is appropriate to employ a panel of immunohistochemical markers (Table 5).

Carcinoma of the breast presents a particular problem since it is common, and metastatic disease may be treated with hormonal therapy. These tumors tend to show solid nodules with patchy necrosis (Fig. 6A). Although breast carcinoma shows similar keratin profiles as lung adenocarcinoma (CK7+, CK20−), several other markers can be used to differentiate between these two lesions (41). Breast carcinoma will often show estrogen and progesterone receptor and S-100 expression. Gross cystic disease fluid protein is expressed in some breast carcinomas, particularly those with apocrine morphology. CEA staining may

Table 5 Immunohistochemical Profile of Lung Adenocarcinoma Vs. Metastatic Carcinomas

	TTF-1	CK7	CK20	CEA	EMA	S100	Vim	Others
Lung	++	++	−	++	++	−	−	
Kidney	−	−	−	−	++	+	++	CD10, RCC, PAX2
Ovary	−	++	−	++	++	−	++	ER, WT-1, CA125
Prostate	−	−	−	−	++	−	−	PSA, PSAP
Endometrium	−	++	−	++	++	−	++	ER
Colon	−	−	++	++	++	−	−	CDX-2
Pancreas	−	++	++	++	++	−	−	CA19-9, DPC-4
Stomach	−	+	++	++	++	−	−	
Breast	−	++	−	+	++	+	−	ER, PR, GCDFP
Thyroid	++	++	−	−	++	++	++	Thyroglobulin
Bladder	−	++	+	++	++	−	−	Uroplakin

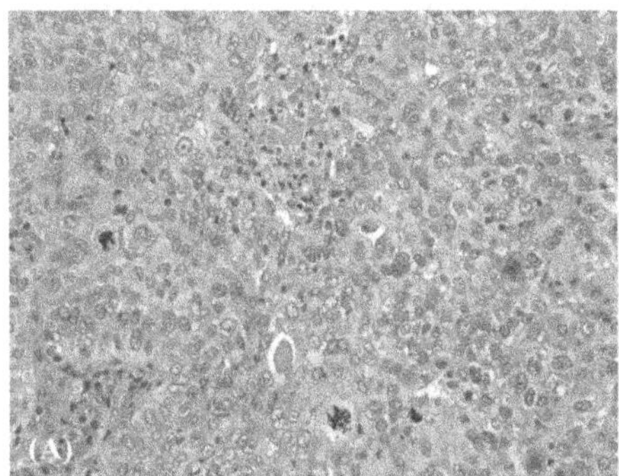

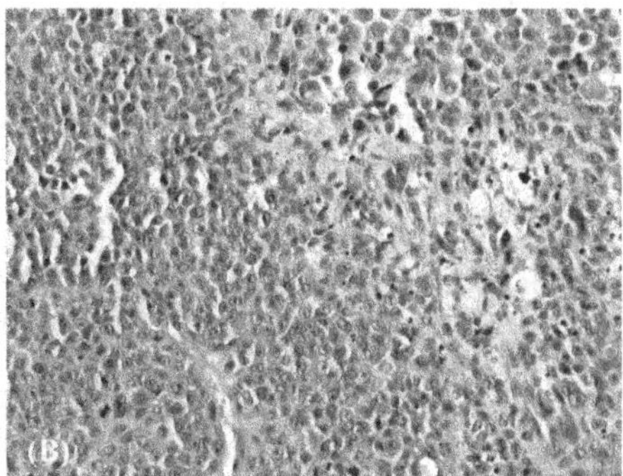

Figure 6 Undifferentiated neoplasms, which can mimic large cell undifferentiated carcinoma. (**A**) Metastatic breast carcinoma showing sheet-like growth of neoplastic cells with focal necrosis. (**B**) Metastatic melanoma showing sheet-like growth with anaplastic cells containing prominent central macronucleoli.

also be helpful as lung adenocarcinomas frequently show diffuse strong positive staining, while breast carcinoma shows patchy variable staining.

D. Poorly Differentiated Epithelial Vs. Epithelioid Tumors

Epithelioid tumors are approached in the same manner as poorly differentiated carcinomas. These tumors often show architectural patterns that may mimic carcinomas, including papillary or solid growth, and are composed of polygonal cells with enlarged nuclei and ample amounts of cytoplasm. Differentiation from carcinomas is supported by clinical, histologic, and immunohistochemical data.

Carcinoma Vs. Melanoma

Metastatic melanoma may metastasize to the lung and thus present a challenging diagnosis (Fig. 6B), particularly if the history of melanoma is not available or if the primary skin lesion has regressed or gone unrecognized. In cases of poorly differentiated neoplasms with predominantly solid growth patterns, an immunohistochemical profile showing lack of keratin staining and staining for S-100 or HMB-45 helps establish the diagnosis (48). Other markers such as melan-A or tyrosinase may be added in difficult cases.

Carcinoma Vs. Mesothelioma

Pleural involvement by adenocarcinoma may be difficult to differentiate from mesothelioma. Epithelioid mesotheliomas frequently show a tubulopapillary growth pattern that has some resemblance to the glandular architecture of adenocarcinoma. The tumor cells show distinct borders and occasionally show perinuclear cytoplasmic densities due to concentration of intermediate filaments (42). As mentioned previously, approximately one-quarter of mesotheliomas will show staining with mucicarmine. This is a result of the mesothelial cell production of glycosaminoglycan hyaluronic acid and is not indicative of epithelial-type mucin production. On the other hand, the vast majority of mesotheliomas are PAS-D negative. This is a relatively inexpensive stain that may be useful in differentiating mesothelioma from adenocarcinoma. Presence of intracytoplasmic mucin droplets is useful in securing a diagnosis of adenocarcinoma. In the not-so-distant past, mesothelioma was differentiated from adenocarcinoma by the absence of staining by numerous immunohistochemical markers (e.g., LeuM1, B72.3, and CEA). Several antibodies that preferentially stain mesothelial cells were developed during the 1990s. This allows for an immunohistochemical panel that contains both epithelial and mesothelial markers. The epithelial markers include MOC-31, CEA, B72.3, Ber-EP4, and E-cadherin. TTF-1 will also be positive in pulmonary adenocarcinoma. The mesothelial markers include D2-40, calretinin, cytokeratin 5/6, WT-1, and HBME-1 (43–47). Many pathologists construct a panel of antibodies containing two or more epithelial markers and two or more mesothelial markers. It is important to recognize the pattern of staining for each stain (Fig. 7). In particular, nuclear staining in calretinin is more specific for the diagnosis of mesothelioma than cytoplasmic staining.

The development of more specific positive markers for mesothelial cells, in combination with high cost and longer turnaround time, has led to the marked decrease in the use of electron microscopy for the diagnosis of mesothelioma. Nevertheless, the highly specific finding of long, bushy, complex, branching microvilli with a length-to-width ratio of 15:1 or greater has kept the technique in use for some complicated cases. The combined histologic, immunohistochemical, and ultrastructural features that differentiate mesothelioma from adenocarcinoma are summarized in Table 6.

Carcinoma Vs. Angiosarcoma and Other Vascular Malignancies

Epithelioid angiosarcoma and epithelioid hemangioendothelioma may mimic pulmonary carcinoma or mesothelioma by virtue of similar growth patterns (solid or tubulopapillary)

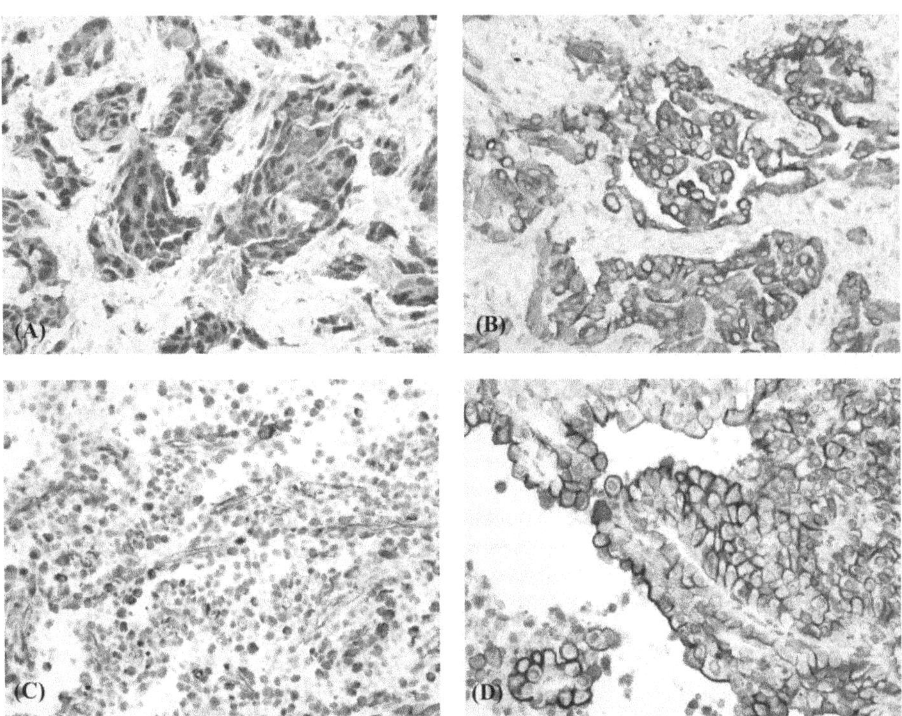

Figure 7 Immunohistochemical staining of mesothelioma. (**A**) Calretinin showing more specific nuclear staining combined with cytoplasmic staining. (**B**) Cytokeratin 5/6 showing crisp membrane staining. (**C**) WT-1 showing strong nuclear staining. (**D**) D2-40 showing staining along the apical cell membrane.

Table 6 Features Differentiating Lung Adenocarcinoma from Epithelioid Mesothelioma

	Adenocarcinoma	Mesothelioma
Distribution	Parenchymal > pleural	Pleural > parenchymal
Histology	Glandular, papillary, solid	Tubulopapillary
Histochemistry	PAS-D (+)	PAS-D (−)
Immunohistochemistry	TTF-1 (+) MOC-31 (+) Ber-EP4 (+) CEA (+) Calretinin (−) WT-1 (−) CK 5/6 (−) Podoplanin (−) Vimentin (−)	TTF-1 (−) MOC-31 (−) Ber-EP4 (−) CEA (−) Calretinin (+) WT-1 (+) CK 5/6 (+) Podoplanin (+) Vimentin (+)
Electron microscopy	Short, thick microvilli Secretory vacuoles	Long branching microvilli Lacks secretory vacuoles

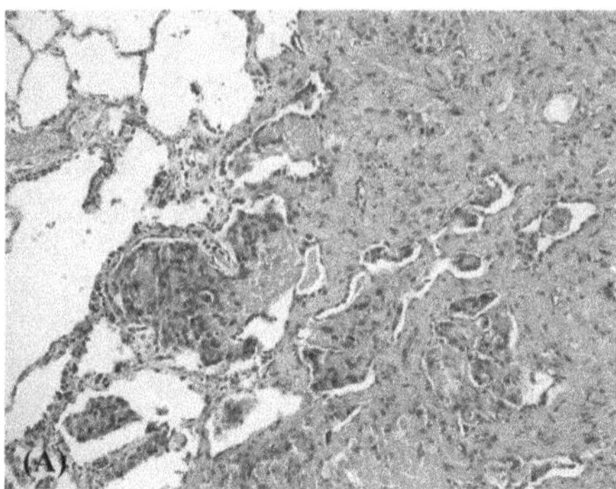

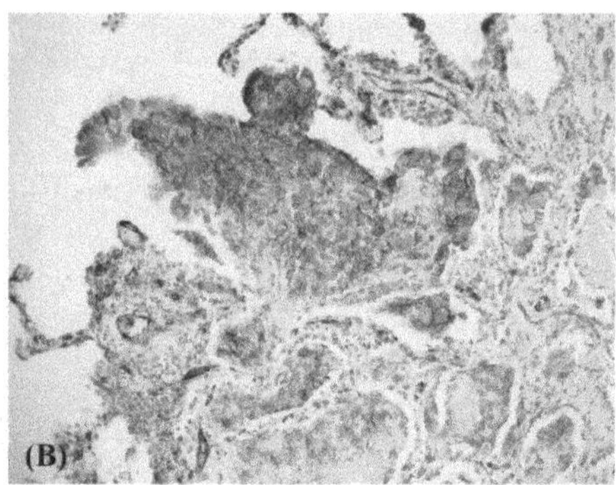

Figure 8 Epithelioid angiosarcoma. (**A**) Peripheral accentuation of anaplastic tumor cells with central paucicellular stroma. (**B**) CD31 staining of tumor cells.

and cytologic appearance (Fig. 8). To add to the diagnostic dilemma, these tumors often show immunohistochemical staining for routine keratin stains. Histologic clues of vascular differentiation include formation of abortive vessels and cystic spaces with micropapillary tufting of tumor cells. These tumors will often show cells with well-defined intracytoplasmic vacuoles containing red blood cells. These so-called blister cells are felt to resemble a single-cell recapitulation of a blood vessel. Hemangioendothelioma frequently shows central regions of paucicellularity with a chondroid or myxoid appearance and peripheral increased cellularity by anaplastic tumor cells. Staining for vascular markers is useful in all large cell epithelioid tumors lacking glandular or squamous differentiation (49,50). Staining for CD31 is more sensitive and specific, but occasionally it is useful to perform this stain in conjunction with CD34. In addition, these tumors show strong diffuse vimentin staining, unlike the majority of lung adenocarcinomas.

References

1. Travis WD, Brambilla E, Muller-Hermelink HK, et al, eds. World Health Organization Classification of Tumors. Pathology and Genetics of Tumours of the Lung, Pleura, Thymus and Heart. Lyon: IARC Press, 2004.
2. Fraire AE, Roggli VL, Vollmer RT, et al. Lung cancer heterogeneity. Prognostic implications. Cancer 1987; 60:370–375.
3. Roggli VL, Vollmer RT, Greenberg SD, et al. Lung cancer heterogeneity: a blinded and randomized study of 100 consecutive cases. Hum Pathol 1985; 16:569–579.
4. Katzenstein AL, Prioleau PG, Askin FB. The histologic spectrum and significance of clear-cell change in lung carcinoma. Cancer 1980; 45:943–947.
5. Chu P, Wu E, Weiss LM. Cytokeratin 7 and cytokeratin 20 expression in epithelial neoplasms: a survey of 435 cases. Mod Pathol 2000; 13:962–972.
6. Chu PG, Weiss LM. Expression of cytokeratin 5/6 in epithelial neoplasms: an immunohistochemical study of 509 cases. Mod Pathol 2002; 15:6–10.
7. Nakamura N, Miyagi E, Murata S, et al. Expression of thyroid transcription factor-1 in normal and neoplastic lung tissues. Mod Pathol 2002; 15:1058–1067.

8. Chang YL, Lee YC, Liao WY, et al. The utility and limitation of thyroid transcription factor-1 protein in primary and metastatic pulmonary neoplasms. Lung Cancer 2004; 44:149–157.
9. Au NH, Gown AM, Cheang M, et al. P63 expression in lung carcinoma: a tissue microarray study of 408 cases. Appl Immunohistochem Mol Morphol 2004; 12:240–247.
10. Wang BY, Gil J, Kaufman D, et al. P63 in pulmonary epithelium, pulmonary squamous neoplasms, and other pulmonary tumors. Hum Pathol 2002; 33:921–926.
11. McCaughey WT, Colby TV, Battifora H, et al. Diagnosis of diffuse malignant mesothelioma: experience of a US/Canadian Mesothelioma Panel. Mod Pathol 1991; 4:342–353.
12. Clayton F. The spectrum and significance of bronchioloalveolar carcinomas. Pathol Annu 1988; 23(pt 2):361–394.
13. Clayton F. Bronchioloalveolar carcinomas. Cell types, patterns of growth, and prognostic correlates. Cancer 1986; 57:1555–1564.
14. Nakano KY, Iyama KI, Mori T, et al. Loss of alveolar basement membrane type IV collagen alpha3, alpha4, and alpha5 chains in bronchioloalveolar carcinoma of the lung. J Pathol 2001; 194:420–427.
15. Yousem SA, Beasley MB. Bronchioloalveolar carcinoma: a review of current concepts and evolving issues. Arch Pathol Lab Med 2007; 131:1027–1032.
16. Noguchi M, Morikawa A, Kawasaki M, et al. Small adenocarcinoma of the lung. Histologic characteristics and prognosis. Cancer 1995; 75:2844–2852.
17. Suzuki K, Yokose T, Yoshida J, et al. Prognostic significance of the size of central fibrosis in peripheral adenocarcinoma of the lung. Ann Thorac Surg 2000; 69:893–897.
18. Yokose T, Suzuki K, Nagai K, et al. Favorable and unfavorable morphological prognostic factors in peripheral adenocarcinoma of the lung 3 cm or less in diameter. Lung Cancer 2000; 29:179–188.
19. Terasaki H, Niki T, Matsuno Y, et al. Lung adenocarcinoma with mixed bronchioloalveolar and invasive components: clinicopathological features, subclassification by extent of invasive foci, and immunohistochemical characterization. Am J Surg Pathol 2003; 27:937–951.
20. Johansson L. Histopathologic classification of lung cancer: relevance of cytokeratin and TTF-1 immunophenotyping. Ann Diagn Pathol 2004; 8:259–267.
21. Saad RS, Liu YL, Han H, et al. Prognostic significance of thyroid transcription factor-1 expression in both early-stage conventional adenocarcinoma and bronchioloalveolar carcinoma of the lung. Hum Pathol 2004; 35:3–7.
22. Lau SK, Desrochers MJ, Luthringer DJ. Expression of thyroid transcription factor-1, cytokeratin 7, and cytokeratin 20 in bronchioloalveolar carcinomas: an immunohistochemical evaluation of 67 cases. Mod Pathol 2002; 15:538–542.
23. Rossi G, Marchioni A, Milani M, et al. TTF-1, cytokeratin 7, 34betaE12, and CD56/NCAM immunostaining in the subclassification of large cell carcinomas of the lung. Am J Clin Pathol 2004; 122:884–893.
24. Colby TV, Koss MN, Travis WD. Tumors of the lower respiratory tract. In: Atlas of Tumor Pathology, 3d series, fascicle 13. Washington, DC: Armed Forces Institute of Pathology, 1995.
25. Filderman AE, Coppage L, Shaw C, et al. Pulmonary and pleural manifestations of extrathoracic malignancies. Clin Chest Med 1989; 10:747–807.
26. Yoneda KY, Louie S, Shelton DK. Approach to pulmonary metastases. Curr Opin Pulm Med 2000; 6:356–363.
27. Negri F, Musolino A, Cunningham D, et al. Retrospective study of resection of pulmonary metastases in patients with advanced colorectal cancer: the development of a preoperative chemotherapy strategy. Clin Colorectal Cancer 2004; 4:101–106.
28. Briccoli A, Rocca M, Salone M, et al. Resection of recurrent pulmonary metastases in patients with osteosarcoma. Cancer 2005; 104:1721–1725.
29. Geurts TW, Nederlof PM, van den Brekel MW, et al. Pulmonary squamous cell carcinoma following head and neck squamous cell carcinoma: metastasis or second primary? Clin Cancer Res 2005; 11:6608–6614.

30. Flint A, Lloyd RV. Pulmonary metastases of colonic carcinoma. Distinction from pulmonary adenocarcinoma. Arch Pathol Lab Med 1992; 116:39–42.
31. Werling RW, Yaziji H, Bacchi CE, et al. CDX2, a highly sensitive and specific marker of adenocarcinomas of intestinal origin: an immunohistochemical survey of 476 primary and metastatic carcinomas. Am J Surg Pathol 2003; 27:303–310.
32. Yousem SA. Pulmonary intestinal-type adenocarcinoma does not show enteric differentiation by immunohistochemical study. Mod Pathol 2005; 18:816–821.
33. Castro CY, Moran CA, Flieder DG, et al. Primary signet ring cell adenocarcinomas of the lung: a clinicopathological study of 15 cases. Histopathology 2001; 39:397–401.
34. Rossi G, Murer B, Cavazza A, et al. Primary mucinous (so-called colloid) carcinomas of the lung: a clinicopathologic and immunohistochemical study with special reference to CDX-2 homeobox gene and MUC2 expression. Am J Surg Pathol 2004; 28:442–452.
35. Ordóñez NG. The diagnostic utility of immunohistochemistry and electron microscopy in distinguishing between peritoneal mesotheliomas and serous carcinomas: a comparative study. Mod Pathol 2006; 19:34–48.
36. Rosai J. Immunohistochemical markers of thyroid tumors: significance and diagnostic applications. Tumori 2003; 89:517–519.
37. McGregor DK, Khurana KK, Cao C, et al. Diagnosing primary and metastatic renal cell carcinoma: the use of the monoclonal antibody 'Renal Cell Carcinoma Marker'. Am J Surg Pathol 2001; 25:1485–1492.
38. Mazal PR, Stichenwirth M, Koller A, et al. Expression of aquaporins and PAX-2 compared to CD10 and cytokeratin 7 in renal neoplasms: a tissue microarray study. Mod Pathol 2005; 18:535–540.
39. Gaffey MJ, Mills SE, Ritter JH. Clear cell tumors of the lower respiratory tract. Semin Diagn Pathol 1997; 14:222–232.
40. Gal AA, Koss MN, Hochholzer L, et al. An immunohistochemical study of benign clear cell ('sugar') tumor of the lung. Arch Pathol Lab Med 1991; 115:1034–1038.
41. Raab SS, Berg LC, Swanson PE, et al. Adenocarcinoma in the lung in patients with breast cancer. A prospective analysis of the discriminatory value of immunohistology. Am J Clin Pathol 1993; 100:27–35.
42. Bedrossian CW, Bonsib S, Moran C. Differential diagnosis between mesothelioma and adenocarcinoma: a multimodal approach based on ultrastructure and immunocytochemistry. Semin Diagn Pathol 1992; 9:124–140.
43. Mimura T, Ito A, Sakuma T, et al. Novel marker D2-40, combined with calretinin, CEA, and TTF-1: an optimal set of immunodiagnostic markers for pleural mesothelioma. Cancer 2007; 109:933–938.
44. Ordóñez NG. Value of thyroid transcription factor-1, E-cadherin, BG8, WT1, and CD44S immunostaining in distinguishing epithelial pleural mesothelioma from pulmonary and nonpulmonary adenocarcinoma. Am J Surg Pathol 2000; 24:598–606.
45. Ordóñez NG. What are the current best immunohistochemical markers for the diagnosis of epithelioid mesothelioma? A review and update. Hum Pathol 2007; 38:1–16.
46. Ordóñez NG. Podoplanin: a novel diagnostic immunohistochemical marker. Adv Anat Pathol 2006; 13:83–88.
47. Ordóñez NG. D2-40 and podoplanin are highly specific and sensitive immunohistochemical markers of epithelioid malignant mesothelioma. Hum Pathol 2005; 36:372–380.
48. Miettinen M, Fernandez M, Franssila K, et al. Microphthalmia transcription factor in the immunohistochemical diagnosis of metastatic melanoma: comparison with four other melanoma markers. Am J Surg Pathol 2001; 25:205–211.
49. Zhang PJ, Livolsi VA, Brooks JJ. Malignant epithelioid vascular tumors of the pleura: report of a series and literature review. Hum Pathol 2000; 31:29–34.
50. Lin BT, Colby T, Gown AM, et al. Malignant vascular tumors of the serous membranes mimicking mesothelioma. A report of 14 cases. Am J Surg Pathol 1996; 20:1431–1439.

34
Differential Diagnosis of Neuroendocrine Lung Neoplasms

ELISABETH BRAMBILLA
Centre Hospitalier Universitaire de Grenoble, INSERM U823, University UJF, Grenoble, France

I. Introduction

Neuroendocrine (NE) lung tumors include four histological types of increasing malignancy: the low-grade typical carcinoids (TCs) (1), the atypical carcinoids (ACs) with an intermediate prognosis (2), the large cell neuroendocrine carcinomas (LCNECs), which have recently been described (3), and the well-known small cell lung carcinoma (SCLC), both of which are high-grade NE carcinomas (1). Increasing degree of malignancy is associated with decreasing degree of differentiation along this tumor spectrum. No detailed criteria for the distinction of ACs from TCs were given in the 1981 WHO classification, where they were presented as "having more anaplastic features than the usual carcinoids." They have been precisely defined by Arrigoni (2) and subsequently referred to under the term of well-differentiated NE carcinoma (4), where Arrigoni's criteria were extended to include all tumors of higher grade than carcinoids between TC and SCLC. In the revised version of the WHO classification of lung cancer, TCs and ACs are distinguished on the basis of objective criteria (5,6).

The previous WHO classification did not consider the entity of LCNEC, which has a large cell appearance and NE features (3,7–9) and fulfills the criteria of tumors of high grade. In addition to this spectrum of NE tumors, there are NE tumor-like hyperplasias called "tumorlets," as well as NSCLC, with NE differentiation. Both entities are discussed with regard to their differential diagnosis from the four common types of NE lung tumors. High-grade NE proliferations are believed to derive from an endodermal stem cell that is common to other types of lung carcinoma but which adopted a NE differentiation characterized by specific enzyme equipment of the amine precursor uptake and decarboxylation (APUD) system (4,10) and present often as component of combined SCLC or LCNEC. In contrast, carcinoid (typical or atypical) are almost never mixed with other NE or non-NE tumors and are believed to derive from another non-pluripotential stem cell assigned to NE differentiation.

All these neoplasms are collectively and phenotypically characterized by the expression of NE markers. Despite the large variety of their histomorphological features using conventional stains on paraffin sections, which are considered as the starting point for their differential diagnosis, we first define their common phenotypical characteristics, allowing their specific differential diagnosis from non-NE lung tumors. While NE differentiation is primarily recognized histologically and is exemplary in carcinoids, the hallmarks of NE differentiation are the expression of specific NE markers, including generalized NE immunohistochemical (IHC) markers, the secretion of specific neurohormonal peptides, and the presence of dense-core neurosecretory granules (NSG) at electron microscopy. The last is considered as the most definitive label of NE origin (11). However, since electron microscopy is not available in all laboratories, we will list the commonly used NE IHC markers that were previously compared with electron microscopy in order to attest their specificity and sensitivity (4).

These IHC markers can be divided in two categories: the neuroectodermal lineage markers and the NE differentiation markers. Neuroectodermic lineage markers are those that typify the family of normal and neoplastic neuronal and NE cells and are the most consistently expressed in normal NE cells and along the spectrum of differentiation in NE tumors. Synaptophysin, neural cell adhesion molecule (NCAM), neuron-specific enolase (NSE), Synaptophysin, NCAM 9.5, and S100 protein belong to this category. Synaptophysin (12), a cytoplasmic antigen, is the most sensitive IHC marker on frozen and paraffin sections. NCAM molecules are recognized by 123C3/CD56 antibody on paraffin sections (13). Almost 100% of NE neoplasms, regardless of grade, express synaptophysin (3,14) and NCAM (15,16) f. NSE is a very unspecific IHC marker present in 30% to 60% of non-NE tumors (3,15). PGP 9.5 and PS100 are neither particularly sensitive nor specific enough to be of help in the differential diagnosis of NE from non-NE tumors (17).

The second category of NE differentiation markers include chomogranin A and argyrophilia (staining with Grimelius silver stain using a reducing agent to develop silver positivity), Leu 7, and neurohormonal peptides. Chromogranin A is a specific protein attached to the external membrane of NSG (18,19). Both chromogranin A and Grimelius staining intensities (argyrophilia) reflect the number and density of NSG observed in tumor cells at electron microscopy, explaining their positivity in 100% of carcinoids and 50% to 60% of LCNEC and SCLC, with a significant decrease in number of stained cells from carcinoids to the less differentiated SCLC. Human bombesin [gastrin-releasing peptide (GRP)], calcitonin, Leu enkephalin, alpha human chorionic gonadotropin (α-hCG), and serotonin (5HT) are considered as eutopic hormones, whereas adrenocorticotropic hormone (ACTH), growth hormone (GH), vasointestinal peptide (VIP), and neurotensin are inappropriate ectopic products (20,21) absent in normal pulmonary NE cells. These secretions (mostly eutopic) are detected with decreasing frequency from carcinoids to SCLC. The more widely expressed hormones are 5HT, GRP, and ACTH, whereas α-hCG is also secreted in numerous non-NE tumors. However, the frequency of positive immunostaining is often low because of the high turnover of these peptides, which are more often excreted in the cell environment than being stocked inside granules (22). Although not mandatory, they can be useful in the differential diagnosis if antibodies are available.

Overall, three NE markers, chromogranin A, synaptophysin, and CD56, the most sensitive and specific NE markers will allow detection of NE differentiation in any situation. In order to avoid false-positive diagnosis, the following guidelines for interpretation should be observed: for chromogranin A and synaptophysin, only strong granular cytoplasmic staining should be interpreted as positive, in contrast to NCAM, where it is characterized by an exclusively membranous staining. Faint cytoplasmic staining should be considered as negative in any case.

It is crucial to decide how many positive markers are required to classify a tumor with an endocrinoid pattern as an NE tumor. This is still a matter of debate but is of clinical importance since the tumor classification and its distinction from other entities, which will result in different clinical management, depends on this criterion. Proliferations expressing NE markers in at least 30% of tumor cells should be considered as NE lung tumor with four exceptions: desmoplastic small round cell tumor, rhabdoid tumor, primitive neuro-ectodermic tumor (PNET), and pulmonary blastoma, which may express NE markers. It is obvious that NSG recognition at electron microscopy by itself obviously imposes the diagnosis of NE tumor. Electron microscopy however, besides being time consuming and confined to a small number of laboratories, may be confounded by tumor heterogeneity, which is common in lung tumors (23). Especially in NE tumors with less differentiation, such as SCLC, the "absence" of NSG, which occurs in 20% of cases (24), is not sufficient to deny their NE differentiation. Since other NE markers, such as NCAM expression and neuropeptide secretion, could be present in SCLC where NSG are absent, only a positive result has value for the diagnosis of NE differentiation.

Since NE proliferations in the lung are of epithelial type, they all harbor cytokeratin (CK) expression, mostly low– and medium–molecular weight (MW) CK. They will not express high-MW CK specific for squamous epidermoid differentiation. The most common expressed in NE tumors are the low-MW 7, 8, 17, and 18 CK, which are recognized by antibodies KL1, Cam 5,2, or a cocktail of anti-CK antibodies AE1/AE3 (25). Most NE tumors express epithelial membrane antigen (EMA), which could help when CK is faintly or not expressed, as it happens in SCLCs. Neurofilaments (NFs) are sometimes coexpressed with CK but IHC reactivity with anti-NF antibodies is relatively infrequent, not exceeding 25% in TC and less than 10% in SCLC (21).

II. Typical Carcinoids

TCs represent less than 1% of lung tumors. They are the most frequent primary lung tumors in the first two decades, and have a younger mean age of occurrence (55 years) than other NE lung tumors. They have an equal male-to-female distribution and are not related to smoking. Most are located in proximal airways, forming smooth red endobronchial polyps. More often, the bulk of the tumor growth is intrapulmonary (iceberg pattern). Ten-year overall survival is 85% to 95% despite regional lymph node metastasis, occurring in 5% to 15%.

Carcinoids display several histological patterns often seen in combination. The most frequent are mosaic and trabecular patterns with cords and ribbons. Palisading of tumor cells along the fibrovascular stroma and perivascular rosettes (pseudorosettes) or true rosettes are the characteristic features and define their organoid or endocrinoid pattern (also called "carcinoid" pattern) (Fig. 1A, B). Tumor cells are uniform, large (15–20 um), polygonal, with eosinophilic, finely granular cytoplasms and round nuclei with an open, clumped chromatin and small nucleoli (Fig. 1A). Mitoses are absent or less than 2 per 10 high-power field (HPF). All of them express chromogranin A, synaptophysin, and NCAM. They all show large number of NSGs of varying shape and size (150–300 nm in diameter), and express CK sometimes as a dot-like pattern. In this classical form, the differential diagnosis is not difficult on surgical samples and is essentially restricted to tumorlets and small cell minute chemo-dectomas on distal bronchial or transbronchial biopsies.

Spindle cell TCs are rare (less than 10%) and more frequent in peripheral locations. Because some lack an easily recognizable carcinoid pattern, they should be distinguished from tumorlets, nerve sheath proliferation such as neurofibroma or schwannoma, and from hemangiopericytoma (Fig. 1C, D). Tumorlets frequently show spindle cells, and are

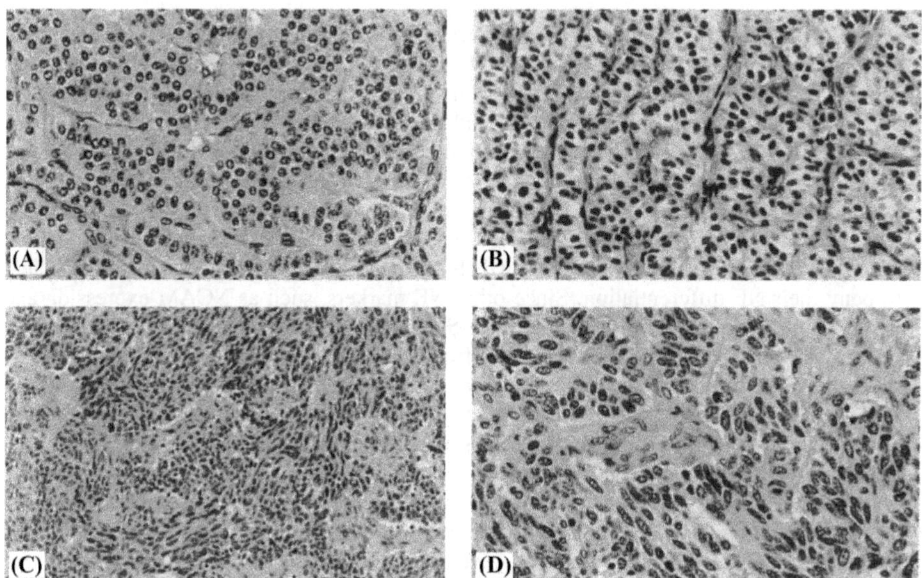

Figure 1 (**A**) TC with mosaic pattern, showing palisading of tumor cells along delicate fibrovascular stroma, perivascular rosettes, and true rosettes (H&E, 200×). (**B**) TC with trabecular pattern showing ribbons of cells forming rosettes in transversal section (H&E, 200×). (**C**) Spindle cell TC. Note the apparent lack of organoid pattern (H&E, 100×). (**D**) At higher magnification of the same case as Figure 1C, some rosettes are seen. Nuclei have a clumped open chromatin and some are dark but not in mitosis (H&E, 200×). *Abbreviations*: TC, typical carcinoid; H&E, hematoxylin and eosin.

differentiated from carcinoids by size (Fig. 2C): tumorlets are smaller than 5 mm by definition (WHO, 1999) (5). Neural lesions have more elongated and wavy cytoplasmic extensions, and are immunoreactive to glial fibrillary acidic protein (GFAP), in contrast with carcinoids. S100 protein positivity will not be of help since it can be positive in both: S100 protein is likely to be expressed in carcinoids, on sustentacular-like cells, and antigen-presenting dendritic cells. Vascular markers (factors VIII, CD31, CD34, smooth muscle actin) will distinguish fusiform carcinoid with hemangiopericytoma-like pattern from true hemangiopericytoma and CD34 from solitary fibrous tumor although this last tumor presents very specific morphologic features. More important is the differential diagnosis of spindle cells carcinoid from SCLC (Fig. 3A) or AC (Fig. 4C), which can also arise as peripheral tumors. Small cell carcinoma with fusiform pattern will be differentiated from AC on the basis of much higher mitotic activity in SCLC [by definition greater than 10 per 10 HPF, although most cases exceed 50 per 10 HPF] than in spindle cell carcinoid [less than 2 mitoses for 10 HPF). Moreover, the nuclear chromatin pattern which is open and clumped in TCs (Fig. 1D) is dark and condensed in SCLC (Fig. 3A). More difficult is the differential diagnosis between spindle cell TCs and ACs, which are discussed below.

Acinar, glandular, or the less frequent adenopapillary patterns (26,27) could lead to misdiagnosis of a carcinoid with adenocarcinoma, especially on bronchial biopsy (Fig. 4A). Mucin secretion has been shown to induce goblet cell, clear cell, or signet-ring cell variant

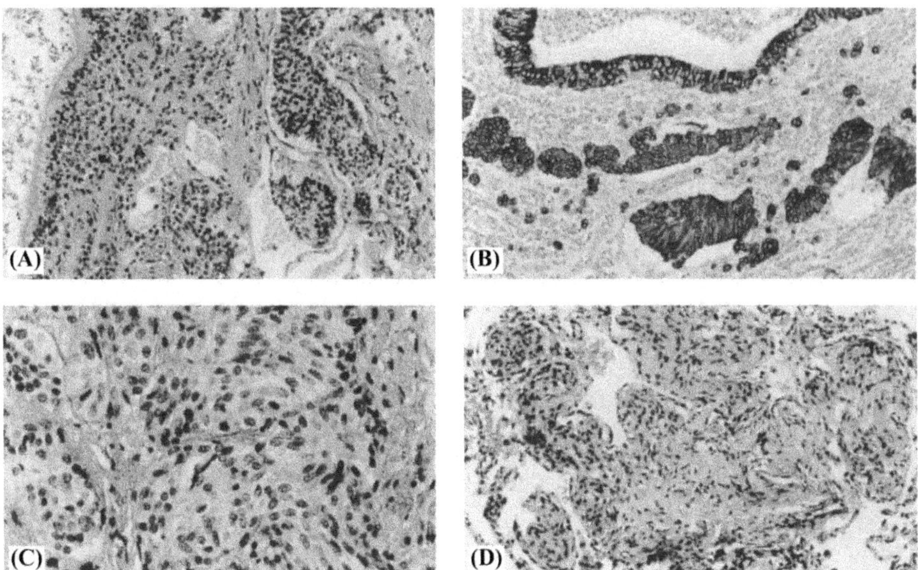

Figure 2 (**A**) Tumorlets (multiple) peripherally located in the wall of a small terminal bronchiole. Some tumorlets are observed inside lymphatic lumens (H&E, 100×). (**B**) Same tumorlets as in Figure 5A positively stained with CK KL1 (H&E, 100×). (**C**) High magnification of a tumorlet in scar tissue showing oval or fusiform cells with more delicate chromatin and smaller size than the spindle cell TC of Figure 1C (H&E, 200×). (**D**) Small minute chemodectoma in the vicinity of a small vein extending to alveolar walls (H&E, 100×). *Abbreviations*: H&E, hematoxylin and eosin; CK, cytokeratin; TC, typical carcinoid.

morphologies in carcinoids. Moreover, 40% of carcinoids, without specific morphological change, may show mucus production in association with NE differentiation (10,27). Thus diastase-digested periodic acid–Schiff (PAS) or alcian blue–positive stainings are not sufficient to rule out the diagnosis of carcinoid. Amphicrine cells, showing both NE and glandular differentiation, occur in normal lung and NE neoplasia (28). NE markers will make the distinction between amphicrine carcinoids and adenocarcinoma, since they are always positive in carcinoids and negative in adenocarcinoma. Amphicrine differentiation also exists in otherwise typical adenocarcinoma but is a rare event.

Sclerosing hemangioma enters in the differential diagnosis of carcinoids with papillary architecture: although the vast majority of sclerosing hemangioma express thyroid transcription factor-1 (TTF-1) in both epithelial and mesenchymal fetal type cells. Most carcinoids (>95%) do not express TTF-1 (29).

Oncocytic change in carcinoids, characterized by abundant eosinophilic granular cytoplasm (Fig. 4B) due to mitochondrial hyperplasia, may be a source of confusion with bronchial gland oncocytic adenoma and acinic cell tumor, which are rare salivary types of bronchial gland tumors also presenting as proximal endobronchial growth, and with granular cell tumors and glomangioma. Oncocytic (or oxyphilic) adenomas show uniform plump polyhedral cells with round central nuclei but a more vesicular chromatin than carcinoids. They show occasional tubular formation. They are more likely to be confused

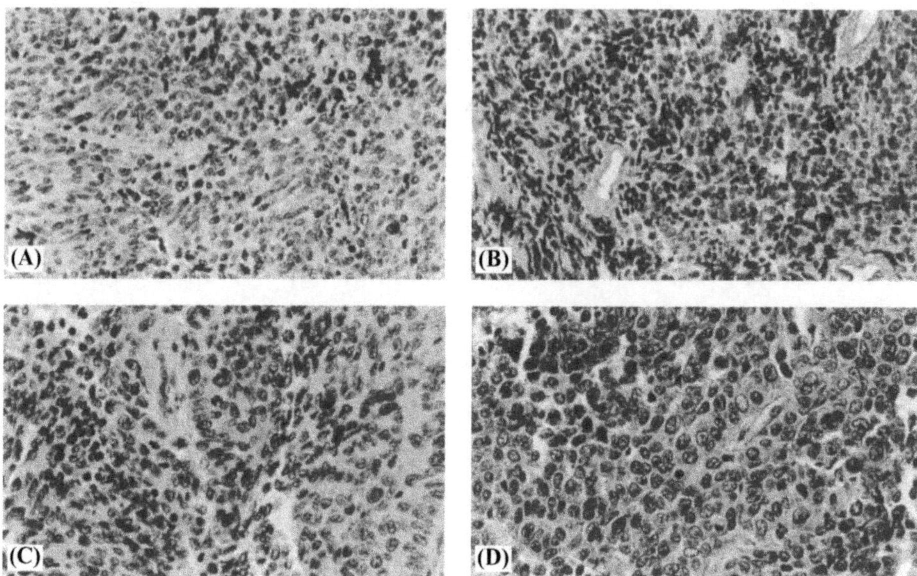

Figure 3 (**A**) Classical SCLC with small, elongated cells with diffuse granular chromatin and tendency to crush artifact. Compare with tumorlets in Figure 5C (H&E, 200×). (**B**) SCLC on a bronchial biopsy with crush artifact. Note the "oat cell" pattern (H&E, 20×). (**C**) SCLC with area of palisading and rosettes. Note at the same magnification the cell-size difference with the case in Figure 2A (intermediate size). Small and large cell types are visible at right (H&E, 200×). (**D**) Small cell and large cell carcinomas with an admixture of small and large cells, but "salt-and-pepper" chromatin, high N/C ratio, and nuclear molding (H&E, 200×). *Abbreviations*: SCLC, small cell lung cancer; H&E, hematoxylin and eosin; N/C, nuclear-to-cytoplasmic.

with carcinoid than acinic cell rumor (a rare type of serous gland tumor), which also has a granular cytoplasm but more dark and basophilic than that of carcinoid. Acinar cells contain typical coarse serous granules well stained by PAS and are arranged in acinar groups. Granular cell tumor is a benign, rare tumor of putative Schwann cell origin arising in proximal bronchi, made of spindle cells showing large eosinophilic granular cytoplasm, which express S100 protein. Glomangioma is even less common and is distinguished from carcinoid by smooth muscle marker positivity (smooth muscle actin and/or desmin). Both granular cell tumor and glomangioma are negative for chromogranin A, synaptophysin, and keratins.

Carcinoids with clear cell changes (Fig. 4C), should not be confused with two rare entities: the meningothelial bodies further discussed and clear cell (sugar) tumor. Sugar (clear cell) tumors are peripheral pericytic proliferations expressing CD34 and HMB45, and do not express NE markers nor do they display NSG at electron microscopy. Rarely, will carcinoids contain melanin (30) granules and must be distinguished from melanoma: melanoma does not express keratin and specific NE markers (SI00 protein can be positive in both) but expresses HMB45, MelanA, and tyrosine hydroxylase which is not found in NE tumors.

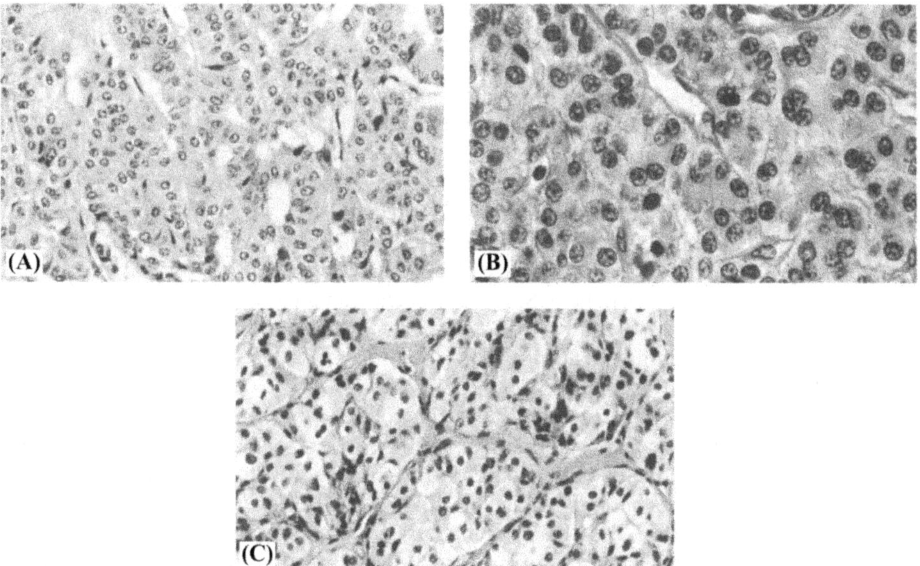

Figure 4 (**A**) TC with a pseudoglandular pattern and typical nuclei with open clumped chromatin (H&E, 200×.) (**B**) TC with oncocytic change and typical nuclei with open clumped chromatin and a small nucleolus (H&E, 400×.) (**C**) TC with clear cell change and gangliocytic pattern (H&E, 200×). *Abbreviations*: TC, typical carcinoid; H&E, hematoxylin and eosin.

Tumorlets are smaller (<5 mm) than carcinoids and are visualized only at histological examination. They can be multiple and associated with carcinoids but are more peripherally located in the wall of small terminal bronchioles (Fig. 2A). They are found in the context of bronchiectasis and scarring flbrosis (Fig. 2C). Large tumorlets (≥5 mm) in normal lung are diagnosed as carcinoid (5,6). They show the same morphology as carcinoids (Fig. 2C). They express the same NE markers and CK (Fig. 2B). They can be observed migrating in lymphatics or even hilar lymph nodes without any clinical import (31) but induce a wrong diagnosis of lymphatic spread of a NE lung tumor. Minute menigothelial-like nodules are described as nodules along small veins (Fig. 2D), and express neither NE markers nor keratins. Paragangliomas typically present only as a miliary metastasis in lung, and the existence of true primary pulmonary paragangliomas is controversial. Like some carcinoids with gangliocytic (paraganglioma-like) patterns (Fig. 4C) (21), they harbor well-defined nests of polygonal or fusiform clear cells separated from vascular and fibrous septa by sustentacular elongated cells stained with SI00 protein and GFAP. Paragangliomas express NE markers but are CK negative.

A pitfall in the diagnosis of carcinoid tumor on a small biopsy can arise from stromal modification including amyloid deposit, calcification, ossification, and cartilage formation, which can displace or hide the carcinoid cells. They should not be confused with a mixed salivary gland type of tumor or with pleomorphic carcinoma or carcinosarcoma. The differential diagnosis with ACs is discussed below.

III. Atypical Carcinoids

The exact frequency of ACs is very difficult to appreciate owing to the inclusion of all cases of large cell NE carcinoma in series reported previously to the revised WHO classification (1999). ACs probably represent about 10% of the carcinoid tumors and have metastatic potential (up to 70%). They have 70% and 50% survival rate at 5 and 10 years, respectively (32). Histologically, TC tumors with hilar node spread (2–10% of carcinoids) should not be considered atypical. They have a 2:3 male-to-female ratio and are more frequently peripheral (50%). They share with TCs a characteristic organoid growth pattern (mosaic, trabecular, palisading, and rosettes). Since they occupy an intermediate place between low-grade carcinoids and high-grade LCNECs and SCLCs, their differential diagnosis must be discussed with those entities first.

ACs must be differentiated from TCs (Table 1) essentially by increased mitotic activity and/or necrosis. Whereas TCs show no mitosis or less than 2 per 10 HPF (2 mm^2), ACs show 2 to 10 mitosis per 10 HPF (2 mm^2), and proliferative markers (Ki67) exceed 5% (Fig. 5A–D). Necrosis, which is never seen in TCs, can occur in AVs as focal, punctate, sharply demarcated areas but rarely as infarct-like necrosis. These atypical features may be missed on small biopsies. Thus, the differential diagnosis between TCs and ACs is mainly achieved on surgical resection, allowing extensive observation of serial sections of the

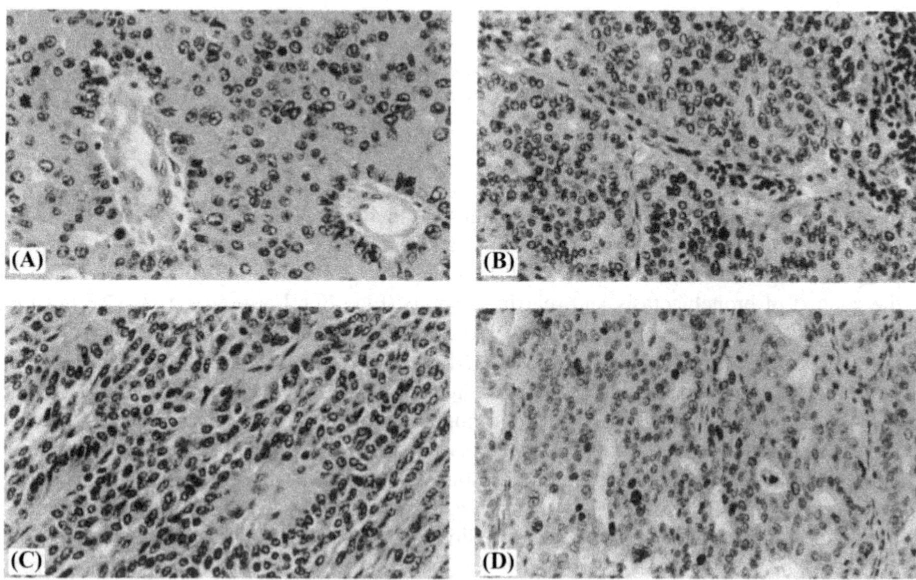

Figure 5 (**A**) AC with oncocytic cells, perivascular rosettes, and palisading. Note two mitoses in the field and some nuclear pleomorphism (H&E, 200×). (**B**) AC with rosettes, palisades, hypercellularity, and mitoses (H&E, 200×). (**C**) AC with spindle cell pattern, rosettes, discrete pleomorphism, and mitosis (H&E, 200×). (**D**) Immunostaining with Ki67 of the same AC as Figure 4B, showing 10% of Ki67-positive cells (Ki67, 200×). *Abbreviations*: AC, atypical carcinoid; H&E, hematoxylin and eosin.

Table 1 Typical and Atypical Carcinoids: Distinguishing Features

Histological features	TCs	ACs
Endocrinoid pattern (organoid, carcinoid)	Characteristic	Characteristic
Mitoses	Absent or less than 2 per 10 HPF	Present 2–10 per 10 HPF
Necrosis	Absent	Focal, punctuate
Nuclear pleomorphism, hyperchromatism	Absent or focal	Often present
Increased cellularity with architectural disorganization	Absent or focal	Often present

Source: From Ref. 2.
Abbreviations: TCs, typical carcinoids; ACs, atypical carcinoids; HPF, high-power field.

tumor. Additional features in ACs, such as focal nuclear pleomorphism (Fig. 5A–C), nuclear hyperchromasia, higher nuclear-to-cytoplasmic (N/C) ratio, increased cellularity (Fig. 5B), or architectural disorganization are not decisive in this differential diagnosis, although significant pleomorphism is almost never seen in TCs. NE markers are less widely distributed in ACs than TCs. IHC NE markers, Grimelius, and NSG are found together in 100% of TCs, and in 80% of ACs (21), which means that some ACs may lack one NE marker. Both TCs and ACs have large numbers of NSGs at ultrastructural analysis.

The differential diagnosis should be made between ACs with spindle cell appearance (Fig. 5C), which is frequent in peripheral tumors, and SCLC. SCLCs are usually centrally located, and it is likely that many peripheral tumors previously labeled as peripheral SCLC are ACs with a spindle cell appearance (33). The mitotic index is definitely higher (>10 mitoses per 10 HPF) in SCLC than AC (between 2–10 per 10 HPF). This is an objective criterion that should be regarded as the best. Proliferative activity, as tested by Ki67 and MIB1 nuclear staining, also reflects these differences in proliferation rate: while less than 30% in ACs (Fig. 5D), it ranges from 30% to 80% in SCLC. The Azzopardi effect (basophilic DNA staining of vessel walls) can be seen in AC. The differential diagnosis resides also in the nuclear chromatin, more uniform as "salt-and-pepper" and dense in SCLCs and more open in ACs (Fig. 5C). The N/C ratio is much higher in SCLCs. Intensity and distribution of NE marker reactivity are greater in ACs than in SCLCs, but this is only statistical and has no value for an individual case.

Many of the differential diagnoses with rare entities already discussed for carcinoid would apply to ACs according to cytological and architectural particularities: oncocytic (Fig. 5A) (oxyphilic adenoma of bronchial glands) or spindle cell (Fig. 5C) (neurilemoma, hemangiopericytoma). Although p53 staining has not been recommended as a way to achieve the differential diagnosis between tumor classes, the differential diagnosis between TCs and ACs may be an exception. Whereas p53 is neither mutant nor stabilized in TC, p53 stabilization and subsequent immunoreactivity occurs in 20% to 30% of ACs. Mutation with stabilization occurs with still higher frequency (50–70%) in SCLCs and LCNEC (34,35). Thus, p53 immunoreactivity in a carcinoid tumor would stress the necessity of a careful search for other signs of malignant potential, such as mitoses and necrosis.

Even more difficult is the distinction of AC from LCNEC, which is discussed below.

Table 2 Atypical Carcinoids and Large Cell Neuroendocrine Carcinomas: Distinguishing Features

Histological features	ACs	LCNECs
Endocrinoid pattern (organoid, carcinoid)	Characteristic	Present, less extensive
Necrosis	Punctate, focal	Punctate or infarct-like
Mitosis	2–10 per 10 HPF	20–200 per 10 HPF
Cell size	Medium to large (20–45 μm)	Medium to large (20–45 μm)
N/C ratio	Moderate or low	Low
Nuclear chromatin	Fine or slightly coarse	Coarse or vesicular
Nucleoli	Small or absent	Present, often prominent
Cellular pleomorphism	Sometimes	Frequent
Azzopardi effect	No	Uncommon
NE markers	Optional	Required

Source: From Ref. 3.
Abbreviations: ACs, atypical carcinoids; LCNECs, large cell neuroendocrine carcinomas; HPF, high-power field; N/C, nuclear-to-cytoplasmic; NE, neuroendocrine.

IV. Large Cell Neuroendocrine Carcinoma

LCNECs are large cell proliferations (20–45 μm in cell diameter) expressing NE differentiation markers. They are probably more frequent than ACs, with which they were confused in many reported series. Their frequency of occurrence is about the same as that of TCs and ACs together (about 5% of lung tumors). LCNECs should be differentiated from ACs, SCLCs, basaloid carcinomas (BCs), and large cell carcinomas.

LCNECs should first be distinguished from ACs, with which they have been confused (Table 2). Like ACs, they show NE histopathological features, including organoid nesting, mosaic, and trabecular pattern, and rosette-like and palisading features (Fig. 6), but these are less widely distributed than in ACs. Some areas can appear undifferentiated with solid and lobular patterns (Fig. 7A). Centrolobular necrosis is frequent, as well as infarct-like necrosis (Fig. 6A). While NE markers are not mandatory for the diagnosis of TCs or ACs because they maintain a diffuse typical organoid pattern, they are required for the diagnosis of LCNEC (Fig. 7B–D). The demonstration of NSG at electron microscopy also allows the diagnosis. These are fewer and more confined to distant cytoplasmic cell processes than in ACs, where they are more numerous and perinuclear. LCNECs as a group show a lower percentage, intensity, and distribution of IHC NE marker positivity and hormonal products than TCs and ACs. LCNECs also differ from ACs by a lower N/C ratio, a larger nucleus with coarse or vesicular chromatic, more frequent prominent nucleoli, and higher nuclear pleomorphism and cytological atypia (Fig. 6B–D). Necrosis is more extensive in LCNECs than in ACs (Fig. 6A). The differential diagnosis resides essentially in a higher proliferation rate, usually of 20 to 100 up to 200 mitosis per 10 HPF compared with 2 to 10 per 10 HPF in ACs (Fig. 7B). This is the most practical and objective criterion to distinguish them from ACs (3). However, mitoses can be difficult to appreciate on a small bronchial biopsy and nuclear differences described above will be of help.

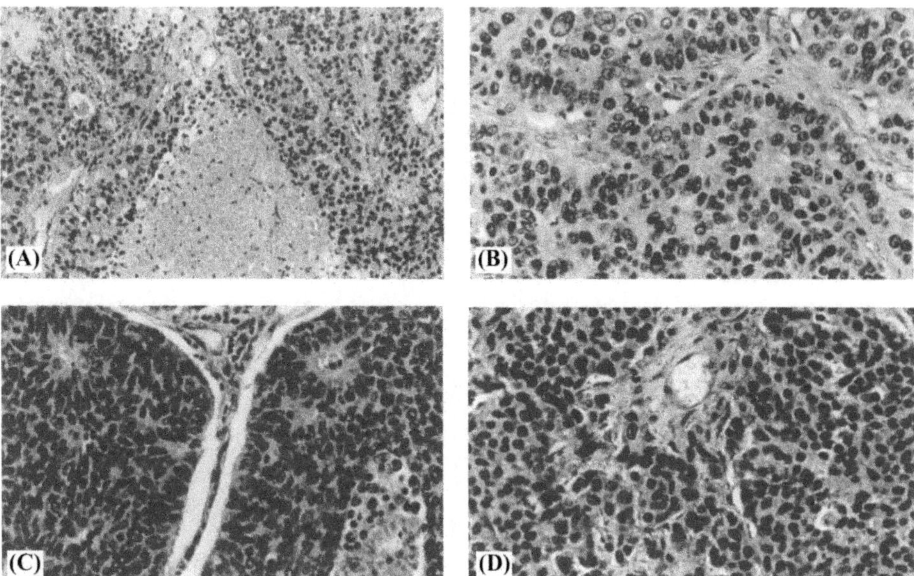

Figure 6 (**A**) LCNEC with organoid trabecular pattern, and infarct-like necrosis (H&E, 100×). (**B**) Higher magnification of the same case as Figure 7A, showing rosettes, palisades, vesicular chromatin, and numerous mitoses (H&E, 200×). (**C**) LCNEC with a lobular pattern, well-defined strands of stroma, rosettes, and centrilobular necrosis (H&E, 200×). (**D**) LCNEC with poorly defined lobular pattern, palisading, coarse or vesicular chromatin, and numerous mitoses. Note a high N/C ratio and a more condensed chromatin (H&E, 200×). *Abbreviations*: LCNEC, large cell neuroendocrine carcinoma; H&E, hematoxylin and eosin; N/C, nuclear-to-cytoplasmic.

Theoretically, LCNECs can be distinguished from SCLCs by a larger cell size (Table 3). However, because of a continuous spectrum and overlap of size range between SCLC and LCNEC, cell size is an unreliable criterion. SCLCs have scantier cytoplasm than LCNECs, most of which have a large eosinophilic cytoplasm (Fig. 6B). Nuclear molding is much more frequent in SCLCs than LCNECs. The Azzopardi effect is far more common in SCLCs than in LCNECs. Moreover, the chromatin, which is usually coarse or vesicular and irregular in LCNEC (Fig. 6B), is more homogeneous and granular, with a "salt-and-pepper" pattern, and condensed in SCLCs. However, some LCNECs have a condensed chromatin (Fig. 6D). The nucleolus, which is prominent in LCNECs, is inconspicuous in SCLCs. A fusiform shape is common in SCLCs and uncommon in LCNEC cells, which are more polygonal. Architectural differences are easy to recognize on large biopsies only: SCLC forms diffuse sheets of tumor cells infiltrating bronchial walls and adjacent lung parenchyma, with poorly developed stroma. In contrast, LCNECs are architecturally organized by well-defined basement membranes and intervening fibrous and inflammatory strands of stroma (Fig. 6C–D). NE markers expressed in both SCLCs and LCNECs are of no help in their differential diagnosis. Keratin is less

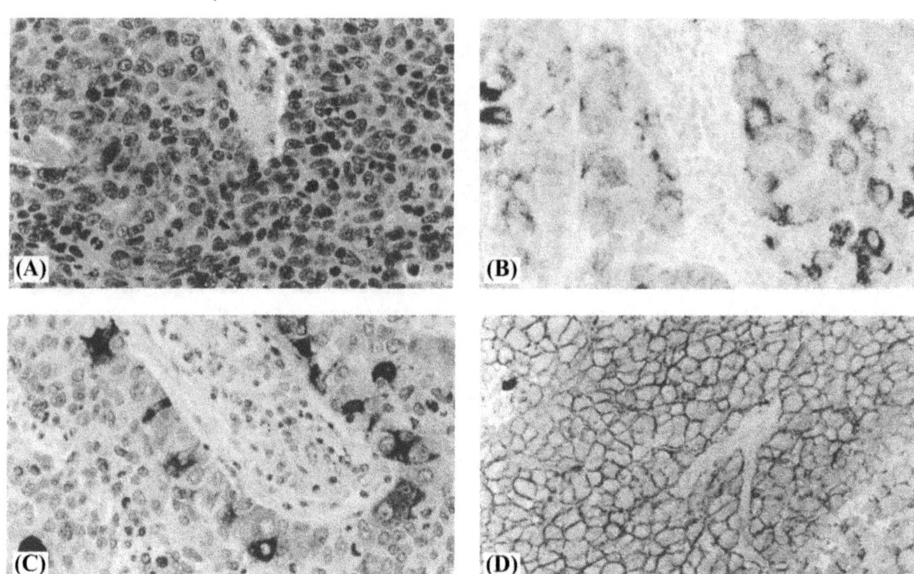

Figure 7 (**A**) LCNEC in an area of poorly defined organoid pattern, cell pleomorphism, and high mitotic rate (H&E, 200×). (**B**) LCNEC immunostained for chromogranine A, showing the specific granular heterogeneous cytoplasmic pattern of staining (chromogranine, 200×). (**C**) LCNEC immunostained for synaptophysin, showing the specific granular heterogeneous cytoplasmic staining (synaptophysin, 200×). (**D**) LCNEC immunostained for NCAM with 123 C3 (CD 56) showing the typical specific membranar pattern of staining (123 C3, 200×). *Abbreviations*: LCNEC, large cell neuroendocrine carcinoma; H&E, hematoxylin and eosin; NCAM, neural cell adhesion molecule.

Table 3 Small Cell Lung Carcinomas and Large Cell Neuroendocrine Carcinomas: Distinguishing Features

Histological features	SCLCs	LCNECs
Cell size	Small (less than three lymphocytes)	Larger, 20–45 μm
N/C ratio	High	Low
Nuclear chromatin	Finely granular, uniform, dense	Coarse or vesicular
Nucleoli	Absent	Present (often), may be prominent
Nuclear molding	Characteristic	Uncommon
Fusiform	Common	Uncommon
Polygonal	Uncharacteristic	Characteristic
Nuclear smear	Frequent	Uncommon
Azzopardi effect	Occasional	Rare

Source: From Ref. 3.
Abbreviations: SCLCs, small cell lung carcinomas; LCNECs, large cell neuroendocrine carcinomas; N/C, nuclear-to-cytoplasmic.

Table 4 Large Cell Neuroendocrine Carcinomas and Basaloid Carcinomas: Distinguishing Features

Histological features	LCNECs	BCs
Cell size	Large (20–40 μm)	Moderate (15–20 μm)
N/C ratio	Lower	Higher
Nuclear chromatin	Coarse and vesicular	Finely granular, uniform, moderately dense
Nucleoli	Present, often prominent	Infrequent, small, inconspicuous
Fusiform	Uncommon	Frequent
NE markers	Required (positive)	Negative

Abbreviations: LCNECs, large cell neuroendocrine carcinomas; BCs, Basaloid Carcinomas; N/C, nuclear-to-cytoplasmic; NE, neuroendocrine.

expressed in frequency, intensity, and distribution in SCLCs than in LCNECs, which have the same rate of p53 mutation and positive immunoreactivity.

LCNECs should be distinguished from BC, another highly malignant lung neoplasm (Table 4). BC, which represents 5% of NSCLCs (non-NE), has been separated from other NSCLCs by cardinal histopathological features: a solid lobular or trabecular pattern of small cuboidal to fusiform cells 12 to 15 μm in diameter with moderately hyperchromatic nuclei, finely granular chromatin, no prominent nuclei, a high N/C ratio, peripheral palisading, and a high rate of mitosis of 25 to 60 per 10 HPF (Fig. 6A). As a source of confusion, rosettes are present in one-third of the cases. BC can present as a pure form in half of the cases, where more than 80% of the tumors show a basaloid pattern, or as a mixed form, where the basaloid component represents at least 60% of the tumor bulk and is juxtaposed with another tumor type of larger size, which can be squamous cell carcinoma (80%), large cell carcinoma (10%), or adeno- or adenosquamous carcinoma (10%). The most difficult differential diagnosis resides in the distinction of the pure form of BC showing rosettes and palisades from LCNEC (Fig. 8B). Most LCNECs have a larger cell size, a higher degree of cellular pleomorphism, more coarsely granular and vesicular chromatin, and more prominent nucleoli, than BCs (Table 4). Palisading in several layers in BC rather than one row of cells in LCNEC. NE markers are required to separate pure BC showing rosettes and palisades from LCNECs. Whereas NE markers (at least three positive markers using frozen and a paraffin sections) are expressed in 50% to 100% of tumor cells in LCNECs, they are not expressed in BC, and NSGs are absent at ultrastractural examination. It should be remembered here that a single

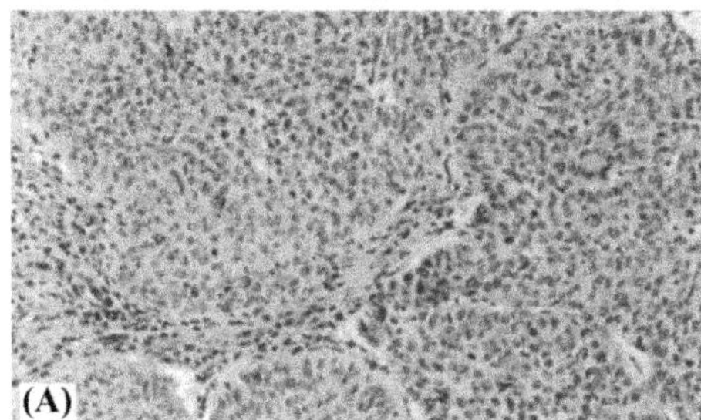

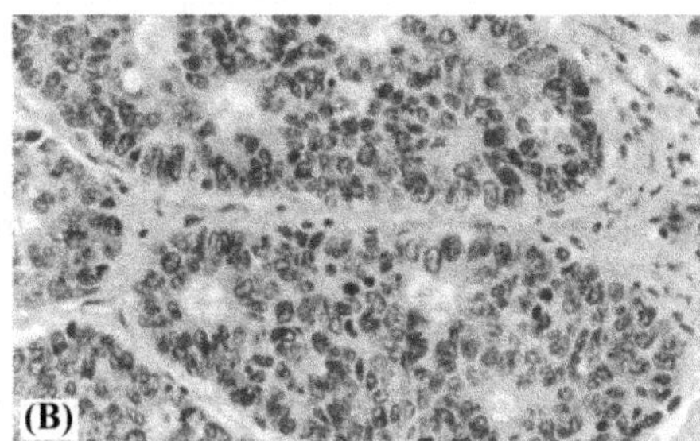

Figure 8 (**A**) BC with typical lobulated pattern, small cells, and peripheral palisading. Note some rosettes (H&E, 100×). (**B**) BC showing numerous rosettes in addition to palisades (H&E, 200×). *Abbreviations*: BC, basaloid carcinoma; H&E, hematoxylin and eosin.

positive NE marker could occasionally be found in 5% to 20% of tumor cells in 20% of tumors not otherwise classified as NE carcinoma (14,15). In accordance with this prevalence, 10% of BCs express one isolated NE marker in 5% to 20% of tumor cells and are not considered to be NE tumors. Basaloid-like tumor expressing multiple NE markers (at least three) on more than 20% of tumor cells should be regarded as authentic NE carcinomas and classified as LCNECs, despite a basaloid pattern. The evidence of NSG at electron microscopy should eliminate the diagnosis of BC and allow that of LCNEC as well. With the exception of pure BC showing rosettes, the NE markers are not required to differentiate BC from LCNEC on surgical samples. However, a diagnosis of BC versus LCNEC on a small bronchial biopsy can be difficult and may be solved only by NE markers, since the mitotic rate and proliferation markers are equally high in both types of tumors.

Differentiating LCNEC from large cell (non-NE) carcinoma is easier. The latter tumors have no endocrinoid pattern and do not express NE markers. As already pointed out, a dissociated expression of one or two NE markers (less than 5% of tumor cells in less than 5% of tumors) can be observed in squamous carcinoma and adenocarcinoma. A more widespread expression of several NE markers would refer to another class of NE lung tumors, which is NSCLC with NE differentiation (3,15,36).

NSCLCs with NE differentiation theoretically embraces all carcinomas with large cell appearance showing NE differentiation, including LCNECs. However, they differ from LCNECs by lack of endocrinoid architecture at light microscopy, whereas NE features are detected at IHC or ultrastructural levels only (3). They can have the histological appearance of large cell carcinomas, squamous cell carcinomas, or adenocarcinomas. These tumors comprise less than 10% of ordinary NSCLCs. In our experience, squamous carcinomas and adenocarcinomas with no evidence of endocrinoid architectural pattern are unlikely to express NE markers to the same extent than that observed in LCNECs. However, a partial expression of NE markers (one or two NE markers) could have clinical importance and could predict chemosensitivity or affect survival, although this has been diversely appreciated (37). At the present time, there is no consensus on the clinical value of the recognition of partial NE differentiation in squamous carcinoma and adenocarcinoma. Amphicrine adenocarcinomas (with multidirectional differentiation) have been described (38). They are tumors showing both glandular and NE differentiation and are very rare. They should be considered non-SCLC with NE differentiation.

The histological similarity between LCNECs and metastatic medullary carcinomas is high, but their differential diagnosis is virtually impossible on the basis of immunohistochemistry, since NE markers are expressed in both and calcitonin can be expressed in LCNECs. The only parameter of value is the high level of serum calcitonin in medullary carcinoma.

The nesting pattern of LCNECs may be confused with that of malignant melanoma. This differential possibility is resolved by HMB-45, MelanA, and tyrosine hydroxylase positivity in melanomas only.

V. Small Cell Lung Carcinoma

SCLCs generally arise in major airways and grow very rapidly. Their chemosensitivity is initially high, and a prompt diagnosis is required from bronchial biopsies. SCLC is made up of uniform, round or elongated small cells ranging from one to three lymphocytes in

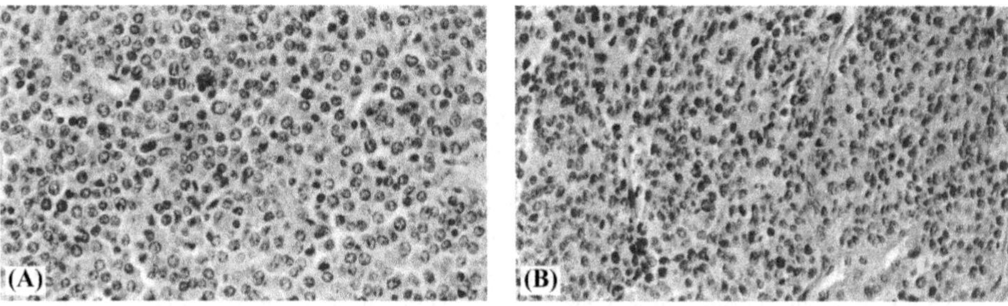

Figure 9 (**A**) Lymphoplasmocytoid lymphoma on a small lung biopsy showing round lymphoid cells with large cytoplasm (H&E, 200×). (**B**) SCLC in an intermediate form, with more cytoplasm than "oat cell" form but more cell cohesion and density than lymphoma shown in Figure 9A (H&E, 200×). *Abbreviations*: H&E, hematoxylin and eosin; SCLC, small cell lung carcinoma.

size (8–20 μm in diameter). They have round or oval nuclei; diffuse homogeneous, finely granular, dense chromatin; and inconspicuous nucleoli. Cytoplasm is very sparse and the N/C ratio is the highest seen in tumors. They form diffuse sheets of loosely connected cells with a minimal amount of intervening stroma (Fig. 3A). Some may palisade around small vessels or make pseudorosettes in transverse sections. True rosettes can be seen (Fig. 3A). The presence of occasional large cells, small tubules, or even mucin substance should not rule out the diagnosis of SCLC. A little mucin can be seen inside rosettes. In the WHO 1981 classification, they were divided into oat cell, intermediate cell type, and combined oat cell carcinoma in which areas of squamous and adenocarcinoma were also present. The distinction of oat cell from intermediate cell groups does not have clinical significance and lacks interobserver reproducibility (39–41). The intermediate cell type differs from the oat cell type by a little more nuclear pleomorphism and more visibility of the cytoplasmic ring. It is likely that the "oat cell" appearance corresponds to an artifact, since this appearance most often occurs in bronchial biopsies where distortion due to crushing commonly occurs (Fig. 3B). In contrast, the intermediate cell type is exclusively seen in well-preserved large biopsies or surgical material (Fig. 9B). Accordingly, it is reasonable to abandon these subgroups and keep SCLC as a single group. Necrosis is frequent and occurs in large infarct-like areas. The NE markers are present with a lesser intensity and smaller percentage of staining than in all other NE tumors. Accordingly, the NSG in SCLC are usually fewer and smaller (100–130 nm) than in AC and TC and are often situated in cytoplasmic processes. They are not required to allow the diagnosis of SCLC. TTF-1 is expressed in 80% of SCLC and of great help in addition to NE markers to distinguish SCLC from any other small, round or fusiform cell proliferation including fusiform-type carcinoids (29). The differential diagnosis of classical SCLC is discussed with lymphoma, inflammatory lymphoid infiltrate, and Askin tumor [peripheral primitive neuroectodermic tumor (PNET)].

SCLC should not be confused with lymphoma, especially on bronchial biopsies with a crush artifact. Both proliferations, because they lack protection of tumor cells by sufficient amounts of cytoplasm and protective stroma, are prone to "crush artifact." On well-preserved tissue, there are nuclear and N/C ratio differences, depending on the class of lymphoma considered. Small cell lymphomas—lymphocytic, lymphoplasmocytoid, and the mucosa-associated lymphoid tissue (MALT) type (centrocytic-like) are more likely to occur primarily in the lung than large cell lymphomas, which occur more frequently at a secondary localization. SCLCs have scantier cytoplasm than any kind of lymphoma, even small cell lymphoma. Giemsa stain shows basophilic cytoplasm in plasmocytoid and MALT lymphomas, whereas SCLCs have inapparent cytoplasm and frequent nuclear molding. SCLCs have more dense, homogenous, granular chromatin than lymphomas, and nucleoli that are always absent in SCLC, are small but present in lymphoma (Fig. 9A). Immunohistochemistry definitely separates both entities: SCLCs express keratin and EMA and are CD45 (common leukocyte antigen)-negative, whereas all lymphomas express CD45, but not keratin, EMA, and NE markers. Fortunately, both keratin and CD45 immunoreactivities are surprisingly well preserved despite crushing artifact and necrosis, which are frequent in both tumor types. Use of several anti-CK antibodies (KL1, Cam 5,2) or cocktails of CK (AE1–AE3) may be recommended if the usual CK available in the laboratory is negative. Exceptional cases of lymphomas appear CD45-negative at least on paraffin section: CD20 for B-cell antigen recognition as well as CD45-Rho (UCHL1) for T-cell recognition can be of help.

In a well-preserved cell population on surgical samples or bronchial biopsy, SCLC can easily be differentiated from inflammatory cell infiltrates. However, these inflammatory infiltrates may also show severe crush artifacts and be difficult to differentiate from SCLC. CD45 positivity and CK negativity of inflammatory cells are the main tools for this differential diagnosis. Some pitfalls should be pointed out: inflammatory infiltrates or lymphomas rich in plasma cells will be stained with EMA, and natural killer (NK) cells will be stained with Leu 7 and NCAM antibodies.

Tumorlets can be confused with SCLC (Fig. 2C) on a small crushed bronchial biopsy since they are composed of small round or oval cells. However, these benign, hyperplastic proliferations are peripherally situated. They have been reported, besides proximal tuberculoma, giving radiological mass density and bronchial compression and deformation. They harbor keratin and NE expression as well as SCLC but are TTF-1 negative, chromatin is less dark and dense than that of SCLC and proliferation markers are quite low in tumorlets (Ki67 $< 2\%$).

SCLC in their classical type (oat cell or intermediate) differ histolopathologically from LCNEC primarily by cell size (10–20 μm in SCLC against 20–45 μm in LCNEC). Other differences have been exposed under the heading of LCNEC and are shown in Table 3.

SCLC can coexist with another squamous or adenocarcinoma component and called combined SCLCs. Their frequency reaches 20% on surgical samples (42). However, occurrence of large cells admixed within the small cell population has been well recognized and previously proposed as a new class under the term small cell and large cell carcinoma (43) (Fig. 3D). They represent 10% to 15% of SCLCs and are now included in the combined SCLC. Cases where SCLCs and LCNECs are associated but topographically segregated, are also encountered. Under recognition of small and large, SCLCs can occur if only the large cell component is present in the area under examination on a bronchial biopsy. Crush artifact or necrosis in a mixed small cell/large cell population overrates large cell which will be preferentially examined. This, of course, overestimates their proportion and leads to a wrong diagnosis of LCNEC or large cell carcinoma. Since therapy depends on the diagnosis of SCLC component, this is a serious pitfall in biopsy analysis. NE markers would not be useful to differentiate small cell from LCNEC but of great help to differentiate LCNEC or SCLC/SL from large cell (non-NE) carcinoma.

Other pitfalls come from the effect of chemotherapy. Chemotherapy in SCLC induces larger cell size, appearance of LCNEC, sometimes squamous or glandular differentiation, with a much higher frequency than that observed spontaneously in the absence of therapy. Such morphological changes occur in about 50% of treated SCLCs, which were otherwise classical before therapy (44). Mucin production and the appearance of higher-MW keratins accompany this differentiation or induction phenomenon. The diagnosis should be proposed as "common changes on post-therapy samples of SCLC" and not as a second metachronous tumor.

Another pitfall results from the high frequency of bronchial squamous metaplasia and dysplasia in contact with SCLC on biopsies (45). Superficial sampling may lead to erroneous histological classification, and cytological material from brushing may contain only these squamous cells. It is thus essential that invasive tumor be examined.

Differential diagnosis of SCLC from BC is less difficult than it was for LCNEC. BCs have a delicate, finely granular chromatin, which is never as dense and compact than that of SCLC. Nuclear molding, which is usual in SCLC, rarely occurs in BC, where cytoplasm is substantial. Importantly, the diffuse sheet-like pattern of SCLC and its paucity of stroma are in contrast with the well-defined lobular and trabecular pattern with abundant stroma of BC. These architectural differences can be missed on bronchial biopsies. NE markers are expected to be positive in SCLC and negative in BC. However, it should be kept in mind that NE markers on bronchial biopsies remain negative in 10% to 40% on reported series in SCLC, in keeping with their low differentiation status. NCAM expression on paraffin section may be of great help, since it is not dependent on differentiation.

Poorly differentiated adenocarcinoma with small cell size, showing solid patterns, ribbons, and trabeculae and small rosette-like acini, can mimic SCLC. Despite nuclear chromatin and cytoplasmic differences, this is a diagnostic problem requiring immunohistochemistry, with the same reservations as for BC.

PNET is a rare tumor that occurs in younger patients than SCLC, in the first two decades. These tumors correspond to Askin tumor, a small, round cell primary tumor of the chest wall invading contiguous lung parenchyma. Askin tumors belong to the PNET family (or Ewing tumor family). Tumor cells form diffuse or cohesive broad sheets of uniform small round cells (12–15 μm) with a round nucleus. The finely dispersed chromatin, one or two small nucleoli, and an eosinophilic scant cytoplasm with indistinct borders all differ from SCLC (Fig. 10A). These tumors are characterized by a common chromosomal

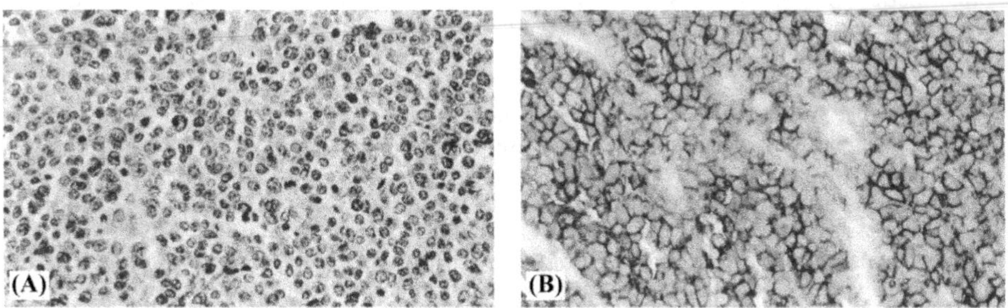

Figure 10 (**A**) PNET to be compared with SCLC of Figure 9B, involving the chest wall and adjacent lung, showing uniform round cells with a dispersed chromatin and two small nucleoli (H&E, 200×). (**B**) Same case of PNET immunostained with MIC 2 antibody, showing a typical membranous staining (MIC 2, 200×) *Abbreviations*: PNET, primitive neuroectodermic tumor; SCLC, small cell lung cancer; H&E, hematoxylin and eosin; MIC2 (CD99).

translocation (t11–22) involving EWS-Fli or EWS-Erg genes recognized by the presence of abnormal fusion chimeric transcripts at molecular analysis. They all stain with MIC2(CD99) antibody recognizing a membrane glycoprotein (Fig. 10B). They are not responsible for a real differential diagnosis problem if their primary chest wall localization is well recognized. They do not arise primarily in bronchi or lung parenchyma. However, since MIC2 is also expressed in about 40% (46–49) of SCLCs and in a variety of others tumors than PNET, a MIC2 positivity in small cell proliferation of peripheral lung or bronchi should not deserve diagnosis of PNET, inasmuch as PNET can express some NE markers.

References

1. Histological typing of lung tumours. In: International Histological Classification of Tumours. 2nd ed. Geneva, Switzerland: World Health Organization, 1981.
2. Arrigoni MG, Woolner LB, Bernatz PE. Atypical carcinoid tumors of the lung. J Thorac Cardiovasc Surg 1972; 44:413–421.
3. Travis WD, Linnoila RI, Tzokos MG, et al. Neuroendocrine tumors of the lung with proposed criterion for large cell neuroendocrine carcinoma. Am J Surg Pathol 1991; 15:529–553.
4. Gould VE, Linnoila I, Memoli VA, et al. Neuroendocrine components of the bronchopulmonary tract in hyperplasias, dysplasias and neoplasms. Lab Invest 1983; 15:519–537.
5. Travis WD, Colby TV, Corrin B, Shimosato Y. Brambilla E. In Collaboration with L.H. Sobin and Pathologists from 14 Countries. World Health Organization. International Histological Classification of Tumors. Histological Typing of Lung and Pleural Tumors. 3rd ed. New York: Springer, 1999.
6. Travis WD, Brambilla E, Muller-Hemerlink HK, Harris CC, eds. World Health Organization Classification of Tumours. Pathology and Genetics of Tumours of the Lung, Pleura, Thymus and Heart. Lyon: IARC Press, 2004.
7. McDowell EM, Wilson TS, Trump BF. Atypical endocrine tumors of the lung. Arch Pathol Lab Med 1981; 105:20–28.
8. Hammond ME, Sause WT. Large cell neuroendocrine tumors of the lung: clinical significance and histopathologic definition. Cancer 1985; 56:1624–1629.
9. Mooi WJ, Dewar A, Springall D, et al. Non small cell lung carcinomas with neuroen docrine features: a light microscopic, immunohistochemical and ultrastructural study of 11 cases. Histopathology 1988; 13:329–337.
10. McDowell DM, Sorokin SP, Hoyt RF, et al. An unusual bronchial carcinoid tumor: light and electron microscopy. Hum Pathol 1981; 12:338–348.
11. Hage E. Histochemistry and fine structure of bronchial carcinoid tumors. Virchows Arch A 1973; 361:121–128.
12. Gould VE, Wiedenmann B, Lee I, et al. Synaptophysin expression in neuroendocrine neoplasms as determined by immunocytochemistry. Am J Pathol 1987; 126:243–257.
13. Schol DJ, Mooi WJ, Vand Der Gugten AA, et al. Monoclonal antibody 123C3, identifying small cell carcinoma phenotype in lung tumours, recognizes mainly, but not exclusively, endocrine and neuron-supporting normal tissues. Int J Cancer Suppl 1988; 2:34–40.
14. Linnoila RI, Mulshine JL, Steinberg SM, et al. Neuroendocrine differentiation in endocrine and non-endocrine lung carcinomas. Am J Clin Pathol 1988; 90:641–652.
15. Brambilla E, Veale D, Moro D, et al. Neuroendocrine phenotype in lung cancers: comparison of immunohistochemistry with biochemical determination of enolase isoenzymes. Am J Clin Pathol 1992; 98:88–97.
16. Lantuejoul S, Moro D, Michalides RJ, et al. NCAM and NCAM-PSA expression in neuro-endocrine lung tumors. Am J Surg Pathol 1998; 22(10):1267–1276.

17. Gosney JR, Gosney MA, Lye M, et al. Reliability of commercially available immunocytochemical markers for identification of neuroendocrine differentiation in bronchoscopic biopsies of bronchial carcinoma. Thorax 1994; 50:116–120.
18. Lauweryns JM, Van Ranst L, Lloyd RV, et al. Chromogranin in bronchopulmonary neuroendocrine cells: immunocytochemical detection in human, monkey, and pig respiratory mucosa. J Histochem Cytochem 1987; 35:113–118.
19. Totsch M, Muller LC, Hittmair A, et al. Immunohistochemical demonstration of chromogranins A and B in neuroendocrine tumors of the lung. Hum Pathol 1992; 23:312–316.
20. Warren WH, Memoli VA, Gould VE. Immunohistochemical and ultrastructural analysis of bronchopulmonary neuroendocrine neoplasms: I. Carcinoids. Ultrastruct Pathol 1984; 6:15–27.
21. Bonato M, Cerati M, Pagani A, et al. Differential diagnosis patterns of lung neuroendocrine tumours: a clinico-pathological and immunohistochemical study of 122 cases. Virchows Arch A 1992; 420:201–211.
22. Addis BJ, Hamid Q, Ibrahim NBN, et al. Immunohistochemical markers of small cell carcinoma and related neuroendocrine tumours of the lung. J Pathol 1987; 153:137–150.
23. Yesner R. Small-cell tumors of the lung. Am J Surg Pathol 1983; 7:775–785.
24. Bolen JW, Thorning D. Histogenetic classification of lung carcinomas. Small cell carcinomas studied by light and electron microscopy. J Submicrosc Cytol 1982; 14:199–514.
25. Blobel GA, Gould VE, Moll R, et al. Coexpression of neuroendocrine markers and epithelial cytoskeletal proteins in bronchopulmonary neuroendocrine neoplasms. Lab Invest 1985; 52: 39–51.
26. Mark EJ, Quay SC, Dickerson GR. Papillary carcinoid tumor of lung. Cancer 1981; 48: 316–324.
27. Wise WS, Bonder D, Aikawa M, et al. Carcinoid tumor of lung with varied histology. Am J Surg Pathol 1982; 6:261–267.
28. Chejfec G, Capella C, Solcia E, et al. Amphicrine cells, dysplasias and neoplasias. Cancer 1985; 56:2683–2690.
29. Sturm N, Rossi G, Lantuejoul S, et al. Expression of thyroid transcription factor-1 (TTF-1) in the spectrum of neuroendocrine cell lung proliferations with special interest in carcinoids. Hum Pathol 2002; 33(2):175–182.
30. Cebelin MS. Melanocytic bronchial carcinoid tumor. Cancer 1980; 46:1843–1848.
31. D'Agati VD, Perzin KH. Carcinoid tumorlets of the lung with metastasis to a peribronchial lymph node: report of a case and review of the literature. Cancer 1985; 55:2472–2476.
32. McCaughan BC, Martini N, Bains MS. Bronchial carcinoids: review of 124 cases. J Thorac Cardiovasc Surg 1985; 89:8–17.
33. Valli M, Fabris GA, Dewar A, et al. Atypical cracinoid tumour of the lung: a study of 33 cases with prognostic features. Histopathology 1994; 24:363–369.
34. Przygodski RM, Finkelstein SD, Langer JC, et al. Analysis of p53, K-ras-2, and C-raf-1 in pulmonary neuroendocrine tumors. Am J Pathol 1996; 148:1531–1541.
35. Brambilla E, Gazzeri S, Moro D, et al. Immunohistochemical study of p53 in human lung carcinomas. Am J Pathol 1993; 143:199–210.
36. Wick MR, Berg LC, Hertz MI. Large cell carcinoma of the lung with neureoendocrine differentiation: a comparison with large cell undifferentiated pulmonary tumors. Am J Clin Pathol 1992; 97:796–805.
37. Schleusener JT, Tazelaar HD, Jung SH, et al. Neuroendocrine differentiation is an independent prognostic factor in chemotherapy treated non small cell lung carcinoma. Cancer 1996; 7: 1284–1291.
38. Sheppard MN, Thurlow NP, Dewar A. Amphicrine differentiation in bronchioloalveolar cell carcinoma. Ultrastruct Pathol 1994; 18:437–441.
39. Hirsch FR, Matthews MJ, Yesner R. Histopathologic classification of small cell carcinoma of the lung: comments based on an interobserver examination. Cancer 1982; 50:1360–1366.

40. Hirsch FR, Osterlind K, Hansen HH. The prognostic significance of histopathologic subtyping of small cell carcinoma of the lung according to the classification of the World Health Organization: a study of 375 consecutive patients. Cancer 1983; 52:2144–2150.
41. Vollmer RT, Birch R, Ogden L, et al. Subclassification of small cell cancer of the lung: the Southeastern Cancer Study Group experience. Hum Pathol 1985; 16:247–252.
42. Nicholson SA, Beasley MB, Brambilla E, et al. Small cell lung carcinoma (SCLC): a clinicopathologic study of 100 cases with surgical specimens. Am J Surg Pathol 2002, 26: 1184–1197.
43. Hirsch FR, Matthews MJ, Aisner S, et al. Histopathologic classification of small cell lung cancer: changing concepts and terminology. Cancer 1988; 62:1973–1977.
44. Brambilla E, Moro D, Gazzeri S, et al. Cytotoxic chemotherapy induces cell differentiation in small cell lung carcinoma. J Clin Oncol 1991; 9:50–61.
45. Yoneda K, Boucher LD. Bronchial epithelial changes associated with small cell carcinoma of the lung. Hum Pathol 1993; 24:1180–1188.
46. Lumadue JA, et al. MIC2 analysis of small cell carcinoma. Am J Clin Pathol 1994; 102:692–694.
47. Rossi G, Cavazza A, Marchioni A, et al. Role of the chemotherapy and the receptor tyrosine kinases KIT, PDGFRα, PDGFRβ and Met in large-cell neuroendocrine carcinoma of the lung. J Clin Oncol 2005, 23(34):8774–8785.
48. Pelosi G, Fraggetta F, Sonzogni A, et al. CD99 immunoreactivity in gastrointestinal and pulmoanry neuroendocrine tumours. Virchows Arch 2000; 437:270–274.
49. Pelosi G, Leon ME, Veronesi G, et al. Decreased immunoreactivity of CD99 is an independent predictor of regional lymph node metastases in pulmonary carcinoid tumors. J Thorac Oncol 2006, 1(5):468–477.

35
Benign Tumors of the Lung

ALBERTO M. MARCHEVSKY and RUTA GUPTA
Cedars Sinai Medical Center, Los Angeles, California, U.S.A.

I. Benign Tumors of the Lung

Benign tumors of the lung include a variety of epithelial and mesenchymal lesions that represent less than 5% of all pulmonary neoplasms. The classification of these lesions listed in the most recent World Health Organization Classifications of Tumors is shown in Table 1 (1).

II. Benign Epithelial Lesions of the Lung

A. Squamous Cell Papilloma

Squamous cell papillomas are rare benign tumors that usually result from the spread of laryngo-tracheal papillomatosis in children and young adults. They can also develop as solitary pulmonary lesions in patients of all ages, with a median age of 54 years (1–22). They are usually detected as incidental lung densities on routine imaging studies in approximately 60% of patients (3,4,6,12,18). Other patients present with cough or other symptoms secondary to airway obstruction. The role of smoking in the pathogenesis of squamous cell papillomas of the lung is unknown, although approximately half of the patients are smokers.

Squamous papillomas of the airways and the lung are frequently associated with infections by the human papilloma virus (HPV), particularly subtypes 6, 11, and 16 (1,8–10,19,22). The presence of HPV-11 DNA has been demonstrated by molecular methods in both the benign and the malignant lesions in several cases of recurrent respiratory papillomatosis progressing to squamous cell carcinoma. Although HPV-11 is uncommonly associated with the development of squamous cell carcinoma in the uterine cervix and other sites, it may be correlated with malignant transformation in the setting of juvenile-onset recurrent respiratory papillomatosis (19). Immunohistochemical studies have shown that the expression of p53, Rb, and p16 remain normal during tumor progression into malignant transformation in cases associated with HPV-11 expression (19). However, molecular studies with polymerase chain reaction (PCR) amplification and restriction fragment length polymorphism (RFLP) analysis have shown the presence of p53 mutations associated with the integration of HPV-11 in malignant lesions (8).

Table 1 Benign Tumors of the Lung

Category	Type	Subtype
Epithelial Lesions		
	Papilloma	
		Squamous cell papilloma
		Glandular papilloma
		Mixed papilloma
	Alveolar adenoma	
	Papillary adenoma	
	Adenomas of salivary gland type	
		Mucous gland adenoma
		Pleomorphic adenoma
	Mucinous cystadenoma	
Mesenchymal Tumors		
	Chondroma	
	Congenital peribronchial myofibroblastic tumor	
	Inflammatory Myofibroblastic Tumor	
Miscellaneous Tumors		
	Hamartoma	
	Sclerosing hemangioma	
	Intrapulmonary thymoma	
	Meningioma	
Clear Cell Tumor		

Gross Pathology

Squamous papillomas usually involve a large bronchus and appear as exophytic, cauliflower-like, tan-gray, soft, single or multiple lesions (23). They are usually small, although large squamous papillomas measuring up to 9 cm in diameter have been described (1). The airways distal to a papilloma can develop postobstructive pneumonia and/or bronchiectasis.

Microscopic Features

Squamous papillomas are composed of a fibrovascular core with multiple papillary fronds lined by a mature squamous epithelium with focal areas of keratinization (Fig. 1 A,B). They can present as exophytic papillomas or inverted papillary lesions.

Differential Diagnosis

Squamous papillomas need to be distinguished from inflammatory endobronchial polyps exhibiting focal squamous metaplasia of the bronchial mucosa. These lesions usually exhibit a more regular surface without papillary excrescences and are considerably more inflamed. Squamous papillomas can rarely progress to well-differentiated squamous cell carcinomas, particularly in patients with recurrent laryngo-tracheal papillomatosis (Fig. 1 C).

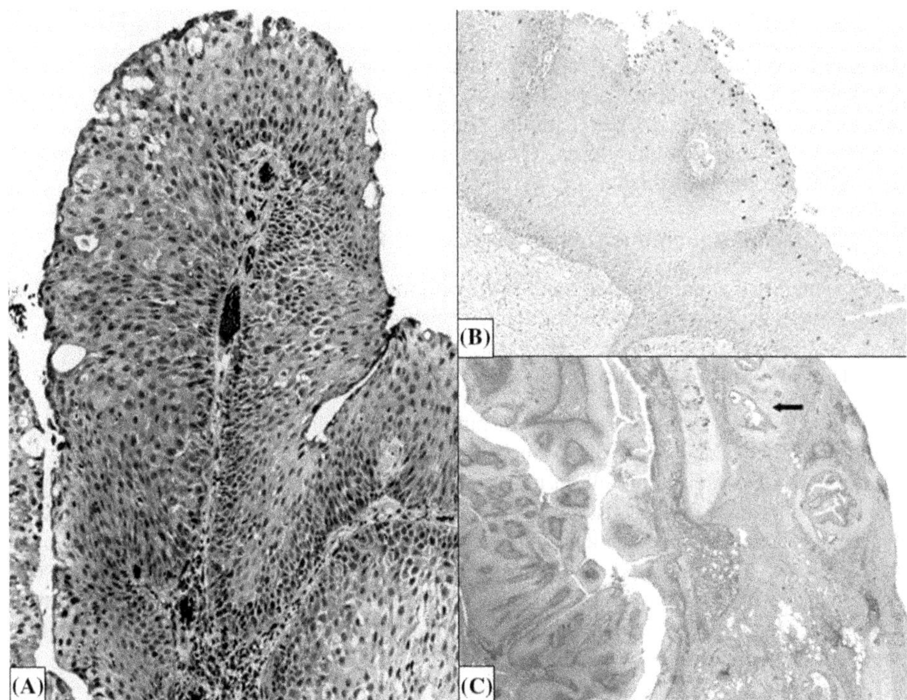

Figure 1 (**A**) Exophytic squamous papilloma composed of stratified squamous epithelium lining a fibrovascular core. The squamous epithelium shows orderly maturation from the basal cell layer to the superficial flattened and occasionally keratinized cells. (**B**) Squamous cell papilloma. In situ hybridization staining for HPV subtypes 6/11 shows nuclear reactivity in many of the nuclei. (**C**) Focally invasive well-differentiated squamous cell carcinoma can be seen arising from a squamous papilloma (*arrow*). *Abbreviation*: HPV, human papilloma virus.

The malignant lesions are usually larger, show loss of polarity of the epithelial cells, anisocytosis, increased mitotic activity above the basal layer and more extensive keratinization with parakeratosis and dyskeratosis. The presence of focal areas of invasion is helpful for the diagnosis of malignancy, but this feature can be difficult to identify in endobronchial biopsies.

Treatment and Prognosis

Solitary squamous papillomas are benign lesions that are usually cured by endoscopic excision (2,7). They can recur in approximately 20% of patients, particularly in patients with multiple papillomas or laryngo-tracheal papillomatosis. Treatment with $\alpha_2\beta$ interferon, isotretinoin and/or methotrexate has been used to slow disease progression. Benign squamous papilloma can also rarely progress into squamous cell carcinoma, lesions that are treated with lobectomy or other surgical procedures (4,19).

B. Glandular Papilloma

Glandular papillomas are very rare pulmonary lesions characterized by the presence of papillary structures composed of a fibrovascular core and an epithelial lining of ciliated columnar epithelium (1,24,25). Patients present with similar clinical findings to those described for squamous papilloma. Glandular papillomas are benign lesions that rarely recur after a complete excision.

C. Mixed Squamous Cell and Glandular Papilloma

Rare examples of endobronchial papillomas with mixed squamous and glandular epithelial lining have been described under the name transitional papilloma in the past (1,25,26).

D. Alveolar Adenoma

Alveolar adenomas are very rare benign pulmonary neoplasms of unknown histogenesis first described by Yousem and Hochholzer in 1986 (27). They are characterized by the proliferation of alveolar epithelium and septal mesenchyme (23,27–35). They have been described in patients from the fourth to eight decade of life (median age of 53 years) (1,36). They can develop in both genders, with slight female predominance. Alveolar adenomas present as a small intrapulmonary nodule visible on chest X ray and CT scan, which can develop in any of the five lobes of the lung (30,32,35). They are generally single neoplasms, and it remains controversial whether cases of presumed multiple alveolar adenomas are true examples of this entity (1).

Gross Pathology

Alveolar adenomas appear as well-demarcated, smooth, multicystic, soft, yellow-tan intrapulmonary lesions that are well circumscribed from the adjacent pulmonary parenchyma (27–30).

Microscopic Features

Alveolar adenomas present as a well-circumscribed nodule composed of multiple spaces lined by a simple low cuboidal epithelium (Fig. 2 A) (27,28,30,31). The spaces are usually filled with granular, proteinaceous eosinophilic material and are lined by epithelial cells with round to elongated nuclei and inconspicuous cytoplasm (Fig. 2 B). The stroma can vary from thin alveolar septae to wider septae showing spindle cells, a variable myxoid matrix and occasional inflammatory cells. The epithelial cells of alveolar adenomas lack any significant cytologic atypia.

Immunohistochemistry and Electron Microscopy

The epithelial cells of alveolar adenomas usually exhibit immunoreactivity for keratin, TTF-1, prosurfactant protein B, and prosurfactant protein C, consistent with pneumocyte type II differentiation (29). Immunostains for CC10, a Clara cell marker is usually negative. The stromal cells are usually positive for smooth muscle-specific actin and negative for desmin (1). The epithelial cells contain lamellar bodies, bland microvilli, and cell junctions, ultrastructural features consistent with type 2 pneumocyte differentiation (28,29).

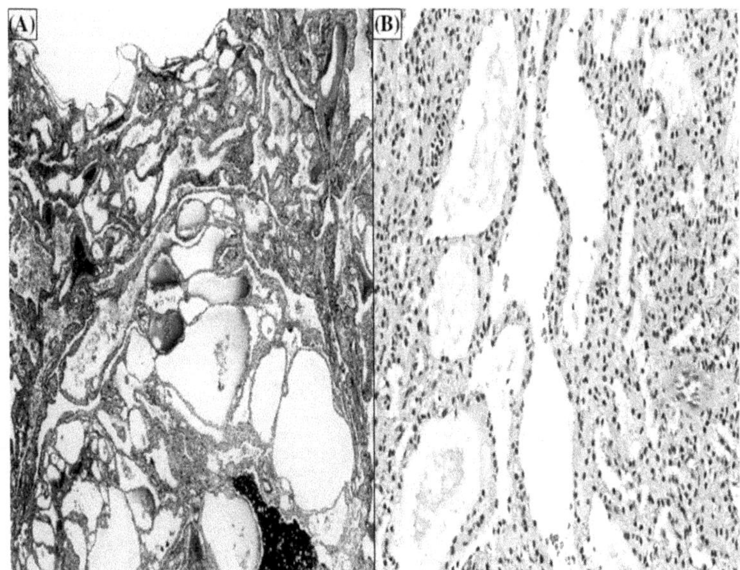

Figure 2 (**A**) Alveolar adenomas are well-circumscribed but unencapsulated lesions composed of dilated, ectatic spaces filled with granular eosinophilic material. The intervening stroma varies from thin alveolar septae to occasionally wider septae. (**B**) The alveoli like spaces are lined by cytologically bland cuboidal or flat pneumocytes.

Differential Diagnosis

Alveolar adenomas can be confused for rare intrapulmonary lymphangiomas, sclerosing hemangiomas, atypical adenomatous hyperplasia (AAH), and bronchioloalveolar carcinoma (BAC). The presence of keratin cytoplasmic immunoreactivity is helpful to distinguish alveolar adenoma from lymphangiomas and hemangiomas (29,30). The absence of stromal proliferation of epithelial cells in alveolar adenomas is helpful to distinguish these lesions from sclerosing hemangiomas (so-called pneumocytoma) (37,38). The cells of alveolar adenomas lack the presence of prominent nucleoli, intranuclear pseudoinclusions, hobnail features, and other atypical cytologic features that are usually present in BAC and AAH (1).

Treatment and Prognosis

Alveolar adenomas area benign tumors that are cured by surgical resection (27–31,35).

E. Papillary Adenoma

Papillary adenoma is a rare benign lung tumor characterized by the presence of a well-localized papillary lesion composed of cuboidal to columnar cells lining a fibrovascular stroma (1,39–42). It has been reported under various names, including bronchiolar

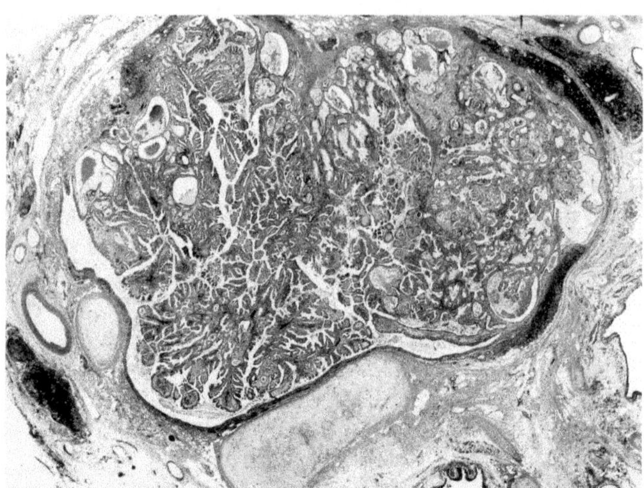

Figure 3 Intraluminal well-circumscribed glandular papilloma.

adenoma, papillary adenoma of type II pneumocytes, type II pneumocyte adenoma, and peripheral papillary pneumocytoma (40–42).

Gross Pathology

Papillary adenomas appear as intrapulmonary, well-circumscribed, occasionally encapsulated, soft to firm nodules (39–43). In contrast to glandular papillomas of the lung (Fig. 3) they do not involve an airway, although they can extend into small bronchioles microscopically.

Microscopic Features

Papillary adenomas are well-circumscribed nodules composed of papillary structures lined by cuboidal, columnar, ciliated, or oxyphilic cells. The epithelial cells lack atypia and can exhibit small nucleoli and/or eosinophilic nuclear inclusions. Intracellular mucin, mitoses, and necrosis are absent.

Immunohistochemistry and Electron Microscopy

The cells of papillary adenomas of the lung exhibit immunoreactivity to keratin, Clara cell protein, TTF-1, CEA, and surfactant apoprotein, features consistent with type II pneumocyte or Clara cell differentiation (40,42). They lack immunoreactivity for neuroendocrine markers, an important feature that help distinguish papillary adenomas from carcinoid tumors exhibiting papillary growth features. Electron microscopy shows the presence of lamellar bodies, membrane-bound electron dense deposits, and surface microvilli (39,40).

Treatment and Prognosis

Papillary adenomas are benign neoplasms that are cured by surgical resection (42). Dessy et al. (42) described the presence of pleural invasion in a papillary adenoma and suggested that these neoplasms have an undetermined malignant potential. To our knowledge, the presence of metastases or recurrences has not been reported in patients with pulmonary papillary adenomas.

III. Adenomas of the Salivary Gland Type: Mucous Gland Adenoma, Pleomorphic Adenomas, and Others

Bronchial adenomas of salivary gland type are extremely rare neoplasms composed of glandular elements that exhibit histopathologic features of bronchial gland or salivary gland differentiation (36).

A. Gross Pathology

Bronchial gland adenomas of salivary gland origin appear as usually small, well-circumscribed, polypoid endobronchial lesions (3,26,43–53). The cut surface is solid and cystic, filled with mucus in cases of mucous gland adenoma.

B. Microscopic Features

Mucous gland adenomas are composed of numerous mucin-filled cystic spaces, microacini, glands, tubules, and papillae lined by mucin-secreting cells (Fig. 4) (53). Oxyphilic and clear cells can also be present. The lesion lacks cellular atypia, mitoses, and necrosis. Pleomorphic adenomas exhibit similar features to their salivary counterparts, with an

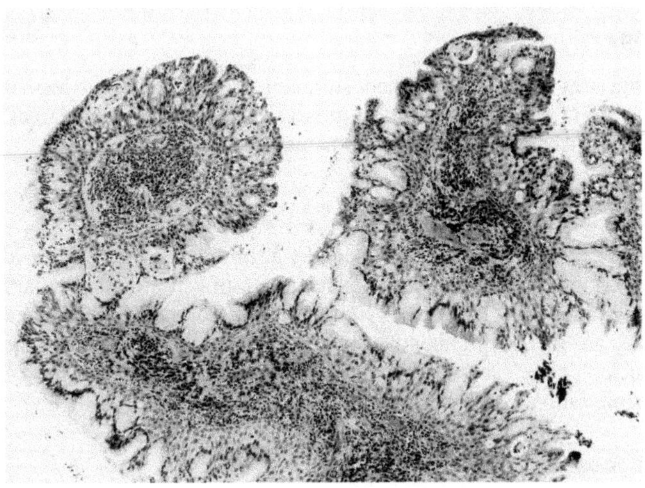

Figure 4 Mucous gland adenoma, composed of papillae lined by mucin-secreting cells. Note the basally aligned bland nuclei and abundant apical mucin.

admixture of epithelial and myoepithelial cells (54–60). The epithelial cells are arranged in cellular sheets, trabeculae, or ducts admixed with a myxoid matrix with myoepithelial cells.

C. Immunohistochemistry

Mucicarmine and D-PAS stains confirm the presence of intracytoplasmic mucin in the cells of mucous gland adenoma. The epithelial cells of both lesions exhibit cytoplasmic immunoreactivity for keratin. Myoepithelial cells can exhibit smooth muscle actin, calponin, and S100 immunoreactivity (29).

D. Differential Diagnosis

Mucous gland adenomas of the lung need to be distinguished from low-grade mucoepidermoid carcinomas. The latter exhibit, in addition to mucin-secreting cells, the presence of intermediate cells (61–63).

E. Treatment and Prognosis

Mucous gland adenomas are benign neoplasms that are cured by surgical resection (3,26,43–53). Pleomorphic adenomas are also benign neoplasms, although few examples of malignant neoplasms arising from a pleomorphic adenoma have been described (55,59).

IV. Mucinous Cystadenoma

Mucinous cystadenoma of the lung is a very rare tumor that has been described in both men and women in their sixth and seventh decades of life. The majority of reported cases have occurred in smokers.

A. Gross Pathology

Mucinous cystadenomas appear as well-circumscribed, soft, nonencapsulated cystic lesions that range in size from 1 to 5 cm (1,64). The cyst wall is grossly thick with no nodular areas. The lesion is filled with thick, viscous, yellow mucoid material.

B. Microscopic Features

The lesions are well circumscribed and usually surrounded by a fibrous wall partially lined by a single layer of columnar epithelial cells (1,36). Nuclear stratification and papillary structures are absent. The tumor cells have basal nuclei and a columnar, vacuolated cytoplasm. The cystic spaces are filled with abundant mucus. The epithelial cells lack the presence of prominent nucleoli, nuclear pseudoinclusions, significant anisocytosis, or increased nuclear: cytoplasmic ratio.

C. Differential Diagnosis

Mucinous cystadenomas need to be distinguished from BAC, mucinous type, mucinous cystadenocarcinoma of the lung, and metastatic mucin-secreting adenocarcinomas from extrapulmonary primary sites (1). The presence of an encapsulated lesion lined by a single layer of mucinous epithelium lacking cytologic atypia is helpful to distinguish mucinous cystadenomas from the malignant neoplasms. Non-neoplastic lesions that also need to be considered in the differential diagnosis include bronchogenic cysts and congenital cystic adenomatoid malformations. A detailed description of the histopathologic features of those conditions is beyond the scope of this chapter.

D. Treatment and Prognosis

Mucinous cystadenomas are benign tumors that are cured by complete surgical excision (64).

V. Congenital Peribronchial Myofibroblastic Tumor

Congenital peribronchial myofibroblastic tumor (CPBMT) is a very rare neoplasm that has been described in fewer than 20 neonates (1). It has been reported using different terms, such as congenital fibrosarcoma, congenital leiomyosarcoma, congenital bronchopulmonary leiomyosarcoma, congenital myofibroblastic tumor, congenital mesenchymal malformation of lung, and/or neonatal pulmonary hamartoma. It has been suggested that CPBMT arise from condensed mesenchyme surrounding respiratory ducts during development (65).

CPBMT are congenital tumors usually detected by prenatal ultrasounds or recognized shortly after birth (65,66). They can be associated with polyhydramnios and nonimmune hydrops fetalis during pregnancy.

A. Gross Pathology

CPBMT appear as well-circumscribed, nonencapsulated tumors with a smooth and/or multinodular surface (1). They are usually large neoplasms that can measure up to 10 cm in maximal diameter and weigh over 100 g. Their cut surface is tan-gray, yellow, and fleshy, with focal areas of hemorrhage and necrosis. They are usually present in association with a distorted or totally obliterated bronchus.

B. Microscopic Features

CPBMT appear as nodules formed by spindle cells that are arranged in intersecting fascicles (1,65). The tumor cells obliterate the pulmonary parenchyma and/or form multiple nodules interspersed with normal lung tissue, exhibit a herringbone pattern, and/or grow along septa and the pleura in a "lymphatic" distribution (Figs. 5 A,B). The tumor cells have elongated nuclei with a finely dispersed chromatin and lack cytologic features of malignancy (Figs. 5 C,D). Mitotic activity is variable, without atypical mitoses.

C. Immunohistochemistry

The tumor cells of CPBMT exhibit cytoplasmic immunoreactivity for vimentin (1). Immunoreactivity for smooth muscle actin and desmin is usually absent or present in only a small number of tumor cells. Occasionally the tumor cells can express S100 protein, CD34, CD57, CD68, CAM 5.2, factor XIIIA, and other epitopes (1).

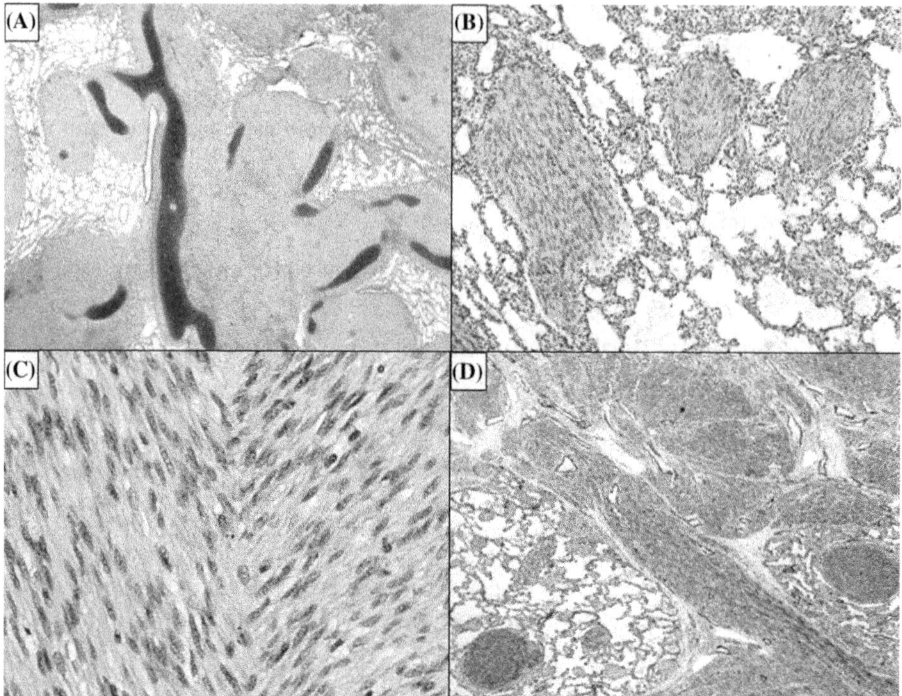

Figure 5 (**A**) Congenital peribronchial myofibroblastic tumor. The lung parenchyma is replaced by nodules of spindle cells arranged in fascicles. The peribronchial cartilage shows abnormal structural development with hypercellularity and immature chondrocytes. (**B**) Interstitial growth of the nodules of CPMT along the septae, reminiscent of "lymphatic" distribution. (**C**) The spindle cells of CPMT are arranged in intersecting fascicles with herringbone pattern. The nuclei are elongated with finely dispersed chromatin. Pleomorphism or anaplasia are absent. (**D**) The tumor cells of CPMT are uniformly immunoreactive for vimentin. *Abbreviation*: CPMT, Congenital peribronchial myofibroblastic tumor.

D. Electron Microscopy

The tumor cells of CPBMT exhibit myofibroblastic differentiation under electron microscopy.

E. Treatment and Prognosis

CPBMT are benign neoplasms that are cured by lobectomy.

VI. Inflammatory Myofibroblastic Tumor

Inflammatory myofibroblastic tumor (IMFT) is a variant of "inflammatory pseudotumors" of the lung, which has been described under various names, including inflammatory pseudotumor, plasma cell granuloma, fibroxanthoma, fibrous histiocytoma, pseudosarcomatous myofibroblastic tumor, and invasive fibrous tumor of the tracheobronchial tree (67–89). It is composed of myofibroblastic cells admixed with variable amounts of collagen and inflammatory cells (1). IMFT occurs in patients of both sexes and in all age groups, with a prevalence for individuals younger than 40 years (74,78,80). It is the most common endobronchial mesenchymal tumor of children (74,76).

In adults, IMFT usually arises as a peripheral lung nodule. Patients can be asymptomatic or present with paraneoplastic problems such as anemia, fever, weight loss, hyperglobulinemia, leukothrombocytosis, and elevated erythrocyte sedimentation rates (74). Rare patients with superior vena syndrome secondary to mediastinal involvement by IMFT have been described (80).

It has been controversial whether IMFT are inflammatory lesions or low-grade mesenchymal neoplasms (67,68,75). Some cases have been associated with viral infections such as HHV-8 (1). In contrast, the description of IMFT that develop recurrences and/or rare metastases favors the concept of a neoplasm of low malignant potential, akin to other "borderline" tumors (80,88,89).

A. Gross Pathology

IMFT appear as solitary, usually well-circumscribed lung masses that can be lobulated or globoid in appearance and develop in the peripheral lung in an endobronchial location (74). Grossly they are well-circumscribed, rubbery, yellow-gray masses that usually measure less than 5 cm in greatest dimension, although they can range in size from 1 to 36 cm (1). The lesions tend to have ill-circumscribed infiltrating margins and can extend into hilar soft tissues or the chest wall in approximately 5% to 10% of cases (80,89). Rare lesions exhibit calcifications and/or cystic degeneration.

B. Microscopic Features

IMFT are composed of spindle cells arranged in fascicles, with or without a storiform architecture that may permeate the adjacent lung parenchyma in an infiltrating pattern that can be unexpected in light of their gross circumscription (Figs. 6 A,B) (68,74,77,81,85). The spindle cells exhibit oval nuclei with fine chromatin, inconspicuous nucleoli, and slightly eosinophilic cytoplasm (Figs. 6 C,D). The spindle cells can rarely infiltrate the blood vessels. Mitoses are infrequent. Cytologic atypia is usually absent. Touton-like giant cells, foamy histiocytes, and lympho-plasmacytic cells are frequently present admixed with the tumor cells (Figs. 7 A–D). Variable amounts of collagen bands are present. Some lesions exhibit a prominent number of plasma cells, often associated with lymphoid follicles; these lesions have been reported as "plasma cell granuloma" of the lung.

C. Immunohistochemistry and Molecular Changes

The spindle cells of IMFT are usually immunoreactive to vimentin, muscle-specific actin, and calponin and exhibit negative immunoreactivity to CD34, keratin, and desmin (74). Cytoplasmic immunoreactivity for anaplastic lymphoma kinase-1 (ALK-1) has been reported in 56% of IFMT (74). Coffin et al. have recently reported that patients with metastatic IMFT are negative for ALK-1 (74).

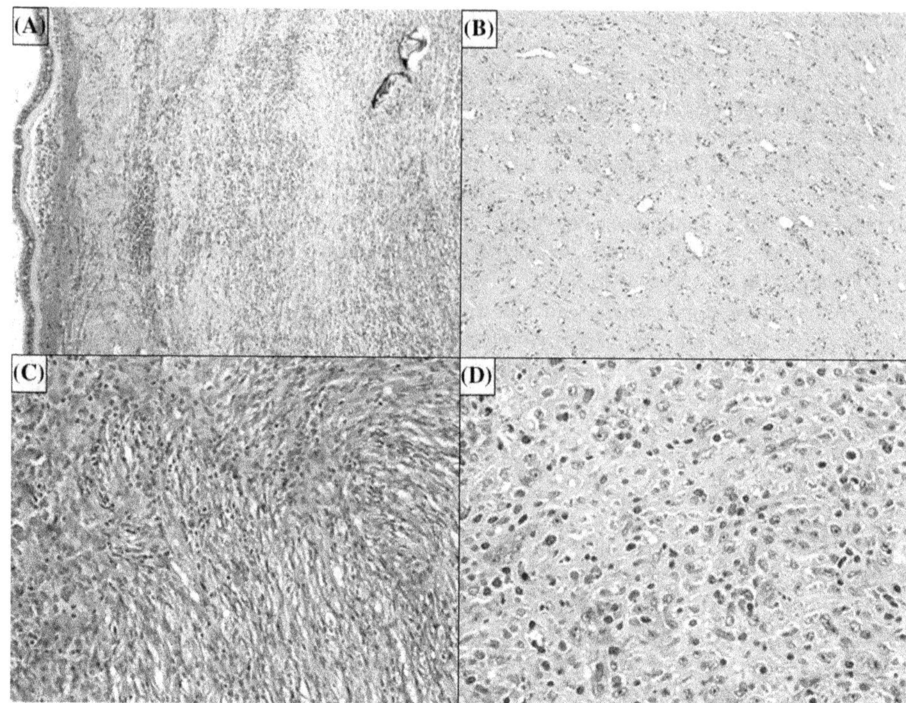

Figure 6 (**A**) Submucosal inflammatory myofibroblastic tumor. Abundant inflammatory cells consisting predominantly of plasma cells are admixed with fascicles of spindle cells and collagen. Foci of dystrophic calcification are also noted. (**B**) IMFT may often show sclerotic, hypocellular areas with dense collagen. (**C**) IMFT is composed of spindle cells arranged in fascicles and storiform pattern. The spindle cells have abundant bipolar cytoplasm, oval nuclei, with fine chromatin and without nucleoli. Foamy macrophages are also present. (**D**) The spindle cells of IMFT have oval nuclei, fine chromatin, inconspicuous nucleoli and eosinophilic bipolar cytoplasm. *Abbreviation*: IMFT, inflammatory myofibroblastic tumor.

Approximately one-third have a translocation between chromosome 2 and 5 and an NPM-ALK gene fusion t(2;5) (p23: q35) (74). The remainder have various molecular changes such as ALK gene rearrangement following translocation (2;11;2)(p23;p15;q31), TPM3-ALK gene fusion, fusion of ALK to the Ran-binding protein 2 (RANBP2) gene, fusion of the SEC31L1 and ALK gene, rearrangement of the HMGIC gene, and others (67–69,71,72,83).

D. Electron Microscopy

The spindle cells of IMFT exhibit the presence of plasmalemmal dense patches, pinocytotic vesicles, cytoplasmic bundles of thin actin-like filaments, and pericellular basal lamina (1).

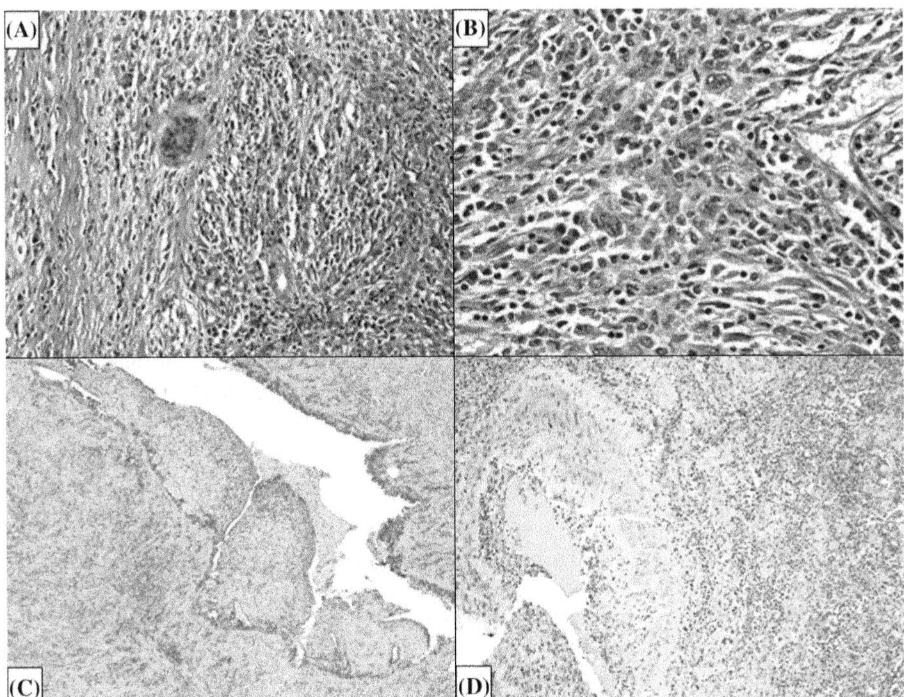

Figure 7 (**A**) Touton like giant cells in IMFT against a background of histiocytes and plasma cells. (**B**) Multinucleate bizarre-looking cells admixed with eosinophils and plasma cells against a background of spindle cells arranged in fascicles. (**C**) Involvement of a bronchiole by IMT. Surface scalloping is noted. (**D**) Invasion of a medium-sized artery by IMT. This is one of the poor prognostic factors in IMT. This case also showed areas of necrosis.

E. Differential Diagnosis

IMFT need to be distinguished from organizing pneumonia and from carcinomas or other neoplasms exhibiting marked inflammation. The presence of a marked spindle cell proliferation, with some atypia and occasional vascular or bronchiolar invasion is helpful to distinguish IMFT from organizing pneumonia with fibrosis. Immunostain for ALK-1 can be helpful to confirm the diagnosis of IMFT. Careful observation to exclude the presence of cytologically malignant cells allows for the distinction between IMFT and neoplasms with severe inflammation. Ritter et al. have reviewed the pathologic features of malignancies with extensive fibroblastic proliferation and inflammation simulating an IMFT (90).

F. Treatment and Prognosis

Patients with IMFT usually have excellent survival with surgical excision (80,88,89). A small proportion of patients ($\sim$5%) can develop extrapulmonary invasion, local recurrence, and/or metastasis (1). Features that have been associated with a more aggressive clinical behavior include incomplete excision, focal invasion, vascular invasion, foci of increased cellularity, nuclear pleomorphism with bizarre giant cells, necrosis, and a mitotic rate greater than three mitoses in 50 HPF (High-power-field) (1,74,85,86).

VII. Hamartoma

Hamartomas of the lung are benign neoplasms composed of mesenchymal tissues such as cartilage, fat, fibrous tissue, and smooth muscle combined with entrapped respiratory epithelium (66,91–128). They have been reported under various names, including benign mesenchymoma, hamartochondroma, chondromatous hamartoma, adenochondroma, and/or fibroadenoma (1).

They are relatively frequent lesions and are more common in male patients (107,108,115). They are usually diagnosed in adult patients with a peak incidence in the sixth decade and are rare in children. The latter finding probably supports the concept that these lesions are not true malformations or hamartomas but benign mesenchymal neoplasms.

A. Gross Pathology

Pulmonary hamartomas are usually peripheral lesions measuring up to 4 cm in diameter, although rare giant lesions have been described (104). Approximately 10% of the lesions arise endobronchially, and are difficult to distinguish from pulmonary chondromas (112,121,129). They appear as multilobulated, firm, white to gray lesions that easily "shell out" from the surrounding parenchyma. The cut surface appears glistening and may contain focal speckled calcification. Endobronchial lesions tend to appear as broad-based polypoid, soft or firm, and tend to be composed of cartilage and fibroadipose tissue.

B. Microscopic Features

Hamartomas appear as well-circumscribed, lobulated masses composed of mature cartilage and variable amounts of adipose tissue, smooth muscle, fibrovascular tissue, and/or bone (Figs. 8 A,B) (92,93,98,102,103,106–108). These mesenchymal elements are frequently associated with entrapped slit-like spaces lined by respiratory-type epithelium. The epithelial cells can undergo metaplasia, papillary proliferation, or rarely, proliferative changes of placental transmogrification of the lung similar to those usually seen in patients with severe emphysema (1). Lesions with prominent smooth muscle, fibrous tissue, or adipose tissue have reported as leiomyomatous, fibroleiomyomatous, or fibrolipomatous hamartomas (102,103). Endobronchial hamartomas are usually composed of cartilage and fibroadipose tissue and may lack the presence of epithelial inclusions.

C. Genetic and Molecular Studies

Pulmonary hamartomas have frequent mutations of high mobility group (HMG) proteins in the regions 6p21 and 12q14-15 (1,91). These chromatin-associated proteins are important in regulating chromatin architecture and gene expression. The presence of these genetic mutations favors the concept that the term hamartoma is probably a misnomer and that these lesions represent benign mesenchymal neoplasms.

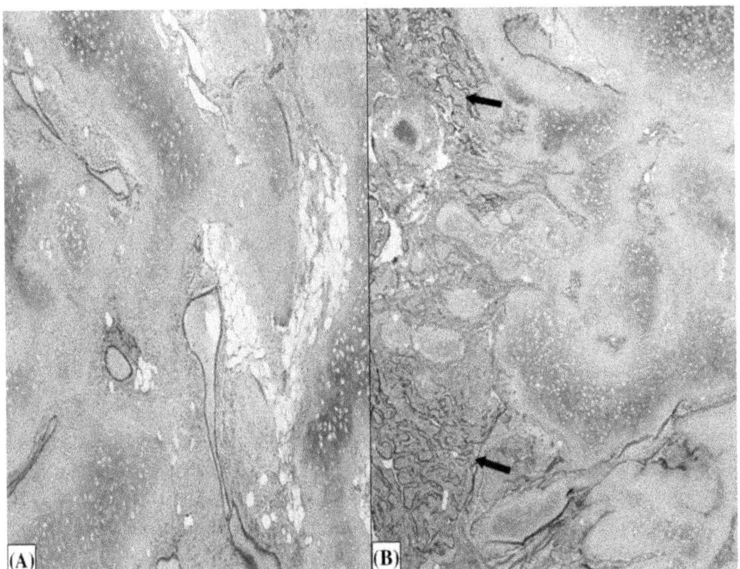

Figure 8 (**A**) Hamartoma composed predominantly of lobulated mass of mature cartilage, with interspersed mature adipose tissue. Clefts lined by respiratory type epithelium extend between the lobules of mesenchymal elements. (**B**) The epithelial cells at the periphery of a hamartoma have undergone papillary proliferation; these may also rarely undergo metaplasia (*arrow*).

D. Differential Diagnosis

Pulmonary hamartomas rarely pose a differential diagnosis problem. They need to be distinguished from bronchopulmonary chondromas and pleuro-pulmonary blastomas. Chondromas are endobronchial lesions composed only of mature cartilage. Pleuro-pulmonary blastomas usually develop in children, an age group where hamartomas are infrequent and are composed of immature mesenchymal tissues (1,66).

E. Treatment and Prognosis

Hamartomas are usually resected by enucleation of wedge resection, though rare examples of recurrence or sarcomatous transformation have been described (1,114).

VIII. Sclerosing Hemangioma

Sclerosing hemangioma of the lung is a benign or very low-grade malignant pulmonary lesion first reported by Liebow and Hubbell in 1956 (130,131). It has also been reported under various names such as pneumocytoma or papillary pneumocytoma (37,38,132–151). The designation of “hemangiomas” is probably incorrect, as these lesions are composed of epithelial cells (40,41,152–157). They affect predominantly middle-aged adults, and approximately 80% of the cases have been reported in women (1). Approximately 1% of sclerosing hemangiomas involve peribronchial lymph nodes (143). Various cellular origins have been proposed for sclerosing hemangiomas, including vascular, mesothelial, mesenchymal, epithelial, and/or neuroendocrine differentiation. The immunophenotype of the lesion suggests an origin from an undifferentiated, primitive respiratory epithelium.

A. Gross Pathology

Sclerosing hemangiomas usually present as well-circumscribed, solid, gray to tan-yellow peripheral lung nodules ranging in size from 0.3 to 8.0 cm (1). Several patients with multiple sclerosing hemangiomas have been described (137,138). The lesions can be rarely cystic, simulating an hydatid cyst (140).

B. Microscopic Features

Sclerosing hemangiomas present as solid, well-circumscribed but not encapsulated lesions composed of round stromal cells and surface cells arranged in a variety of growth patterns, including papillary, solid, sclerotic, and hemorrhagic cellular arrangements (Figs. 9 A,B) (37,134,147,156). Lesions with a hemorrhagic pattern exhibit large spaces lined by epithelial cells and filled with red blood cells. The tumor cells have round nuclei, with finely distributed chromatin, inconspicuous nucleoli, and occasional pseudoinclusions (Figs. 9 C,D). The cytoplasm is usually amphophilic, with indistinct cellular borders, although cells with clear, vacuolated, or foamy cytoplasm can also be present. Focal multinucleated cells can be present. Nuclear atypia is usually absent. Mitoses are infrequent, usually less than one mitosis per 10 HPF. The stroma may contain hemosiderin-laden histiocytes, foamy macrophages, cholesterol clefts, focal calcifications, and focal cholesterol granulomas.

C. Immunohistochemistry

The neoplastic cells of sclerosing hemangiomas exhibit nuclear immunoreactivity for TTF-1, cytoplasmic immunoreactivity for epithelial membrane antigen (EMA), surfactant protein A, and pancytokeratin (37,38,134,150). Immunostains for vascular markers (CD31, CD34) are negative.

D. Differential Diagnosis

Sclerosing hemangiomas need to be distinguished from metastatic renal cell carcinomas and clear cell tumors of the lung, carcinoid tumors, and papillary adenocarcinomas (1). The absence of cytologic atypia and mitoses in the presence of a dual population of round cells and surface cells are helpful for the diagnosis.

E. Treatment and Prognosis

Sclerosing hemangiomas are most often benign lesions that are cured by a resection (138,145,152,156). However, as some cases have presented with pulmonary, hilar, and/or mediastinal lymph node involvement, the concept of very low malignant potential has been proposed (143,144,147). To our knowledge, there are no reports of patients with metastatic sclerosing hemangiomas of the lung.

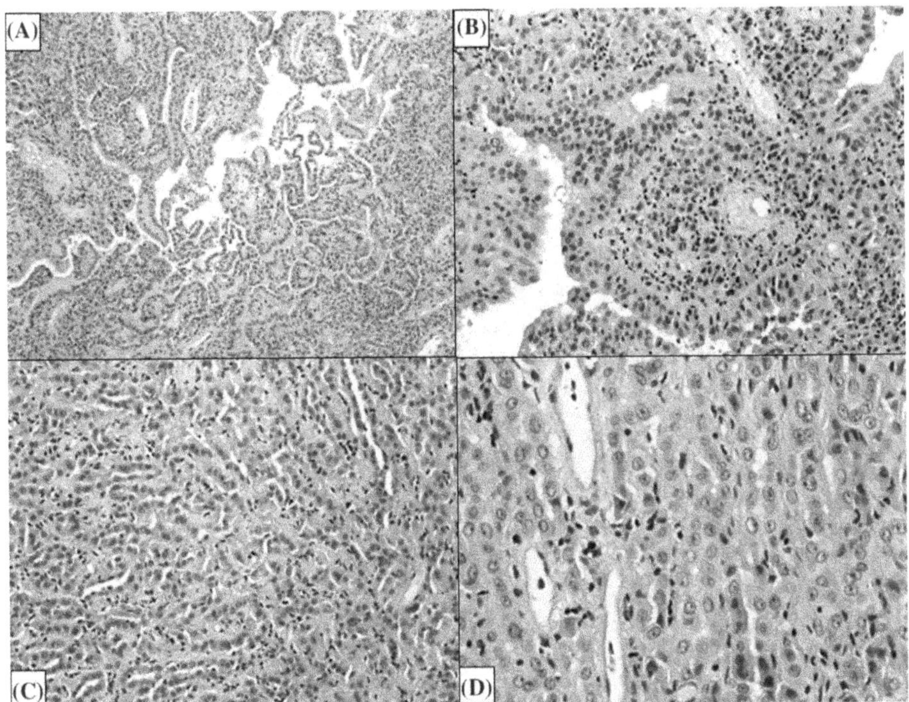

Figure 9 (**A**) Sclerosing hemangioma with solid and papillary patterns and occasional foci of sclerosis. (**B**) Complex papillae of sclerosing hemangioma lined by cuboidal surface cells. The cells resemble bronchiolar epithelium and activated type II pneumocytes. These can occasionally show nuclear atypia and multinucleation. Few round cells with centrally located round to oval bland nuclei can be noted within the stalk. (**C**) Solid pattern of sclerosing hemangioma, the round cells with distinct cell borders, and centrally located round to oval nuclei are dispersed against a sclerotic background. The cuboidal surface cells are forming tubules. (**D**) The cells of sclerosing hemangioma have an epithelioid appearance.

IX. Intrapulmonary Thymoma

Primary thymomas of the lung are very unusual neoplasms that have identical histopathologic features to mediastinal thymomas (158–166). They have been described in patients of both sexes of ages ranging from 17 to 77 years, with a median age of 50 years; there is a slight predominance in female patients (1). Primary thymomas of the lung are thought to arise from ectopic thymic rests within pulmonary tissues.

Patients with intrapulmonary thymomas rarely exhibit findings of myasthenia gravis and usually develop nonspecific findings such as cough, weight loss, chest pain, fever, and/or dyspnea or are discovered incidentally on imaging studies of the chest (158–166). Ryman described an unusual patient with primary pulmonary thymoma and Good syndrome (158).

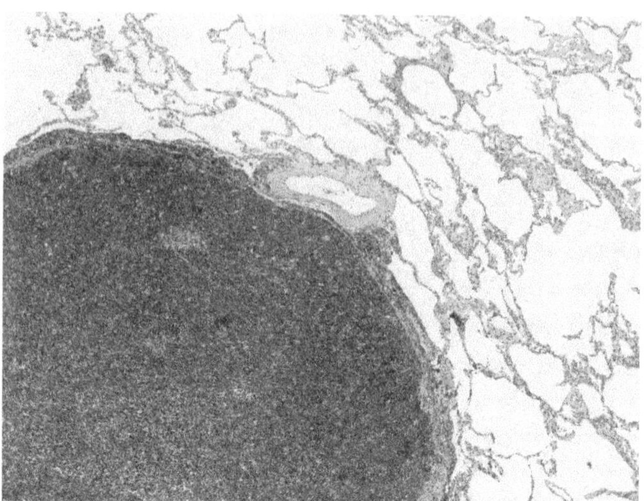

Figure 10 Well-circumscribed intrapulmonary thymoma. The tumor resembles the predominantly cortical lymphocyte rich type B1 thymoma known to occur in the thymus.

A. Gross Pathology

Intrapulmonary thymomas appear as well-circumscribed nodules ranging in size from 0.5 to 12.0 cm (164). The cut surface is characteristically lobulated. They may exhibit focal cystic changes and/or calcification.

B. Microscopic Features

Intrapulmonary thymomas are composed of lobules of epithelial cells admixed with variable amounts of mature lymphocytes (Fig. 10) (164). The tumor lobules are surrounded by fibrous septae. The tumor cells can be round or spindled with variable amounts of lymphocytes (Fig. 11). A rare case of primary pulmonary thymoma presenting with extensive granulomatous reaction has been reported by Srivastava et al. (163).

C. Immunohistochemistry

The neoplastic epithelial cells of intrapulmonary thymomas usually exhibit cytoplasmic immunoreactivity for keratin and EMA and can exhibit immunoreactivity for CD5 (164). The lymphocytes of the lesion usually exhibit immunoreactivity for various T cell markers, according to the cell type.

D. Differential Diagnosis

Intrapulmonary thymomas need to be distinguished from carcinomas of the lung, spindle cell carcinoid tumors, small cell carcinoma, and lymphomas (1,167). The characteristic septation of thymomas, lack of cytologic atypia, and presence of a biphasic population of

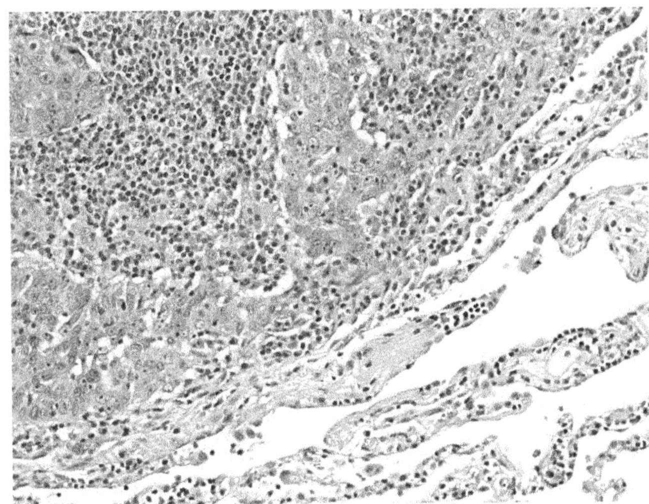

Figure 11 Well-circumscribed intrapulmonary thymoma resembling type B3 thymoma of the thymus with its solid epidermoid appearing epithelial nests separated by lymphocytes.

neoplastic epithelial cells and mature lymphocytes are usually helpful in the differential diagnosis.

E. Treatment and Prognosis

Intrapulmonary thymomas are treated with surgical excision (158–166). As their mediastinal counterparts, they are currently regarded as low-grade malignant neoplasms that can recur and/or metastasize, usually many years after initial therapy. Primary thymomas of the lung are too unusual to determine whether the World Health Organization classification proposed for mediastinal thymomas has a prognostic role (1).

X. Intrapulmonary Meningiomas

Primary intrapulmonary meningiomas are unusual lesions that have identical histopathologic features to those of central nervous system meningiomas (167–172). They have been described in middle age patients, usually detected as solitary pulmonary nodules on routine chest X rays. They are thought to develop from heterotopic embryonal nests of arachnoid cells or from pluripotential cells of the subpleural mesenchyme (1).

A. Gross Pathology

Intrapulmonary meningiomas appear as well-circumscribed soft, white lesions ranging in size from 1.5 to 4.0 cm in greatest dimension (1).

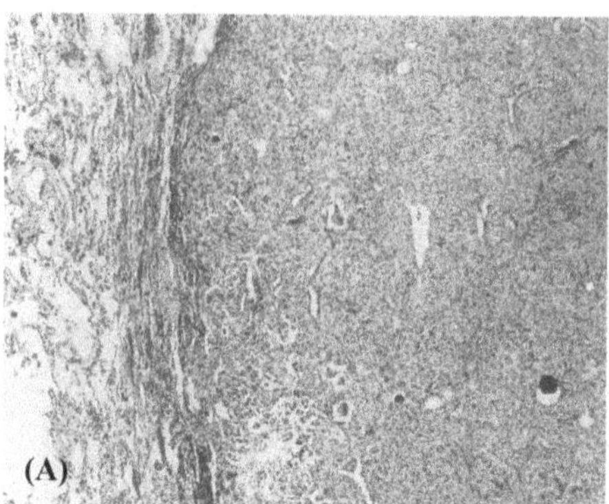

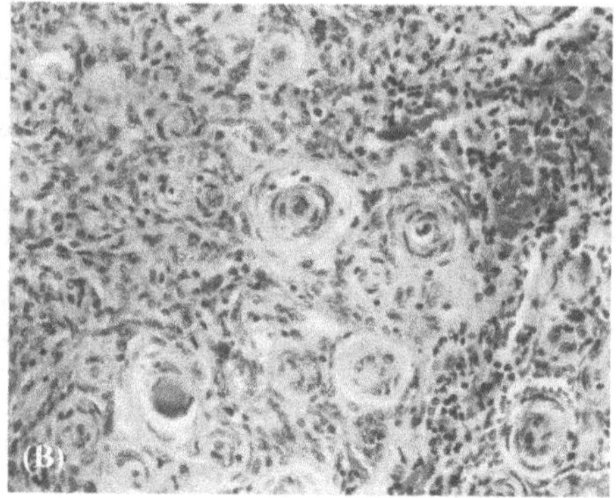

Figure 12 (**A**) Primary meningioma of the lung usually presenting as small, well-circumscribed tumors. Psammoma bodies are readily seen at low magnification. (**B**) Pulmonary meningiomas are composed of spindle cells in whorls and swirls with occasional psammoma bodies. Transitional types of meningiomas are more frequent in the lung. *Source*: Courtesy of Dr. Samuel A. Yousem.

B. Microscopic Features

Intrapulmonary meningiomas are composed of spindle cells arranged in the characteristic growth patterns of central nervous system lesions, primarily transitional and fibrous cells (Figs. 12 A,B). The tumor cells have round, oval, or spindle cell nuclei and are arranged in focal fascicles and cellular whorls. Psammoma bodies can be present.

C. Immunohistochemistry

The tumor cells of meningiomas exhibit cytoplasmic immunoreactivity for EMA and vimentin (1). Immunostains for keratin, desmin, S100 protein, and SMA are usually negative.

D. Electron Microscopy

The cells of meningiomas exhibit ultrastructurally numerous interdigitating cell processes that are attached by prominent desmosomes and skeins of well-developed tonofilaments that insert into the attachment complexes (1,168–172).

E. Differential Diagnosis

Intrapulmonary meningiomas need to be distinguished from the much more frequent meningothelial-like nodules, solitary fibrous tumor, spindle cell carcinoid, and other spindle cell tumors involving the lungs. To our knowledge, there is no convention regarding the acceptable largest size of a meningothelial-like nodule. The diagnosis of small meningothelial lesions is left to the judgment of individual pathologists. Solitary fibrous tumors are composed of spindle cells arranged in a patternless growth arrangement with more abundant collagenous bands. The tumor cells exhibit a different immunophenotype than meningiomas, with immunoreactivity for CD34 and Bcl-2 (1).

F. Treatment and Prognosis

Intrapulmonary meningiomas are benign lesions cured by surgical excision (167). To our knowledge, no examples of recurrent or metastatic primary pulmonary meningiomas have been described.

XI. Clear Cell Tumor (Sugar Tumor)

Clear cell tumors ("sugar cell") of the lung (STL) are low-malignant potential neoplasms composed of clear or eosinophilic cytoplasm (173–191). They are currently thought to be derived from perivascular epithelioid cells (PEC) and have also been described as PEComas or myomelanocytomas (1,184). They are extremely rare neoplasms that occur in patients of all ages, ranging from 8 to 73 years. They occur in patients of both sexes, with a slight female predominance. STL has been reported in patients with tuberous sclerosis and lymphangiomyomatosis (189).

A. Gross Pathology

STL usually appear as well-circumscribed, soft, red-tan, peripheral solitary nodules usually ranging in size from 1.0 mm to 6.5 cm (183). They can also appear in tracheal, bronchial, or extrapulmonary locations (181,190,192).

B. Microscopic Features

STL appear as well-circumscribed, frequently hemorrhagic tumors that can contain dilated ectatic vessels (Fig. 13 A). The cells of STL of the lung have round or oval nuclei with granular chromatin, frequent cytoplasmic invaginations with pseudoinclusions, and indistinct nucleoli (Fig. 13 B) (179,183,185,186). The cytoplasm is abundant, clear, and/or eosinophilic. The tumor cells are arranged in an organoid pattern with broad trabeculae and rounded cellular nests separated by variable amount of stroma or in solid sheets. Necrosis and mitoses are infrequent. Rare clear cell tumors with marked cytologic atypia simulating a malignancy have been recently reported (186). The stroma of clear cell tumors can exhibit sclerotic blood vessels in some cases.

C. Histochemistry, Immunohistochemistry, and Genetic Studies

Periodic acid-Schiff (PAS), with and without diastase, shows the presence of abundant intracytoplasmic glycogen in clear cell tumors (173–179). The neoplastic cells also exhibit cytoplasmic immunoreactivity for HMB-45 and may exhibit immunoreactivity for CD1a, vimentin, CD117, smooth muscle actin, neuron-specific enolase, and S100 protein (180,183,185,189). Genetic studies show the loss of heterozygosity (LOH) in the TSC2 region of chromosome 16p13 in STL of the lung in patients with tuberous sclerosis, lymphangioleiomyomatosis, and multifocal micronodular pneumocyte hyperplasia (193,194).

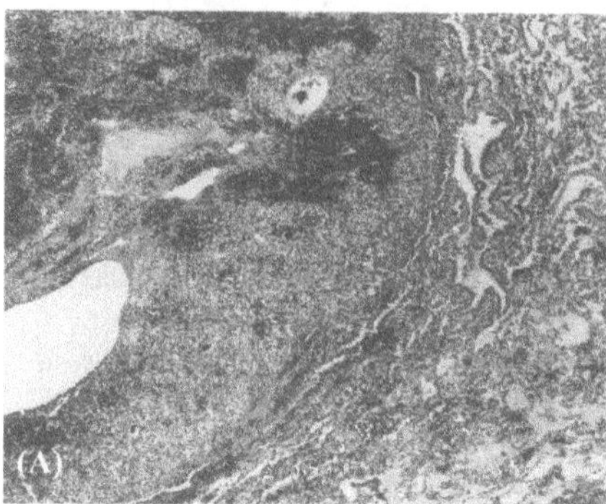

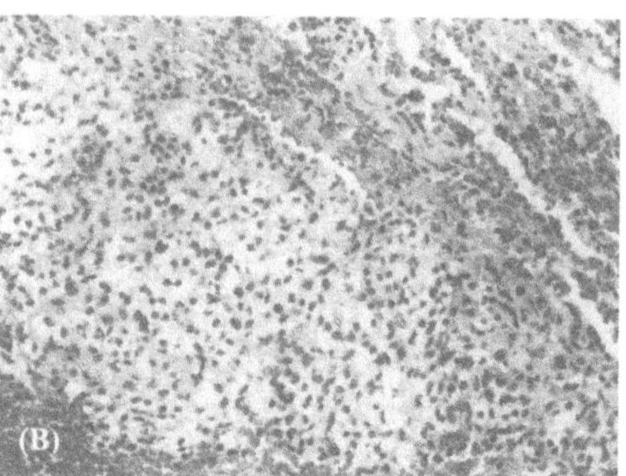

Figure 13 (**A**) Clear cell tumors of the lung are well-circumscribed, frequently hemorrhagic tumors and contain dilated ectatic vessels. (**B**) Clear cell tumors are composed of cytologically bland cells with clear cytoplasm, which are rich in glycogen. Occasional cells have intranuclear inclusions, suggesting type II alveolar pneumocyte differentiation. *Source*: Courtesy of Dr. Samuel A. Yousem.

D. Electron Microscopy

Electron microscopy confirms the presence of abundant free and membrane-bound glycogen and can show premelanosomes, interdigitating cellular processes, pericellular basal lamina, primitive intercellular attachment complexes, and plasmalemmal pinocytosis (185).

E. Differential Diagnosis

STL needs to be distinguished from metastatic clear cell carcinomas (e.g., renal, ovary, other origin), melanomas, and primary carcinomas of the lung with prominent clear cell component. The absence of cytologic atypia, mitoses and necrosis and the immunophenotype of the lesion, aid in the differential diagnosis from carcinomas. Melanomas exhibit nuclear atypia, necrosis, and/or increased mitotic atypia, features that are absent in STL.

F. Treatment and Prognosis

STL are usually cured by excision (183,188,191). However, a few patients with metastatic STL have been reported, indicating the low malignant potential of these lesions (183). Gaffey et al. have suggested that tumor larger than 2 cm and exhibiting focal necrosis should be regarded as potentially malignant neoplasms (183).

References

1. World Health Organization Classification of Tumors. Tumors of the Lung, Pleura, Thymus and Heart. Lyon: IARC Press, 2004.
2. Kozower BD, Javiden-Nejad C, Lewis JS, et al. Clinical-pathologic conference in general thoracic surgery: malignant transformation of recurrent respiratory papillomatosis. J Thorac Cardiovasc Surg 2005; 130:1190–1193.

3. Brightman I, Morgan JA, von ZD, et al. Cytological appearances of a solitary squamous cell papilloma with associated mucous gland adenoma in the lung. Cytopathology 1992; 3:253–257.
4. Silver RD, Rimell FL, Adams GL, et al. Diagnosis and management of pulmonary metastasis from recurrent respiratory papillomatosis. Otolaryngol Head Neck Surg 2003; 129:622–629.
5. Katial RK, Ranlett R, Whitlock WL, et al. Human papilloma virus associated with solitary squamous papilloma complicated by bronchiectasis and bronchial stenosis. Chest 1994; 106:1887–1889.
6. Glikman D, Baroody FM, Glikman D, et al. Images in clinical medicine. Recurrent respiratory papillomatosis with lung involvement. N Engl J Med 2005; 352:E22.
7. Gerein V, Rastorguev E, Gerein J, et al. Incidence, age at onset, and potential reasons of malignant transformation in recurrent respiratory papillomatosis patients: 20 years experience. Otolaryngol Head Neck Surg 2005; 132:392–394.
8. Rady PL, Schnadig VJ, Weiss RL, et al. Malignant transformation of recurrent respiratory papillomatosis associated with integrated human papillomavirus type 11 DNA and mutation of p53. Laryngoscope 1998; 108:735–740.
9. Xu H, Lu DW, El-Mofty SK, et al. Metachronous squamous cell carcinomas evolving from independent oropharyngeal and pulmonary squamous papillomas: association with human papillomavirus 11 and lack of aberrant p53, Rb, and p16 protein expression. Hum Pathol 2004; 35:1419–1422.
10. Lele SM, Pou AM, Ventura K, et al. Molecular events in the progression of recurrent respiratory papillomatosis to carcinoma. Arch Pathol Lab Med 2002; 126:1184–1188.
11. Veale A, Jurisevic C, Pieterse S, et al. 'Papillomatization' and 'malignant transformation' of an abscess cavity in a 25-year old man with recurrent respiratory papillomatosis who may have had Lemierre syndrome. Chron Respir Dis 2004; 1:229–231.
12. Abe K, Tanaka Y, Takahashi M, et al. Pulmonary spread of laryngeal papillomatosis: radiological findings. Radiat Med 2006; 24:297–301.
13. Yantsos VA, Farr GH Jr., McFadden PM, et al. Recurrent juvenile-onset laryngotracheal papillomatosis with transformation to squamous cell carcinoma of the lung. South Med J 1999; 92:1013–1016.
14. Bhat SP, Sundaram P, Kamble RT, et al. Recurrent respiratory papillomatosis. Indian J Chest Dis Allied Sci 2000; 42:35–37.
15. Derkay CS, Rimell FL, Thompson JW, et al. Recurrent respiratory papillomatosis. Head Neck 1998; 20:418–424.
16. Orphanidou D, Dimakou K, Latsi P, et al. Recurrent respiratory papillomatosis with malignant transformation in a young adult. Respir Med 1996; 90:53–55.
17. Katz SL, Das P, Ngan BY, et al. Remote intrapulmonary spread of recurrent respiratory papillomatosis with malignant transformation. Pediatr Pulmonol 2005; 39:185–188.
18. Harada H, Miura K, Tsutsui Y, et al. Solitary squamous cell papilloma of the lung in a 40-year-old woman with recurrent laryngeal papillomatosis. Pathol Int 2000; 50:431–439.
19. Cook JR, Hill DA, Humphrey PA, et al. Squamous cell carcinoma arising in recurrent respiratory papillomatosis with pulmonary involvement: emerging common pattern of clinical features and human papillomavirus serotype association. Mod Pathol 2000; 13:914–918.
20. Armbruster C, Kreuzer A, Vorbach H, et al. Successful treatment of severe respiratory papillomatosis with intravenous cidofovir and interferon alpha-2b. Eur Respir J 2001; 17:830–831.
21. Sakopoulos A, Kesler KA, Weisberger EC, et al. Surgical management of pulmonary carcinoma secondary to recurrent respiratory papillomatosis. Ann Thorac Surg 1995; 60:1806–1807.
22. Auborn KJ. Therapy for recurrent respiratory papillomatosis. Antivir Ther 2002; 7:1–9.
23. Marchevsky AM, Changsri C, Gupta I, et al. Frozen section diagnoses of small pulmonary nodules: accuracy and clinical implications. Ann Thorac Surg 2004; 78:1755–1759.
24. Basheda S, Gephardt GN, Stoller JK. Columnar papilloma of the bronchus. Case report and literature review. Am Rev Respir Dis 1991; 144:1400–1402.

25. Flieder DB, Koss MN, Nicholson A, et al. Solitary pulmonary papillomas in adults: a clinicopathologic and in situ hybridization study of 14 cases combined with 27 cases in the literature. Am J Surg Pathol 1998; 22:1328–1342.
26. Spencer H. Bronchial mucous gland tumours. Virchows Arch A Pathol Anat Histol 1979; 383:101–115.
27. Yousem SA, Hochholzer L, Yousem SA, et al. Alveolar adenoma. Hum Pathol 1986; 17:1066–1071.
28. Hartman MS, Epstein DM, Geyer SJ, et al. Alveolar adenoma. Ann Thorac Surg 2004; 78:1842–1843.
29. Burke LM, Rush WI, Khoor A, et al. Alveolar adenoma: a histochemical, immunohistochemical, and ultrastructural analysis of 17 cases. Hum Pathol 1999; 30:158–167.
30. Cavazza A, Paci M, De ML, et al. Alveolar adenoma of the lung: a clinicopathologic, immunohistochemical, and molecular study of an unusual case. Int J Surg Pathol 2004; 12:155–159.
31. Halldorsson A, Dissanaike S, Kaye KS, et al. Alveolar adenoma of the lung: a clinicopathological description of a case of this very unusual tumour. J Clin Pathol 2005; 58:1211–1214.
32. Fujimoto K, Muller NL, Sadohara J, et al. Alveolar adenoma of the lung: computed tomography and magnetic resonance imaging findings. J Thorac Imaging 2002; 17:163–166.
33. Oliveira P, Moura Nunes JF, Clode AL, et al. Alveolar adenoma of the lung: further characterization of this uncommon tumour. Virchows Arch 1996; 429:101–108.
34. Roque L, Oliveira P, Martins C, et al. A nonbalanced translocation (10; 16) demonstrated by FISH analysis in a case of alveolar adenoma of the lung. Cancer Genet Cytogenet 1996; 89:34–37.
35. Bohm J, Fellbaum C, Bautz W, et al. Pulmonary nodule caused by an alveolar adenoma of the lung. Virchows Arch 1997; 430:181–184.
36. Marchevsky AM. Surgical Pathology of Neoplasms of the Lung: In Lung Biology in Health and Disease. New York, NY: Marcel Dikker, 1990.
37. Iyoda A, Hiroshima K, Shiba M, et al. Clinicopathological analysis of pulmonary sclerosing hemangioma. Ann Thorac Surg 2004; 78:1928–1931.
38. Wu CT, Chang YL, Lee YC, et al. Expression of the estrogen receptor beta in 37 surgically treated pulmonary sclerosing hemangiomas in comparison with non-small cell lung carcinomas. Hum Pathol 2005; 36:1108–1112.
39. Fantone JC, Geisinger KR, Appelman HD. Papillary adenoma of the lung with lamellar and electron dense granules. An ultrastructural study. Cancer 1982; 50:2839–2844.
40. Heikkila P, Salminen US. Papillary pneumocytoma of the lung. An immunohistochemical and electron microscopic study. Pathol Res Pract 1994; 190:194–200.
41. Baldi A, Santini M, Vicidomini G, et al. Papillary pneumocytoma of the lung simulating a pleomorphic adenoma. In Vivo 2002; 16:387–390.
42. Dessy E, Braidotti P, Del CB, et al. Peripheral papillary tumor of type-II pneumocytes: a rare neoplasm of undetermined malignant potential. Virchows Arch 2000; 436:289–295.
43. Delpiano C, Claren R, Sironi M, et al. Cytological appearance of papillary mucous gland adenoma of the left lobar bronchus with histological confirmation. Cytopathology 2000; 11:193–196.
44. Kroe DJ, Pitcock JA, Kroe DJ, et al. Benign mucous gland adenoma of the bronchus. Arch Pathol Lab Med 1967; 84:539–542.
45. Dickstein PJ, Amaral SM, Silva AM, et al. Bronchial mucous gland adenoma presenting as bronchogenic cyst. Pediatr Pulmonol 1993; 16:370–374.
46. Payne WS, Fontana RS, Woolner LB. Bronchial tumors originating from mucous glands. Current classification and unusual manifestations. Med Clin North Am 1964; 48:945–960.
47. Dambara T, Dambara T. Endoscopic laser treatment of mucous gland adenoma arising in the trachea. Int Med 1996; 35:841.
48. Edwards CW, Matthews HR, Edwards CW, et al. Mucous gland adenoma of the bronchus. Thorax 1981; 36:147–148.

49. Key BM, Pritchett PS, Key BM, et al. Mucous gland adenoma of the bronchus. South Med J 1979; 72:83–85.
50. Emory WB, Mitchell WT Jr., Hatch HB Jr., et al. Mucous gland adenoma of the bronchus. Am Rev Respir Dis 1973; 108:1407–1410.
51. Kwon JW, Goo JM, Seo JB, et al. Mucous gland adenoma of the bronchus: CT findings in two patients. J Comput Assist Tomogr 1999; 23:758–760.
52. Ishida T, Kamachi M, Hanada T, et al. Mucous gland adenoma of the trachea resected with an endoscopic neodymium: yttrium aluminum garnet laser. Int Med 1996; 35:890–893 (comment).
53. England DM, Hochholzer L, England DM, et al. Truly benign "bronchial adenoma". Report of 10 cases of mucous gland adenoma with immunohistochemical and ultrastructural findings. Am J Surg Pathol 1995; 19:887–899.
54. Hayes MM, van der Westhuizen NG, Forgie R, et al. Malignant mixed tumor of bronchus: a biphasic neoplasm of epithelial and myoepithelial cells. Mod Pathol 1993; 6:85–88.
55. Moran CA, Suster S, Askin FB, et al. Benign and malignant salivary gland-type mixed tumors of the lung. Clinicopathologic and immunohistochemical study of eight cases. Cancer 1994; 73:2481–2490.
56. Moran CA, Suster S, Carter D. Benign mixed tumors (pleomorphic adenomas) of the breast. Am J Surg Pathol 1990; 14:913–921.
57. Berho M, Moran CA, Suster S. Malignant mixed epithelial/mesenchymal neoplasms of the lung. Semin Diagn Pathol 1995; 12:123–139.
58. Sakamoto H, Uda H, Tanaka T, et al. Pleomorphic adenoma in the periphery of the lung. Report of a case and review of the literature. Arch Pathol Lab Med 1991; 115:393–396.
59. Takeuchi E, Shimizu E, Sano N, et al. A case of pleomorphic adenoma of the lung with multiple distant metastases–observations on its oncogene and tumor suppressor gene expression. Anticancer Res 1998; 18:2015–2020.
60. Takeuchi J, Sobue M, Yoshida M, et al. Pleomorphic adenoma of the salivary gland. With special reference to histochemical and electron microscopic studies and biochemical analysis of glycosaminoglycans in vivo and in vitro. Cancer 1975; 36:1771–1789.
61. Shimizu J, Watanabe Y, Oda M, et al. Clinicopathologic study of mucoepidermoid carcinoma of the lung. Int Surg 1998; 83:1–3.
62. Yousem SA, Hochholzer L. Mucoepidermoid tumors of the lung. Cancer 1987; 60:1346–1352.
63. Yang CS, Kuo KT, Chou TY, et al. Mucoepidermoid tumors of the lung: analysis of 11 cases. J Chin Med Assoc 2004; 67:565–570.
64. Kragel PJ, Devaney KO, Meth BM, et al. Mucinous cystadenoma of the lung. A report of two cases with immunohistochemical and ultrastructural analysis. Arch Pathol Lab Med 1990; 114:1053–1056.
65. McGinnis M, Jacobs G, el-Naggar A, et al. Congenital peribronchial myofibroblastic tumor (so-called "congenital leiomyosarcoma"). A distinct neonatal lung lesion associated with nonimmune hydrops fetalis. Mod Pathol 1993; 6:487–492.
66. Van PH, Duponselle E, Gruwez J, et al. Congenital cystic adenomatoid malformation or adenomatoid hamartoma of the lung. A new case in a neonate review of the literature. Acta Paediatr Belg 1981; 34:83–88.
67. Sirvent N, Hawkins AL, Moeglin D, et al. ALK probe rearrangement in a t(2; 11; 2)(p23; p15; q31) translocation found in a prenatal myofibroblastic fibrous lesion: toward a molecular definition of an inflammatory myofibroblastic tumor family? Genes Chromosomes Cancer 2001; 31:85–90.
68. Kinoshita Y, Tajiri T, Ieiri S, et al. A case of an inflammatory myofibroblastic tumor in the lung which expressed TPM3-ALK gene fusion. Pediatr Surg Int 2007; 23:595–599.
69. Cessna MH, Zhou H, Sanger WG, et al. Expression of ALK1 and p80 in inflammatory myofibroblastic tumor and its mesenchymal mimics: a study of 135 cases. Mod Pathol 2002; 15:931–938.

70. Hannah CD, Oliver DH, Liu J, et al. Fine needle aspiration biopsy and immunostaining findings in an aggressive inflammatory myofibroblastic tumor of the lung: a case report. Acta Cytol 2007; 51:239–243.
71. Ma Z, Hill DA, Collins MH, et al. Fusion of ALK to the Ran-binding protein 2 (RANBP2) gene in inflammatory myofibroblastic tumor. Genes Chromosomes Cancer 2003; 37:98–105.
72. Panagopoulos I, Nilsson T, Domanski HA, et al. Fusion of the SEC31L1 and ALK genes in an inflammatory myofibroblastic tumor. Int J Cancer 2006; 118:1181–1186.
73. Kaya S, Aydin E, Sirmali M, et al. A huge intrathoracal mass in a 1-year-old infant: an inflammatory myofibroblastic tumor. Eur J Cardiothorac Surg 2003; 24:1031–1032.
74. Coffin CM, Hornick JL, Fletcher CD, et al. Inflammatory myofibroblastic tumor: comparison of clinicopathologic, histologic, and immunohistochemical features including ALK expression in atypical and aggressive cases. Am J Surg Pathol 2007; 31:509–520.
75. Su LD, tayde-Perez A, Sheldon S, et al. Inflammatory myofibroblastic tumor: cytogenetic evidence supporting clonal origin. Mod Pathol 1998; 11:364–368.
76. Coffin CM, Dehner LP, Meis-Kindblom JM, et al. Inflammatory myofibroblastic tumor, inflammatory fibrosarcoma, and related lesions: an historical review with differential diagnostic considerations. Semin Diagn Pathol 1998; 15:102–110.
77. Privitera S, Hwang DM, Darling GE, et al. Inflammatory myofibroblastic tumor of the left main stem bronchus. J Thorac Oncol 2006; 1:726–728.
78. Sakurai H, Hasegawa T, Watanabe S, et al. Inflammatory myofibroblastic tumor of the lung. Eur J Cardiothorac Surg 2004; 25:155–159.
79. Zennaro H, Laurent F, Vergier B, et al. Inflammatory myofibroblastic tumor of the lung (inflammatory pseudotumor): uncommon cause of solitary pulmonary nodule. Eur Radiol 1999; 9:1205–1207.
80. Yamaguchi M, Yoshino I, Osoegawa A, et al. Inflammatory myofibroblastic tumor of the mediastinum presenting as superior vena cava syndrome. J Thorac Cardiovasc Surg 2003; 126:870–872.
81. Makimoto Y, Nabeshima K, Iwasaki H, et al. Inflammatory myofibroblastic tumor of the posterior mediastinum: an older adult case with anaplastic lymphoma kinase abnormalities determined using immunohistochemistry and fluorescence in situ hybridization. Virchows Arch 2005; 446:451–455.
82. Dehner LP. Inflammatory myofibroblastic tumor: the continued definition of one type of so-called inflammatory pseudotumor. Am J Surg Pathol 2004; 28:1652–1654.
83. Kazmierczak B, Dal CP, Sciot R, et al. Inflammatory myofibroblastic tumor with HMGIC rearrangement. Cancer Genet Cytogenet 1999; 112:156–160.
84. Priebe-Richter C, Ivanyi P, Buer J, et al. Inflammatory pseudotumor of the lung following invasive aspergillosis in a patient with chronic graft-vs.-host disease. Eur J Haematol 2005; 75:68–72.
85. Nakamura H, Kawasaki N, Taguchi M, et al. Pulmonary inflammatory myofibroblastic tumor resected by video-assisted thoracoscopic surgery: Report of a case. Surg Today 2007; 37:137–140.
86. Farris AB III, Mark EJ, Kradin RL, et al. Pulmonary inflammatory myofibroblastic" tumors: a critical examination of the diagnostic category based on quantitative immunohistochemical analysis. Virchows Arch 2007; 450:585–590.
87. Kim TS, Han J, Kim GY, et al. Pulmonary inflammatory pseudotumor (inflammatory myofibroblastic tumor): CT features with pathologic correlation. J Comput Assist Tomogr 2005; 29:633–639.
88. Omasa M, Kobayashi T, Takahashi Y, et al. Surgically treated pulmonary inflammatory pseudotumor. Jpn J Thorac Cardiovasc Surg 2002; 50:305–308.
89. Lee HJ, Kim JS, Choi YS, et al. Treatment of inflammatory myofibroblastic tumor of the chest: the extent of resection. Ann Thorac Surg 2007; 84:221–224.

90. Ritter JH, Humphrey PA, Wick MR. Malignant neoplasms capable of simulating inflammatory (myofibroblastic) pseudotumors and tumefactive fibroinflammatory lesions: pseudotumors. Semin Diagn Pathol 1998; 15:111–132.
91. Johansson M, Heim S, Mandahl N, et al. t(3; 6; 14)(p21; p21; q24) as the sole clonal chromosome abnormality in a hamartoma of the lung. Cancer Genet Cytogenet 1992; 60: 219–220.
92. Dempster AG, Dempster AG. Adenomatoid hamartoma of the lung in a neonate. J Clin Pathol 1969; 22:401–406.
93. Takeshima Y, Furukawa K, Inai K, et al. 'Adenomyomatous' hamartoma of the lung. Pathol Int 2000; 50:984–986.
94. Yamazaki Y, Yasukawa S, Mizuno R, et al. The adult type pulmonary hamartoma in an 11-year-old boy. Zeitschrift fur Kinderchirurgie 1986; 41:109–111.
95. Palvio D, Egeblad K, Paulsen SM, et al. Atypical lipomatous hamartoma of the lung. Virchows Arch A Pathol Anat Histopathol 1985; 405:253–261.
96. Kleinman J, Zirkin H, Feuchtwanger MM, et al. Benign hamartoma of the lung presenting as massive hemoptysis. J Surg Oncol 1986; 33:38–40.
97. Darke CS, Day P, Grainger RG, et al. The bronchial circulation in a case of giant hamartoma of the lung. Br J Radiol 1972; 45:147–150.
98. Naresh KN, Mohan G, Murthy SC, et al. Chondroid hamartoma of the lung–an underdiagnosed entity in fine needle aspiration cytology. Indian J Pathol Microbiol 1994; 37(suppl):S17–S18.
99. Demos TC, Armin A, Chandrasekhar AJ, et al. Cystic hamartoma of the lung. J Can Assoc Radiol 1983; 34:149–150.
100. Chou TF, Lee YC, Shiao CS, et al. Cystic hamartoma of the lung: report of two cases. J Formos Med Assoc 1991; 90:705–707.
101. Chadwick SL, Corrin B, Hansell DM, et al. Fatal haemorrhage from mesenchymal cystic hamartoma of the lung. Eur Respir J 1995; 8:2182–2184.
102. Hassani SN, Nuba R, Bard RL, et al. Fibroleiomyomatous hamartoma of the lung. Respiration 1979; 37:238–240.
103. Taniyama K, Sasaki N, Yamaguchi K, et al. Fibrolipomatous hamartoma of the lung: a case report and review of the literature. Jpn J Clin Oncol 1995; 25:159–163.
104. Fujino S, Tezuka N, Sawai S, et al. Giant hamartoma of the lung. Jpn J Thorac Cardiovasc Surg 1998; 46:1229–1231.
105. Okabayashi K, Hiratsuka M, Noda Y, et al. Giant hamartoma of the lung with a high production of carbohydrate antigen 19-9. Ann Thorac Surg 1993; 55:511–513.
106. Koutras P, Urschel HC Jr., Paulson DL, et al. Hamartoma of the lung. J Thorac Cardiovasc Surg 1971; 61:768–776.
107. Olsen P. Hamartoma of the lung. Dan Med Bull 1968; 15:117–120.
108. Oldham HN Jr., Young WG Jr., Sealy WC, et al. Hamartoma of the lung. J Thorac Cardiovascu Surg 1967; 53:735–742.
109. Krishna BM, Rajagopala SK, Saraswathy K, et al. Hamartoma of the lung. (A case report). Indian J Pathol Bacteriol 1966; 9:201–205.
110. Munsakul N, Areechon W, Hongthiamtong P, et al. Hamartoma of the lung. A report of 4 cases. J Med Assoc Thai 1970; 53:898–904.
111. Gluck MC, Moser KM, Gluck MC, et al. Hamartoma of the lung presenting as a mediastinal mass. Am Rev Respir Dis 1968; 98:281–286.
112. Bergh NP, Hafstrom LO, Schersten T, et al. Hamartoma of the lung: with special reference to the endobronchial localization. Scand J Respir Dis 1967; 48:201–207.
113. Karasik A, Modan M, Jacob CO, et al. Increased risk of lung cancer in patients with chondromatous hamartoma. J Thorac Cardiovasc Surg 1980; 80:217–220.
114. Torikata C, Ishiwata K, Fukai S, et al. Malignant change in a solitary hamartoma of the lung. A case report. Acta Pathol Jpn 1977; 27:541–546.

115. Hayward RH, Carabasi RJ. Malignant hamartoma of the lung: fact or fiction? J Thorac Cardiovasc Surg 1967; 53:457–466.
116. Leroyer C, Quiot JJ, Dewitte JD, et al. Mesenchymal cystic hamartoma of the lung. Respiration 1993; 60:305–306.
117. Mark EJ. Mesenchymal cystic hamartoma of the lung. New Engl J Med 1986; 315:1255–1259.
118. van Klaveren RJ, Hassing HH, Wiersma-van Tilburg JM, et al. Mesenchymal cystic hamartoma of the lung: a rare cause of relapsing pneumothorax. Thorax 1994; 49:1175–1176.
119. Cottin V, Thomas L, Loire R, et al. Mesenchymal cystic hamartoma of the lung in Cowden's disease. Respir Med 2003; 97:188–191.
120. Yalcin S, Kars A, Firat P, et al. Multiple bilateral chondromatous hamartomas of the lung. A rare entity mimicking metastatic carcinoma. Respiration 1997; 64:364–366.
121. Lahiri TK, Pandey S. Multiple fibrochondromatous hamartoma of the lung. Indian J Chest Dis Allied Sci 1991; 33:161–164.
122. Uzaslan E, Ebsen M, Freudenberg N, et al. Reactive alveolar epithelium in chondroid hamartoma of the lung. Acta Cytol 2005; 49:154–156.
123. Bateson EM. So-called hamartoma of the lung–a true neoplasm of fibrous connective tissue of the bronchi. Cancer 1973; 31:1458–1467.
124. Itoh H, Yanagi M, Setoyama T, et al. Solitary fibroleiomyomatous hamartoma of the lung in a patient without a pre-existing smooth-muscle tumor. Pathol Int 2001; 51:661–665.
125. de Rooij PD, Meijer S, Calame J, et al. Solitary hamartoma of the lung: is thoracotomy still mandatory? Neth J Surg 1988; 40:145–148.
126. Narita T, Takahashi H, Narita T, et al. Unusual cystadenomatous hamartoma of the lung. Histopathology 1996; 28:285–287.
127. Oei TK, Wouters EF, Visser R, et al. The value of conventional radiography and computed tomography (CT) in diagnosis of pulmonary hamartoma. Rontgenblatter 1983; 36:324–327.
128. Varma BN. Vascular hamartoma of the lung. Lancet 1966; 86:183–186.
129. Sampath KA, Panda RK, Pande JN, et al. Primary chondroma of the lung. Indian J Chest Dis Allied Sci 1984; 26:114–118.
130. Dail DH, Liebow AA, Gmelich JT, et al. Intravascular, bronchiolar, and alveolar tumor of the lung (IVBAT). An analysis of twenty cases of a peculiar sclerosing endothelial tumor. Cancer 1983; 51:452–464.
131. Liebow AA, Hubbell DS. Sclerosing hemangioma (histiocytoma, xanthoma) of the lung. Cancer 1956; 9:53–75.
132. Hanaoka J, Ohuchi M, Inoue S, et al. Bilateral multiple pulmonary sclerosing hemangioma. Jpn J Thorac Cardiovasc Surg 2005; 53:157–161.
133. Sakamoto I, Tomiyama N, Sugita A, et al. A case of sclerosing hemangioma surrounded by emphysematous change. Radiat Med 2004; 22:123–125.
134. Dai SD, Zhang XW, Qi FJ, et al. Expression of E-cadherin, beta-catenin and p120ctn in the pulmonary sclerosing hemangioma. Lung Cancer 2007; 57:54–59.
135. Yoo SH, Jung KC, Kim JH, et al. Expression patterns of markers for type II pneumocytes in pulmonary sclerosing hemangiomas and fetal lung tissues. Arch Pathol Lab Med 2005; 129:915–919.
136. Dacic S, Sasatomi E, Swalsky PA, et al. Loss of heterozygosity patterns of sclerosing hemangioma of the lung and bronchioloalveolar carcinoma indicate a similar molecular pathogenesis. Arch Pathol Lab Med 2004; 128:880–884.
137. Soumil VJ, Navin B, Sangeeta D, et al. Multiple sclerosing hemangiomas of the lung. Asian Cardiovasc Thorac Ann 2004; 12:357–359.
138. Hishida T, Yoshida J, Nishimura M, et al. Multiple sclerosing hemangiomas with a 10-year history. Jpn J Clin Oncol 2005; 35:37–39.
139. Jin LJ, Shin BK, Jung WY, et al. Proteomic analysis of pulmonary sclerosing hemangioma. Proteomics 2006; 6:4877–4883.

140. Pekcolaklar A, Turna A, Urer N, et al. Pulmonary sclerosing haemangioma mimicking hydatid cyst: a case report. Acta Chir Belg 2007; 107:328–330.
141. Takatani H, Ashizawa K, Kawai K, et al. Pulmonary sclerosing hemangioma manifesting as a nodule with irregular air clefts on high-resolution CT. Am J Roentgenol 2007; 189:W26–W28.
142. Chung MJ, Lee KS, Han J, et al. Pulmonary sclerosing hemangioma presenting as solitary pulmonary nodule: dynamic CT findings and histopathologic comparisons. AJR. 2006; Am J Roentgenol 187:430–437.
143. Katakura H, Sato M, Tanaka F, et al. Pulmonary sclerosing hemangioma with metastasis to the mediastinal lymph node. Ann Thorac Surg 2005; 80:2351–2353.
144. Komatsu T, Fukuse T, Wada H, et al. Pulmonary sclerosing hemangioma with pulmonary metastasis. Thorac Cardiovasc Surg 2006; 54:348–349.
145. Neuman J, Rosioreanu A, Schuss A, et al. Radiology-pathology conference: sclerosing hemangioma of the lung. Clin Imaging 2006; 30:409–412.
146. Stafford CM, Crawford SW, Bradshaw DA, et al. Sclerosing hemangioma. South Med J 2005; 98:580.
147. Jungraithmayr W, Eggeling S, Ludwig C, et al. Sclerosing hemangioma of the lung: a benign tumour with potential for malignancy? Ann Thorac Cardiovasc Surg 2006; 12:352–354.
148. Kim GY, Kim J, Choi YS, et al. Sixteen cases of sclerosing hemangioma of the lung including unusual presentations. J Korean Med Sci 2004; 19:352–358.
149. Tan HW, Goh SG, Yap WM, et al. Test and teach. Number fifty-three. Diagnosis: Sclerosing haemangioma. Pathology 2006; 38:66–70.
150. Nicholson AG, Magkou C, Snead D, et al. Unusual sclerosing haemangiomas and sclerosing haemangioma-like lesions, and the value of TTF-1 in making the diagnosis. Histopathology 2002; 41:404–413.
151. Robbins P, Holthouse D, Newman M, et al. An unusually large pulmonary sclerosing haemangioma. Pathology 2006; 38:267–268.
152. Chan KW, Gibbs AR, Lo WS, et al. Benign sclerosing pneumocytoma of lung (sclerosing haemangioma). Thorax 1982; 37:404–412.
153. Tanaka I, Inoue M, Matsui Y, et al. A case of pneumocytoma (so-called sclerosing hemangioma) with lymph node metastasis. Jpn J Clin Oncol 1986; 16:77–86.
154. Grayson W, Leiman G, Cooper K. Exuberant fibroadenomatoid proliferation in a pulmonary mesenchymoma (hamartoma): report of a lesion mimicking a sclerosing pneumocytoma. Gen Diagn Pathol 1997; 142:247–252.
155. van WQ, Suvarna SK. Frozen section diagnosis of fibrotic sclerosing pneumocytoma with psammomatous calcification. Histopathology 2003; 43:504–505.
156. Satoh Y, Tsuchiya E, Weng SY, et al. Pulmonary sclerosing hemangioma of the lung. A type II pneumocytoma by immunohistochemical and immunoelectron microscopic studies. Cancer 1989; 64:1310–1317.
157. Papla B. Sclerosing hemangioma of the lung–benign sclerosing pneumocytoma. Pol J Pathol 1999; 50:99–106.
158. Ryman NG, Burrow L, Bowen C, et al. Good's syndrome with primary intrapulmonary thymoma. J R Soc Med 2005; 98:119–120.
159. James CL, Iyer PV, Leong AS, et al. Intrapulmonary thymoma. Histopathology 1992; 21:175–177.
160. Green WR, Pressoir R, Gumbs RV, et al. Intrapulmonary thymoma. Arch Pathol Lab Med 1987; 111:1074–1076.
161. Yeoh CB, Ford JM, Lattes R, et al. Intrapulmonary thymoma. J Thorac Cardiovasc Surg 1966; 51:131–136.
162. Kung IT, Loke SL, So SY, et al. Intrapulmonary thymoma: report of two cases. Thorax 1985; 40:471–474.

163. Srivastava A, Padilla O, Alroy J, et al. Primary intrapulmonary spindle cell thymoma with marked granulomatous reaction: report of a case with review of literature. Int J Surg Pathol 2003; 11:353–356.
164. Moran CA, Suster S, Fishback NF, et al. Primary intrapulmonary thymoma. A clinicopathologic and immunohistochemical study of eight cases. Am J Surg Pathol 1995; 19:304–312.
165. Stefani A, Boulenger E, Mehaut S, et al. Primary intrapulmonary thymoma associated with congenital hyperhomocysteinemia. J Thorac Cardiovasc Surg 2007; 134:799–801.
166. Ishibashi H, Takahashi S, Tomoko H, et al. Primary intrapulmonary thymoma successfully resected with vascular reconstruction. Ann Thorac Surg 2003; 76:1735–1737.
167. Marchevsky AM. Lung tumors derived from ectopic tissues. Semin Diagn Pathol 1995; 12:172–184.
168. Gardiman M, Altavilla G, Marchioro L, et al. Metastasis to intracranial meningioma as first clinical manifestation of occult primary lung carcinoma. Tumori 1996; 82:256–258.
169. Rowsell C, Sirbovan J, Rosenblum MK, et al. Primary chordoid meningioma of lung. Virchows Arch 2005; 446:333–337.
170. Picquet J, Valo I, Jousset Y, et al. Primary pulmonary meningioma first suspected of being a lung metastasis. Ann Thorac Surg 2005; 79:1407–1409.
171. de PM, Kurt AM, Robert J, et al. Primary pulmonary meningioma presenting as lung metastasis. Scand Cardiovasc J 1999; 33:121–123.
172. Maiorana A, Ficarra G, Fano RA, et al. Primary solitary meningioma of the lung. Pathologica 1996; 88:457–462.
173. Hashimoto T, Oka K, Hakozaki H, et al. Benign clear cell tumor of the lung. Ultrastruct Pathol 2001; 25:479–483.
174. Zolliker A, Jacques J, Goldstein AS, et al. Benign clear cell tumor of the lung. Arch Pathol Lab Med 1979; 103:526–530.
175. Wills JS, Hewes AC, Wills JS, et al. Benign clear cell tumor of the lung: a cautionary tale. Urol Radiol 1980; 2:255–257.
176. Nakanishi K, Kawai T, Suzuki M, et al. Benign clear cell tumor of the lung. A histopathologic study. Acta Pathol Jpn 1988; 38:515–522.
177. Hoch WS, Patchefsky AS, Takeda M, et al. Benign clear cell tumor of the lung. An ultrastructural study. Cancer 1974; 33:1328–1336.
178. Fukuda T, Machinami R, Joshita T, et al. Benign clear cell tumor of the lung in an 8-year-old girl. Arch Pathol Lab Med 1986; 110:664–666.
179. Harbin WP, Mark GJ, Greene RE, et al. Benign clear-cell tumor ("sugar" tumor) of the lung: a case report and review of the literature. Radiology 1978; 129:595–596.
180. Adachi Y, Kitamura Y, Nakamura H, et al. Benign clear (sugar) cell tumor of the lung with CD1a expression. Pathol Int 2006; 56:453–456.
181. Hirata T, Otani T, Minamiguchi S, et al. Clear cell tumor of the lung. Int J Clin Oncol 2006; 11:475–477.
182. Seo JB, Im JG, Seo JW, et al. Clear cell tumor of the lung. AJR Am J Roentgenol 1996; 166:730–731.
183. Gaffey MJ, Mills SE, Askin FB, et al. Clear cell tumor of the lung. A clinicopathologic, immunohistochemical, and ultrastructural study of eight cases. Am J Surg Pathol 1990; 14:248–259 (comment).
184. Lantuejoul S, Isaac S, Pinel N, et al. Clear cell tumor of the lung: an immunohistochemical and ultrastructural study supporting a pericytic differentiation. Mod Pathol 1997; 10:1001–1008.
185. Gaffey MJ, Mills SE, Zarbo RJ, et al. Clear cell tumor of the lung. Immunohistochemical and ultrastructural evidence of melanogenesis. Am J Surg Pathol 1991; 15:644–653.
186. Kavunkal AM, Pandiyan MS, Philip MA, et al. Large clear cell tumor of the lung mimicking malignant behavior. Ann Thorac Surg 2007; 83:310–312.

187. Chuah KL, Tan PH, Chuah KL, et al. Multifocal micronodular pneumocyte hyperplasia, lymphangiomyomatosis and clear cell micronodules of the lung in a Chinese female patient with tuberous sclerosis. Pathology 1998; 30:242–246.
188. Santana AN, Nunes FS, Ho N, et al. A rare cause of hemoptysis: benign sugar (clear) cell tumor of the lung. Eur J Cardio-Thorac Surg 2004; 25:652–654.
189. Hironaka M, Fukayama M, Hironaka M, et al. Regional proliferation of HMB-45-positive clear cells of the lung with lymphangioleiomyomatosislike distribution, replacing the lobes with multiple cysts and a nodule. Am J Surg Pathol 1999; 23:1288–1293.
190. Gora-Gebka M, Liberek A, Bako W, et al. The "sugar" clear cell tumor of the lung-clinical presentation and diagnostic difficulties of an unusual lung tumor in youth. J Pediatr Surg 2006; 41:E27–E29.
191. Takanami I, Kodaira S, Imamura T, et al. The use of transbronchial lung biopsy to establish a diagnosis of benign clear cell tumor of the lung: report of a case. Surg Today 1998; 28:985–987.
192. Tazelaar HD, Batts KP, Srigley JR. Primary extrapulmonary sugar tumor (PEST): a report of four cases. Mod Pathol 2001; 14:615–622.
193. Flieder DB, Travis WD. Clear cell "sugar" tumor of the lung: association with lymphangioleiomyomatosis and multifocal micronodular pneumocyte hyperplasia in a patient with tuberous sclerosis. Am J Surg Pathol 1997; 21:1242–1247.
194. Urban T. Clinical and molecular epidemiology of lymphangioleiomyomatosis and pulmonary pathology in tuberous sclerosis. Rev Mal Respir 2000; 17:597–603.

36
Spindle Cell Neoplasms of the Lung and Pleura

MARY BETH BEASLEY
Mount Sinai Medical Center, New York, New York, U.S.A.

I. Introduction

Pure spindle cell malignancies occurring in the lung are relatively rare. Most spindle cell tumors presenting as an intraparenchymal mass lesion will represent a sarcomatoid carcinoma. Spindle morphology may also be observed in neuroendocrine tumors, such as carcinoids, and these are discussed in chapter 34. Sarcomas as a group tend to metastasize hematogenously and therefore may involve the lungs secondarily. True primary pulmonary sarcomas are exceedingly rare.

II. Sarcomatoid/Spindle Cell Carcinoma

In the World Health Organization (WHO) classification of pulmonary neoplasms, sarcomatoid carcinomas are defined as "a group of poorly differentiated non–small cell carcinomas that contain a component of sarcoma or sarcoma-like (spindle or giant cell) differentiation." This category includes pure spindle cell and giant cell carcinomas as well as "pleomorphic carcinomas," which contain an identifiable component of squamous cell carcinoma, adenocarcinoma, or large cell carcinoma admixed with the spindle or giant cell component. Carcinosarcoma and pulmonary blastoma are also included in this category (1). Spindle cell carcinomas will be discussed herein, while pleomorphic carcinoma, carcinosarcoma, and pulmonary blastoma will be discussed in chapter 37 on biphasic neoplasms.

Sarcomatoid carcinomas are rare and account for approximately 1% of all pulmonary malignancies. In spite of this, a spindle cell malignancy encountered in the lung is most likely going to be a sarcomatoid carcinoma. The average age at diagnosis is 60, and there is a 4:1 male to female predominance. Over 90% of these carcinomas are associated with tobacco smoking. They typically present as a large peripheral mass but may occur centrally (1,2).

Pure spindle cell carcinomas are rare, and the majority of tumors will contain an identifiable component of squamous cell carcinoma, adenocarcinoma, or large cell carcinoma and should therefore be classified as pleomorphic carcinomas (2). The WHO classification recommends that the sarcomatoid or carcinomatous component comprise at least 10% of the tumor to warrant a diagnosis of pleomorphic carcinoma, but this is admittedly arbitrary (1).

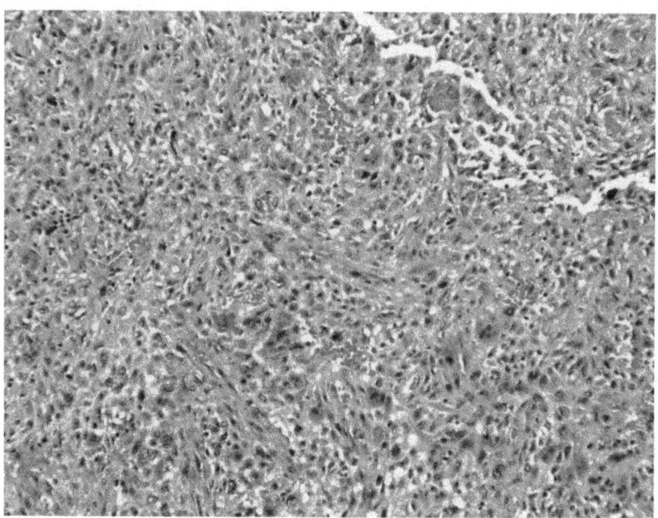

Figure 1 Spindle cell carcinoma with pleomorphic spindle cells and occasional giant cells. [hematoxylin and eosin stain (H&E, 200×)].

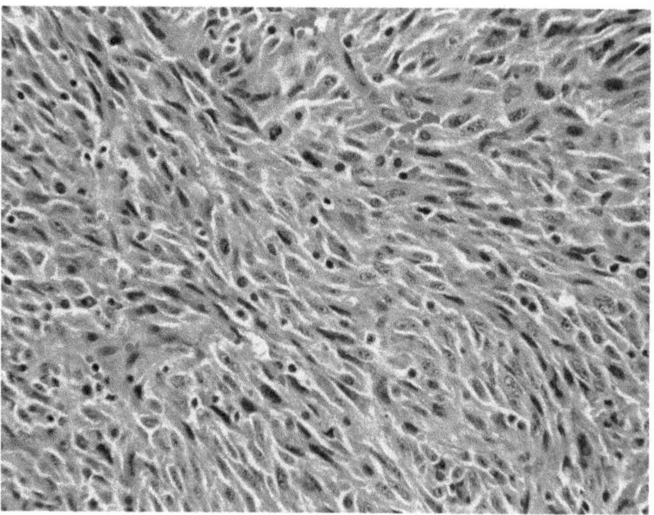

Figure 2 Spindle cell carcinoma with a relatively uniform appearance of spindle cells. (H&E, 200×).

The spindle cells are overtly malignant and are arranged in a haphazard fascicular or storiform pattern (Fig. 1). The cells are usually fairly pleomorphic and have identifiable mitoses, although they may sometimes have a comparatively uniform appearance (Fig. 2). Necrosis is frequently a feature. Expression of epithelial markers such as keratin or

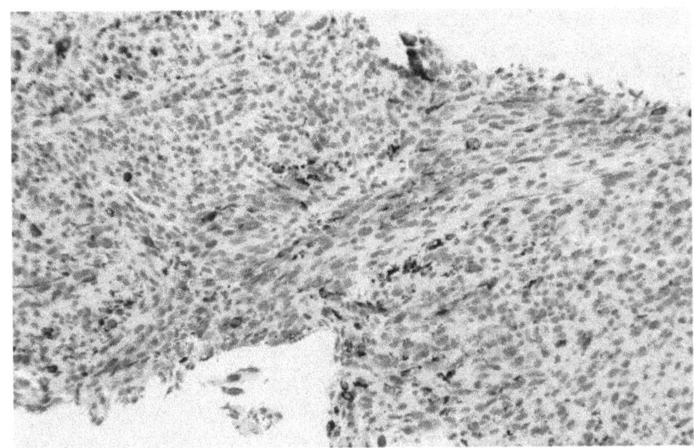

Figure 3 Keratin stains are frequently weakly positive in spindle cell carcinoma. (AE1/AE3, 200×).

epithelial membrane antigen (EMA) is usually sufficient to support a diagnosis of spindle cell carcinoma in the clinical presence of a lung mass. Keratin staining may be focal and may require the use of multiple markers to demonstrate positive staining (Fig. 3) (2). On a small biopsy, it may not always be possible to demonstrate keratin staining. For this reason, a sarcomatoid/spindle cell carcinoma should not be definitively ruled out in a keratin-negative spindle cell malignancy occurring in a clinical setting otherwise typical for lung cancer.

III. Inflammatory Myofibroblastic Tumor

Inflammatory myofibroblastic tumor (IMT) is the current nomenclature in the WHO classification used to encompass the entities previously known as inflammatory pseudotumor and plasma cell granuloma (1). While many of these lesions do appear to be true neoplasms and contain a mutation of the ALK gene, there is continuing controversy regarding whether all of the lesions formerly in the inflammatory pseudotumor group are truly neoplastic or whether some of them are indeed reactive processes.

Grossly, IMT is typically well circumscribed and peripheral in location, although it may occasionally occur in an endobronchial location (3).

IMT is characterized by a proliferation of plump spindled cells admixed with varying numbers of chronic inflammatory cells and foamy macrophages (Fig. 4). The cells are usually fairly uniform in appearance and mitotic activity is usually low. IMT is negative for cytokeratin (3). The finding of a positive cytokeratin stain implies a sarcomatoid carcinoma with a prominent inflammatory reaction, although care must be taken not to misinterpret entrapped pneumocytes as keratin-positive tumor cells. Approximately 40% of IMT are positive for ALK protein. Otherwise, the immunohistochemical staining pattern is not specific, with reports showing varying percentages of positive staining with actin and S-100 (1,3).

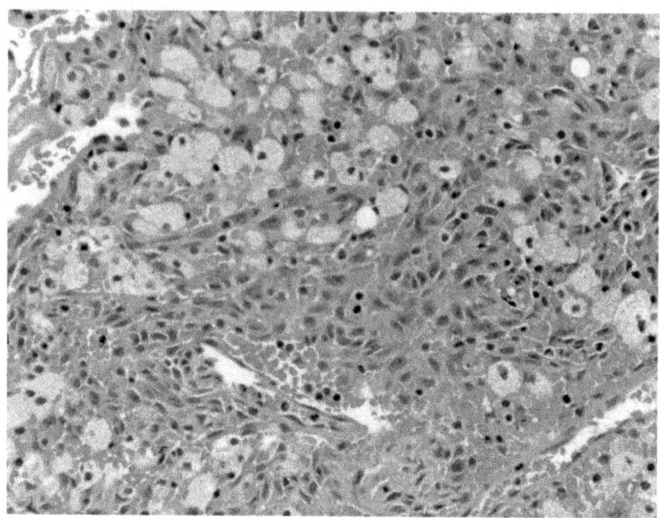

Figure 4 Inflammatory myofibroblastic tumor is composed of spindle cells admixed with foamy macrophages. (H&E, 200×).

IV. Sarcomatoid Mesothelioma

Sarcomatoid mesothelioma is a subtype of mesothelioma composed of malignant spindled cells, in contrast to the epithelioid variant, which is discussed in chapter 31. Biphasic mesotheliomas, consisting of both epithelioid and sarcomatoid elements, are discussed in chapter 37. Like their epithelioid counterparts, sarcomatoid mesotheliomas characteristically involve the pleura diffusely. The spindle cells resemble those seen in other sarcomas, and may range from relatively uniform to markedly pleomorphic (Fig. 5). Heterologous elements such as malignant chondroid or osseous elements may occasionally be present (1,4).

In contrast to epithelioid mesothelioma, in which the differential diagnosis is largely with adenocarcinomas, the differential diagnosis for sarcomatoid mesothelioma is with sarcomatoid carcinomas and true sarcomas. As such, the choice of immunohistochemical stains will be different. In a patient with diffuse pleural thickening, a positive cytokeratin stain is generally sufficient to support a diagnosis of sarcomatoid mesothelioma. Sarcomatoid carcinomas of the lung typically produce a large intraparenchymal mass lesion, and have only rarely been reported to produce pleural thickening mimicking mesothelioma. Differentiating sarcomatoid mesothelioma from metastatic sarcomatoid renal cell carcinoma may, however, prove to be particularly problematic.

Cytokeratin staining in sarcomatoid mesothelioma is usually strong and diffuse, although this is not uniformly the case (5,6). Sarcomatoid mesothelioma may be positive for calretinin in anywhere from 30% to 60% of cases, and this finding is extremely helpful in supporting a diagnosis of sarcomatoid mesothelioma over sarcomatoid carcinoma when present. Other markers which are typically positive in epithelioid mesothelioma such as CK5/6, WT-1, and thrombomodulin are only rarely positive in sarcomatoid mesothelioma

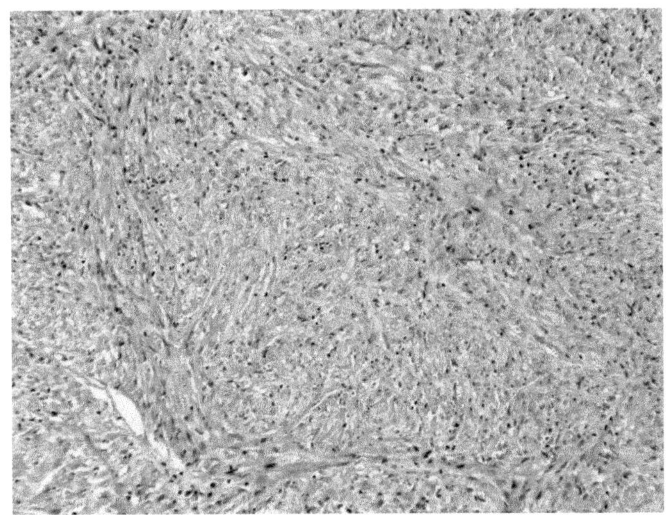

Figure 5 Sarcomatoid mesothelioma is composed of pleomorphic spindle cells resembling those seen in true sarcomas. (H&E, 200×).

(5,6). D2-40 has been reported to be positive in sarcomatoid mesothelioma in one study thus far (7).

Desmoplastic mesothelioma (DMM) is a subtype of sarcomatoid malignant mesothelioma (SMM) in which atypical mesothelial cells are present in a dense collagenous stroma arranged in a storiform pattern (Figs. 6 and 7). The WHO recommends that this pattern be present in at least 50% of the tumor to warrant this diagnosis (1). The cellularity of DMM is deceptively low, and the differential diagnosis is primarily with fibrosing pleuritis or pleural plaque rather than with other malignancies. Fibrous pleuritis and pleural plaque both show a linear pattern of collagen deposition rather than the storiform pattern seen in DMM. Mangano et al. (8) proposed criteria to separate DMM from fibrous pleuritis, which included (*i*) the presence of frankly sarcomatoid areas; (*ii*) bland necrosis; (*iii*) invasion of adipose tissue, skeletal muscle, or lung; and (*iv*) distant metastases. Special stains are of little utility in this differential diagnosis, although keratin staining is useful to highlight the storiform pattern of growth and demonstrate areas of invasion (8).

V. True Sarcomas of the Lung and Pleura

Most sarcomas have been reported as occurring as primary pulmonary tumors, usually as scattered case reports, and sarcomas may involve the lung as metastases. The most common primary sarcomas of the lung and pleura are synovial sarcoma and vascular sarcomas. Primary liposarcomas and leiomyosarcomas have been reported as small case series (9,10).

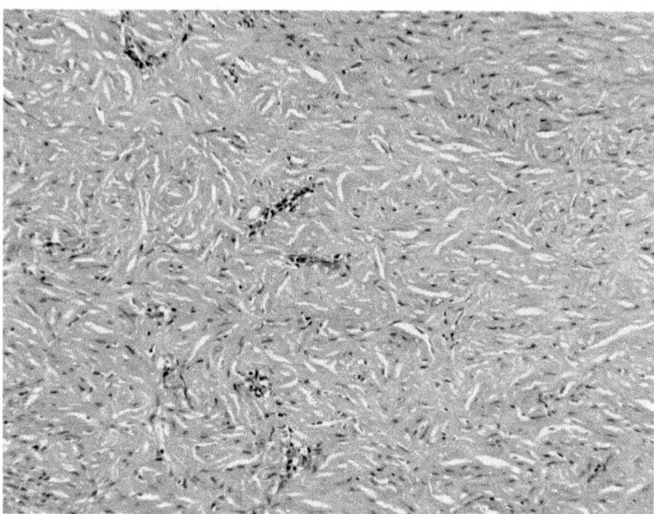

Figure 6 Desmoplastic mesothelioma is deceptively hypocellular but exhibits a storiform growth pattern rather than the linear pattern seen in fibrous pleuritis or pleural plaque. (H&E, 200×).

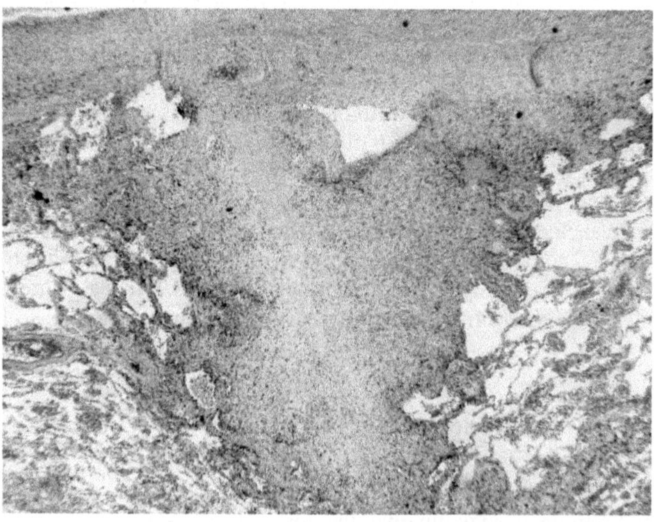

Figure 7 Desmoplastic mesothelioma invading the underlying lung parenchyma. When identifiable, this feature is supportive of the malignant nature of the otherwise deceptively bland appearance of the tumor. (H&E, 100×).

VI. Synovial Sarcoma

Synovial sarcoma may occur as a primary lung or pleural tumor and both monophasic and biphasic subtypes have been reported. Synovial sarcoma is discussed in detail in chapter 37.

VII. Vascular Tumors or the Lung and Pleura

Primary vascular tumors of the lung and pleura include epithelioid hemangioendothelioma (EH), angiosarcoma, and Kaposi's sarcoma (KS).

EH may present as a pulmonary parenchymal tumor, most often forming multiple small parenchymal nodules in females, or it may occur as a primary pleural tumor (1). In the pleura, EH may present as a mass or as diffuse pleural thickening mimicking mesothelioma. EH in both locations is characterized by polygonal shaped epithelioid cells arranged individually or in cords in a myxoid background (Fig. 8). The background may have a chondroid appearance. Careful examination of the epithelioid cells will reveal intracytoplasmic lumen formation, which represents attempted vascular lumen formation. On occasion, red blood cells may be observed within the lumens. EH is typically negative for cytokeratin, although weak, focal staining may occasionally be present. EH is positive for CD34, CD31, Factor VIII, and Ulex Europaeus. In contrast to EH occurring in the soft tissues, where it is considered a low-grade angiosarcoma with a relatively good prognosis, the clinical course of EH in the lung is variable and associated with a worse prognosis, overall, than those of the soft tissue (11–13). EH occurring in the pleura, in spite of a bland morphologic appearance, behaves in an aggressive fashion and has an extremely poor prognosis (13).

Angiosarcoma may occur as a primary pleural tumor, where, like EH, it may produce diffuse pleural thickening mimicking mesothelioma. Angiosarcomas occurring in this location typically have an epithelioid morphology, but may contain a spindle cell

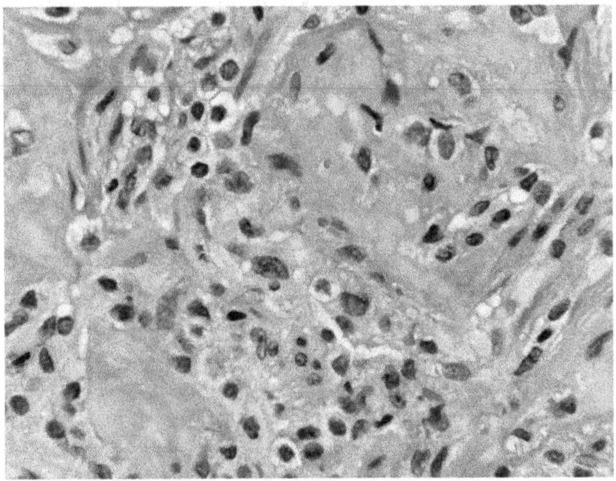

Figure 8 Epithelioid hemangioendothelioma is composed of relatively bland polygonal cells set in a myxoid background (H&E, 400×).

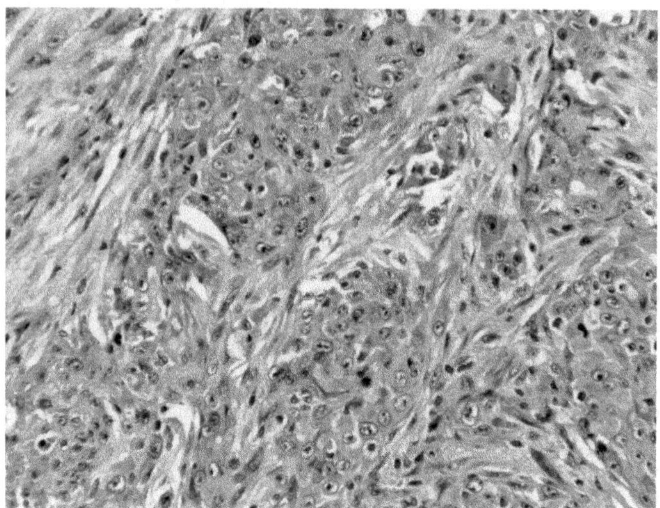

Figure 9 Epithelioid angiosarcoma typically shows a solid growth pattern with only vague vasoformative features. (H&E, 200×).

component. The tumor is usually overtly malignant and mitotic figures may be numerous. The cells tend to grow in relatively solid sheets and the vasoformative nature of the tumor is generally subtle morphologically (Fig. 9). Like EH, angiosarcoma is typically negative or only weakly/focally positive for cytokeratin, and is positive for endothelial markers, distinguishing it from mesothelioma (12,13).

KS may involve the lung in advanced cases of AIDS. The tumor forms blue-red plaques along the airways which are recognizable at bronchoscopy. KS may also involve the pleura. The bronchoscopic picture of KS is fairly characteristic, and the lesions are not usually biopsied given the risk of bleeding. Histologically, KS occurring in the lung is identical to that seen in other sites and consists of hyperchromatic spindle cells arranged in fascicles. Extravasated red blood cells are present and slit-like vascular spaces may be present (14).

VIII. Solitary Fibrous Tumor

Solitary, or localized, fibrous tumor (SFT) typically produces a well-circumscribed pedunculated mass arising from the visceral pleura, but may occur as an intraparenchymal mass. It is characterized by relatively uniform hyperchromatic spindled cells arranged in what has been described as a "patternless pattern". Cellularity may vary from field to field, and the background is characterized by a "wire-like" or "ropey" collagen (Fig. 10). A "hemagiopericytomatous" vascular pattern is usually present. Most tumors are benign, although malignant variants have been described. In the series by England and Hochholzer, criteria supporting malignancy include size greater than 10 cm, mitotic activity greater than 4/10 high-power field (HPF), and necrosis. SFT, in general, is negative for cytokeratin and is positive for CD34 and bcl-2.

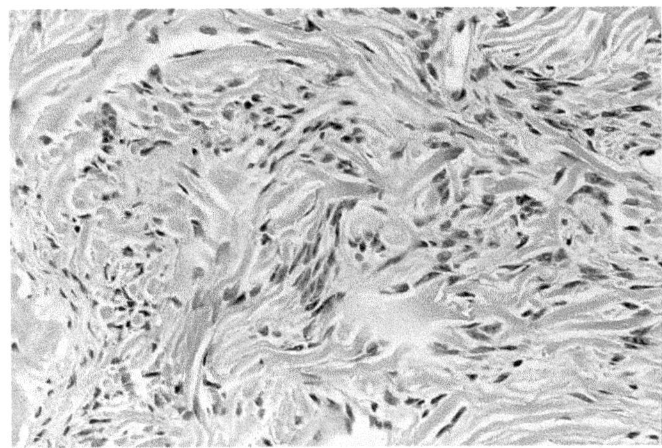

Figure 10 Solitary fibrous tumor showing a typical background of wire-like collagen interspersed among relatively bland, uniformly appearing spindle cells. (H&E, 200×).

IX. Desmoid Tumors

Primary desmoid tumors of the pleura are rare and resemble their soft tissue and abdominal counterparts. Spindle cells of low to moderate cellularity occur as a poorly circumscribed mass that shows interdigitation of spindle cells between adjacent adipocytes or skeletal muscle fibers (Fig. 11). Mitotic activity and necrosis are absent. Desmoid tumors are negative for cytokeratins and CD34, which distinguishes them from mesothelioma and solitary fibrous tumor, respectively (15,16). β-Catenin is characteristic of desmoid tumors in other sites, and has also been found in desmoid tumors of the pleura (15).

X. Calcifying Fibrous Pseudotumor of the Pleura

Only a few examples of calcifying fibrous pseudotumor have been reported in the pleura. These tumors consist of well-circumscribed masses of virtually acellular collagenous tissue containing readily observable psammomatous type calcifications (Fig. 12) (17). The calcifications are usually observable radiographically (18).

XI. Small Blue Cell Tumors of the Pleura

Small blue cell tumors of the lung and pleura are rare and occur primarily in childhood and adolescence. Such tumors include primitive neuroectodermal tumor (PNET), desmoplastic small round cell tumor (DSRCT) and pleuropulmonary blastoma.

PNET was originally described by Askin in 1979 (19) and termed "malignant small blue cell tumor of thoracopulmonary origin". Also referred to as "Askin tumor," this neoplasm was later determined to be a member of the PNET family (20). These tumors

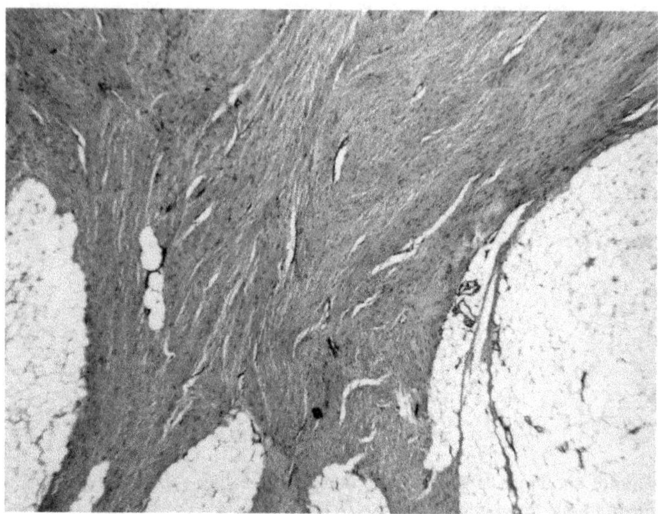

Figure 11 Desmoid tumor of the pleura demonstrates the same features as desmoid tumors of other sites. This example is characterized by bland spindled cells infiltrating the chest wall adipose tissue. (H&E, 100×).

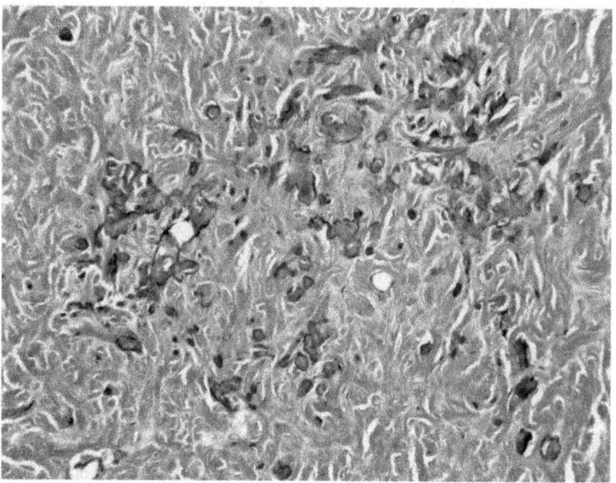

Figure 12 Calcifying fibrous pseudotumor of the pleura showing hypocellular areas of fibrosis containing scattered areas of calcification. (H&E, 200×).

present as a chest wall mass in children and adolescents. In spite of their frequently large size, many cases are asymptomatic, but chest pain or dyspnea may also occur.

The tumor cells of PNET are small and oval to spindle in shape with smooth chromatin and inconspicuous nucleoli (Fig. 13). Mitotic activity is variable. Glycogen may or may not be detectable. The tumor cells are classically positive for vimentin and CD99,

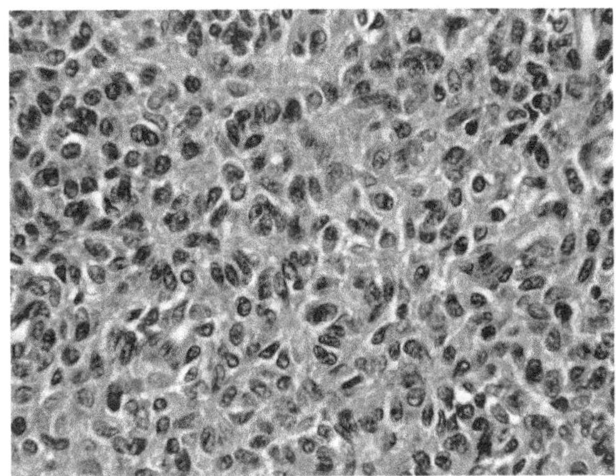

Figure 13 Primitive neuroectodermal tumor demonstrating relatively uniform population of small blue cells with scant cytoplasm and inconspicuous nucleoli. (H&E, 400×).

and will also stain for β2-microglobulin. Like other PNET, Askin tumor contains the characteristict(11:22)(q24;q12) translocation resulting in FLI-1-EWS gene fusion (1,20).

DSRCT occurs primarily in the abdomen but a small number of pleural cases have also been reported. These tumors have occurred almost exclusively in young males and present as either a single mass or multiple pleural nodules. These tumors are composed of small blue cells similar to those seen in Askin tumor, but are separated into irregularly shaped nests by a dense fibrocollagenous stroma (Fig. 14A, B). DSRCT is positive for CD99, but is also positive for keratins, desmin, and WT-1. DSRCT also contains t(11;22) (p13;q12), resulting in WT1-EWS fusion, which differs from the translocation present in Askin tumor (21,22).

Pleuropulmonary blastoma is a tumor of infancy and childhood which may be either cystic or solid. Tumors are divided into subtypes on the basis of the presence of cystic or solid components. Type 1 (purely cystic) tumors consist of multiple cysts lined by

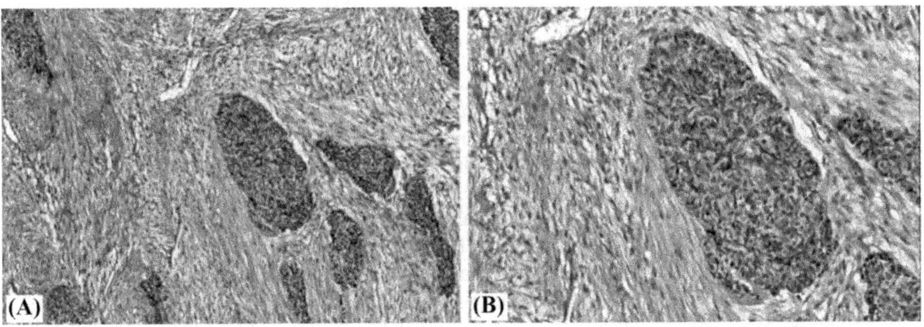

Figure 14 (**A**) and (**B**): Desmoplastic small round cell tumor showing irregular nests of small blue cells in a fibrocollagenous background. (H&E, 100× and 200×).

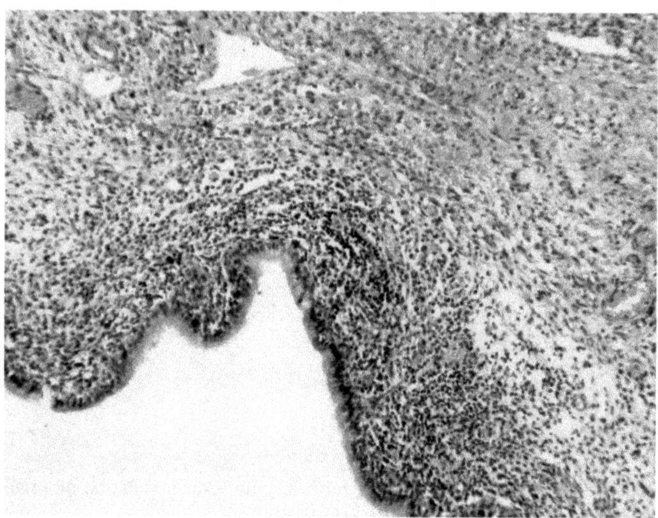

Figure 15 Pleuropulmonary blastoma characterized by a cyst lined by respiratory-type epithelium. Small blue cells coalesce underneath the epithelium in a fashion reminiscent of a cambium layer. (H&E, 200×).

respiratory-type epithelium. Primitive small blue cells underlie the epithelium in a fashion reminiscent of a cambium layer (Fig. 15). These cells may or may not show rhabdomyoblastic differentiation. Type 2 tumors contain areas of identifiable type 1 morphology but additionally contain a solid component of spindle cells with a sarcomatoid appearance typically resembling those of fibrosarcoma. Type 3 tumors are completely solid and exhibit a mixed sarcomatous and blastemous appearance (20,23,24).

References

1. Travis WD, Brambilla E, Muller-Hermerlink HK, et al. Pathology and Genetics. Tumours of the Lung, Pleura, Thymus and Heart. Lyon: IARC Press, 2004.
2. Fishback NF, Travis WD, Moran CA, et al. Pleomorphic (spindle/giant cell) carcinoma of the lung. A clinicopathologic correlation of 78 cases. Cancer 1994; 73(12):2936–2945.
3. Coffin CM, Hornick JL, Fletcher CD. Inflammatory myofibroblastic tumor: comparison of clinicopathologic, histologic, and immunohistochemical features including ALK expression in atypical and aggressive cases. Am J Surg Pathol 2007; 31(4):509–520.
4. Attanoos RL, Gibbs AR. Pathology of malignant mesothelioma. Histopathology 1997; 30(5): 403–418.
5. Attanoos RL, Dojcinov SD, Webb R, et al. Anti-mesothelial markers in sarcomatoid mesothelioma and other spindle cell neoplasms. Histopathology 2000; 37(3):224–231.
6. Cagle PT, Truong LD, Roggli VL, et al. Immunohistochemical differentiation of sarcomatoid mesotheliomas from other spindle cell neoplasms. Am J Clin Pathol 1989; 92(5):566–571.
7. Hinterberger M, Reineke T, Storz M, et al. D2-40 and calretinin—a tissue microarray analysis of 341 malignant mesotheliomas with emphasis on sarcomatoid differentiation. Mod Pathol 2007; 20(2):248–255.

8. Mangano WE, Cagle PT, Churg A, et al. The diagnosis of desmoplastic malignant mesothelioma and its distinction from fibrous pleurisy: a histologic and immunohistochemical analysis of 31 cases including p53 immunostaining. Am J Clin Pathol 1998; 110(2):191–199.
9. Okby NT, Travis WD. Liposarcoma of the pleural cavity: clinical and pathologic features of 4 cases with a review of the literature. Arch Pathol Lab Med 2000; 124(5):699–703.
10. Al-Daraji WI, Salman WD, Nakhuda Y, et al. Primary smooth muscle tumor of the pleura: a clinicopathological case report with ultrastructural observations and a review of the literature. Ultrastruct Pathol 2005; 29(5):389–398.
11. Crotty EJ, McAdams HP, Erasmus JJ, et al. Epithelioid hemangioendothelioma of the pleura: clinical and radiologic features. AJR Am J Roentgenol 2000; 175(6):1545–1549.
12. Suster S. Primary sarcomas of the lung. Semin Diagn Pathol 1995; 12(2):140–157.
13. Zhang PJ, Livolsi VA, Brooks JJ. Malignant epithelioid vascular tumors of the pleura: report of a series and literature review. Hum Pathol 2000; 31(1):29–34.
14. Aboulafia DM. The epidemiologic, pathologic, and clinical features of AIDS-associated pulmonary Kaposi's sarcoma. Chest 2000; 117(4):1128–1145.
15. Andino L, Cagle PT, Murer B, et al. Pleuropulmonary desmoid tumors: immunohistochemical comparison with solitary fibrous tumors and assessment of beta-catenin and cyclin D1 expression. Arch Pathol Lab Med 2006; 130(10):1503–1509.
16. Wilson RW, Gallateau-Salle F, Moran CA. Desmoid tumors of the pleura: a clinicopathologic mimic of localized fibrous tumor. Mod Pathol 1999; 12(1):9–14.
17. Pinkard NB, Wilson RW, Lawless N, et al. Calcifying fibrous pseudotumor of pleura. A report of three cases of a newly described entity involving the pleura. Am J Clin Pathol 1996; 105(2): 189–194.
18. Erasmus JJ, McAdams HP, Patz EF Jr., et al. Calcifying fibrous pseudotumor of pleura: radiologic features in three cases. J Comput Assist Tomogr 1996; 20(5):763–765.
19. Askin FB, Rosai J, Sibley RK, et al. Malignant small cell tumor of the thoracopulmonary region in childhood: a distinctive clinicopathologic entity of uncertain histogenesis. Cancer 1979; 43(6): 2438–2451.
20. Askin FB, Perlman EJ. Neuroblastoma and peripheral neuroectodermal tumors. Am J Clin Pathol 1998; 109(4 suppl 1):S23–S30.
21. Parkash V, Gerald WL, Parma A, et al. Desmoplastic small round cell tumor of the pleura. Am J Surg Pathol 1995; 19(6):659–665.
22. Syed S, Haque AK, Hawkins HK, et al. Desmoplastic small round cell tumor of the lung. Arch Pathol Lab Med 2002; 126(10):1226–1228.
23. Priest JR, McDermott MB, Bhatia S, et al. Pleuropulmonary blastoma: a clinicopathologic study of 50 cases. Cancer 1997; 80(1):147–161.
24. Priest JR, Hill DA, Williams GM, et al. Type I pleuropulmonary blastoma: a report from the International Pleuropulmonary Blastoma Registry. J Clin Oncol 2006; 24(27):4492–4498.

37
Biphasic Neoplasms of the Lung and Pleura

MARY BETH BEASLEY
Mount Sinai Medical Center, New York, New York, U.S.A.

PHILIP S. HASLETON
Clinical Sciences Block, Manchester Royal Infirmary, Manchester, U.K.

I. Introduction

Biphasic tumors of the lung and pleura overlap considerably with the spindle cell neoplasms discussed in chapter 36, although there are some unique tumors in this category. In many cases, the incidence of biphasic tumor morphology increases with the number of sections taken.

Most biphasic pulmonary tumors do not pose a considerable diagnostic burden on the pathologist, except for malignant pleural mesothelioma. Biphasic tumors typically consist of a mixture of histologically identifiable "epithelial" and "mesenchymal" elements, which in most tumors are thought to represent divergent differentiation of a single cell type.

The World Health Organization (WHO) classification of pulmonary tumors divides sarcomatoid carcinoma into the subtypes of pleomorphic carcinoma, spindle cell carcinoma, giant cell carcinoma, carcinosarcoma, and pulmonary blastoma (1). Spindle cell carcinoma is covered in chapter 36, while pleomorphic carcinoma, carcinosarcoma, and pulmonary blastoma are discussed in this chapter. Biphasic mesothelioma (BMM) and synovial sarcoma (SS) are also covered in this chapter. Pulmonary hamartoma and certain salivary gland tumors, such as pleomorphic adenoma, may also have a biphasic morphology and are discussed in chapter 38.

II. Biphasic Tumors of the Pulmonary Parenchyma

A. Pleomorphic Carcinoma

Pleomorphic carcinoma of the lung is defined in the current WHO classification as a subtype of sarcomatoid carcinoma, which contains a spindle or giant cell component in addition to an identifiable component of squamous cell carcinoma, adenocarcinoma, or large cell carcinoma. The WHO classification recommends that the sarcomatoid or carcinomatous component comprise at least 10% of the tumor to warrant a diagnosis of pleomorphic carcinoma, but this figure is arbitrary (1).

Clinically, the average age at diagnosis for pleomorphic carcinoma is 60 years, and there is a 4:1 male to female predominance. Over 90% of these carcinomas are associated

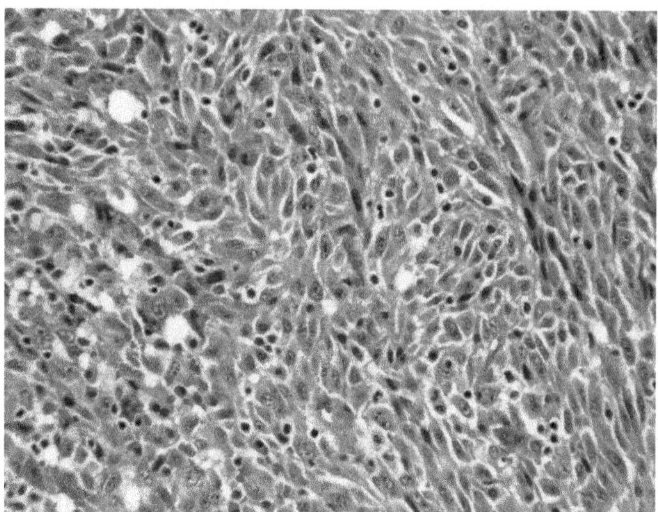

Figure 1 The spindle component of pleomorphic carcinoma typically resembles other high-grade sarcomas (H&E, 200×). *Abbreviation*: H&E, hematoxylin and eosin.

with tobacco smoking. They typically present as a large peripheral mass but may occur centrally up to 20% of tumors may be asymptomatic (1,2).

The spindle cells of pleomorphic carcinoma are overtly malignant and are arranged in a haphazard fascicular or storiform pattern (Fig. 1). The cells are usually fairly pleomorphic and have easily identifiable mitoses, although they may sometimes have a comparatively uniform appearance. Necrosis is frequently a feature. The carcinomatous component will appear the same as conventional pulmonary squamous cell carcinoma, adenocarcinoma, or large cell carcinoma (Fig. 2) (2). A component of giant cell carcinoma may also be observed, comprised of large multinucleate giant cells, which have a propensity to be associated with numerous neutrophils (Fig. 3) (1). When an identifiable epithelial component is present, the diagnosis is readily apparent and does not require immunohistochemical stains. Difficulties may arise if only the sarcomatoid component is present on a small biopsy. Expression of epithelial markers, such as keratin or epithelial membrane antigen (EMA), support a diagnosis of sarcomatoid carcinoma in the presence of an intraparenchymal lung mass. Keratin staining may be focal and may require the use of multiple markers to demonstrate positivity (2,3). On a small biopsy, it may be impossible to demonstrate keratin staining. For this reason, a sarcomatoid carcinoma cannot be excluded in a keratin-negative spindle cell malignancy occurring in a clinical setting otherwise typical for lung cancer. It should be noted that keratin and EMA are both positive in mesothelioma, and "mesothelial" markers may be of limited help in the pleomorphic or sarcomatoid variant. For this reason, correlation with the radiographic findings is always prudent in the situation of a keratin-positive spindle or biphasic tumor encountered on a lung biopsy.

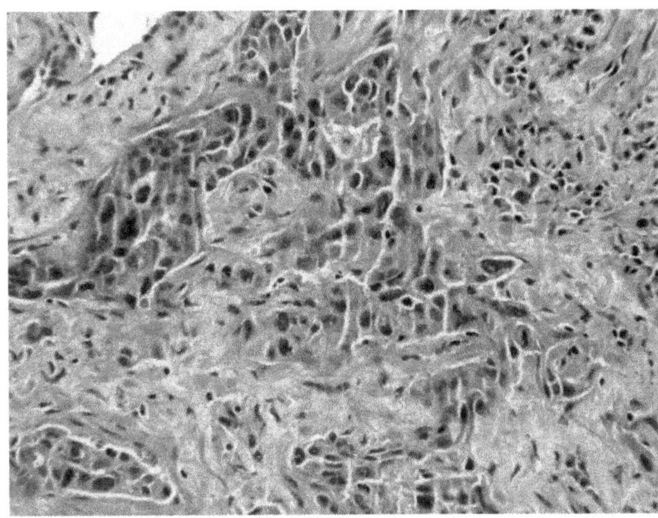

Figure 2 The carcinomatous component of pleomorphic carcinoma consists of otherwise typical appearing squamous cell carcinoma, large cell carcinoma, or, as demonstrated in this example, adenocarcinoma (H&E, 200×). *Abbreviation*: H&E, hematoxylin and eosin.

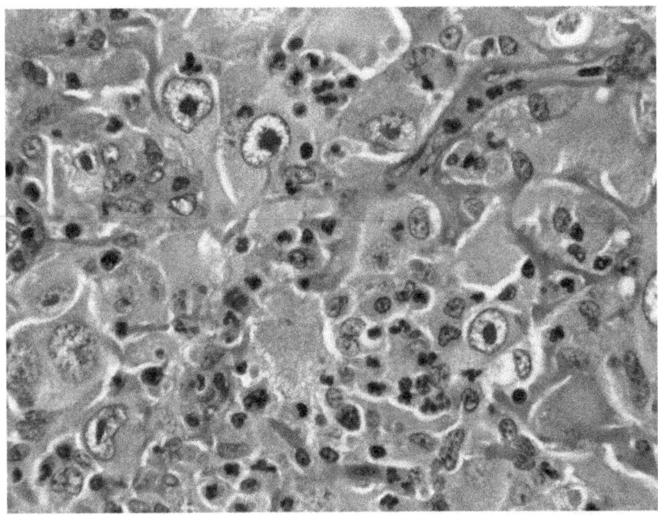

Figure 3 Giant cell carcinoma is composed of extremely large bizarre-appearing tumor cells, which frequently exhibit neutrophilic emperipolesis (H&E, 200×). *Abbreviation*: H&E, hematoxylin and eosin.

B. Carcinosarcoma

The WHO defines carcinosarcoma as a tumor with a mixture of carcinomatous and sarcomatous elements, in which the sarcomatous elements also show heterologous differentiation, such as malignant bone, cartilage, or skeletal muscle (1). The retention of the carcinosarcoma nomenclature, distinct from spindle cell/pleomorphic carcinoma, is largely academic as there is no difference in prognosis for these high-grade tumors. Mesenchymal differentiation may be detected via immunohistochemical methods or by electron microscopy; however, the view taken in this chapter mirrors the WHO definition and restricts a diagnosis of carcinosarcoma to tumors with heterologous elements identified by light microscopy rather than with immunohistochemistry. Some non-small cell lung cancers (NSCLC), without a sarcomatoid pattern, can stain positively for mesenchymal markers. Thus, special stains can confuse the diagnoses.

Carcinosarcomas are usually endobronchial and polypoid and seen most commonly in male smokers. They may also be well-demarcated lobulated masses. The cut surface is gray or white with hemorrhage or necrosis.

The carcinomatous component of carcinosarcoma may consist of squamous cell carcinoma, adenocarcinoma, or large cell carcinoma, with squamous cell being most frequent. The sarcomatoid component consists of plump, overtly malignant pleomorphic spindled cells, identical to those in pleomorphic carcinoma. Carcinosarcomas, by definition, will show heterologous differentiation, most frequently in the form of malignant cartilage, bone, or skeletal muscle formation (Figs. 4 and 5). The diagnosis is usually made on morphologic grounds and does not require immunohistochemical stains. Similar to pleomorphic carcinoma, the spindle component of carcinosarcoma may be positive for cytokeratin, although weak or focal in many cases. Positive cytokeratin staining in the setting of

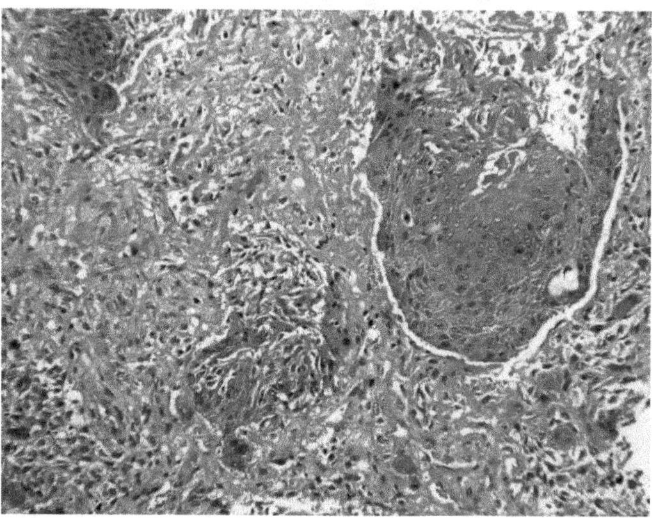

Figure 4 Carcinosarcoma demonstrating squamous cell carcinoma admixed with a malignant mesenchymal component showing osteoid formation (H&E, 200×). *Abbreviation*: H&E, hematoxylin and eosin.

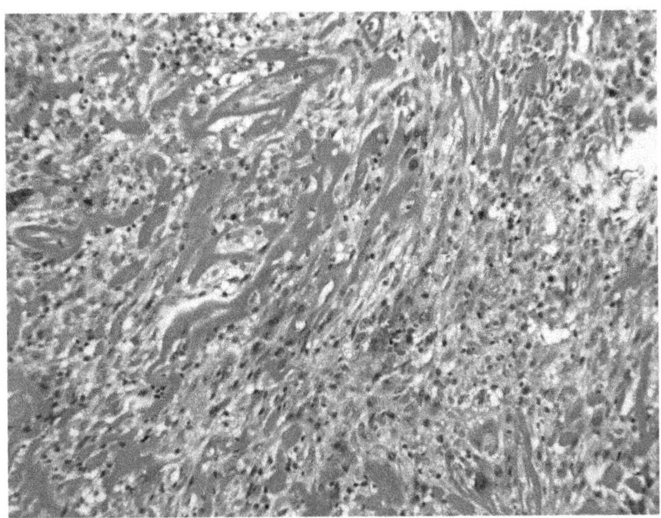

Figure 5 Carcinosarcoma. By definition, the mesenchymal component of carcinosarcoma must contain identifiable heterologous differentiation, in this case exemplified by prominent osteoid formation (H&E, 200×). *Abbreviation*: H&E, hematoxylin and eosin.

a pulmonary mass lesion showing malignant chondroid or osteoid should be regarded as evidence of carcinosarcoma. Evaluation of the radiographic distribution of disease is important as mesothelioma may also show heterologous differentiation and positive staining for cytokeratin as discussed below.

C. Pulmonary Blastoma

Pulmonary blastoma is a tumor found in adults and typically presents as a large mass lesion. Pulmonary blastoma is a biphasic tumor containing a primitive epithelial component resembling the pseudoglandular phase of fetal lung admixed with a primitive mesenchymal stroma. The two components (epithelial and mesenchymal) are present to varying degrees. When a tumor consists of only the glandular component, it is classified as well-differentiated fetal adenocarcinoma (WDFA) which is considered a subtype of adenocarcinoma. Tumors consisting of only the mesenchymal component typically occur as pleural tumors in the pediatric population and are termed "pleuro-pulmonary blastoma" (1). It is essential to sample a WDFA well, since it may contain blastomatous areas, altering the prognosis.

The glandular component of pulmonary blastoma consists of well-differentiated tubules lined by columnar epithelium with varying degrees of stratification. Perinuclear vacuoles are generally visible, imparting an "endometrioid" appearance to the glands. Nuclei are typically hyperchromatic, oval, and relatively uniform and cytoplasm is eosinophilic to clear (Fig. 6). Morule formation may also be present (Fig. 7). The mesenchymal component, as the name implies, has a primitive blastemous appearance and a "small blue cell pattern." The cells tend to condense around the glandular component. The mesenchymal component may occasionally contain elements of chondrosarcoma,

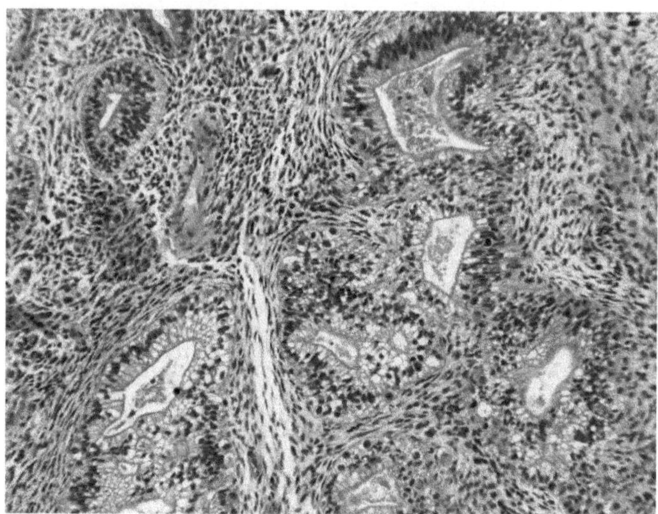

Figure 6 Pulmonary blastoma consists of an embryonic-appearing glandular component exhibiting perinuclear vacuoles admixed with a primitive mesenchymal stromal component (H&E, 100×). *Abbreviation*: H&E, hematoxylin and eosin.

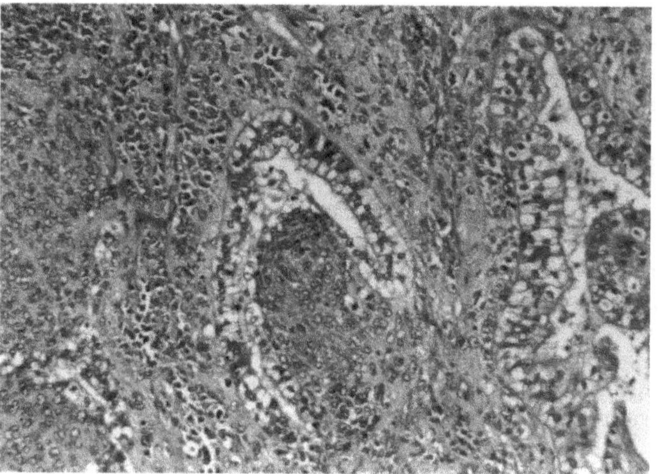

Figure 7 Pulmonary blastoma with a central morula and acini with clear cytoplasm (H&E, 313×). *Abbreviation*: H&E, hematoxylin and eosin.

osetosarcoma (Fig. 8), or rarely rhabdomyosarcoma. The diagnosis of pulmonary blastoma is typically made histologically, and immunohistochemical studies are of limited use. The glandular component is positive for epithelial markers, and morules may also be positive for neuroendocrine markers. The mesenchymal component is positive for vimentin and,

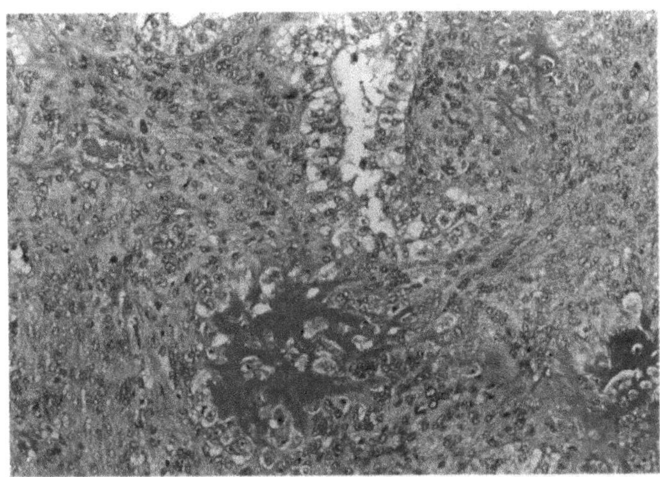

Figure 8 Pulmonary blastoma with well-marked osteoid (H&E, 313×). *Abbreviation*: H&E, hematoxylin and eosin.

depending on whether heterologous differentiation is present, may also be positive for actin, desmin, and S-100 (1).

III. Biphasic Tumors of the Pleura

A. Biphasic Mesothelioma

Biphasic Mesothelioma (BMM) is a subtype of mesothelioma, which consists of both epithelioid and a sarcomatoid components, with at least 10% of one cell type. These may be present in varying proportions, and this subtype comprises roughly 30% of mesotheliomas. The epithelioid component of BMM is identical to that in pure epithelioid mesothelioma, consisting of cuboidal or polyhedral cells with mainly regular nuclei having an open vesicular pattern with one or two nucleoli and a fairly consistent nuclear/cytoplasmic ratio (Figs. 9 and 10). The cells may be arranged in tubulopapillary structures or complex acinar patterns. Psammoma bodies may be seen. Microcystic foci with a lacelike pattern and flattened epithelioid cells may be identified (Fig. 11). Similarly, the sarcomatoid component exhibits the same range of morphologic features found in sarcomatoid mesothelioma, and may show storiform morphology or exhibit osseous or cartilaginous differentiation (Fig. 12). Desmoplastic areas may also be encountered (Fig. 13). Like pure epithelioid mesothelioma, the epithelioid component of BMM will be positive for mesothelial markers, such as calretinin, CK5/6, WT-1, and D2-40, and negative for glycoprotein markers, such as CEA, Leu-M1, MOC-31, BG-8, and BER-EP4. (BER-EP4 is, however, focally positive in 10% of epithelioid mesotheliomas and therefore undue reliance should not be placed on this marker.) The sarcomatoid component will be positive for keratin and may, in a variable percentage of cases (up to 60% depending on the study), show expression of calretinin, but staining for CK5/6 or WT-1 is rare (3–6).

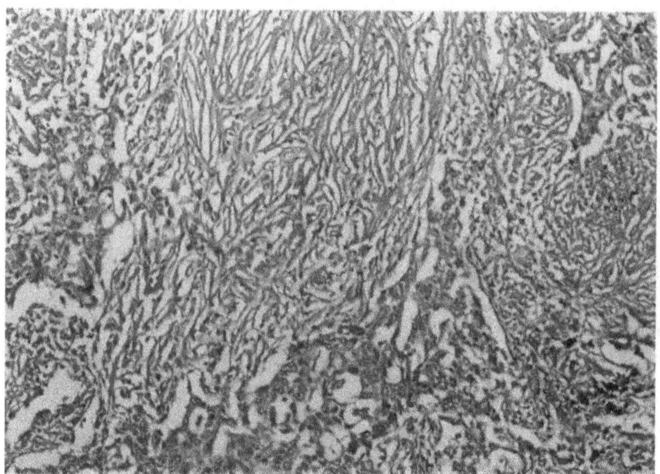

Figure 9 Biphasic pleural mesothelioma with a prominent epithelial content (H&E, 125×). *Abbreviation*: H&E, hematoxylin and eosin.

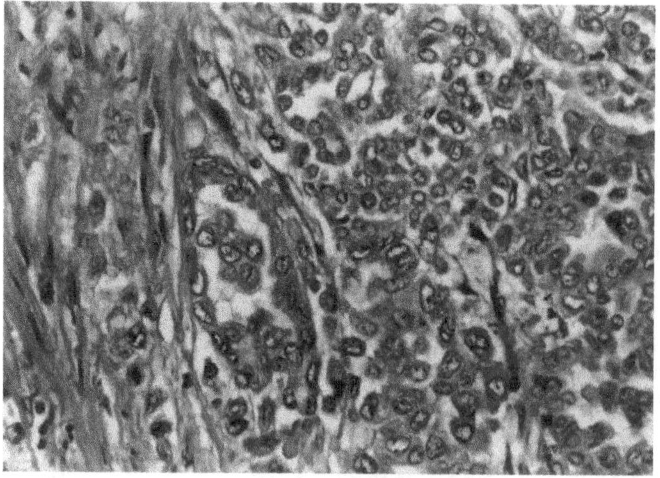

Figure 10 Epithelial content of a biphasic mesothelioma showing regular open vesicular nuclei (H&E, 313×). *Abbreviation*: H&E, hematoxylin and eosin.

B. Synovial Sarcoma

Synovial Sarcoma (SS) may occur as a primary pleural neoplasm and may produce diffuse pleural thickening, mimicking mesothelioma, but may present as a mass lesion. SS may also occur as a primary lung parenchymal tumor. Both monophasic and biphasic subtypes have been reported, with the monophasic subtype being slightly more frequent (7–9).

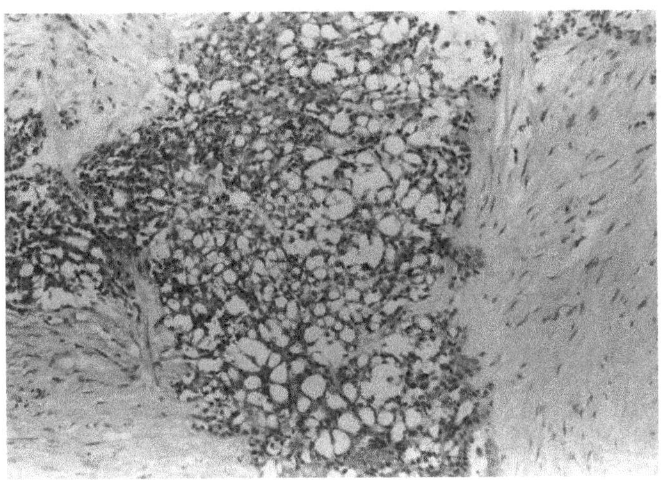

Figure 11 Microcystic focus in a mesothelioma (H&E, 125×). *Abbreviation*: H&E, hematoxylin and eosin.

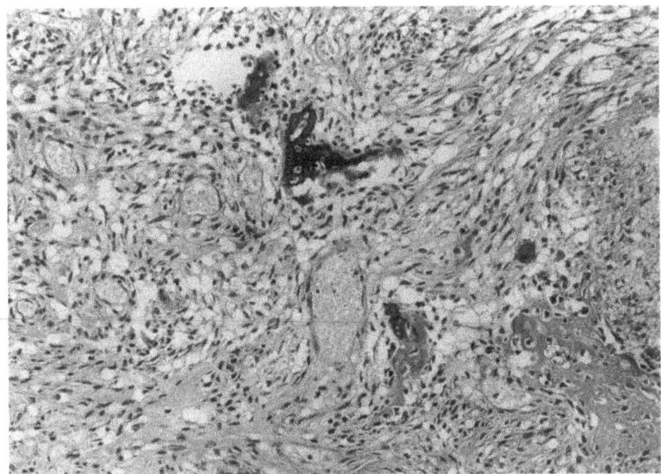

Figure 12 Pleural mesothelioma with prominent bone formation (H&E, 125×). *Abbreviation*: H&E, hematoxylin and eosin.

The spindle component of SS is typically a relatively monotonous population of hyperchromatic spindle cells with hyperchromatic nuclei. The cells are arranged in densely packed fascicles but often show alternating areas of lower cellularity, which frequently have a myxoid background (Fig. 14). A "hemangiopericytomatous" vascular pattern is often present, and there may be areas of collagenous fibrosis or calcification. The epithelial

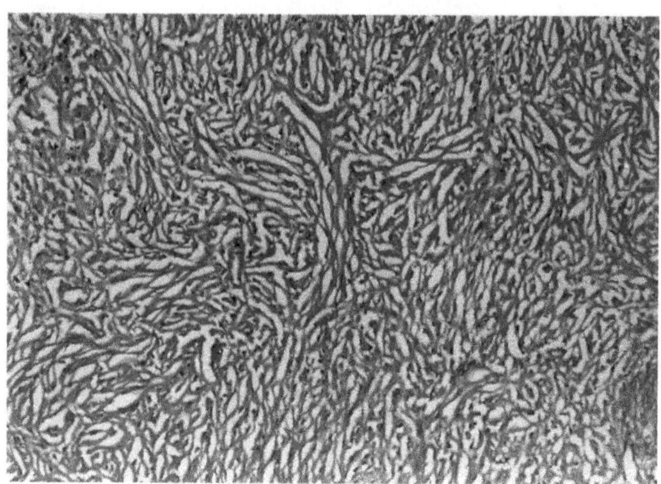

Figure 13 Storiform area in a fibrous component of a biphasic pleural mesothelioma (H&E, 125×). *Abbreviation*: H&E, hematoxylin and eosin.

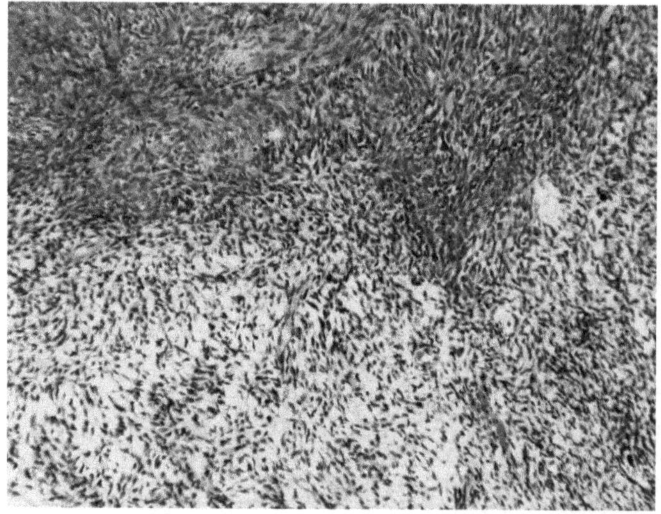

Figure 14 The spindle component of SS consists of relatively uniform hyperchromatic spindled cells with a fascicular growth pattern. Alternating areas of densely packed and hypocellular regions are often present (H&E, 100×). *Abbreviations*: SS, synovial sarcoma; H&E, hematoxylin and eosin.

component may be subtle and consists of slitlike glandular spaces lined by cuboidal cells with eosinophilic cytoplasm (Fig. 15). Mitotic activity is variable.

SS is positive for EMA and cytokeratins, including cytokeratin 7 and cytokeratin 19. This staining is better seen in the epithelial component and may be focal in the spindle component. SS is also frequently positive for calretinin, a finding causing misdiagnosis as a

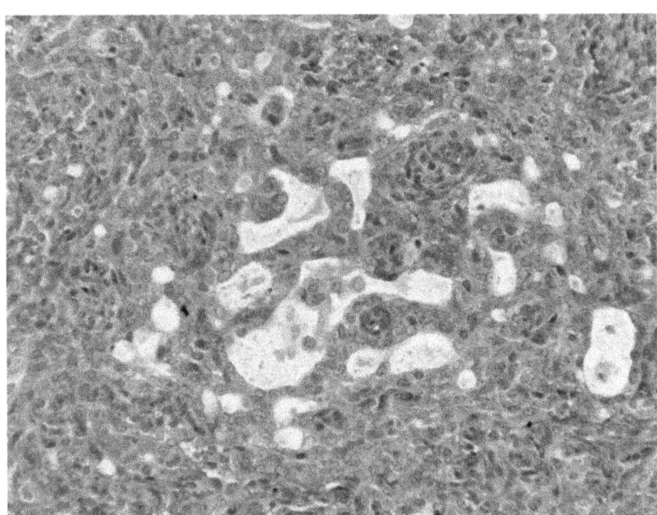

Figure 15 The epithelial component of SS consists of glandular spaces, which may be slitlike, lined by cuboidal cells (H&E, 200×). *Abbreviations*: SS, synovial sarcoma; H&E, hematoxylin and eosin.

mesothelioma, but is negative for CK 5/6 and WT-1 (9,10). SS is also positive for bcl-2, which is usually negative in mesothelioma. The spindle component of SS may be positive for S-100 and is rarely focally positive for actin and desmin. The epithelial component may contain mucinous material within glandular lumina and may show positive staining with glycoprotein markers, such as CEA or BER-EP4 (8). Molecular analysis for the t(X;18) translocation supports this diagnosis in difficult cases (11).

IV. Other Sarcomas Involving the Lung and Pleura

Other sarcomas may involve the lung and pleura as mestastses, or rarely as primary tumors. The vast majority of sarcomas are keratin negative, and thus immunohistochemical studies typically separate most sarcomas from sarcomatoid or biphasic carcinoma or mesothelioma. Certain sarcomas may however express cytokeratins, either consistently or with a high degree of frequency, which creates difficulties in this discrimination. The main sarcomas that express cytokeratins and involve the lung or pleura with any regularity are synovial sarcoma (discussed above) and vascular sarcomas (discussed in chapter 36). Others include epithelioid sarcoma, leiomyosarcoma, primitive neuroectodermal tumor (PNET), and chordoma. Epithelioid sarcoma is classically keratin positive and may involve the lung or pleura as a metastasis. Approximately half of all epithelioid sarcomas will stain with CD34, which is a helpful feature absent of appropriate clinical information regarding a previous soft tissue diagnosis (12). Leiomyosarcoma may also involve the lung and pleura secondarily or rarely as a primary pleural tumor (13). Epithelioid morphology may occasionally be encountered, imparting a biphasic appearance. Keratin staining in leiomyosarcomas, when present, is usually focal, in contrast to the diffuse staining typically seen in biphasic/sarcomatoid mesothelioma or the epithelial component of pleomorphic carcinoma (3,5). Muscle markers such as actin, desmin, and h-caldesmon are also positive in leiomyosarcoma. These markers may also be encountered in sarcomatoid carcinomas and a significant number of sarcomatoid mesotheliomas, which is a noteworthy pitfall (6,14,15). PNET may occasionally show positive staining with cytokeratin, but the small blue cell morphology does not usually create a diagnostic dilemma with carcinoma or mesothelioma (16). Finally, chordoma, while very rare, is characteristically cytokeratin positive and not infrequently metastasizes to the lungs. While the myxoid background may lead to confusion with more common lung or pleural tumors, chordoma is characterized by large "physaliphorous" cells with multiple cytoplasmic vacuoles, reminiscent of lipoblasts. Chordomas are also typically positive for S-100 (12).

References

1. Travis WD, Brambilla E, Muller-Hermerlink HK, et al. Pathology and Genetics. Tumours of the Lung, Pleura, Thymus and Heart. Lyon, France: IARC Press, 2004.
2. Fishback NF, Travis WD, Moran CA, et al. Pleomorphic (spindle/giant cell) carcinoma of the lung. A clinicopathologic correlation of 78 cases. Cancer 1994; 73(12):2936–2945.
3. Cagle PT, Truong LD, Roggli VL, et al. Immunohistochemical differentiation of sarcomatoid mesotheliomas from other spindle cell neoplasms. Am J Clin Pathol 1989; 92(5):566–571.
4. Roggli VL, Sporn TS, Oury T. Pathology of Asbestos-Associated Diseases. 2nd ed. Berlin, Germany: Springer-Verlag, 2004.
5. Attanoos RL, Dojcinov SD, Webb R, et al. Anti-mesothelial markers in sarcomatoid mesothelioma and other spindle cell neoplasms. Histopathology 2000; 37(3):224–231.
6. Lucas DR, Pass HI, Madan SK, et al. Sarcomatoid mesothelioma and its histological mimics: a comparative immunohistochemical study. Histopathology 2003; 42(3):270–279.
7. Aubry MC, Bridge JA, Wickert R, et al. Primary monophasic synovial sarcoma of the pleura: five cases confirmed by the presence of SYT-SSX fusion transcript. Am J Surg Pathol 2001; 25(6): 776–781.
8. Gaertner E, Zeren EH, Fleming MV, et al. Biphasic synovial sarcomas arising in the pleural cavity. A clinicopathologic study of five cases. Am J Surg Pathol 1996; 20(1):36–45.
9. Nicholson AG, Goldstraw P, Fisher C. Synovial sarcoma of the pleura and its differentiation from other primary pleural tumours: a clinicopathological and immunohistochemical review of three cases. Histopathology 1998; 33(6):508–513.
10. Miettinen M, Limon J, Niezabitowski A, et al. Calretinin and other mesothelioma markers in synovial sarcoma: analysis of antigenic similarities and differences with malignant mesothelioma. Am J Surg Pathol 2001; 25(5):610–617.
11. Weinbreck N, Vignaud JM, Begueret H, et al. SYT-SSX fusion is absent in sarcomatoid mesothelioma allowing its distinction from synovial sarcoma of the pleura. Mod Pathol 2007; 20(6): 617–621.
12. Fletcher CD, Unni KK, Mertens F. World Health Organization Classification of Tumours. Pathology and Genetics. Tumours of the Soft Tissue and Bone. Lyon, France: IARC Press, 2002.
13. Moran CA, Suster S, Abbondanzo SL, et al. Primary leiomyosarcomas of the lung: a clinicopathologic and immunohistochemical study of 18 cases. Mod Pathol 1997; 10(2):121–128.
14. Comin CE, Dini S, Novelli L, et al. h-Caldesmon, a useful positive marker in the diagnosis of pleural malignant mesothelioma, epithelioid type. Am J Surg Pathol 2006; 30(4):463–469.
15. Hurlimann J. Desmin and neural marker expression in mesothelial cells and mesotheliomas. Hum Pathol 1994; 25(8):753–757.
16. Folpe AL, Goldblum JR, Rubin BP, et al. Morphologic and immunophenotypic diversity in Ewing family tumors: a study of 66 genetically confirmed cases. Am J Surg Pathol 2005; 29(8): 1025–1033.

38
Uncommon Endobronchial Neoplasms

N. PAUL OHORI
UPMC-Presbyterian, Pittsburgh, Pennsylvania, U.S.A.

I. Introduction

Primary endobronchial neoplasms arise in the large airways and produce obstructive signs and symptoms (e.g., cough, wheezing, dyspnea, hemoptysis, bronchiectasis, atelectasis, hyperinflation, mediastinal shift, pneumonia). They are much less common than metastases; therefore, integration of the clinical information (especially the history of previous neoplasms and radiographical imaging studies) with the histomorphology and ancillary studies is important in arriving at the correct diagnosis. Endobronchial neoplasms are often visible and amenable to fine needle aspiration or biopsy through a bronchoscope. Most benign neoplasms are slow growing, while malignant neoplasms are variable in their growth rate. In evaluating these neoplasms, it is important to be aware that the histological features of many of the neoplasms discussed in this chapter are not unique to the lung or bronchial tree. Therefore, clinical correlation is important in excluding the possibility of metastasis.

II. Epithelial Neoplasms

Historically, the term "adenoma of the bronchus" was applied to what we know today as carcinoid tumors and adenoid cystic carcinoma (AdCC) (1). Carcinoid tumors are the most common bronchial neoplasm and are recognized as neuroendocrine neoplasms, discussed in Chapter 34. The remaining neoplasms are those of epithelial, mixed epithelial-mesenchymal, mesenchymal, or other differentiation. Among the epithelial type neoplasms, those of salivary gland type [e.g., AdCC, mucoepidermoid carcinoma (MEC)] are more common than those of surface epithelial type (e.g., squamous papilloma, basal cell adenoma/carcinoma) (Table 1).

A. Adenoid Cystic Carcinoma

Like its counterpart in the salivary gland, bronchial AdCC is a slow-growing, well-differentiated adenocarcinoma (2,3). While they are the most common salivary gland type neoplasm in the lung, they comprise less than 0.2% of all primary lung neoplasms (4). They are more common in women and in nonsmokers (5). AdCC usually grows as an exophytic, endobronchial, tan, soft, well-circumscribed mass in the lower trachea or mainstem bronchus, infiltrates into the adjacent bronchial wall, and demonstrates perineural invasion. Due

Table 1 Epithelial Endobronchial Neoplasms

Neoplasm	Gross features	Microscopical features	Special studies	DDx	References
AdCC	Exophytic (polypoid, intraluminal) or endophytic, soft, tan, well circumscribed, 0.9–4 cm	Cribriform, tubular, solid	S100+ Actin+ CAM 5.2+ CD117+	Metastatic AdCC, adenocarcinoma, small cell carcinoma, basal cell carcinoma, pleomorphic adenoma	2–7
MEC	Exophytic, with smooth or papillary contours, soft, cytic, solid and mucoid, 0.6–6.0 cm	Low grade: abundant mucinous cysts with sheets of epidermoid areas High grade: sheets of intermediate cells giving an epidermoid appearance	PAS+ D/PAS+ Mucicarmine+	Adenosquamous carcinoma, MGA, mucinous cystadenoma, cystadenocarcinoma, squamous cell carcinoma, mucin-producing adenocarcinoma	8–11
MGA	Exophytic or endophytic with growth above the cartilaginous plates, 2–6.5 cm	Tubular, papillary, cystic	PAS+ Mucicarmine+	Mucinous cystadenoma, low-grade MEC	12–16
ACC	Exophytic, well circumscribed, tan-white, soft to rubbery, 1.2–4 cm; others may be intraparenchymal	Solid sheets of acinar cells with granular basophilic cytoplasm; some microacinar or papillocystic structures may be present	PAS+ D/PAS+ Mucicarmine +/– CAM 5.2+ EMA+ S100– Chromogranin–	"Sugar" tumor, oncocytoma, oncocytic carcinoid, granular cell tumor, primary and metastatic clear cell carcinoma	17–21
EMC	Exophytic, white, nonencapsulated, 2–2.5 cm	Myoepithelioma: sheets of spindle-shaped myoepithelial cells EMC: tubules and cysts of epithelial cells surrounded by clear myoepithelial cells and compact masses of myoepithelial cells	Epithelial cells: Cytokeratin+ S100– Actin– Myoepithelial cells: Cytokeratin– S100+ Actin+	AdCC, pleomorphic adenoma, "sugar" tumor	22–27

Squamous papilloma	Exophytic, papillary, and endophytic into bronchial wall; often multiple and may show extensive spread along airways	Nonkeratinizing or minimally keratizing squamous epithelial proliferation; not invasive	HPV+ by immunohistochemistry and/or in situ hybridization	Squamous cell carcinoma, benign reactive squamous metaplastic reactions	28–31
Basaloid carcinoma	Exophytic, endobronchial tumors, 1–6 cm	Lobular growth of small cells surrounded by a rim of palisading oval basal cells; high mitotic count	Chromogranin– Synaptophysin– Mucicarmine –	Carcinoid, poorly differentiated squamous cell carcinoma, solid variant of AdCC	32–34
Sarcomatoid carcinoma	Polypoid endobronchial tumors, average 6 cm	Spindle cell proliferation with/without heterologous features such as rhabdoid, chondroid, or osteoid differentiation	Cytokeratin+ Desmin+/– Actin+/–	Sarcoma, melanoma	35

Abbreviations: DDx, differential diagnosis; AdCC, adenoid cystic carcinema; MEC, mucoepidermoid carcinoma; PAS, periodic acid–Schiff; MGA, mucous gland adenoma; ACC, acinic cell carcinomas; D/PAS, diastase-digested PAS; EMA, epithelial membrane antigen; EMC, epithelial-myoepithelial carcinoma; HPV, human papillomavirus.

to the submucosal location, the overlying epithelial is often smooth and intact. Therefore, tissue diagnosis requires invasive procedures such as fine needle aspiration or bronchial biopsy (6). Among the histological patterns—cribriform, tubular, and solid—the cribriform pattern is most common and the solid pattern is the least common pattern. As a reflection of its slow-growing behavior, usually no mitosis, necrosis, or angiolymphatic invasion is seen. The cribriform structures show the typical intraluminal hyaline basement membrane material. AdCCs with a predominantly solid pattern are poorly differentiated and tend to be larger, with more extensive extraluminal growth, necrosis, nuclear atypia, and prominent nucleoli. Fine needle aspiration or bronchial biopsy of the solid component results in a wide differential diagnosis and the final diagnosis of AdCC may be achieved only by complete resection of the neoplasm that shows focal areas of the more typical low-grade cribriform and tubular patterns.

Immunohistochemically, the neoplastic cells of most cases mark with CAM 5.2. Immunostains for S100 and actin are less sensitive but more specific in marking the neoplastic cells. While not a specific marker, CD117 (c-kit) is positive in the vast majority of cases. Staining by the proliferation marker, Ki-67 does not correlate with the grade of the neoplasm (5) unless the neoplasm shows dedifferentiated areas (7).

The differential diagnosis of pulmonary AdCC includes metastasis from a head and neck site, conventional adenocarcinoma, small cell carcinoma, and basal cell carcinoma. Since the histomorphology is not site specific, the distinction of a primary AdCC from a metastasis requires clinical correlation with the history of previous salivary gland neoplasms and radiological imaging studies of the chest. Distinction of AdCC from conventional adenocarcinoma in the endobronchial location is based on the recognition of the characteristic cribriform growth pattern of AdCC and the intraluminal basement membrane type material. The glands of AdCC are relatively monotonous and the neoplastic cells demonstrating the cribriform pattern appear "rigid." AdCC with a predominantly solid growth pattern may be difficult to distinguish from other "small cell" neoplasms. The key features are the lack of a "salt-and-pepper" chromatin pattern, mitoses, individual cell necrosis, and nuclear molding in AdCC. It is important to recognize that the characteristic growth patterns (cribriform and tubular) are found at least focally in AdCC.

B. Mucoepidermoid Carcinoma

After AdCC, MEC is the second most common bronchial neoplasm (8,9). Grossly, these are exophytic and polypoid, and endobronchial lesions with solid and cystic areas. The defining criteria for a bronchial MEC include origin in the conducting airways, evidence of squamous differentiation with intermediate cells, and evidence of glandular differentiation. The proportion of the components may differ greatly and the types of cells include basaloid, intermediate (transitional), squamous, clear, nonmucinous columnar, and mucin-producing goblet cells. In most series, the majority of MECs are low-grade neoplasms with predominance of the glandular component. This is particularly true in the pediatric population where conservative resection is recommended (10).

The main issues regarding the histopathological diagnosis of MEC are distinguishing low-grade from high-grade tumors and differentiating MEC from other non–small cell carcinomas, particularly adenosquamous carcinoma. The subclassification of low- and high-grade MECs is based on mitotic count, necrosis, and nuclear pleomorphism. Low-grade MECs often exhibit glandular and cystic growth patterns as the predominant

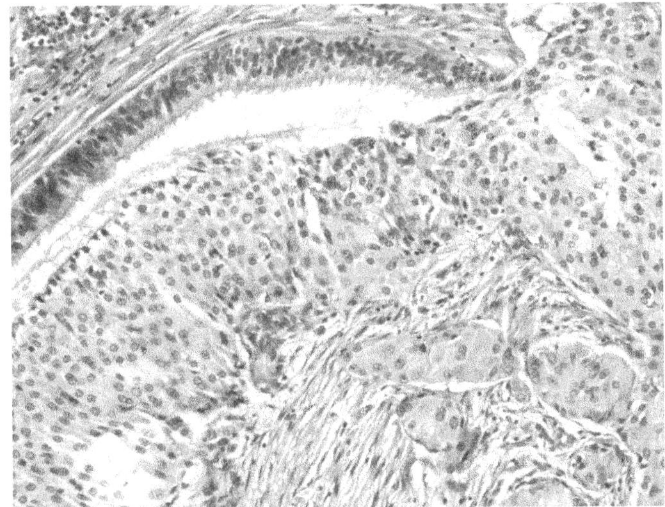

Figure 1 Like its counterpart in the salivary glands, endobronchial mucoepidermoid carcinoma is often composed of intermediate cells and epidermoid cells.

components (Fig. 1). On the other hand, high-grade MECs have more solid areas consisting of squamoid and intermediate cells that invade into the adjacent pulmonary parenchyma. Necrosis, high mitotic count (greater than 4 per 10 high-power fields), and atypical mitotic figures are seen only in high-grade MECs.

The distinction between MEC (particularly high-grade MEC) and adenosquamous carcinoma may be difficult, since both tumors exhibit glandular and epidermoid differentiation. However, MECs are typically centrally located, exophytic endobronchial tumors with an admixture of solid, sheet-like, and glandular areas and transitional areas. They lack changes of in situ squamous cell carcinoma. Foci of low-grade MEC are often identified if sampled adequately. By contrast, adenosquamous carcinomas are often peripheral tumors associated with scars and derived from terminal bronchioles. The distinction may be somewhat academic, since high-grade MECs are often localized stage I neoplasms with a prognosis comparable to that of other non–small cell carcinomas of the same stage.

Recently, pulmonary MEC with a prominent lymphoplasmacytic component has been described. With the heavy lymphoplasmacytic infiltrate, there is accompanying multinucleated giant cells and clear cell change. The differential diagnosis includes inflammatory myofibroblastic tumor, lymphoma, mucous gland adenoma (MGA), and other lesions with a lymphoid component. When carefully searched, areas of more typical MEC are identified in these neoplasms (11).

C. Mucous Gland Adenoma

In contrast to the two endobronchial neoplasms above, MGA is a benign neoplasm and does not have a counterpart in the salivary gland (12–14). By definition, MGAs are exophytic cystic neoplasms arising above the level of the cartilaginous plates. The constituent cells resemble normal mucous glands of the bronchus (cuboidal, columnar, and goblet cells). The solid pattern of intermediate (transitional) cells seen in MECs is not appreciated. Grossly, MGAs are solitary, soft to firm, exophytic polypoid endobronchial neoplasms ranging from 2 to 6.5 cm. On cut section, these neoplasms are mostly solid, with small cysts containing gelatinous material. Histologically, the cysts are composed of a coalescence of microacini, tubules, and glands. Within some cysts, papillary structures are apparent. The lining cells range from cuboidal to tall columnar with varying mucin content. Nuclear pleomorphism is minimal and nucleoli are small and inconspicuous. Mitotic figures are rare. The intraluminal mucinous material may be stained with periodic acid–Schiff (PAS) with and without diastase and mucicarmine. The immunohistochemical profile of MGA is similar to that of non-neoplastic bronchial glands. Immunostains for cytokeratin, epithelial membrane antigen (EMA), and carcinoembryonic antigen are positive in most cases. However, these markers are not helpful in distinguishing MGA from other endobronchial lesions in the differential diagnosis.

Endobronchial neoplasms that are most often considered in the differential diagnosis of MGA include MEC, mucinous cystadenoma, and inflammatory myofibroblastic tumor. The key features used in distinguishing MGAs from MECs are the lack of intermediate cells and squamous cell differentiation in the former. In contrast to MGA, mutinous cystadenoma is not an endobronchial neoplasm but arises beneath the bronchus and is composed of macrocysts predominantly lined by columnar mucin-secreting cells (15,16). However, the mucinous material of mucinous cystadenomas may dissect into the bronchial lumen. With adequate sampling, the relationship of MGA to a bronchus can be observed. MGAs with a rich lymphoplasmacytic component may resemble inflammatory myofibroblastic tumors. Indeed, upon focal sampling, an MGA rich in inflammatory cells may be difficult to distinguish from an inflammatory myofibroblastic tumor. The distinction depends on identifying the characteristic features of MGA, consisting of the small cystic glands, tubules, and microacini. In other cases, inflammatory cell infiltration may also produce an appearance similar to that of Warthin's tumor. In contrast to Warthin's tumor, uniform oncocytic epithelial cell changes are lacking in MGA. Interestingly, a bona fide case of Warthin's tumor has not yet been reported in the lung.

D. Acinic Cell Carcinoma (Fechner Tumor)

Acinic cell carcinomas (ACCs) are rare pulmonary neoplasms that are histologically similar to their counterparts in the salivary glands (17–19). Fewer than 20 cases have been reported in the literature. In general, they are low-grade malignant neoplasms that occasionally show lymph node metastasis or recurrence (20,21). Distant metastasis has not been reported. Endobronchial ACCs are well-circumscribed, tan-white, soft to rubbery nodules covered by a smooth mucosal surface. Histologically, the predominant growth pattern is solid with sheets of cells that may be divided into discrete nests by bands of fibrous tissue. In addition to solid growth, foci of acinar, microcystic, or papillocystic patterns may be seen. The cells constituting ACCs are polygonal with basophilic granular to clear cytoplasm and small, round, eccentrically placed nuclei. Nucleoli are inconspicuous. Histochemical findings are variable; the neoplastic cells may or may not stain with PAS, diastase-digested PAS (D/PAS), or mucicarmine. Ultrastructural studies demonstrate the abundance of electron-dense zymogen granules.

Immunohistochemical profile on ACC demonstrates positivity with cytokeratin, CAM 5.2, and EMA. Immunostains for S100, chromogranin, and vimentin are negative.

These features may assist in the distinction of ACCs from other neoplasms, including "sugar" tumor, oncocytic carcinoid, oncocytoma, granular cell tumor, primary clear cell carcinoma of the lung, and metastatic clear cell carcinoma (particularly from the kidney). Sugar tumors and granular cell tumors demonstrate S100-positivity and sugar tumors are further distinguished by their HMB45-positivity. Oncocytomas show an intensely eosinophilic cytoplasm and ultrastructurally demonstrate abundant intracytoplasmic mitochondria. The clear cell areas of ACCs may appear similar to clear cell carcinomas (primary or metastatic) at low-power examination. However, clear cell carcinomas characteristically harbor pleomorphic nuclei with prominent nucleoli. The nuclei of ACCs are small, round, and bland with inconspicuous nucleoli.

E. Epithelial-Myoepithelial Carcinoma

Primary endobronchial neoplasms with histological features of epithelial-myoepithelial carcinoma (EMC) of the salivary glands were initially reported by Hayes et al. (22) and Nistal et al. (23). To date, only 22 cases have been reported in the literature (24–27). They have been variably reported as epithelial myoepithelial tumor, adenomyoepithelioma, and EMC. Like their salivary gland counterpart, bronchial EMC is an indolent neoplasm with rare cases with distant metastases. Due to the potentially malignant behavior, the term EMC is preferred. Grossly, the tumors are white to gray, exophytic, and measure 1 to 5 cm in greatest dimension. Histologically, the base of the polypoid tumor is often between two cartilaginous rings. The neoplastic proliferation consists of epithelial cells that formed tubules and sheets of myoepithelial cells with clear cytoplasm surrounding the tubules. Like their salivary gland counterparts, the inner epithelial cells mark positively with cytokeratin and are negative for S100 and actin. In contrast, the outer myoepithelial cells are positive for S100 and actin and negative for cytokeratin. The cases that have demonstrated aggressive behavior show predominance of the spindle-cell component, high mitotic count, necrosis, and significant nuclear pleomorphism.

F. Squamous Papilloma and Invasive Papillomatosis

Endobronchial squamous papillomas are rare. They may be a part of an extensive involvement of the airways (laryngeal and tracheobronchial papillomatosis) or a primary and solitary lesion in the bronchus (28–30). Tracheolaryngeal papillomatosis occurs most commonly in the pediatric population and 2% to 4% of the cases extend down into the bronchi. These endobronchial squamous papillomas are multiple and histologically composed of nonkeratinizing or minimally keratinizing squamous epithelium. There is a strong association with human papillomavirus (HPV) serotypes 6 and 11 and some of the lesions will demonstrate koilocytic changes. While most are cytologically bland, some show atypia ranging to that of squamous-cell carcinoma in situ. Regardless of the degree of atypia, it is important to assess the lesions for evidence of parenchymal extension, which would satisfy the criterion for invasive papillomatosis. These lesions may have bland cytological features, but the extensive squamous proliferation produces morbidity by airway obstruction and alveolar filling.

Solitary squamous papillomas are much less common and occur most often in male adults in their sixth decade of life with a positive smoking history. Just as in the squamous papillomas above, it is important to assess the degree of atypia in the surface squamous cells and whether invasion is present. In situ hybridization studies have shown that HPV is involved in some but not all solitary squamous papillomas (31).

The differential diagnosis of squamous papilloma and invasive papillomatosis includes other endobronchial lesions with a squamous component. These include squamous-cell carcinoma, MEC, and neoplasms with adjacent metaplastic squamous epithelial cells. Due to the focality of diagnostic areas, endobronchial or transbronchial biopsies may not be representative (i.e., stromal or angiolymphatic invasion may be missed). Therefore, it is best to be descriptive and comment on the differential diagnosis when evaluating squamous proliferations without obvious invasion in small biopsy or cytology specimens.

G. Basaloid Carcinoma

Exophytic neoplasms lined on the surface by basaloid (transitional) cells that invade the underlying stroma are classified as basaloid carcinoma of the lung (32,33). Most of these neoplasms arise in the lobar segmental bronchial mucosa and demonstrate nodular protrusion by anastomosing cords and lobules of proliferating basal cells. At the periphery, the basal cells are radially arranged and exhibit peripheral palisading (Fig. 2). The nuclei are slightly enlarged, with moderate hyperchromasia and inconspicuous nucleoli. These changes may be focal and it is important to determine whether the basaloid features are present in throughout the neoplasm or whether these represent focal changes of a non–small cell carcinoma. The non–basal cell component may consist of squamous cell carcinoma, adenocarcinoma, or large cell carcinoma and a tumor is considered mixed when at least 60% of the neoplasm is composed of basaloid cells. While earlier reports documented the poor prognosis of basaloid carcinoma when compared to other non–small cell carcinomas, more recent studies have shown no significant difference in behavior (34).

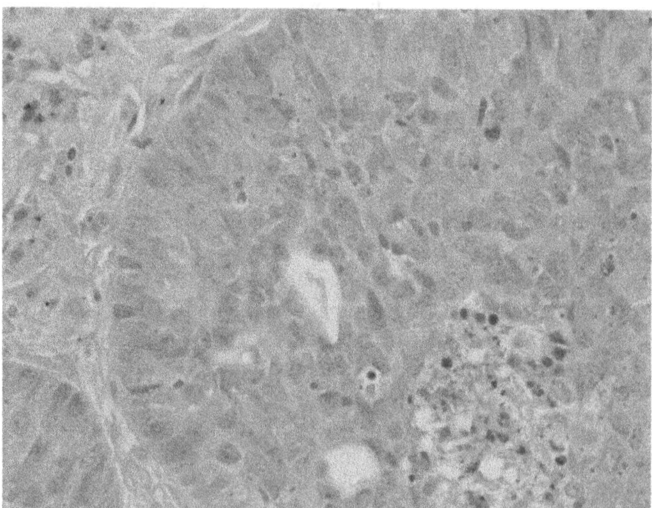

Figure 2 Basaloid carcinoma demonstrates solid growth pattern of monomorphic cells and peripheral palisading. The nuclei are moderately hyperchromatic and finely granular and show absent or occasional nucleoli.

In addition to non–small cell carcinoma with a basaloid component, other entities in the differential diagnosis include AdCC (solid component) and neuroendocrine neoplasms (small cell carcinoma, large cell neuroendocrine carcinoma, and carcinoid tumor). The solid areas of AdCC can be difficult to distinguish from basaloid carcinoma. In small biopsy samples, the high mitotic count, individual cell necrosis, lack of mucin production, and negative S100 immunoreactivity favors basaloid carcinoma over AdCC. Evidence of neuroendocrine differentiation by electron microscopy or immunohistochemistry favors a neuroendocrine neoplasm over basaloid carcinoma.

H. Sarcomatoid Carcinoma

The current "World Health Organization (WHO) Classification of Lung Tumours" defines sarcomatoid carcinoma as a group of non–small cell carcinoma with a sarcoma or sarcoma-like component (35). Depending on the degree of sarcoma or sarcoma-like differentiation, this group is further subdivided into pleomorphic carcinoma, spindle cell carcinoma, giant cell carcinoma, carcinosarcoma (CS), and pulmonary blastoma. Pleomorphic carcinoma is a non–small cell carcinoma (e.g., squamous cell carcinoma, adenocarcinoma, or large cell carcinoma) with a spindle or giant cell component (Fig. 3). Otherwise, pleomorphic carcinoma may be a carcinoma composed of spindle and giant cells only. Spindle cell carcinoma is a carcinoma composed of spindle cells only. Likewise, giant cell carcinoma is a carcinoma composed of giant cells only. Since these carcinomas are poorly differentiated, multiple keratin and EMA immunostains may be necessary to demonstrate the epithelial differentiation. Furthermore, smooth muscle markers may be coexpressed. CS and pulmonary blastoma are discussed in section III.

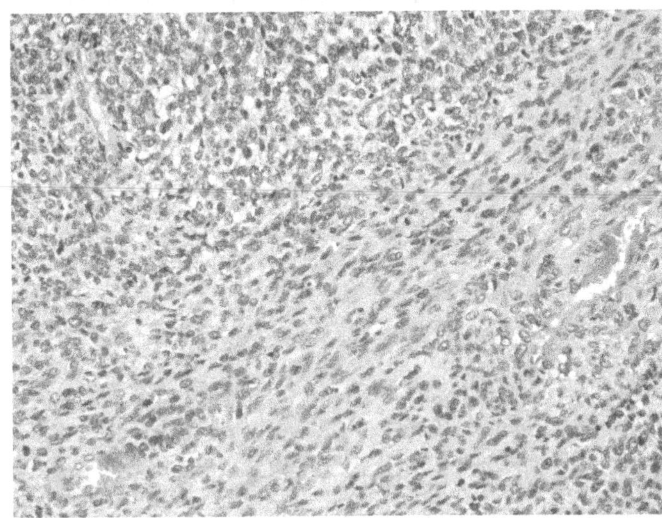

Figure 3 Pleomorphic carcinoma is a poorly differentiated non–small cell carcinoma with a spindle cell and/or giant cell component. In this case, the spindle cell component is seen in the right side of the image.

III. Neoplasms with Mixed Epithelial and Mesenchymal Components

Due to the multipotential nature of the stem cells in the lung, some pulmonary neoplasms show divergent differentiation. Whether this represents two independent clones or one cellular lineage giving rise to a subclass is an area of current investigation and debate. The epithelial and mesenchymal components may be histologically distinct from one another, or the two components may be distinguished only by the use of immunohistochemical or other ancillary studies (Table 2).

A. Pleomorphic Adenoma

Since the bronchial submucosal glands give rise to a number of salivary gland type neoplasms, it is not surprising to find pleomorphic adenomas in this region as well (36,37). Endobronchial pleomorphic adenomas are rare with morphological features that are similar to those of the more common salivary gland counterpart. They are usually soft to rubbery polypoid nodular masses ranging from 2 to 16 cm in diameter and are covered by bronchial mucosa. The cut surface is gray-white and myxoid. Three histological types of pleomorphic adenomas are recognized in the lung: classic (glandular and chondromyxoid elements), solid (predominantly myoepithelial with a myxoid background), and cytologically malignant (frank necrosis and numerous mitotic figures). However, in the case of endobronchial polypoid pleomorphic adenomas, the classic histological type is predominant. This pattern is virtually identical to the classic type of pleomorphic adenoma in the salivary gland (Fig. 4). The differential diagnosis includes other biphasic neoplasms: hamartoma, blastoma, and CS. The mesenchymal component of pleomorphic adenoma is not as well developed as in hamartomas, which contain mature chondroid elements. Furthermore, the population of myoepithelial cells is lacking in hamartomas. However, the presence of adipose tissue and osteoid has been documented in the stroma of pleomorphic adenoma (38,39). Pulmonary blastoma contains a "fetal" type of epithelium that resembles secretory epithelium of the endometrium. This feature is lacking in the glands of pleomorphic adenoma. Distinction from CS can be made by recognizing the frankly sarcomatous element, which is absent in pleomorphic adenoma. Due to the limited number of cases, the biological behavior of bronchial pleomorphic adenoma is not well characterized. Most appear to behave in a similar fashion as the salivary gland pleomorphic adenomas. However, two cases have been reported to behave aggressively. Histologically, these aggressive tumors showed infiltrative borders, poor circumscription, and high mitotic counts.

B. Hamartoma

Approximately 10% of pulmonary hamartomas are endobronchial while others are intraparenchymal (40). Regardless of the location, they usually range in size from 1 to 3 cm and are gray-white, rubbery to firm, and well demarcated. The endobronchial hamartomas are polypoid; histologically, they are composed of mature hyaline cartilage, adipose tissue, and occasionally bone. Interestingly, only 18% of endobronchial hamartomas contain a canalicular network of epithelium separating lobular cartilaginous proliferations. These benign proliferations form a spectrum from those that are predominantly cartilaginous (chondromatous) to those predominantly composed of adipocytes (lipomatous). The

Table 2 Mixed Epithelial and Mesenchymal Neoplasms

Neoplasm	Gross features	Microscopical features	Special studies	DDx	References
Pleomorphic adenoma	Exophytic and endophytic, well-circumscribed, soft to rubbery mass with a gray-white myxoid cut surface, 2–16 cm	Biphasic with glandular epithelial component and chondomyxoid stroma	CAM 5.2+ Actin+ S100+ GFAP+	Hamartoma, blastoma, CS, AdCC	36,37
Endobronchial hamartoma	Exophytic polypoid or sessile lesions with a thin pedicle	Mature hyaline cartilage, adipose tissue, bone, smooth muscle and entrapped glandular cells		Metastatic chondrosarcoma, pleomorphic adenoma	38–41
Teratoma/ teratocarcinoma	Cystic lesions with solid and extracellular debris	Three germ-cell layers represented; most common components include skin, appendages, adipose tissue, gastrointestinal and respiratory tract, thymus, pancreas, bone, cartilage, smooth muscle, and brain		CS, blastoma, hamartoma	42–44
CS	Homogeneous gray-tan mass with focal areas of necrosis and hemorrhage. Tendency to spread endobronchially	Carcinoma component: squamous cell carcinoma, adenocarcinoma, or large cell undifferentiated carcinoma. Sarcoma component: fibrosarcoma, malignant fibrous histiocytoma, other sarcoma	Cytokeratin+ Desmin+/– Actin+/–	Sarcoma, teratoma, blastoma	45–47
Pulmonary blastoma	Variegated, soft to rubbery, tan-white, and well circumscribed, 5–10 cm	Glandular component consists of endometrioid glands and the stroma consists of an adult type sarcoma	Cytokeratin+ (in glands)	Sarcoma, CS, teratoma	48–52

Abbreviations: DDx, differential diagnosis; AdCC, adenoid cystic carcinema; CS, carcinosarcoma.

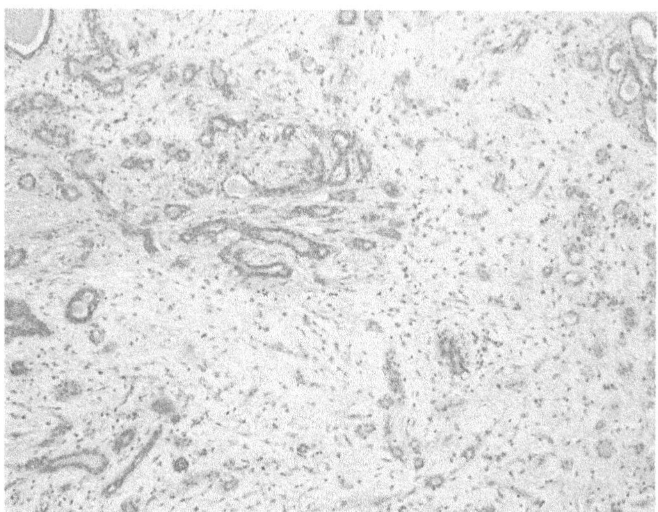

Figure 4 Endobronchial pleomorphic adenoma is similar to its salivary gland counterpart. The proliferating ductal structures are seen in the chondromyxoid stroma.

predominantly cartilaginous type of hamartoma, especially when multiple, should alert one to the possibility of Carney's syndrome (41). The differential diagnosis includes other benign, biphasic neoplasms such as pleomorphic adenoma and teratoma. As mentioned above, the cartilaginous proliferation is mature in hamartoma, whereas pleomorphic adenoma demonstrates a myxoid mesenchymal component. Representation of the three germ-cell layers is absent in hamartomas.

C. Teratoma/Teratocarcinoma

Teratomas and teratocarcinomas are rarely found in the endobronchial location (42,43). Rupture of mediastinal cystic teratomas may result in invasion into the tracheobronchial tree (44). Teratomas involving the bronchus are similar to those of other sites in that tissue from the three germinal layers is represented in the neoplasm. The types of tissues reported include pancreas, thymus, skin and adnexa, intestines, cartilage, respiratory tract, and brain. Bronchiectatic changes may be present due to the polypoid and obstructive nature of this lesion. The differential diagnosis includes other tumors that may show divergent differentiation, such as hamartomas and pulmonary blastomas.

D. Carcinosarcoma

Carcinosarcomas (CSs) may be found as an endobronchial or peripheral lung neoplasm (45–47). The majority (approximately 60%) are endobronchial or central neoplasms. Approximately 90% are amenable to surgical resection and 50% are found to be stage I. The most frequent epithelial component is squamous cell carcinoma followed by adenocarcinoma and adenosquamous carcinoma. The common sarcomatous elements are rhabdomyosarcoma, chondrosarcoma, and osteosarcoma. In the endobronchial type of CS, the carcinomatous component is usually squamous cell carcinoma, although adenocarcinoma and large cell carcinoma are sometimes encountered. Interestingly, the endobronchial CSs have a better prognosis than their peripheral counterparts. This may be related to the limited invasion of these neoplasms into the underlying submucosa.

As expected, the carcinomatous component is positive with cytokeratin and EMA immunostains. However, the finding may be very focal. In addition, since the spindle-cell (sarcomatoid) component is occasionally positive for cytokeratin, some authors prefer to categorize CSs as sarcomatoid carcinomas. However, by the current WHO criteria, sarcomatoid carcinomas do not contain such heterologous components. Entities in the differential diagnosis include primary pulmonary sarcoma [e.g., fibrosarcoma, leiomyosarcoma, rhabdomyosarcoma, osteosarcoma, chondrosarcoma, and Kaposi sarcoma (KS)], which are cytokeratin-negative or only weakly positive. Although angiosarcomas are often cytokeratin-positive, they show histological evidence of vascular differentiation (e.g., intracytoplasmic lumen formation) and are positive for endothelial markers (factor VIII, CD34, CD31) by immunostaining.

E. Pulmonary Blastoma

Pulmonary blastomas are biphasic tumors with a primitive epithelial component (resembling fetal adenocarcinoma) and a primitive mesenchymal component with a blastematous mesenchymal component that may show rhabdomyosarcomatous, smooth muscle, or chondroid differentiation (48). Approximately 20% of pulmonary blastomas demonstrate involvement of small or large airways and may present as endobronchial masses (49–52). A prospective biopsy or cytology diagnosis may be difficult. Their distinction from other non–small cell carcinomas can be made by the recognition of the immature fetal type of glandular epithelium with clear cytoplasmic vacuoles.

IV. Mesenchymal Neoplasms

Primary mesenchymal endobronchial neoplasms are much less common than epithelial neoplasms. The diagnosis of soft tissue neoplasms has been influenced by the advent of electron microscopy, immunohistochemistry, cytogenetics, and molecular analysis. Primary sarcomas do occur in the lung and may occasionally present as endobronchial lesions. As discussed earlier, the first step in making this diagnosis is to obtain a thorough clinical history to rule out the possibility of a metastatic process. Regarding the histopathological assessment of primary soft tissue neoplasms, three major issues confront the diagnostic pathologist: (1) Where is the tumor's primary site? (2) What type or types of differentiation are evident? and (3) Is it benign or malignant? (Table 3).

A. Granular Cell Tumor

Approximately 6% to 10% of all granular cell tumors arise in the tracheobronchial system (53–57). Most of these present as endobronchial plaques or polypoid masses partially or completely occluding the central and peripheral airway lumen. Patients often present with atelectasis, recurrent pneumonia, and other obstructive symptoms. Up to 20% of them are

Table 3 Mesenchymal Endobronchial Neoplasms

Neoplasm	Gross features	Microscopical features	Special studies	DDx	References
Granular cell tumor	Soft to rubbery, tan-gray, and limited to the bronchial wall, 2–6 cm	Monotonous population of large polygonal cells with granular cytoplasm and eccentrically placed small nuclei; infiltrates among submucosal glands	S100+ PAS+ Alcian blue+	Mycobacterial infection, malakoplakia, Whipple's disease	53–57
Lipoma	Soft, exophytic polypoid intrabronchial lesion	Vascularized mature adipose tissue, as in other soft tissue lipomas		Teratoma, hamartoma	(58–61)
Hemangioma	Small, soft, pinhead-sized (1 mm) lesion	Cavernous with thrombosis or recanalization	Factor VIII+ CD34+ CD31+	Pyogenic granuloma	62,63
Peripheral nerve sheath tumors	Small, submucosal nodules, 0.2 cm	Compact bundles of spindle cells with nuclear palisading	S100+ Electron microscopy showing interdigitating cell processes, cytoplasmic tonofilament, long spacing collagen, desmosomes	KS, leiomyoma, fibrous tumor, inflammatory myofibroblastic tumor	64,65
Leiomyoma	Rubbery nodules, 1–2.5 cm	Intersecting bundles of spindle cells with entrapped glands	Trichrome (fuchsinophilic), Desmin+, Actin+ S100–	KS, peripheral nerve sheath tumor, fibrous tumor, inflammatory myofibroblastic tumor	66,67

Fibrous tumor	Spherical, dense, rubbery spherical nodules	Long spindle cells with variable cellularity arranged in a haphazard array; background consists of dense fibrous collagenous or loose myxoid stroma	Trichrome, Desmin– Actin– S100–	KS, peripheral nerve sheath tumor, leiomyoma, inflammatory myofibroblastic tumor	68–70
KS	Mucosal nodules or plaques	Slit-like vascular spaces, eosinophilic globules, extravasation of red blood cells, and mild cytological atypia of the spindle cells	Factor VIII+ CD34+ CD31+	Hemangioma, other spindle cell neoplasms	71,72
Other sarcomas	Large endobronchial lesions with or without ulceration	Specific histological changes depend on differentiation and grade of neoplasm	Desmin Actin S100	Metastatic sarcoma, melanoma, spindle cell carcinoma	73–77

Abbreviations: DDx, differential diagnosis; PAS, periodic acid–Schiff; KS, Kaposi sarcoma.

multifocal. The histological features are similar to those of granular cell tumors from more conventional sites. The neoplasm is primarily composed of large polygonal cells with granular eosinophilic cytoplasm and small vesicular nuclei. While 3% to 6% of extrapulmonary granular cell tumors demonstrate malignant behavior, all endobronchial granular cell tumors reported have bland nuclear and cytoplasmic features and to date, none have behaved in a malignant fashion. The differential diagnosis includes other neoplasms with eosinophilic cytoplasm such as oncocytic carcinoid tumor, renal cell carcinoma, alveolar soft part sarcoma, histiocytic lesion, and smooth muscle tumor. By histochemical and immunohistochemical studies, granular cell tumor is S100-positive, cytokeratin-negative, and contains PAS-positive granules in the cytoplasm.

B. Lipoma and Liposarcoma

Most pulmonary lipomas are endobronchial and protrude into the lumen as pedunculated or polypoid mass (58,59). The larger lipomas occlude the bronchial lumen and produce obstructive signs and symptoms and may result in atelectasis or bronchiectasis of the distal pulmonary parenchyma. Histologically, the lesion resembles lipomas from other sites. They are composed of mature adipose tissue and may have spindle cells in areas. Primary liposarcoma of the lung is exceedingly rare; in a report by Petrov et al., only one liposarcoma was documented among 48 primary pulmonary sarcomas (60). The differential diagnosis of an endobronchial lipoma includes a lipomatous hamartoma that contains areas of cartilage and/or bone (61).

C. Hemangioma

Bronchial hemangiomas are more commonly seen in children than in adults and may be associated with other hemangiomas in the body or a syndrome such as hereditary hemorrhagic telangiectasia or Osler-Weber-Rendu syndrome (62). In children, hemangiomas are predominantly found in the subglottic area and less commonly in the distal airways (63). Typical symptoms include stridor, dyspnea, and hemoptysis. The lung parenchyma is also diffusely involved. In contrast, adult hemangioma is usually limited to the tracheobronchial tree. The lesions are often small (1 mm), cavernous, and show thrombosis or recanalization. Histologically, the distinction from a pyogenic granuloma may be difficult. While inflammation and edema are characteristics of pyogenic granulomas, deep-seated lesions may lack these features. The lobular capillary vascular architecture is perhaps the most distinctive feature of pyogenic granuloma that separates it from other vascular proliferations. If the vascular nature of the lesion is questioned, immunostains for factor VIII, CD34, or CD31 may be utilized.

D. Peripheral Nerve Sheath Tumors

Pulmonary endobronchial neurofibromas and neurilemomas may occur with or without an association with von Recklinghausen's disease (64). The syndromic lesions are multiple and circumferentially located in the intramucosal or submucosal regions of the bronchi. Histologically, the neoplasms are composed of compact bundles of spindle cells with focal nuclear palisading. These features are comparable to those occurring in the soft tissues. Malignant peripheral nerve sheath tumors behave aggressively and demonstrate multiple intrapulmonary metastases (65).

E. Leiomyoma

Leiomyoma of the lung are rare and account for less than 2% of all benign lung tumors (66). Approximately one-third of these arise in the bronchi and produce obstructive complications including atelectasis, mediastinal shift, or bronchiectasis (67). Histologically, they are composed of intersecting bundles of smooth muscle that entrap neighboring glands. The spindle-cell proliferation may be difficult to distinguish from other neoplasms, and use of trichrome stain and immunostains for muscle markers (desmin, actin) may be helpful.

F. Solitary Fibrous Tumor

While pleural solitary fibrous tumors are not uncommon, endobronchial pulmonary solitary fibrous tumors are rare (68–70). They are spherical, dense, rubbery well-circumscribed masses that are separate from the pleura. Histologically, they are composed of a haphazard array of spindle cells. Most lesions show low cellularity and the intervening stroma is densely collagenized. As expected, these tumors mark with CD34 immunostain. To date, only the benign type of solitary fibrous tumor has been described in the bronchus.

G. Kaposi Sarcoma

With improved management of organ transplantation recipients and acquired immunodeficiency syndrome (AIDS) patients, the incidence of KS has declined. Lymphangitic dissemination along the bronchial tree and the interlobular septa with pleural involvement is the characteristic manifestation of KS in the lung (71–73). Some KSs may form endobronchial nodules, and these are relatively easily recognized by the bronchoscopist. On the other hand, others grow diffusely along the tracheobronchial mucosa and may be apparent to the bronchoscopist as erythematous macular or papular mucosal plaques (74,75).

Histologically, bronchial KSs are similar to those in the skin and soft tissue and are seen in two forms: classic and inflammatory KS. The classic type is characterized by loosely organized spindle cells with slit-like vascular spaces, eosinophilic globules, extravasation of red blood cells, and mild cytological atypia of the spindle cells. The neoplasm tracks along the bronchopulmonary tree and the interlobular septa. The inflammatory type of pulmonary KS is characterized by a vascular proliferation along with a heavy lymphoplasmacytic infiltrate. The differential diagnosis includes vascular processes (capillary hemangiomatosis, lymphangiomatosis), reactive and myofibroblastic processes (granulation tissue, inflammatory pseudotumor). The slit-like vascular spaces, extravasation of red blood cells, and the eosinophilic globules distinguish KS from other vascular processes. In contrast to reactive and myofibroblastic lesions, KS demonstrates a lymphangitic pattern of dissemination that is a useful feature in its diagnosis. Immunohistochemical stains for human herpesvirus 8, CD34, and CD31 marks the neoplastic cells of KS.

H. Other Sarcomas

A variety of sarcomas including leiomyosarcomas, malignant fibrous histiocytomas, fibrosarcomas, chondrosarcomas, osteosarcomas, malignant peripheral nerve sheath tumors, rhabdomyosarcomas, and synovial sarcoma have been reported to occur in the lung as primary malignancies (73,76,77). A subset of these neoplasms present as endobronchial lesions that ulcerate and subsequently produce hemoptysis. Since the lung is a fertile site for metastatic disease, the possibility of a metastatic sarcoma must be excluded before the diagnosis of a primary sarcoma is made. The histological differential diagnosis includes other neoplasms that may demonstrate a spindle-cell component, such as spindle-cell carcinoma and malignant melanoma.

V. Others

A. Melanoma

Malignant melanoma usually involves the lung as a metastatic neoplasm. In a study by Miyake et al., 95% pulmonary melanomas were metastases (78). Metastatic melanomas are often multiple as well as bilateral and involve the parenchyma. Endobronchial involvement by metastatic melanoma is seen in only 6% of these cases. In contrast, primary pulmonary melanomas (79,80) are extremely rare (less than 0.01% of all lung neoplasms) and require rigorous exclusion of metastatic disease by obtaining a thorough history and performing an extensive dermatological examination. In the largest series of primary pulmonary melanoma by Wilson and Moran, the inclusion criteria were strictly defined as follows: (1) A solitary lung tumor, (2) A malignant melanoma confirmed by immunohistochemistry and/or electron microscopy, (3) No past history of excision or fulguration of a cutaneous, mucous membrane, or ocular lesion, (4) A central pulmonary lesion, and (5) No demonstrable tumor elsewhere at the time of diagnosis (81). Since primary pulmonary melanomas are thought to arise from the bronchus, the majority (55–88%) of these neoplasms present with an endobronchial component. Many primary bronchial melanomas are pigmented and therefore are detected by bronchoscopy (Fig. 5). Knowledge of the radiological imaging studies

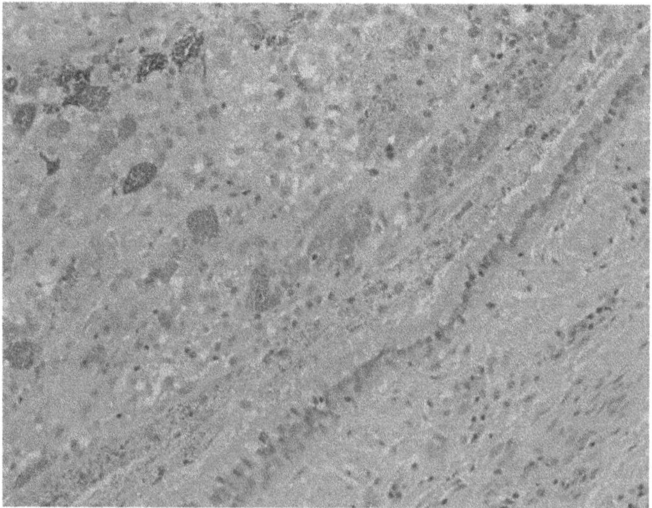

Figure 5 Primary endobronchial melanoma is a diagnosis that is made after the possibility of metastasis is excluded. Melanin pigment is seen in the neoplastic cells in the upper left corner.

is important, since peripheral nodular melanomas are virtually always metastatic. Cases of bronchial melanoma reported in the literature emphasize the relationship of the melanocytic cells to the bronchial mucosa and the demonstration of junctional activity as a sign of the neoplasm arising at that site. The histological features of primary pulmonary melanomas are similar to those of melanomas from other sites (large polygonal discohesive cells with prominent nucleoli). The differential diagnosis includes other poorly differentiated malignant neoplasms. Of particular interest are carcinoid tumors (chromogranin- and synaptophysin-positive), which may contain melanin pigment, and "sugar" tumors, which are positive for S100 and HMB45 by immunohistochemistry. The latter is a peripheral lesion and is not found endobronchially. Additional immunohistochemical stains such as Melan A and tyrosinase assist in the diagnosis of melanoma.

B. Lymphoma

Most endobronchial lymphomas occur in the setting of systemic disease. Low-, intermediate-, and high-grade lymphomas characteristically present with a lymphangitic distribution or nodular masses (82–85). Although not typically endobronchial, a variety of non-Hodgkin's lymphomas may involve the bronchovascular bundle. Infiltration and necrosis of the bronchial epithelium, vascular infiltration, and invasion of the cartilage are features reflecting the malignant nature of the lymphoid population. The criteria for diagnosis are identical to those of nodal and other extranodal sites. The low-grade lymphomas may be difficult to distinguish from reactive lymphoid hyperplasia or lymphoid interstitial pneumonia; the use of immunohistochemistry or flow cytometry to demonstrate a clonal population is often required to make a definitive diagnosis. Immunophenotypically, most are of B-cell origin; the histological subtypes include small lymphocytic, plasmacytoid, and cleaved follicular center cell types. Tracking along the lymphatics of the airways, vasculature, and pleura is a common feature of low-grade lymphomas. Bronchial wall involvement with invasion of the cartilage is seen in approximately two-thirds of the cases. Architecturally and cytologically, these lesions are similar to lymphomas of mucosa-associated lymphoid tissues (so-called MALTomas) and foci of necrosis are uncommon. In addition to demonstrating clonality by immunohistochemical or in situ hybridization methods, the coexpression of a B-cell marker (e.g., CD20) and an aberrant T-cell marker (CD43) is useful in establishing the presence of a neoplastic lymphoid population. High-grade lymphomas are readily recognized as malignant neoplasms but may be difficult to distinguish from other poorly differentiated malignancies. Necrosis, vascular invasion, and regional lymph node involvement are common features. Immunophenotyping with lymphoid markers differentiates these lymphomas from other poorly differentiated neoplasms. On rare occasion, non-Hodgkin's lymphomas present as an endobronchial mass (86). These lymphomas most likely arise from bronchial-associated lymphoid tissue. These are usually B-cell lymphomas and remain localized. Primary Hodgkin's disease of the lung typically presents as nodular sclerosis or mixed cellularity types. The criteria are identical to those of nodal disease, and immunohistochemistry (Leu-Mi, Ki-1) is valuable in recognizing Reed-Sternberg cells (87).

As in the case of other neoplasms mentioned above, the issue of primary versus secondary involvement of the lung must be addressed. Secondary involvement of the lung by lymphoma is more common than primary disease. Interestingly, intermediate and high-grade lymphomas more readily involve the lung secondarily than low-grade lymphomas.

Leukemic infiltrations are also possible. Pulmonary involvement by chronic lymphocytic leukemia is morphologically identical to pulmonary involvement by small lymphocytic lymphoma and primary low-grade lymphoma. The differential diagnosis of the low-grade lymphomas includes bronchus-associated lymphoid tissue and follicular bronchitis/ bronchiolitis.

C. Inflammatory Myofibroblastic Tumor (Plasma Cell Granuloma, Inflammatory Pseudotumor, Fibroxanthoma, Histiocytoma)

Most inflammatory myofibroblastic tumors are solitary, peripheral, circumscribed, and lobulated mass. In approximately 10% of cases, this uncommon lesion involves the bronchus (88–91). By definition, these inflammatory myofibroblastic tumors are composed of spindle-cell (myofibroblastic) proliferation, inflammatory cells, and macrophages (Fig. 6). The majority of them are thought to be neoplastic; some cases are reactive, inflammatory processes. Subtypes include plasma cell granuloma type, fibrous histiocytoma type, and organizing pneumonia type. The spindle-cell population lacks atypia and the lymphoplasmacytic component is polymorphous and polyclonal if studied by flow cytometry. Some inflammatory myofibroblastic tumors show abnormalities in chromosomes 1, 2 (ALK gene), 4, and/or 5. The differential diagnosis depends on the component in question. Atypia in the spindle-cell population raises an issue with regard to distinction from sarcomas. An immunohistochemical stain panel using cytokeratin, mesenchymal markers (desmin, actin), S100, HMB45, and ALK-1 markers may assist in differentiating other spindle-cell neoplasms such as sarcomatoid carcinoma and melanoma (Table 4).

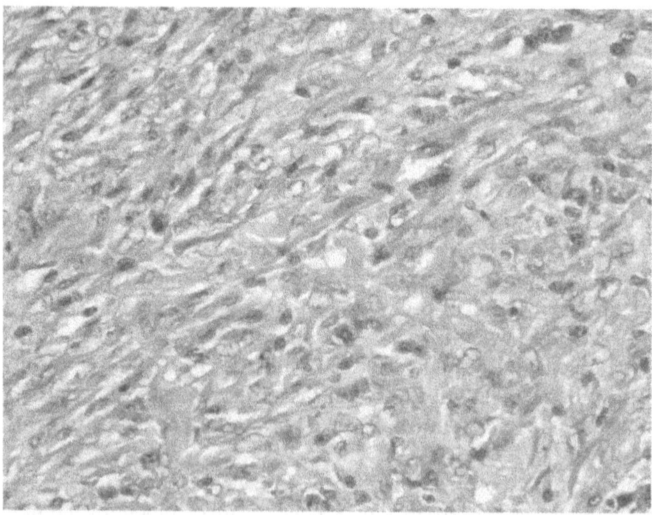

Figure 6 Inflammatory myofibroblastic tumor shows interlacing fascicles of spindle cells. No significant cytologic atypia is noted.

Table 4 Other Endobronchial Neoplasms

Neoplasm	Gross features	Microscopical features	Special studies	DDx	References
Melanoma	Black or nonpigmented endobronchial nodules or plaques	Large polygonal discohesive cells with prominent nucleoli	Cytokeratin-S100+ HMB45+	Sarcoma, spindle cell carcinoma	78–81
Lymphoma	Nodular parenchymal lesions surrounding airways; intra/submucosal tracking of lymphoma	Depends on type and grade of lymphoma	Atypical lymphoid population marking with B-cell marker (e.g., L-26, CD20); Coexpression of B-cell marker and CD43; monoclonality by demonstrating light chain expression by immunohistochemistry or in situ hybridization; flow cytometry and immunophenotyping	Low-grade lymphomas: bronchial-associated lymphoid tissue; follicular bronchitis/bronchiolitis High-grade lymphomas: poorly differentiated carcinoma, sarcoma, melanoma	82–86
Inflammatory myofibroblastic tumor	Firm, gray-white, well circumscribed but no true capsule	Spindle cell (myofibroblastic) proliferation, inflammatory cells, and macrophages	Cytokeratin–(marks entrapped glands) Sl00-factor VIII–(marks endothelial cells of vessels) LCA–(marks lymphoid component) ALK-1	Sarcoma, sarcomatoid carcinoma, melanoma	87–91

Abbreviation: DDx, differential diagnosis.

References

1. Kramer R. Adenoma of bronchus. Ann Otol Rhinol Laryngol 1930; 39:698–695.
2. Moran CA, Suster S, Koss MN. Primary adenoid cystic carcinoma of the lung: a clinicopathologic and immunohistochemical study of 16 cases. Cancer 1994; 73:1390–1397.
3. Nomori H, Kaseda S, Kobayashi K, et al. J Thorac Cardiovasc Surg 1988; 96:271–277.
4. Inoue H, Iwashita A, Kanegae H, et al. Peripheral pulmonary adenoid cystic carcinoma with substantial extension to the proximal bronchus. Thorax 1991; 46:147–148.
5. Albers E, Lawrie T, Harrell JH, et al. Tracheobronchial adenoid cystic carcinoma: a clinicopathologic study of 14 cases. Chest 2004; 125:1160–1165.
6. Qui S, Nampoothiri MM, Zaharopoulos P, et al. Primary pulmonary adenoid cystic carcinoma: report of a case diagnosed by fine-needle aspiration cytology. Diagn Cytopathol 2004; 30:51–56.
7. Nagao T, Gaffey TA, Serizawa H, et al. Dedifferentiated adenoid cystic carcinoma: a clinicopathologic study of 6 cases. Mod Pathol 2003; 16:1265–1272.
8. Yousem SA, Hochholzer L. Mucoepidermoid tumors of the lung. Cancer 1987; 60:1346–1352.
9. Heitmiller RF, Mathisen DJ, Ferry JA, et al. Mucoepidermoid lung tumors. Ann Thorac Surg 1989; 47:394–399.
10. Dinopoulos A, Lagona E, Stinios I, et al. Mucoepidermoid carcinoma of the bronchus. Pediatr Hematol Oncol 2000; 17:401–408.
11. Shilo K, Foss RD, Franks TJ, et al. Pulmonary mucoepidermoid carcinoma with prominent tumor-associated lymphoid proliferation. Am J Surg Pathol 2005; 29:407–411.
12. Edwards CW, Matthews HR. Mucous gland adenoma of the bronchus. Thorax 1981; 36:147–148.
13. Heard BE, Corrin B, Dewar A. Pathology of seven mucous cell adenomas of the bronchial glands with particular reference to ultrastructure. Histopathology 1985; 9:687–701.
14. England DM, Hochholzer L. Truly benign "bronchial adenoma": report of 10 cases of mucous gland adenoma with immunohistochemical and ultrastructural findings. Am J Surg Pathol 1995; 19:887–899.
15. Kragel PJ, Devaney KO, Meth BM, et al. Mucinous cystadenoma of the lung. A report of two cases with immunohistochemical and ultrastructural analysis. Arch Pathol Lab Med 1990; 114:1053–1056.
16. Roux FJ, Lantuéjoul S, Brambilla E, et al. Mucinous cystadenoma of the lung. Cancer 1995; 76:1540–1544.
17. Fechner RE, Bentinck BR, Askew JB. Acinic cell tumor of the lung: a histologic and ultrastructural study. Cancer 1972; 29:501–508.
18. Kay S, Schatzki PF. Ultrastructure of acinic cell carcinoma of the parotid salivary gland. Cancer 1972; 29:235–244.
19. Moran CA, Suster S, Koss MN. Acinic cell carcinoma of the lung ("Fechner tumor"): a clincopathologic, immunohistochemical and ultrastructural study of five cases. Am J Surg Pathol 1992; 16:1039–1050.
20. Lee HY, Mancer K, Koong HN. Primary acinic cell carcinoma of the lung with lymph node metastasis. Arch Pathol Lab Med 2003; 127(4):e216–e219.
21. Chuah KL, Yap WM, Tan HW, et al. Recurrence of pulmonary acinic cell carcinoma. Arch Pathol Lab Med 2006; 130:932–933.
22. Hayes MMM, van der Westhuizen NG, Forgie R. Malignant mixed tumor of the bronchus: a biphasic neoplasm of epithelial and myoepithelial cells. Mod Pathol 1993; 6:85–88.
23. Nistal M, Garcia-Viera M, Martinez-Garcia C, et al. Epithelial-myoepithelial tumor of the bronchus. Am J Surg Pathol 1994; 18:421–425.
24. Fulford LG, Kamata Y, Okudera K, et al. Epithelial-myoepithelial carcinomas of the bronchus. Am J Surg Pathol 2001; 25:1508–1514.
25. Doganay L, Bilgi S, Ozdil A, et al. Epithelial-myoepithelial carcinoma of the lung. A case report and review of the literature. Arch Pathol Lab Med 2003; 127:e177–e180.

26. Ru K, Srivastava A, Tischler AS. Bronchial epithelial-myoepithelial carcinoma. Arch Pathol Lab Med 2004; 128:92–94.
27. Chao TY, Lin AS, Lie CH, et al. Bronchial epithelial-myoepithelial carcinoma. Ann Thorac Surg 2007; 83:689–691.
28. Barzo P, Molnar L, Minik K. Bronchial papillomas of various origins. Chest 1987; 92:132–136.
29. Al-Saleem T, Peale AR, Morris CM. Multiple papillomatosis of the lower respiratory tract. Cancer 1968; 22:1173–1184.
30. Gaylis B, Hayden RE. Recurrent respiratory papillomatosis: progressing to invasion and malignancy. Am J Otolaryngol 1991; 12:104–112.
31. Flieder DB, Koss MN, Nicholson A, et al. Solitary pulmonary papillomas in adults: a clinicopathologic and in situ hybridization study of 14 cases combined with 27 cases in the literature. Am J Surg Pathol 1998; 22:1328–1342.
32. Brambilla E, Moro D, Veale D, et al. Basal cell (basaloid) carcinoma of the lung. Hum Pathol 1992; 23:993–1003.
33. Moro D, Brichon PY, Brambilla E, et al. Basaloid bronchial carcinoma. A histologic group with a poor prognosis. Cancer 1994; 73:2734–2739.
34. Kim DJ, Kim KD, Shin DH, et al. Basaloid carcinoma of the lung: a really dismal histologic variant? Ann Thorac Surg 2003; 76:1833–1837.
35. Travis WD, Brambilla E, Muller-Hermelink HK, et al. Pathology and Genetics: Tumours of the Lung, Pleura, Thymus and Heart. Lyon: IARC, 22004.
36. Moran CA, Suster S, Askin FB, et al. Benign and malignant salivary gland-type mixed tumors of the lung: clinicopathologic and immunohistochemical study of eight cases. Cancer 1994; 73: 2481–2490.
37. Mori M, Furuya K, Kimura T, et al. Mixed tumor of salivary gland type arising in the bronchus. Ann Thorac Surg 1991; 52:1322–1324.
38. Sweeny EC, McDermott M. Pleomorphic adenoma of the bronchus. J Clin Pathol 1996; 49:87–89.
39. Demirag F, Topcu S, Kurul C, et al. Malignant pleomorphic adenoma (malignant mixed tumor) of the trachea: a case report and review of the literature. Eur Arch Otorhinolaryngol 2003; 260:96–99.
40. Tomashefski JF. Benign endobronchial mesenchymal tumors. Am J Surg Pathol 1982; 6:531–540.
41. Kiyru T, Kawaguchi S, Matsui E, et al. Multiple chondromatous hamartomas of the lung: a case report and review of the literature with special reference to Carney syndrome. Cancer 1999; 85: 2557–2561.
42. Bateson EM, Hayes JA, Woo-Ming M. Endobronchial teratoma associated with bronchiectasis and bronchiolectasis. Thorax 1968; 23:69–76.
43. Jamieson MPG, McGowan AR. Endobronchial teratoma. Thorax 1982; 37:157–159.
44. Cheung Y-C, Ng S-H, Wan Y-L, et al. Ruptured mediastinal cystic teratoma with intrapulmonary bronchial invasion: CT demonstration. Br J Radiol 2001; 74:1148–1149.
45. Davis MP, Eagan RT, Weiland LH, et al. Carcinosarcoma of the lung: Mayo clinic experience and response to chemotherapy. Mayo Clin Proc 1984; 59:598–603.
46. Ludwigsen E. Endobronchial carcinosarcoma. Virchows Arch [A] 1977; 373:293–302.
47. Koss MN, Hochholzer L, Frommelt RA. Carcinosarcomas of the lung: a clinicopathologic study of 66 patients. Am J Surg Pathol 1999; 23:1514–1526.
48. Heckman CJ, Truong LD, Cagle PT, et al. Pulmonary blastoma with rhabdomyosarcomatous differentiation: an electron microscopic and immunohistochemical study. Am J Surg Pathol 1988; 12:35–40.
49. Sawada K, Yamada G, Shijubo N, et al. Biphasic pulmonary blastoma presenting as endobronchial polyp with a long stalk. Intern Med 2005; 44:516–517.
50. Nakashima M, Inagaki T, Kunimura T, et al. Cytopathologic and histologic features of biphasic pulmonary blastoma: a case report. Acta Cytol 2005; 49:87–91.
51. Lee HJ, Goo JM, Kim KW, et al. Pulmonary blastoma: radiologic findings in five patients. Clin Imaging 2004; 28:113–118.

52. Yokoyama S, Hayashida Y, Nagahama J, et al. Pulmonary blastoma. A case report. Acta Cytol 1992; 36(3):293–298.
53. Ostermiller WE, Comer TP, Barker WL. Endobronchial granular cell myoblastoma: a report of three cases and review of the literature. Ann Thorac Surg 1970; 9:143–148.
54. Oprah SS, Subramanian VA. Granular cell myoblastoma of the bronchus: report of 2 cases and review of the literature. Ann Thorac Surg 1976; 22:199–202.
55. Young CD, Gay RM. Multiple endobronchial granular cell myoblastomas discovered at bronchoscopy. Hum Pathol 1984; 15:193–194.
56. Deavers M, Guinee D, Koss MN, et al. Granular cell tumors of the lung. Clinicopathologic study of 20 cases. Am J Surg Pathol 1995; 19:627–635.
57. Abdulhamid I, Rabah R. Granular cell tumor of the bronchus. Pediatr Pulmonol 2000; 30:425–428.
58. Crutcher RRN, Waltuch TL, Ghosh AK. Bronchial lipoma: report of a case and literature review. J Thoracic Cardiovasc Surg 1968; 55:422–425.
59. Palvio D, Egeblod K, Paulsen SM. Atypical lipomatous hamartoma of the lung. Virchows Arch [Pathol Anat] 1985; 405:253–261.
60. Petrov DB, Vlassov VI, Kalaydjiev GT, et al. Primary pulmonary sarcomas and carcinosarcomas—postoperative results and comparative survival analysis. Eur J Cardiothorac Surg 2003; 23:461–466.
61. Stey CA, Vogt P, Russi EW. Endobronchial lipomatous hamartoma: a rare cause of bronchial occlusion. Chest 1998; 113:254–255.
62. Harding JR, Williams J, Seal RME. Pedunculated capillary hemangioma of the bronchus. Br J Dis Chest 1978; 72:336–342.
63. Rose AS, Mathur PN. Endobronchial capillary hemangioma: case report and review of the literature. Respiration 2007 Jan 24 [Epub ahead of print].
64. Unger PD, Geller SA, Anderson PJ. Pulmonary lesions in a patient with neurofibromatosis. Arch Pathol Lab Med 1984; 108:654–657.
65. McCluggage WG, Bharucha H. Primary pulmonary tumours of nerve sheath origin. Histopathology 1995; 26:247–254.
66. Bilgin S, Yilmaz A, Okur E, et al. Primary endobronchial leiomyoma: a case report. Tuberk Toraks 2004; 52(3):272–274.
67. Yellin A, Rosenman Y, Lieberman Y. Review of smooth muscle tumor of the lower respiratory tract. Br J Dis Chest 1984; 78:337–351.
68. Corona FE, Okeson GC. Endobronchial fibroma. Am Rev Respir Dis 1974; 110:350–353.
69. Tan-Liu NS, Matsubara O, Grille HC, et al. Invasive fibrous tumor of the tracheobronchial tree: clinical and pathologic study of seven cases. Hum Pathol 1989; 20:180–184.
70. Sagawa M, Ueda Y, Matsubara F, et al. Intrapulmonary solitary fibrous tumor diagnosed by immunohistochemical and genetic approaches: report of a case. Surg Today 2007; 37:423–425.
71. Miller RF, Tomlinson MC, Cottrill CP, et al. Bronchopulmonary Kaposi's sarcoma in patients with AIDS. Thorax 1992; 47:721–725.
72. Mitchell DM, McCarty M, Fleming J, et al. Bronchopulmonary Kaposi's sarcoma in patients with AIDS. Thorax 1992; 47:726–729.
73. Suster S. Primary sarcomas of the lung. Semin Diagn Pathol 1995; 12:140–157.
74. Chin R Jr., Jones DF, Pegram PS, et al. Complete endobronchial occlusion by Kaposi's sarcoma in the absence of cutaneous involvement. Chest 1994; 105(5):1581–1582.
75. Judson MA, Sahn SA. Endobronchial lesions in HIV-infected individuals. Chest 1994; 105 (5):1314–1323.
76. Guccion JG, Rosen SH. Bronchopulmonary leiomyosarcoma and fibrosarcoma: a study of 32 cases and review of the literature. Cancer 1972; 30:836–847.
77. Niwa H, Masuda S, Kobayashi C, et al. Pulmonary synovial sarcoma with polypoid endobronchial growth: a case report, immunohistochemical and cytogenetic study. Pathol Int 2004; 54:611–615.

78. Miyake M, Tateishi U, Maeda T, et al. Pulmonary involvement of malignant melanoma: thin-section CT findings with pathologic correlation. Radiat Med 2005; 23:497–503.
79. Gephardt GN. Malignant melanoma of the bronchus. Hum Pathol 1981; 12:671–673.
80. Carstens PHB, Kuhns JG, Ghazi C. Primary malignant melanomas of the lung and adrenal. Hum Pathol 1984; 15:910–914.
81. Wilson RW, Moran CA. Primary melanoma of the lung: a clinicopathologic and immunohistochemical study of eight cases. Am J Surg Pathol 1997; 21:1196–1202.
82. Koss MN, Hochholzer J, Nichols PW, et al. Primary non-Hodgkin's lymphoma and pseudolymphoma of lung: a study of 161 patients. Hum Pathol 1983; 14:1024–1038.
83. Yousem S, Weiss L, Colby T. Primary pulmonary Hodgkin's disease: a clinicopathologic study of 15 cases. Cancer 1986; 57:1217–1224.
84. Radin A. Primary pulmonary Hodgkin's disease. Cancer 1990; 65:550–563.
85. Koss MN. Pulmonary lymphoid disorders. Semin Diagn Pathol 1995; 12:158–171.
86. Jang M, Choi YW, Jeon SC, et al. Endobronchial non-Hodgkin's lymphoma presenting as an isolated endobronchial mass. Clin Radiol 2006; 61:202–205.
87. Kiani B, Magro CM, Ross P. Endobronchial presentation of Hodgkin lymphoma: a review of the literature. Ann Thorac Surg 2003; 76:967–972.
88. Pettinato G, Manivel JC, DeRosa N, et al. Inflammatory myofibroblastic tumor (plasma cell granuloma): clinicopathologic study of 20 cases with immunohistochemical and ultrastructural observations. Am J Clin Pathol 1990; 94:538–546.
89. Matsurbara O, Tan-Liu NS, Kenney RM, et al. Inflammatory pseudotumor of the lung: progression from organizing pneumonia to fibrous histiocytoma or to plasma cell granuloma in 32 cases. Hum Pathol 1988; 19:807–814.
90. Kim TS, Han J, Kim GY, et al. Pulmonary inflammatory pseudotumor (inflammatory myofibroblastic tumor): CT features with pathologic correlation. J Comput Assist Tomogr 2005; 29:633–639.
91. Coffin CM, Hornick JL, Fletcher CD. Inflammatory myofibroblastic tumor: comparison of clinicopathologic, histologic, and immunohistochemical features including ALK expression in atypical and aggressive cases. Am J Surg Pathol 2007; 31:509–520.

39
Localized Pleural Tumors

ANDREW CHURG
University of British Columbia, Vancouver, British Columbia, Canada

TIMOTHY C. ALLEN
The University of Texas Health Science Center at Tyler, Tyler, Texas, U.S.A.

I. Introduction

The vast majority of tumors involving the pleura appear as multiple nodules or diffuse pleural thickening, representing most commonly metastases from another site or, occasionally, diffuse malignant mesothelioma. Uncommonly, pleural tumors present as discrete localized nodular lesions without evidence of diffuse pleural involvement. Diagnostic confusion occurs with these tumors due to their infrequency, confusion over their nomenclature, and lack of a set of definitive rules for separating these various entities. Table 1 presents a classification of localized pleural tumors.

Radiographically and grossly, all of these lesions are circumscribed (except for the occasional malignant tumor that has grown into surrounding structures), more or less nodular (sometimes ovoid or discoid) masses attached to the pleural surface. Figure 1 shows a computed tomography (CT) scan of a localized pleural tumor; this particular example happens to be a solitary fibrous tumor, but the same CT image could be seen with any of the entities discussed in this chapter.

II. Solitary Fibrous Tumor

Solitary fibrous tumors are by far the most common tumor of this whole group. Two large series have been published by Briselli et al. in 1981 (1) and England et al. in 1989 (2). About 800 cases have been reported in the literature overall (3). Nomenclature has been a source of considerable confusion in this area (Table 2), since solitary fibrous tumor has previously been called *localized fibrous mesothelioma, fibrous mesothelioma, benign mesothelioma, submesothelial fibroma*, and various other combinations of these terms. The evidence for a mesothelial origin has always been dubious and recent reports of identical tumors in the retroperitoneum and orbit, as well as the elucidation of their immunohistochemical and ultrastructural features, make it clear that these are not mesothelial proliferations but rather tumors arising from submesothelial connective tissue (4–7). Equally important, the use of any diagnostic term containing the word *mesothelioma* implies to most physicians a diffuse malignant mesothelioma. Since a vast majority of solitary fibrous tumors are benign, this distinction is vital, and terms such as *localized mesothelioma* and

Table 1 Localized Pleural Tumors

Solitary fibrous tumor
Malignant solitary fibrous tumor
Localized malignant mesothelioma
Localized sarcoma
Benign pleural plaque
Lipoma of the chest wall
Schwannoma

Table 2 Synonyms for Solitary Fibrous Tumor

Submesothelial fibroma
Fibrous mesothelioma
Localized mesothelioma
Benign mesothelioma
Benign fibrous mesothelioma

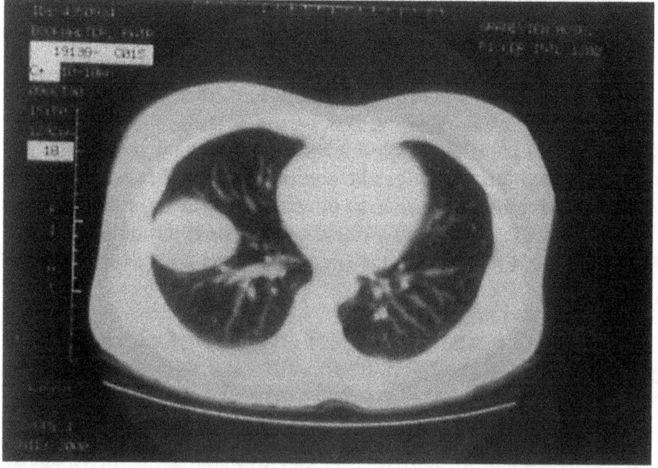

Figure 1 Computed tomography scan showing a nodular pleura-based mass; this particular example is a solitary fibrous tumor, but most of the entities discussed in this paper would have the same radiographical appearance.

fibrous mesothelioma should definitely be avoided, the more so as a few pathologists continue to refer to sarcomatous diffuse malignant mesotheliomas as *fibrous mesotheliomas*.

The clinical features of solitary fibrous tumors are listed in Table 3. Because most of these lesions are asymptomatic, presentation with symptoms should raise concerns about malignancy. The majority (70% or 80%) of solitary fibrous tumors are attached to the

Table 3 Clinical Features of Solitary Fibrous Tumor

Age range: childhood to eighth decade
Not associated with asbestos exposure
Majority of benign lesions asymptomatic
Chest pain, shortness of breath much more common with malignant forms
Pleural effusion much more common with malignant forms
Clubbing, hypoglycemia seen with both benign and malignant forms
Radiographically nodular pleural-based lesions

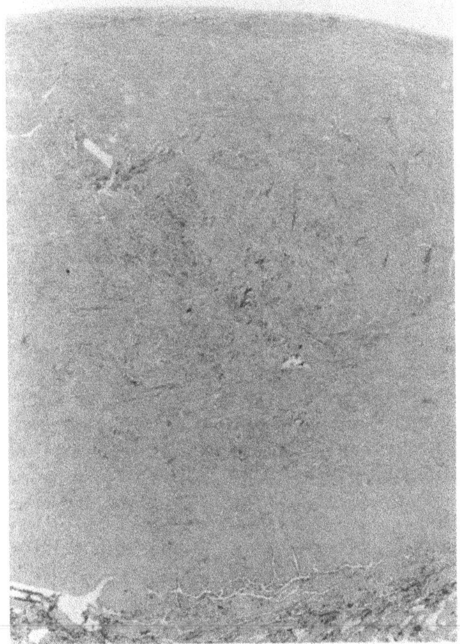

Figure 2 Low-power view of a solitary fibrous tumor. Note the sharply circumscribed appearance of the free (pleural space) surface and the broad peg-like attachment to the underlying lung.

visceral pleura; in about half of the cases, the pleural attachment is by a thin stalk, and about half the cases are sessile (Figs. 2 and 3). Solitary fibrous tumors can also be attached to the parietal pleura, diaphragm, or fissural pleura, or they may be intrapulmonary. Reported tumor sizes range up to 40 cm, but most are in the range of 5 to 10 cm; very large tumors are more likely to be malignant.

Microscopically, solitary fibrous tumors show a variety of patterns including the "patternless pattern of Stout" (Figs. 2–5), a hemangiopericytoma-like pattern, and a cellular pattern (Figs. 6 and 7). A given tumor may show any or all of these patterns. The patternless pattern is distinctive, while the hemangiopericytoma-like pattern is identical to

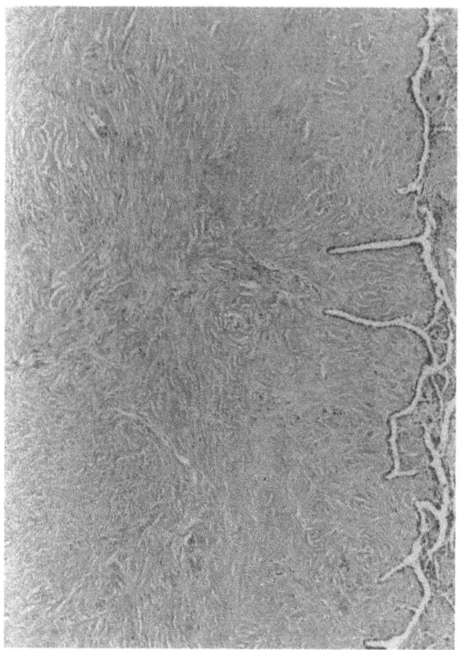

Figure 3 Higher-power view of the attachment of tumor shown in Figure 2 to the underlying lung. The peg-like interface is characteristic of sessile solitary fibrous tumors and is not a sign of malignancy. Note the invaginations lined by pulmonary epithelial cells. These may become trapped in the tumor and form gland-like structures. As opposed to the tumor itself, the entrapped elements are keratin-positive. This view also shows the "patternless pattern."

that seen in benign hemangiopericytomas in other organs, including the lung. The cellular areas tend to be composed of nondescript, usually bland-appearing spindle cells (Figs. 6 and 7), but high cellularity accompanied by cytological atypia and numerous mitoses should raise a question of malignancy. Occasional cases have epithelial-appearing areas, although immunochemical staining confirms that there is no true epithelial differentiation in these lesions, and this finding has no prognostic significance. These foci should be distinguished from the inclusions of pulmonary epithelial cells (Figs. 2 and 3), a common finding in sessile tumors attached to the visceral pleura. In distinction to the actual cells of the solitary fibrous tumor, these inclusions are keratin-positive (see below). Benign solitary fibrous tumors that are attached to the visceral pleura typically show a peg-like pattern of pushing growth into the underlying lung (Figs. 2 and 3); this is not a true invasion and is not by itself a sign of malignancy.

The characteristic immunochemical profile is immunopositivity with CD34 (Fig. 8), vimentin, CD99, and Bcl-2; and immunonegativity with S-100, actin, desmin, and keratin (4,5); the latter is a particularly crucial observation for separating these tumors from localized or diffuse malignant mesotheliomas. The immunoprofile might also help distinguish solitary fibrous tumor from its differential diagnoses such as fibrosarcoma, hemangiopericytoma, and fibrous histiocytoma (7). While it appears that almost all of these

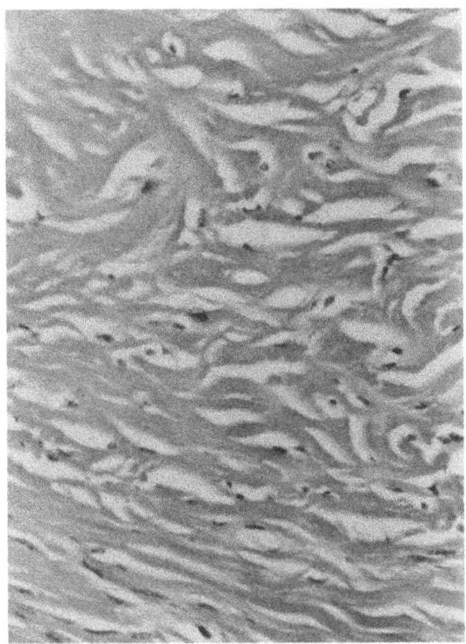

Figure 4 Higher-power view of the same tumor to illustrate the "patternless pattern" and the inconspicuous tumor cells in slit-like spaces.

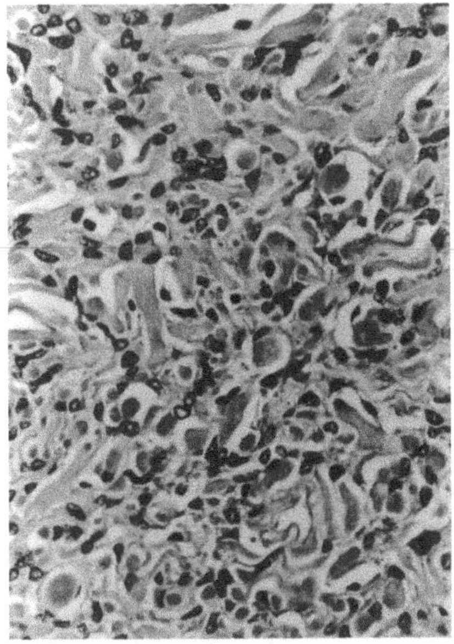

Figure 5 Another solitary fibrous tumor showing an area with features transitional between the patternless pattern and the cellular pattern.

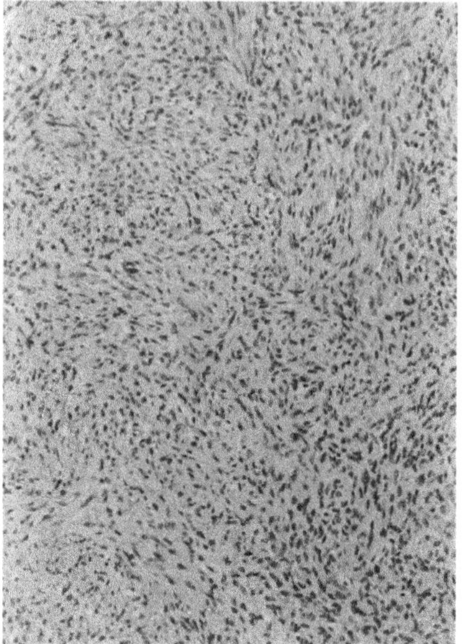

Figure 6 Low-power view of a cellular area from the same tumor as in Figure 5.

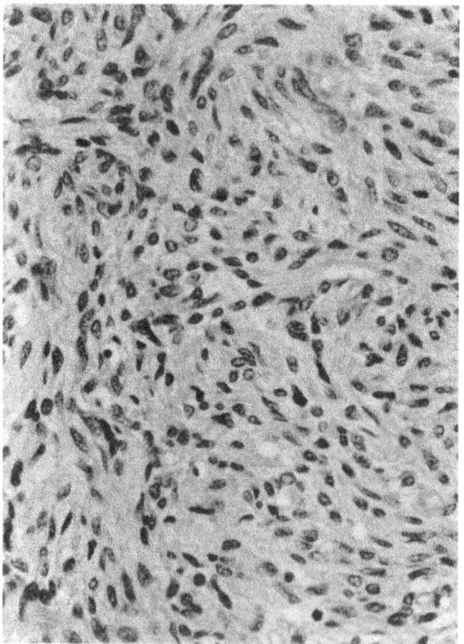

Figure 7 High-power view of a cellular area from the same tumor as in Figure 5. Although cellular foci are common in perfectly benign solitary fibrous tumors, they should nonetheless always be carefully inspected for mitotic figures and cytological atypia.

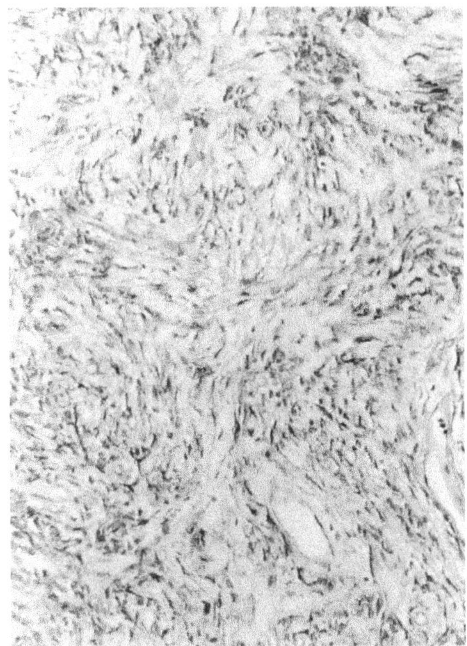

Figure 8 CD34 staining is diffusely positive in a solitary fibrous tumor.

tumors are CD34-positive (4,5), care should be taken in interpreting this stain as CD34 positivity is not specific to solitary fibrous tumor and can be seen in schwannomas (which may present as localized pleural tumors, see below), neurofibromas, and some smooth muscle tumors (5). However, diffuse malignant mesotheliomas are CD34-negative. By electron microscopy, solitary fibrous tumor show nondescript spindled cells.

A vast majority of typical-appearing solitary fibrous tumors are benign; the criteria for malignancy are described below.

Some solitary fibrous tumors present as intrapulmonary masses attached to the visceral pleura; the distinction between an intrapulmonary solitary fibrous tumor and an intrapulmonary hemangiopericytoma may be extremely difficult in such instances, even with the assistance of immunostains.

III. Malignant Solitary Fibrous Tumor

A number of features suggest that a solitary fibrous tumor is malignant (1,2) (Table 4). Clinically, these include presentation with chest pain, shortness of breath, and pleural effusion. Pathologically, large (>10 cm) tumors, tumors attached to the parietal pleura, mediastinum, or inverted into the lung are at greater risk of being malignant. Solitary fibrous tumors that recur are usually malignant, and tumors that show invasion (Figs. 9 and 10) of surrounding structures are almost always malignant.

Table 4 Features Associated with Malignancy in Solitary Fibrous Tumor

Symptomatic at presentation (especially shortness of breath, chest pain, pleural effusion)
Invasion of surrounding structures
Recurrence after resection
Tumor attached to parietal pleura, fissure, mediastinum, in lung
Tumor sessile, size >10 cm
Gross hemorrhage and necrosis
Microscopic cellularity, cytological atypia, mitoses >4 per 10 high-power fields
Overt microscopic foci of sarcoma

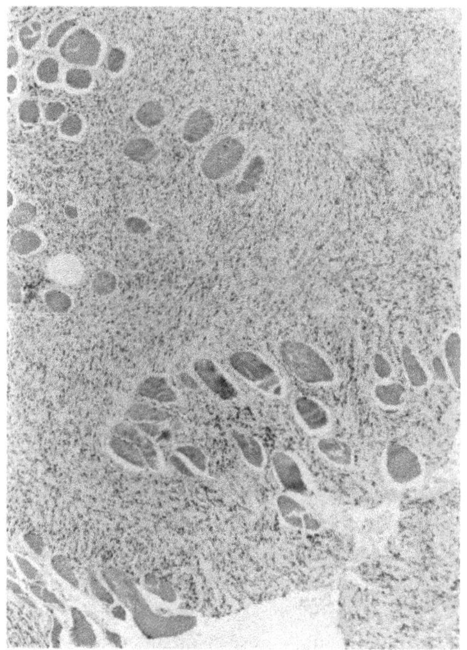

Figure 9 Low-power view of a malignant solitary fibrous tumor showing cellular tumor with muscle invasion.

Histologically, malignant features include increased cellularity, nuclear pleomorphism, hemorrhage and necrosis, and more than 4 mitoses per 10 high-power fields (1,2). The immunochemical staining pattern of a malignant solitary fibrous tumor is similar to that of benign solitary fibrous tumor; however, CD34 expression has been shown to be reduced in malignant solitary fibrous tumors (4,5,8). Microscopically, some malignant solitary fibrous tumors appear to arise from otherwise benign-appearing solitary fibrous tumors, with the malignant tumor showing the same basic histology as the benign areas but with obvious histologically malignant features described above. Other malignant solitary fibrous tumors histologically exhibit high grade, frankly sarcomatous tumor adjacent to otherwise benign-appearing solitary fibrous tumor (Figs. 10 and 11). Still other malignant

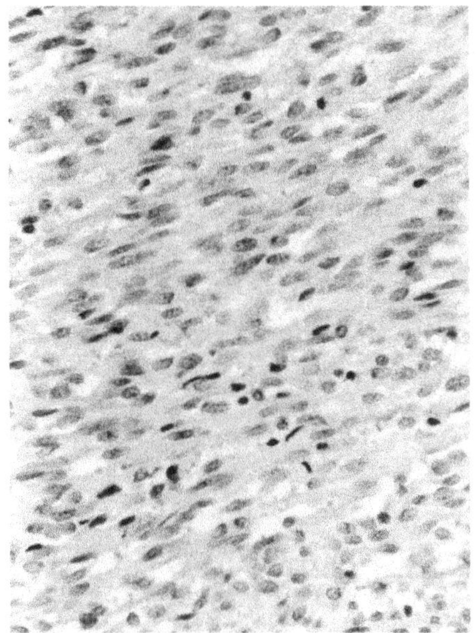

Figure 10 Higher-power view of the same tumor. Mitoses are present and mild cytological atypia, but this portion of the tumor is not histologically very different from the benign tumor shown in Figures 6 and 7. This tumor was CD34-positive.

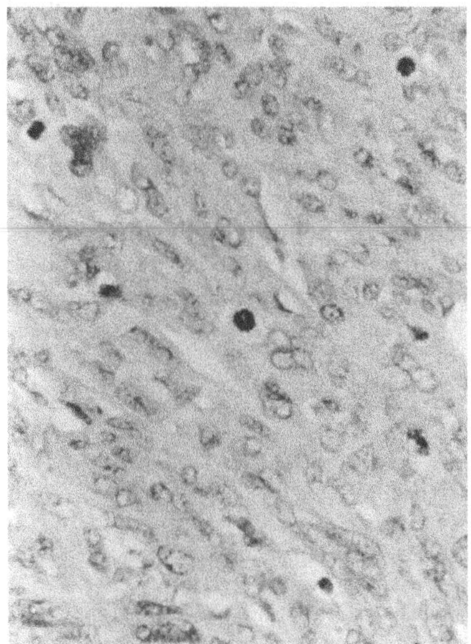

Figure 11 High-grade focus of another malignant solitary fibrous tumor.

solitary fibrous tumors appear to arise *de novo* with histologically and immunohistochemically identifiable malignant solitary fibrous tumor unaccompanied by any benign component of solitary fibrous tumor. Because of the variety of potential patterns of tumor, including presence of a benign solitary fibrous tumor component (possibly widespread), careful and extensive sampling of the lesion is necessary for proper diagnosis.

Malignant solitary fibrous tumors often recur locally and may metastasize but do not spread over the pleural surface. The proportion of solitary fibrous tumors considered malignant has been reported to range from 7% to 60%; however, in their series, England et al. (1) noted 37% were malignant, and Briselli et al. (2) noted 12% were malignant. Referral patterns and problems of definition may bias these numbers. England et al. (1) concluded that about half the tumors that they called malignant ultimately led to the death of the patient. Incomplete tumor resection is associated with poor prognosis, so wide surgical excision of the lesion is necessary.

IV. Localized Malignant Mesothelioma

Localized malignant mesothelioma was recognized by Crotty et al. (9) in 1994, although it is clear from the literature that occasional cases have been reported previously as examples of solitary fibrous tumor and some have probably been classified as diffuse malignant mesotheliomas (9). Clinical features of localized malignant mesothelioma are noted in Table 5. The tumor is extremely rare; the United States-Canadian Mesothelioma Reference Panel (USCMRP) reported 23 such cases in a 2005 study (10). Localized malignant mesotheliomas are discrete, circumscribed masses, which may be attached to the pleura by a pedicle or may be sessile. Many of the reported patients have been asymptomatic and the tumor has been an incidental finding on chest radiograph. The male-female ratio is about 60:40, and the median age has been reported to be 62 years, with almost all the patients over the age of 40 (10). The role of asbestos exposure in these patients has not been defined; only 4 of the 23 patients in the USCMRP study had a history of asbestos exposure (10).

Table 6 summarizes the pathological features of these tumors. Their size ranges from about 2 to 15 cm, with a median of about 6 cm; size does not appear to affect prognosis. Localized malignant mesotheliomas (Figs. 12 and 13) are histologically, immunohistochemically, and ultrastructurally identical to ordinary diffuse malignant mesotheliomas; and clinical, radiographic, and gross pathological correlation is required to separate these two entities, particularly since occasional diffuse malignant mesotheliomas have a dominant

Table 5 Clinical Features of Localized Malignant Mesothelioma

Age range: Almost all over age 40
Association with asbestos exposure undefined
Majority are asymptomatic or present with nonspecific symptoms
Male-female ratio—60:40
As opposed to diffuse malignant mesothelioma, substantial number of patients have prolonged survival and many are apparently cured with surgical excision
Can recur and metastasize in a manner similar to sarcomas, but does not diffusely spread over the pleura
Radiographically nodular pleural-based lesion

Table 6 Pathological Features of Localized Malignant Mesothelioma

Nodular lesions arising from visceral or parietal pleura
No gross or microscopic evidence of widespread tumor on the pleural surface
May be pedunculated or sessile
Histologically, immunohistochemically, and ultrastructurally identical to diffuse malignant mesothelioma
Epithelial, sarcomatous, and biphasic subtypes

local mass. Diffuse malignant mesotheliomas exhibit widespread tumor on the serosal surface, either as tumor nodules or a rind-like pattern around the lung; however, localized malignant mesotheliomas do not spread over the pleura in the fashion of diffuse malignant mesothelioma. Epithelial, biphasic, and sarcomatous subtypes occur (epithelial subtype is the most common); but histological subtype does not correlate with survival. Keratin positivity, helpful in separating localized malignant mesothelioma from benign and malignant solitary fibrous tumor and from other sarcomas in the pleura, does not assist in differentiating localized malignant mesothelioma from diffuse malignant mesothelioma. Unlike diffuse malignant mesotheliomas, localized malignant mesotheliomas recur and metastasize in a manner similar to sarcomas (10). The prognosis of localized malignant mesothelioma is variable and many cases are apparently cured by surgical excision. Half of the patients with follow-up in the USCMRP study were alive, some with many years of follow-up (10).

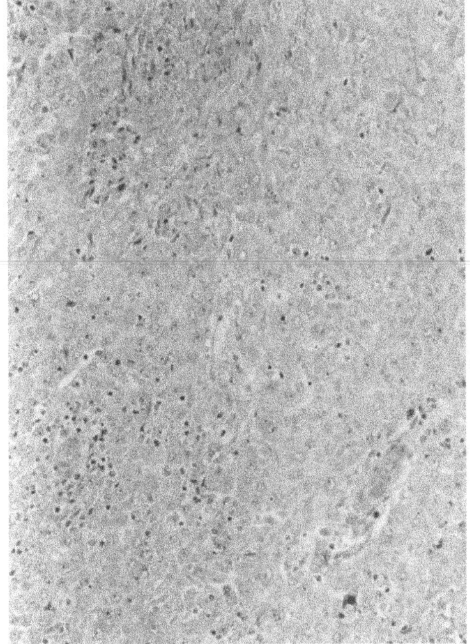

Figure 12 Low-power view of a localized malignant mesothelioma.

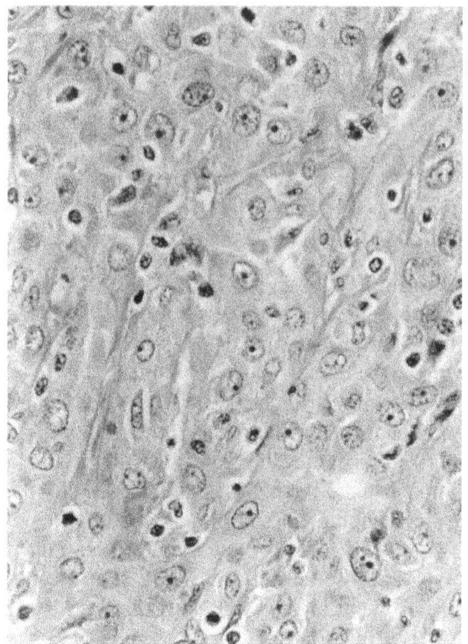

Figure 13 High-power view of the same localized malignant mesothelioma as in Figure 12. The histological appearance is that of an ordinary diffuse epithelial malignant mesothelioma, but the tumor was a circumscribed nodule with no diffuse pleural spread.

V. Localized Sarcoma

This is a poorly defined and somewhat exclusionary group composed of nodular, pleural-based, malignant-appearing spindle-cell tumors that are keratin-negative (otherwise they would be classified as sarcomatous variants of localized malignant mesothelioma), and CD34-negative (otherwise they would be classified as malignant solitary fibrous tumors). Few series exist, but some specifically differentiated localized pleural sarcomas have been reported. For example, Moran et al. (11) reported four tumors that were immunochemically marked as smooth muscle tumors (positive for smooth muscle actin and desmin), but one was also keratin-positive, raising the question of whether this was really a localized malignant mesothelioma. Of interest, despite microscopic evidence of malignancy, none of the three tumors that could be resected has recurred at time periods of up to eight months. Synovial sarcoma may rarely occur in the pleura as a localized mass (10,12).

VI. Miscellaneous Tumors and Tumor-like Lesions

Schwannomas lying in the paravertebral gutter may mimic localized pleural-based tumors, although they are generally classified as posterior mediastinal tumors. Histologically, such lesions have the usual features of Schwannomas and are S-100-positive and CD34-negative, so that their distinction from the solitary fibrous tumor is usually obvious. Asbestos-induced pleural plaques are usually flattened collagenous structures located on the posterior lower zone parietal pleural and superior surface of the diaphragm, but on occasion, a plaque can have a more nodular structure and mimic a localized pleural tumor on radiographical examination; such plaques have sometimes been mistaken for a malignancy (13). Microscopically, nodular plaques show the usual, virtually acellular basket weave pattern of pleural plaques (14). Lipomas arising in the fat of the chest wall are relatively common and may have a dumbbell-shaped structure, with part of the lesion within the chest wall and part protruding between the ribs into the pleural cavity to form a localized mass; microscopically, they appear as ordinary lipomas (15).

VII. Conclusions

A variety of nodular tumors can occur in the pleura. A vast majority are solitary fibrous tumors and most of these are benign. Epithelial forms of localized malignant mesothelioma are microscopically distinctive, but the distinction between malignant solitary fibrous tumor, sarcomatous forms of localized malignant mesothelioma, and other localized sarcomas depend on a combination of histological and immunohistochemical features. From a clinical point of view, many of the pathologically malignant tumors can be cured if they can be completely resected; other than resectability, however, there are no certain criteria to predict which of these malignant forms will recur or metastasize.

References

1. England DM, Hochholzer L, McCarthy MJ. Localized benign and malignant fibrous tumors of the pleura. Am J Surg Pathol 1989; 13:640–658.
2. Briselli M, Mark EJ, Dicersin GR. Solitary fibrous tumors of the pleura. Cancer 1981; 47:2678–2689.
3. de Perrot M, Fischer S, Brundler MA, et al. Solitary fibrous tumors of the pleura. Ann Thorac Surg 2002; 74:285–293.
4. van de Rijn M, Lombard CM, Rouse RV. Expression of CD34 by solitary fibrous tumors of the pleura, mediastinum, and lung. Am J Surg Pathol 1994; 18:814–820.
5. Westra WH, Gerald WL, Rosai J. Solitary fibrous tumor. Consistent CD34 immunoreactivity and occurrence in the orbit. Am J Surg Pathol 1994; 18:992–998.
6. Hanau CA, Miettinen M. Solitary fibrous tumor: histological and immunohistochemical spectrum of benign and malignant variants presenting at different sites. Hum Pathol 1995; 26:440–449.
7. Mitchell JD. Solitary fibrous tumor of the pleura. Semin Thorac Cardiovasc Surg 2003; 15:305–309.
8. Brozzetti S, D'Andrea N, Limiti MR, et al. Clinical behavior of solitary fibrous tumors of the pleura. An immunohistochemical study. Anticancer Res 2000; 20:4701–4706.
9. Crotty TB, Myers JL, Katzenstein A-LA, et al. Localized malignant mesothelioma. Am J Surg Pathol 1994; 18:357–363.
10. Allen TC, Cagle PT, Churg AM, et al. Localized malignant mesothelioma. Am J Surg Pathol 2005; 29:866–873.
11. Moran CA, Suster S, Koss NM. Smooth muscle tumours presenting as pleural neoplasms. Histopathology 1995; 27:227–234.

12. Dalton, WT, Zolliker AS, McCaughey WTE, et al. Localized primary tumors of the pleura: an analysis of 40 cases. Cancer 1979; 44:1465–1475.
13. Funahashi A, Kumar UN, Varkey B. Multiple pleural plaques simulating metastatic lung tumor. Postgrad Med 1977; 61:262–273.
14. Churg A. Nonneoplastic asbestos-induced disease. In: Churg A, Green FHY, eds. Pathology of Occupational Lung Disease, 2nd ed. New York: Igaku Shoin, 1998.
15. Krause LG, Ross Ca. Intrathoracic lipomas. Arch Surg 1962; 84:82–87.

40
Molecular Diagnostics of Pulmonary Neoplasms

SANJA DACIC
University of Pittsburgh, Pittsburgh, Pennsylvania, U.S.A.

I. Introduction

Translational research focused on potential diagnostic and particularly prognostic markers of lung carcinoma using techniques of molecular biology at different levels of resolution from the whole chromosome down to the specific nucleotide sequence, has resulted in a large number of studies that have significantly improved our understanding of pulmonary carcinogenesis. However, only a few DNA or RNA based diagnostic tests have been implemented in clinical practice. RNA based tests usually require fresh or frozen tissue, while DNA based tests can be successfully performed on formalin-fixed paraffin-embedded tissue (FFPE). Fixatives that have a low pH (e.g., picric acid containing Bouin's fixative or decalcifying solutions) or that contain heavy metals (e.g., B5 with mercury) should be avoided when molecular testing is considered as they may interfere with testing (1). The majority of molecular tests are very sensitive and can detect abnormalities from a very small amount of tissue. Therefore, the first requirement for most molecular tests is to obtain a relatively pure cell population by tissue microdissection, which is an excellent method that leads to more accurate test results. Microdissection can be performed in a variety of ways, all of which have different advantages and disadvantages that have been reviewed elsewhere (1–6). Basically, these methods range from simple and inexpensive manual methods to laser-capture microdissection (LCM) methods that require expensive and complex equipment (7,8). Microdissection of target tissue, either frozen or paraffin embedded, is followed by DNA or RNA extraction. In molecular anatomic pathology laboratories, genetic material is often analyzed at the nucleic acid level with polymerase chain reaction (PCR). Other methods commonly used include in situ hybridization (ISH) or fluorescence in situ hybridization (FISH). This chapter provides a short general overview of major areas of molecular testing in lung cancer, which are employed by clinical diagnostic laboratories.

II. Molecular Testing for Diagnosis of Lung Tumors

Many pathologists were using the clinical term non–small cell lung carcinomas (NSCLC) in their surgical pathology reports, because of the historical lack of distinct treatment regimens for the different histologic types of NSCLC. However, with the development of new targeted therapies in lung adenocarcinoma, pathologists are now expected to report the exact histologic subtype of NSCLC. From the diagnostic standpoint, there is a little need for molecular testing that would help to classify histologic subtypes of NSCLC precisely. Morphologic diagnostic criteria and tumor immunoprofiles are well established for different subtypes of NSCLC and for experienced surgical pathologists precise subclassification of NSCLC usually does not present a diagnostic dilemma in most cases.

Mesenchymal or hematopoietic neoplasms usually represent a metastasis or direct spread of mediastinal disease into lung parenchyma. As recognized by the 2004 WHO classification of tumors of the lung and pleura, tumors from both groups may represent a primary lung disease and may cause a diagnostic dilemma. Immunohistochemistry is helpful in many instances, but frequently other ancillary studies are necessary to make a definitive diagnosis. In contrast to epithelial malignancies, the most common genetic abnormalities detected in these two groups of neoplasms are translocations. These tumorigenic translocations often reposition an oncogene partner next to a constitutively active gene. The oncogene is then aberrantly and constitutively activated in the cells harboring the translocation. Depending on the clustering of breakpoints, translocation assays can use reverse-transcription polymerase chain reaction (RT-PCR), PCR alone or ISH. The most common translocations applicable to diagnostic lung pathology are summarized in Table 1.

There are certain advantages and disadvantages of each approach. FISH methods are less sensitive than PCR-based assays for detecting small alterations. FISH probes are typically 20 kb and most average 100 to 200 kb in size, so alterations need to be relatively large for reliable detection. It is estimated that for RT-PCR sample, purity must be at least 70% of the tumor cells, which could be difficult to achieve in infiltrative tumors or tumors with abundant inflammation and stroma (9). On the other hand, FISH assay can detect translocations in as few as 5% of the cells within the sample. RT-PCR is reliable for identifying translocations in fresh frozen tissue, while FFPE tissue may cause false positive or false negative results. This is in contrast to FISH, which gives reliable results on FFPE tissue. This is a very important observation, because if the diagnosis is not suspected clinically, fresh tissue may not be sampled at the time of surgical procedure.

Table 1 Translocations Detected by FISH in Lymphoid and Mesenchymal Tumors of the Lung

Tumor type	FISH probe
Lymphoma	
MALT lymphoma	API2-MALT1
	IGH-MALT1
Follicular lymphoma	IGH-BCL2
Anaplastic large cell lymphoma	ALK
Mantle cell lymphoma	IGH-CCND1
Mesenchymal tumors	
IMT	ALK-TPM3
	ALK-TPM4
Synovial sarcoma	ALK-CARS
	ALK
	SYT-SSX

Abbreviations: FISH, fluorescence in situ hybridization; IMT, inflammatory myofibroblastic tumor.

A. Primary Tumor Vs. Metastasis

A very tough diagnostic challenge is the presence of a solitary lung nodule in a patient with a prior history of extrathoracic carcinoma (10–12). This is a particularly difficult question in a patient with a history of a squamous cell carcinoma of the head and neck. Head and neck squamous cell carcinomas are morphologically indistinguishable from primary squamous cell carcinomas of the lung. In contrast to adenocarcinoma, no immunohistochemical marker can differentiate between head and neck squamous cell carcinoma and pulmonary squamous cell carcinoma, which has important prognostic and therapeutic implications. PCR-based, DNA clonality assays using loss of heterozygosity (LOH) analysis of microsatellite markers located on different chromosomal loci may be very helpful in this clinical scenario (13,14). Comparison of patterns of LOH between two tumors can help to determine whether the tumors are similar (metastases) or different (independent primaries) (15–18). Although this is a clinically very useful test, which may be easily performed on FFPE tissue, there are several issues that should be addressed (19). First, LOH assay requires matched normal DNA in order to determine whether an individual is heterozygous (informative) or homozygous (noninformative) for a particular chromosomal locus. Normal DNA may be obtained from morphologically normal appearing tissue or the patient's leukocytes, which may not be readily available. The second issue is reliability of the results. Some authors report that LOH assay can definitely establish whether tumor represents a metastasis or a new primary lung cancer in 91% of cases (11). In our experience, a number of selected microsatellite markers and selection of chromosomal loci may influence the results and interpretation. Other considerations include tumor cell heterogeneity, sample size, tissue control, and artifactual allelic dropout (19,20). Recently, Vachani et al. reported a panel of 10 genes obtained by gene expression analysis that accurately determine the origin of squamous cell carcinoma in the lungs of patients with previous history of head and neck malignancy (21). The current cDNA chips remain expensive for routine clinical use. Already available, cheaper, and automated methods such as immunohistochemistry, FISH or RT-PCR methods may be a good alternative to test the significance of these markers.

III. Molecular Testing for Targeted Therapies

A. Epidermal Growth Factor Receptor Inhibitors

The epidermal growth factor receptor (EGFR, HER-1/ErbB1) is a member of the ErbB family of tyrosine kinase receptors (TK), which includes HER-1/ErbB1, HER-2/neu/ErbB2, HER-3/ErbB3, and HER-4/ErbB4. Upon ligand binding and receptor homodimerization or heterodimerization and activation, activated EGFR signals downstream to the PI3K/AKT and RAS/RAF/MAPK pathways. These intracellular signaling pathways regulate key processes such as apoptosis, proliferation, and angiogenesis. EGFR is expressed in a large proportion of epithelial tumors and its role in lung cancer has been known for decades.

The development of inhibitors of EGFR resulted in new therapeutic options for patients with advanced lung cancer. It was clear from the experience with targeted therapy for breast cancer that new standardized assay procedures for assessing and predicting the effects of therapeutic agents must be developed. Following the breast cancer model, using a cost-benefit approach and based on method availability in clinical laboratories, the status of the EGFR gene was initially explored by immunohistochemistry and FISH (22–25).

Although there was a good correlation between the two methods, these were not able to predict a patient's response to EGFR inhibitors. In addition, impact of EGFR status on the patient's survival as assessed by these two methods was controversial. Initial clinical trials in unselected NSCLC patients failed to show response to anti-EGFR therapies in a majority of patients. However, a minority showed dramatic tumor shrinkage and survival benefits. It was noted that patients who responded to anti-EGFR therapies were Asian women, never smokers with adenocarcinoma showing features of bronchioloalveolar carcinoma (BAC) (26). These observations resulted in three milestone studies in 2004, demonstrating that tumor response to the EGFR TKIs gefitinib and erlotinib is associated with somatic mutations in exons 18–21 of the TK domain of EGFR (27–29). The most common are in-frame deletions in exon 19 (45%), followed by a point mutation (CTG to CGG) in exon 21 at nucleotide 2573 which results in substitution of leucine by arginine at codon 858 (L858R) (41%). Other less common mutations which are associated with sensitivity to EGFR TKIs include G719 mutations in exon 18 and the L861 mutations in exon 21. It seems that EGFR mutations are limited to lung cancer, and initially no mutations have been identified in other types of cancer. However, recently rare missense mutations in exons 19 and 21 were detected in colorectal carcinoma (30,31). The same deletions in exon 19 as seen in lung cancer were also detected in squamous cell carcinoma of the head and neck (32).

All these observations resulted in the implementation of DNA direct sequencing as a clinical screening test for common EGFR mutations in patients with lung adenocarcinomas. This assay can be performed on fresh, frozen, and archival FFPE tissue, including surgical resection specimens or fine needle biopsies (33,34). The pathologist's role in EGFR testing is to ensure that testing is performed only on adenocarcinomas or adenosquamous carcinomas unless specifically requested by the oncologist (35,36). Mucinous type BAC should not be tested for EGFR mutations. Pathologists should select the most cellular areas usually containing >50% tumor cells. Even though microdissection is the first step in sample analysis, it is known that DNA direct sequencing may not detect mutations if tumor cells represent <25% of the sample. Many other more sensitive mutation detection techniques have been reported including mutation-specific PCR assays, PCR with hybridization in real time with mutation-specific fluorescent probes, and single-strand conformational polymorphism among others (37–40). As these techniques do not significantly improve diagnostic yield, direct sequencing is still considered the gold standard.

It is known that mutations in EGFR, KRAS, BRAF, and HER2 genes are mutually exclusive in lung adenocarcinoma (41). KRAS mutations are predictors of failure of EGFR TKI therapy (42). They occur in adenocarcinomas of smokers and are adverse prognostic factors. HER2 mutations are very similar to EGFR mutations, affecting adenocarcinomas with BAC morphology in women, never smokers and may predict sensitivity to other targeted therapies. Therefore, clinical testing in lung adenocarcinomas goes beyond EGFR mutation status, and some clinical laboratories are putting into practice comprehensive mutational profiles for lung adenocarcinoma since each of the above mentioned mutations have some impact on treatment selection.

EGFR mutations strongly correlate with the clinical response to TKIs, but the correlation is not absolute and patients who initially responded may develop recurrent disease resistant to further TKIs therapy. Acquired resistance to EGFR TKIs has been associated with a second EGFR mutation in about 50% of cases, most frequently T790M in exon 20 of the TK domain (43). The frequency of this mutation may be underestimated particularly in cases with EGFR amplification of the EGFR allele with the first mutation. However, mechanisms for resistance in patients negative for this second mutation are unknown. Molecular analysis of repeat biopsies from relapsed tumors in patients initially treated with TKIs may lead to the discovery of other possible mutations or other genetic alterations responsible for patient relapse.

Despite the fact that most laboratories accepted direct sequencing or other mutational methods as the most reliable assays that predict good responders to TKI, there is still ongoing discussion about the most appropriate clinical testing for establishing EGFR status in lung adenocarcinomas, particularly gene copy number analysis [FISH or chromogenic in situ hybridization (CISH)] (44,45). This has resulted in a proposal for combined clinical testing for assessment of EGFR status in lung adenocarcinoma patients. EGFR mutations are frequently associated with increased EGFR gene copy numbers, but recent evidence supports EGFR mutation status as the most relevant marker for treatment selection (46,47).

In summary, discovery of activating mutations in EGFR as a molecular basis for a patient's response to EGFR TKI revolutionized molecular diagnostics of lung adenocarcinoma. EGFR mutation analysis is currently accepted as the most accurate test for prediction of response to EGFR TKI. Combining EGFR mutation analysis with EGFR FISH or CISH may provide additional useful information. Other genes involved in lung adenocarcinoma carcinogenesis which may represent new targets for therapies, most likely will be tested in a similar way as EGFR in the near future.

IV. Molecular Testing for Origin of Tumors in Lung Allografts

The origins of malignancies that develop after transplantation of lung allografts are not always clear. In our experience, the most common malignancies in lung allografts are primary lung carcinomas. However, more challenging cases are metastatic carcinomas to the lung, which may represent either incidentally transmitted occult tumors from clinically healthy donors to the recipients or metastasis of a recipient's primary tumor outside of the lung. To resolve the question of donor versus recipient tumor origin, DNA typing can be performed. In this type of molecular testing, specific parts of DNA are examined for polymorphisms (differences) that are unique to the individual. These parts of the DNA strand are referred to as microsatellites or minisatellites and are composed of repeated subunits of the DNA strand. Sometimes these repeated units are called short tandem repeats (STRs) or variable number of tandem repeats (VNTRs). Population statistics for these genetic loci have been determined and are used in the calculation of genetic profile frequencies. In our laboratory, DNA typing is performed using the Applied Biosystems AmpFLSTR Identifier PCR Amplification Kit, which tests for 16 different polymorphic loci in one PCR reaction. The kit also includes the amelogenin gene, which is located on the X and Y chromosomes and is useful in determining the sex of an individual. The kit has been internally validated and is optimized for use with small samples with potentially low DNA concentrations. The first step is to obtain DNA from the tumor in question and the recipient DNA (either from tissue or peripheral blood). Allograft biopsies (donor tissue) usually available in pathology archives represent an excellent source of donor's DNA, although this is not necessary for this type of analysis since the results of DNA typing are compared. If tumor and recipient DNA match, then the tumor is of recipient origin; if they are different, the tumor came from the donor.

Interpretation of DNA amplification in tumors in allograft recipients is usually complicated by a mixture of donor and recipient alleles. In addition, the DNA profile of malignant tissue should be interpreted with caution because of possible LOH, which may lead to loss of one allele. Other chromosomal abnormalities could also occur that may alter the allele pattern in tumor tissue. DNA typing can be technically performed in any molecular laboratory, but results of analysis are not always clear-cut and medicolegal issues may arise.

V. Other Potential Molecular Tests

The focus of this chapter is on clinical molecular tests currently available for assessment of lung neoplasia. There are several areas of development that need more validation before tests can be implemented in clinical practice.

Clinical and pathologic staging of lung carcinoma is not always reliable, and several studies have evaluated whether molecular studies of lymph nodes or peripheral blood can provide more accurate staging for patients with lung carcinomas. Most assays are RNA based RT-PCR (48,49). There are several issues with this assay that should be mentioned. RT-PCR assay is very sensitive and can detect a very small amount of nucleic acid, but the clinical significance of these findings is uncertain, particularly if molecular results are not supported by morphology. Another issue is specificity of the markers used for testing. Some markers (e.g., cytokeratin 19 or cytokeratin 20) can be detected in tissues or peripheral blood of patients without cancer. At the present, it seems that no single marker is sensitive and specific enough to be used in clinical practice for diagnostic or prognostic purposes. Another dilemma is whether one or multiple markers should be tested. Before this kind of testing is considered for clinical application, prospective studies are needed to determine whether the presence of submicroscopic disease detected by molecular testing alone has any prognostic significance.

The largest area for molecular testing represents development of molecular testing to predict patient's response to targeted therapies. The availability of drugs that interfere with DNA methylation or demethylation in lung cancer suggests that DNA methylation analysis may have a role in identifying lung cancer patients who may benefit from these types of therapies (50).

There is a great need to develop molecular tests for lung cancer screening in high-risk patients. However, presently it is uncertain what type of specimen should be used and what are the markers of early disease. Results of gene expression analysis may provide some insight into early markers of different types of lung carcinomas, but the current cDNA chips are too expensive for routine clinical use. An alternative would be to test the significance of these biomarkers using already available, cheaper, and automated methods such as immunohistochemistry, FISH or RT-PCR.

References

1. Hunt JL, Finkelstein SD. Microdissection techniques for molecular testing in surgical pathology. Arch Pathol Lab Med 2004; 128:1372–1378.
2. Emmert-Buck MR, Bonner RF, Smith PD, et al. Laser capture microdissection. Science 1996; 274:998–1001.

3. Bonner RF, Emmert-Buck M, Cole K, et al. Laser capture microdissection: molecular analysis of tissue. Science 1997; 278:1481–1483.
4. Curran S, McKay JA, McLeod HL, et al. Laser capture microscopy. Mol Pathol 2000; 53:64–68.
5. Ohyama H, Zhang X, Kohno Y, et al. Laser capture microdissection-generated target sample for high-density oligonucleotide array hybridization. Biotechniques 2000; 29:530–536.
6. Fend F, Raffeld M. Laser capture microdissection in pathology. J Clin Pathol 2000; 53:666–672.
7. Eltoum IA, Siegal GP, Frost AR. Microdissection of histologic sections: past, present, and future. Adv Anat Pathol 2002; 9:316–322.
8. Simone NL, Paweletz CP, Charboneau L, et al. Laser capture microdissection: beyond functional genomics to proteomics. Mol Diagn 2000; 5:301–307.
9. Perry A, Nobori T, Ru N, et al. Detection of p16 gene deletions in gliomas: a comparison of fluorescence in situ hybridization (FISH) versus quantitative PCR. J Neuropathol Exp Neurol 1997; 56:999–1008.
10. Askin FB. Something old? Something new? Second primary or pulmonary metastasis in the patient with known extrathoracic carcinoma. Am J Clin Pathol 1993; 100:4–5.
11. Leong PP, Rezai B, Koch WM, et al. Distinguishing second primary tumors from lung metastases in patients with head and neck squamous cell carcinoma. J Natl Cancer Inst 1998; 90:972–977.
12. Schwartz LH, Ozsahin M, Zhang GN, et al. Synchronous and metachronous head and neck carcinomas. Cancer 1994; 74:1933–1938.
13. Rolston R, Sasatomi E, Hunt J, et al. Distinguishing de novo second cancer formation from tumor recurrence: mutational fingerprinting by microdissection genotyping. J Mol Diagn 2001; 3:129–132.
14. Diaz-Cano SJ, Blanes A, Wolfe HJ. PCR techniques for clonality assays. Diagn Mol Pathol 2001; 10:24–33.
15. Shimizu S, Yatabe Y, Koshikawa T, et al. High frequency of clonally related tumors in cases of multiple synchronous lung cancers as revealed by molecular diagnosis. Clin Cancer Res 2000; 6:3994–3999.
16. Dacic S, Ionescu DN, Finkelstein S, et al. Patterns of allelic loss of synchronous adenocarcinomas of the lung. Am J Surg Pathol 2005; 29:897–902.
17. Lichy JH, Dalbegue F, Zavar M, et al. Genetic heterogeneity in ductal carcinoma of the breast. Lab Invest 2000; 80:291–301.
18. Heinmoller E, Dietmaier W, Zirngibl H, et al. Molecular analysis of microdissected tumors and preneoplastic intraductal lesions in pancreatic carcinoma. Am J Pathol 2000; 157:83–92.
19. Tomlinson IP, Lambros MB, Roylance RR. Loss of heterozygosity analysis: practically and conceptually flawed? Genes Chromosomes Cancer 2002; 34:349–353.
20. Newton MA, Gould MN, Reznikoff CA, et al. On the statistical analysis of allelic-loss data. Stat Med 1998; 17:1425–1445.
21. Vachani A, Nebozhyn M, Singhal S, et al. A 10-gene classifier for distinguishing head and neck squamous cell carcinoma and lung squamous cell carcinoma. Clin Cancer Res 2007; 13:2905–2915.
22. Hirsch FR, Varella-Garcia M, Bunn PA Jr., et al. Epidermal growth factor receptor in non-small-cell lung carcinomas: correlation between gene copy number and protein expression and impact on prognosis. J Clin Oncol 2003; 21:3798–3807.
23. Nakamura H, Kawasaki N, Taguchi M, et al. Survival impact of epidermal growth factor receptor overexpression in patients with non-small cell lung cancer: a meta-analysis. Thorax 2006; 61:140–145.
24. Suzuki S, Dobashi Y, Sakurai H, et al. Protein overexpression and gene amplification of epidermal growth factor receptor in nonsmall cell lung carcinomas. An immunohistochemical and fluorescence in situ hybridization study. Cancer 2005; 103:1265–1273.
25. Dacic S, Flanagan M, Cieply K, et al. Significance of EGFR protein expression and gene amplification in non-small cell lung carcinoma. Am J Clin Pathol 2006; 125:860–865.

26. Blons H, Cote JF, Le Corre D, et al. Epidermal growth factor receptor mutation in lung cancer are linked to bronchioloalveolar differentiation. Am J Surg Pathol 2006; 30:1309–1315.
27. Lynch TJ, Bell DW, Sordella R, et al. Activating mutations in the epidermal growth factor receptor underlying responsiveness of non-small-cell lung cancer to gefitinib. N Engl J Med 2004; 350:2129–2139.
28. Paez JG, Janne PA, Lee JC, et al. EGFR mutations in lung cancer: correlation with clinical response to gefitinib therapy. Science 2004; 304:1497–1500.
29. Pao W, Miller V, Zakowski M, et al. EGF receptor gene mutations are common in lung cancers from "never smokers" and are associated with sensitivity of tumors to gefitinib and erlotinib. Proc Natl Acad Sci U S A 2004; 101:13306–13311.
30. Nagahara H, Mimori K, Ohta M, et al. Somatic mutations of epidermal growth factor receptor in colorectal carcinoma. Clin Cancer Res 2005; 11:1368–1371.
31. Ogino S, Meyerhardt JA, Cantor M, et al. Molecular alterations in tumors and response to combination chemotherapy with gefitinib for advanced colorectal cancer. Clin Cancer Res 2005; 11:6650–6656.
32. Lee JW, Soung YH, Kim SY, et al. Somatic mutations of EGFR gene in squamous cell carcinoma of the head and neck. Clin Cancer Res 2005; 11:2879–2882.
33. Sequist LV, Joshi VA, Janne PA, et al. Epidermal growth factor receptor mutation testing in the care of lung cancer patients. Clin Cancer Res 2006; 12:4403s–4408s.
34. Shih JY, Gow CH, Yu CJ, et al. Epidermal growth factor receptor mutations in needle biopsy/aspiration samples predict response to gefitinib therapy and survival of patients with advanced nonsmall cell lung cancer. Int J Cancer 2006; 118:963–969.
35. Marchetti A, Buttitta F, Pellegrini S, et al. Bronchioloalveolar lung carcinomas: K-ras mutations are constant events in the mucinous subtype. J Pathol 1996; 179:254–259.
36. Marchetti A, Martella C, Felicioni L, et al. EGFR mutations in non-small-cell lung cancer: analysis of a large series of cases and development of a rapid and sensitive method for diagnostic screening with potential implications on pharmacologic treatment. J Clin Oncol 2005; 23:857–865.
37. Sasaki H, Endo K, Konishi A, et al. EGFR Mutation status in Japanese lung cancer patients: genotyping analysis using LightCycler. Clin Cancer Res 2005; 11:2924–2929.
38. Pan Q, Pao W, Ladanyi M. Rapid polymerase chain reaction-based detection of epidermal growth factor receptor gene mutations in lung adenocarcinomas. J Mol Diagn 2005; 7:396–403.
39. Asano H, Toyooka S, Tokumo M, et al. Detection of EGFR gene mutation in lung cancer by mutant-enriched polymerase chain reaction assay. Clin Cancer Res 2006; 12:43–48.
40. Zhou C, Ni J, Zhao Y, et al. Rapid detection of epidermal growth factor receptor mutations in non-small cell lung cancer using real-time polymerase chain reaction with TaqMan-MGB probes. Cancer J 2006; 12:33–39.
41. Shigematsu H, Gazdar AF. Somatic mutations of epidermal growth factor receptor signaling pathway in lung cancers. Int J Cancer 2006; 118:257–262.
42. Eberhard DA, Johnson BE, Amler LC, et al. Mutations in the epidermal growth factor receptor and in KRAS are predictive and prognostic indicators in patients with non-small-cell lung cancer treated with chemotherapy alone and in combination with erlotinib. J Clin Oncol 2005; 23: 5900–5909.
43. Kobayashi S, Boggon TJ, Dayaram T, et al. EGFR mutation and resistance of non-small-cell lung cancer to gefitinib. N Engl J Med 2005; 352:786–792.
44. Johnson BE, Janne PA. Selecting patients for epidermal growth factor receptor inhibitor treatment: a FISH story or a tale of mutations? J Clin Oncol 2005; 23:6813–6816.
45. Cappuzzo F, Hirsch FR, Rossi E, et al. Epidermal growth factor receptor gene and protein and gefitinib sensitivity in non-small-cell lung cancer. J Natl Cancer Inst 2005; 97:643–655.
46. Han SW, Kim TY, Jeon YK, et al. Optimization of patient selection for gefitinib in non-small cell lung cancer by combined analysis of epidermal growth factor receptor mutation, K-ras mutation, and Akt phosphorylation. Clin Cancer Res 2006; 12:2538–2544.

47. Endo K, Sasaki H, Yano M, et al. Evaluation of the epidermal growth factor receptor gene mutation and copy number in non-small cell lung cancer with gefitinib therapy. Oncol Rep 2006; 16:533–541.
48. Herrera LJ, Raja S, Gooding WE, et al. Quantitative analysis of circulating plasma DNA as a tumor marker in thoracic malignancies. Clin Chem 2005; 51:113–118.
49. Xi L, Coello MC, Litle VR, et al. A combination of molecular markers accurately detects lymph node metastasis in non-small cell lung cancer patients. Clin Cancer Res 2006; 12:2484–2491.
50. Fang MZ, Wang Y, Ai N, et al. Tea polyphenol (–)-epigallocatechin-3-gallate inhibits DNA methyltransferase and reactivates methylation-silenced genes in cancer cell lines. Cancer Res 2003; 63:7563–7570.

41
Molecular Diagnosis of Pleural Neoplasms

ALAIN C. BORCZUK
Columbia University Medical Center, New York, New York, U.S.A.

I. Introduction

Molecular pathology is playing an increasing role as a critical adjunct to morphologic diagnosis in the diagnosis of neoplastic disease. In hematopoietic tumors, pediatric tumors, and soft tissue tumors, the understanding of molecular pathogenesis of disease has led not only to improvements in diagnosis, but also to the possibility of molecular classification of neoplasia. Such new methods of classification may provide insight into treatment and prognostic categories beyond what can be achieved through conventional morphology. Furthermore, understanding of molecular pathology and pathogenesis may provide testing opportunities for early detection/screening for disease as well as sensitive tests for disease monitoring after therapy.

The impact of these observations on pleural neoplasia has yet to achieve its full potential, but there remains significant utility to molecular diagnostics, especially in soft tissue tumors that involve pleura/chest wall.

A. Diagnostic Immunohistochemistry in Pleural Neoplasia

Immunohistochemistry has become a critical adjunct to morphologic diagnosis. In many instances, it is the first set of molecular tests that a pathologist performs to define a set of protein expression patterns that are characteristic of a cell lineage or tissue of origin. In some cases, while such a pattern is not unique, the combination of morphologic differential diagnosis and immunohistochemistry profile is sufficient to properly classify a tumor.

A detailed description of diagnostic immunohistochemistry is beyond the scope of this chapter, but given its importance in the diagnosis of pleural neoplasia, some summary points are relevant. If we examine the WHO classification of pleural neoplasia, we can separate these neoplasms into epithelial/epithelioid tumors, biphasic tumors, and spindled cell/sarcomatous tumors. With morphologic assessment, many problems of differential diagnosis can be resolved using immunohistochemistry profiles. Commonly used antibodies in this setting are summarized in Table 1 (1–29).

Reviewing the immunohistochemistry options, several points are relevant. In the diagnosis of epithelial-type malignant mesothelioma (MM), distinction from lung adenocarcinoma has many potentially useful markers. While fewer markers are available that reliably distinguish MM from squamous carcinoma, the relative rarity of "pseudomesotheliomatous" squamous carcinoma makes this a less frequent diagnostic dilemma. Among

Table 1 Differential Diagnosis and Common Immunohistochemistry Markers in Pleural Neoplasms

Pleural neoplasms

Epithelial/epithelioid

Mesothelioma, epithelial

Positive	Negative
Calretinin	MOC31
WT1	BerEP4 (10–20% focal +)
CK5/6	CEA
D240	BG8
	B72.3
	CD15
	TTF1
	P63 (<10% focal+)

Lung adenocarcinoma

Positive		Negative
TTF1	B72.3	Calretinin (10% +)
MOC31	CEA	CK5/6 (<20% focal +)
BG8	CD15	WT1
BerEp4	p63	D240 (7% +)

Squamous carcinoma

Positive		Negative
CK5/6	BG8	WT1
p63	BerEp4	
MOC31	D240	
Calretinin (40%)		

Biphasic

Mesothelioma, biphasic

The epithelial component stains as indicated in the left column

Synovial sarcoma, biphasic

Positive	Negative
Pan-CK	WT1
EMA	
CD56	
Calretinin	
CK5/6	
BerEp4	
CD99	
Bcl 2	

Sarcomatoid carcinoma

Use similar markers as mesothelioma vs. carcinoma markers listed on left, except calretinin is frequently positive and not useful

Sarcomatous/spindled

Mesothelioma, sarcomatous

Positive	Negative
Pan-CK	WT1 (<10% +)
CK 5/6 (few cases, focal)	BerEP4
Calretinin (<50%)	B72.3
Bcl 2 (20%)	BG8
	MOC31
	CD15
	CEA

Synovial sarcoma, monophasic/poorly differentiated

Positive (high %)	Positive (lower %)	Negative
CD99	Pan-CK	WT1
Bcl 2	EMA	
CD56	Calretinin	
	CK5/6	

Ewing's sarcoma/PNET

Positive	Negative
CD99	WT1 (nuclear)
FLI-1	Calretinin (15%)
Bcl 2 (50%)	EMA (17%)
Synaptophysin (34%)	
Pan-CK (25%)	

Desmoplastic small round cell tumor

Positive	Negative
Pan-CK	CD99 (23% +)
NSE	
Desmin	
WT1	

the biphasic tumors, there can be significant morphologic overlap between MM, sarcomatoid carcinoma, and biphasic synovial sarcoma (SS). An examination of positive immunohistochemistry markers also reveals significant overlap, especially with regard to calretinin immunoreactivity. Use of the traditional carcinoma markers in sarcomatoid carcinoma and WT1 for MM assists in the diagnosis; the distinctive morphology of biphasic SS and a panel approach (including BerEP4 and WT1) can be useful in separating SS from MM. Perhaps the most challenging category is the spindle cell/sarcomatous category. Morphologic overlap between sarcomatous mesothelioma, monophasic and poorly differentiated SS (more common than biphasic pattern in pleuropulmonary disease), and other sarcomas can be significant, and overlap between Ewing's/primitive neuroectodermal tumor (PNET) and monophasic and poorly differentiated SS can also be diagnostically challenging. Examination of markers useful in these differential diagnoses reveals relatively fewer options; importantly, WT1 is often negative in sarcomatous mesothelioma, and cytokeratin and BerEp4 is more frequently negative in monophasic and poorly differentiated SS. The significant overlap in both morphology and immunohistochemistry profiles in the spindle cell group increases the potential utility of molecular testing in that subgroup.

For the remainder of the chapter, the discussion will focus on molecular diagnostics as applied to pleural neoplasms as an adjunct to morphology and immunohistochemistry, in testing related to prognostication for early detection or screening, and to monitor therapeutic success. In some instances, these categories may have overlap.

B. Malignant Mesothelioma

While several studies have examined gene expression profiling of MM, this approach is not currently in use in the diagnostic arena. Gordon et al. described gene expression ratios obtained through real-time polymerase chain reaction (PCR)/quantitative RT-PCR (qRT-PCR) analysis that may discriminate between mesothelioma and adenocarcinoma (30). This approach may have future promise; however, immunohistochemistry for the protein products of some of the genes in the ratio approach are already in common use (calretinin, TTF1). In addition, studies of gene expression profiles have led to gene expression assays that may have utility in prognostication (31,32).

Other than immunohistochemistry, there is no specific molecular test to confirm the diagnosis of MM, and this is reflected by some challenging cases in which it is difficult to distinguish reactive mesothelial proliferations from MM. In addition, there is no tumor specific fusion gene to allow for monitoring of disease progression or early detection.

The observation of mesothelin expression in MM has led to interest in enzyme-linked immunosorbent assay (ELISA) testing for mesothelin, soluble mesothelioma related peptide (SMRP), and megakaryocyte potentiating factor in serum and pleural fluid (33–35). It appears that patients with MM have higher levels of detectable SMRP in serum and that asbestos exposed individuals may also have higher levels than the nonexposed population. While further study is needed to determine optimal cutoff levels for this type of testing as a screening tool, it does show promise in the early detection of MM. In addition, testing for serum tumor markers specific for MM may aid in monitoring treatment efficacy and disease recurrence in both pleural and peritoneal disease.

Molecular markers associated with prognosis continue to be investigated. In a set of 99 pleural mesotheliomas, Lopez-Rios et al. (36) determined that expression of aurora kinases and the deletion of p16 were associated with poor prognosis. Loss of p16 expression has been a long recognized mechanism of tumorigenesis in MM, and prior studies in both pleural and peritoneal mesothelioma indicated an association of p16 loss with biphasic and sarcomatous histology (a poor prognosis parameter), and p16 loss as an independent parameter of poor prognosis (37–39). As p16 loss by deletion is the most frequent mechanism in MM, it is possible to test for deletion of p16 by fluorescent in situ hybridization (FISH) as a potential prognostic marker.

C. Synovial Sarcoma

Differentiating biphasic and spindled cell SS from MM can, in some cases, be challenging (40). Whether biphasic, monophasic, or poorly differentiated, SSs frequently possess an X;18 translocation [t(X;18)(p11;q11)] that results in a fusion gene between SYT and either SSX1 or SSX2, and very rarely SSX4 (41,42). The identification of a translocation and a fusion transcript allows for various strategies that allow for diagnostic confirmation and some with utility for disease monitoring. Whether all suspected cases of SS require molecular confirmation is controversial; it has been suggested that in many cases the combination of morphology, clinical data, and immunohistochemistry is sufficient. Therefore for diagnostic purposes, it may be appropriate to reserve molecular testing for challenging cases (43).

Karyotyping remains a common methodology to detect tumor translocations, and if fresh tissue is available, cultured cells are used for this technique. Cells arrested in metaphase are Giemsa stained and the chromosomes visualized and sorted. The chromosome structure and banding pattern is studied, and translocations such as the X;18 translocation of SS can be detected. This method of direct visualization has the advantage of providing definitive evidence of large translocations, and also any other associated cytogenetic abnormality that in the future may be predictive of tumor subtypes or prognostic outcome. It has the disadvantage of requiring fresh tissue and facilities for cell culture. In addition, tumor cell culture can be challenging, and the interpretation of results requires highly skilled individuals. Finally, some translocation events are too small in fragment size to be reliably visualized by this technique. All these factors combine to reduce the sensitivity of this approach, and the diagnostic success is reduced by technical complexity.

Another common strategy for diagnostic testing is FISH. There are two strategies in this setting, fusion and break apart. The fusion strategy uses fluorescent-labeled probes from each translocation partner, for example, orange for SYT and green for SSX1, using regions of these genes known to be involved in the translocation. In a normal cell or in nontranslocated tumor cells, two orange signals and two green signals are present reflecting the normal diploid complement on chromosomes 18 and X (in females). If a translocation has occurred, the two probes are brought into proximity with each other, resulting in a fused yellow signal. The break-apart strategy is based on the fact that translocations in SS always involve the SYT gene. Probes have been developed that flank either side of the SYT gene. Commonly used probes choose an orange color for one end of the gene and a green fluorescent color for the other end. In a normal cell and in tumors other than SS, the two signals by FISH will be adjacent to each other and appear yellow. Two yellow signals in a cell indicate that no translocation is present. If a cell contains separate orange and green signals, the SYT gene has been split or broken apart, indicating that a translocation has occurred. As the name suggests, an SYT split probe or break-apart probe tests for this translocation event. The advantage of this strategy over fusion is that SYT break apart avoids the need to separately test for each translocation partner.

RT-PCR is another commonly used technique for the detection of a fusion mRNA transcript that results from a translocation. By choosing primers that flank the region of a fused mRNA transcript, reverse transcription is performed, and the resultant cDNA is amplified by PCR. This DNA product can be resolved on an agarose gel, and its size can be compared with markers of known DNA size. Since the primers are chosen to flank a region of known size that crosses the area of translocation in the fusion transcript, the resultant PCR product should produce a band of the correct molecular weight, and should not be present in normal cells or cells lacking the specific translocation. Other methods of analyzing the PCR product include restriction enzyme digestion or sequencing. This technique is sensitive and does not usually require prior microdissection of tumor to achieve the sensitivity in fresh tissue. In addition, it can be reliably performed on formalin-fixed paraffin-embedded tissue, although success rates differ depending on fixation and possibly age of the paraffin blocks/slides. The disadvantage of this technique is that it can produce false-positive results, and controls must be carefully evaluated. Also, it only detects one translocation, and primers need to be developed for each different potential translocation. In the case of SS, the associated translocations are commonly either SYT-SSX1 or SYT-SSX2, allowing for the feasibility of a PCR based approach.

Studies have examined qRT-PCR in the diagnosis of SS (44) (also known as real-time PCR). This technique also uses primers that target the fusion transcript from a translocation, as does RT-PCR. However, rather than postreaction evaluation of the product, this technique monitors the accumulation of a measurable signal that increases with each PCR cycle when the target is present in the sample, and this measurement is proportional to the amount of the target RNA message. One example of qRT-PCR links combinations of primers and sequence-specific probes that contain a dye at the 5′ end and a quencher at the 3′ end, preventing fluorescent signal release when the probe is intact. When the target cDNA is bound by primer and DNA polymerase is active, the probe is cleaved releasing the dye from the quencher and allowing for a fluorescent signal. After multiple cycles of the PCR reaction, fluorescent signal will increase in proportion to the number of target cDNA in the original specimen. Therefore, a fusion transcript can be detected using appropriate primers, and if compared with a control mRNA, an estimate of quantity can be made. Given the possibility for different primer-probe dye combinations, reactions can be run simultaneously to separately detect and quantify more than one translocation-derived fusion transcript per sample. In addition, this technique is less prone to contamination as it exploits uracil incorporation during PCR of the product to distinguish it from thymidine containing target cDNA. It is also less time consuming than RT-PCR. The disadvantage of this technique is that it is more sensitive to RNA degradation, and both detection and accurate quantification may be affected by poor quality RNA. It is of note that Hostein et al. (44) demonstrated comparable results from fresh and paraffin tissue thereby addressing this disadvantage as applied to paraffin tissue.

Various studies have examined the molecular diagnosis of SS in general, as well as, in the specific setting of chest wall and pleural disease. In a series of 243 patients, Ladanyi (45) examined 243 SSs using a combination of RT-PCR and FISH, with both fresh and paraffin embedded tissues. SYT-SSX1 translocations were seen in 61% of cases, and a greater proportion of SYT-SSX2 SS were monophasic. They also demonstrated that SYT-SSX1 tumor patients had decreased metastasis-free survival and SYT-SSX2 tumor patients had better overall survival. This has not been a universal finding, however, as grade, not presence of a particular fusion, was associated with survival in a European multicenter study of 165 patients (46). Guillou (47) used RT-PCR in SS and non-SS tumors and found 100% specificity, with an assay success rate of just under 90%. The sensitivity was over 90% with successful amplification, with the observation that Bouin's fixative was detrimental to the assay.

Focusing on pulmonary SS, a study of 11 cases of SS (48) showed 9 of 11 with SYT-SSX1 translocation and all cases with a detectable fusion by RT-PCR. In a study of 60 cases of pulmonary and mediastinal SS using paraffin RT PCR, 92% had a detectable SYT-SSX fusion, with SYT-SSX1 as the majority (60%). While follow-up was not obtained in all cases, a higher proportion of patients with less than five-year survival had SYT-SSX1 fusion (12). In a comparison of difficult spindled cell pleural tumors, Weinbreck et al. (18) confirmed the presence of SYT-SSX in SS and importantly the absence of this fusion in sarcomatoid mesothelioma.

A recent series analyzed RT-PCR, FISH, and qRT-PCR methods of detection in 134 cases of SS. In 131 of 134 cases, RNA quality from formalin fixed paraffin embedded tissue was suitable. In this series, qRT-PCR had a sensitivity of 96% and conventional PCR 92%. Break-apart probe FISH sensitivity was lower (86%), but of note, it did allow for detection in one of the three cases that failed PCR because of RNA quality. FISH testing had a higher failure rate with only 101 interpretable cases. All five cases that were molecular negative were also FISH negative. Of the five molecular negative cases, it was acknowledged that one case was likely a mesothelioma on comprehensive review of all data. Overall, qRT-PCR testing had a higher sensitivity and low rate of failure. It also suggested that FISH testing was less sensitive while equally specific.

D. Ewing's Sarcoma/PNET

When confronted with the category of "small round blue cell tumor," morphology and immunohistochemistry can serve an important role in narrowing down the diagnostic possibilities, thus resolving them. However, molecular testing in Ewing sarcoma/PNET can be critical in confirming the diagnosis.

Classical cytogenetics led to the recognition of a reciprocal translocation involving chromosome 22 and chromosome 11 that was a consistent finding in Ewing's sarcoma (49,50). While karyotyping remains a potential methodology to identify Ewing's/PNET tumors, the limitations previously mentioned for SS apply in this case as well, specifically the need for fresh tissue, cell culture and expertise in interpretation of G-banding. In addition, while other techniques confirm the results of classic cytogenetics, there are cases detected by break-apart FISH and RT-PCR not detected by classic cytogenetics. This can be due to growth of normal cells in culture, but may also reflect cases with complex rearrangements or small rearrangements, not easily resolved by G-banding.

The identification of translocations that involve the EWS gene has allowed for similar strategies for detection of EWS fusion genes as for SYT in SS. The characteristic translocation is a t(11;22) (q24;q12) found in about 85% of these tumors with a resultant EWS-FLI1 gene fusion. This is more complicated than SYT-SSX, as the EWS-FLI1 fusion can occur in different forms based on variable site of translocation, called type 1, 2, and 3. The fusion protein derived from this fusion gene may have different abilities to transform cells, and the resultant tumors may have different growth rates. An additional 10% of cases show t(21;22)(q22;q12) with an EWS-ERG gene fusion. Rarer translocations account for the remaining 5% (51). Therefore, the constellation of translocations in Ewing's/PNET is greater than in SS, and various partners are possible in fusion genes (FLI1, ERG, ETV, E1AF, FEV). Therefore, the use of break-apart probes for the EWS gene has an advantage as the vast majority of Ewing's/PNET related translocations involve split of the EWS gene and can be identified by FISH detection of break-apart probes.

Importantly and in contrast to SS, the diagnostic specificity is partly determined by other tumors that possess EWS translocation; desmoplastic small round cell tumor (DSRCT) with EWS-WT1 translocation, clear cell sarcoma with EWS-AFT1 fusion, myxoid chondrosarcoma with EWS-CHN fusion, and myxoid liposarcoma with EWS-CHOP fusion. Also, EWS-ETS gene fusion has been seen in other types of sarcomas (52–54). Therefore, both break-apart FISH and molecular testing can lead to a positive result in tumors other than Ewing's/PNET, emphasizing the need for integrated diagnostics in these tumors. DSRCT of the pleura is rare, and characteristically is cytokeratin, desmin (dot-like), WT1, and non-specific enolase positive (24,55,56). Since the WT1 in DSRCT is truncated and part of a fusion protein, it is important to select antibodies for WT1 that target the correct part of the protein.

The sensitivity of break-apart FISH in Ewing's/PNET is about 90% (57,58). While in a small number of cases a non-EWS translocation has been reported in Ewing's/PNET (FUS-ERG fusion) (59), this does not account for the entire 10% of cases not detected by break-apart probe. In the series by Bridge et al. (58), comparison of the fusion approach with the break-apart approach yields similar sensitivity in the detection of a single translocation, but the complexity of the EWS translocation favors a break-apart approach. In addition, these authors conclude that break-apart FISH was qualitatively better and therefore easier to interpret. FISH was noninformative in about 15% of cases.

RT-PCR techniques in Ewing's/PNET require a search for multiple different translocations, and is therefore less practical. Also, lower sensitivity has been reported for this technique when using archival and consultation material (58). However, when including challenging cases that were morphologically undifferentiated round cell sarcomas and FISH break apart negative or noninformative, RT-PCR technique identified fusion transcripts in 3 of the 10 cases studied, suggesting that FISH negative or noninformative cases may be complemented by RT-PCR technique.

Given the previously mentioned problems of RT-PCR, qRT-PCR technique allows for the simultaneous evaluation of multiple translocations. In one series (60), the testing was 81% sensitive and 100% specific, and detected 4 EWS fusions among 43 samples, including 2 different EWS-FLI1 fusions.

The use of molecular studies to stratify patients into prognostic categories remains a focus of research. In a meta-analysis conducted in 2003, EWS-FLI1 type 1 fusion transcript containing tumors were associated with improved disease-free survival (61). The suggestion that different chimeric proteins have varied impact on cellular growth leads to an expectation that future studies will result in prognosis stratification on the basis of type of fusion transcript. This may favor a molecular technique that allows for detection of the specific fusion transcript type such as qRT-PCR. This technique also provides the potential for quantitation. While fusion transcript detection in blood (62) and bone marrow (63) is possible, it is not clear that identification of fusion transcripts in serum or bone marrow predicts tumor progression (64); such identification in longer-term survivors may predict recurrence (65).

E. Molecular Aspects of Pleural Lymphoid Neoplasms

The description of body cavity based lymphomas in AIDS patients and its association with KSHV/HHV8 in 1996 by Nador et al. warrants a category of primary effusion lymphoma that can occur in pleura or peritoneum. It has also been identified in HIV seronegative patients. KSHV/HHV8 can be identified by RT-PCR with the caveat that this technique can produce false-positive results. In addition, immunohistochemistry for latency associated nuclear antigen, a viral derived protein, can confirm HHV8 infection (66,67).

Patients with chronic pleural infections resulting in pyothorax can also develop a large cell lymphoma. This entity of pyothorax-associated lymphoma is associated with Epstein-Barr virus (EBV) infection. These cases are positive for EBV RNA by in situ hybridization (EBER); EBV-associated proteins such as LMP-1 can be detected by immunohistochemistry (68).

II. Summary

The correct diagnosis in pleural neoplasia hinges on a combination of morphologic differential diagnosis, diagnostic immunohistochemistry, and use of molecular tests in challenging cases for diagnosis or to introduce molecular subtyping for possible prognostic utility. Break-apart FISH probes may provide evidence for translocation in SS and Ewing/PNET with excellent sensitivity and specificity for diagnostic purposes. PCR approaches, including qRT-PCR, may add diagnostic sensitivity in FISH-negative or noninformative cases, and may be further developed as the clinical significance of translocation subtypes is further elucidated, and as the significance of detection of fusion transcripts as part of disease monitoring is further explored.

References

1. Folpe AL, Schmidt RA, Chapman D, et al. Poorly differentiated synovial sarcoma: immunohistochemical distinction from primitive neuroectodermal tumors and high-grade malignant peripheral nerve sheath tumors. Am J Surg Pathol 1998; 22(6):673–82.
2. Chu PG, Weiss LM. Expression of cytokeratin 5/6 in epithelial neoplasms: an immunohistochemical study of 509 cases. Mod Pathol 2002; 15(1):6–10.
3. Chu AY, Litzky LA, Pasha TL, et al. Utility of D2-40, a novel mesothelial marker, in the diagnosis of malignant mesothelioma. Mod Pathol 2005; 18(1):105–110.
4. Doglioni C, Tos AP, Laurino L, et al. Calretinin: a novel immunocytochemical marker for mesothelioma. Am J Surg Pathol 1996; 20(9):1037–1046.
5. Loy TS, Nashelsky MB. Reactivity of B72.3 with adenocarcinomas. An immunohistochemical study of 476 cases. Cancer 1993; 72(8):2495–2498.
6. Miettinen M, Sarlomo-Rikala M. Expression of calretinin, thrombomodulin, keratin 5, and mesothelin in lung carcinomas of different types: an immunohistochemical analysis of 596 tumors in comparison with epithelioid mesotheliomas of the pleura. Am J Surg Pathol 2003; 27(2):150–158.
7. Ordonez NG. Value of thyroid transcription factor-1, E-cadherin, BG8, WT1, and CD44S immunostaining in distinguishing epithelial pleural mesothelioma from pulmonary and non-pulmonary adenocarcinoma. Am J Surg Pathol 2000; 24(4):598–606.

8. Ordonez NG. The immunohistochemical diagnosis of mesothelioma: a comparative study of epithelioid mesothelioma and lung adenocarcinoma. Am J Surg Pathol 2003; 27(8):1031–1051.
9. Ordonez NG. D2-40 and podoplanin are highly specific and sensitive immunohistochemical markers of epithelioid malignant mesothelioma. Hum Pathol 2005; 36(4):372–380.
10. Sheibani K, Shin SS, Kezirian J, et al. Ber-EP4 antibody as a discriminant in the differential diagnosis of malignant mesothelioma versus adenocarcinoma. Am J Surg Pathol 1991; 15(8): 779–784.
11. Miettinen M, Limon J, Niezabitowski A, et al. Calretinin and other mesothelioma markers in synovial sarcoma: analysis of antigenic similarities and differences with malignant mesothelioma. Am J Surg Pathol 2001; 25(5):610–617.
12. Hartel PH, Fanburg-Smith JC, Frazier AA, et al. Primary pulmonary and mediastinal synovial sarcoma: a clinicopathologic study of 60 cases and comparison with five prior series. Mod Pathol 2007; 20(7):760–769.
13. Montag AG, Pinkus GS, Corson JM. Keratin protein immunoreactivity of sarcomatoid and mixed types of diffuse malignant mesothelioma: an immunoperoxidase study of 30 cases. Hum Pathol 1988; 19(3):336–342.
14. Cagle PT, Truong LD, Roggli VL, et al. Immunohistochemical differentiation of sarcomatoid mesotheliomas from other spindle cell neoplasms. Am J Clin Pathol 1989; 92(5):566–571.
15. Ordonez NG. What are the current best immunohistochemical markers for the diagnosis of epithelioid mesothelioma? A review and update. Hum Pathol 2007; 38(1):1–16.
16. Attanoos RL, Dojcinov SD, Webb R, et al. Anti-mesothelial markers in sarcomatoid mesothelioma and other spindle cell neoplasms. Histopathology 2000; 37(3):224–231.
17. Ordonez NG. The diagnostic utility of immunohistochemistry in distinguishing between mesothelioma and renal cell carcinoma: a comparative study. Hum Pathol 2004; 35(6):697–710.
18. Weinbreck N, Vignaud JM, Begueret H, et al. SYT-SSX fusion is absent in sarcomatoid mesothelioma allowing its distinction from synovial sarcoma of the pleura. Mod Pathol 2007; 20(6): 617–621.
19. Pelmus M, Guillou L, Hostein I, et al. Monophasic fibrous and poorly differentiated synovial sarcoma: immunohistochemical reassessment of 60 t(X;18)(SYT-SSX)-positive cases. Am J Surg Pathol 2002; 26(11):1434–1440.
20. Ordonez NG. The diagnostic utility of immunohistochemistry in distinguishing between epithelioid mesotheliomas and squamous carcinomas of the lung: a comparative study. Mod Pathol 2006; 19(3):417–428.
21. Lae ME, Roche PC, Jin L, et al. Desmoplastic small round cell tumor: a clinicopathologic, immunohistochemical, and molecular study of 32 tumors. Am J Surg Pathol 2002; 26(7): 823–835.
22. Gu M, Antonescu CR, Guiter G, et al. Cytokeratin immunoreactivity in Ewing's sarcoma: prevalence in 50 cases confirmed by molecular diagnostic studies. Am J Surg Pathol 2000; 24(3): 410–416.
23. Barnoud R, Sabourin JC, Pasquier D, et al. Immunohistochemical expression of WT1 by desmoplastic small round cell tumor: a comparative study with other small round cell tumors. Am J Surg Pathol 2000; 24(6):830–836.
24. Hill DA, Pfeifer JD, Marley EF, et al. WT1 staining reliably differentiates desmoplastic small round cell tumor from Ewing sarcoma/primitive neuroectodermal tumor. An immunohistochemical and molecular diagnostic study. Am J Clin Pathol 2000; 114(3):345–353.
25. Lugli A, Forster Y, Haas P, et al. Calretinin expression in human normal and neoplastic tissues: a tissue microarray analysis on 5233 tissue samples. Hum Pathol 2003; 34(10):994–1000.
26. Weidner N, Tjoe J. Immunohistochemical profile of monoclonal antibody O13: antibody that recognizes glycoprotein p30/32MIC2 and is useful in diagnosing Ewing's sarcoma and peripheral neuroepithelioma. Am J Surg Pathol 1994; 18(5):486–494.

27. Folpe AL, Goldblum JR, Rubin BP, et al. Morphologic and immunophenotypic diversity in Ewing family tumors: a study of 66 genetically confirmed cases. Am J Surg Pathol 2005; 29(8): 1025–1033.
28. Olsen SH, Thomas DG, Lucas DR. Cluster analysis of immunohistochemical profiles in synovial sarcoma, malignant peripheral nerve sheath tumor, and Ewing sarcoma. Mod Pathol 2006; 19(5): 659–668.
29. Shanfelt RL, Edelman J, Willis JE, et al. Immunohistochemical analysis of neural markers in peripheral primitive neuroectodermal tumors (pPNET) without light microscopic evidence of neural differentiation. Appl Immunohistochem 1997; 5:78–86.
30. Gordon GJ, Jensen RV, Hsiao LL, et al. Translation of microarray data into clinically relevant cancer diagnostic tests using gene expression ratios in lung cancer and mesothelioma. Cancer Res 2002; 62(17):4963–4967.
31. Gordon GJ, Jensen RV, Hsiao LL, et al. Using gene expression ratios to predict outcome among patients with mesothelioma. J Natl Cancer Inst 2003; 95(8):598–605.
32. Pass HI, Liu Z, Wali A, et al. Gene expression profiles predict survival and progression of pleural mesothelioma. Clin Cancer Res 2004; 10(3):849–859.
33. Scherpereel A, Grigoriu B, Conti M, et al. Soluble mesothelin-related peptides in the diagnosis of malignant pleural mesothelioma. Am J Respir Crit Care Med 2006; 173(10):1155–1160.
34. Scherpereel A, Lee YC. Biomarkers for mesothelioma. Curr Opin Pulm Med 2007; 13(4): 339–443.
35. Beyer HL, Geschwindt RD, Glover CL, et al. MESOMARK: a potential test for malignant pleural mesothelioma. Clin Chem 2007; 53(4):666–672.
36. Lopez-Rios F, Chuai S, Flores R, et al. Global gene expression profiling of pleural mesotheliomas: overexpression of aurora kinases and P16/CDKN2A deletion as prognostic factors and critical evaluation of microarray-based prognostic prediction. Cancer Res 2006; 66(6): 2970–2979.
37. Borczuk AC, Taub RN, Hesdorffer M, et al. P16 loss and mitotic activity predict poor survival in patients with peritoneal malignant mesothelioma. Clin Cancer Res 2005; 11(9):3303–3308.
38. Cheng JQ, Jhanwar SC, Klein WM, et al. p16 alterations and deletion mapping of 9p21-p22 in malignant mesothelioma. Cancer Res 1994; 54(21):5547–5551.
39. Xio S, Li D, Vijg J, et al. Codeletion of p15 and p16 in primary malignant mesothelioma. Oncogene 1995; 11(3):511–515.
40. Carbone M, Rizzo P, Powers A, et al. Molecular analyses, morphology and immunohistochemistry together differentiate pleural synovial sarcomas from mesotheliomas: clinical implications. Anticancer Res 2002; 22(6B):3443–3448.
41. Oliveira AM, Fletcher CD. Molecular prognostication for soft tissue sarcomas: are we ready yet? J Clin Oncol 2004; 22(20):4031–4034.
42. de Leeuw B, Balemans M, Olde Weghuis D, et al. Identification of two alternative fusion genes, SYT-SSX1 and SYT-SSX2, in t(X;18)(p11.2;q11.2)-positive synovial sarcomas. Hum Mol Genet 1995; 4(6):1097–1099.
43. Coindre JM, Pelmus M, Hostein I, et al. Should molecular testing be required for diagnosing synovial sarcoma? A prospective study of 204 cases. Cancer 2003; 98(12):2700–2707.
44. Hostein I, Menard A, Bui BN, et al. Molecular detection of the synovial sarcoma translocation t(X;18) by real-time polymerase chain reaction in paraffin-embedded material. Diagn Mol Pathol 2002; 11(1):16–21.
45. Ladanyi M, Antonescu CR, Leung DH, et al. Impact of SYT-SSX fusion type on the clinical behavior of synovial sarcoma: a multi-institutional retrospective study of 243 patients. Cancer Res 2002; 62(1):135–140.
46. Guillou L, Benhattar J, Bonichon F, et al. Histologic grade, but not SYT-SSX fusion type, is an important prognostic factor in patients with synovial sarcoma: a multicenter, retrospective analysis. J Clin Oncol 2004; 22(20):4040–4050.

47. Guillou L, Coindre J, Gallagher G, et al. Detection of the synovial sarcoma translocation t(X;18) (SYT;SSX) in paraffin-embedded tissues using reverse transcriptase-polymerase chain reaction: a reliable and powerful diagnostic tool for pathologists. A molecular analysis of 221 mesenchymal tumors fixed in different fixatives. Hum Pathol 2001; 32(1):105–112.
48. Okamoto S, Hisaoka M, Daa T, et al. Primary pulmonary synovial sarcoma: a clinicopathologic, immunohistochemical, and molecular study of 11 cases. Hum Pathol 2004; 35(7):850–856.
49. Turc-Carel C, Philip I, Berger MP, et al. Chromosome study of Ewing's sarcoma (ES) cell lines. Consistency of a reciprocal translocation t(11;22)(q24;q12). Cancer Genet Cytogenet 1984; 12(1):1–19.
50. Aurias A, Rimbaut C, Buffe D, et al. Translocation involving chromosome 22 in Ewing's sarcoma. A cytogenetic study of four fresh tumors. Cancer Genet Cytogenet 1984; 12(1):21–25.
51. Burchill SA. Ewing's sarcoma: diagnostic, prognostic, and therapeutic implications of molecular abnormalities. J Clin Pathol 2003; 56(2):96–102.
52. Sorensen PH, Shimada H, Liu XF, et al. Biphenotypic sarcomas with myogenic and neural differentiation express the Ewing's sarcoma EWS/FLI1 fusion gene. Cancer Res 1995; 55(6): 1385–1392.
53. Burchill SA, Wheeldon J, Cullinane C, et al. EWS-FLI1 fusion transcripts identified in patients with typical neuroblastoma. Eur J Cancer 1997; 33(2):239–243.
54. Thorner P, Squire J, Chilton-MacNeil S, et al. Is the EWS/FLI-1 fusion transcript specific for Ewing sarcoma and peripheral primitive neuroectodermal tumor? A report of four cases showing this transcript in a wider range of tumor types. Am J Pathol 1996; 148(4):1125–1138.
55. Syed S, Haque AK, Hawkins HK, et al. Desmoplastic small round cell tumor of the lung. Arch Pathol Lab Med 2002; 126(10):1226–1228.
56. Parkash V, Gerald WL, Parma A, et al. Desmoplastic small round cell tumor of the pleura. Am J Surg Pathol 1995; 19(6):659–665.
57. Jambhekar NA, Bagwan IN, Ghule P, et al. Comparative analysis of routine histology, immunohistochemistry, reverse transcriptase polymerase chain reaction, and fluorescence in situ hybridization in diagnosis of Ewing family of tumors. Arch Pathol Lab Med 2006; 130(12): 1813–1818.
58. Bridge RS, Rajaram V, Dehner LP, et al. Molecular diagnosis of Ewing sarcoma/primitive neuroectodermal tumor in routinely processed tissue: a comparison of two FISH strategies and RT-PCR in malignant round cell tumors. Mod Pathol 2006; 19(1):1–8.
59. Shing DC, McMullan DJ, Roberts P, et al. FUS/ERG gene fusions in Ewing's tumors. Cancer Res 2003; 63(15):4568–4576.
60. Lewis TB, Coffin CM, Bernard PS. Differentiating Ewing's sarcoma from other round blue cell tumors using a RT-PCR translocation panel on formalin-fixed paraffin-embedded tissues. Mod Pathol 2007; 20(3):397–404.
61. Riley RD, Burchill SA, Abrams KR, et al. A systematic review of molecular and biological markers in tumours of the Ewing's sarcoma family. Eur J Cancer 2003; 39(1):19–30.
62. West DC, Grier HE, Swallow MM, et al. Detection of circulating tumor cells in patients with Ewing's sarcoma and peripheral primitive neuroectodermal tumor. J Clin Oncol 1997; 15(2): 583–588.
63. Zoubek A, Ladenstein R, Windhager R, et al. Predictive potential of testing for bone marrow involvement in Ewing tumor patients by RT-PCR: a preliminary evaluation. Int J Cancer 1998; 79(1):56–60.
64. Fagnou C, Michon J, Peter M, et al. Presence of tumor cells in bone marrow but not in blood is associated with adverse prognosis in patients with Ewing's tumor. Societe Francaise d'Oncologie Pediatrique. J Clin Oncol 1998; 16(5):1707–1711.
65. Avigad S, Cohen IJ, Zilberstein J, et al. The predictive potential of molecular detection in the nonmetastatic Ewing family of tumors. Cancer 2004; 100(5):1053–1058.

66. Rainbow L, Platt GM, Simpson GR, et al. The 222- to 234-kilodalton latent nuclear protein (LNA) of Kaposi's sarcoma-associated herpesvirus (human herpesvirus 8) is encoded by orf73 and is a component of the latency-associated nuclear antigen. J Virol 1997; 71(8):5915–5921.
67. Parravicini C, Chandran B, Corbellino M, et al. Differential viral protein expression in Kaposi's sarcoma-associated herpesvirus-infected diseases: Kaposi's sarcoma, primary effusion lymphoma, and multicentric Castleman's disease. Am J Pathol 2000; 156(3):743–749.
68. Copie-Bergman C, Niedobitek G, Mangham DC, et al. Epstein-Barr virus in B-cell lymphomas associated with chronic suppurative inflammation. J Pathol 1997; 183(3):287–292.

Index

Milton Keynes UK
Ingram Content Group UK Ltd.
UKHW020001071024
449327UK00031B/2611

9 780367 452636